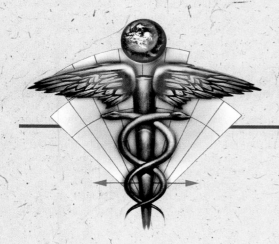

BRADY

Essentials of Medical Assisting

Administrative and Clinical Competencies

Bonnie F. Fremgen, PhD

Advisory Team

Ursula Backner, CMA
Mary King, CMA, EMT-A, BS
Fred Pearson, PhD
Janice M. Simon, MS, EdD
Kathleen Wallington, RN, BSN, CMA

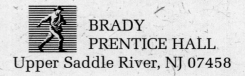

BRADY
PRENTICE HALL
Upper Saddle River, NJ 07458

Library of Congress Cataloging-in-Publication Data

Fremgen, Bonnie F.
    Essentials of medical assisting : administrative and clinical
competencies / Bonnie F. Fremgen ; advisory team, Ursula Backner . . .
[et al.].
        p.   cm.
    Includes bibliographical references and index.
    ISBN 0-8359-5122-7
    1. Medical assistants.   2. Medical offices--Management.
3. Clinical competence. I. Title.
    [DNLM: 1. Physician Assistants.   2. Practice Management,
    Medical.
3. Clinical Competence.   W 21.5 F869e 1998]
R728.8.F725 1998
610.69'53--dc21
DNLM/DLC
for Library of Congress   97-41972
                                                                          CIP

Publisher: *Susan Katz*
Acquisitions editor: *Barbara Krawiec*
Development managing editor: *Marilyn C. Meserve*
Project editor: *Elizabeth Egan-Rivera*
Marketing manager: *Judy Streger*
Director of production and manufacturing: *Bruce Johnson*
Managing production editor: *Patrick Walsh*
Editorial/production supervision: *Julie Boddorf*
Senior production manager: *Ilene Sanford*
Creative director: *Marianne Frasco*
Interior design: *Amy Rosen*
Cover design: *Bruce Kenselaar*
Cover art: *Cary Henrie*
Managing photography editor: *Michal Heron*
Assistant photography editors: *Baylen Leonard, Nancy Soares*
Photographers: *Michal Heron, Brian Warling*
Composition: *Carlisle Communications*
Printing and binding: *Von Hoffman*

© 1998 by Prentice-Hall, Inc.
Simon & Schuster / A Viacom Company
Upper Saddle River, New Jersey 07458

Printed in the United States of America
10 9 8 7 6 5 4 3 2 1

ISBN 0-8359-5122-7

Prentice-Hall International (UK) Limited, *London*
Prentice-Hall of Australia Pty. Limited, *Sydney*
Prentice-Hall Canada, Inc., *Toronto*
Prentice-Hall Hispanoamericana, S.A., *Mexico*
Prentice-Hall of India Private Limited, *New Delhi*
Prentice-Hall of Japan, Inc., *Tokyo*
Simon & Schuster Asia Pte. Ltd., *Singapore*
Editora Prentice-Hall do Brasil, Ltda., *Rio de Janeiro*

NOTICE

The procedures described in this textbook are based on consultation with medical authorities. The author and publisher have taken care to make certain that these procedures reflect currently accepted clinical practice; however, they cannot be considered absolute recommendations.

The material in this textbook contains the most current information available at the time of publication. However, federal, state, and local guidelines concerning clinical practices, including without limitation, those governing infection control, universal precautions, and standard precautions, change rapidly. The reader should note, therefore, that new regulations may require changes in some procedures.

It is the responsibility of the reader to familiarize himself or herself with the policies and procedures set by federal, state and local agencies, as well as the institution or agency where the reader is employed. The authors and the publishers of this textbook, and the supplements written to accompany it, disclaim any liability, loss, or risk resulting directly or indirectly from the suggested procedures and theory, from any undetected errors, or from the reader's misunderstanding of the text. It is the reader's responsibility to stay informed of any new changes or recommendations made by any federal, state, and local agency as well as by his or her employing health care institution or agency.

NOTE ON GENDER USAGE

The English language has historically given preference to the male gender. Among many words, the pronouns "he" and "his" are commonly used to describe both genders. The male pronouns still predominate our speech, however, in this text "he" and "she" have been used interchangeably when referring to the Nursing Assistant and/or the patient. The repeated use of "he or she" is not proper in long manuscript, and the use of "he or she" is not correct in all cases. The authors have made great effort to treat the two genders equally. Throughout the text, solely for the purpose of brevity, male pronouns and female pronouns are often used to describe both males and females. This is not intended to offend any reader of the female or male gender.

NOTICE RE "ON THE JOB"

The names used in the case studies throughout this text are fictitious.

Brief Contents

Detailed Contents

Procedures

The number of the chapter in which the procedure appears is in parentheses.

Guidelines

The number of the chapter in which the guideline appears is in parentheses.

Preface

Essentials of Medical Assisting: Administrative and Clinical Competencies provides an explanation of the administrative and clinical procedures that the medical assisting student will find in the office or clinic setting. A description of the process or procedure is accompanied with an explanation of the rationale for the performance standard. This comprehensive guide to medical assisting prepares students for success in the classroom, on the certification exam, and in the workplace. It reflects the latest techniques, guidelines, psychology, and terminology throughout its in-depth coverage of administrative and clinical essentials.

The book includes the latest Role Delineation Study from the American Association of Medical Assistants which updates and replaces DACUM. The Role Delineation Study is presented in chart form at the beginning of each chapter. The topics covered within that chapter are highlighted in yellow for easy reference. The opportunity to use this format will encourage students to become familiar with the new guidelines.

Success in the classroom is stressed throughout the book using a variety of techniques. **Med Tips,** placed at strategic points in the narrative, provide helpful hints and useful information relating to the discussion within the text. **Strategies for Success** from instructors follow chapters 2, 6, 8, and 11. **Workplace Wisdom** from employers follow chapters 12, 18, 24, 28, and 30. A special interest section called **On the Job** appears at the end of each chapter to profile the real-life experiences of practicing medical assistants and to allow students to work through the dilemmas presented. A **Test Taking Tip** to help the students perform well on their certification examination and ten multiple choice **Examination Review Questions** are included at the end of each chapter as well. **Legal and Ethical Issues** and a **Patient Education** information section are a part of each chapter.

The book is presented in a format that takes the medical assistant student from beginning administrative through clinical teachings in preparation for work in the medical office. In the first few chapters the students are presented with an overview of the medical profession and ethics. Then, the student is moved into the office setting for such administrative skills as telephone use, scheduling, record keeping, medical transcription, billing, and insurance work. Administrative chapters include both theory and procedures relating to vital signs and measurement, assisting with physical examinations and minor surgical procedures, microbiology, hematology, urinalysis, x-rays and related procedures, electrocardiography and pulmonary function, physical therapy and rehabilitation, pharmacology and the administration of medications, patient education, nutrition, psychology, emergency first aid, and handling the patient who has special needs.

Special emphasis is placed on the concept of asepsis as mandated by the Occupational Safety and Health Administration (OSHA) and the Center for Disease Control (CDC). A chapter on Quality Assurance prepares the student to handle many dimensions of a quality assurance program in the medical office. Patient education techniques are explained in-depth in a chapter including information on nutrition. A unit on career planning and the externship experience provides valuable information on obtaining and keeping a job.

The textbook is organized so that each chapter is self-sufficient. This allows the instructor to have flexibility regarding how the material is covered. This method of organization also allows each instructor to link the text material to their school's particular curriculum in a comfortable manner. For instance, the instructor may wish to present the chapters on microbiology and urinalysis testing after the students have covered the urinary system in their anatomy and physiology course.

Essentials of Medical Assisting: Administrative and Clinical Competencies can be used successfully by students in a community college, a technical training program, or as an independent study. Since the book provides photographs and information on the latest equipment, it also serves as an up-to-date reference tool for staff in physicians' offices and clinics.

About the Author

Bonnie F. Fremgen, PhD

Bonnie F. Fremgen is a former associate dean of the Allied Health program at Robert Morris College. She has taught clinical and administrative topics as well as medical terminology, and anatomy and physiology to medical assisting students. In addition, she has served as an advisor for students' career planning.

Dr. Fremgen holds a nursing degree as well as a masters in health care administration. She received her Ph.D. from the College of Education at the University of Illinois.

She has broad interests and experiences in the health care field which include physician's offices, nursing homes, hospitals, and responsibility for departments of social services, home health care, discharge planning, quality assurance, and hospital-wide education.

Dr. Fremgen is currently an adjunct associate professor at the University of Notre Dame in South Bend, Indiana.

Advisory Team

Ursula Backner, CMA
Medical Assisting Program Coordinator
Clarian Health Partners—Educational Services
Methodist Hospital
Indianapolis, Indiana

Mary King, CMA, EMT-A, BS
Curriculum Development Consultant
Lake Geneva, Wisconsin

Fred Pearson, PhD
Health Science Department
Ricks College
Rexburg, Idaho

Janice M. Simon, MS, EdD
Adjunct Professor
National-Louis University
Department of Healthcare
and Leadership Policy Studies
Evanston, IL
Formerly Education Director
National Education Center
Chicago, IL

Kathleen Wallington, RN, BSN, CMA
Formerly Medical Assisting Instructor
American Career College
Irvine, California

DEDICATION
To my husband for his love and encouragement.
This book is also dedicated
to Dr. William Kristy and Dr. James Faulkner,
whose dedication to patient care in the medical office
has been inspirational.

Acknowledgments

Program Development

This book would not have been possible without the assistance and guidance of many people. I am grateful to the editorial and production staff of Brady/Prentice Hall for their skill and patience with this project.

Brady/Prentice Hall Editorial Team   Susan Katz, publisher, for her enthusiastic support of this project; Barbara Krawiec, acquisitions editor, for her continued understanding and leadership throughout this project; Stephanie Camangian, editorial assistant, whose courtesy and follow-through are greatly appreciated; and in particular, Marilyn Meserve, managing development editor, whose encouragement and quiet efficiency kept everyone moving in the right direction.

Brady/Prentice Hall Production Team   Pat Walsh, managing production editor, whose calm presence was always available; Julie Boddorf, production editor, whose quiet effectiveness moved the book through the production process.

Brady/Prentice Hall Marketing and Sales Team   Judy Streger, marketing manager, for her quick responsiveness to all questions; Judy Stamm, Brady sales manager, and the Brady sales team for their suggestions and support.

Editorial, Photography, and Production Support Staff Elizabeth Egan-Rivera, project editor, for her unique editing ability, understanding of a technical topic, stamina, and wonderful support throughout this entire project; Michal Heron, managing photography editor, whose unerring eye for preciseness turned the abstract idea into instructive photos; Thanks to Mark Ammerman and his artists at North Market Street Graphics for their ability to turn an idea into art.

Special Consultants and Contributors   Special thanks to Mary King, CMA, EMT-A, BS for her excellent technical advice throughout the project, and in particular, during the photography sessions. Special thanks to Janice M. Simon, MS, EdD, for her unique suggestions, review of manuscript, and her contribution of special interest features throughout the text, especially the On the Job features. Special thanks to Karen Mcgrath, BS, MA, for her motivational insights of success strategies and her special way of speaking and writing to the student regarding success in the classroom and on the job.

Organizations   Thanks go out to the staff at Robert Morris College in Orland Park, Illinois and Lincoln Park Family Physicians for their assistance in setting up scenes for photography.

Contributing Writers

Chapters 12, 17
Ursula Backner, CMA
Medical Assisting Program Coordinator

Clarian Health Partners—Educational Services
Methodist Hospital
Indianapolis, IN
Chapter 29
Susan Buboltz, RN, BSN, MS, CMA
Program Director and Instructor
Medical Assistant Program
Madison Area Technical College
Madison, Wisconsin
Chapter 27
Susanne Ezzo, AST, BS, RN
Ultrasound Diagnostic School
Pittsburgh, Pennsylvania
Chapter 14
Irene Figliolina, AAS, CMA
Medical Programs Director
Berdan Institute
Totowa, New Jersey
Chapter 34
Thom Hillson, BA
Retired Paramedic of 23 years
Lakeside, California
Chapter 25
Catherine Schoen, CMA
Medical Assisting Clinical Instructor
Clarian Health Partners—Educational Services
Methodist Hospital
Indianapolis, Indiana

Reviewers

The following reviewers provided valuable feedback during the writing process. We thank all these professionals for their contribution and attention to detail.

Jerri Adler, CMA, CMT
Instructor, Health Records Technology/Medical Transcription
Family & Health Careers Department
Lane Community College
Eugene, Oregon
Nadine Anderson, CMA-C
Vice Speaker
Board of Trustees
American Association of Medical Assistants
Chicago, Illinois
Mary M. Andrus, BA
Medical Assistant Instructor
Spencer Business & Technical Institute
Schenectady, New York
Lynn Augenstern, CMA, MA
Program Director/Instructor
Medical Assisting Program
Ridley-Lowell Business & Technical Institute
Binghamton, New York

Linda Bednar, CMA
Medical Assisting Instructor
McCarrie Schools of Health Sciences & Technology
Philadelphia, Pennslyvania

Wendy M. Blume, EdD, MT (ASCP)
Associate Professor
Clinical Laboratory Sciences
Community College of Philadelphia
Philadelphia, Pennsylvania

Susan Buboltz, RN, BSN, MS, CMA
Program Director/Instructor
Medical Assistant Program
Madison Area Technical College
Madison, Wisconsin

Linda Burke, CMA, CPT
Instructor/Assistant Director
Star Technical Institute
Lakewood, New Jersey

Mary F. Chiaravalloti, RN, CMA, BA, MEd, MS
Medical Assistant Instructor
Bryant & Stratton Business Institute
Buffalo, New York

Melody Crawford, RMA, LT
Medical Instructor/Department Head
Missouri College
St. Louis, Missouri

Michael L. Decker, MA, BS
Director of Education
Omaha College of Health Careers
Omaha, Nebraska

Bonnie L. Deister, MA, MS, BSN, RN, CMA-C
Department Chair/Assistant Professor
Medical Assisting/ Paramedic Program
Broome Community College
Binghamton, New York

Sandra Dickerson, BS, MT (ASCP)
Former Instructor
Medical Assistant Program
Bryan Institute
Wichita, Kansas

Kathleen Corbett-Duncan, RRT, CMA
Dominion Business School
Roanoke, Virginia

Linda C. Ermshar, RN, AA, LPT
Director/Director of Education
Modern Technology School of X-ray
Anaheim, California

Suzanne Ezzo, AST, BS, RN
Ultrasound Diagnostic School
Pittsburgh, Pennsylvania

Irene Figliolina, AAS, CMA
Medical Programs Director
Berdan Institute
Totowa, New Jersey

Margaret S. Frazier, RN, CMA, BS
Medical Assistant Department Chair
Health & Human Services Division
Ivy Tech State College, Northeast
Fort Wayne, Indiana

Eugenia M. Fulcher, RN, BSN, MEd, CMA
Medical Assistant Instructor
Swainsboro Technical Institute
Swainsboro, Georgia

Kris Gaiero, AS, CMA
Silicon Valley College
Fremont, California

Martha Garrels, BS, MSA, MT (ASCP), CMA-C
Medical Assistant Technologies Chair
Ivy Tech State College, North Central
South Bend, Indiana

Joanna E. George, CMA
Director, Medical Secretary/Transcriptionist
Program
Office Administration Program
Somerset County Technical Institute
Bridgewater, New Jersey

Rona E. Goldman, CMA-AC, CCVT, CPT
Instructor/Externship Coordinator
Medix School
Towson, Maryland

Ann M. Gray, AS, CMA-AC, BS, MSA
Clinical Office Coordinator
Department of Surgery
Division of Urology
Fletcher Allen Health Care
Burlington, Vermont

Debra L. Grieneisen, BS, MT (ASCP), CMA
Instructor, Health Professions, MLT/PBT
Harrisburg Area Community College
Harrisburg, Pennsylvania

Laurie Guest, CMA
Instructor
Occupational Training Services
San Diego, California

Judy White Harris, RN, CMA-C
Former Department Chairman Allied Health
Sarasota County Technical Institute
Sarasota, Florida

Jan Hasselbar, RN
Medical Programs Coordinator
AIBT
Phoenix, Arizona

Lisa Hutchison, CMA/RMA
Clinical Instructor
Apollo College
Phoenix, Arizona

Elizabeth Keene, RN, BSN, CMA
Medical Assistant Instructor
Lansdale School of Business
North Wales, Pennsylvania

Mary King, CMA, EMT-A, BS
Curriculum Development Consultant
Lake Geneva, Wisconsin

Cynthia K. Lundgren, BS, CMA
Manager
Colon & Rectal Clinic
Houston, Texas
Instructor
CMA Study Course
Bay Area Galveston County
Houston, Texas
Past President
Texas Society of Medical Assistants
Proctor
AAMA CMA Exam

Liza McMahon, RN, BSN, CMA
Education Supervisor
Medical Assistant Program
Porter & Chester Institute
Chicopee, Massachusetts

Cris A. McTighe, CMA, RMA
Program Director
Medical Program Director
Western Career College
San Leandro, California

Paula Michal, RN, BSN
Program Director, Medical Assisting
Santa Barbara Business College
Santa Barbara, California

Karen Minchella, CMA, PhD
Instructional Designer/Trainer
Consulting Management Associates, Inc.
Fraser, Michigan
Allied Health Director
Warren Woods Public Education
Warren, Michigan

Pat G. Moeck, MBA, CMA
Director, Medical Assisting Program
Continuing Education
El Centro College
Dallas, Texas
Director
Medical Assisting Program/Workforce
Development
Mountain View College
Dallas, Texas

Marilyn Pooler, RN, CMA-C, MEd
Professor
Medical Assistant Program
Springfield Technical Community College
Springfield, Massachusetts

Vicki Prater, CMA, RMA, RAHA
Medical Program Director
Concorde Career Institute
San Bernardino, California

Linda K. Ramge, MT (ASCP), CMA
Program Director, Medical Office Assisting
King's College
Charlotte, North Carolina

Catherine Rogers, RN, BSN, MBA, CMA
Health Occupations Department Chair
Rockford Business College
Rockford, Illinois

Diane Samuelson, RN, CMA
Medical Assistant Instructor
Grand Island College
Grand Island, Nebraska

Tanya Shelton, RN, ADA, CMA
Medical Assisting Program
Pitt Community College
Greenville, North Carolina

Janet R. Sesser, RMA, BS Ed. Admin.
Corporate Training Director Allied Health
High-Tech Institute, Inc.
Phoenix, Arizona

Lois M. Smith, RN, CMA
Department Chair, Allied Health
Medical Office Assisting
Arapahoe Community College
Littleton, Colorado

Dee A. Stout, BA, MS
Academic Dean
Concorde Career Institute
Kansas City, Missouri

Shirley A. Stasiak, CMA
Health Sciences/Medical Assisting Program
Winter Park Tech
Winter Park, Florida

Becky Thomason, RN, CMA, CPUR
Former Medical Program Director
Phillips Junior College
Springfield, Missouri

Kathleen Tozzi, CLPN/RMA
Director of Education
Cleveland Institute of Dental/Medical Assistants, Inc.
Mentor, Ohio

Angelina C. Urquhart, EMT, NRMA
Medical Program Director
Medical Assistant Dept.
Corinthian Schools, Inc.
Bryman Campus
Winnetka, California

Kathleen Wallington, RN, BSN, CMA
Former Medical Assisting Instructor
American Career College
Irvine, California

Melanie J. Wilhelm, RN, BSN
Instructor
School of Practical Nursing
Norfolk Vocational Technical School
Norfolk, Virginia

Supplements Team

Thanks to the team of authors who assisted in the development of the supplements. Kathleen Wallington, RN, BSN, CMA co-authored the student workbook with Bonnie Fremgen, PhD. Janice M. Simon, MS, EdD co-authored the instructor's guide, and authored the test item file and the interactive study guide. Thanks also goes to Fred Pearson, PhD who authored the software. And thanks to all the additional writers, reviewers, and development team members of the supplement components.

Photo Acknowledgments

Technical Advisor

Our grateful appreciation to Mary King, CMA, EMT-A, BS for providing excellent and untiring technical support during the photo shoots.

Organizations

We wish to thank the following organizations for their assistance in creating the photo program for this book.

Robert Morris College, Orland Park Campus, Orland Park, IL 60462—Nancy Rotunno, Lora Saner; Doctor's Medical Center, 6240 West 55th Street, Chicago, IL 60636—Ehlma Mendez, CMA, EMT-A; Lincoln Park Family Physicians, Chicago, IL 60614—Stephen A. Leedy, MD, Steven H. Rube, MD; MacNeal HealthCare Center, Oak Park, IL 60301—Belita Smith.

Companies

We wish to thank the following companies for their cooperation in providing us with photos:

Abbott Laboratories, Diagnostic Division, Abbott Park, IL; Aetna/US Healthcare, Wayne, PA; Allegiance Healthcare Corp, McGaw Park, IL; American Medical Technologists, Park Ridge, IL; American Association of Medical Assistants, Chicago, IL; American Cancer Society, Atlanta, GA; Andwin Scientific, Canoga Park, CA; Bausch & Lomb, Rochester, NY; Bayer Corporation, Tarrytown, NY; Becton Dickinson and Company; Microbiology Systems and VACUTAINER Systems, Franklin Lakes, NJ; BlueCross BlueShield Association, Chicago, IL; Boehringer Mannheim Diagnostics, Indianapolis, IN; Burdick, Rolling Meadows, IL; Cardinal Scale Manufacturing Co., Webb City, MO; Carter-Wallace Wampole, Cranbury, NJ; Chattanooga Group, Inc., Hixson, TN; Chematics Inc., North Webster, IN; Coulter Corporation, Miami, FL; Forrest Medical, LLC, East Syracuse, NY; The Harloff Company, Inc., Colorado Springs, CO; Hollister Inc., Libertyville, IL; International Remote Imaging Systems, Inc., Chatsworth, CA; Johnson & Johnson Clinical Diagnostics, Rochester, NY; Kendall Healthcare Products Co., Mansfield, MA; Lifescan, Inc., Milpitas, CA; Lucent Technologies, Inc., Basking Ridge, NJ; Lukens Medical Corporation, Rio Rancho, NM; Medi-Ject Corporation, Minneapolis, MN; Midmark Corporation, Versailles, OH; Miltex Instrument Company, Inc., Lake Success, NY; Mita Copystar America, Inc., Fairfield, NJ; Omron Healthcare, Inc., Vernon Hills, IL; Profex Medical Products, St. Louis, MO; Propper Manufacturing Company, L.I.C., NY; Sage Products, Inc., Crystal Lake, IL; Seca Corporation, Columbia, MD; Seiler Instrument & Manufacturing Co., Inc., St. Louis, MO; Sherwood Davis & Geck, St. Louis, MO; Tecnol Medical Products, Inc., Fort Worth, TX; 3M Health Care, St. Paul, MN; Vee Gee Scientific, Inc., Kirkland, WA; W.A. Baum Co., Inc., Copiague, NY; Welch Allyn, Skaneateles Falls, NY; Winfield Medical, San Diego, CA.

Photo Sources

The following photos are credited as:

02-01 Brian Warling/International Museum of Surgical Science, Chicago, IL; 02-02 Brian Warling/International Museum of Surgical Science, Chicago, IL; 02-05 Brian Warling/International Museum of Surgical Science, Chicago, IL; 02-11 Brian Warling/International Museum of Surgical Science, Chicago, IL; 02-06 Tom Stewart/The Stock Market; CO-06 Jose Pelaez /The Stock Market; 04-01 Brian Warling/International Museum of Surgical Science, Chicago, IL; 04-02 Brian Warling/International Museum of Surgical Science, Chicago, IL; 04-03 Brian Warling/International Museum of Surgical Science, Chicago, IL; 04-07a Paul Barton/The Stock Market; 04-07b Mug Shots/The Stock Market; CO-04 Paul Steel/The Stock Market; 03-05 Pete Saloutos/The Stock Market; 08-01 Jose Pelaez/The Stock Market; CO-08 Jose Pelaez/The Stock Market; 12-01 Matt Meadows /Science Photo Library/Photo Researchers Inc.; 12-06 William Taufic/The Stock Market; 12-02 Chris Priest/Science Photo Library/Photo Researchers; 12-07 Index Stock/Phototake; 16-01 William Taufic/The Stock Market; CO-16 Craig Hammell/The Stock Market; 17-02 The Blue Cross and Blue Shield Names and Symbols are registered marks of the Blue Cross and Blue Shield Association, an association of independent Blue Cross and Blue Shield Plans. Used by permission.; 18-01 Michal Heron Photography; 18-2a Michal Heron Photography; 18-04 Michal Heron Photography; 18-2b Michal Heron Photography; 20-09 Michal Heron Photography; 20-22 Michal Heron Photography; 20-25 Ron Sutherland/Science Photo Library/Photo Researchers; 20-26 Michal Heron Photography; CO-20 Michal Heron Photography; 22-15 Jose Pelaez/The Stock Market; 22-01 Michal Heron Photography; CO-25 The Stock Shop, Inc./Medichrome; 27-20 Harry J. Przekop/The Stock Shop, Inc./ Medichrome; 28-06 Brownie Harris/The Stock Market; 28-02 Index Stock Photography, Inc.; 29-09 David Scott Smith/David Scott Smith, Photographer; CO-29 ATC Productions/The Stock Market; 30-11 Michal Heron Photography; 30-06 Michal Heron Photography; CO-30 Michal Heron Photography; 31-03 Michal Heron Photography; 31-05 Jose Pelaez/The Stock Market; 32-02 Michal Heron Photography; 32-21a Michal Heron Photography; 24-09 Michal Heron Photography; 36-09 Michal Heron Photography; CO-36 Michal Heron Photography

Successful Starts

Congratulations! You have crossed a main threshold in your life. An important step has been taken that will impact the rest of your life. You have entered school to receive the instruction that will enable you to be a skilled medical assistant.

Instructors from throughout the fifty states have shared their words of wisdom that will impact your successful completion of this course of study. You can read some of their suggestions following chapters 2, 5, 8, and 11. They compiled these suggestions from many years of experience in working with students and have had the opportunity to determine which habits lend to success in their classes. Their suggestions are easy to remember and follow if you think of them as the ABC's of Classroom Success.

Attendance . . . It is necessary for you to attend class to truly benefit from your educational experience. So much happens in that classroom. The flow of information is so dynamic! This text will certainly give you information and impart that to you. However, your instructor will take that information and apply it to real life situations and show you how to apply the techniques, theories, etc. to actual daily activities. Your classmates will add their experiences to the discussion so that the class time becomes an active, challenging, exciting event where information is shared and understanding and enlightenment has occurred. Unless you are there, you can not share all of this wonderful experience.

Actively participate! There certainly will be times that you need to sit quietly in the classroom and absorb all that is being said, done, and communicated. However, if you don't share your thoughts, questions, ideas, and experiences, something is lost and you are the one who loses the most. You must ask questions, make suggestions for solutions, and share experiences that are pertinent to the discussion.

Benefit from your peers! Join and establish study groups. Learn to work as a team to accomplish goals and objectives. Help each other.

Contribute to class discussions. Contribute to the lab classes. Contribute to projects.

Commit! Commit yourself to this new adventure. You are taking time out of your life and away from family and others. Get the most out of this that you can. If you don't, you have wasted your time, effort, and dollars.

Communicate! Your instructor can't read your mind so help out here. Let your instructor know when you don't understand or when you are confused. You, the student, are the customer. The instructor is there because of and for you. Go ahead . . . make his or her day. Your instructor wants to hear from you. Communicate with your family what is going on in this new world you have entered. Let them be a part of it. Share some experiences and things that you have learned with them.

The results of your full participation in the classroom setting will be to enrich your knowledge and life. As you strive to possess the skills and knowledge that will make you a valued employee in the job market, you will find you have become a better person. You will have something to offer others. Your expertise will be used to aid the medical office in which you are employed to service its patients. It will lend itself to adjusting those situations that will be difficult and trying. It will help you work together with other employees to do the job.

Success in the classroom can be measured by your efforts. Attend, benefit, and communicate. Enter this threshold with a willingness to do whatever it takes to reap the full benefit. You are the key that opens the door. You will determine the extent of the success.

A feast is being set for you. Pick up the fork and dig in.

Karen Mcgrath, BS, MA
NAHCHS Board of Directors
Accreditation Reviewer, ABHES and ACCSCT

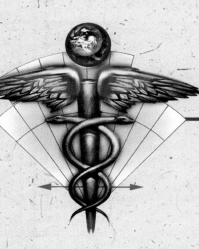

Unit One

Introduction
to Health Care

MEDICAL ASSISTANT ROLE DELINEATION CHART

Highlight indicates material covered in this chapter

ADMINISTRATIVE

ADMINISTRATIVE PROCEDURES

- Perform basic clerical functions
- Schedule, coordinate, and monitor appointments
- Schedule inpatient/outpatient admissions and procedures
- Understand and apply third party guidelines
- Obtain reimbursement through accurate claims submission
- Monitor third-party reimbursement
- Perform medical transcription
- Understand and adhere to managed care policies and procedures
- *Negotiate managed care contracts (adv)*

PRACTICE FINANCES

- Perform procedural and diagnostic coding
- Apply bookkeeping principles
- Document and maintain accounting and banking records
- Manage accounts receivable
- Manage accounts payable
- Process payroll
- *Develop and maintain fee schedules (adv)*
- *Manage renewals of business and professional insurance policies (adv)*
- *Manage personal benefits and maintain records (adv)*

CLINICAL

FUNDAMENTAL PRINCIPLES

- Apply principles of aseptic technique and infection control
- Comply with quality assurance practices
- Screen and follow up patient test results

DIAGNOSTIC ORDERS

- Collect and process specimens
- Perform diagnostic tests

PATIENT CARE

- Adhere to established triage procedures
- Obtain patient history and vital signs
- Prepare and maintain examination and treatment areas

- Prepare patient for examinations, procedures, and treatments
- Assist with examinations, procedures, and treatments
- Prepare and administer medications and immunizations
- Maintain medication and immunization records
- Recognize and respond to emergencies
- Coordinate patient care information with other health care providers

GENERAL (TRANSDISCIPLINARY)

PROFESSIONALISM

- Project a professional manner and image
- Adhere to ethical principles
- Demonstrate initiative and responsibility
- Work as a team member
- Manage time efficiently
- Prioritize and perform multiple tasks
- Adapt to change
- Promote the CMA credential
- Enhance skills through continuing education

COMMUNICATION SKILLS

- Treat all patients with compassion and empathy
- Recognize and respect cultural diversity
- Adapt communications to individual's ability to understand
- Use professional telephone technique
- Use effective and correct verbal and written communications
- Recognize and respond to verbal and nonverbal communications
- Use medical terminology appropriately
- Receive, organize, prioritize, and transmit information
- Serve as liaison
- Promote the practice through positive public relations

LEGAL CONCEPTS

- Maintain confidentiality
- Practice within the scope of education, training, and personal capabilities
- Prepare and maintain medical records
- Document accurately
- Use appropriate guidelines when releasing information
- Follow employer's established policies dealing with the health care contract
- Follow federal, state, and local legal guidelines
- Maintain awareness of federal and state health care legislation and regulations
- Maintain and dispose of regulated substances in compliance with government guidelines
- Comply with established risk management and safety procedures
- Recognize professional credentialing criteria
- Participate in the development and maintenance of personnel, policy, and procedure manuals
- *Develop and maintain personnel, policy, and procedure manuals (adv)*

INSTRUCTION

- Instruct individuals according to their needs
- Explain office policies and procedures
- Teach methods of health promotion and disease prevention
- Locate community resources and disseminate information
- *Orient and train personnel (adv)*
- *Develop educational materials (adv)*
- *Conduct continuing education activities (adv)*

OPERATIONAL FUNCTIONS

- Maintain supply inventory
- Evaluate and recommend equipment and supplies
- Apply computer techniques to support office operations
- *Supervise personnel (adv)*
- *Interview and recommend job applicants (adv)*
- *Negotiate leases and prices for equipment and supply contracts (adv)*

SOURCE: Reprinted by permission of the American Association of Medical Assistants from the *AAMA Role Delineation Study: Occupational Analysis of the Medical Assisting Profession.*

1

Medical Assisting: The Profession

CHAPTER OUTLINE

LEARNING OBJECTIVES

After completing this chapter, you should:
1. Define and spell the glossary terms for this chapter.
2. Discuss the history of medical assisting as a profession.
3. Identify career opportunities available to medical assistants and give six examples of areas in which you may choose to work.
4. List ten administrative duties of the medical assistant.
5. List ten clinical skills medical assistants need to know.
6. List ten qualities usually found in a good medical assistant.
7. Discuss the professional organizations that certify medical assistants.

Glossary

accreditation   Process in which an institution (school) voluntarily completes an extensive self-study after which an accrediting association visits the school to verify the self-study statements.

administrative   Relating to the business functions of the physician's office.

American Association of Medical Assistants (AAMA)   Professional association for medical assistants that oversees program accreditation, graduate certification, and provides a forum for issues of concern to the physician.

American Medical Association (AMA) Professional association for physicians which maintains directories of all qualified physicians, evaluates prescription and non-prescription drugs, advises congressional and state legislatures regarding proposed health care laws, and publishes a variety of scientific journals.

American Medical Technologists (AMT) Professional association that oversees the registration of medical technologists.

certification   The issuance by an official body of a certificate to a person indicating that he or she has been evaluated and has met certain standards.

Certified Medical Assistant (CMA)   A multiskilled health care professional who assists providers in an allied health care setting and who has successfully completed the CMA certification examination validating his or her credentials.

clinical   Relating to the medical treatment and care of patients.

confidentiality   Keeping private information about a person (patient) and not disclosing it to a third party without the patient's written consent.

continuing education units (CEUs)   Credit awarded for additional course work beyond certification in order to remain current in one's field or for recertification.

group practice   A practice in which at least three physicians are joined in order to share the workload and expenses.

health maintenance organization (HMO)   An organization established to provide comprehensive health care to an enrolled group of people at a fixed price.

managed care organization (MCO)   An organization that acts as a "gatekeeper," such as the insurance company, to approve all non-emergency services, hospitalization, or tests before they can be provided.

Registered Medical Assistant (RMA)   A multiskilled health care professional who assists providers in an allied health setting, has taken and successfully completed the RMA examination, and is registered with a national association.

solo practice   A physician practicing alone.

The health care field has experienced rapid growth and significant change during the past decade. In this environment, the role of the medical assistant continues to evolve in response to expressed needs. Likewise the duties of the medical assistant have multiplied and become varied from setting to setting. No matter how varied the roles or duties of the medical assistant, the essential skills and personal qualities needed in all good medical assistants are quite similar.

A well trained multiskilled health care professional, the medical assistant, fulfills many roles in the allied health field where the challenges of every day are balanced by opportunities for advancement, personal growth, and satisfaction. Professional organizations that oversee or regulate the education, training, and certification of medical assistants are also discussed in this chapter along with current career opportunities and the future of the medical assisting field.

History of Medical Assisting

Years ago men and women assisted the physician in the office as untrained workers. They became skilled through the day-to-day education and training provided by the physician. However, advances in medical technology and the expansion of the heath care field created a need for more formally trained personnel. Many physicians had become familiar with the clinical skills of nurses while working closely with nurses in the hospital setting, so they chose to hire registered nurses to work in their offices. When a shortage of nursing personnel occurred physicians had to look elsewhere for professionally trained office personnel who could handle both the administrative and clinical responsibilities of a medical office practice. The administrative responsibilities are the "front office" or business functions of the office while the clinical responsibilities relate to the direct care and treatment of the patient.

Over the years, the education and training of medical assistants has undergone many changes and today medical assistants are well-trained and respected practitioners in the allied health field.

The American Association of Medical Assistants (AAMA) (Figure 1-1), organized in 1956 to oversee the education, training, and certification of this broad group of medical professionals offers the following definition of medical assisting:

Medical assisting is a multi-skilled allied health profession whose practitioners work primarily in ambulatory settings such as medical offices and clinics. Medical assistants function as members of the health care delivery team and perform administrative and clinical procedures.

(From Essentials and Guidelines for an Accredited Educational Program for the Medical Assistant, adopted by the AAMA's Endowment and the American Medical Association in 1969, revised 1971, 1977, 1984, and 1991. Copyright by the American Association of Medical Assistants, Inc. Reprinted by permission.)

The American Medical Association (AMA), composed of physicians, welcomed the professional education and training of their office and clinic personnel and saw a need to expand the number of people entering the field.

Role of the Medical Assistant

The medical assistant's role developed in response to the demand for well trained medical office staff. Medical assistants have become expert at keeping medical offices and clinics running smoothly (Figure 1-2). They assist physicians with

many administrative and clinical aspects of the practice, including taking vital signs, preparing patients for procedures, taking patient history, and preparing and maintaining the examination and treatment area. The medical assistant's main function is to assist the physician. *Note:* The role of the medical assistant should not be confused with that of the physician's assistant who actually examines, diagnoses, and treats patients under the supervision of a physician.

The field of medical assisting is open to both men and women in a variety of work settings such as: physicians' offices, ambulatory care clinics, government agencies, extended care centers, hospitals, free-standing facilities and managed care organizations (MCOs) including health maintenance organizations (HMOs) and insurance companies. Managed care provides a mechanism for a "gatekeeper" such as the insurance company to approve all non-emergency services, hospitalization, or tests before they can be provided. This approval process is an attempt to eliminate all unnecessary costs.

Job Opportunities

The wide range of health care settings presents many opportunities for the medical assistant who is trained in both clinical and administrative duties.

Table 1-1 lists several inpatient and ambulatory care (outpatient) facilities or settings with

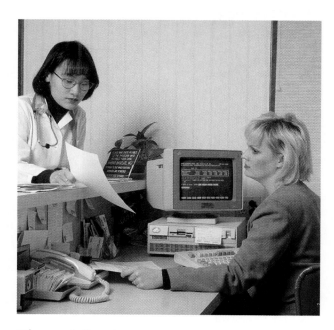

Figure 1-2 Physicians employ medical assistants to assist with the many administrative and clinical aspects of physician's practice.

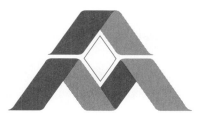

Figure 1-1 LOGO of the American Association of Medical Assistants (AAMA). (Copyright by the American Association of Medical Assistants, Inc. Reprinted by permission.)

TABLE 1-1 Job Opportunities for Medical Assistants in Inpatient and Ambulatory Care Settings

Inpatient Setting	Description of Job
Rehabilitation facility	Perform both clinical and administrative tasks in medical setting focused on rehabilitation and physical therapy.
Extended care center	Work with patients who require a protective environment.
Hospital	Perform both clinical and administrative tasks as a member of the health care team.
Nursing home	Perform clinical and administrative tasks working with older adult patients.
Ambulatory Care Setting	Description of Job
Clinic	Use clinical and administrative skills to schedule and assist with patients who require special medical attention (for example, eye clinic, orthopedic clinic, mental health clinic).
Free-standing facility	Care for patients who require immediate medical treatment.
Physician's office	Use clinical and administrative skills in the private office setting for physicians of all specialties.
Rehabilitation center	Provide care for patients recovering from illness or injury.

TABLE 1-2 Job Opportunities for Medical Assistants in Healthcare Departments and Specialties

Department/Specialty	Description of Job
Admissions	Handle pre-admission interviews, schedule laboratory testing, and document insurance coverage.
Billing and Insurance	Work with patients, third-party payers, insurance companies to process insurance forms, claims forms, and DRG, ICD9, CPT, and HCPC coding.
EKG/ECG Tech	Perform electrocardiogram studies on patients.
Medical Records	Use administrative skills of transcription, medical terminology, and insurance coding. Requires use of the computer.
Phlebotomy	Use clinical skills to draw blood samples for testing and blood bank use.
Surgery	Use clinical skills to sterilize surgical instruments and set up surgical trays, and assist when needed.
Treatment/Procedure/ Emergency Room (ER)	Assist with minor surgeries and procedures performed in physicians' offices, hospitals, rehabilitation centers, and emergency rooms (ER).

descriptions of some possible job opportunities for medical assistants in each setting. Table 1-2 lists departments or specialties in which medical assistants may seek employment in either inpatient or ambulatory care settings. In some states and settings, additional education and training may be required for medical assistants to fulfill certain responsibilities.

Since your education and training includes general, administrative, and clinical skills, you can seek employment in many different types of work. Then, too, you may work for a physician who practices alone in a **solo practice** or one who participates in a **group practice** with other physicians. If you choose to work for a physician, he or she may specialize in an area of medicine such as family practice, internal medicine, pediatrics, surgery, gerontology, psychiatry, obstetrics and gynecology, sports medicine, or dermatology, just to name a few.

Many medical assistants become certified and then continue their education into areas such as laboratory technology, x-ray, nursing, and medical transcription. Transcription refers to the preparation of written, printed, or typed notes usually prepared from a recording.

Responsibilities of the Medical Assistant

The list of responsibilities that medical assistants perform is extensive. For this reason, the education and training for this field is carefully designed and must involve both theory and hands-on-experience. The actual duties of the medical assistant vary from office to office (Figure 1-3). However, a good medical assistant, who has received a well-rounded education, will be able to adjust to different work environments. Never perform duties that are beyond your level of responsibility—education and training.

Medical assistants' responsibilities will also vary according to the size and type of setting and state laws that apply. Always familiarize yourself with the regulations governing the procedures medical assistants are allowed to perform in whatever environment you work. Generally, the medical assistants' duties are grouped into two categories: administrative and clinical.

Administrative Responsibilities—Business and Front Office
- Scheduling patients, including referrals to specialists
- Greeting and receiving patients
- Screening nonpatients and visitors
- Making arrangements for patient admissions to hospitals, patient tests, and procedures such as x-rays and laboratory tests
- Providing patient instruction regarding procedures and tests performed in the physician's office and hospitals
- Updating and filing patient medical records
- Coding diagnoses and procedures for insurance purposes
- Computer skills
- Handling financial arrangements with patients
- Transcribing medical dictation
- Handling the telephone, reports, correspondence, and filing
- Handling mail, billing, insurance claims, credit, and collections
- Operating office equipment
- Preparing and maintaining employee records
- Handling petty cash
- Reconciling bank statements
- Maintaining records for license renewals, membership fees, and insurance premiums
- Handling the office in the physician's absence
- Assisting the physician with articles, lectures, and manuscripts
- Utilization review of necessary procedures and referrals
- Coordinating managed-care coverage for patients and physicians

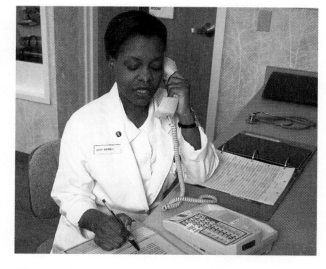

Figure 1-3 Medical assistants take care of many patient related needs on the telephone.

Clinical Responsibilities—Care and Treatment of Patients

- Assisting patients in preparation for physical examinations and for procedures
- Obtaining a medical history
- Performing routine clinical and laboratory procedures under the supervision of a physician
- Collecting, preparing, and transporting laboratory specimens
- Venipuncture, where permitted
- Assisting the physician with procedures
- Instructing and educating patients on treatments and procedures
- Cleaning and sterilizing equipment
- Obtaining patient's height, weight, and vital signs (Figures 1-4 and 1-5)
- Preparing and maintaining examination and treatment rooms
- Inventory control—ordering and storing of supplies
- Disposing of hazardous waste and other materials
- Administering medications under the supervision and orders of the physician, where permitted
- Changing bandages and dressings, and suture removal, where permitted
- Handling drug refills as directed by the physician
- Performing EKG's

- Occupational Safety and Health Administration (OSHA) guidelines compliance and employee instruction
- Performing skills relevant to a particular practice (for example audiometry, spirometry, halter monitor)
- Disposing of contaminated supplies
- Sterilizing medical instruments
- Authorizing drug refills as directed by the supervising physician
- Telephoning prescriptions to pharmacies
- Preparing patients for x-rays

Medical assistants who specialize will have additional duties. Some of these specialties include pediatric medical assistants, ophthalmic medical assistants, and surgical medical assistants.

Role Delineation

The AAMA analyzed the medical assisting field in 1979 to determine the responsibilities of the medical assistant. As a result of this survey and analysis, the AAMA used a process for developing a curriculum called DACUM based on the skills performed daily by medical assistants. In 1984 and 1990, the DACUM list was revised to reflect the major changes in medicine and the health care delivery system.

The Role Delineation Study released in 1997 by the AAMA updates and replaces DACUM. This study is the result of a composite of current competencies essential for medical assistants based upon the prac-

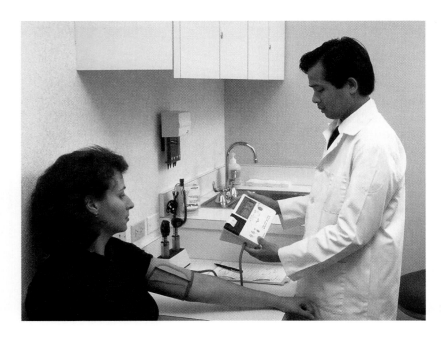

Figure 1-4 Measuring a patient's blood pressure using a digital unit.

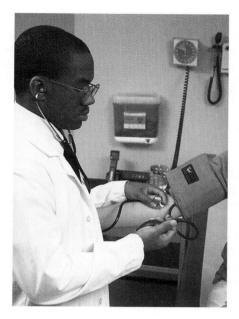

Figure 1-5 Measuring a patient's blood pressure using a wall unit.

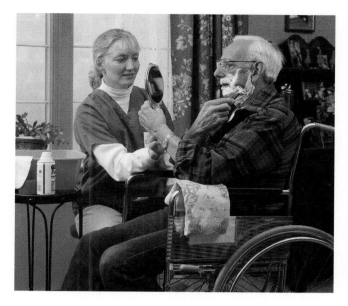

Figure 1-6 Medical assistants spend much time caring for older adult patients.

tice experience of an expert panel. A Role Delineation Chart, which outlines the study, identifies three major categories of competence—administrative, clinical, and general, or interdisciplinary—for entry-level medical assistants. These areas are further expanded to include competencies that should be taught in medical assisting programs. (See Role Delineation Chart included with each chapter.)

Characteristics of a Good Medical Assistant

In addition to having a general medical knowledge, including medical terminology, and being able to perform their administrative and clinical responsibilities, medical assistants must genuinely care about others (Figure 1-6). The nature of the patient/health care worker relationship demands medical assistants be able to communicate effectively and get along with others. Qualities or characteristics regularly found in good medical assistants are integrity, discretion, empathy, and the ability to safeguard the patient's right to confidentiality.

- Integrity—A medical assistant with integrity will do what is expected, when it is expected, for the simple reason that it is expected. Someone with integrity is usually honest, dependable, punctual, and dedicated to high standards.
- Empathy—Patience, a sense of humor, and the ability to work with the sick and the

infirm depend on one's ability and willingness to show empathy. For example, when a medical assistant has some insight or understanding of the pain or distress a patient is feeling and acts in a kindly way that expresses sensitivity to the patient's feelings.

- Discretion—The use of good judgment and prudence make it possible for the medical assistant to offer timely and efficient instruction to the unwilling patient or to remain calm in emergencies and instill confidence in the patient.
- Confidentiality—The ability to safeguard patient confidences, particularly information in the medical record regarding family history, past or current diseases or illnesses, test results, and medications is vital to the patient/health care professional relationship. No information about the patient is to be disclosed without the written permission of the patient. This is a legal and ethical issue with penalties for violating patient confidentiality. Without this trust there can be no relationship. As the person with most frequent access to patient records and verbal confidences, the medical assistant has a serious professional responsibility to safeguard the patient's right to confidentiality.

In many cases, the medical assistant will be the first health professional with whom the patient interacts and on whom the patient bases his or her opinion of the physician. It is important to present a confident, professional image which helps put the patient at ease. A calm, pleasant speaking voice conveys a professional attitude. Remember, eating, drinking, or chewing gum while working are not appropriate in areas open to the public. Along with a basic understanding of human behavior and good communication skills—written, spoken, and non-verbal—the medical assistant must be able to handle tasks requiring basic mathematics, grammar and spelling skills.

Daily habits of good personal hygiene and good grooming are expected in the medical assistant. The use of strong perfumes and showy jewelry is not professional and may even be harmful. For example, strong perfume may actually trigger headaches in some individuals and loose dangling jewelry may get in the way while treating a patient. Long hair and nails should be avoided.

Medical assistants provide the quality of care that they would wish to have given to themselves or to members of their families. The medical assistant must have the ability to see beyond the gruff or complaining manner of the patient who is not feeling well and project a professional, pleasant, and caring attitude.

Med Tip: It helps to focus on the most caring health care worker you have encountered and then try to mirror that behavior.

Professional Organizations

The American Association of Medical Assistants (AAMA), founded in 1959, is the key association in the field of medical assisting. Chicago, Illinois is national headquarters for the AAMA. This organization is responsible for the certification process and offers the certification examination in January and in June. **Certification** indicates that a candidate has met the standards of the AAMA by achieving a satisfactory test result. A certificate, or legal document, is issued to such a person. The first examination given to certify medical assistants was administered in 1963.

After the January 1998 examination, the certification examination will only be offered to graduates of programs accredited by the Commission on **Accreditation** of Allied Health Education Programs (CAAHEP). Accreditation is the process in which an institution completes an extensive self-study af-

ter which an accrediting association visits the school to verify the self-study statements. Upon successful completion of the certification examination, candidates will receive a certificate, confirming them as certified medical assistants. At this time, a medical assistant is able to wear the official pin of the **Certified Medical Assistant (CMA)** (Figure 1-7). A registry is maintained by the AAMA to verify the CMAs credential is current.

Membership in the AAMA is not necessary to take the Certification Examination. For the credential to remain current, it must be revalidated every five years, either by earning **continuing education units (CEUs)** or through reexamination. The American Association of Medical Assistants requires 6.0 CEUs over a five-year period. CEUs are broken down into points with each point (0.1) representing one hour. It takes sixty (60) points (or hours) to equal 6.0 CEUs. The breakdown of units is 20 hours general, 20 hours administrative, and 20 hours clinical. The AAMA sponsors workshops, seminars, and county, state, and national conferences to assist medical assistants to remain current in their field.

The AAMA accredits medical assisting education/training programs and has set the minimum standards for the entry-level in this profession. Since the AAMA is so closely allied with the medical assisting profession, it is able to monitor the needs and the skill education/training of the students. Education programs are periodically reevaluated by the AAMA to assure that the curriculum is adequate and maintained. Recommendations for re-accreditation are then made by the AAMA to the new accrediting agency, Commission on Accreditation of Allied Health Education Program (CAAHEP).

As members of the AAMA, medical assistants can participate in workshops, attend regional,

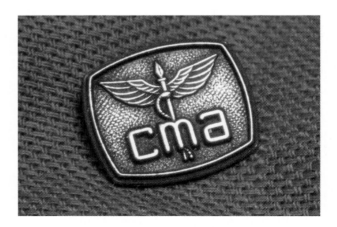

Figure 1-7   Certified Medical Assistant (CMA) pin.

state, and local meetings, interact with other medical assistants, and receive the bimonthly journal, *PMA (Professional Medical Assistant)*. This bimonthly magazine provides articles that discuss current medical issues with the latest information on developments in the field and on continuing education.

The American Medical Technologists (AMT) association provides oversight for the registration and testing of medical technologists. This association, in cooperation with the AMT Institute for Education (AMTIE) has developed a continuing education (CE) program and recording system.

The AMT, a nonprofit certifying body, provides a Registered Medical Assistant (RMA) Certification Examination for medical assistants who meet the eligibility requirements and who can prove their competency to perform entry level skills through written examination. The RMA is awarded to candidates who pass the AMT certification examination (Figure 1–8). The RMA certification examination is formed around the following parameters:

I. General Medical Assisting Knowledge
   A. Anatomy and Physiology
   B. Medical Terminology
   C. Medical Law
   D. Medical Ethics
   E. Human Rights
   F. Patient Education

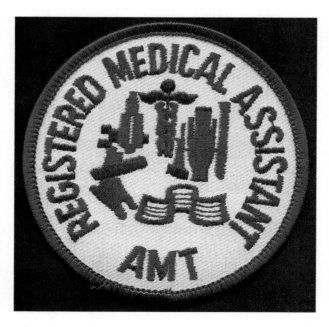

Figure 1-8 Insignia of the Registered Medical Assistant.

II. Administrative Medical Assisting
   A. Insurance
   B. Financial Bookkeeping
   C. Medical Secretarial—Receptionist

Education and Training for the Medical Assistant

The US Department of Education recognizes three agencies to accredit programs in medical assisting:

• The Commission on Accreditation of Allied Health Education Programs (CAAHEP)
• The Accrediting Bureau of Health Education Schools (ABHES)
• The Accrediting Commission of Career Schools and Colleges of Technology (ACCSCT).

The Joint Review Committee for Ophthalmic Medical Personnel accredits programs in ophthalmic medical assisting.

The American Association of Medical Assistants (AAMA) and local chapters of the American Medical Association (AMA) have provided leadership in guiding and directing the formal training requirements for the medical assistant. Courses to prepare medical assistants are offered in community colleges and in private colleges and vocational schools. The certificate or diploma may take from ten months to two years to complete. In many cases the student will go on to receive an associate degree in allied health or nursing from a two or four year college. The programs leading to an associate degree will include general education requirements such as mathematics, English, communications and humanities.

The CAAHEP Essentials state that to provide for student attainment of "*Entry-Level Competencies for the Medical Assistant*" the curriculum—"shall include, but is not limited to the following units, modules, and/or courses of instruction"

   a. Anatomy and Physiology
   b. Medical Terminology
   c. Medical Law and Ethics
   d. Psychology
   e. Communication (oral and written)
   f. Medical Assistant Administrative Procedures
   g. Medical Assistant Clinical Procedures
   h. Externship

An externship experience is required in which students work without payment in a physician's office, clinic or hospital setting for 160 to 190 hours over several weeks during the final stage of their training.

Career Opportunities

According to US Department of Labor Statistics (1992-1993 edition) medical assistants held about 165,000 jobs in 1990. Three out of five workers were employed in physicians' offices, and one in five worked in the offices of other health care practitioners such as optometrists, podiatrists, and chiropractors. Moreover, the US Bureau of Labor Statistics indicates there are more than 800,000 jobs, particularly in physician's offices, which require the expertise of trained paramedical persons such as medical assistants. [Bureau of Labor Statistics, US Department of Labor: Employment by Occupation and Industry, 1990, Washington, DC, US Government Printing Office.]

The medical assistant is the most frequently employed allied health professional in the physician's office and most physicians have more than

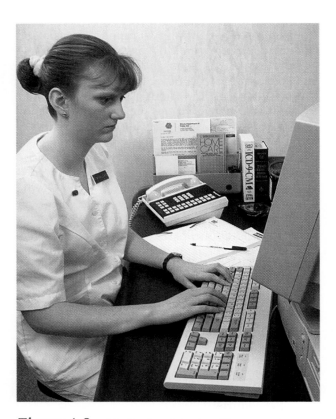

Figure 1-9 Medical assistants with computer skills have many career opportunities.

one medical assistant working in their office. The US Bureau Of Labor Statistics lists medical assisting as one of the top 30 fastest growing occupations with a 59% increase in the number of medical assistants expected between 1994 and the year 2005. (Bureau of Labor Statistics, Office of Employment Projections, 1995.)

The anticipated need for more health professionals is based on the expected increase in the numbers of older adults who will require the care of a physician and the tremendous growth in the number of outpatient facilities.

The variety and numbers of jobs available, requiring the skills learned in medical assistant training programs, grow daily. While the general category, "medical assistant," may be used in some career ads, some of the job title opportunities may include:

- Data processing clerk
- Billing or collection assistant
- Insurance claim coder
- Medical records clerk
- Medical records transcriptionist
- Office manager
- Physician's administrative or clinical assistant
- Receptionist

With Additional Education and Credentials, You May Even Respond to Ads For:
- A medical laboratory assistant
- An electrocardiography technician, where allowed
- A phlebotomist

Experienced medical assistants may find work as office managers, medical records managers, hospital ward clerks, and EKG technicians and teachers of medical assistants. With additional schooling, medical assistants can enter other health care occupations such as nursing, occupational therapists, physical therapists, medical and x-ray technologists (Figure 1-9).

The Future of the Medical Assisting Field

The future is bright for medical assistants. There are more than 600,000 physicians in the nation, so there is always a demand for formally educated medical assistants in the medical offices. In addition, awareness of the variety of tasks that a qualified medical assistant can perform is growing along with the actual need for such skills. For example, people are living longer due to advances in medical technology, and so the size of the general population who require medical care is increasing.

It is also quite true that the future will hold new opportunities for medical assistants to expand their skill base. The expectation is that by the year 2000 the number of medical assistants working in hospitals and nursing homes will have increased in great numbers.

As government involvement increases in health care so does the need for good documentation and records maintenance. Medical records management and insurance coding, professions that require some additional credentials, are growing fields in which the medical assistant has training. Medical assistants with computer skills—word processing, data bases, and spreadsheets are in great demand.

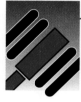 ## LEGAL AND ETHICAL ISSUES

It is important to fully understand what your credentials allow you to do. The medical assistant is uniquely qualified to perform the administrative and clinical procedures associated with responsibilities assigned in the particular setting by the physician. In fulfilling these responsibilities, however, you must always be aware that the potential for psychological, financial, and physical injury to the patient exists. It is your ethical responsibility to patients and

your employer that you do your utmost to maintain a high level of skill performance in all that you do. The medical assistant always works as an agent of the physician.

Many of the jobs/careers discussed in this chapter require additional education, including passing a written certification examination. Be mindful that patients understand what your title—Certified Medical Assistant (CMA) or Registered Medical Assistant (RMA)—means. Never be afraid to say, "I am not qualified to do that."

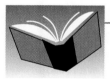 ## PATIENT EDUCATION

Patients do not always clearly understand the distinctions among the professions of medical assistant, physician's assistant, and nurse. It is your responsibility to clarify

for the patients what you are permitted to do. Do not accept being addressed as "nurse," since the nursing license carries different responsibilities and standards than does the medical assistant's certificate.

Summary

The field of medical assisting is growing in response to increasing health care needs of consumers. The profession of medical assistant offers many opportunities—roles, responsibilities, and settings for employment. Most medical assistants work in ambulatory settings such as physicians' offices where they fulfill the administrative and clinical responsibilities associated with running medical offices. The size and nature of the medical office practice will determine the

number of medical assistants and the actual work they will do.

Caring individuals, who are dedicated professionals with a commitment to maintain their skills through continuing education make the best medical assistants. The important thing to remember is that the opportunities presented are many and the future of medical assisting looks attractive. A career in medical assisting is emotionally and professionally challenging as well as financially satisfying.

Competency Review

1. Define and spell the glossary terms for this chapter.
2. List several health care facilities or specialties in which you may choose to work as a medical assistant.
3. Explain the difference between administrative and clinical functions of medical assisting.
4. Name a medical assistant's professional organization.

5. What qualities are regularly found in good medical assistants?

6. Explain what the curriculum in medical assisting should include.

7. What is the future for medical assisting?

8. Interview a working medical assistant about his or her duties.

9. Ask to "shadow" a working medical assistant for a day.

PREPARING FOR THE CERTIFICATION EXAM

Test Taking Tip — Come into an exam with a positive attitude. You know more than you think you do!

Examination Review Questions

1. What is the AAMA?
   (A) All American Medical Association
   (B) Allied American Medical Association
   (C) Administrative (division) of the American Medical Association
   (D) American Association of Medical Assistants
   (E) American Association of Medical Assistance

2. What are the two general categories that would BEST describe the responsibilities of a medical assistant?
   (A) administrative and laboratory
   (B) secretarial and direct patient care
   (C) assisting the physician and secretarial
   (D) clinical and secretarial
   (E) administrative and clinical

3. What refers to the preparation of a written form of an audio recorded medical report?
   (A) medical transcription
   (B) coding
   (C) decoding
   (D) word processing
   (E) documentation

4. Which of the following administrative tasks falls beyond the scope of practice for a medical assistant?
   (A) coordinating managed care coverage
   (B) handling petty cash
   (C) assisting the physician with a journal article
   (D) utilization review of necessary procedures
   (E) none of the above

5. Which of the following clinical tasks falls beyond the scope of practice for a medical assistant?
   (A) vital signs
   (B) patient education
   (C) phlebotomy
   (D) handling drug refills
   (E) none of the above

6. The AAMA certifies, through examination, that a medical assistant has met the standards of the AAMA. In addition, to the certificate that a CMA receives upon the successful completion of the examination, what might the CMA automatically be entitled to?
   (A) the CMA pin
   (B) the letters RMA after his or her name
   (C) the AAMA journal, *PMA*
   (D) advanced placement in a nursing program
   (E) none of the above

7. Which of the following statements is TRUE?
   (A) a medical assistant is equivalent to a nurse
   (B) a medical assistant is equivalent to a physician assistant
   (C) it is acceptable for a medical assistant to allow patients to refer to him or her as a "nurse"
   (D) an advertisement for a medical assistant might include "medical records clerk"
   (E) an advertisement for a medical assistant might include "x-ray technician"

8. As per the CAAHEP Essentials, in order to provide for student attainment of "entry-level competencies for the medical assistant," at a minimum the curriculum of a medical assisting school must include

(A) medical assistant administrative procedures

(B) medical assistant clinical procedures

(C) medical law and ethics

(D) externship of 160 to 190 hours

(E) all of the above

9. Necessary characteristics of a good medical assistant should include all EXCEPT

(A) confidentiality

(B) discretion

(C) empathy

(D) integrity

(E) physical attractiveness

10. Which of the following statements is TRUE?

(A) with over 600,000 physicians practicing in the US, the demand for medical assistants is great

(B) by the year 6000 the number of medical assistants will have reached the demand

(C) irrespective of experience, a medical assistant is equivalent to a CMA

(D) all of the above

(E) none of the above

ON THE JOB

Darlene Smith, a CMA, has been employed for six years by a practice of three physicians specializing in Cardiology. She is a graduate of a CAAHEP accredited medical assisting school. Furthermore, Darlene received extensive hands-on training performing EKGs while doing her required externship.

One of the clinical duties Darlene has just completed was an EKG on Mrs. Warner, a 76 year old patient. This test was ordered by Darlene's boss, Dr. Patel.

Dr. Patel has just telephoned Darlene, explaining he was behind schedule as he was still doing rounds at one of the hospitals the practice services. He asked her to do him a favor and interpret Mrs. Warner's EKG, sign his name, and FAX the report to Mrs. Warner's referring Internist who is expecting the results.

What is your response?

1. Given the scope of Darlene's education, training, and years of experience as a CMA, would this "favor" fall within the AAMA guidelines as one of her responsibilities?

2. Would any portion of Dr. Patel's request fall within the guidelines, if so, which portion(s)? Is there ever a case for an exception to these guidelines?

3. What, if anything, should Darlene say to Dr. Patel?

References

Allied Health Education Directory. Chicago: American Medical Association, 1996.

American Association of Medical Assistants Bylaws. Chicago: American Association of Medical Assistants.

Badash, S. and Chesebro, D. *Introduction to Health Occupations.* Upper Saddle River, NJ: Brady/Prentice Hall, 1997.

Fremgen, B. *Medical Terminology.* Upper Saddle River, NJ: Brady/Prentice Hall, 1997.

"Results of the 1991 AAMA Employment Survey." *PMA.* November/December, 1991, pp. 23-26.

Statistical Abstract of the United States 1996: The National Data Book. Washington, DC: US Bureau of Census, 1996.

Tabor's Cyclopedic Medical Dictionary, 17th ed. Philadelphia: F.A. Davis, 1989.

US Department of Labor, Bureau of Labor Statistics. Occupational Outlook Handbook. Washington: US. Government Printing Office, 1993.

Professional Organizations

American Association of Medical Assistants (AAMA), 20 North Wacker Drive, Suite 1575, Chicago, IL, 60606.

American Association for Medical Transcription (AAMT), PO Box 576187, Modesto, CA 95357.

American Medical Technologists (AMT), Registered Medical Assistant (RMA), 710 Higgins Road, Park Ridge, IL 60068-5765.

MEDICAL ASSISTANT ROLE DELINEATION CHART

Highlight indicates material covered in this chapter

ADMINISTRATIVE

ADMINISTRATIVE PROCEDURES

- Perform basic clerical functions
- Schedule, coordinate, and monitor appointments
- Schedule inpatient/outpatient admissions and procedures
- Understand and apply third party guidelines
- Obtain reimbursement through accurate claims submission
- Monitor third-party reimbursement
- Perform medical transcription
- Understand and adhere to managed care policies and procedures
- *Negotiate managed care contracts (adv)*

PRACTICE FINANCES

- Perform procedural and diagnostic coding
- Apply bookkeeping principles
- Document and maintain accounting and banking records
- Manage accounts receivable
- Manage accounts payable
- Process payroll
- *Develop and maintain fee schedules (adv)*
- *Manage renewals of business and professional insurance policies (adv)*
- *Manage personal benefits and maintain records (adv)*

CLINICAL

FUNDAMENTAL PRINCIPLES

- Apply principles of aseptic technique and infection control
- Comply with quality assurance practices
- Screen and follow up patient test results

DIAGNOSTIC ORDERS

- Collect and process specimens
- Perform diagnostic tests

PATIENT CARE

- Adhere to established triage procedures
- Obtain patient history and vital signs
- Prepare and maintain examination and treatment areas

- Prepare patient for examinations, procedures, and treatments
- Assist with examinations, procedures, and treatments
- Prepare and administer medications and immunizations
- Maintain medication and immunization records
- Recognize and respond to emergencies
- Coordinate patient care information with other health care providers

GENERAL (TRANSDISCIPLINARY)

PROFESSIONALISM

- Project a professional manner and image
- Adhere to ethical principles
- Demonstrate initiative and responsibility
- Work as a team member
- Manage time efficiently
- Prioritize and perform multiple tasks
- Adapt to change
- Promote the CMA credential
- Enhance skills through continuing education

COMMUNICATION SKILLS

- Treat all patients with compassion and empathy
- Recognize and respect cultural diversity
- Adapt communications to individual's ability to understand
- Use professional telephone technique
- Use effective and correct verbal and written communications
- Recognize and respond to verbal and non-verbal communications
- Use medical terminology appropriately
- Receive, organize, prioritize, and transmit information
- Serve as liaison
- Promote the practice through positive public relations

LEGAL CONCEPTS

- Maintain confidentiality
- Practice within the scope of education, training, and personal capabilities
- Prepare and maintain medical records
- Document accurately
- Use appropriate guidelines when releasing information
- Follow employer's established policies dealing with the health care contract
- Follow federal, state, and local legal guidelines
- Maintain awareness of federal and state health care legislation and regulations
- Maintain and dispose of regulated substances in compliance with government guidelines
- Comply with established risk management and safety procedures
- Recognize professional credentialing criteria
- Participate in the development and maintenance of personnel, policy, and procedure manuals
- *Develop and maintain personnel, policy, and procedure manuals (adv)*

INSTRUCTION

- Instruct individuals according to their needs
- Explain office policies and procedures
- Teach methods of health promotion and disease prevention
- Locate community resources and disseminate information
- *Orient and train personnel (adv)*
- *Develop educational materials (adv)*
- *Conduct continuing education activities (adv)*

OPERATIONAL FUNCTIONS

- Maintain supply inventory
- Evaluate and recommend equipment and supplies
- Apply computer techniques to support office operations
- *Supervise personnel (adv)*
- *Interview and recommend job applicants (adv)*
- *Negotiate leases and prices for equipment and supply contracts (adv)*

SOURCE: Reprinted by permission of the American Association of Medical Assistants from the *AAMA Role Delineation Study: Occupational Analysis of the Medical Assisting Profession.*

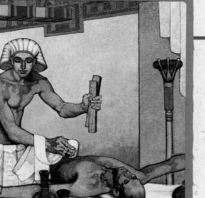

2

Medical Science: History and Practice

LEARNING OBJECTIVES

After completing this chapter, you should:
1. Define and spell the glossary terms for this chapter.
2. Describe the history of medicine from early man to the present time.
3. Identify the major achievements during each of these periods: early medicine, 18th century, 19th century, and 20th century or modern medicine.
4. Identify who discovered anesthetics, aseptic technique, cure for yellow fever, insulin, microscope, penicillin, polio vaccine, radium, stethoscope, treatment for syphilis, and x-ray.
5. Name and explain the benefit to medicine of contributions made by each of these women: Clara Barton, RN; Elizabeth Blackwell, MD; and Florence Nightingale, RN.
6. Describe the difference between an internship and a residency in relationship to the training of physicians.
7. List six medical professionals who are addressed by the title "Doctor."
8. Name and describe four types of medical practice.
9. State which type of medical practice is addressed under the medical and surgical specialties.

Glossary

anesthesia   Partial or complete loss of sensation.

anthrax   A deadly infectious disease caused by *Bacillus anthracis*. Humans contract the disease from infected animal hair, hides, or waste.

autopsy   An examination of organs and tissues in a deceased body to determine the cause of death.

bacteria   Microorganism capable of causing disease.

cadaver   A dead body; a corpse.

caduceus   Symbol for healing made up of a staff with two snakes coiled around it which has become the recognized symbol for medicine.

chemotherapy   Use of chemicals, including drugs to treat or control infections and diseases.

cholera   Acute infection involving the small bowel which causes severe diarrhea.

homeopathy   Treatment and prevention of disease based on the premise that large doses of drugs which cause symptoms in healthy people will cure the same symptoms when given in small doses.

immunology   Study of immunity—resistance to or protection from disease.

medicinal   Plants and other substances that have a therapeutic value for the body.

microbes   One-celled form of life such as bacteria.

microorganism   Minute living organisms such as bacteria, virus, protozoa, and fungus that are not visible to the human eye without a microscope.

morbidity rate   Number of sick persons or cases of a disease within a certain population.

mortality rate   Death rate; the ratio of the number of deaths in a given population.

pasteurization   Process of heating substances, such as milk or cheese, to a certain temperature in order to destroy bacteria.

pathology   Study of the nature and cause of disease.

puerperal sepsis   Severe infection of the genital tract during the postpartum period or as a complication of an abortion. Also called childbed fever.

syphilis   An infectious, chronic, venereal disease with lesions that can affect many organs. It is treated with antibiotics.

The healing art of medicine was taught and practiced before humans kept written records. This chapter describes the science and practice of medicine from the earliest evidence of healing when disease was considered to be of supernatural origin or the field of demons to the present—a time of astounding research, discovery, and healing. Contributions of many ancient peoples still influence medicine today. The discussion of present day medical codes of ethics, rules about sanitation, personal hygiene, herbal cures, acupuncture and other medical and surgical practices highlights the specific contributions of ancient peoples and the men and women whose accomplishments catapulted the science of medicine along in leaps and bounds.

The chapter provides a picture of today's medical practice—issues of licensure, including evaluation, credentials, reciprocity, renewals, and suspension; doctor's titles; and types of practice, for example solo practice and partnership. Also covered in the chapter are the numerous medical and surgical specialties.

History of Medicine

Drawings, bony remains, and some surgical tools are evidence of early man's attempt to practice medicine. Folk medicine using plants adopted a trial and error method to determine which plants were poisonous and which had medicinal value. Early man attributed supernatural origins to some ailments. In early medicine, some diseases were considered the work of a demon, evil spirit, or an offended god who had placed some object, such as a worm, into the body of the patient. Treatment consisted of trying to remove the evil intruder.

Med Tip: One means used in ancient times to remove evil demons from a patient was called trepanning. The practice consisted of making a hole in the patient's skull. Trepanned skulls from prehistoric man have been found in parts of Europe and Peru. Today, burr holes are drilled into the skull when a surgeon performs a craniotomy to relieve pressure.

The first doctors, "medicine men," were witch doctors or sorcerers (Figure 2-1). In 3000 BC, Babylonian physicians practiced using the written "Code of Hammurabi." This code, named after Hammurabi, an early king of Babylon, has laws relating to the practice of medicine which included severe penalties for errors. For example, according to the code, if the doctor killed the patient while opening an abscess, his hands would be cut off.

Contributions of Ancient Civilizations

A study of medical practice in early Egypt offers greater insight into the basis of modern medicine. The Egyptians left behind lists of remedies and surgical treatments of wounds and injuries.

Records for rules of sanitation go back as far as the Egyptians. Personal hygiene, the sanitary preparation of food and other matters of public health were pioneered by the practices of the Jewish religion. Other cultures contributed to moving the practice forward.

The early Greeks have records of using non-poisonous snakes to treat the wounds of patients. The caduceus, which has become the recognized symbol for medicine, depicts a healing staff with two snakes coiled around the staff.

Herbal medical remedies from ancient India are recorded from 800 BC. The Chinese culture wrote about pulses around the time of 250 AD. Early Japanese and Chinese cultures practiced acupuncture successfully.

Ancient Cures Today's Legacy

Early medicine, while often based on superstition, actually provided medicinal remedies that are still used today. The effect of opium produced by the poppy plant was known in ancient times and even now is used to relieve severe pain when used in the medication morphine. Other remedies include using:

- *Nitroglycerin* to treat heart patients
- *Digitalis* from the foxglove plant to regulate and strengthen the heartbeat
- *Sulfur* and *cayenne pepper* to stop bleeding
- *Chamomile* and *licorice* to aid digestion
- *Cranberry* to treat urinary tract infections

Early Medicine

Early medicine began with Hippocrates and the shift from the belief in magical sources of illness and disease to more scientific study which looked to physical causes of disease. This period concludes with the introduction of the microscope and the ability to see and measure bacteria previously not observed with the naked eye.

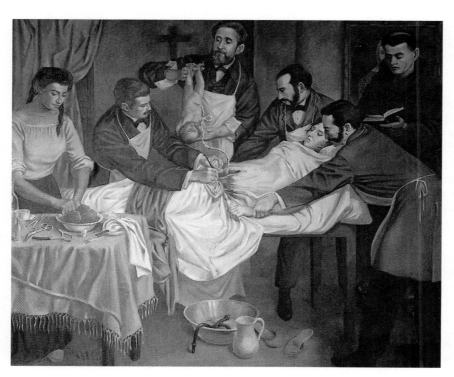

Figure 2-1 Cesarean section from old medical textbook.

Hippocrates (Father of Medicine)

Historically, the first scientific system of medicine is of Greek origin and is usually associated with Hippocrates (460–377 BC) who has since become known as the "Father of Medicine." Hippocrates shifted medicine from the realm of mysticism and into the area of scientific practice. He stressed the body's healing nature, clinical descriptions of diseases and the ability to discover some diseases by listening to the chest. He practiced medicine at a time in history when little was known about anatomy and physiology. Nevertheless, his writings and descriptions of symptoms remain accurate today.

The Hippocratic Oath is part of the writings of this fifth century physician. The oath serves as a widely used ethical guide for physicians who pledge to work for the good of the patient, to do him or her no harm, to prescribe no deadly drugs, to give no advice that could cause death, and to keep confidential medical information regarding the patient. The oath is still often administered as part of graduation ceremonies in medical schools.

Med Tip: The term "oath" should not be interpreted too narrowly. The Hippocratic Oath was an ethical code and not a law. It is actually an appeal for correct conduct but contains no threat of punishment.

Galen

Galen (130–201 AD), a Greek physician who practiced in Rome, followed the Hippocratic method. He stressed the value of anatomy and founded experimental physiology. He stated that arteries contained blood and not air as previously believed. Since the dissection of humans was illegal during Galen's time, he based his theories on the examination of pigs and apes. While some of his work is inaccurate due to the lack of human cadavers, or dead bodies, from which to study the human anatomy, he is still known as the "Prince of Physicians." Galen was an early believer in the value of preventive medicine.

Vesalius

Anatomy as a science was developed by Andreas Vesalius (1514–1564). He is known as the "Father of Modern Anatomy." Vesalius is responsible for naming many of the anatomical terms we use today.

One of his students, Gabrielle Fallopius (1523–1562), went on to identify and name many anatomical parts. He gave his name to the fallopian tubes. Today we find that anatomical designations, surgical instruments, procedures, and even diseases are often named after the physician or scientist who first described them.

William Harvey

In England during the 17th century, William Harvey (1578–1657) began writing on the topic of blood circulation and using the experimental method in medicine. Unfortunately for Harvey the microscope had not yet been invented and he was never able to view capillaries.

Harvey's work was enhanced when Marcello Malpighi (1628–1694), from Italy, began using a crude microscope to see small vessels in the lungs of frogs.

Galileo

Galileo (1564–1642), who stressed the value of measurement in medicine rather than using guesswork, was the first to use a telescope to study the skies. Zacharias Janssen in Holland, was an eyeglass maker who invented the microscope.

Anton van Leeuwenhoek

Anton van Leeuwenhoek (1632–1723), also in Holland, devoted his life to microscopic studies. He is known as the first person to observe and describe bacteria which he referred to as "tiny little beasties." He is also responsible for describing spermatozoa (mature male sex cells) and protozoa. Protozoa are simplest forms—usually one cell—of animals.

Medicine During the 18th Century

In England, formal medical training began when it was required that anyone wishing to become a doctor must first become an apprentice. Medical schools in Edinburgh and Glasgow, Scotland were developed.

Med Tip: The term "surgeon" comes from the Greek word "cheir" which means hand and "ergon" meaning work. Some of the early surgeons were barbers.

John Hunter

John Hunter (1728–1793) developed surgery and surgical pathology into a science. He is noted as the "Founder of Scientific Surgery." Some of his contributions to medical science include the introduction of a flexible feeding tube into the stomach.

Med Tip: The term "vaccination" comes from the Latin term "vacca" meaning cow. Cowpox was referred to as "vaccinia." Today the term vaccine means a live or attenuated material given to a person for the purpose of establishing resistance to disease. Vaccines come from animals other than cows today and synthetic sources.

Edward Jenner

Public health and hygiene began to attract attention during the 18th century. A country doctor, Edward Jenner (1749–1823), a pupil of John Hunter, observed that dairy maids who had become infected with the disease cowpox would not become infected with the deadly disease smallpox. Jenner overcame ridicule from the medical community and went on to perform the first vaccination using the smallpox vaccine.

Rene Laennec

Another major advancement in medicine was made by Rene Laennec (1781–1826) who invented the stethoscope. His invention was based on the use of a paper wrapped into a cone shape which was then placed over the patient's chest to listen to the heart.

Samuel Hahnemann

Samuel Hahnemann (1755–1843) developed the practice of homeopathy, the use of small doses of drugs to treat symptoms and diseases. He acted on the premise that "like cures like" and used minute doses of quinine to treat patients and put their bodies into the proper rhythm. Homeopathy gained respect during the great influenza epidemic in England when calendula from the marigold flower was used to successfully treat victims.

Benjamin Franklin

The American statesman, Benjamin Franklin (1706–1790), was also an inventor and, in addition to the discovery of electricity, he invented bifocals. One of his most important contributions to medical science was the discovery that colds could be passed from one person to another.

Medicine During the 19th Century

During the 19th century, the practice of medicine advanced rapidly. The documentation of accurate anatomy and physiology allowed the human body to be known and understood by physicians. The use of sophisticated microscopes, injection materials, and instruments such as the ophthalmoscope all moved the practice of medicine forward.

The discovery of the cell was one of the most enlightening discoveries of this era. Many believe that the greatest achievement of the 19th century was the knowledge that certain diseases, as well as surgical wound infections, were directly caused by microorganisims—minute living organisms. The practice of surgery changed as a result of this knowledge along with the advances in the use of anesthetics.

Louis Pasteur

Louis Pasteur (1822–1895) is credited for establishing the science of bacteriology. His experiments determined that putrefaction, or decay, was caused by living organisms known as bacteria. His work solved many medical problems during his day including rabies, anthrax in sheep and cattle, and chicken cholera. Cholera was determined to be a bacillus transmitted through water, milk, or food contaminated with excreta of carriers. The process of pasteurization is named after Pasteur. Pasteurization is the process during which substances, such as milk and cheese, are heated to a certain temperature to eliminate bacteria.

Joseph Lister

Joseph Lister (1827–1912) borrowed Pasteur's theories and eventually introduced the antiseptic system in surgery (Figure 2-2). Until that time, surgeons and obstetricians did not wash their hands between patients. Disease was being spread from one patient to another. Lister advised placing an antiseptic barrier between the wound and the germ-containing atmosphere. Present day aseptic techniques can be attributed to Lister's work.

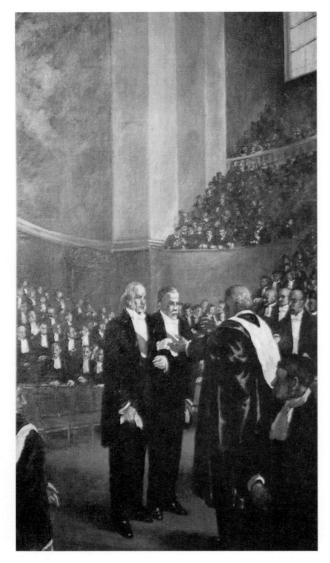

Figure 2-2   Louis Pasteur and Joseph Lister.

Ignaz Semmelweiss

Ignaz Semmelweiss (1818–1865), an obstetrician in Vienna, was already advising medical students to disinfect the hands and clothing of anyone who attended a birth. He noted that the medical students would attend a mother in childbirth immediately after having participated in an autopsy. An autopsy is an examination of the organs and tissues of a deceased body to determine the cause of death. When he advised the students to disinfect their hands before attending a childbirth, the incidence of disease went down dramatically.

Today, it is commonly known that disease can be spread from person to person if careful washing and disinfection does not take place. But, in the 1800s, the men who advocated disinfection were ridiculed.

Robert Koch

Robert Koch (1843–1910) showed how bacteria could be cultivated and stained. He discovered the tubercle bacillus, the cause of the dreaded disease tuberculosis. His investigation into the cause of cholera led us to the knowledge that contaminated food and water can cause disease.

Paul Ehrlich

Paul Ehrlich (1854–1915) was a pioneer in the study of microbiology. He was a pioneer in the fields of immunology, bacteriology, and the use of chemotherapy. He developed a method for staining bacteria and cells which eventually led to a means for providing a differential diagnosis based on classifying organisms. He was one of the original "microbe hunters." Microbes are one-celled forms of life such as bacteria. His greatest achievement was the discovery, on his 606th attempt, of the "magic bullet" to treat syphilis. He originally called the drug "salvarsan" since it offered a salvation from this dreaded disease. However, he later discovered a milder drug, neosalvarsan, to treat syphilis.

Other Major Advances During This Period

William Roentgen (1845–1923) discovered x-rays, Pierre (1859–1906) and Marie (1867–1934) Curie discovered radium, and Sigmund Freud (1856–1939) worked in the field of psychiatry.

Several physicians have given their names to diseases they are credited with discovering. Richard Bright (1789–1858) advanced the knowledge of kidney disease including Bright's disease. Thomas Addison (1793–1860) discovered a disease named after him caused by a deficiency of adrenocortico hormones from the adrenal gland.

American Medicine During This Period

Significant contributions were made to medicine through the work of William Norton, Crawford Long, Walter Reed, and William Beaumont. The specific work of each of these individuals is highlighted here.

William Morton and Crawford Long The most famous contribution by the United States to the practice of medicine during this period was the discovery of anesthesia. William Morton (1819–1868), a dentist at Massachusetts General Hospital, and Crawford Long (1815–1878), a Georgia physician, are generally credited with having first demonstrated the use of ether as a general anesthetic. Anesthesia refers to the absence of partial or complete sensation. An anesthetic is a substance used to produce anesthesia. These two men worked independently of each other and made possible life-saving operations that previously could not be performed without anesthetics.

Walter Reed Walter Reed (1851–1902) and others helped to conquer yellow fever which allowed for completion of the Panama canal by reducing the death rate for the workers. Dr. Reed gathered volunteers who allowed him to inject them with yellow fever in order to find a cure.

William Beaumont The surgeon William Beaumont (1785–1853) aided the study of the digestive process when he carefully documented his observation of a patient's gastrointestinal process through a stomach wound that would not heal.

Medicine During the 20th Century

The first half of the 20th century resulted in major medical advances. The death rates from diseases such as tuberculosis and diphtheria dropped dramatically. The overall mortality rates (death rates) decreased due to improved medical care and new emphasis was placed on morbidity rates (rates of disease and illness). Four major developments dominate this period:

- The development of chemotherapy and the specialty of oncology
- The development of immunology
- The progress in endocrinology
- The progress in nutrition

Alexander Fleming

One of the most dramatic episodes of the modern era was the discovery of antibiotics. Sir Alexander Fleming (1881–1955) accidentally discovered that a stray mold on his culture plate of staphylococci would cause the bacteria to stop growing. He called this mold *Penicillium* and this became known throughout the world as penicillin. Fleming's discovery took place in 1928. He, along with two other scientists, won the Nobel prize for their work with penicillin.

Med Tip: The use of penicillin was one of the first examples of using chemicals to treat infections. This has become known as **chemotherapy.** Today the term chemotherapy generally refers to drugs used to treat forms of cancer.

Gerhard Domagk

In 1932 a German pathologist, Gerhard Domagk (1895–1964) developed sulfa drugs from a dye called Prontosil red. The sulfonamide compounds ushered in the chemotherapeutic era in medicine. This discovery helped to change the way that medicine was practiced. Lives could now be saved from deadly diseases.

Jonas Salk and Albert Sabin

The study of immunology advanced with the discovery of vaccines against typhoid, tetanus, diphtheria, tuberculosis, yellow fever, influenza and measles. During the 1950s Drs. Jonas Salk (1914–1996) and Albert Sabin (1906–1993) developed vaccines which eradicated the crippling disease polio.

Sir Frederick Banting

Endocrinology made advances when hormones were identified. Sir Frederick Banting (1891–1941), a Canadian physician, along with two other physicians discovered insulin for controlling diabetes mellitus in 1921. Scientists at the Mayo Clinic in Rochester, Minnesota isolated cortisone as an anti-inflammatory agent.

The outstanding discovery in the field of nutrition was the vitamin. Deficiency diseases, such as scurvy due to lack of vitamin C, rickets due to lack of vitamin D, and beriberi due to lack of vitamin B1, almost disappeared with the discovery and use of these vitamins.

Women in Medicine

Few women were allowed to practice medicine in the early years. In part, this was due to social constraints against women appearing in public. However, many women did practice as midwives and became skilled at delivering babies. There are also some remarkable female physicians and nurses who overcame great odds to practice in their profession.

Elizabeth Blackwell

Elizabeth Blackwell (1821–1910) was the first female physician in the United States. After being turned down by several medical schools she was finally awarded a degree in 1849 in New York. She went on to open a medical college for women and her own dispensary.

Florence Nightingale

Florence Nightingale (1820–1910) is considered the founder of modern nursing (Figure 2-3). She studied nursing in Europe and nursed wounded soldiers during the Crimean War (1850–1853). Florence Nightingale and her fellow nurses were treated poorly by the doctors at that time.

Her attention to detail, record keeping and compassionate nursing care changed the way nursing was practiced. She advocated the use of the nursing process and elevated nursing to an honored profession. She is referred to as "The Lady with the Lamp" due to her tireless work night and day to supervise the nursing care of wounded soldiers. She started the first school of nursing in 1860 at St. Thomas Hospital in London.

Clara Barton

Clara Barton (1821–1912) was a contemporary of Florence Nightingale, but nursed soldiers in a different war, the Civil War. She established the American Red Cross when she became aware of the need for support services for the soldiers (Figures 2-4 and 2-5). She also established the Federal Bureau of Records to help track injured and dead soldiers.

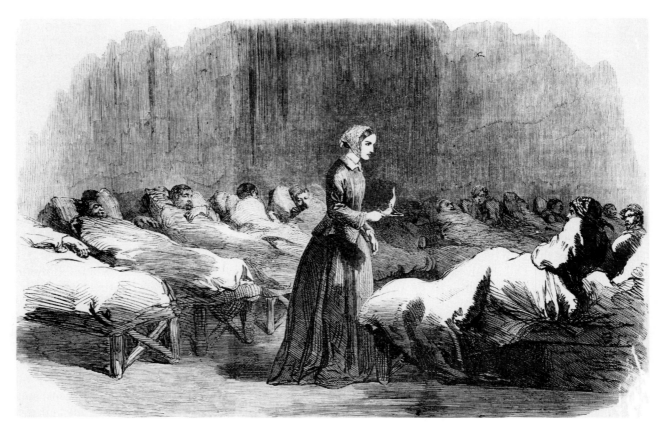

Figure 2-3   Florence Nightingale, founder of modern nursing.

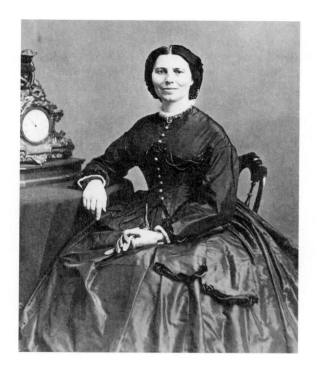

Figure 2-4   Clara Barton, founder of the Red Cross.

Lillian Wald

Another nurse, Lillian Wald (1867–1940), established public health nursing at the Henry Street Settlement House in New York City. She believed the patient's social as well as physical needs were important.

Marie Curie

Marie Curie (1867–1934), a Polish born scientist, won the Nobel Prize along with her husband, Pierre, for the discovery of radium. She overcame great hardships to become a scientist. She later went on to win the Nobel Prize in chemistry by herself. Marie Curie's work is the basis for the present-day treatment of cancer with the element radium.

Table 2-1 provides a summary of major discoveries and achievements by men and women in medicine from the early history of medicine to the present era.

Medical Practice

Today's medical practice for physicians includes family, or general, practice as well as a strong emphasis on specialization. Areas covered in this section include: education requirements, the Medical Practice Act, and licensure issues, such as examination, reciprocity, and suspension.

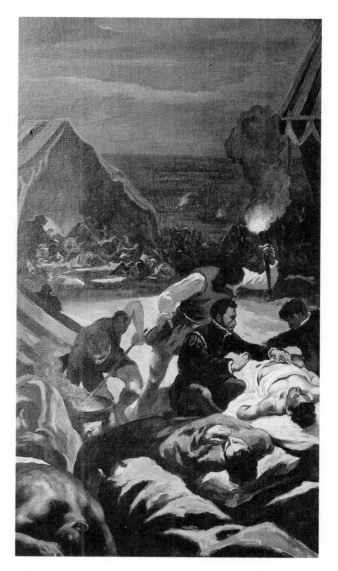

Figure 2-5   Healing wounded on the battlefield.

Medical Education

The practice of medicine, which is the science of diagnosis, treatment, and prevention of disease, requires a minimum of nine years of training. The training and education to become a physician generally includes a four-year college degree in pre-med, four years of medical school, and a one year internship. A state board examination is then completed. If the person passes the board exam, they then become licensed to practice.

Medical Practice Acts

Each state has regulations that direct the practice of medicine in that state. While there are some slight differences from state to state, in general,

TABLE 2-1 Summary of Medical Discoveries and Achievements

Dates	Person	Discovery/Achievement
3000 BC	Hammurabi	"Code of Hammurabi"—code of medical ethics
460–377 BC	Hippocrates, Father of Medicine	Hippocratic Oath
130–201 AD	Galen	Experimental physiology
1514–1564	Andreas Vesalius	Father of Modern Anatomy
1578–1657	William Harvey	Described blood circulation
1628–1694	Marcello Malpighi	Microscopic anatomy
1632–1723	Anton van Leeuwenhoek	Founder of microbiology
1706–1790	Benjamin Franklin	Bifocal lens
1728–1793	John Hunter	Founder of scientific surgery
1749–1823	Edward Jenner	Discovered smallpox vaccine
1755–1843	Samuel Hahnemann	Introduction of homeopathy
1781–1826	Rene Laennec	Invented the stethoscope
1785–1853	William Beaumont	Studied the digestive process
1789–1858	Richard Bright	Discovered Bright's disease (kidney)
1793–1860	Thomas Addison	Discovered Addison's disease (adrenal gland)
1818–1865	Ignaz Semmelweiss	Theory of childbed fever and disinfection of hands
1815–1878	Crawford Long	Discovered anesthesia
1819–1868	William Morton	Discovered anesthesia
1820–1910	Florence Nightingale	Founder of nursing
1821–1912	Clara Barton	Founder of American Red Cross
1821–1910	Elizabeth Blackwell	First woman in US to receive a medical degree
1822–1895	Louis Pasteur	Father of bacteriology
1827–1912	Joseph Lister	Developed sterile techniques in surgery
1843–1910	Robert Koch	Bacteriologist who discovered tubercle bacillus
1845–1922	Wilhelm Roentgen	Discovered x-ray in 1895
1851–1902	Walter Reed	Helped to conquer yellow fever
1854–1915	Paul Ehrlich	"Magic bullet" to treat syphilis
	Sigmund Freud	Introduced psychiatry

TABLE 2-1 (Continued)

Dates	Person	Discovery/Achievement
1859–1906	Pierre Curie	Discovered radium with his wife, Marie
1867–1934	Marie Curie	Discovered radium with husband, Pierre
1867–1940	Lillian Wald	Founded Henry Street Settlement House
1881–1955	Alexander Fleming	Discovered penicillin
1891–1941	Frederick Banting	Discovered insulin
1895–1964	Gerhard Domagh	Discovered sulfa drugs
1906–1993	Albert Sabin	Discovered oral polio vaccine
1914–1996	Jonas Salk	Discovered polio vaccine

these practice acts state who must be licensed to perform certain procedures. These acts also state the requirements for licensure, duties of that license, grounds on which the license can be revoked or taken away and reports that must be made to the government. The Medical Practice Act also states the penalties for practicing without a valid license.

If a physician moves to another state, he or she must obtain a license to practice in that state also. It may mean that another state medical examination will have to be taken and passed. See the section Reciprocity later in this chapter.

Generally physicians in different states may consult with each other without being licensed in each other's states. Physicians who practice only in governmental institutions, such as Veteran's Administration hospitals, or in military service may practice without the local licensure of the state they are in.

Licensure

The Board of Medical Examiners in each state grants a license to practice medicine. Licensure may be granted through one of three ways: examination, endorsement, or through reciprocity.

Examination

Each state will offer its examination for licensure or instead of taking a state board examination to become licensed as a physician, some states ac-

cept or endorse the completion of the National Board Medical Examination (NBME) for licensure. This examination is usually taken before the end of medical school. Within the United States the official medical licensing examination is called the Federation Licensing Examination (FLEX). The license is then issued after an internship is completed. Successful performance on this exam entitles one to set up private practice as a general practitioner. A general practitioner may treat any aged male or female patient with medical problems. They are frequently referred to as family practitioners. Family practice is now a recognized specialty, American Board of Family Practice (ABFP).

The United States Medical Licensing Examination (USMLE) which began in 1992 provides a single licensing examination for graduates from accredited medical schools.

Endorsement

Endorsement, meaning an approval or sanction, is granted to applicants who have successfully passed the National Board Medical Examination. In fact most physicians in the United States are licensed by endorsement. Any medical school graduate who is not licensed by endorsement is required to pass the state board examination (FLEX). Graduates of foreign medical schools must pass the same requirements as American graduates.

Reciprocity

In some cases, the state to which the physician is applying for a license will accept the state licensing requirements of the state from which the physician already holds a license and the physician will not have to take another examination. This practice is known as reciprocity.

Registration

It is necessary for physicians to maintain their license by periodic re-registration either annually or bi-annually. The physician is notified by mail when to re-register and must submit the registration fee within a designated time period.

In addition to payment of a fee to re-register, 75 hours in a three year period of continuing medical education (CME) units are required to assure that the physician is remaining current in the field of practice.

Suspending or Revoking a Medical License

A physician's license may be revoked in cases of severe misconduct which include unprofessional conduct, commission of a crime, or personal incapacity to perform one's duties. Unprofessional conduct relates to behavior which fails to meet the ethical standards of the profession such as inappropriate use of drugs or alcohol. Crimes include rape, murder, larceny and narcotics convictions. Personal incapacity relates to the physician's inability to perform due to physical or mental incapacities.

Residency for Specialization

In spite of a strong movement back to the licensure as a family practitioner, specialization in medicine continues to be important. New technology developed as a result of the treatment of patients with unusually severe injuries during World War II. The US Army Medical Corps fostered specialization such as neurosurgery and orthopedics. Interest in medical and surgical specialties still continues to grow.

These specialties all require residency training. Residency refers to that period during which the physician works under the guidance of another specialist to gain further experience within the chosen specialty. Residency, which may last anywhere from two to six years and is usually associated with a particular medical institution, generally follows the licensure examination.

Title of Doctor

The designation doctor may be used by someone who holds a doctoral degree. The initials designating the degree that the person holds are written after the person's name, for example, Michael Smith, MD or Anna Reyes, DO.

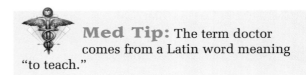 **Med Tip:** The term doctor comes from a Latin word meaning "to teach."

The designation doctor is also used as a proper way of addressing—verbally or in writing—someone who holds a doctoral degree of any kind. The abbreviation for doctor is "Dr." In the medical field, the title "Doctor/Dr." indicates that a person is qualified to practice medicine. In other fields, the title "Doctor/Dr." means that a person has attained the highest educational degree in his or her field. Several designations for doctor are listed in Table 2-2 with the corresponding initials.

Both MDs and DOs are licensed physicians. Both categories of physicians use similar approaches to medicine including the use of drugs, therapy and radiation. Both groups must pass the state board examinations to become licensed in their states. Doctors of osteopathy (DO) learn the skill of manipulation therapy in schools of osteopathy. The osteopath places great emphasis on the relationship between the musculoskeletal systems

TABLE 2-2 **Designations and Initials for Doctors**

Term	Initials
Doctor of Chiropractic	DC
Doctor of Dental Medicine	DMD
Doctor of Dental Surgery	DDS
Doctor of Education	EdD
Doctor of Medicine	MD
Doctor of Optometry	OD
Doctor of Osteopathy	DO
Doctor of Philosophy	PhD
Doctor of Podiatric Medicine	DPM

and the organs of the body. In most states, the osteopath is able to perform the same procedures as a medical doctor (MD).

A chiropractor (DC) is trained in the manipulation of the spinal cord and other areas of the body. This field requires two years of premedical studies and four years of training in a licensed chiropractic school.

A medical assistant can work for a medical doctor (MD), an osteopath (DO), a chiropractor (DC), a psychologist (PD), or a podiatrist (DPM), a physican who treats conditions of the foot. However, some additional training would be necessary to work for a dentist (DMD or DDS) or an optometrist (OD).

Types of Medical Practice

In the early part of the 20th century, the main form of medical practice was the solo practice. In this type of practice, a family practitioner set up a medical practice within a designated town and geographic area. Over the years, the practice of medicine and the legal environment have changed. Few physicians make house calls any longer. Patient's now expect to be able to reach their physicians on a 24 hour basis. In addition to these changes, the marked increase in the numbers of patients who have initiated lawsuits charging malpractice has necessitated increased insurance coverage costs for physicians.

Other forms of medical practice have become popular to meet patient needs for around-the-clock medical coverage. Also, alternative forms of practice provide the opportunity for a group of physicians to share insurance premium costs, staff and facilities investments.

Solo Practice

In a solo practice a physician practices alone. This is a common type of practice for dentists. However, physicians generally enter into agreements with other physicians to provide coverage for each other's patients and to share office expenses.

Sole Proprietorship

In a sole proprietorship, one physician is still responsible for making all the administrative decisions. However, this physician may employ other physicians and pay them a salary. The physician-owner will pay all expenses and retain all assets.

In the sole proprietorship form of practice, the owner is responsible and liable for the actions of all the employees. This is also referred to as solo practice. This form of practice is diminishing rapidly due to increasing expenses and a lack of someone to share the patient load.

Partnership

A partnership is a legal agreement to share in the business operation of a medical practice. A partnership is between two or more physicians. In this legal arrangement, each of the partners becomes responsible for the actions of all the partners. This refers to debts and all legal actions unless otherwise stipulated in the legal partnership agreement. It is always advisable to have partnership agreements in writing.

Associate Practice

The associate practice is a legal arrangement in which physicians agree to share a facility and staff. They do not, as a general rule, share responsibility for the legal actions of each other as in the partnership. The legal contract of agreement stipulates the responsibilities of each party. The physicians act as if their practice is a sole proprietorship.

The legal arrangement must be carefully described and discussed with patients. In some cases, patients have mistakenly believed that there was a shared responsibility by all the physicians in the practice. This can lead to legal difficulties if one physician is accused of committing an error. Physicians must be careful about the signage on the offices, their letterhead stationary, and the manner in which staff answer the telephone if they wish to avoid confusion over the type of practice.

Group Practice

A group practice consists of three or more physicians who share the same facility (office or clinic) and practice medicine together. This is a legal form of practice in which the physicians share all expenses and income, personnel, equipment, and records. Some areas of medicine frequently found in group practice are anesthesiology, rehabilitative or obstetrical services, radiology, and pathology.

A group practice can also be designated as a health maintenance organization (HMO) or as an independent practice association (IPA). Group practices have grown rapidly during the last decade. Large groups with over 100 doctors are not uncommon. A large group practice will often form a legal corporation.

Professional Corporation

During the l960s state legislatures passed laws (statutes) allowing professionals, for example physicians, lawyers, and accountants, to incorporate. A corporation is managed by a board of directors and there are legal and financial benefits from incorporating.

Professional corporation members are known as shareholders. Therefore, the physician-members become the shareholders in the corporation. Some of the benefits that can be offered to employees of a corporation include medical expense reimbursement, profit-sharing, pension plans, and disability insurance. These fringe benefits would not be taxable to the employee and are generally tax deductible to the employer. While a corporation can be sued, the individual assets of the members cannot be touched (as in a solo practice).

A corporation will remain after a member leaves or dies. Other forms of practice, such as the sole proprietorship, may die with the death of the owner. Today, most medical practices are corporations.

Physician Distribution

Of the 9 million people employed in the health care system, there are approximately 600,000 physicians, 35,000 doctors of osteopathy, and 150,000 dentists. Of the 600,000 physicians, only 150,000 practice primary patient care: family medicine, internal medicine, obstetrics, and pediatrics. The majority of physicians work in such specialty fields as surgical specialty, anesthesiology, or psychiatry. Physicians are scarce in some areas of the country, including slum areas in big cities and sparsely populated rural areas.

Physicians are becoming increasingly reluctant to enter solo practice, due to the large burden of debt they incur during their medical training and the high cost of operating an independent office. Many physicians are now working at salaried staff positions in hospitals, as members of group practices, for a corporate-sponsored medical care firm, or for community clinics.

American Board of Medical Specialties

Currently, there are 23 specialty boards that are covered by the American Board of Medical Specialists. The purpose of the board includes improving the quality of medical care and treatment by encouraging physicians to seek further education and training. The board evaluates the qualifications of candidates who apply and successfully pass an examination. Those physicians who successfully pass the board review then become certified as diplomates. These physicians are then referred to as being board certified. They are then able to use this designation after their name. For instance, Beth Williams, MD, Diplomate of the American Board of Pediatrics. See Table 2-3 for a listing of the 23 approved specialty boards.

TABLE 2-3 **Approved Specialty Boards**

Approved Specialty Boards
American Board of Allergy and Immunology
American Board of Anesthesiology
American Board of Colon and Rectal Surgery
American Board of Dermatology
American Board of Emergency Medicine
American Board of Family Practice
American Board of Internal Medicine
American Board of Neurological Surgery
American Board of Nuclear Medicine
American Board of Obstetrics and Gynecology
American Board of Ophthalmology
American Board of Orthopedic Surgery
American Board of Otolaryngology
American Board of Pathology
American Board of Pediatrics
American Board of Physical Medicine and Rehabilitation
American Board of Plastic Surgery
American Board of Preventive Medicine
American Board of Psychiatry and Neurology
American Board of Radiology
American Board of Surgery
American Board of Thoracic Surgery
American Board of Urology

American College of Surgeons

The American College of Surgeons also confers a fellowship degree upon its applicants who have completed additional training and have submitted documentation of 50 surgical cases in which they were chief surgeon during the past three years. A successful candidate then becomes a Fellow of the American College of Surgeons (FACS).

American College of Physicians

The American College of Physicians offers a similar fellowship and entitles the applicant to become a Fellow of the College of Physicians (FACP) in a nonsurgical specialty area.

Medical and Surgical Specialties

Due to the dramatic advances in medicine over the past two decades there continues to be an interest in specialization among physicians. Transplant surgery, including liver, kidneys, lungs, and pancreas, has expanded the need for medical and surgical specialties.

Medical Specialties

A description of some of the more common medical specialties follows.

Adolescent Medicine

Adolescent medicine is a relatively new medical specialty. Physicians who practice in this area treat patients from puberty to maturity who range in age from 11 to 21. The physicians have special training in adolescent psychiatry. Patients who seek this service may have drug dependency, behavioral, self-image, or perhaps psychiatric problems. In some cases, the physician will admit the patient to an adolescent unit in a hospital setting for acute treatment of their condition.

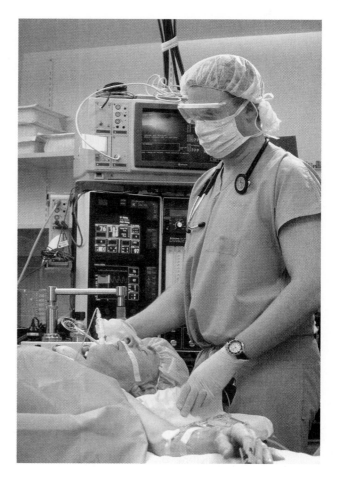

Figure 2-6   Anesthesiologist.

Allergy and Immunology

An allergist treats abnormal responses or acquired hypersensitivity to substances with medical methods including testing and desensitization. Pediatricians and internists may sit for the board examination in allergy and immunology after taking several years of additional training.

Anesthesiology

An anesthesiologist is trained to administer both local and general drugs to induce a complete or partial loss of feeling (anesthesia) during a surgical procedure (Figure 2-6). This physician also provides respiratory and cardiovascular support during surgery. The anesthesiologist meets with the patient before the surgical procedure to explain the type of anesthetic that will be used. Certified registered nurse anesthesiologists (CRNA) also may administer anesthetics.

An anesthesiologist will either work directly for a hospital or else as a member of a group of anesthesiologists who contract with a hospital or other health care facility.

Cardiology

A cardiologist is trained to treat cardiovascular disease. This physician has received special training in the diseases and disorders of the heart and blood vessels.

A cardiologist specializing in the treatment of children's heart disease would receive special training as a pediatric cardiologist.

Dermatology

A dermatologist treats injuries, growths, and infections relating to the skin, hair, and nails. This physician may treat patients either medically or surgically. A dermatologist may remove growths such as warts, moles, benign cysts, birthmarks, and skin cancers. In some cases, they have received additional training in cosmetic surgery including skin grafts, dermabrasion, hair transplants, and use of the laser.

Emergency Medicine

The physician who specializes in emergency medicine has received additional training as an emergency medical resident. Emergency medicine specialists typically work in hospital emergency rooms and free-standing walk-in emergency centers. They possess the ability or skills, to quickly recognize and prioritize (triage) acute injuries, trauma, and illnesses. They also supervise paramedic prehospital care.

Family Practice (Primary Medicine)

The family practitioner physician will treat the entire family regardless of age and sex. In some cases they will refer patients to other specialists such as nephrologists for the treatment of renal (kidney) diseases.

Geriatric Medicine

The practice of geriatrics is focused on the care of diseases and disorders of the elderly. Gerontology is a relatively new field of medicine and is the direct result of the larger aging population.

Hematology

Hematology is the study of blood and blood-forming tissues.

Infection Control

Infection control is the prevention of infectious disease by maintaining medical asepsis, practicing good hygiene, and obtaining immunizations.

Oncology

Oncology is the study of cancer and cancer related tumors.

Internal Medicine (Primary Medicine)

The internist is a physician who treats adult patients with medical problems. This physician is skilled in diagnosis and treatment of nonsurgical problems. There are subspecialties within the area of internal medicine including: cardiology, endocrinology, gastro-enterology, hematology, immunology, nephrology, oncology, and pulmonary medicine.

Neurology

The neurologist treats the nonsurgical patient who has a disorder or disease of the nervous system.

Nephrology

A nephrologist specializes in pathology of the kidney including disorders and diseases. A nephrologist is skilled in both medical and surgical treatments including kidney dialysis (Figure 2-7).

Nuclear Medicine

The physician specializing in this field uses radioactive substances for the diagnosis and treatment of diseases such as cancer.

Obstetrics and Gynecology

An obstetrician treats the female as she begins pre-natal care and continues through labor, delivery, and the postpartum period (Figure 2-8). A gynecologist provides both medical and surgical treatment of diseases and disorders of the female reproductive system. This is a sub-specialty which deals with infertility, the study of a diminished capacity or inability to produce offspring.

Ophthalmologist

An ophthalmologist treats disorders of the eye. The study of ophthalmology includes the diagno-

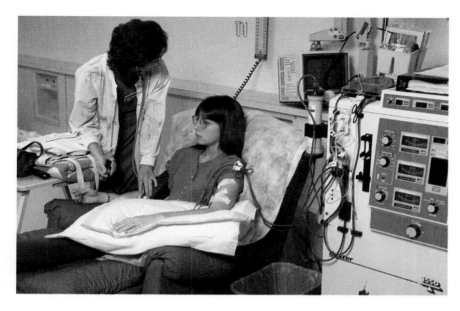

Figure 2-7   Nephrologist.

sis and treatment of vision problems using both medical and surgical procedures.

Orthopedics

An orthopedist or orthopod specializes in the branch of medicine that deals with the prevention and correction of disorders of the musculoskeletal system (Figure 2-9). An orthopedic surgeon specializes in surgical procedures relating to this specialty.

Otorhinolaryngologist (ENT)

The otorhinolaryngologist specializes in the medical and surgical treatment of ear, nose, and throat disorders. This includes the study of otology (ear), rhinology (nose), and laryngology (throat) and it is also known as otorhinolaryncology.

Pathology

A pathologist specializes in diagnosing the abnormal changes in tissues that are removed during a surgical operation and in postmortem examinations. A forensic pathologist is an expert in determining the identity of a person based on such evidence as body parts, dental records, and tissue samples.

Pediatrics

The pediatrician specializes in the development and care of children from birth to maturity. (Figure 2-10).

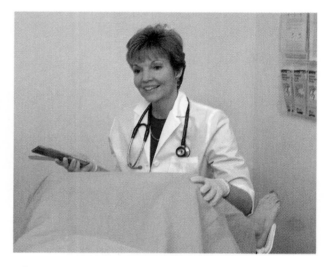

Figure 2-8   Obstetrician.

Physical Medicine/Rehabilitative Medicine

Physical medicine and/or rehabilitative medicine specialists treat patients after they have suffered an injury or disability. The purpose of treatment is to return patients to their former state of physical health if possible. This rapidly growing field is closely associated with sports medicine in which the physician treats athletes using preventive and diagnostic medicine.

Preventative Medicine

The preventive medicine specialist focuses treatment on the prevention of both physical and mental illness or disability.

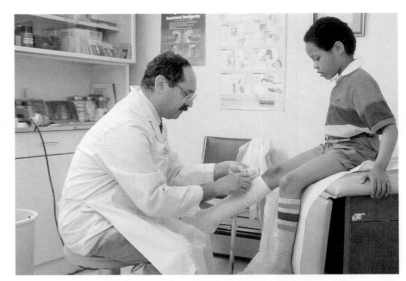

Figure 2-9 Orthopedist putting cast on young boy.

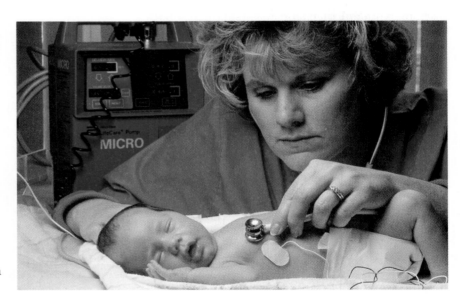

Figure 2-10 Pediatrician with baby.

Psychiatry

The psychiatrist specializes in the diagnosis and treatment of patients with mental, behavioral, or emotional disorders. A psychiatrist is qualified to administer and prescribe medications. This specialist may also practice psychotherapy.

Radiology

A radiologist specializes in the study of tissue and organs that is based on x-ray visualization. This physician has been tested and approved by the American Board of Radiology.

Rheumatology

A rheumatologist treats disorders and diseases characterized by inflammation of the joints such as arthritis.

Surgery

A surgeon corrects illness, trauma, and deformities using an operative procedure (Figure 2-11). Surgery is any invasive procedure which requires entering the body by making an incision or passing instruments through the skin and organs.

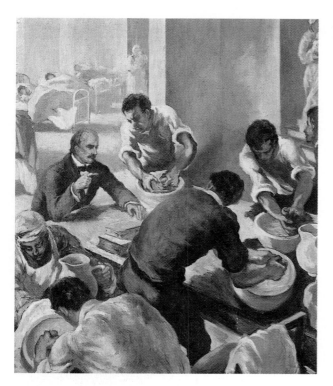

Surgical Specialties

General surgery includes all areas of surgery. General surgeons may restrict their practices to abdominal surgical procedures. However, many surgeons specialize in areas such as neurosurgery, cardiovascular surgery and orthopedic surgery. Some of the more common surgical subspecialties are described in Table 2-4.

Figure 2-11 Surgical procedures are safer today because of handwashing and disinfection techniques introduced by Semmelweiss.

TABLE 2-4 Surgical Specialties and Their Descriptions

Surgical Specialty	Description
Cardiovascular	Cardiovascular surgery is the surgical treatment of the heart and blood vessels.
Colorectal	Colorectal surgery involves the surgical treatment of the lower intestinal tract (colon and rectum).
Cosmetic Surgery/Plastic	Cosmetic surgery involves the reconstruction of underlying tissues. This surgical intervention is used to correct structural defects or remove scars and signs of aging.
Hand	Hand surgery is orthopedic surgery that involves surgical treatment of defects, traumas, and disorders of the hand. Hand surgeons may employ physical therapy staff and have x-ray equipment at their disposal.
Neurosurgery	Neurosurgery involves surgical intervention for diseases and disorders of the central nervous system.
Orthopedic	Orthopedic surgery treats musculoskeletal injuries and disorders, congenital deformities, and spinal curvatures through surgical means.
Oral (Periodontics, Orthodontics)	Oral surgery involves treatment of disorders of the jaws and teeth by means of incision and surgery as well as the extraction of teeth.
Thoracic	Thoracic surgery involves treatment of disorders and diseases of the chest with surgical intervention.

LEGAL AND ETHICAL ISSUES

Licensure and continuing medical education (CME) are two areas in which you can assist the physician. The renewal of licenses is usually dependent on the completion of re-registration forms and the filing of these forms on time with the necessary fees. Always take care to maintain accurate records of continuing medical education units earned by the physician since CME is an important part of the licensing process. Be alert to this legal obligation and remind your employing physician in advance of such renewals.

Medical assistants dedicate themselves to the care and well being of all patients, according to the American Association of Medical Assistant's code of ethics. In addition, medical assistants should take the Oath of Hippocrates, ". . . to do no harm to the patient . . . ," as seriously as the physicians who state it at the time of their graduation from medical school. As a medical assistant, you will act as a representative of the physician and must be well versed on all legal issues that affect the physician's practice.

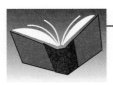

PATIENT EDUCATION

Some patients require information about the physician's specialty and credentials. Patients often have questions regarding the skill level of the physician or the amount of their bill. The medical assistant is the one who discusses these concerns with the patient. Explaining the physician's credentials, including the years of education and training required to become a doctor, particularly if the doctor specializes, often increases the patient's level of confidence in the physician.

Patients welcome an explanation of the reasons they are being referred to a specialist by their physician. In many cases, you will provide them with a list of referral specialists approved by your employer.

Summary

The medical profession contains a rich history of achievement and progress. The history of medicine can be broken into four categories: early medicine going back to 3000 BC, the 18th century, the 19th century, and the 20th century. Major advancements include the eradication of many deadly diseases with the advent of vaccines, the decrease of infections due to the discovery of aseptic technique and antibiotics, the harnessing of radium to treat disease, the inventions of the microscope and surgical instruments, discovery of anesthesia, and an understanding of anatomy and physiology.

Contemporary licensed physicians must maintain their knowledge base by completing 75 continuing medical education (CME) units over a period of three years. There are 23 medical specialty boards for the purpose of improving the quality of care by encouraging physicians to seek further education and training. The medical assistant will have the opportunity to pursue a career working for physicians in all areas of specialization.

Competency Review

1. Define and spell the glossary terms for this chapter.
2. State some of the major achievements in medicine during each of these periods: early medicine, 18th century, 19th century, and 20th century or modern medicine.
3. List the three methods by which a physician can become licensed.
4. Explain three circumstances which would justify the suspension or revocation of a physician's license.
5. Describe four types of medical practice.
6. Identify and explain issues in this chapter that might require patient education.
7. Find examples of board certified physicians in your local telephone directory.
8. Describe the role of the MA as it relates to patient education concerning the physician's credentials.

PREPARING FOR THE CERTIFICATION EXAM

Test Taking Tips — Come into an exam well rested. "Cramming" for an exam does not generally result in good test performance or retention of knowledge.

Examination Review Questions

1. What is the name of the symbol for healing made up of a staff with two coiled snakes?
   (A) colliculus
   (B) caisson
   (C) cachination
   (D) choleretic
   (E) caduceus

2. The number of individual cases of a disease within a defined population is known as the
   (A) morbidity rate
   (B) mortality rate
   (C) illness factor
   (D) disease factor
   (E) none of the above

3. The name of the first written source of medical ethics for the first doctors in history is called the
   (A) Code of Medical Conduct
   (B) Code of Hammurabi
   (C) Hippocratic Oath
   (D) Code of Caduceus
   (E) none of the above

4. One of the sources of medicine to treat pain in early times was
   (A) the poppy plant
   (B) cayenne pepper
   (C) chamomile tea
   (D) licorice
   (E) the foxglove plant

5. The "father of medicine" is
   (A) Caduceus
   (B) Galen
   (C) Hippocrates
   (D) Vesalius
   (E) Galileo

6. Who developed the practice of homeopathy?
   (A) Laennec
   (B) Pasteur
   (C) Lister
   (D) Hahnemann
   (E) Ehrlich

7. Which physician, in the late 1800s, helped find a cure for yellow fever?
   (A) Morton
   (B) Reed
   (C) Long
   (D) Hahnemann
   (E) Beaumont

8. Who discovered penicillin?
   (A) Sabin
   (B) Salk
   (C) Fleming
   (D) Banting
   (E) Nightingale

9. The name of the state law which governs the licensure of physicians is the
   (A) Medical Licensure Act
   (B) Code of Medical Conduct and Licensure
   (C) Medical Practice Act
   (D) Physicians' Practice Act
   (E) none of the above

10. The type of medical doctor that specializes in the diagnosis and treatment of patients with mental disorders is
    (A) psychologist
    (B) physiatrist
    (C) psychobiologist
    (D) psychiatrist
    (E) none of the above

ON THE JOB

One of the important characteristics of a medical assistant is to have a concrete foundation in the practice of medicine. This would include a complete understanding of the many medical and surgical specialties and subspecialties a physician can be board certified in.

An important responsibility for the medical assistant is to have the ability to convey this information about the treating physician to the anxious patient and the patient's family. This is part of patient education.

Mary is employed as a medical assistant for a physician who is a pediatric cardiovascular surgeon. She is taking a history on the patient, a newborn, by interviewing the parents, Mr. and Mrs. Appleby. They are extremely anxious and upset over the condition of their newborn who

was diagnosed, shortly after birth, with a serious, yet quite treatable, heart defect. The prognosis, should the parents agree to the corrective surgery, is quite good. However, the parents are having a difficult time understanding how the physician could help their newborn. They are not even quite sure why they were referred to this specialist and why their pediatrician could not treat the infant.

What is your response?

1. How could Mary comfort and reassure these parents?
2. What could she possibly say about the physician that might help the parents to understand why they were referred and how their newborn could be helped?

References

Badasch, S. and Chesebro, D. *Introduction to Health Occupations*. Upper Saddle River, NJ: Brady/Prentice Hall, 1993.

Current Opinions of the Judicial Council of the American Medical Association. Chicago: American Medical Association, 1992.

Dubler, N. and Nimmons, D. *Ethics on Call*. Harmony Books, 1992.

Fremgen, B. *Medical Terminology*. Upper Saddle River, NJ: Brady/Prentice Hall, 1997.

Lipman, M. *Medical Law & Ethics*. Upper Saddle River, NJ: Brady/Prentice Hall, 1994.

Stanfield, P. *Introduction to the Health Professions*. Boston: Jones and Bartlett Publishers, 1990.

Taber's Cyclopedic Medical Dictionary, 18th ed. Philadelphia: F.A. Davis, 1997.

The American Medical Association Home Medical Encyclopedia. New York: Random House, 1989.

The Professional Medical Assistant. Chicago: American Association of Medical Assistants.

Strategies for Success

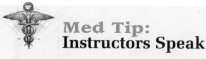

Med Tip:
Instructors Speak

Learn to focus on your goals and set priorities. When you're in school, remember the goals and commitments you have made.

Schedule time for study each day.

Diane Samuelson, RN, CMA
Grand Island, Nebraska

Take time to assess how you learn, then practice what works.

Dee A. Stout, BA, MA
Kansas City, Missouri

Prepare to *sacrifice* for success. Often times, your private time becomes school time. Make your training count; remember, it is for only a limited and relatively short period of time.

Lois Smith, CMA
Littleton, Colorado

Get a *study buddy* or join a *study group*—write tests for each other.

Shirley A. Stasiak, CMA
Orlando, Florida

Prepare yourself *for* class *before* class. If there is a reading assignment, read through the assigned pages. Much of the terminology used in the medical field is acquired through constant use. The more you read it, hear it, say it, and write it, the more the vocabulary becomes yours and the more likely you are to remember the term and its meaning.

When you review material before class, mark pertinent passages in the book with questions or ideas. That way, when the topic is presented by your instructor, you are able to participate. Participation in the learning process is another key to success in the classroom and in real life.

Ursula Backner, CMA
Debra Hampton, BSPH
Dede Schaeffer, CMA, RN
Catherine Schoen, CMA
Indianapolis, Indiana

Sit toward the front of the classroom. Ask questions. Answer questions.

Take notes in the classroom. Go over your notes right after class, or as soon as possible after class.

Mary M. Andrus, BA
Albany, New York

Especially during the days or weeks when you are involved with tests, make a special effort to avoid contacts, activities, or any engagements that are likely to create unwanted stress and anxiety prior to taking the test.

Melody Crawford, RMA, LT
St. Louis, Missouri

Part of being a successful learner is being in class everyday. Attendance is essential to understanding the material being presented, and regular attendance is also a good practice for your future jobs.

Take notes; don't just *highlight* a chapter. An active learner listens *and* writes to more clearly understand what is being presented.

Participate fully in group activities in class. You will learn from your classmates and your ability to understand the perspectives of other people will help you become a lifelong learner.

Elizabeth Keene, BSN, RN, CMA
North Wales, Pennsylvania

Allow yourself time to study. Many students are surprised at the amount of time needed for homework and studying. Plan for the time that you need.

Don't be afraid to ask questions . Your instructor is there for you. Take advantage of the experience and expertise that is available to you through your instructor.

Lisa Hutchison, CMA/RMA
Peoria, Arizona

MEDICAL ASSISTANT ROLE DELINEATION CHART

Highlight indicates material covered in this chapter

ADMINISTRATIVE

ADMINISTRATIVE PROCEDURES

- Perform basic clerical functions
- Schedule, coordinate, and monitor appointments
- Schedule inpatient/outpatient admissions and procedures
- Understand and apply third party guidelines
- Obtain reimbursement through accurate claims submission
- Monitor third-party reimbursement
- Perform medical transcription
- Understand and adhere to managed care policies and procedures
- *Negotiate managed care contracts (adv)*

PRACTICE FINANCES

- Perform procedural and diagnostic coding
- Apply bookkeeping principles
- Document and maintain accounting and banking records
- Manage accounts receivable
- Manage accounts payable
- Process payroll
- *Develop and maintain fee schedules (adv)*
- *Manage renewals of business and professional insurance policies (adv)*
- *Manage personal benefits and maintain records (adv)*

CLINICAL

FUNDAMENTAL PRINCIPLES

- Apply principles of aseptic technique and infection control
- Comply with quality assurance practices
- Screen and follow up patient test results

DIAGNOSTIC ORDERS

- Collect and process specimens
- Perform diagnostic tests

PATIENT CARE

- Adhere to established triage procedures
- Obtain patient history and vital signs
- Prepare and maintain examination and treatment areas

- Prepare patient for examinations, procedures, and treatments
- Assist with examinations, procedures, and treatments
- Prepare and administer medications and immunizations
- Maintain medication and immunization records
- Recognize and respond to emergencies
- Coordinate patient care information with other health care providers

GENERAL (TRANSDISCIPLINARY)

PROFESSIONALISM

- Project a professional manner and image
- Adhere to ethical principles
- Demonstrate initiative and responsibility
- Work as a team member
- Manage time efficiently
- Prioritize and perform multiple tasks
- Adapt to change
- Promote the CMA credential
- Enhance skills through continuing education

COMMUNICATION SKILLS

- Treat all patients with compassion and empathy
- Recognize and respect cultural diversity
- Adapt communications to individual's ability to understand
- Use professional telephone technique
- Use effective and correct verbal and written communications
- Recognize and respond to verbal and non-verbal communications
- Use medical terminology appropriately
- Receive, organize, prioritize, and transmit information
- Serve as liaison
- Promote the practice through positive public relations

LEGAL CONCEPTS

- Maintain confidentiality
- Practice within the scope of education, training, and personal capabilities
- Prepare and maintain medical records
- Document accurately
- Use appropriate guidelines when releasing information
- Follow employer's established policies dealing with the health care contract
- Follow federal, state, and local legal guidelines
- Maintain awareness of federal and state health care legislation and regulations
- Maintain and dispose of regulated substances in compliance with government guidelines
- Comply with established risk management and safety procedures
- Recognize professional credentialing criteria
- Participate in the development and maintenance of personnel, policy, and procedure manuals
- *Develop and maintain personnel, policy, and procedure manuals (adv)*

INSTRUCTION

- Instruct individuals according to their needs
- Explain office policies and procedures
- Teach methods of health promotion and disease prevention
- Locate community resources and disseminate information
- *Orient and train personnel (adv)*
- *Develop educational materials (adv)*
- *Conduct continuing education activities (adv)*

OPERATIONAL FUNCTIONS

- Maintain supply inventory
- Evaluate and recommend equipment and supplies
- Apply computer techniques to support office operations
- *Supervise personnel (adv)*
- *Interview and recommend job applicants (adv)*
- *Negotiate leases and prices for equipment and supply contracts (adv)*

SOURCE: Reprinted by permission of the American Association of Medical Assistants from the *AAMA Role Delineation Study: Occupational Analysis of the Medical Assisting Profession.*

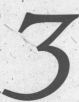

Health Care Environment

LEARNING OBJECTIVES

After completing this chapter, you should:
1. Define and spell the glossary terms for this chapter.
2. Name and describe the three categories of hospitals.
3. Explain the different type of care provided in a skilled nursing facility, an intermediate nursing facility, an extended care facility, and an assisted living facility.
4. List and describe three ambulatory care facilities.
5. Discuss ten allied health fields and the educational requirements for each of them.
6. Discuss the role of managed care as it relates to medical services for patients.

Glossary

acquired immune deficiency syndrome (AIDS)
Series of infections that occur as a result of infection by the human immunodeficiency virus (HIV) which causes the immune system to break down.

ambulatory care   Refers to health service facility which provides health care to individuals who are not hospitalized.

Diagnostic Related Groups (DRGs)
Designations used to identify reimbursement per condition in a hospital. Used for Medicare patients.

hospice   Patient-centered interdisciplinary program of care and supportive services for terminally ill patients and their families.

inpatient   Patient who remains within the medical facility at least overnight for care and/or treatment.

Legionnaires' disease   Severe, sometimes fatal disease, caused by a bacillus that is inhaled. First occurrence was at the Legionnaires' convention in 1976.

medical privileges   Ability of a physician to admit patients and practice medicine at a particular hospital.

outpatient   Patient undergoing medical treatment which does not necessitate staying overnight in the facility. Also referred to as ambulatory or a "23 hour hold."

primary care   Basic or general health care a person receives for common illnesses. A primary care physician is the one to whom the patient and/or family will go to seek most medical care.

proprietary hospital   A hospital that operates on a for-profit basis.

Health care has changed dramatically in the past fifteen years. The growth rate of the older adult population, the increase in physician specialization, and the remarkable technological discoveries and applications, such as heart and kidney transplants and mobile mammogram units are just a few of the developments that have caused the rapid expansion of the health care system. In addition, insurance companies, managed care plans, such as health maintenance organizations (HMOs) which stress preventive care and patient education, **Diagnostic Related Groups (DRGs)**, and government legislation have had a significant impact on the way health care services are delivered.

Med Tip: In 1983 Medicare instituted a hospital payment system—Diagnostic Related Groups (DRGs)—which classifies each Medicare patient according to his or her illness. There are 467 illness categories. Under this system hospitals receive a preset sum for treatment, regardless of the actual number of "bed days" of care used by the patient. This method of payment provides a further incentive to keep costs down. However, it has also discouraged the treatment of severely ill patients.

Health care institutions are more diversified and offer a range of inpatient and outpatient services. Outpatient services are frequently referred to as ambulatory care services and they are delivered in a variety of settings or facilities. It is important that you understand the functions of the various types of health care facilities and organizations in order to be able to assist your patients as they select caregivers and services, remembering always that the focus of care and treatment is the patient.

Health Care Costs and Payments

The cost of health care has been rising steeply over the past decade. For example, in 1981 total medical costs for the nation were $286 billion; in 1991 they rose to $750 billion of which physicians received 20% and hospitals 40%. The remainder of the expenses were spent on government and private-funded research, public-health services, on construction and equipment purchases, and other health-related expenditures. Private insurance covered about 50% of individual medical costs; the federal and state governments spent close to $120 billion for reimbursement of Medicare and Medicaid.

Insurance coverage is very uneven or fragmented. While most of the population is covered for much of the hospitalization costs as a result of private insurance plans through employment or Medicare, only about half are covered for the costs of physicians' services. Insurance coverage for home care of the chronically ill or mentally and physically challenged is virtually nonexistent.

Health Insurance

Health insurance includes all forms of insurance against financial loss resulting from illness or injury. These losses may include the expenses of hospitalization, surgery, and other medical services. In 1991 private health insurance was more than a $200 billion business. A large amount of US medical insurance is sold by the nationally organized, privately operated nonprofit plans such as Blue Cross and Blue Shield.

Commercial insurance companies sell various types of medical policies. Both commercial and nonprofit programs offer essentially the same types of coverage, which are divided into four categories: regular medical expenses, hospitalization, surgery, and major medical expenses. Hospitalization insurance includes expenses such as the cost of the hospital room and meals, use of the operating room, x-ray and laboratory fees for tests done while the insured patient is in the hospital as well as some medications and supplies.

Hospitalization benefits, under insurance plans, are usually limited to a total monetary amount or a maximum number of days. Insurance covering surgical procedures may change according to the city or state where the surgery is performed. These limits are based on "customary" charges for various types of surgery within the region. Thus insurance payments for a hysterectomy will be higher in New York City than in Moline, Illinois.

Health insurance covering hospital care is the most common type of health insurance. The policyholder (insured) must usually pay a percentage, for example 20%, of all costs above the deductible amount. Some major-medical policies protect the insured against charges due to major medical catastrophes after the insured has paid an initial deductible amount. This type of policy may pay a total that ranges from $10,000 to even $2,000,000. Physicians' charges are not always covered entirely by insurance which results in the patient paying a large out-of-pocket amount.

Relatively new types of insurance are the fixed payment plans. These are offered by organizations that operate their own health-care facilities or that have made arrangements with a hospital or health care provider within a city or region. The fixed-payment plan offers subscribers, or members, complete medical care in return for a fixed monthly fee. For example, health maintenance organizations (HMOs) base their operations on fixed prepayment plans. More and more employers are offering this type of plan to their employees.

Medicare

Medicare is health insurance for the elderly which is provided by the US government. The Medicare system is operated by the Social Security Administration and paid for largely through Social Security funds. It is designed for persons 65 years old and older and for the severely disabled. Medicare pays for the services of physicians, inpatient hospital care, some outpatient hospital services, and limited home care after hospital discharge.

Medicare covers approximately 32 million elderly citizens as well as 2 million permanently disabled persons. Medicare Part A pays hospital costs and covers all enrollees. Part B, called Supplemental Medical Insurance, is an optional plan the patient may purchase. This part pays 80 percent of the fee for each office visit to a doctor, although it will not pay beyond what the Social Security Administration considers "customary and reasonable" fees.

Medicare covers all expenses for the first 60 days of hospitalization, except for an initial amount, or deductible, that is paid by the patient. Medicare will also pay for a proportion of hospital costs for an additional 30 days. Medicare does not cover prescription drugs, extended nursing-home care, or the costs of lengthy or chronic illnesses.

A new fee standard was issued in 1989 that increased payments for preventive medicine and reduced fees for surgery and such diagnostic specialties as radiology.

Health Care Institutions

Hospitals are one of the largest employers in the nation. In recent years, there has been increased demand from the public, the government, and insurance companies to curb hospital expenses. The result has been an increased emphasis on **outpatient** rather than **inpatient** care especially in the area of minor surgery. Outpatient care refers to services provided to patients on a walk-in basis where no overnight stay is required; inpatient care refers to services provided to patients who are in a facility overnight or on a long term basis. A patient may be referred to as an inpatient or outpatient.

Same day surgery sites, home health agencies, and physical therapy/rehabilitative and sports medicine are all growing rapidly. Also, care that can be provided to older adults in their own homes is encouraged.

Hospitals

The hospital is still considered the key resource for health care in America. While the patient's **primary care** is delivered in the physician's office, hospitals deliver care for acute illnesses, are sites for major surgical procedures, train and educate health care professionals, conduct research and provide educational resources to the public. Hospital sizes vary depending on the needs within the community where the hospital was built. The size is based on the number of patient beds.

The length of stay in the hospital has been decreasing steadily over the past decade as a result of the DRG system of payment and better medical procedures and surgery. Consequently there are many patients who have been discharged from the hospital who still need care and attention. There are three categories of hospitals:

1. *General hospital*—provides both routine care and special care as found in intensive care units and emergency rooms (Figure 3-1). They range in size from fifty beds to several hundred beds and are usually found in most towns and communities.
2. *Teaching hospital*—provides the same type of care as in a general hospital. Teaching hospitals are generally located near a university medical school and have medical students, interns, and residents who treat patients under the supervision of staff physicians. Teaching hospitals may have more specialists on staff in order to educate and train the interns and residents.
3. *Research hospital*—provides patient care as well as conducting research to combat disease. Veteran's Administration hospitals throughout the nation and Shriner's hospitals for crippled children are examples of research hospitals.

Many larger hospitals provide all three services: general patient care, teaching, and research. Hospitals can also be categorized according to the type of service they provide, length of stay, and ownership. See Table 3-1 for a description of these categories.

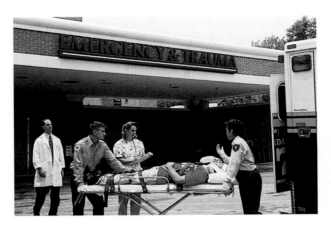

Figure 3-1   Emergency room.

The hospital organization contains many departments which interact to provide a comprehensive health care for the patient. Hospital departments include emergency services, laboratory, radiology, oncology, nuclear medicine, psychiatry, pathology, immunology, respiratory, physical and occupational therapy, nursing, dietary, pharmacy, central supply, housekeeping, engineering, and medical records. See Figure 3-2 for an example of a medical records department. The social services department will assist in locating medical care,

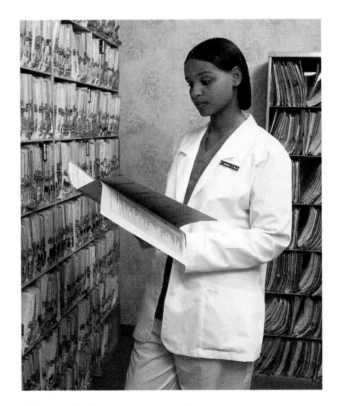

Figure 3-2   Medical records department.

TABLE 3-1 **Categories of Hospitals**

Category	Description	Example
Type of service	Single disease	Cancer
	Teaching hospital	Multiple specialties
	Same day surgery (ambulatory surgery)	Cataract removal Hernia repair Dilatation and curettage (D&C) Tonsillectomy Laparoscopic cholecystectomy
Length of Stay	Short term	1-5 days (acute care)
	Long term	Psychiatric hospital Rehabilitation hospital
Ownership	Government	Veteran's hospitals
	Proprietary (private)	For profit
	Voluntary (or religious)	Nonprofit

treatment and/or placement for the patient after discharge from the hospital.

Physicians generally serve on the staff of more than one hospital but seldom more than three. Physicians will then refer their patients to one of these hospitals in which they have medical privileges. Medical privileges refer to the physician's right to practice medicine in a particular hospital or other health care facility. Physicians may also have "courtesy" or "visiting privileges" at a hospital in which they may be called in to see a patient on a referral basis but in which the physicians do not have admitting privileges.

Nursing Homes

Nursing homes were established in the nineteenth century to provide food, clothing, and shelter for the poor. Over the past century the quality of care has improved in nursing homes and most homes that care for the elderly. Many homes are owned and operated by church groups, but the majority of homes are run on a for-profit basis by nursing home corporations. There is much tighter control over the quality of care due to stricter regulations by the state public health departments and Medicare. Due to the increased costs of nursing home care some patients have to convert to Medicaid, the national health insurance for the poor, when their funds are depleted.

The present day nursing home is a long-term facility that cares for elderly persons who are sick, too feeble to care for themselves, and have no other source of care. There are approximately 23,000 long-term-care institutions within the United States which house more than 1.3 million persons, 85% of them over 65 years old.

The number of residents in nursing homes has doubled since 1960 due to several factors: an increase in the over 65 population; changes in living styles that now separate the elderly from their families; and, since 1965, the payment of over half the costs of nursing-home care through federal programs such as Medicaid and Medicare. Both the state and federal governments regulate the levels of care and minimum staff skills in nursing homes. If these regulations are not observed, the home can lose its Medicaid reimbursement for each patient. Currently, very few private insurance companies pay for nursing home care which may range from $36,000 to over $50,000 per year.

The US Department of Health and Human Services require that nursing homes provide their patients all possible privacy, allow them to receive visitors and guarantee certain other basic rights. Patients in nursing homes may also receive a regular physician's examination and be given routine dental care.

Types of Long-Term-Care Institutions

Long-term-care institutions are classified by federal regulations either as skilled nursing facilities (SNF); intermediate-care facilities (ICF); and extended-care facilities (ECF). A description of each of these facilities and of assisted living follows.

1. Skilled-nursing facility (SNF)—provides around-the clock supervision of patients by skilled nurses assisted by physicians as mandated by law. This care is similar to the care given to patients in a hospital setting. Care includes: 24-hour nursing, medical supervision, rehabilitation, physical therapy, dietetic, and pharmacy services. Skilled care is for patients who are convalescing from a major illness or surgery and those patients with a long-term illness such as a stroke (Figure 3-3). Patients must be re-certified every 100 days to allow them to remain in a skilled care facility.

2. Intermediate-care facility (ICF)—intended for patients who are no longer able to live alone and care for themselves but who do not require skilled nursing care on a 24-hour basis. Many ICFs also have occupational and rehabilitative therapists on their staff. Intermediate care facilities must meet federal guidelines in order to receive federal funds for services provided to Medicare patients.

3. Extended-care facility (ECF)—provides services to patients who no longer need the skilled nursing care of a hospital but are still too ill or incapacitated to return home. Many hospitals have opened extended-care facilities for such patients (Figure 3-4). An extended-care facility provides custodial care and thus does not employ skilled personnel.

4. Assisted-living facility—offers living arrangements for the older adult in which each resident or couple has a separate apartment and pays a fixed fee to have some meals and services provided. Older adults who are able to care for themselves and require a minimum of supervision are living in this relatively new environment.

Hospice

Through the hospice movement begun in medieval England, the wounded, sick, and dying were cared for by religious communities of sisters. Today's modern hospice movement emphasizes improved quality of care for the dying. Most hospice care is provided at home but some programs also provide care in centers. This interdisciplinary program of care and supportive services facilitates the care of the patient by family members or significant others in the privacy of the patient's home or in a hospice facility.

On home visits, hospice personnel provide nursing care for the special needs of the dying patient, including pain management, but not necessarily treatment for the disease. These visits often provide great emotional support to the patient and the patient's family. Often the visiting health care worker can offer suggestions that might make the patient more comfortable. Most patients in a hospice facility are suffering from terminal illnesses like cancer and Medicare currently covers part of this care in a hospice setting. Medicare (Part B) will cover a part of home care if there is a qualifying diagnosis.

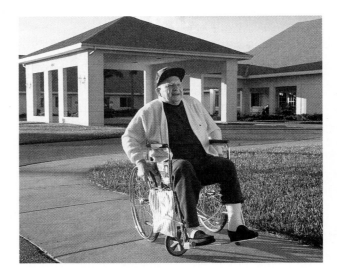

Figure 3-3   Skilled nursing facilities provide care for patients requiring longer stays than hospitals allow.

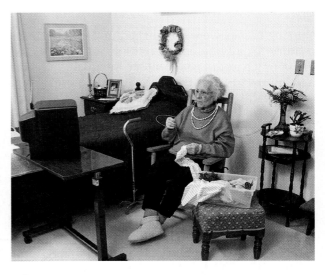

Figure 3-4   Extended care facility.

Patients who are in the last stages of a terminal illness may have prepared a living will. In such cases, there is more often than not a "do not resuscitate" (DNR) order. This means that cardiopulmonary resuscitation (CPR) will not be given if the person goes into cardiac arrest. See the discussion of living wills, DNR orders, and medical power of attorney in Chapter 5.

Ambulatory Care

Health care delivered outside of an institutional setting is referred to as ambulatory care or outpatient care. Most people receive health care in this type of setting and they are referred to as outpatients. Ambulatory care settings include medical offices with solo, partnership, or group practices as well as clinics. These clinics include surgery, radiology, mental health, and rehabilitative centers. Public health care centers which offer immunization programs are considered part of this large ambulatory care system.

Emergency medicine is a fast growing specialty area for physicians. Trauma centers, established to serve large regions, may be hospital-based but are managed as free-standing centers. Many hospitals have established fully staffed ambulatory care centers. Primary care as well as specialties such as ophthalmology, orthopedics, endoscopic GI lab, and neurology are provided in some hospital-sponsored ambulatory care centers. In its broadest sense, an ambulatory care center could include pharmacies staffed with registered pharmacists and optical shops with optometrists and opticians providing vision care.

A variety of practitioners—physicians, medical assistants, nurses, dentists, technicians, therapists, and aides—function in ambulatory care settings. Centers that provide same-day surgery have anesthesiologists on staff while community health and mental health centers employ psychologists and social workers. Nurses and nursing aides staff home health agencies. Paramedics and emergency medical technicians, too, are considered part of this growing network of practitioners providing services in ambulatory care settings.

Clinics

Clinics, covering many specialty areas such as allergy and immunology, rheumatology, ophthalmology, pediatrics, and mental health, are established by teaching facilities to serve the general public and some patients who cannot afford to pay for health care. In many cases, the clinic setting is an opportunity for medical students to receive additional training and experience.

Laboratories

A laboratory is a facility that is equipped for testing, research, scientific experimentation, or clinical studies of materials, fluids, or tissues taken from patients. Medical teaching and research institutions will have an experimental laboratory on the premises.

Independent laboratories provide routine analysis of patient's blood, urine, tissue and other materials (Figure 3-5). Material sent to these labs for testing must be packaged carefully in specially designed containers. In some instances, a physician's office will contain a small laboratory where routine tests can be conducted. These are referred to as POLs, physician operated laboratories. Many

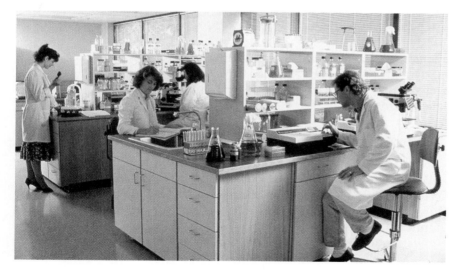

Figure 3-5 Hospital laboratory.

clinics have laboratories in their facilities to do routine testing.

Centers for Disease Control (CDC)

The Centers for Disease Control (CDC), a federal agency that is part of the United States Public health service, was established in 1946. The CDC's main headquarters and laboratories are in Atlanta, Georgia. This is a governmental agency that employs over 4000 people. The purpose of the CDC is to safeguard health by preventing and controlling disease. It seeks information about causes of disease in order to find cures and acts as a resource for the medical profession. The CDC alerts the medical profession to potential outbreaks of diseases such as influenza, describes the group who will be the most at risk during an outbreak of disease such as the aged, and recommends the proper treatment.

The CDC has divisions that conduct disease research, prevention, control and education programs nationally and in several other countries; help to train doctors; provide public health information; develop immunization services with state and local agencies; and establish standards for healthful working conditions. The CDC's past work has included a determination of the nature and cause of Legionnaires' disease and of toxic shock syndrome; the agency is currently engaged in the study of acquired immune deficiency syndrome (AIDS). The CDC has conducted research into disease conditions such as:

- Acquired immune deficiency syndrome (AIDS)—The series of infections that occur as a result of infection by the human immunodeficiency virus (HIV) which causes the immune system to break down.
- Legionnaires' disease—A severe, sometimes fatal disease, caused by a bacillus that is inhaled.
- Toxic shock syndrome—A rare and sometimes fatal disease caused by toxins produced by *staphlococcus* bacterium. It is most often associated with menstruating women who are using tampons.

Public Health

Public health, as defined by the World Health Organization, is "the science and art of preventing disease, prolonging life, and promoting health and efficiency through organized community efforts." Public health efforts are directed toward sanita-tion of the environment, control of communicable infections, education of individuals regarding personal hygiene, and the organization of medical and nursing services for the early diagnosis and preventive treatment of disease.

The emphasis in public health may be either personal or environmental or both. Personal public health applies to principles of hygiene; it consists of preventive medicine, social hygiene, social medicine, and social insurance. Environmental public health is concerned with the community's physical surroundings; it consists of epidemic disease control and sanitary hygiene. These two elements of public health are illustrated below:

Personal Public Health	Environmental Public Health
Cancer Prevention	Atmospheric Pollution
Care of the Aged	Epidemiological Services
Epidemiological Studies	
Health Education	
Immunization	Housing
Infant Health	Radiation Hazards
Maternal Health	Safe Food
Nutritional Measures	Sewage Disposal
Preventive Examinations	Water Supplies
Rehabilitation	
Social Surveys	
Social Welfare	
Vital Statistics	

Managed Care Organizations (MCOs)

Managed care provides a mechanism for a "gatekeeper," such as the insurance company, to approve all non-emergency services, hospitalization, or tests before they can be provided. This mechanism is an attempt to eliminate all unnecessary costs.

Health Maintenance Organizations (HMOs)

A health maintenance organization (HMO) is a type of managed care plan in which a range of health care services are made available to plan members for a predetermined fee (the capitation rate) per member, by a limited group of providers (such as physicians and hospitals). The HMO concept was started to control the cost explosion in health care due to an over utilization of services. Before HMOs were popular, insurance companies reimbursed providers (physicians and hospitals) for all their charges without questioning whether the services were necessary. There was little incentive for providers to control costs. HMOs operate on a budget that is the total of their member patients' fees. For this reason, HMOs attempt to control the length of hospital stays or unnecessary surgery for their members. Two important components of an HMO are:

1. All medical services are provided based upon a predetermined (per capita) fee and not on a fee-for-service basis. If the actual cost of services exceeds this predetermined (or capitation) amount, then the provider must absorb the excess in costs. This provides the incentive for the provider to control costs.
2. A member patient must use the physicians and hospitals that are identified by the HMO. The HMO will not pay for any services that are provided by an unaffiliated provider. Therefore pre-approval must be granted when and if a patient has to seek consultation or medical services elsewhere. The exception to this is in the case of an emergency.

HMOs place an emphasis on maintaining health. Regular physical examinations and patient education are encouraged. The advantage of HMOs is the control of health costs by encouraging providers to limit unnecessary tests and procedures. The disadvantage is that providers may decide not to provide services patients need in order to cut costs.

A member patient who joins an HMO may either choose a personal physician from a list of provider physicians or be assigned a "primary care physician" (PCP) who is generally an internist, family practitioner, or pediatrician. The PCP must provide all primary care services, except in the case of an emergency, since the HMO will not pay for the costs of a non-member provider.

HMOs are required to tell members, in the documents regarding their coverage, of the patient's right to ask for an investigation of any problems concerning care or coverage under the HMO. The toll-free number for complaints is (800) 400-0815.

Preferred Provider Organizations (PPOs)

The "preferred provider option" means that the patient must use a medical provider (physician or hospital) who is under contract with the insurer for an agreed-on-fee. A Preferred Provider Organization (PPO) is similar to an HMO, but differs in two main areas:

1. The PPO is a fee-for-service program and not based on a prepayment or capitation program such as with the HMO. Thus the physicians and hospitals who are designated as a PPO are reimbursed for each medical service they provide.
2. The PPO members/enrollees are not restricted to certain designated physicians or hospitals. The PPO member may receive care from a non-PPO provider, however they will generally have to pay more when they do this.

PPOs manage cost containment in the following ways:
- They negotiate fees with providers which are less than the current market fees
- There are financial incentives for PPO members to use a PPO provider
- The quality and type of services offered by PPO providers is carefully monitored to maintain cost containment.

Exclusive Provider Organizations (EPOs)

Exclusive Provider Organizations (EPOs) are a relatively new managed care concept. They are a combination of concepts developed by HMOs and PPOs. The EPO is defined as a "managed care system that limits the patient's selection of providers to a defined panel and reimburses these providers not on the basis of capitation, as in an HMO, but on a modified fee-for-service method." The EPO differs from a PPO since no insurance reimbursement is made if there is a non-emergency service provided by a non-EPO provider.

Allied-Health Careers

Careers in the health care field involve both administrative work and patient care. In some professions, such as medical assisting, both areas are studied and practiced. An extensive list of possible career choices follows.

Dental Assistant

A dental assistant works under the direct supervision of a dentist to prepare the patient for treatment, take dental x-rays, hand instruments to the dentist, teach oral health, and take impressions and casts of the mouth. Dental assistants receive on-the-job training or attend a one or two year program in a private vocational school or community college.

Dental Hygienist

A dental hygienist works directly with the patient to clean teeth, take oral x-rays, teach oral health, and discusses results of dental examinations with the dentist. The dental hygienist must graduate from either a 2-year community college program or a 4-year bachelor's program and pass both a state written and clinical examination.

Electrocardiograph Technologist

Electrocardiograph (ECG/EKG) technicians operate an electrocardiograph machine to record the electrical heart activity. ECG technicians work in hospitals, physicians' offices, and some ambulatory care facilities. They receive training on-the-job or in a specialized training program.

Electroencephalograph Technologist

Electroencephalography (EEG) is the field devoted to recording and studying the electrical activity of the brain. An EEG tech operates an electroencephalograph which records the activity of the brain with a written tracing of the brain's electrical impulses. EEG technologists work primarily in hospitals. Some are employed in the private practice of neurologists and neurosurgeons.

Emergency Medical Technicians (EMTs)-Paramedics

Emergency medical technicians-paramedics (EMTs-paramedics) are trained in providing emergency care and transporting injured patients to a medical facility. They are skilled in recognizing emergency conditions such as cardiac arrhythmias, airway obstruction, and psychological crisis. There are different levels of EMTs:

1. *Basic:* The beginner EMT who performs basic life support.
2. *Advanced:* This EMT has more training and advanced skills beyond the basic level.
3. *Paramedic:* This highest level EMT is able to treat cardiac arrest, perform defibrillation, and administer certain drugs.

Emergency Medical Technicians/Paramedics always work under the direct supervision of a physician and follow a physician's orders. In some cases, they are employed in fire fighter and ambulance services. EMTs receive certification after completion of an approved EMT program. They must be recertified every two years and receive ongoing education and training in their field.

Health Care/Patient Care Careers

Following are descriptions of some careers in health care that are associated with daily hands-on care of patients. This care may be provided in a variety of health care facilities—hospitals, nursing homes, medical offices to name a few. The unique factor here is that person-to-person contact between the patient and the health care provider is a regular occurrence.

Nurse

The term nurse refers to a diversified group of health care professionals with a range of qualifications. A description follows of a certified nursing assistant (CNA), licensed practical nurse (LPN), registered nurse (RN), and nurse practitioner (NP).

Certified Nursing Assistant (CNA)

A certified nursing assistant is a member of the health care team who has completed a training program and taken a state examination to qualify to assist nurses in nursing homes. The CNA provides such patient care as bed baths, vital signs, feeding, and ambulation.

Licensed Practical Nurse (LPN)

A licensed practical nurse performs some of the same, but not all, clinical nursing tasks as a registered nurse. The LPN must have graduated from a recognized 1-year program and become licensed by the National Federation of Licensed Practical Nurses. In some states, the LPN is known as a licensed vocational nurse (LVN).

Registered Nurse (RN)

A nursing career is ideal for the person who wishes to provide hands-on patient care. Nurses work in hospitals, physicians offices, industry, governmental agencies, ambulatory care units, emergency services, and schools. Their work ranges from managed care organizations providing direct patient care, to teaching and supervising other staff, performing research and managing agencies. Nurses receive their education and training in either a 2-year or 4-year program. To become licensed as a registered nurse requires successful completion of a national licensure examination known as the National Council Licensure Examination (NCLEX).

Nurse Practitioner (NP)

A nurse practitioner is a registered nurse who has received additional training in a specialty area such as obstetrics and gynecology, gerontology or community health. A nurse practitioner must complete an accredited course in Nurse Practitioner Training. This nurse is a masters-degree-trained individual.

Occupational Therapist (OT)

Occupational therapy provides treatment to people who are physically, mentally, developmentally, or emotionally disabled. Occupational therapists evaluate the patient's ability for self-care, work, and leisure skills. The goal of the occupational therapist is to develop programs that will help to restore the patient's ability to manage activities of daily living (ADL).

An occupational therapy assistant must complete a 2-year vocational training program and be certified by the American Occupational Therapy Association (AOTA).

Occupational therapists require a bachelor's degree from a 4-year approved program in occupational therapy. In addition, certification by the AOTA and six months of on-the-job training are needed.

Physical Therapist (PT)

Physical therapy is the treatment of diseases or disabilities of the joints, bones, and nerves by massage, therapeutic exercises, and heat and cold treatments, just to name a few. Conditions treated by means of physical therapy include: multiple sclerosis, cerebral palsy, arthritis, fractures, spinal cord injuries, and heart disease. Practitioners work in a variety of facilities including hospitals, ambulatory care, rehabilitation centers, private practice, and schools for the physically challenged.

A physical therapy assistant may be required to have a degree from an accredited 2-year college and pass a written licensure examination in some states.

A physical therapist is required to hold a 4-year degree in physical therapy, participate in a

4-month clinical internship, and successfully pass the state licensure examination. After obtaining a master's degree, some physical therapists set up private practices and provide services on a contract basis.

Physician's Assistant (PA)

The field of physician's assistant is relatively new since the 1970s. The goal of this profession is to assist the physician in the primary care of patients. The job description for a physician's assistant includes evaluation, monitoring, diagnostics, therapeutics, counseling, and referral skills. The profession has expanded to include surgeon's, pathologist's, anesthesiologist's, and radiologist's assistant and others. The general educational program is similar to a master's level program with two years education after a bachelor's degree. In most programs, the student must have work and/or internship experience and pass an accreditation examination.

Respiratory Therapist

Respiratory therapy (RT) deals with patients who have breathing problems. A respiratory therapist evaluates, treats, and cares for patients with these problems. Therapists test lung capacity, administer breathing treatments, teach self-care to patients, and provide emergency care. They are employed in hospitals, cardiopulmonary laboratories, nursing homes, health maintenance organizations (HMOs), and ambulatory care facilities.

A respiratory therapy technician receives training to become a certified respiratory therapy technician (CRTT). A CRTT must complete a 1-year internship and pass a written examination given by the National Board of Respiratory Therapy.

To become a registered respiratory therapist (RRT) requires the completion of a college program, an approved training program, one year's experience in the field, and the successful completion of a written examination given by the National Board of Respiratory Therapy.

Ultrasound Technologist (AART)

An ultrasound technologist receives training in the use of equipment which uses inaudible sound waves to outline shapes of tissues and organs. Ultrasound also produces pictures of fetal development in the uterus to assist with fetal monitoring.

X-ray Technologist (Radiologic Technologist)

An x-ray or radiologic technologist must hold a bachelor's degree in radiologic technology, have experience in two or more radiologic disciplines (for example, nuclear medicine and radiation therapy), and be a registered radiologic technologist (ARRT).

Health-Related Occupations

Health care offers varied opportunities in such diverse fields as medical illustration, secretarial work (unit clerk), public relations, hospital administration, computer operations, and other related technologies.

Diagnostic Imaging

Diagnostic Imaging Technicians are trained in the operation of x-ray equipment such as ultrasound, CT scan, MRI, and many computer assisted diagnostic machines. Radiology practitioners include: darkroom attendants with a minimum of education/training; radiologic technicians who are graduates of an accredited program; radiologists, who are graduates of an accredited medical school; and licensed physicians with specialized training in radiology. Employment opportunities are available in physician's office, hospitals, trauma centers, and other ambulatory care facilities.

Dietetics

Dietitians are skilled in applying the principles of good nutrition to food selection and meal preparation. A clinical dietitian will work closely with the patient's physician to coordinate a patient's diet with other treatments such as medications. Dietitians also provide consulting services and offer seminars, author books, counsel patients, plan food service systems, and design nutrition plans within fitness programs for athletes.

A dietitian must have a bachelor's degree with a major in foods and nutrition. In addition an internship in a dietary department is required. To become registered requires successful completion of an examination.

Dietitians work in a variety of settings including hospitals, long-term care facilities, schools, and prisons. The employment opportunities for dietitians are currently excellent.

Medical Illustration

Medical illustrators are skilled artists who create visual material to assist health care professionals and educators. Their work can include drawings, paintings, designs, sculpting, computer graphics and electronic imaging techniques. Schools of medical illustration usually require four years of college before admission into a program.

Medical Laboratory

The medical laboratory performs a variety of tests on blood, tissues and other body specimens. The laboratory obtains, handles, studies and analyzes the specimens.

Phlebotomist or Venipuncture Technician

A phlebotomist is skilled in drawing blood from patients. This requires the ability to maintain Standard Precautions, aseptic technique, excellent venipuncture technique, and good communication skills. Training in a vocational educational program is required. In some cases, certification as a phlebotomist is required.

Laboratory Technician (MLT and CLT)

The Medical Laboratory Technician (MLT) and the Clinical Laboratory Technician (CLT) are laboratory technicians skilled in testing blood, urine, lymph, and body tissues. The lab tech must have the ability to pay close attention to detail, have an understanding of computer technology, and an understanding of medical terminology. This career requires two years training in a vocational education program and certification by the National Certification Agency for Medical Laboratory Personnel.

Laboratory Technologist MT (ASCP)

A laboratory or medical technologist (MT) must complete a 4-year medical technology program in a college or university and receive certification as a certified medical technologist (CMT). This person directs the work of other laboratory staff, is responsible for maintaining the quality assurance standards for all equipment, and also performs laboratory analysis. The examination is prepared by the Board of Registry of the American Society of Clinical Pathologists (ASCP).

Blood Bank Technologist

Specialists in blood bank technology perform routine and specialized tests relating to hematology studies. They must be proficient in testing for blood groups, antigens, and antibody identification and compatibility. Technologists must also investigate abnormalities such as hemolytic anemia and diseases of the newborn. They provide support for the physician with transfusion therapy and blood drawing.

A blood bank technologist may work in a blood bank facility or independent laboratory. The technologist must use standards that conform to the "Standards for Blood Banks and Transfusion Services" of the American Association of Blood Banks. In addition, a blood bank technologist must be certified in medical technology by the Board of Registry and receive a baccalaureate degree from a regionally accredited school.

Health Information Technology (Medical Records Technician)

Health information technology refers to the massive data base known as medical records. Every person seen by a health care professional has a medical record. Medical records technicians, now more commonly referred to as health information technologists, maintain the permanent records relating to a patient's condition and treatment. The medical record is a legal document that can be used in a court of law. These records have to be carefully indexed and filed. The records are also used by insurance companies to determine who will pay the medical bills.

A medical records technician (ART) must graduate from an accredited program in medical records, have a 2-year associates degree, several years experience as a medical records clerk, and 30 credit hours from an accredited college. Successful completion of the accredited Record Technical examination allows the technician to use the initials ART after his or her name.

A registered medical records administrator (RRA) requires a bachelor's degree in Health Information Technology and the successful completion of an examination.

Medical Transcription

A medical transcriptionist types, or enters as data into the computer, dictation that is taken from a recording machine or tape. This dictation consists of medical reports from physicians and surgeons. Skills required for this profession include typing ability, good spelling skills, understanding of medical terminology and data processing equip-ment. Dictation can also be dictated directly into a computer.

Office Management

The role of office manager is a choice open to some allied health professionals, including medical assistants and nurses. Office managers supervise the entire support staff. The position requires someone with a sound knowledge of the type of work performed in the office or institution, strong supervisory skills, and the ability to work closely with top management. It is the responsibility of the office manager to provide inservice training, hire and dismiss staff, and to document personnel records. The office manager interacts with all vendors and works to ensure the best price and quality for supplies and services. Excellent time management and communication skills are a must for office managers.

Pharmacy

Pharmacy deals with the ordering, maintaining, preparing, and distributing (with prescription) of medications. Several pharmacy roles are described here along with the education requirements.

A pharmacy clerk assists the pharmacist with typing prescription labels, assigning prescription numbers, and maintaining supplies and records. A high school degree is necessary for this position. There is also a 1-year diploma program for pharmacy technicians available in some states.

Pharmacy technicians receive on-the-job training or can attend a community college or private vocational program. They are able to assist the pharmacist in preparing medications. In some states they are issued a Pharmacy Technician Certificate upon completion of an examination.

A pharmacist must complete five years of education in an accredited pharmacy program. In addition a pharmacy student must serve a 1-year internship and become licensed in the state in which they are employed. A registered pharmacist can work in a variety of institutions including hospitals, drug stores, or may own their own pharmacy.

Social Work

Social work involves programs and services that are developed to meet the special needs of the ill, physically and mentally challenged, and older adults. A medical social worker cares for the total person, including the emotional, cultural, social, and physical needs of the patient. Social workers are skilled at working with members of the patient's family, other health care professionals, and public agencies to find the best sources of help for the patient.

Medical social workers assist patients and their families in handling problems associated with a long illness or disability. They may even work closely with the patient's employer to assure an easy transition back to work. Social workers need a thorough understanding of a community's resources for the disabled.

A medical social worker requires a bachelor's degree. Many states require licensing or registration for social workers and a master's degree.

Unit Clerk/Communications Clerk

The unit clerk, or ward secretary, is responsible for clerical duties, reception work, and other communication duties in hospitals, long-term care facilities, and clinics. The unit clerk in the hospital setting performs varied tasks, for example taking physician's orders from the charts and assisting the nursing staff. This work requires skills in typing, handling communications both in person and over the phone, interpersonal skills for handling patient and staff requests, and excellent time management skills. Also, a knowledge of medical terminology is required.

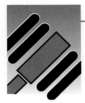

LEGAL AND ETHICAL ISSUES

As a medical assistant, you are cross-trained in administrative and clinical areas, for example typing, medications administration, and physical therapy. Many offices and facilities have regulations regarding procedures and tasks the medical assistant may perform. For instance, only a registered nurse (RN) may give intravenous medications in *all* states. The regulation that only the RN may administer medications applies in *some* states but not all.

It is the medical assistant's responsibility to learn and to follow the policies of your specific office or facility as well as the federal/state regulations governing your work as a medical assistant in your specific setting.

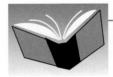

PATIENT EDUCATION

You will find that patients will seek you out as their personal information resource for health care. Therefore, you must be knowledgeable about the various types of health care settings and of the wide range of services available so that you can correctly advise patients seeking information. Perhaps an explanation which you provide of the difference between two types of nursing homes—"skilled nursing" and "assisted living"—may prevent the patient or patient's family from wasting time needlessly in seeking the proper type of health care facility.

Providing new patients with a written explanation, preferably a brochure, describing the services your office/facility offers, an explanation of payment options, and the staff members credentials is an excellent means of patient education.

Summary

The health care environment can be confusing and intimidating to the patient. It is important to have an understanding of the health care system and the diversity of institutions that deliver health care services. The descriptions provided in this chapter of inpatient facilities including hospitals, nursing homes, hospices, as well as the less traditional ambulatory care settings and services provide a basic explanation of a rather complex structure. Patients need to know the options available as they seek out services and follow up on the referrals made by their primary physician for treatment, procedures, or further diagnosis. The medical assistant's understanding of the system is key to providing clear explanations to the patient. Understanding managed care plans and using the proper insurance codes (CPT and ICD-9 in Chapter 17) for services provided to patients is necessary to assure insurance claims reimbursement.

Competency Review

1. Define and spell the glossary terms for this chapter.
2. Using the local telephone directory find examples of the names and addresses of three hospitals, a hospice, an extended care facility, and a medical laboratory.
3. Write to an association and request information for one of the allied health fields discussed in this chapter.
4. Discuss the role of the medical assistant in relationship to other health care providers.
5. Call a managed care group in your area and request information relating to the group's policies.

PREPARING FOR THE CERTIFICATION EXAM

Test Taking Tip — Many students score lower than they should on a long multiple choice exam simply because they do not get to many of the easier questions. Precious time is lost puzzling over the difficult questions. Usually, the difficult questions cover some of the same points as the easy questions, so it makes sense not to do the hard questions until you have answered the easy ones.

Examination Review Questions

1. The type of health facility which provides health care to individuals who are not hospitalized is referred to as
   (A) hospice
   (B) primary care
   (C) ambulatory care
   (D) proprietary care
   (E) intermediate care
2. The three categories of hospitals are
   (A) primary, secondary, and tertiary
   (B) general, specialty, and teaching
   (C) teaching, ICF, and ECF
   (D) ICF, primary, and specialty
   (E) general, research, and teaching
3. Hospitals can be categorized by the type of service they provide. An example of a long term care hospital might be a
   (A) psychiatric
   (B) rehabilitation
   (C) proprietary
   (D) A and B
   (E) A, B, and C
4. Health care that is provided solely outside of an institutional setting is referred to as
   (A) ambulatory care
   (B) hospice

   (C) intermediate care
   (D) extended care
   (E) assisted living
5. Which government agency was established to safeguard health by preventing and controlling disease through research?
   (A) ICF
   (B) ECF
   (C) FDA
   (D) HMO
   (E) CDC
6. DRG stands for
   (A) Diagnostic Related Group
   (B) Diagnostic Research Group
   (C) Delivery Related Group
   (D) Drug Related Group
   (E) Drug Reactive Group
7. Which of the following allied health professionals is trained in providing emergency care in the field?
   (A) basic EMT
   (B) advanced EMT
   (C) paramedic
   (D) all of the above
   (E) none of the above

8. Which of the following statements is TRUE?
   (A) an LPN is essentially the same as a medical assistant
   (B) an LPN and an RN basically have the same training
   (C) a nurse practitioner is a registered nurse
   (D) a PT and a PA are equivalent as far as training
   (E) an RT and a PT are equivalent as far as training

9. A phlebotomist is a technician that is skilled, and possibly certified, in
   (A) drawing blood
   (B) starting IVs
   (C) performing clinical laboratory testing
   (D) food selection and preparation
   (E) creating visual materials in order to assist health care professionals

10. Which of the following statements is TRUE?
   (A) the regulation that only a registered nurse may administer medication applies in some, but not all, states
   (B) medical assistant becomes certified in either administrative or clinical areas
   (C) it is not the function of a medical assistant to provide patient education
   (D) a medical assistant has the equivalent training to a pharmacy technician
   (E) all of the above

ON THE JOB

Elizabeth is a medical assistant who has worked in a very large HMO in California, where they originated, for more than 6 years. One of her duties is to facilitate the provision of care as the HMO subscribers transition from one type of patient care environment to another. For example, an elderly subscriber may at first be under the primary care of one of the HMO physicians on an outpatient basis. The patient may then be under the care of a physician specialist in an inpatient setting. He/she may then, as the years progress, require an assisted living facility, then an intermediate care facility, then extended care, and then possibly skilled care.

This week Elizabeth has been working with the family of a 22 year old man who is about to be discharged from the hospital following acute care for depression, drug, and alcohol abuse. The patient has a history of progressively worsening reactive violence and depression. He is unable to live on his own and care for himself at this time. In addition, the family is afraid of him and do not want to assume responsibility for his care.

The primary physician, medical social worker, and clinical psychologist assigned to his case have recommended that he be placed in a suitable long term care facility.

Is it beyond the scope of her training for Elizabeth to arrange for such care and the physical transition for this patient?

What is your response?

1. If yes, how could Elizabeth handle this situation with the physician and other providers that are involved in this case?
2. If no, what options could Elizabeth investigate in order to help facilitate the placement of this patient?
3. Is patient and family education merited in this particular situation or as some sort of intervention?
4. Does the fact that alcohol and drug abuse are involved alter potential treatment options?
5. Because the patient has a history of violent behavior should this fact limit the placement options?

Inquiries regarding careers can be made to:

American Association of Medical Assistants
20 N. Wacker Drive, Suite 1575
Chicago, IL 60606-2903
1-800-ACT-AAMA

American Association for Medical Transcription
P. O. Box 6187
Modesto, CA 95355
1-800-982-2182

American Association for Respiratory Therapy
1720 Regal Row
Dallas, TX 75235

American Health Information Management Association (AHIMA)
919 N. Michigan Avenue
Chicago, IL 60611-1683
1-312-787-2672

American Dietetic Association
430 N. Michigan Ave.
Chicago, IL 60611

American Medical Record Association
875 N. Michigan Ave.
Chicago, IL 60611

American Occupational Therapy Certification Board
1383 Piccard Dr. Suite 300
Rockville, MD 20852

American Society for Medical Technologists
2021 L St., NW, Suite 400
Washington, DC 20056

American Society of Clinical Pathologists
Board of Registry
2100 W. Harrison
Chicago, IL 60612

American Society of Radiologic Technologists
15000 Central Ave., SE
Albuquerque, NM 87123

Association of Medical Illustrators
2692 Hugerot Sprint Rd.
Midlothian, VA 23113

Association of Physician Assistant Programs
1117 North 19th St.
Arlington, VT 22209

Council on Social Work Education
345 E. 46th St.
New York, NY 10017

National League for Nursing
Career Information Services
10 Columbus Circle
New York, NY 10009

National Society for Cardiopulmonary
Technology Suite 307
1 Bank Street
Gaithersburg, MD 20760

Registered Medical Technologist
710 Higgins Road
Park Ridge, IL 60068-5765
1-847-823-5169

References

Abrahamson, B., et. al. *Mastering the Medicare Maze.* Madison, WI: Center for Public Representation, Incorporated, 1991.

Anderson, O. *Health Services in the US* 2nd ed. Chicago: Health Administration Press, 1990.

A Patient's Bill of Rights. Chicago: American Hospital Association, 1992.

Badasch, S. and Chesebro, D. *Introduction to Health Occupations.* Upper Saddle River, NJ: Brady/Prentice Hall, 1997.

Dubler, N. and Nimmons, D. *Ethics on Call.* Harmony Books, 1992.

"Results of the 1991 AAMA Employment Survey." *PMA.* November/December, 1991, pp. 23–26.

Richards, C. *Managing Managed Care for the Physician's Office.* Chicago: American Association of Medical Assistants, 1991.

Shortell, S., Morrison, E., and Friedman, B. *Strategic Choices for America's Hospitals.* San Francisco: Jossey-Bass Publishers, 1990.

Stanfield, P. *Introduction to the Health Professions.* Boston: Jones and Bartlett Publishers, 1990.

Statistical Abstract of the United States 1996: The National Data Book. Washington, DC: US Bureau of the Census.

Taber's Cyclopedic Medical Dictionary, 18th ed. Philadelphia: F.A. Davis, 1997.

The Professional Medical Assistant. Chicago: American Medical Association.

US Department of Labor, Bureau of Labor Statistics, *Occupational Outlook Handbook.* Washington: US. Government Printing Office, 1993.

Wirth, A. *Education and Work in the Year 2000.* San Francisco: Jossey-Bass Publishers, 1992.

MEDICAL ASSISTANT ROLE DELINEATION CHART

Highlight indicates material covered in this chapter

ADMINISTRATIVE

ADMINISTRATIVE PROCEDURES

- Perform basic clerical functions
- Schedule, coordinate, and monitor appointments
- Schedule inpatient/outpatient admissions and procedures
- Understand and apply third party guidelines
- Obtain reimbursement through accurate claims submission
- Monitor third-party reimbursement
- Perform medical transcription
- Understand and adhere to managed care policies and procedures
- *Negotiate managed care contracts (adv)*

PRACTICE FINANCES

- Perform procedural and diagnostic coding
- Apply bookkeeping principles
- Document and maintain accounting and banking records
- Manage accounts receivable
- Manage accounts payable
- Process payroll
- *Develop and maintain fee schedules (adv)*
- *Manage renewals of business and professional insurance policies (adv)*
- *Manage personal benefits and maintain records (adv)*

CLINICAL

FUNDAMENTAL PRINCIPLES

- Apply principles of aseptic technique and infection control
- Comply with quality assurance practices
- Screen and follow up patient test results

DIAGNOSTIC ORDERS

- Collect and process specimens
- Perform diagnostic tests

PATIENT CARE

- Adhere to established triage procedures
- Obtain patient history and vital signs
- Prepare and maintain examination and treatment areas

- Prepare patient for examinations, procedures, and treatments
- Assist with examinations, procedures, and treatments
- Prepare and administer medications and immunizations
- Maintain medication and immunization records
- Recognize and respond to emergencies
- Coordinate patient care information with other health care providers

GENERAL (TRANSDISCIPLINARY)

PROFESSIONALISM

- Project a professional manner and image
- Adhere to ethical principles
- Demonstrate initiative and responsibility
- Work as a team member
- Manage time efficiently
- Prioritize and perform multiple tasks
- Adapt to change
- Promote the CMA credential
- Enhance skills through continuing education

COMMUNICATION SKILLS

- Treat all patients with compassion and empathy
- Recognize and respect cultural diversity
- Adapt communications to individual's ability to understand
- Use professional telephone technique
- Use effective and correct verbal and written communications
- Recognize and respond to verbal and non-verbal communications
- Use medical terminology appropriately
- Receive, organize, prioritize, and transmit information
- Serve as liaison
- Promote the practice through positive public relations

LEGAL CONCEPTS

- Maintain confidentiality
- Practice within the scope of education, training, and personal capabilities
- Prepare and maintain medical records
- Document accurately
- Use appropriate guidelines when releasing information
- Follow employer's established policies dealing with the health care contract
- Follow federal, state, and local legal guidelines
- Maintain awareness of federal and state health care legislation and regulations
- Maintain and dispose of regulated substances in compliance with government guidelines
- Comply with established risk management and safety procedures
- Recognize professional credentialing criteria
- Participate in the development and maintenance of personnel, policy, and procedure manuals
- *Develop and maintain personnel, policy, and procedure manuals (adv)*

INSTRUCTION

- Instruct individuals according to their needs
- Explain office policies and procedures
- Teach methods of health promotion and disease prevention
- Locate community resources and disseminate information
- *Orient and train personnel (adv)*
- *Develop educational materials (adv)*
- *Conduct continuing education activities (adv)*

OPERATIONAL FUNCTIONS

- Maintain supply inventory
- Evaluate and recommend equipment and supplies
- Apply computer techniques to support office operations
- *Supervise personnel (adv)*
- *Interview and recommend job applicants (adv)*
- *Negotiate leases and prices for equipment and supply contracts (adv)*

SOURCE: Reprinted by permission of the American Association of Medical Assistants from the *AAMA Role Delineation Study: Occupational Analysis of the Medical Assisting Profession.*

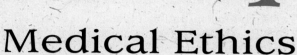

4

Medical Ethics

LEARNING OBJECTIVES

After completing this chapter, you should:

1. Define and spell the glossary terms for this chapter.
2. Explain the difference between medical ethics and medical law.
3. Explain the importance of the Hippocratic Oath today.
4. Describe measures that can be taken when a physician engages in unethical behavior.
5. List the 7 main points under the AMA Principles of Medical Ethics.
6. List and discuss the main points of the AAMA Principles of Medical Ethics.
7. Discuss what is meant by the medical assistant's standard of care.
8. Describe the Patient's Bill of Rights.
9. List and discuss 10 ethical issues addressed by the Council on Ethical and Judicial Affairs of the AMA.
10. Explain what is meant by medical etiquette.

Glossary

agent Person who represents or acts on behalf of another person.

alleged Asserted or declared without proof.

artificial insemination Placement of semen into the vagina by means other than through sexual intercourse.

artificial insemination donor (AID) An insemination procedure that uses the semen of a man other than the husband or partner.

artificial insemination husband (AIH) An insemination procedure that uses the husband's semen.

censure To find fault with, criticize, or condemn.

code of ethics Statement of principles or guidelines for moral behavior.

ethics Principles and guides for moral behavior.

expulsion The act of forcing out.

fee splitting Unethical sharing of a fee with another physician based on services other than medical services performed, for example patient referral.

gene therapy Replacement of a defective or malfunctioning gene with one that functions properly. Gene therapy is being researched as a means of correcting medical conditions caused by defective genes.

legally binding Form of contract that must be honored by law.

licensure An authorization to practice one's profession usually issued after successful completion of an examination.

medical ethics Moral conduct based on principles regulating the behavior of health care professionals.

medical etiquette Courtesy physicians extend to one another.

revocation The act of taking away or recalling, for example, taking away a license to practice medicine.

statutes Laws and regulations.

subpoena Court order for a person to appear in court. Documents as well as persons may be subpoenaed.

Ethics is a branch of philosophy relating to morals or moral principles. It involves the examination of human character and conduct, the distinction between right and wrong, and a person's moral duty and obligations to the community. Ethics, then, has been a part of the medical profession from the early beginning of the profession (Figure 4-1).

The earliest code of ethics, or principles to govern conduct, that we know about for those who practiced medicine goes back 4000 years (around 1800 BC) to the Code of Hammurabi. In 400 BC, Hippocrates, a Greek physician referred to as the "father of medicine," wrote a statement of principles for his medical students to follow that is still important today. Figure 4-2 offers an artist's interpretation of Hippocrates. Called the Oath of Hippocrates, the code reminds medical students of the importance of their profession, the need to teach others, and the obligation they have to act in such a way as to never knowingly harm a patient or divulge a confidence. The Oath of Hippocrates, which has been recited at graduation by medical students for centuries, still has an important ethical message for physicians today.

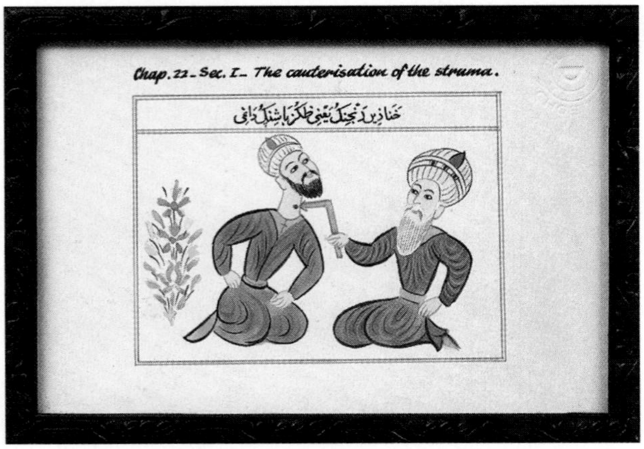

Modern codes of ethics have been developed by physicians due to advances in medical science, technology, and changes in the medical profession itself. Figure 4-3 illustrates medical students being taught about amputation by a physician.

Medical Ethics and the Law

Medical ethics refers to the moral conduct of people in medical professions. This moral conduct of medical professionals is governed by the high

Figure 4-1 Mohammed cauterizing a wound.

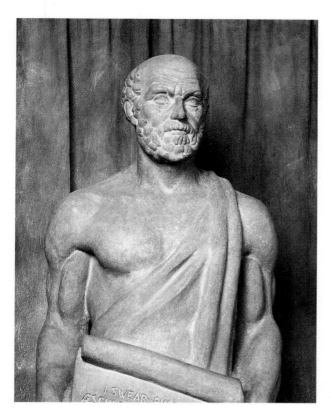

Figure 4-2 An artist's interpretation of Hippocrates.

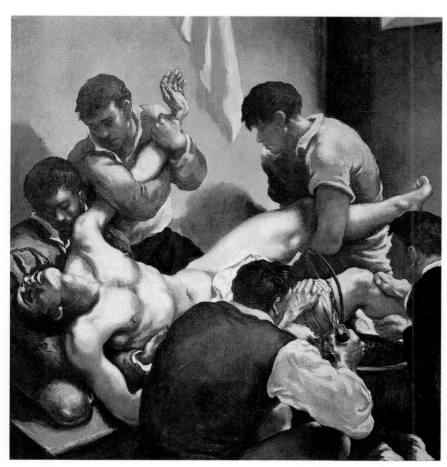

Figure 4-3 Medical students being taught about amputation by a physician.

principles and standards that these professionals set for themselves and willingly choose to follow through personal dedication. Medical law, on the other hand, refers to the regulations and standards set up by federal, state, and local governments. These two areas—medical ethics and medical law—overlap sometimes making it difficult to tell the difference between the two.

Med Tip: An illegal act or one that is against the law, is always unethical. However, an unethical act may not be illegal. For instance, when an employee looks at a neighbor's medical record out of curiosity, it is not necessarily against the law, but it is unethical.

Ethical Standards and Behavior

Ethical standards are generally more severe than those standards that are required by law. In many cases, ethical standards are more demanding than the law. A violation of an ethical standard could mean the loss of the physician's reputation.

Ethical behavior, according to the American Medical Association (AMA), refers to moral principles or practices, the customs of the medical profession, and matters of medical policy. Unethical behavior would be any actions that did not follow these ethical standards. When a physician is accused of unethical behavior or conduct in violation of these standards, he or she can be issued a warning or **censure** (criticism) by the AMA. The AMA Board of Examiners may recommend the **expulsion** or suspension of a physician from membership in the association. Expulsion, or being put out of the association, is a severe penalty for physicians since it limits the physician's ability to practice medicine. Not all physicians are members of the AMA, however. In cases dealing with members, the AMA does not have authority to bring legal action against them for unethical conduct.

If it is **alleged** that a physician has committed a criminal act, the medical society is required to report it to the state board or governmental agency. Allege means assert or declare without proof. Violation of the law, which is followed by a conviction for the crime, may result in a fine, imprisonment, and/or **revocation** of the physician's license. Revocation means the li-

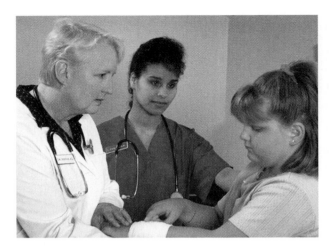

Figure 4-4 Medical assistant assists physician with a patient.

cense to practice medicine is recalled or taken away.

AMA Principles of Medical Ethics

In the United States, the AMA has taken a leadership role in setting standards for the ethical behavior of physicians. The AMA was organized in New York City in 1846 and the first Code of Ethics was formed shortly after that in 1847. Figure 4-4 shows a patient with a physician being assisted by a medical assistant.

The AMA Principles of Medical Ethics discuss human dignity, honesty, responsibility to society, confidentiality, the need for continued study, freedom of choice, and a responsibility of the physician to improve the community. Table 4-1 presents this statement of principles in its entirety.

Council on Ethical and Judicial Affairs

The Council on Ethical and Judicial Affairs of the AMA is a group of nine members who interpret the Principles (see Table 4-2). Their interpretation or clarification is then published for AMA members. As a member of the medical team, it is important for you to be familiar with these ethical principles since you will be asked to cooperate with the physician in his or her practice.

A few opinions of the Council on Ethical and Judicial Affairs of the AMA are adapted and summarized in Table 4-2.

TABLE 4-1 AMA Principles of Medical Ethics

Preamble

The medical profession has long subscribed to a body of ethical statements developed primarily for the benefit of the patient. As a member of this profession, a physician must recognize responsibility not only to patients, but also to society, to other health professionals, and to self. The following principles adopted by the American Medical Association are not law, but standards of conduct which define the essentials of honorable behavior for the physician.

Human Dignity

I. A physician shall be dedicated to providing competent medical service with compassion and respect for human dignity.

Honesty

II. A physician shall deal honestly with patients and colleagues, and strive to expose those physicians deficient in character or competence, or who engage in fraud or deception.

Responsibility to Society

III. A physician shall respect the law and recognize a responsibility to seek changes in those requirements which are contrary to the best interests of the patient.

Confidentiality

IV. A physician shall respect the rights of patients, of colleagues, and of other health professionals, and shall safeguard patient confidence within the constraints of the law.

Continued Study

V. A physician shall continue to study, apply and advance scientific knowledge, make relevant information available to patients, colleagues, and the public, obtain consultation, and use the talents of other health professionals where needed.

Freedom of Choice

VI. A physician shall, in the provision of appropriate patient care, except in emergencies, be free to choose whom to serve, with whom to associate, and the environment in which to provide service.

Responsibility to Improved Community

VII. A physician shall recognize a responsibility to participate in activities contributing to an improved community.

Source: Code of Medical Ethics, *American Medical Association, copyright 1996–97.*

Medical Assistant's Principles of Medical Ethics

As a medical assistant, you may not be involved with the life and death ethical decisions that face the physician, but you will face many dilemmas regarding right or wrong behavior on an almost daily basis. For example, what do you do when another employee violates patient confidentiality or uses foul language in front of a patient? How do you treat a patient whose body may smell of urine or alcohol? How do you choose between arriving at work on time and sleeping late when you are responsible for opening the office? All these issues involve ethics or doing the right thing at the right time.

Code of Ethics of the AAMA

The Code of Ethics of the American Association of Medical Assistants (AAMA) is a standard that medical assistants are expected to follow. The Code, which describes ethical and moral conduct for the medical assistant, is similar to the AMA's Principles of Medical Ethics. As a medical assistant, you assume a position of trust and you must try to live up to the standards of your profession as stated in the Code (Table 4-3).

TABLE 4-2   Summary of Opinions of the Council on Ethical and Judicial Affairs of the AMA

Issue	Opinion
Abuse	In some cases you and the physician will learn that a child or parent is being abused. Under the law this must be reported. If it were not reported it might mean further abuse or even death for the victim.
Accepting patients	A physician may decline to accept a patient if the medical condition of that patient is not within the area of the physician's expertise and practice. However, a physician may not decline a patient due to race, color, religion, national origin, or any other basis for discrimination.
Artificial insemination	Artificial insemination, the insertion of semen by the physician into a woman's vagina from the woman's husband or partner or a donor by means other than sexual intercourse. This procedure requires the consent of the woman and her husband. Artificial insemination husband (AIH) refers to a procedure in which sperm from the woman's husband or partner is used. Artificial insemination donor (AID) refers to a procedure in which sperm from a donor is used. If the artificial insemination is from a donor (AID) the physician is ethically bound to carefully screen the donor for any defects. The physician or physician's staff may not reveal the identity of the donor to anyone.
Confidential care for minors	Physicians who treat minors have an ethical duty to promote the autonomy of minor patients by involving them in the medical decision-making process to a degree equal with their abilities.
Euthanasia	Euthanasia is the administration of a lethal agent by another person to a patient for the purpose of relieving the patient's intolerable and incurable suffering. Instead of engaging in euthanasia, physicians must aggressively respond to the needs of patients at the end of life. Patients should not be abandoned once it is determined that cure is impossible.
Fee splitting	The practice of a physician accepting payment from another physician for the referral of another patient is known as fee splitting and is considered unethical.
Financial incentives for organ donation	The voluntary donation of organs in appropriate circumstances is to be encouraged. However, it is not ethical to participate in a procedure to enable a living donor to receive payment, other than for the reimbursement of expenses necessarily incurred in connection with removal, for any of the donor's non-renewable organs.
Gene therapy	The Council's position is that gene therapy, the replacement of a defective or malfunctioning gene, is acceptable as long as it is used for therapeutic purposes and not for altering human traits.
Ghost surgery	A surgeon cannot substitute another surgeon to perform a procedure without the consent of the patient.
HIV testing	Physician should ensure that HIV testing is conducted in a way that respects patient autonomy and assures patient confidentiality as much as possible.
Mandatory parental consent to abortion	Physicians should ascertain the law in their state on parental involvement to ensure that their procedures are consistent with their legal obligations.

TABLE 4-2 (Continued)

Issue	Opinion
Medical application of fetal tissue transplantation	The principal ethical concern in the use of human tissue for transplantation is the degree to which the decision to have an abortion might be influenced by the decision to donate the fetal tissue.
Organ donation	The physician is encouraged to seek the donation of patient organs when advisable. However, it is considered unethical to receive any payment for donating organs. In addition, the death of the donor must be decided by a physician other than the patient's physician.
Physician-assisted suicide	Instead of assisting in assisted suicide, physicians must aggressively respond to the patients at the end of life.
Sexual harassment and exploitation between medical supervisors and trainees	Sexual relationships between medical supervisors and their medical trainees raise concerns because inherent inequalities in the status and power that medical supervisors wield in relation to medical trainees and may adversely affect patient care. Sexual relationships between a medical trainee and a supervisor, even if consensual, are not acceptable regardless of the degree of supervision in any given situation. The supervisory role should be eliminated if the parties involved wish to pursue their relationship.
Withholding or withdrawing life-prolonging treatment	Patients must be able to make decisions concerning their lives. Physicians are committed to saving life and relieving suffering. When these two objectives are in conflict, the wishes of the patient must be given preference.

Adapted from: Code of Medical Ethics, *American Medical Association, copyright 1996–97.*

TABLE 4-3 Code of Ethics of the American Association of Medical Assistants

Preamble

The Code of Ethics of AAMA shall set forth principles of ethical and moral conduct as they relate to the medical profession and the particular practice of medical assisting.

Members of the AAMA dedicated to the conscientious pursuit of their profession, and thus desiring to merit the high regard of the entire medical profession and the respect of the general public which they serve, do hereby pledge themselves to strive always to:

Human Dignity

I. Render service with full respect for the dignity of humanity;

Confidentiality

II. Respect confidential information obtained through employment unless legally authorized or required by responsible performance of duty to divulge such information;

Honor

III. Uphold the honor and high principles of the profession and accept its disciplines;

Continued Study

IV. Seek to continually improve the knowledge and skills of medical assistants for the benefit of patients and professional colleagues;

Responsibility for Improved Community

V. Participate in additional service activities aimed toward improving the health and well-being of the community (see Figure 4-6 on page 70).

Copyright by the American Association of Medical Assistants, Inc. Reprinted by permission.

Creed of the AAMA

The Creed of the American Association of Medical Assistants can be best followed by the medical assistant who spends time reading about and discussing ethical problems such as transplants, artificial insemination, the right to die with dignity, and AIDS. To be true to this Creed, the medical assistant must know about the ethical issues the patient faces and be committed to treat the patient with respectful care regardless of the patient's religious beliefs or cultural practices.

Creed of the American Association of Medical Assistants

I believe in the principles and purposes of the profession of medical assisting.
I endeavor to be more effective.
I aspire to render greater service.
I protect the confidence entrusted to me.
I am dedicated to the care and well-being of all people.
I am loyal to my employer.
I am true to the ethics of my profession.
I am strengthened by compassion, courage, and faith.

Copyright by the American Association of Medical Assistants, Inc. Reprinted by permission.

Medical Assistant's Standard of Care

As a medical assistant, you must remember that your actions can have legal consequences for the physician who employs you. You are not held to the same standard of care as a physician due to differing credentials—licensure and education. However, you will carry out your duties under the direction of a physician and, therefore, you must use the same approved methods that a physician would use. For example, you must have the same quality standard as any physician would use when taking an electrocardiogram, drawing blood, and collecting specimens.

A medical assistant is not expected to diagnose medical conditions, interpret electrocardiograms, or prescribe medications since these are all within the area of the physician's standard of care. In fact, medical assistants must continually use caution and not take on any tasks or duties for which they are not trained within the scope of their practice.

Your actions as a medical assistant reflect upon the physician who employs you. Many duties carried out by you could result in harm to the patient if not done properly. There have been lawsuits in which the physician has been found guilty of negligence due to improper performance of his or her medical assistant (Figure 4-5).

Patient's Bill of Rights

The American Hospital Association developed a statement called "The Patient's Bill of Rights" which describes the patient-physician relationship. Medical assistants also follow these guidelines when working with the physician's patients. Table 4-4 states these rights.

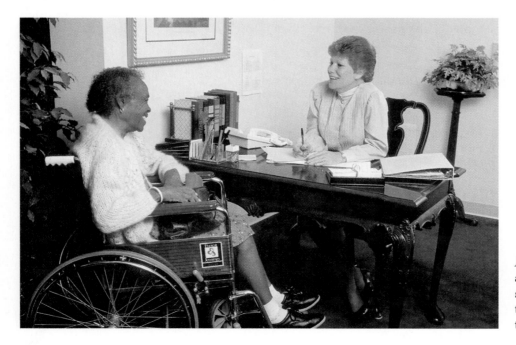

Figure 4-5 Medical assistant explaining a sheet of written instructions before giving them to the patient.

Confidentiality

According to the Medical Patients Rights Act, all patients have the right to have their personal privacy respected and their medical records handled with confidentiality. Any information such as test results, patient histories and even the fact that the patient is a patient cannot be told to another person. No information can be given over the telephone without the person's permission. No patient records can be given to another person or physician without the patient's written permission or unless the court has subpoenaed it. A subpoena is a court order for a person to appear in court or for documents to be presented to the court.

Your treatment and concern for the patient reflects the physician's high standards of care. The human dignity of each patient must be preserved regardless of the patient's socioeconomic background, race, age, nationality, sexual orientation or gender (Figure 4-6). Any promise or commitment that you make to a patient can be legally binding to the physician who employs you. This means that the physician can be held responsible for something you have said or implied with regard to the physician improving the patient's condition. Keep all matters relating to patients in confidence. If you believe that any health professional is acting in an unethical or unprofessional manner, you should discuss this with your employer or another physician.

TABLE 4-4 Patient's Bill of Rights

1. The patient has the right to considerate and respectful care.

2. The patient has the right to and is encouraged to obtain from physicians and other direct caregivers relevant, current, understandable information concerning diagnosis, treatment, and prognosis.

3. The patient has the right to make decisions about the plan of care prior to and during the course of treatment and to refuse a recommended treatment or plan of care to the extent permitted by law and hospital policy and to be informed of the consequences of this action.

4. The patient has the right to have an advance directive (such as a living will, health care proxy, or durable power of attorney for health care) concerning treatment or designating a surrogate decision maker with the expectation that the hospital will honor the intent of that directive to the extent permitted by law and hospital policy.

5. The patient has the right to every consideration of privacy.

6. The patient has the right to expect that all communications and records pertaining to his/her care will be treated as confidential by the hospital, except in cases such as suspected abuse and public health hazards when reporting is permitted or required by law.

7. The patient has the right to review the records pertaining to his/her medical care and to have the information explained or interpreted as necessary, except when restricted by law.

8. The patient has the right to expect that, within its capacity and policies, a hospital will make reasonable response to the request of a patient for appropriate and medically indicated care and service.

9. The patient has the right to ask and be informed of the existence of business relationships among the hospital, educational institutions, other health care providers, or payers that may influence the patient's treatment or care.

10. The patient has the right to consent to or decline to participate in proposed research studies or human experimentation affecting care and treatment or requiring direct patient involvement, and to have those studies fully explained prior to consent.

11. The patient has the right to expect reasonable continuity of care when appropriate and to be informed by physicians and other caregivers of available and realistic patient care options when hospital care is no longer appropriate.

12. The patient has the right to be informed of hospital policies and practices that relate to patient care, treatment, and responsibilities.

Reprinted with permission of the American Hospital Association, copyright 1992.

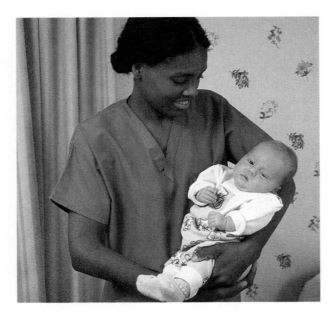

Figure 4-6 Patients of all socioeconomic backgrounds should be given quality care.

Any information that is given to a physician by a patient is considered confidential and it may not be given to an unauthorized person. As the physician's medical assistant, you are considered to be an authorized person. Therefore, you will have access to the patient's file and information. You may not divulge any of this information without permission of the doctor or patient. You must also inform the physician of any information the patient gives you. For instance, you may become aware that the patient is not taking prescribed medications or complying with treatment. As a member of the medical team, you would inform the physician.

Med Tip: Be careful about discussing anything relating to a patient within earshot of others. A comment such as "Did Miss Jones come in for her pregnancy test?" can result in a breach-of-confidentiality lawsuit against the physician.

Ethical Issues and Personal Choice

In some cases, you may have a personal, religious or ethical reason for not wishing to be involved in a particular procedure such as artifi-

cial insemination husband (AIH) or artificial insemination donor (AID). This preference should be stated before you are hired, so that your prospective employer can make a decision on hiring that is compatible with his or her practice. In the event that the situation arises after you are hired, communicate your concerns regarding your participation in such procedures by speaking openly and frankly with your employer. Do not judge what your employer is doing since he or she is acting within ethical guidelines. Rather, request that you be allowed to refrain from participating in this procedure. In the event that your inability to assist the physician would jeopardize the health and safety of the patient or the operation of the practice, it may be necessary to seek other employment.

Scientific Discovery and Ethical Issues

There are still many areas of medical ethics for which there are no conclusive answers. For instance, when should life support be withdrawn; when does a life begin; is euthanasia ever permissible; and should the unborn baby's life be sacrificed to save the mother? Scientific discoveries daily present new medical possibilities and choices. (Figure 4-7 A and B). With these possibilities there are often more complicated ethical issues to be addressed before choices can be made. The medical assistant has a responsibility to keep current on medical advances and form opinions based on sound medical ethics and practice.

Medical Etiquette

There are certain rules of medical etiquette that physicians practice in their relationship or conduct with other physicians. These are general points of behavior or etiquette and are not considered to be medical ethics issues. For instance, physicians expect that their calls to fellow physicians will be taken promptly and that they will be taken into the physician's office immediately when they visit.

There is also an unwritten practice among some physicians that they will not charge each other for professional services. This practice is losing favor since many physicians are concerned about the lack of documentation when seeing a fellow physician free of charge. Many physicians only charge fellow physicians what the insurance company will reimburse.

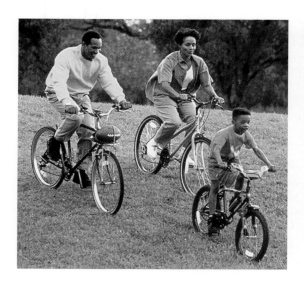

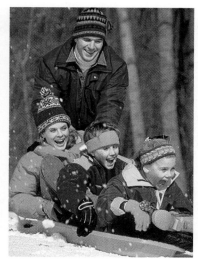

Figure 4-7
Families must be allowed to make their own personal choices.

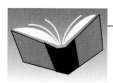

PATIENT EDUCATION

As an **agent** or representative of the physician, it is your responsibility to understand ethical standards so that you can respond to patient questions relating to advertising, physician specializations, the Patient's Bill of Rights, and fees. When patients inquire about other patients under the care of your physician, remind the inquiring patient firmly, but kindly, that patient confidentiality does not permit you to discuss any patient. This is also true in the case of family members seeking information about a loved one. Unless the patient has made it perfectly clear, preferably in writing, that the information is to be shared, the family member should be directed to speak with the patient.

Summary

The medical ethics discussed in this chapter date back to the Code of Hammurabi, and more specifically, to the Oath of Hippocrates which is still used today. The codes of ethics for physicians and medical assistants generated by the AMA, the AAMA, and the RMA set patient care as a priority. Each code addresses the specific principles or moral conduct expected of the physician or the medical assistant as each fulfills his or her responsibilities. The physician is held to a higher standard than the medical assistant due to education, training, and credentials. As a medical assistant, you will be the agent of the physician and you will be expected to know and protect the rights of every patient as described in the "Patient's Bill of Rights." Patient confidentiality is a key point of this chapter and a major responsibility of the medical assistant.

Competency Review

1. Define and spell the glossary terms for this chapter.
2. Explain the difference between medical ethics and medical law.
3. What is the Oath of Hippocrates? Why do we still discuss it?
4. Compare the principles of your organization, the AAMA or RMA, with the AMA Principles of Medical Ethics.
5. Just before surgery begins, a surgeon finds another surgeon to do the surgery without the patient's knowledge or consent. Discuss this in terms of the AMA Council on Ethical and Judicial Affairs guidelines.
6. Jim Bailey is being treated in your office after having fallen off a ladder at work. His employer calls to find out how Jim is doing. What do you say?
7. What is the difference between medical etiquette and medical ethics?
8. Describe the medical assistant's responsibilities concerning medical ethics.
9. A reporter calls to verify that your physician is treating a popular performer who attempted suicide. What do you say?

Test Taking Tip — Always read all the answer choices on a multiple choice exam even though you believe you know the correct response.

Examination Review Questions

1. Which of these statements is TRUE?
   (A) (AID) is an autoimmune disease.
   (B) Censure is the procedure whereby a physician is suspended from membership in the AMA.
   (C) Fee splitting refers to the unethical practice of, for example, a physician sharing a fee-for-service for a patient referral.
   (D) Licensure is equivalent to certification.
   (E) A subpoena is strictly an order for a person, for example a physician, to appear in court.

2. The earliest principles of ethical conduct, established to govern the practice of medicine, were known as the
   (A) Code of Hammurabi
   (B) Code of Ethical Medical Practice
   (C) Hippocratic Oath
   (D) AMA Principles of Medical Ethics
   (E) Code of Medical Practice and Conduct

3. Medical Ethics, by definition, refers to the
   (A) regulations and standards established by the government
   (B) moral conduct of medical professionals
   (C) standard by which medical practice is deemed illegal
   (D) ethical standards that are less severe than those required by law
   (E) revocation of a physician's license to practice medicine

4. The AMA Principles of Medical Ethics include
   (A) compassion and respect for human dignity
   (B) safeguarding patient confidentiality within the constraints of the law
   (C) a responsibility to society for a physician to expose the medical malpractice of another physician
   (D) A and B

   (E) A, B, and C

5. According to the AMA Principles of Medical Ethics, a physician may choose
   (A) regardless of the situation, to treat or not treat a patient
   (B) to refer, rather than treat, a non-emergency patient
   (C) the environment in which to provide medical service
   (D) A and B
   (E) B and C

6. The Code of Ethics of the AAMA describes
   (A) ethical conduct for the medical assistant
   (B) moral conduct for the medical assistant
   (C) a commitment to patients to maintain their dignity and confidentiality
   (D) a responsibility to improve the health and well-being of the community
   (E) all of the above

7. Which of the following requires medical assistants to keep current in ethical issues, for example organ transplantation and the right for a patient to die with dignity?
   (A) Creed of the AAMA
   (B) Credo of the AAMA
   (C) Code of Ethics of the AAMA
   (D) AMA Principles of Medical Ethics
   (E) Patient's Bill of Rights

8. Of the following, which falls OUTSIDE the medical assistant's standard of care?
   (A) all medical assisting duties should always be under the direction of the treating physician
   (B) the same standard of quality that is applicable to a physician in performing a procedure, for example, an EKG, is applicable to the medical assistant
   (C) the medical assistant is allowed to, for example, prescribe over-the-counter medication

(D) all of the above

(E) none of the above

9. The Patient's Bill of Rights

(A) was developed by the AMA

(B) was developed by the AHA

(C) is the same as the Medical Patient's Rights Act

(D) includes the provision that a patient's medical records become the domain of the attending physician to distribute as he/she deems necessary

(E) is designed to inform a patient that a physician has the right, at any time, to discontinue treating the patient as long as the patient is informed within 30 days by certified mail

10. Which of the following is in accordance with the Medical Patient's Rights Act?

(A) complete patient confidentiality, unless directed by a court of law, in regards to their medical records

(B) all except telephone conversations in regard to patient confidentiality and their medical records

(C) a promise a medical assistant makes to a patient is never legally binding to the employing physician

(D) patient confidentiality regarding the disclosure, for example, that a patient is being non-compliant with a medication treatment regime

(E) the rules of medical etiquette

ON THE JOB

Dr. Barnes is a board certified oncologist. Although in a solo practice, she employs a staff of five—an office manager, insurance administrator, receptionist, registered nurse, and medical assistant. They have worked in the practice together for more than 3 years.

Dr. Barnes has asked the medical assistant, Sue Halt, to take over the insurance administrator's duties in her absence. Since the medical assistant is multi-skilled, she is the best choice on staff.

Sue was surprised to discover that insurance companies were being billed for medication that is, according to the FDA, experimental. She also was troubled by the fact that insurance companies were being billed as if the patients were being treated on an outpatient basis. In reality, many of the patients resided out of state and had been shipped the experimental medication for self-administration.

What is your response?

1. Should Sue
   • report the situation to the FDA?
   • inform the physician of the situation?
   • wait until the insurance administrator returns from vacation and confront her?
   • continue the same billing practice?
2. Would Sue be required by any Code of Ethics to report the physician?
4. Might she be legally responsible if she chooses to continue the billing practice?

References

American Association of Medical Assistants Bylaws. Chicago: American Association of Medical Assistants.

Code of Medical Ethics: Current Opinions with Annotations. Chicago: Council on Ethical and Judicial Affairs of the American Medical Association, 1997.

Dubler, N. and Nimmors, D. *Ethics on Call.* Harmony Books, 1992.

Garrett, T., Baillie, H. and Garrett, R. *Health Care Ethics.* Upper Saddle River, NJ: Brady/Prentice Hall, 1993.

Health Care Law and Ethics. Chicago: American Association of Medical Assistants, 1996.

Judson, K. and Blesie, S. *Law and Ethics for Health Occupations.* New York: Macmillan/McGraw, 1994.

Lewis, M. and Tamparo, C. *Medical Law, Ethics, and Bioethics in the Medical Office.* Philadelphia: F. A. Davis Company, 1993.

Lipman, M. *Medical Law & Ethics.* Upper Saddle River: Brady/Prentice Hall, 1994.

McConnell, T. *Moral Issues in Health Care.* New York: Wadsworth Publishing Company, 1997.

Munson, R. *Intervention and Reflection: Basic Issues in Medical Ethics.* New York: Wadsworth Publishing Company, 1996.

Newton, L. and Schmidt, D. *Wake Up Calls: Classic Cases in Business Ethics.* New York: Wadsworth Publishing Company, 1996.

MEDICAL ASSISTANT ROLE DELINEATION CHART

Highlight indicates material covered in this chapter

ADMINISTRATIVE

ADMINISTRATIVE PROCEDURES

- Perform basic clerical functions
- Schedule, coordinate, and monitor appointments
- Schedule inpatient/outpatient admissions and procedures
- Understand and apply third party guidelines
- Obtain reimbursement through accurate claims submission
- Monitor third-party reimbursement
- Perform medical transcription
- Understand and adhere to managed care policies and procedures
- *Negotiate managed care contracts (adv)*

PRACTICE FINANCES

- Perform procedural and diagnostic coding
- Apply bookkeeping principles
- Document and maintain accounting and banking records
- Manage accounts receivable
- Manage accounts payable
- Process payroll
- *Develop and maintain fee schedules (adv)*
- *Manage renewals of business and professional insurance policies (adv)*
- *Manage personal benefits and maintain records (adv)*

CLINICAL

FUNDAMENTAL PRINCIPLES

- Apply principles of aseptic technique and infection control
- Comply with quality assurance practices
- Screen and follow up patient test results

DIAGNOSTIC ORDERS

- Collect and process specimens
- Perform diagnostic tests

PATIENT CARE

- Adhere to established triage procedures
- Obtain patient history and vital signs
- Prepare and maintain examination and treatment areas

- Prepare patient for examinations, procedures, and treatments
- Assist with examinations, procedures, and treatments
- Prepare and administer medications and immunizations
- Maintain medication and immunization records
- Recognize and respond to emergencies
- Coordinate patient care information with other health care providers

GENERAL (TRANSDISCIPLINARY)

PROFESSIONALISM

- Project a professional manner and image
- Adhere to ethical principles
- Demonstrate initiative and responsibility
- Work as a team member
- Manage time efficiently
- Prioritize and perform multiple tasks
- Adapt to change
- Promote the CMA credential
- Enhance skills through continuing education

COMMUNICATION SKILLS

- Treat all patients with compassion and empathy
- Recognize and respect cultural diversity
- Adapt communications to individual's ability to understand
- Use professional telephone technique
- Use effective and correct verbal and written communications
- Recognize and respond to verbal and non-verbal communications
- Use medical terminology appropriately
- Receive, organize, prioritize, and transmit information
- Serve as liaison
- Promote the practice through positive public relations

LEGAL CONCEPTS

- Maintain confidentiality
- Practice within the scope of education, training, and personal capabilities
- Prepare and maintain medical records
- Document accurately
- Use appropriate guidelines when releasing information
- Follow employer's established policies dealing with the health care contract
- Follow federal, state, and local legal guidelines
- Maintain awareness of federal and state health care legislation and regulations
- Maintain and dispose of regulated substances in compliance with government guidelines
- Comply with established risk management and safety procedures
- Recognize professional credentialing criteria
- Participate in the development and maintenance of personnel, policy, and procedure manuals
- *Develop and maintain personnel, policy, and procedure manuals (adv)*

INSTRUCTION

- Instruct individuals according to their needs
- Explain office policies and procedures
- Teach methods of health promotion and disease prevention
- Locate community resources and disseminate information
- *Orient and train personnel (adv)*
- *Develop educational materials (adv)*
- *Conduct continuing education activities (adv)*

OPERATIONAL FUNCTIONS

- Maintain supply inventory
- Evaluate and recommend equipment and supplies
- Apply computer techniques to support office operations
- *Supervise personnel (adv)*
- *Interview and recommend job applicants (adv)*
- *Negotiate leases and prices for equipment and supply contracts (adv)*

SOURCE: Reprinted by permission of the American Association of Medical Assistants from the *AAMA Role Delineation Study: Occupational Analysis of the Medical Assisting Profession*.

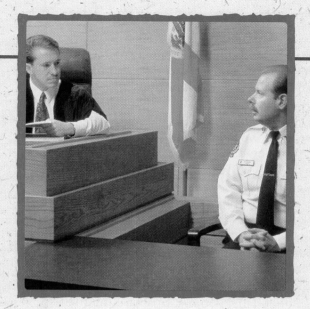

5

Medicine and the Law

LEARNING OBJECTIVES

After completing this chapter, you should:
1. Define and spell the glossary terms for this chapter.
2. Differentiate between criminal and civil law.
3. List and discuss the 4 D's of negligence.
4. Describe contract law and how it applies in the physician's office.
5. Discuss what can be done to avoid a claim of abandonment.
6. Name and describe four laws that apply to the collections process.
7. Describe how the Good Samaritan Law affects a medical assistant.
8. Describe the patient/physician relationship.
9. Discuss informed consent.
10. Discuss the role of medical assistant relating to legal issues in the medical office.

Glossary

abandonment To desert or leave a person, for example, when a physician discontinues treatment of a patient without providing coverage or sufficient notice of withdrawal.

appellant A person who appeals a court decision by going to a higher court.

arraignment Calling someone before a court of law to answer a charge.

breach of contract Failure to comply with all the terms in a valid contract.

breach (neglect) of duty Neglect or failure to perform an obligation.

case law Law that is based on precedent—principles established in prior cases.

civil case Court action between private parties, corporations, or government bodies not involving a crime.

competent Qualified to make decisions about one's affairs.

consent To give permission, approve, or allow as when a person gives permission to be examined and/or treated by authorized medical personnel. Consent may be written, verbal, informed, or implied (for example, rolling up one's sleeve to have blood drawn).

consent, informed Patient's consent to undergo surgery or treatment based on knowledge and understanding of the potential risks and benefits provided by the physician before the procedure is performed.

consent, implied Inference by signs, inaction, or silence that consent has been granted.

consideration Inducement or benefit that compels a person to enter into a contract.

contract Agreement between two or more persons which creates an obligation to perform or not perform some action or service.

criminal case Court action brought by the state against persons or groups of people accused of committing a crime, resulting in a fine or imprisonment if found guilty.

damages Compensation for a loss or injury.

defendant Person or group of persons who are accused in a court of law.

deposition Written statement of oral testimony that is made before a public officer of the court to be used in a lawsuit.

duty Obligation or responsibility.

emancipated minors Persons under the age of 18 who is free of parental care and financially responsible for herself or himself.

expert witness A medical practitioner who through education, training, or experience has special knowledge about a subject and gives testimony about that subject in court usually for a fee.

felony A crime more serious than a misdemeanor carrying a penalty of death or imprisonment.

guardian ad litem Court-appointed guardian to represent a minor or unborn child in litigation.

interrogation Questioning by authorities of a person, often a witness, to obtain information.

liable Compelled or responsible under the law to make satisfaction, restitution, or compensation because a wrong has occurred.

libel False statements placed in writing about another person.

litigation Lawsuit tried in court.

malpractice Professional negligence.

mature minor Person, usually under 18 years of age, who possesses an understanding of the nature and consequences of proposed treatment.

minor Person under the age of 18.

misdemeanor Crime that is less serious than a felony carrying a penalty of up to one year imprisonment and/or a fine.

neglect Failure to perform some action.

negligence Injury or harm to a patient caused by the performance of an act that a responsible and prudent physician would not have done or the failure to do some act that a responsible and prudent physician would have done.

plaintiff Person or group of persons who bring an action into litigation.

precedent Law that is established in a prior case.

proximate cause Natural continuous sequence of events, without any intervening cause, which produces an injury. Also referred to as the direct cause.

public duty Physician's responsibility to provide birth and death certificates and report cases of communicable diseases and abuses.

res ipsa loquitur Latin phrase which means "The thing speaks for itself." This is a doctrine of negligence law.

respondeat superior Latin phrase which means "Let the master answer." This means the physician/employer is responsible for acts of the employee.

rule of discovery The statute of limitations begins to run at the time the injury is discovered or when the patient should have known of the injury.

settle Act of determining the outcome of a case outside a courtroom. Settling a case is not an indication of guilt or innocence.

slander False, malicious spoken words about another person.

standard of care The ordinary skill and care that medical practitioners such as physicians, nurses, and medical assistants must use which is commonly used by other medical practitioners when caring for patients.

statutes Acts of a federal, state, or county legislature.

statute of limitations Maximum time period set by federal and state governments during which certain legal actions can be brought forward.

subpoena Court order for a person to appear in court. Documents as well as persons may be subpoenaed.

subpoena duces tecum Court order requiring a witness to appear in court and to bring certain records or other material to a trial or deposition.

termination End as in the end of a contract.

tort Wrongful act (other than a breach of contract) committed against another person or property that results in harm.

Today's health care consumer demands more of a partnership with the physician and the rest of the health care team. Patients expect to be a part of the decision-making process regarding their care and treatment. This chapter addresses the impact of law, specifically civil law, on current medical practice: the rights and obligations of consumers and medical employees alike. The discussion includes issues such as malpractice, abandonment, and litigation as well as specific regulations and documents protecting the consumer (patient), the consumer's family, physicians and medical staff involved in care and treatment. Some examples are the Uniform Rights of the Terminally Ill Act of 1989, the Living Will, and the Durable Power of Attorney. Other topics presented include the public duties of the physician, documentation of medical records, regulations relating to controlled substances, and the medical assistant's role in preventing liability suits.

Classification of the Law

Laws are controlled by the three branches of government: legislative, executive, and judicial. Written laws are the result of statutes (legislative), administrative (executive) laws, and case (judicial) law which is based on precedent. Precedent refers to law established in a prior case. Statutes are acts of legislative bodies at the federal, state, and county levels. Laws are classified into four types:

- criminal
- civil
- international
- military

Only criminal and civil law are discussed here.

Criminal Law

Criminal laws are made to protect the public as a whole from the harmful acts of others. State and federal laws are in place as a protection from crime for the average citizen. A violation of a state or federal law means that the government will bring criminal charges against the person who committed the crime.

Federal criminal offenses include illegal actions that cross state lines—kidnapping, treason, or other actions that affect national security. Crimes involving the borders of the United States, for example illegal transport of drugs, and any illegal act against a federally regulated business such as banks are criminal offenses.

State criminal offenses include murder, robbery, burglary, larceny, rape, sodomy, and practicing medicine without a license.

Criminal acts fall into two categories: felony and misdemeanor. A felony carries a punishment of death or imprisonment in a state or federal prison. These crimes include murder, rape, robbery, tax evasion, and practicing medicine without a license. A misdemeanor carries a punishment of fines or imprisonment in jail for up to a year. Misdemeanors are less serious offenses. They include traffic violations, disturbing the peace, and thefts.

A physician's license may be revoked or taken away if he or she is convicted of a crime. **Criminal cases** have included revocation of a license for sexual misconduct, income tax evasion, counterfeiting, murder, violating narcotics laws, and wrongful death.

Med Tip: Remember that practicing medicine without a license is a state criminal offense. A medical assistant may not diagnose or treat patients. Use particular care when patients ask you for advice. Always refer their questions to the physician.

Civil Law

Civil law concerns relationships between individuals or between individuals and the government. It generally does not involve the crimes which are handled by criminal law. (An exception would be the example of murder which can be tried under both criminal and civil law.) An individual can sue another person, a business, or the government. Some **civil (law) cases** include divorce, child custody, child support, auto accidents, slander, libel, and trespassing.

Civil law includes contract law, tort law, and administrative law. Contract law includes enforceable promises and agreements between two or more persons to do or not do a particular thing. Tort law covers acts that result in harm to another. These acts may be intentional or unintentional. An administrative law covers regulations that are set by governmental agencies. Health care employees are most frequently involved in cases of civil law, in particular, tort and contract law.

Tort Law

A **tort** is a wrongful act which is committed against another person or property that results in harm. In order to meet the definition of a tort, there must be damage or injury to the patient that was caused by the physician or the physician's employee. Torts can be either intentional or unintentional (accidental).

Med Tip: According to tort law, if a wrongful act has been committed to another person and there is no harm done then there is not a tort. However, in medical practice every wrongful act or error must be reported since patients may experience harm sometime later than when the tort occurs. For instance, if a woman in the first trimester (first 3 months) of her pregnancy has an x-ray procedure, the fetus may not demonstrate any harmful effects until several months later at birth. As a medical assistant, every unusual occurrence must be reported to your supervisor or employer.

Intentional Torts Intentional torts include assault, battery, false imprisonment, defamation of character, fraud, and invasion of privacy. Table 5-1 provides a description and example of each of these.

Unintentional Torts Unintentional torts, such as negligence, occur when the patient is injured as a result of the health care professional not exercising the ordinary standard of care. The health care professional must exercise the type of care that a "reasonable" person would use in a similar circumstance.

Med Tip: In terms of the law, actions are compared to those of a "reasonable person." This means that behavior or action which a peer would do in a similar circumstance.

Negligence is the failure to perform professional duties to an accepted standard of care. Negligence and malpractice are the same thing. As a health care professional, you should know that it is easier to prevent negligence than it is to defend it. Physicians do not knowingly indulge in acts that are negligent. Physicians can take steps to avoid negligence suits by:

- Protecting the physician-client relationship.
- Being above any reproach in the performance of their medical duties.

TABLE 5-1   **Intentional Torts**

Tort	Description	Example
Assault	The threat of bodily harm to another. There does not have to be actual touching (battery) or injury for assault to take place.	Threatening to harm a patient or to perform a procedure for which they do not consent.
Battery	Actual bodily harm to another person without permission. This is also referred to as unlawful touching or touching without consent.	Performing surgery or a procedure without the informed consent (permission) of the patient.
False imprisonment	A violation of the personal liberty of another person through unlawful restraint.	Refusing to allow a patient to leave an office, hospital, or medical facility, when they request.
Defamation of character	Damage caused to a person's reputation through spoken or written word.	Making a negative statement about another physician's ability.
Fraud	Deceitful practice.	Promising a miracle cure.
Invasion of privacy	The unauthorized publicity of information about a patient.	Allowing personal information, such as test results for HIV, to become public without the patient's permission.

Today's health care consumers (patients) are much more aware of their rights than in past years. In order to obtain a judgment for negligence against a physician, the patient must be able to show what is referred to as the "four Ds"—duty, dereliction or neglect of duty, direct cause, and damages.

In legal terms, a plaintiff is a person or group of people who file a law suit. The defendant is the person, or group of people, who are accused of wrong doing in a court of law. The person losing a case, whether a plaintiff or defendant, has the right to appeal the case to a higher court (Figure 5-1). This person would then be referred to as the appellant.

The Four D's Of Negligence

1. *Duty* refers to the physician-client relationship. The patient must prove that this relationship has been established. When the patient has made an appointment and been seen by the physician a relationship has been established. Further office visits and treatment will establish that the physician had a duty or obligation to the patient. (Contract)

2. *Dereliction or neglect of duty* refers to a physician's failure to act as any ordinary and prudent physician (a peer) within the same community would act in a similar circumstance when treating a patient. To prove dereliction or neglect of duty, a patient would have to prove that the physician's performance or treatment did not comply with the acceptable standard of care based on the norm of the ordinary and prudent physician described above. (Standard of Care)

3. *Direct cause* requires the patient to prove that the physician's derelict or breach of duty was the direct cause for the injury that resulted.

4. *Damages* refers to any injuries that were received by the patient. The court may award compensatory damages to pay for the patient's injuries.

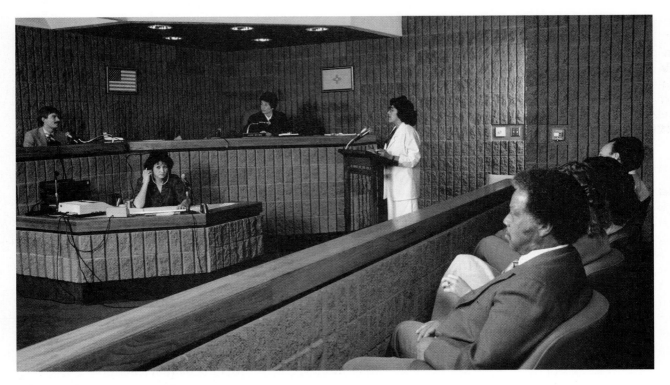

Figure 5-1   Cases lost in a lower court may be appealed to a higher court.

The plaintiff must prove proximate cause in a case of negligence. This means that the plaintiff must prove there was a continuous, natural sequence of events without interruption that produced an injury. For example, if a patient returns to his room after having prostate surgery and experiences severe headaches that were not present before having the surgery, the patient must prove that the physician's performance of the prostate surgery was the cause of the headaches.

Contributory negligence relates to the patient's contribution to the injury which, if proven, would release the physician as the direct cause (for example, the patient didn't keep an appointment causing an undetected infection to advance).

Contract Law

The branch of law known as contract law is generally concerned with a breach or neglect of an understanding between two parties. This breach can relate to insurance, sales, business, real estate, and services such as health care.

A contract is a voluntary agreement that two parties enter into with the intent of mutual benefit for both parties. Something of value which is termed consideration is part of the agreement. In the medical profession, the consideration might

be the performance of a hysterectomy for a specific fee. An agreement would take place between the two parties which would include the offer ("I will perform the hysterectomy") and the acceptance of the offer ("I will allow you to perform a hysterectomy"). In order for the contract to be valid, both parties must be competent.

In order for a contract to be legal, there are several considerations. For one thing, the concerned party (patient) must be mentally competent at the time the contract is made. For example, the patient must not be under the influence of drugs or alcohol at the time the contract is entered into. The classifications of competence are presented in Table 5-2.

A breach of contract occurs when either party fails to comply with the terms of the agreement. In the previous example, a breach of contract would occur if the physician removed the appendix along with the uterus during a hysterectomy without the expressed consent of the patient.

Abandonment Once a physician has agreed to take care of a patient that contract may not be terminated improperly. The physician may be charged with abandonment of the patient if he or she does not give formal notice of withdrawal from the case. In addition, the physician must al-

TABLE 5-2 Classifications of Competence

Classification	Definition
mentally incompetent	A person who is legally insane, one under the influence of drugs or alcohol, or an older adult suffering from an incapacitating illness such as a stroke is considered mentally incompetent. Such a person cannot enter into a contract.
minor	A person under the age of 18 is considered a minor (termed "infant" under the law). The signature of a parent or legal guardian is needed for consent to perform a medical treatment in nonemergency situations.
mature minor	A person described by the "mature minor" doctrine is one judged to be mature enough to understand the physician's instructions. Such a minor may seek medical care for treatment of drug or alcohol abuse, contraception, venereal disease, and pregnancy.
emancipated minor	A person between the ages of 15 and 18 who is either married, in the military, self-supporting and no longer lives under the care of a parent. Parental consent for medical care is not required. Proof of the emancipation (for example, marriage certificate) should be included in the medical record.

TABLE 5-3 Premature Termination of the Physician-Patient Contract

Office should document any of the incidents below with a certified letter.

1. Failure to pay for service.

2. Missed appointments.

3. Failure to follow instructions.

4. The patient states (orally or in writing) that he or she is seeking the care of another physician. Reasons for seeking another physician are many. For example, the patient's insurance may have changed and the patient's physician may not be covered by the new insurance, or the patient may move.

low the patient enough time to seek the services of another physician. The best method to protect the physician from a charge of abandonment is to send a letter by certified mail.

An example of abandonment is the patient who is under treatment for a heart ailment but has canceled appointments for periodic check-ups to assess his condition. The physician may decide that he or she can no longer accept responsibility for the medical treatment of this patient without periodic physical examinations to assess medication dosage and other factors. In this case the physician makes a decision to no longer treat this patient. Abandonment would occur if the physician did not provide enough notice to the patient of withdrawal from the case. This notice must be sufficient for the patient to find another physician

who will provide treatment. The time varies from state to state.

Termination of the Contract The termination of the contract between a physician and a patient generally occurs when the treatment has ended and the fee has been paid. However, there are serious issues which arise causing premature termination of a contract between the physician and the patient. It should be noted that both physicians and patients have the right to terminate the contractual relationship. Letters from the physician should indicate the date the physician's services will be terminated. The medical assistant needs to understand these situations and handle them correctly. Table 5-3 lists some of the reasons for premature termination of a medical contract.

Collections Several laws have been enacted to provide protection against unscrupulous collection practices that harm individuals. The medical assistant needs to be familiar with these laws since they are responsible for following the administrative procedures these laws require. The laws relating to the collection process are discussed in Table 5-4.

Professional Liability

Lawsuits related to health care have greatly increased during the past decade and the average liability award granted to plaintiffs in medical malpractice cases is now over one million dollars. Professional liability is determined by the federal, state, and local laws governing the patient/physician relationship and relates to the standard of care, legal contracts, and informed consent. An important issue in the question of liability is the physician/employee relationship. Some factors impacting on this relationship are discussed here. They include: *respondeat superior*, standard of care, malpractice, *res ipsa loquitur*, statute of limitations, Good Samaritan laws, and defamation of character.

Respondeat Superior

Your physician/employer is especially concerned that you have a complete understanding of the law. The Latin term *respondeat superior* literally means "Let the master answer." What this means to your employer, the physician, is that he or she is liable for the negligent actions of anyone working for him or her. In some cases and in some states, both the physician and the employee may be liable.

In effect, under respondeat superior, the physician delegates certain duties to you and if you perform them incorrectly then the ultimate liability rests with the physician/employer. However, you should know that medical assistants and other health care workers are also named in malpractice suits.

For example, if you are authorized by your employer to draw a sample of blood from a patient and you inadvertently enter a nerve causing permanent damage to the patient's arm, then you may also be liable for that patient's injury. Since the physician's medical license is in jeopardy when errors are made, it is vital that you understand the law.

Med Tip: These statements are not meant to frighten you or deter you from your chosen profession. A cautious, careful approach to the practice of your profession can help you to avoid any legal actions.

TABLE 5-4 **Laws Governing Collection**

Law	Description
Equal Credit Opportunity Act of 1975	Prohibits discrimination—unfair treatment—in the granting of credit. This law mandates that women and minorities must be issued credit if they qualify for it, based on the premise that if credit is given to one patient it should be given to all patients that request it.
Fair Debt Collection Practices Act of 1978	Provides a guide for determining what are considered the fair collections practices for creditors.
Fair Credit Reporting Act of 1971	Provides guidelines for collecting an individual's credit information. Individuals are able to learn what credit information is available about them. Consumers can correct and update this credit information.
Notice on "Use of Telephone for Debt Collection" from the Federal Communications Commission	Provides guidelines for the specific times that credit collection phone calls can be made. It prohibits using the telephone for harassment and threats. Telephone calls for the purposes of collections must be made between the hours of 8 AM and 9 PM.
Truth in Lending Act of 1969	Requires a full written disclosure concerning the payment of any fee that will be collected in more than 4 installments. Also referred to as Regulation Z of the Consumer Protection Act.

Understand, that if you are aware that a crime is taking place or if you actually participate in a crime, you can be named as either an accessory contributing to the crime or an accomplice who actually participates in the crime.

Standard of Care

While a physician is under no obligation to treat everyone, once he or she does accept a patient for treatment the physician has then entered into the physician/patient relationship and must provide a certain standard of care. This means that the physician must then provide the same knowledge, care, and skill that a similarly trained physician would provide under the same circumstances in the same locality. This is important to know since the law is not stating that the physician's skill must be extraordinary. The law requires only reasonable, ordinary care and skill.

The physician is expected to perform the same acts that a "reasonable and prudent" physician would. This standard also states that a physician will not perform any acts that a "reasonable and prudent" physician would not. Physicians are expected to exhaust all the resources available to them when they are treating a patient. This would include:

- Taking a thorough medical history
- Giving a complete physical examination
- Conducting the necessary laboratory tests/ x-rays

Physicians are not expected to expose their patients to undue risk. If the physician violates this standard of care he or she is liable for negligence.

As an employee of the physician, the medical assistant must also adhere to a standard of care for the patient. This standard will depend on your training, skills, education, and the responsibility the physician has given to you. If you act outside the area of your competency and the patient is injured as a result, you are liable for negligence.

Malpractice

Professional misconduct or demonstration of an unreasonable lack of skill with the result of injury, loss, or damage to the patient is considered malpractice. It means the physician was negligent. Every mistake or error, however, is not considered malpractice. Therefore, when a treatment or diagnosis does not turn out well, the physician is not necessarily liable. You and your physician/employer must each act within the "standard of care" appropriate for your particular levels of medicine. All other health care providers are held to this same standard.

Med Tip: Remember that both actions and inactions (omissions) can be considered negligence. Failure to provide clear instructions regarding treatment or the use of medications is an omission that could have a disastrous outcome for the patient. On the other hand, the action of providing incorrect information is also considered negligent.

Malpractice Insurance

In most cases, employers carry insurance to cover acts of their employees during the course of carrying out their duties. This is general liability coverage. You should request to see your employer's "certificate of insurance" to determine what the policy covers. For example, some policies cover the theft of a patient's coat, purse, or other personal items while a patient is in the office. Other policies cover professional liability; and still others cover both types of liability.

Some physicians carry a rider, or addition, to their professional liability or malpractice policy to cover any negligence on the part of their clinical assistants. An example of this is the patient who slips and falls while getting off the exam table even though you had warned the patient to sit up slowly and use the foot stool. If this type of fall were to result in a broken bone the insurance company might settle the case even though negligence was not found.

Med Tip: Remember that you can be sued even if you are right. Patients can be injured through no fault of the medical personnel.

The time taken away from the job to hire and meet with a lawyer, in order to discuss a case prior to appearing in court, as well as the court appearance itself, could become quite costly. So, if you are not covered by your employer's malpractice policy, then you must purchase your own professional liability coverage from an insurance carrier who specializes in this type of coverage.

Res Ipsa Loquitur

The doctrine of *res ipsa loquitur*, meaning "The thing speaks for itself," applies to the law of negligence. This doctrine tells us that the **breach (neglect) of duty** is so obvious that it doesn't need further explanation or "it speaks for itself." For instance, leaving a sponge in the patient during abdominal surgery, dropping a surgical instrument causing injury to the patient, and operating on the wrong body part are all examples of *res ipsa loquitur*. None of these examples would have occurred without the negligence of someone.

Statute of Limitations

The **statute of limitations** refers to the period of time during which a patient has to file a law suit. The court will not hear a case that is filed after the time limit has run out. This varies from state to state. In some states, the time period is one or two years.

The statute of limitations doesn't always start "running" when the treatment is administered. It may begin when the problem is discovered which may be some time after the actual treatment. This is known as the **rule of discovery**. For instance, there is a case in which a physician accidentally left a surgical sponge in a patient's body during an abdominal operation. After sixteen years of abdominal discomfort, the patient required more surgery but the physician who had performed the original operation had died. So, the second surgery was performed by another surgeon who found the sponge and removed it. The patient then sued the estate of the original surgeon for malpractice and won because the statute of limitations, which was two years in that state, started running when the sponge was discovered.

The reverse of a statute "running" is a situation in which the statute is stopped from running. This occurs when the injury is to a minor child. Generally, the court will appoint a "guardian ad litem," an adult who will act in the court on behalf of the child. However, the child does not have to sue through a "guardian ad litem" as a minor but may wait until he or she reaches adulthood. In such a case, an obstetrician and his or her assistants can be sued twenty-one years and nine months (plus the statute of limitations period in that state) after a birth injury has occurred.

Good Samaritan Laws

Good Samaritan laws are state laws which help to protect a health care professional from liability while giving emergency care to an accident victim. Such laws are in effect in most states to encourage physicians and other health care professionals to offer aid.

No one is required to provide aid in the event of an emergency (Figure 5-2), except in the state of Vermont. Someone responding in an emergency situation, is only required to act within the limits of his or her skill and training. A medical assistant, would not be expected, nor

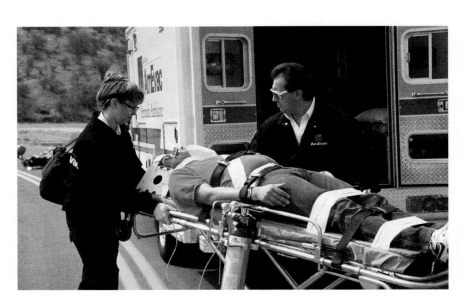

Figure 5-2 Emergency care at the scene of an accident.

advised, to perform emergency treatment that is within the area practiced by physicians and nurses.

Defamation of Character

Defamation of character is a scandalous statement about someone which can injure the person's reputation. Defamation can result even when the statement is true. Slander occurs when the defaming statement is spoken. Libel is written defamation.

As a medical assistant, you will have access to privileged information about patients that may seem harmless, but, in reality, the information could be very damaging to their reputation. For instance, a patient who has a test for an infectious disease, such as hepatitis or AIDS, may not wish an employer to know the test took place even if the test result is negative. If you call the patient's place of employment and leave a message regarding a test result of this nature, the action could be considered a breach of confidentiality and/or defamation.

The fact that a patient was seen by a physician must be kept confidential. The medical assistant should not fax information or leave messages on answering machines unless specifically instructed to do so in writing by the patient. Such instructions should be documented.

In order to protect yourself and avoid involvement in lawsuits, you must practice your caregiving skills with care, be concerned about maintaining good public relations with patients and other staff members, and understand the law.

Patient/Physician Relationship

Both physician and patient must agree to form a relationship if there is to be a contract for service and treatment. In order to receive proper treatment, the patient must confide truthfully in the physician. Failure to state all the facts may result in serious consequences for the patient. The physician is not liable if the patient has withheld

critical information. Patients can expect to be treated as long as necessary.

Physician Rights

Physicians have the right to select the patients they wish to treat. They also have the right to refuse service to patients. From an ethical standpoint, most physicians do treat patients who need their skills. This is particularly true in cases of emergency.

Physicians may also state the type of services they will provide, the hours their offices will be open and where they will be located. The physician has the right to expect payment for treatment given.

Physicians have a right to take vacations and time off from their practice. Care must be taken to inform patients if their physician will be unavailable. In most cases another physician will "cover" or take care of a colleague's patients while he or she is away.

Patient Rights

The patient has the right to approve or give consent—permission—for all treatment. In giving consent for treatment, the patient reasonably expects that his or her physician will use the appropriate "standard of care" in providing care and treatment. That is, that the physician will use the same skill that is used by other physicians in treating patients with the same ailments. Patients also expect that all information and records about their case will be kept confidential by the physician and staff. The patient's right to privacy prohibits the presence of unauthorized persons during physical examinations or treatments. See the Patient's Bill of Rights in Chapter 4 for more information on patient rights.

In addition to these rights, the patient also has certain obligations. For example, patients are expected to follow the instructions given by the physician. And finally, the patient is expected to pay the physician for medical services.

Informed Consent

The patient can expect to receive information concerning the advantages and potential risks of all treatments. Informed consent means just that. The patient is informed about the possible consequences of both having and not having certain procedures and treatment. The physician must carefully explain that in some cases the treatment may even make the patient's condition worse.

The Doctrine of Informed Consent includes the following:

1. Explanation of advantages and risks to the treatment
2. Alternatives available to the patient
3. Potential outcomes to the treatment
4. What might occur if there is no treatment
5. The use of understandable language

Touching someone without the person's consent is referred to as battery. Since consent means to give permission or approval for something, for example for medical treatment, then when a patient is seen for a routine examination, there is implied consent that the physician will touch the person during the examination. Therefore, the "touching" required for the examination would not be considered a crime of battery.

It is very difficult to "fully" inform a patient about all the things that can go wrong with a treatment. In an emergency situation in which the patient is not able to understand the explanation, nor sign a consent form, a physician is protected by law to provide care. The process of obtaining consent cannot be delegated by the physician to someone else except in emergency situations.

Does the signed informed consent protect the physician and staff (Figure 5-3)? If after the physician has carefully explained the treatment, the patient acknowledges understanding the explanation and risks involved and signs the consent form, then, generally speaking, there is some protection from law suits. However, patients have

sued and won cases in which they were presented the risks of a procedure, signed the form, and then proceeded to sue the physician when the treatment failed.

Med Tip: As a medical assistant, you may become aware of a situation in which the patient is not fully informed regarding the treatment. You need to bring this to the attention of your supervisor or the physician. Do not take it upon yourself to obtain informed consent from the patient. This is the physician's responsibility. Table 5-5 explains what is included in a typical surgical consent form.

Outpatient surgical forms or procedure forms used in clinic settings may be shorter in content. There are exceptions to the informed consent doctrine that are unique to each state. Some of the more general exceptions follow.

1. A physician does not have to inform a patient about risks that are commonly known. For example, a patient could choke swallowing a pill.
2. If the physician feels the disclosure of risks may be detrimental to the patient then he or she is not responsible for disclosing them. This might occur if a patient has a severe heart condition which may be worsened by an announcement of risks.
3. If the patient requests the physician not to disclose the risks then the physician is not responsible for failing to do so.

Patients have the right to refuse treatment. Some members of religious groups, such as Jehovah's Witnesses and Christian Scientists, do not wish to receive blood transfusions or certain types of medical treatment. The adults would not receive the treatment against their wishes. In the case of a minor child, the court may appoint a guardian who can then give consent for the procedure.

Rights of Minors

A minor is considered a person who has not reached the age of maturity, which in most states is 18. In most states minors are unable to give consent

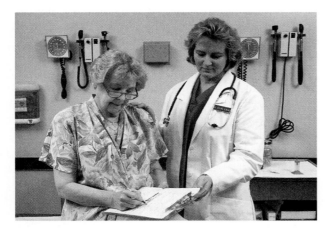

Figure 5-3 The patient's signature on the consent form indicates that the patient understands the limits or risks involved in the pending treatment or surgery as explained by the physician.

TABLE 5-5 Content of Surgical Consent Form

A consent form must include the following:

1. Consent to perform a particular operation and any other procedure that might be medically necessary (for example, removal of inflamed ovary during hysterectomy). The exact name of the procedure with a listing of all the organs to be removed is necessary. In addition, the location (left or right and so on) must be stated. A disclosure of risks associated with the surgical procedure is included.

2. Name of the surgeon performing the operation. If other staff physicians, residents, and medical students may be present to assist this must be stated.

3. Consent for anesthesia. The anesthetist will discuss the type of anesthesia with the patient prior to surgery. A disclosure of the risks associated with the anesthesia is included.

4. Consent to dispose of all tissue or organ parts which are removed.

5. Consent to be photographed if necessary.

6. Consent to be observed by qualified personnel such as medical students.

7. Consent to be examined by medical students during the recovery period.

8. Signature of the patient. If the patient is a minor then a parent or guardian may sign. In addition to signing a consent form, the patient may give consent either verbally or nonverbally. Nonverbal consent, a form of implied consent, is legally binding if the patient understands what he or she is agreeing to.

for treatment. Exceptions are special cases involving pregnancy, request for birth control information, abortion, testing and treatment for sexually transmitted diseases, problems with substance abuse, and a need for psychiatric care. There are two types of minors who can give consent for treatment:

- mature minors
- emancipated minors.

A mature minor is a young person generally under the age of 18 but who possesses a maturity to understand the nature and consequences of the treatment in spite of his or her young age. Emancipated minors actually have the same legal capacity as an adult under any of the following five conditions:

1. They live on their own.
2. They are married.
3. They are self-supporting.
4. They are in the armed forces.
5. Any combination of the above conditions.

Since not all states recognize the categories of mature and emancipated minors it is wise to handle consent on a case-by-case basis.

Legal Implications to Consider when Treating a Minor:

1. *Right to confidentiality.* A 16-year old who is seeking birth control information has a right to have her records remain confidential.
2. *Financial responsibility.* The 16-year old girl seeking birth control information may not be able to pay for the office visit. Contacting her parents for payment may breach confidentiality.
3. *Minor's legal guardian.* This is sometimes difficult to determine if the child lives with the mother but the father is financially responsible for care and treatment.

Patient Self-determination Acts

Several documents executed by the patient provide protection for the patient and physician. Such documents also provide direction for the patient's caregiver or proxy to make health-care-related decisions according to the patient's wishes at a point in time when the patient is unable to do so. These documents include living wills, durable power of attorney, and organ donations.

Living Will The living will allows patients to request that life-sustaining treatments and nutritional support not be used to prolong their life. This document gives patients the legal right to direct the type of care they wish to receive when their death is imminent. The document provides protection for physicians and hospitals when they follow the patients wishes. This process is often discussed in the office with patients when they are capable of making the decision. Other family members or significant others can also be part of the discussion/decision. One copy of the living will should be kept with the patient's record.

Durable Power of Attorney The durable power of attorney, when signed by the patient, allows an agent or representative to act on behalf of the patient. If the durable power of attorney is for health care only, then the agent may only make health-care-related decisions on behalf of the patient. The agent may be a spouse, grown child, friend or, in some cases, an attorney.

The durable power of attorney is a safeguard that someone will be able to act on the patient's behalf if he or she becomes physically or mentally unable. This document is in effect until it is canceled by the patient. A copy of the durable power of attorney should be kept with the patient's record.

Uniform Anatomical Gift Act The Uniform Anatomical Gift Act allows persons 18 years or older and of sound mind to make a gift of any or all parts of their body for purposes of organ transplantation or medical research (Figure 5-4). One of the regulations of the act is that the time of death will be determined by a physician who is not involved in the transplant. No money is allowed to change hands for organ donations.

The donor will carry a card that has been signed in the presence of two witnesses. In some states, the back of the driver's license has a space to indicate the desire to be an organ donor with space for a signature.

In some cases, the family will make the decision for the donor if this was not done while the donor was alive. It is generally agreed that if a member of the family opposes the donation of organs, then the physician and hospital do not insist upon it.

Documentation

Carefully document all calls, visits, treatments, no shows, appointment cancellations, medications, prescription refills, vital signs and other pertinent information in the patient's chart. Do not write notes regarding any patient on pieces of paper that are then filed with the patient's chart. These can be easily misplaced. If an action is not recorded on the medical chart, then it is considered by most courts not to have been performed.

In some health care facilities, a notice of information regarding the use of medical records is posted for their patients. Following is an example of one type of notice.

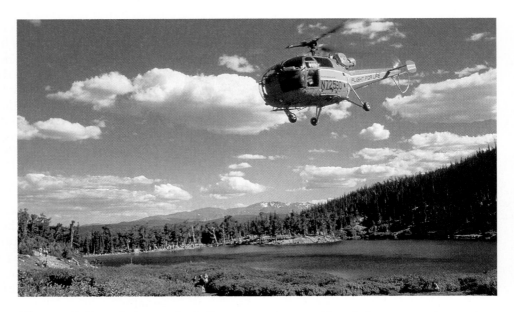

Figure 5-4 "Flight to Life" helicopter service provides vital transportation, making possible organ transplants which would otherwise have been impossible due to factors of time and distance.

Notice of Use of Medical Records

We keep a record of the health care services we provide you. We will not disclose your record to others unless directed by you to do so or unless the law compels us to do so. You may see your record and request a copy of specific notes, reports, or the entire record. You may also ask us to correct information in your medical record. *Note:* Minimum fees are usually charged for copies of patient records.

The patient's chart is not the place to document your opinion or internal office problems. Statements such as, "Patient not administered injection due to lack of staffing" or "Patient very angry with physician" can lead to trouble in court.

Errors in documentation on the medical record must be carefully corrected. Write legibly in black ink. Do not erase or totally obliterate the original error with commercial products like correcting fluid. Altered documents are always suspect in court. If the error is made during the typing process then it should be corrected as any other errors are corrected. However, if the error is noted later then you must draw a line through the error, write "correction" or "corr.," your initials, the date, and write in the correction. Handwritten errors on the medical chart are handled in the same manner. Figure 5-5 is an example of a corrected chart notation.

Use of Records in Litigation

Litigation refers to a lawsuit tried in court. For this purpose a court of law may subpoena a medical record. When this is done, only the parts of the record that are requested should be copied and sent to the requesting attorney. Unless the original record is subpoenaed, a certified photocopy may be sent. If the original record is subpoenaed, then make a copy and return the copy to the locked file. A receipt for the subpoenaed record should then be placed in the patient's file. The patient should also be notified that his or her record has been subpoenaed. Both the subpoenaed record and the notification to the patient should be sent by certified mail.

Be especially careful when using a FAX transmission for medical records. You should be assured by the person receiving the FAX that the machine is located in a restricted area. Confidential material is not generally sent over a FAX transmission. Of course, a FAX is not usable when an original record is requested. A disclaimer should be placed on the FAX cover sheet explaining the records are confidential.

The patient's medical record is considered a confidential document. No records may be released without consent in writing from the patient and the physician's approval. An example of a release form is seen in Figure 5-6 .

Should you or your employing physician receive a subpoena duces tecum, meaning an order to appear in court and to bring certain records or other materials to a trial or deposition, remember *only* the records specifically stated in the subpoena are required.

Court Testimony

Not everyone who has information relating to a case will be called into court to testify. An attorney may interrogate, or ask questions, of a witness. Another means of obtaining information from a witness to be used during a court case is to submit a deposition. In this case a written statement is taken of oral testimony given in front of a court officer. The person who gives the oral testimony and then signs a deposition does not have to actually appear in court. The deposition is submitted by an attorney during the court case. Arraignment occurs when a defendant is called before the court to answer a charge.

Date	Time	Order	Doctor	Administered by
9/9/98	3 pm	Erythromycin ~~500 mg~~ 250 mg BT 9/9	Williams	B. Fremgen RN.

Figure 5-5 Example of corrected chart notation.

WINDY CITY CLINIC
Beth Williams, M.D.
123 Michigan Avenue
Chicago, IL 60610
(312) 123-1234

RECORDS RELEASE

Date _____

To _____

_____Doctor_____

_____Address_____

I hereby authorize and request you to release

to _____

_____Doctor_____

_____Address_____

all medical records in your possession concerning any
examination, diagnosis, and/or treatment rendered to me
during the period from _____ to _____

_____
Signature of patient or closest relative

_____
Relationship

_____
Signature of witness

_____
Address

Figure 5-6   Records release form.

An **expert witness** is a person called upon to testify in court regarding what standard of care for a patient is in a similar community. An expert witness in a medical malpractice suit is generally a physician (Figure 5-7).

In the event that you are called upon to appear in court, you will want to be as comfortable as you can when giving testimony. It will be well to remember a few pointers.

- *Be professional.* You will be judged by your appearance and behavior as well as by what you say. Your attorney can advise you on this more fully.
- *Remain calm, dignified, and serious at all times.* The opposing attorney may try to make you nervous.
- *Do not answer questions you do not understand.* Simply ask the attorney to repeat the question or state, "I don't know."
- *Just present the facts surrounding the case.* Do not give any information that is not asked for. Do not insert your opinion. "The patient was shouting" is stating a fact. Stating "He was angry" is your opinion.
- *Do not memorize your testimony ahead of time.* You will generally be allowed to take

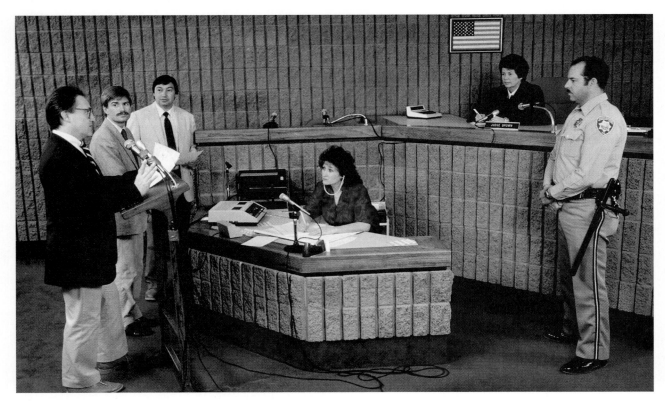

Figure 5-7   A physician giving testimony in a courtroom.

some notes with you to refresh your memory concerning dates.
- Always tell the truth.

Giving testimony in court is a crucial and sensitive matter. It is best to consult an attorney if you have any questions.

Public Duties of Physicians

There are responsibilities the physician has to the public—**public duties**—that include reports of births, stillbirths and deaths, communicable illnesses or diseases, drug abuse, certain injuries such as rape; abuse of children, spouses, and older adults; gunshot and knife wounds; and animal bites.

Many of the duties that relate to these responsibilities are carried out by office personnel including the medical assistant. Refer to Table 5-6 for a description of the physician's public duties.

Drug Regulations

The Food and Drug Administration (FDA) is the agency within the federal government that has jurisdiction over testing and approving drugs for public use. The Drug Enforcement Agency (DEA), a branch of the Justice Department, regulates the sale and use of schedule drugs.

The Controlled Substances Act of 1970 requires physicians to handle controlled drugs— drugs that are highly addictive—in very specific ways. The physician who dispenses, purchases, administers, prescribes or handles drugs is required to register with the Drug Enforcement Administration. The physician then receives a DEA registration number which must appear on all prescriptions for controlled substances. A DEA number is required for every location in which controlled drugs are stored. If a physician practices in two states then two DEA numbers must be obtained. DEA registration numbers are generally printed on physicians' prescription blanks. See Chapter 31, for the visual of a sample prescription form.

Controlled drugs must be kept in a locked or even double-locked cabinet and any theft must be immediately reported to both the regional DEA office and the local police. In addition, the physician's black bag and prescription blanks should always be stored in a secure locked location.

Records must be kept documenting the administering and dispensing of controlled drugs. In addition, federal regulations require a written inventory of drug supplies on a triplicate form based on daily use be made every two years and be kept for two more years.

Controlled drugs are classified into five schedules, or categories, which indicate levels of potential abuse. Schedule I drugs have the highest potential for addiction and abuse while Schedule V drugs have the least. See Chapter 31, Table 31-1 Schedule for Controlled Substances for the meaning of each classification and examples of drugs for each category.

The physician's medical assistant may not dispense controlled substances, however, she or he must be knowledgeable about the regulations governing the documentation and control of drugs. Only licensed personnel are permitted to dispense drugs. Be sure to report to the physician any unusual patient behavior indicating addictive drug use.

The potential for drug use/abuse by physicians and other health care professionals always has been and continues to be a serious problem. Refer to Chapter 4 for more information on the topic of substance abuse by health care professionals.

Role of the Medical Assistant

The role of the medical assistant in preventing liability suits is of paramount importance to both you and your employer. Remember that in many cases you are the only one in the office who will hear a patient's complaint. Your ability to handle the complaint professionally and efficiently may eliminate a potential lawsuit for the physician.

Acting under a code of ethics that compels you to safeguard any patient whose care and safety are affected by the negligent action of someone else, you must follow the chain of command, the authority structure within your office, and report to your immediate supervisor any negligent action you observe. It goes without saying that if you accidentally make an error, you will bring this to your supervisor's attention so that it can be corrected immediately.

You can help your employer and protect yourself, by remembering the recommendations and cautions that follow. These recommendations and cautions are clustered around major areas of responsibility you address daily in your role as a medical assistant.

Confidentiality/Privacy
- Never make any statements about your employing physician that could be interpreted as an admission of fault. On the

TABLE 5-6 **Public Duties of the Physician**

Duty	Description
Births	Issuing of a legal certificate which will be maintained during a person's life as proof of age. Many benefits including social security, passport, and driver's license depend on having a valid birth certificate.
Deaths	Physicians sign a certificate indicating the cause of a natural death. Check with your state public health department to determine specific requirements. For example, in the case of a stillbirth before the 20th week of gestation you will have to determine if both a birth and death certificate are required.
	A coroner or health official will have to sign a certificate in the following cases: • No physician present at the time of death • Violent death, unlawful death • Death as a result of criminal action • Death from an undetermined cause.
Reportable communicable diseases	Physicians must report all diseases that can be transmitted from one person to another and are considered a general threat to the public. The list of reportable diseases differs from state to state. The report can be either by mail or phone. The following childhood vaccines and toxoids are required by law (The National Childhood Vaccine Injury Act of 1986): • Diphtheria, tetanus toxoids, pertussis vaccine (DTP) • Pertussis vaccine (whooping cough) • Measles, mumps, rubella (MMR) • Poliovirus vaccine, live • Poliovirus vaccine, inactivated • Hepatitis B vaccine • Tuberculosis test
Reportable injuries	Certain injuries are reportable according to state requirements. These injuries include gun or knife wounds, rape and battered persons injuries, and spousal, child, and elder abuse.
Child abuse	Questionable injuries of children including bruises, fractured bones, and burns must be reported. Signs of neglect such as malnutrition, poor growth, and lack of hygiene are reportable in some states.
Elder abuse	Physical abuse, neglect, and abandonment of older adults is reportable in most states. The reporting agency varies by state but generally includes social service agencies.
Drug abuse	Abuse of prescription drugs is reportable according to the law. Such abuse can be difficult to determine since the abuser may seek prescriptions for the same drug from several different physicians. A physician will want to see a patient before prescribing a medication.

other hand, you as a medical assistant, cannot remain silent if you are aware that your employing physician is doing something illegal. You can then be held liable for remaining silent.

• Do not participate in negative or critical discussions of the physician(s) or other practitioners in your office with your patients. Do not comment on a patient's negative criticism of a current or former physician.

• Never discuss anything about the patient outside of the office.

• Make sure that a female medical assistant is present when the physician (male or female) examines a female patient.

- Treat all patients with dignity and respect.

Office Management

- Treat all patients with the same courtesy and dignity you would expect to receive. Log and return telephone calls promptly. Explain any delays to patients who are waiting to see the physician. Offer to set up another appointment if the delay will be very long.
- Never make promises regarding what the physician can do for the patient.
- Carefully explain all fees and responsibilities for bills to the patient, relating any concerns the patient may have to the physician.
- Relay any dissatisfied patient's comments to the physician.
- If the physician will be out of town or absent from the office, post these dates. Include this announcement in the monthly billing envelopes. Also provide the name and telephone number of the physician available for patients who need care when their own physician is absent.
- If a physician is withdrawing from a case then a certified letter must be sent to the patient declaring this. Send the letter certified mail with return receipt requested and keep a copy of the letter and receipt with the patient's record. The physician can be brought up on charges of "abandonment" if there is no documentation or evidence that there was a formal withdrawal.

Documentation

- Carefully sign or initial every documentation. Remember: medical documents are considered legal documents and may be used in a court of law.
- If the patient did not keep an appointment be sure to document the fact as a "no show." Document canceled appointments and follow-up to determine why the patient missed the appointment.
- Document when a patient is referred to another physician and follow-up to make sure the patient did see the referral physician.
- Document all patient contacts including telephone prescription refills and tests and procedures that have been ordered. Call all patients the day after surgery to check on their progress. Document this phone call.
- Record all care and treatment given as soon as possible after the patient's visit. This will

keep patient records current and insure appropriate follow-up treatment if it is required.

- Be sure the physician sees and initials all diagnostic reports before they are filed.
- Provide all instructions to patients in writing.

Drug Regulations

- A medical assistant may administer medication ONLY under the direct supervision of a physician. Follow the Controlled Substances Act by careful procedure and documentation. This may vary from state to state.
- Secure the supply of prescription pads from theft at all times.
- When preparing medications for administration, check the medication three times. Remember the "three befores." Check the medication *before* removing it from the shelf; check the name and dosage again *before* preparing the dosage; and check the label again *before* returning the medication to the shelf.

Certification and Licensing

- Have a thorough understanding of the limits of certification and standards of care for the medical assisting profession. Never perform any procedure for which you are not trained or qualified.
- Do not diagnose or prescribe over the telephone. This applies to all drugs even those that can be obtained over the counter. You could be charged with practicing medicine without a license.
- Do not call yourself a "nurse" or allow anyone else to refer to you as the nurse. You must be held to your own standard of care and not that of a nurse.
- Participate in continuing education and training programs to maintain your skill levels.

Informed Consent

- The physician must thoroughly explain all procedures to the patient. The medical assistant is responsible for making sure there is a signed consent form. Never have the patient sign a document they do not understand.
- Obtain a parent or guardian's signature before any procedure is performed on a minor. The only exception is in a case of emergency when the parent or guardian

cannot be reached. File the signed consent form immediately.

Safety

- Maintain a safe environment in the office or work site for the patients and staff. Handle requests for maintenance repairs. Report any safety hazards at once. If you knowingly overlook a hazard that a "reasonable person" would report and eliminate you can be guilty of negligence.

- Carefully check and document medical waste disposal. Be concerned about the safety of maintenance personnel who must handle the waste containers. Always dispose of syringes and needles correctly in designated hazardous waste containers.
- Maintain and document careful quality checks on laboratory testing equipment.

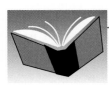

PATIENT EDUCATION

Both the physician and medical assistant are responsible for the patient education relating to legal issues. The medical assistant can assist the physician in providing good patient care and avoiding litigation by following practical recommendations. Patients must understand all papers they sign, including permission for treatment, insurance payments, and other billing matters. You may have to read and explain this material to patients if you have any doubts about their comprehension of the written materials.

Summary

Even though health care consumers of today are more informed, medical costs—particularly medical insurance—and the advanced state of medical technology pose new financial, moral, ethical, and legal problems for the consumer. The medical practitioner also faces the same problems. Today, more than previously, court cases and rulings have a greater impact on the way health care professionals practice business in the medical field.

The legal issues presented here will form the basis of your understanding of your responsibility to the patients you will care for as well as the physician/employer for whom you will work. As a medical assistant you must be aware of federal, state, and local regulations governing the care and treatment of patients. If the patient's care and safety are your most important responsibility, it is possible that you may be able to save your physician/employer from needless lawsuits.

Competency Review

1. Define and spell the glossary terms for this chapter.
2. What is the difference between criminal and civil law?
3. List and describe the 4 D's of negligence.
4. What is contract law? What application does it have in a physician's office?
5. What are Good Samaritan Laws and how do they apply to you?
6. Describe the patient/physician relationship.
7. Why do you need thorough understanding of the law as it impacts your employer's practice?
8. State 10 steps that can be taken to help protect the physician and staff from liability.

PREPARING FOR THE CERTIFICATION EXAM

Test Taking Tip — Pay careful attention to quantifiers such as some, none, never, always, everywhere, and sometimes.

Examination Review Questions

1. What are the four types of written laws?
   (A) misdemeanor, felony, civil, tort
   (B) felony, tort, negligence, contract
   (C) civil, tort, multi-national, governmental
   (D) criminal, civil, tort, military
   (E) civil, criminal, international, military

2. Performing surgery on a patient without the proper informed consent of the patient is an example of
   (A) intentional tort
   (B) battery
   (C) assault
   (D) A and B
   (E) A and C

3. What might a physician be guilty of when, for example, a treatment that was below an acceptable standard of care, was the direct cause of an injury?
   (A) negligence
   (B) malpractice
   (C) battery
   (D) A and B
   (E) A, B and C

4. According to the laws governing the collection of an accounts receivable, telephone calls must only be made between the hours of
   (A) 7 AM and 7 PM
   (B) 8 AM and 8 PM
   (C) 8 AM and 9 PM
   (D) 7 AM and 6 PM
   (E) 8 AM and 6 PM

5. The doctrine which applies to the law of negligence that means "The thing speaks for itself" is
   (A) respondeat superior
   (B) res ipsa loquitur
   (C) standard of care
   (D) informed consent
   (E) statute of limitations

6. Which of the following statements regarding patient/physician relationships is TRUE?
   (A) Physicians have the right to select the patients they wish to treat.
   (B) Patients expect that their physicians will use the appropriate "standard of care" in providing treatment.
   (C) Consent refers to giving permission to treat.
   (D) Patients can expect to receive information concerning both the advantages and potential risks of a given treatment.
   (E) All of the above

7. What, when signed by a patient, allows a representative to act on behalf of the patient in regards to medical treatment and care?
   (A) durable power of attorney
   (B) living will
   (C) advanced directives
   (D) the Uniform Anatomical Gift accord
   (E) the Good Samaritan accord

8. All actions must be carefully documented in a patient's medical chart. This would include
   (A) calls and office visits
   (B) office visits and treatments
   (C) appointments and appointment cancellations
   (D) prescribed medications and their refills
   (E) all of the above

9. Public duties of the physician would include the reporting of
   (A) births and deaths
   (B) communicable diseases
   (C) injuries such as those that are caused by battery and/or assault
   (D) child and elder (or older adult) abuse
   (E) all of the above

10. The Controlled Substance Act, which requires physicians and their representatives

to handle controlled substances in specific ways, includes

(A) storing these substances in a locked cabinet

(B) reporting the theft of any controlled substance to the police

(C) detailed record keeping regarding the administration and dispensing of these substances

(D) A and B

(E) A, B, and C

ON THE JOB

Dr. Spring, a board certified obstetrician and gynecologist, has been in practice for more than 10 years. He is licensed to practice medicine in both New York and Pennsylvania. Dr. Spring employs a staff that includes two medical assistants.

On Monday one of the medical assistants, Nancy Watts, took a history on a new patient that was referred to Dr. Spring by her internist. The 40 year old and married patient, has had vaginal spotting for more than 6 weeks.

As part of the history, Nancy learned that the patient has been under the care and supervision of a fertility specialist for more than 2 years. In fact, although not always compliant, the patient has been on a medication treatment regime for fertility problems.

*After examining the patient, Dr. Spring ordered a uterine biopsy to be performed in the office. The patient returns the following week, undergoes the biopsy and is sent home. However, the patient's husband has just telephoned the office, requesting to speak to Dr. Spring immedi-*ately. His wife had just been admitted because of intense vaginal bleeding.*

What is your response?

1. Was there anything in the patient's history that should have caused Nancy to alert the physician about performing a uterine biopsy?
2. What laboratory test(s) would have been appropriate prior to the uterine biopsy?
3. Should Nancy have given this patient special instructions prior to the biopsy because of her history?
4. How should Nancy handle the husband's telephone call?
5. Would it violate patient confidentiality to FAX the patient's records to the emergency room physician, if requested?
6. Is this a potential case of medical negligence and malpractice? Could Nancy, as the medical assistant, have complicity in this particular case?

References

A Patient's Bill of Rights. Chicago: American Hospital Association, 1992.

Black, H. *Black's Law Dictionary.* St. Paul: West Publishing Co., 1991.

Brody, B. and Engelhardt, H. *Bioethics: Readings and Cases.* Upper Saddle River, NJ: Brady/Prentice Hall, 1987.

Code of Medical Ethics: Current Opinions with Annotations. Chicago: Council on Ethical and Judicial Affairs of the American Medical Association, 1997.

Dubler, N. and Nimmons, D. *Ethics on Call.* Harmony Books, 1992.

Hall, M. and Ellman, I. *Health Care Law and Ethics in a Nutshell.* St. Paul: West Publishing Co., 1990.

Health Care Law and Ethics. Chicago: American Association of Medical Assistants, 1996.

Judson, K. and Blesie, S. *Law and Ethics for Health Occupations.* New York: Macmillan/McGraw, 1994.

Lewis, M. and Tamparo, C. *Medical Law, Ethics, and Bioethics in the Medical Office.* Philadelphia: F. A. Davis Company, 1993.

Lipman, M. *Medical Law & Ethics.* Upper Saddle River, NJ: Brady/Prentice Hall, 1994.

Locher, C. "How to Make the Most of Your Charting." *Journal of Practical Nursing.* 42:2, 1992.

McConnell, T. *Moral Issues In Health Care.* New York: Wadsworth Publishing Company, 1997.

Munson, R. *Intervention and Reflection: Basic Issues in Medical Ethics.* New York: Wadsworth Publishing Company, 1996.

Neubauer, M. "Careful Charting—Your Best Defense." *RN.* 53:11, 1990.

Newton, L. and Schmidt, D. *Wake Up Calls: Classic Cases in Business Ethics.* New York: Wadsworth Publishing Company, 1996.

Snell, M. *Bioethical Dilemmas in Health Occupations.* Lake Forest, IL: Macmillan/McGraw, 1991.

Veatch, R. *Medical Ethics.* Boston: Jones and Bartlett Publishers, 1989.

MEDICAL ASSISTANT ROLE DELINEATION CHART

Highlight indicates material covered in this chapter

ADMINISTRATIVE

ADMINISTRATIVE PROCEDURES

- Perform basic clerical functions
- Schedule, coordinate, and monitor appointments
- Schedule inpatient/outpatient admissions and procedures
- Understand and apply third party guidelines
- Obtain reimbursement through accurate claims submission
- Monitor third-party reimbursement
- Perform medical transcription
- Understand and adhere to managed care policies and procedures
- *Negotiate managed care contracts (adv)*

PRACTICE FINANCES

- Perform procedural and diagnostic coding
- Apply bookkeeping principles
- Document and maintain accounting and banking records
- Manage accounts receivable
- Manage accounts payable
- Process payroll
- *Develop and maintain fee schedules (adv)*
- *Manage renewals of business and professional insurance policies (adv)*
- *Manage personal benefits and maintain records (adv)*

CLINICAL

FUNDAMENTAL PRINCIPLES

- Apply principles of aseptic technique and infection control
- Comply with quality assurance practices
- Screen and follow up patient test results

DIAGNOSTIC ORDERS

- Collect and process specimens
- Perform diagnostic tests

PATIENT CARE

- Adhere to established triage procedures
- Obtain patient history and vital signs
- Prepare and maintain examination and treatment areas

- Prepare patient for examinations, procedures, and treatments
- Assist with examinations, procedures, and treatments
- Prepare and administer medications and immunizations
- Maintain medication and immunization records
- Recognize and respond to emergencies
- Coordinate patient care information with other health care providers

GENERAL (TRANSDISCIPLINARY)

PROFESSIONALISM

- Project a professional manner and image
- Adhere to ethical principles
- Demonstrate initiative and responsibility
- Work as a team member
- Manage time efficiently
- Prioritize and perform multiple tasks
- Adapt to change
- Promote the CMA credential
- Enhance skills through continuing education

COMMUNICATION SKILLS

- Treat all patients with compassion and empathy
- Recognize and respect cultural diversity
- Adapt communications to individual's ability to understand
- Use professional telephone technique
- Use effective and correct verbal and written communications
- Recognize and respond to verbal and non-verbal communications
- Use medical terminology appropriately
- Receive, organize, prioritize, and transmit information
- Serve as liaison
- Promote the practice through positive public relations

LEGAL CONCEPTS

- Maintain confidentiality
- Practice within the scope of education, training, and personal capabilities
- Prepare and maintain medical records
- Document accurately
- Use appropriate guidelines when releasing information
- Follow employer's established policies dealing with the health care contract
- Follow federal, state, and local legal guidelines
- Maintain awareness of federal and state health care legislation and regulations
- Maintain and dispose of regulated substances in compliance with government guidelines
- Comply with established risk management and safety procedures
- Recognize professional credentialing criteria
- Participate in the development and maintenance of personnel, policy, and procedure manuals
- *Develop and maintain personnel, policy, and procedure manuals (adv)*

INSTRUCTION

- Instruct individuals according to their needs
- Explain office policies and procedures
- Teach methods of health promotion and disease prevention
- Locate community resources and disseminate information
- *Orient and train personnel (adv)*
- *Develop educational materials (adv)*
- *Conduct continuing education activities (adv)*

OPERATIONAL FUNCTIONS

- Maintain supply inventory
- Evaluate and recommend equipment and supplies
- Apply computer techniques to support office operations
- *Supervise personnel (adv)*
- *Interview and recommend job applicants (adv)*
- *Negotiate leases and prices for equipment and supply contracts (adv)*

SOURCE: Reprinted by permission of the American Association of Medical Assistants from the *AAMA Role Delineation Study: Occupational Analysis of the Medical Assisting Profession.*

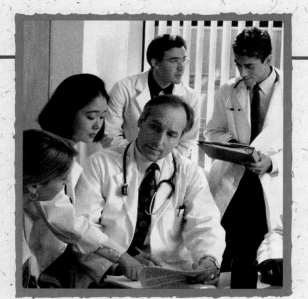

6

Quality Assurance and the Medical Assistant

CHAPTER OUTLINE

LEARNING OBJECTIVES

After completing this chapter, you should:
1. Define and spell the glossary terms for this chapter.
2. Explain the AMA's eight essentials of quality care.
3. Describe the difference between quality of life and quality assurance.
4. Explain the basic components of a quality assurance program.
5. State 4 ways in which the medical assistant can participate in the quality assurance process.
6. Define and describe the peer review process.
7. State 4 issues that a Peer Review Organization might review.
8. Describe the work of the Joint Commission on Accreditation of Health Organizations.

Glossary

criteria Standards against which something is compared to make a decision or judgment.

data Statistics, figures, or information.

evaluation Assessment or judgment.

health care consumer Individual who engages the services of a physician or other health care practitioner.

incident report Formal written description of an incident, such as a patient falling, occurring in a medical setting.

Medicare Federal health care insurance program for adults over 65 and disabled persons who qualify.

mortality rate Death rate; the ratio of the number of deaths in a given population.

non-invasive procedure Procedure or treatment in which the skin and body is not entered or invaded.

norm Standard, criterion, or the ideal measure for a specific group.

occurrence Any event or incident.

Peer Review Organization (PRO) A professional organization that reviews a physician's conduct.

procedure manual A collection of policies and procedures for carrying out day-to-day operations in an office or facility.

quality assurance program (QAP) A program in which hospitals and medical practices evaluate the services they provide by comparing their services with accepted standards.

The medical assistant works in a diverse range of health care institutions each requiring a good understanding and practice of quality assurance (QA) and quality improvement. This chapter identifies what quality assurance is, why it is needed, and what health care institutions and their employees can do to maintain or improve quality of care standards. Learning where and how the medical assistant fits into the quality assurance picture will help to safeguard patients and to assist employers in the delivery of quality patient-centered care. Organizations like the Peer Review Organization and the Joint Commission on Accreditation of Health Organizations continually monitor quality assurance in health care organizations such as hospitals, nursing homes, ambulatory care settings, and clinics.

Quality Medical Care

Quality medical care is an expectation of all patients. This care requires the health care team to use procedures and techniques that result in the best possible outcome for the patient. In addition, the patient must be satisfied with the care.

The major parameters or attributes of health care that are regularly examined include treatment, benefit of treatment, cost-benefit, accessibility to health care, and delivery location. The outcome factor actually requires a measurable change in the health status of the patient that is a direct result of the care received. Cost/benefit refers to the expenditure or cost in terms of time, money and effort and the relationship of this cost to the actual benefit the patient receives. Accessibility to health care refers to the effort a patient must make to receive health care.

The American Medical Association (AMA) has defined quality care by listing eight essential elements (Table 6-1).

> **Med Tip:** "Quality of life" is a phrase used to indicate the physician's responsibility to always do what is in the best interest of the patient. Quality of life issues become important factors in determining treatment for critically injured accident victims, newborns with multiple birth defects, and patients with terminal diseases. In determining "quality of life" issues, the physician is cautioned to consider the patient's needs first and foremost and not to focus on whether the patient is or is not a burden to the family or society.

What Is Quality Assurance?

In the early 1960s, the health care industry began to feel an increasing demand from the public for accountable quality care. From that initial swell of public pressure developed a continuing effort on the part of health care providers to deliver optimal

TABLE 6-1 **The AMA's Eight Essentials of Quality Care**

1. Bring about the optimal in the patient's condition within the earliest time frame possible based on the patient's comfort and physical condition.

2. Have an emphasis on early detection and treatment as well as health promotion and disease prevention.

3. Receive treatment in a timely fashion without unnecessary delay, termination, interruption, or prolongation.

4. Encourage the patient's participation in the decision process regarding his or her treatment.

5. Base the treatment on skillful use of technology and health professionals using accepted principles of medical science.

6. Demonstrate concern for the patient, patient's family with a sensitivity to the stress caused by illness.

7. Achieve the treatment goal through the wise use of technology and other resources.

8. Provide adequate documentation in the patient's medical record to facilitate peer evaluation and continuity of care.

Printed with permission of the AMA, House of Delegates, 1996.

achievable excellence in care. Quality assurance is gathering and evaluating information about the services provided as well as the results achieved compared with an accepted standard.

Med Tip: Some patients just assume they will receive high quality medical care when they enter a medical office. Other patients are informed health care consumers. They are aware of the term "quality assurance" from their own work experience or as consumers in general. It is the medical assistant's task to educate and assist patients in their efforts to obtain quality care.

Quality assessment measures consist of formal, systematic evaluations, or assessments, of overall patterns of care. The actual programs and activities of quality assurance have as a goal a desired degree, or level, of care in a health care setting. The results of the evaluation are then compared to standard results and as deficiencies are identified recommendations for improvement in care are made (Figure 6-1). So it is that Quality Improvement Programs (QIPs) utilize the data gathered by quality assurance/assessment to effect quality improvement in health care.

Quality Assurance Program

A **quality assurance program (QAP)** in a hospital, ambulatory health care setting, long-term care facility or health maintenance organization (HMO) consists of a system for reviewing records maintained by staff. These records may consist of medical or nursing records, data regarding days of hospitalization or treatment, progress reports, and other statistics that provide a firm indication of the care received by patients. A quality assurance program must include evaluation and educational components to identify and correct problems. Quality assurance programs such as these are required in order for the facility to receive funding by the Public Health Act as well as to achieve and maintain accreditation. The basic components of a quality assurance program include the following:

1. *Establish a QA Committee:* Representatives from the entire patient care team (such as physician, nurse, and medical assistant) should be part of a QA committee (Figure 6-2).
2. *Review all clinical and administrative services and procedures:* Committee members or an assigned individual can conduct the review. All team members should have a role in the QA process— from designing the QA forms to selecting

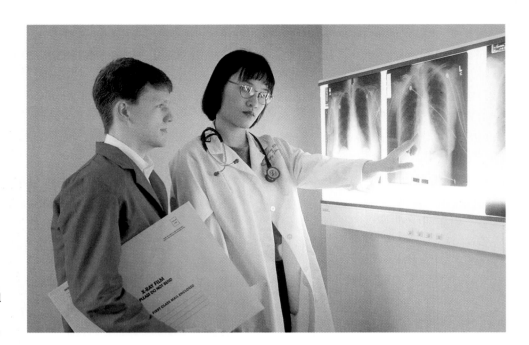

Figure 6-1 Medical assistant speaking with physician about patient.

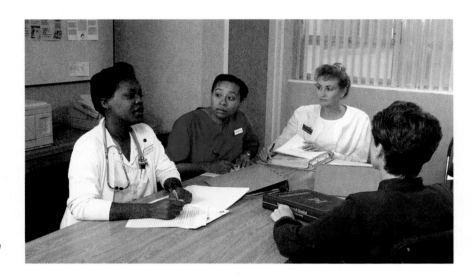

Figure 6-2 Quality assurance health care team meeting.

issues for review. Procedure and policy manuals are also subject to review during this process.

3. *Set up structure for identifying items to review:* Pay particular attention to problem issues.

4. *Quantify all issues:*
   For example:
   - Average length of waiting time in minutes to see physician.
   - Number of errors in writing items on patient records.
   - Number of insurance claims disallowed per 100 filed.
   - Number of failed "needle sticks" per 50 attempts.

5. *Limit the number of issues:* A limit should be set on the number of issues or problems reviewed at any one session. Emphasis should be placed on taking corrective measures.

6. *Maintain careful records:* Review all records, such as incident reports and committee records, and progress or improvement with the entire medical team.

Table 6-2 lists examples of issues that a QA committee might review in a physician's office.

TABLE 6-2   Issues Reviewed By a QA Committee in a Physician's Office

Issues reviewed or evaluated

1. Disallowed insurance claims
2. Errors in dispensing medications (use incident reports)
3. Errors in labeling of laboratory specimens
4. Incorrect coding of diagnosis for insurance claims
5. Long waiting time for patient
6. Adverse reactions to treatments and/or medications (use incident reports)
7. Inability to obtain venous blood on the first attempt
8. Member satisfaction (from survey/questionnaire results)
9. Patients who leave the office without seeing the physician
10. Patient complaints relating to confidentiality
11. Appearance of office
12. Handicapped parking availability
13. Safety
14. Provider availability
15. Emergency preparations
16. Treatment areas
17. Safety/monitoring practices for radiology and laboratory
18. Medications
19. Infection control
20. Patient education/rights
21. Medical records
22. Collection procedures
23. Telephone and reception behaviors

Implementing a Quality Assurance Program (QAP)

The ultimate goal of a formal quality assurance program is to improve the quality of care so that there is no difference between what should be done and what is actually being done. These norms or standards are developed by professionals in the field who are expert in a particular health care area.

Implementation of such a QAP requires the development of patient-centered criteria based on acceptable standards of care. Criteria are standards against which to compare something in order to make a decision. For example, years ago some patients were discharged from a hospital without being given any formal information or education about what to do when they returned home. Now all hospitalized patients should receive instructions at discharge regarding medications, diet, activity, and a follow-up appointment with the physician. This discharge plan is explained to the patient who then signs the plan and keeps a copy. A copy of the signed plan is also put in the patient's chart indicating this instruction took place. A quality assurance program would monitor the discharge planning process.

Incident Report

One means of documenting problem areas within the office or facility is through the incident report. In Chapter 10 an example of a typical incident report is provided. This report should be completed whenever there is an unusual occurrence such as a fall, error in medication dispensing, or patient complaint. An occurrence is any event or incident out of the norm. Other incidents that require documentation are fire, flood, theft, computer crash, and improper needlesticks just to name a few. The purpose is to objectively document exactly what happened with the goal of preventing another episode. Incident report forms are generally designed to meet the individual needs of each facility. Details on completing an incident report are usually included in every office's procedure manual—a collection of policies and procedures for carrying out the day-to-day operations in an office or facility.

The incident report like all other information relating to the patient is subject to subpoena in litigation. After the report is filed, a copy is placed in the patient file and the original is kept in the main office file where incident files are stored or another secure place.

Medical Assistant's Role in a QAP

The medical assistant is trained in clinical and administrative skills with the expectation for the highest level of performance. To assist the physician/employer, pay rigorous attention to the quality of care given to patients. Patient satisfaction is a key element in quality of care. The medical assistant may be the first person to respond to a patient's complaint or discomfort. Medical assistants have the opportunity to present patients' concerns and/or complaints at a team QA meeting so that corrective measures can be taken (Figure 6-3). Some of the areas in which to assist the physician with quality assurance are noted in Table 6-3.

Measures to Assure Quality Assurance

Quality of patient care can be assessed from within the medical profession by organized groups of physicians. It is also monitored and assessed from outside the profession through governmental or insurance provider intervention.

Peer Review Organizations

Peer Review Organizations (PROs) are professional organizations that review a physician's conduct. The Peer Review Organizations (PROs) program is an example of a government-directed program to assess and affect the quality of medical care. This program was established under the Tax Equity and Fiscal Responsibility Act (TEFRA) of 1982. The purpose of this law is to carefully monitor both the cost and quality of hospital and physician services for Medicare patients. The program is administered by the Health Care Financing Administration (HCFA) which oversees PROs throughout the United States.

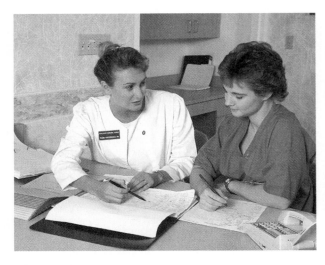

Figure 6-3   Medical assistant at a QA team meeting.

Peer Review

Hospital peer review, in which physicians reach a judgment on the nature and length of hospital care provided by their colleagues, has had the effect of reducing medical costs. The purpose is to reduce the number of unnecessary admissions, surgery and other invasive and **non-invasive procedures**. An invasive procedure refers to a technique or method of treatment in which the skin and body is entered or invaded, for example surgery. The body is not entered or invaded during a non-invasive procedure. A PRO looks at the utilization of services by examining admissions and invasive procedures. In addition, it monitors medical services that are provided when needed to prevent complications. Issues reviewed by Peer Review Organizations (PROs) include:

- Death rate due to poor care
- Discharge planning

TABLE 6-3 Medical Assistant's Role in QA

1. Resolving patient complaints about items such as billing questions and long waiting times in the reception room.

2. Patient education regarding diet, laboratory and procedure instructions, and personal care.

3. Telephone follow-up regarding a patient's condition and progress.

4. Double-checking laboratory tests performed in the office.

5. Verifying the results of laboratory tests given over the telephone. Always ask the laboratory to repeat any results that are abnormal or unclear. Request to have a written report sent by mail or FAX.

6. Bringing patient complaints to the attention of the physician.

- Medical stability of patient at the time of discharge
- Nosocomial—hospital-acquired—infection rate
- Re-admission to hospital within 31 days after discharge which indicates that the patient may have been discharged too soon
- Trauma actually suffered during hospitalization (for example medication errors, bed sores, and falls)
- Unscheduled returns to surgery (which generally require emergency surgery)
- Length of hospital stay

Peer Review Process

The peer review process is conducted by physicians and nurses. There are around 2000 physicians who participate in reviewing the work of other physicians. A hospitalized patient's case automatically may come up for review after a particular number of days have passed. In addition, the review process is started when the insurance claim is filed for Medicare reimbursement.

PRO nurse reviewers examine hospital records and discharge plans. The attending physician has an opportunity to explain the case more fully to the reviewers. However, if the review determines that a procedure was unnecessary or could have been performed in a more cost-effective setting, a payment denial notice is issued. In serious cases of quality issues, the physician may be barred from participating in the Medicare program. In some severe cases, physicians have lost their license to practice.

The PRO process is expanding to include health care facilities other than hospitals such as ambulatory care settings and health maintenance organizations (HMOs). The medical assistant is becoming increasingly involved in the review process either by gathering data or by providing the high quality patient care the employer requires.

Joint Commission on Accreditation of Health Organizations (JCAHO)

The Joint Commission on Accreditation of Health Organizations (JCAHO), headquartered in Chicago, Illinois, is a private, nongovernmental agency that establishes guidelines for hospitals and health care agencies to follow regarding quality of care. It is supported by representatives of the American Hospital Association (AHA), American College of Surgeons, American College of Physicians, and the American Dental Association. In addition to forming guidelines for the operation of health care institutions, such as hospitals, ambulatory care facil-

ities, and long-term care institutions, the JCAHO conducts surveys and accreditation programs.

JCAHO inspectors visit the health care institutions such as hospitals by invitation and review patient medical records, organization of the medical staff, and the general operation of the facility. Some indicators that are used during the survey and accreditation process are mortality rate, frequency of complication, nosocomial infection rate, and autopsy rate. The mortality rate refers to the number of deaths in a given population. Based on their assessment, the inspectors will issue either a "full accreditation" or "provisional accreditation" report. The Commission works with the institution to correct any deficiencies within a specified time frame.

The JCAHO does not actually have authority or power to take punitive action against a physician or hospital for poor patient treatment. However, the survey results of the JCAHO are used by other agencies, such as the Department of Health and Human Services, that do have the authority to impose a sanction or penalty.

Competitive Performance Reports (CPRs)

In order to better control the Medicare program, Congress mandates that Competitive Performance Reports (CPRs) be done. These reports are compiled by selecting a large number of physicians, up to 5000, whose Medicare claims have a higher frequency of certain medical services when compared with the claims of other physicians in the same locality and specialty. A Competitive Performance Report (CPR) is sent to these physicians in order for them to see how they compare with others. The expectation of Congress is that the CPRs will result in favorable practice changes by the physicians to eliminate the overuse of Medicare. However, there is little follow-up to CPRs and physicians are not required to respond. The medical assistant may be asked to assist in gathering data—statistics, figures, or information—for this report.

Health Plan Employer Data and Information Set 3.0 (HEDIS)

Under HEDIS managed care plans that serve Medicare patients must collect data relating to eight categories of performance:

1. Effectiveness of care
2. Access to/availability of care
3. Member satisfaction
4. Informed health care choices

5. Health plan descriptive information
6. Cost of care
7. Health plan stability
8. Use of service

Medicare HMOs and other plans seeking accreditation from the National Committee for Quality Assurance (NCQA) must also report data. Eventually, most of the health plans (HMOs and PPOs) a physician contracts with will be collecting data for medical practice.

Occupational Safety and Health Administration (OSHA)

The Occupational Safety and Health Administration (OSHA) was established by the U.S. Congress in the Occupational Safety and Health Act of 1970 "to assure so far as possible every working man and woman in the nation safe and healthful working conditions." This act covers every employer whose business affects interstate commerce.

OSHA is the federal agency that has the power to enforce regulations concerning the health and safety of employees. Every office and health care institution must be aware of OSHA recommendations and carefully monitor potential violations. For instance, the Centers for Disease Control (CDC) has issued recommendations for a set of universal precautions that all health care workers must follow when dealing with hazardous materials. The CDC has authorized OSHA to enforce these precautions.

OSHA, in cooperation with other agencies, carries out research to establish basic safety standards. OSHA inspectors carry out frequent, surprise inspections of workplaces to see that standards are maintained. OSHA safety regulations include standards for exposure to noise, asbestos, toxic chemicals, lead, pesticides, and cotton dust. Violators of OSHA standards must pay fines if found guilty.

Since July 6, 1992, OSHA standards mandate that all health care employers must provide a means for protecting their employees from potential exposure to *Hepatitis B*. In fact, every employee must be given the choice to elect or refuse immunization. If refused, the employee has the right to change his or her mind and receive immunization at no charge. All costs associated with this immunization must be provided by the employer.

Clinical Laboratory Improvement Amendment (CLIA)

The federal government now mandates that all clinical laboratories that test human specimens must be controlled. The Clinical Laboratories Improvement Amendment of 1988 (CLIA88) divides laboratories into three categories. These are described in Table 6-4.

Refer to Chapter 25 for further discussion of the Clinical Lab Improvement Act (CLIA) which mandates quality control of lab tests by categories and documentation.

TABLE 6-4   **Clinical Laboratory Improvement Amendment (CLIA)**

Category	Explanation
1. Simple testing	Incorrect test results pose little risk for the patient.
	Laboratory subject to random inspectors only.
	Some physician laboratories fall in this category.
2. Intermediate-level testing (Level II)	Risk to patient if there is an incorrect test result.
	Must be certified by approved accrediting agency.
	Must be staffed by credentialed personnel.
	Must meet quality assurance standards.
3. Complex testing (Level III)	High risk to patient if there is an incorrect test result.
	Must be certified by approved accrediting agency.
	Must be staffed by credentialed personnel.
	Must meet quality assurance standards.

LEGAL AND ETHICAL ISSUES

All health care personnel have a responsibility for quality assurance. There is an ethical and moral responsibility to report to your superior or employer issues that you believe are a potential for harm either to the patients or other employees. Responsibility for maintaining records requires the medical assistant to be extremely careful. Medical records are legal documents and form the basis for data used in the quality assurance process.

PATIENT EDUCATION

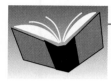

While today's health care consumers are quite knowledgeable about many medical issues, they may not understand the quality assurance process. Health care consumers are individuals who engage the services of a physician or other health care practitioner. Some consumers may resent being a statistic or number in a quality assurance report. It should be stressed that quality assurance is meant to improve the quality of health care for a patients. When the necessity for maintaining accurate, current data is explained, patients and their families are usually willing to cooperate.

Summary

It is important to understand that the patient is the central figure at the core of the health care delivery system and that the medical assistant along with all other health care professionals must place the patient's interests first. Quality assurance programs are means for assuring quality patient care. Organizations like Peer Review Organizations, the Joint Commission on Accreditation of Health Organizations, and OSHA monitor quality assurance in health care organizations such as hospitals, nursing homes, and ambulatory care settings including clinics and physicians' offices. In addition, other controls such as the Competitive Performance Report and the Clinical Lab Improvement Act regulate the behavior of physicians and the quality levels of laboratories throughout the country.

Competency Review

1. Spell and define the glossary terms for this chapter.
2. What is meant by quality assurance (QA)?
3. Describe the basic components of a quality assurance program.
4. How is an incident report used in quality assurance?
5. List 5 situations in which an incident report must be filed.
6. What 4 things can the medical assistant do to assist in the QA process?
7. What 4 issues might be reviewed by a PRO?
8. What is the JCAHO?
9. Define and discuss the purpose of TEFRA.

PREPARING FOR THE CERTIFICATION EXAM

Test Taking Tips — If your exam contains several pages, be careful not to turn over two pages at once. Your answers on the answer card would then be entered in the wrong spaces.

Examination Review Questions

1. The ratio of the number of deaths in a defined population versus the number in the population is the

(A) morbidity rate
(B) mortality rate
(C) occurrence rate

(D) normative rate

(E) quality assurance rate

2. The major parameters of health care that are regularly examined regarding quality medical care are

(A) treatment protocols

(B) benefit and cost-benefit of treatment

(C) accessibility to health care

(D) location for the delivery of health care

(E) all of the above

3. Which of the following is NOT one of the AMA's 8 Essentials of Quality Care?

(A) the cost-effectiveness of health care

(B) the encouragement of patient involvement in treatment options

(C) the demonstration of concern for the patient's family

(D) the prudent use of technology and other resources

(E) the provision for adequate documentation of treatment

4. The evaluation of information about the health care services provided, as well as the results, in comparison with the acceptable standard of care is

(A) quality care

(B) quality assurance

(C) systematic evaluation

(D) formative evaluation

(E) summative evaluation

5. What type of program utilizes data gathered and analyzed by quality assurance for the purpose of positively effecting the overall quality improvement in a health care setting?

(A) Quality of Life Program

(B) Quality Involvement Program

(C) QAP

(D) QIP

(E) None of the above

6. A quantification issue, as part of a quality assurance program, might include the

(A) average waiting time for a patient to see a physician

(B) number of prescription errors

(C) number of disallowed insurance claims

(D) number of failed "needle sticks"

(E) all of the above

7. Which of the following would NOT be an example of an issue that may be reviewed by a Quality Assurance Committee in a physician's office?

(A) a breach of confidentiality

(B) the incorrect CPT and/or ICD-9 coding

(C) a prolonged waiting time for a physician

(D) an adverse reaction to a prescribed medication

(E) physician accreditation and licensure

8. One acceptable method for the documentation of problem areas in a physician's office is through a/an

(A) procedure manual

(B) normative report

(C) incident report

(D) occurrence report

(E) health care consumer's report

9. Which of the following is a private, nongovernment agency that establishes guidelines for hospital and health care agencies regarding the quality of care?

(A) JCAHO

(B) AHA

(C) AMA

(D) AAMA

(E) OSHA

10. Which of the following is the federal agency that has the power to enforce regulations concerning the health and safety of employees?

(A) CDC

(B) CLIA

(C) JCAHO

(D) OSHA

(E) none of the above

ON THE JOB

Jean Simon has been a medical assistant for more than five years. Most of her career has been spent doing administrative rather than clinical tasks in the practice of Dr. John Klean, an infectious disease specialist. However, she is a skilled phlebotomist.

Today, while doing a differential smear off of a specimen of blood that she had drawn from a patient earlier, Jean has broken a microscope slide and cut the middle finger of her left hand. She was wearing surgical gloves at the time, but they did not prevent the incident from happening, and, in fact, she is bleeding quite severely.

What is your response?

1. What should Jean immediately do?
2. In terms of quality assurance, what needs to be done?

3. What if Jean is alone in the office at the time of the incident?
4. Does the fact that she was relatively inexperienced play a major role in this incident and, if so, how could this incident have been prevented?
5. Is this a procedure that should have been performed in D. Klean's office by a medical assistant? Does the history of the patient help to determine the answer to this question?
6. Does any follow-up course of action need to be taken?
7. Does the patient need to be advised of the incident?

References

A Patient's Bill of Rights. Chicago: American Hospital Association, 1992.

Black, H. *Black's Law Dictionary*. St. Paul: West Publishing Co., 1991.

Code of Medical Ethics. Chicago: American Medical Association, 1996–97.

Wedding, M. and Toenjes, S. *Medical Laboratory Procedures*. Philadelphia: F. A. Davis Company, 1992.

Strategies for Success

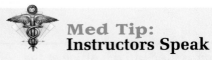

Med Tip:
Instructors Speak

Strive for mastering as much as possible in each class. Don't settle for a "C" grade. The medical field demands more than "average."

Take your assignments seriously! Stay caught up with your assignments and homework.

Martha Garrels,
BS, MSA, MT (ASCP), CMA-C
Granger, Indiana

After class, go home and study the lesson of that particular day for at least one hour.

Don't be afraid to ask for help.

Mary F. Chiaravalloti, RN, CMA
Lackawanna, New York

Develop and then designate a special place for studying. Try to find enough space so that you can leave your reference books and other materials handy for your next study session.

Catherine Rogers, BSN, MBA, CMA
Davis, Illinois

Sometimes it is helpful to consider one word or paragraph at a time. For example, check the dictionary for words you don't understand and rewrite the paragraph in your own words, if necessary.

Jan Hasselbar, RN
Phoenix, Arizona

Be proactive! Show initiative! For example, during idle time make requests that will help you learn something new.

John P. Cody, MPH, MBA, CMA
Richfield, Minnesota

Don't be afraid to ask questions. The only *dumb* question is the one that is not asked. Often times, the same question you have in your mind is one that other people in the class also have. So, don't be afraid to *speak up.*

Recognize that it is not necessary to try to learn all alone. Form a study group or make use of the instructor's office hours. There is a great advantage to verbalizing your concepts in order to share them with others.

Jerri Adler, CMA, CMT
Eugene, Oregon

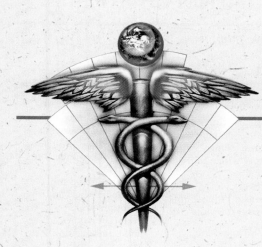

Unit Two

Administrative

MEDICAL ASSISTANT ROLE DELINEATION CHART

Highlight indicates material covered in this chapter

ADMINISTRATIVE

ADMINISTRATIVE PROCEDURES

- Perform basic clerical functions
- Schedule, coordinate, and monitor appointments
- Schedule inpatient/outpatient admissions and procedures
- Understand and apply third party guidelines
- Obtain reimbursement through accurate claims submission
- Monitor third-party reimbursement
- Perform medical transcription
- Understand and adhere to managed care policies and procedures
- *Negotiate managed care contracts (adv)*

PRACTICE FINANCES

- Perform procedural and diagnostic coding
- Apply bookkeeping principles
- Document and maintain accounting and banking records
- Manage accounts receivable
- Manage accounts payable
- Process payroll
- *Develop and maintain fee schedules (adv)*
- *Manage renewals of business and professional insurance policies (adv)*
- *Manage personal benefits and maintain records (adv)*

CLINICAL

FUNDAMENTAL PRINCIPLES

- Apply principles of aseptic technique and infection control
- Comply with quality assurance practices
- Screen and follow up patient test results

DIAGNOSTIC ORDERS

- Collect and process specimens
- Perform diagnostic tests

PATIENT CARE

- Adhere to established triage procedures
- Obtain patient history and vital signs
- Prepare and maintain examination and treatment areas

- Prepare patient for examinations, procedures, and treatments
- Assist with examinations, procedures, and treatments
- Prepare and administer medications and immunizations
- Maintain medication and immunization records
- Recognize and respond to emergencies
- Coordinate patient care information with other health care providers

GENERAL (TRANSDISCIPLINARY)

PROFESSIONALISM

- Project a professional manner and image
- Adhere to ethical principles
- Demonstrate initiative and responsibility
- Work as a team member
- Manage time efficiently
- Prioritize and perform multiple tasks
- Adapt to change
- Promote the CMA credential
- Enhance skills through continuing education

COMMUNICATION SKILLS

- Treat all patients with compassion and empathy
- Recognize and respect cultural diversity
- Adapt communications to individual's ability to understand
- Use professional telephone technique
- Use effective and correct verbal and written communications
- Recognize and respond to verbal and non-verbal communications
- Use medical terminology appropriately
- Receive, organize, prioritize, and transmit information
- Serve as liaison
- Promote the practice through positive public relations

LEGAL CONCEPTS

- Maintain confidentiality
- Practice within the scope of education, training, and personal capabilities
- Prepare and maintain medical records
- Document accurately
- Use appropriate guidelines when releasing information
- Follow employer's established policies dealing with the health care contract
- Follow federal, state, and local legal guidelines
- Maintain awareness of federal and state health care legislation and regulations
- Maintain and dispose of regulated substances in compliance with government guidelines
- Comply with established risk management and safety procedures
- Recognize professional credentialing criteria
- Participate in the development and maintenance of personnel, policy, and procedure manuals
- *Develop and maintain personnel, policy, and procedure manuals (adv)*

INSTRUCTION

- Instruct individuals according to their needs
- Explain office policies and procedures
- Teach methods of health promotion and disease prevention
- Locate community resources and disseminate information
- *Orient and train personnel (adv)*
- *Develop educational materials (adv)*
- *Conduct continuing education activities (adv)*

OPERATIONAL FUNCTIONS

- Maintain supply inventory
- Evaluate and recommend equipment and supplies
- Apply computer techniques to support office operations
- *Supervise personnel (adv)*
- *Interview and recommend job applicants (adv)*
- *Negotiate leases and prices for equipment and supply contracts (adv)*

SOURCE: Reprinted by permission of the American Association of Medical Assistants from the *AAMA Role Delineation Study: Occupational Analysis of the Medical Assisting Profession.*

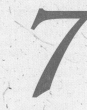

Communication: Verbal and Nonverbal

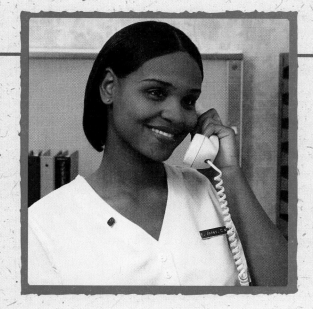

LEARNING OBJECTIVES

After completing this chapter, you should:
1. Define and spell the glossary terms for this chapter.
2. Describe the communication process.
3. List several examples of nonverbal communication conveying impatience.
4. State six types of directive communication giving an example for each.
5. Describe the difference between assertive and aggressive behavior.
6. Make a statement which communicates loyalty for your employer.
7. List six guidelines for effective listening.
8. Describe the three types of listening.
9. State six types of defensive behavior giving an example for each.
10. List seven things to avoid when placing a caller on hold.
11. Describe the steps to take when handling a prescription refill request.
12. What are the eight questions you would ask when handling an emergency telephone caller.
13. Describe several ways in which effective communication skills can be useful for patient education.

ADMINISTRATIVE PERFORMANCE COMPETENCIES

After completing this chapter, you should perform these tasks:
1. Use assertive behavior with a classmate.
2. Answer a telephone using good communication technique.
3. Communicate an idea to a classmate using only body language.
4. Talk to a co-worker using effective communication techniques.
5. Place a second caller on "hold" correctly.
6. Record a telephone message accurately.
7. Telephone triage.

Glossary

aggressive The practice of using a bold or pushy style when trying to convince the other person to agree with you.

assertive The practice of declaring a point in a positive manner.

assessment Evaluation.

condescending Assume an air of superiority.

defensive behavior Conscious or unconscious reaction to a perceived threat.

empathy The ability to imagine how another person is feeling.

feedback Any response to a communication.

nonverbal communication The information conveyed by the way a person acts over and

above (or in place of) the message conveyed by his words.

open-ended questions Questions which require an explanatory answer rather than a yes or no response.

reflecting Directing the conversation back to the patient by repeating the words. Also called mirroring.

restating Directing the conversation back to the patient by stating what the patient has said in different terms.

sympathy Feeling sorry for a patient.

Communication is a necessary requirement in any field, but is particularly essential in the health care field. As a medical assistant, you will relate to a variety of people, including sick and worried patients, your physician/employer, fellow staff members, vendors, and even personal acquaintances of the physician. Some individuals you will interact with will be angry, frustrated or simply ill and tired. It is not enough for the medical assistant to have excellent technical skills. Good interpersonal skills as well as good oral and written communication skills are needed to relate well to patients and fellow staff members.

It has been said that the most important piece of equipment in the doctor's office is the telephone. But, the telephone is useless without an effective communicator at each end. In this chapter, you will learn about the communication process, including good directive techniques to improve effective communication, barriers to good communication, and defensive behaviors. This knowledge along with the information presented on telephone techniques, long-distance calling, and using an answering service will give you a basic understanding of the value of effective communication.

The Communication Process

The basic units of the communication process are the source, message, channel, and receiver. Think of this as S-M-C-R.

S   stands for the source of the communication. Who is sending the message?

M   represents the actual message or the actual words that are placed on paper if the message is in writing.

C   indicates the channel or channels through which the message moves from the source to the receiver. These channels include the senses: sight, smell, taste, hearing, and touch. Another set of channels consists of pathways such as the telephone or interoffice mail.

R   stands for the receiver of the message.

For example, a physician (S) writes a prescription (M) which the medical assistant then reads over the telephone (C) to the pharmacist (R). If any link in this chain is broken, then an incorrect message is relayed. The same holds true when you relay a message to a patient. If the medical assistant, (S) explains a procedure (M) to a patient who has a hearing loss (C) then the patient (R) will not hear the message as it was intended.

The communication process then is a chain effect that requires a source (S) and a receiver (R). The source (S) acts upon a stimulus to encode or transmit a message (M) in a particular form. The actual message can be transmitted in a variety of ways (C), including face-to-face, over the telephone, or in written form. The receiver (R) decodes or translates the message based on his or her emotional state, perceptions, education, socioeconomic background, and many other factors.

Add to this process the ever present background noises that are part of the daily functioning of a medical office, for example, conversations between patients or patients and staff, background music, ringing telephones, or requests for assistance, and it is very possible that the receiver may not receive the message the sender intended.

Channels of Communication

Channels of communication include the various means by which the spoken or written word is communicated from one person to another. Information is said to be "rich" if it conveys to the listener or reader the intent of the speaker. The greatest amount of information richness is gained from face-to-face discussion (Figure 7-1). The least amount of information is generally gained from formal numeric documents such as budget reports. When you wish to convey an important message to someone, it is better to do it face-to-face than to place the information into writing. This becomes important to remember when determining how to adequately educate patients regarding their medications. If you place all the important facts into a

TABLE 7-1   **Information Richness of Channels**

Information Channel	Level Richness
Face-to-face discussion	Highest
Telephone conversations	High
Written letters/memos (individually addressed)	Moderate
Formal written documents (general bulletins or reports)	Low
FAX (facsimile)	Low
E-mail	Low
Internet	Low
Formal numeric document (printouts, budget reports)	Lowest

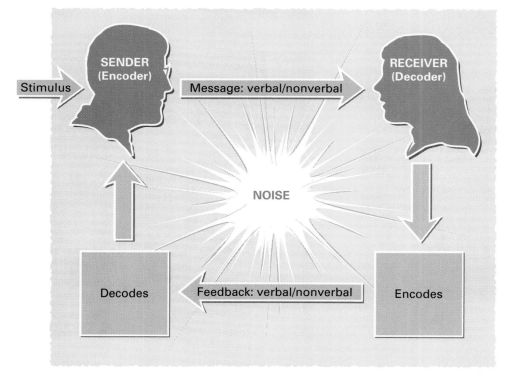

Figure 7-1   After face-to-face discussion, telephone conversations are probably the most frequently used channel of communication.

pamphlet they may never read it or might not understand your meaning. Yet, it is important to give written instructions to follow-up after any verbal explanation you give the patient. Table 7-1 illustrates the information richness of various channels of information.

Verbal and Nonverbal Information

Virtually everything a person does from birth to death is a form of communication. Smiling is a form of nonverbal communication while talking "with a smile in your voice" is verbal communication.

Nonverbal communication is the language of gesture and actions including body language. In many cases, people are not even aware of the image they project with their bodies. The way a person holds his or her arms, makes eye contact, gestures, frowns, or turns toward or away from the speaker, frequently conveys more than just words

Med Tip: The gesture of touching is considered a form of nonverbal communication referred to as body language. Gently touching a distraught patient's arm can reassure and comfort the patient. However, one must be cautious that a touch is not misinterpreted by the receiver. In some cultures, for instance, it is considered rude to touch a child's head without permission. Also, abused children can be fearful of even innocent touching. Use caution when touching to console a patient unless you know the patient well.

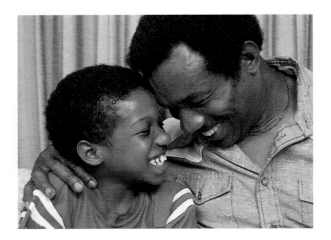

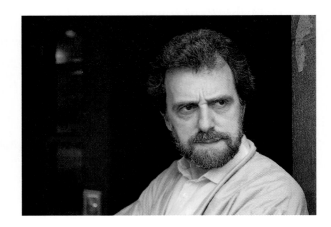

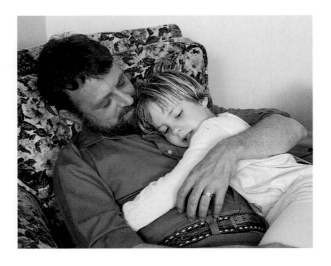

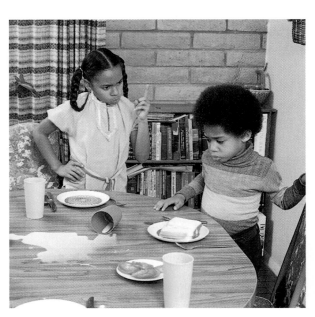

Figure 7-2 Nonverbal communications convey strong, powerful messages that may be negative or positive.

could convey (Figure 7-2). Table 7-2 offers some examples of messages that convey impatience.

Conveying a Positive Attitude

The ability to convey a positive attitude is so important in working with people. Smiling immediately reassures the patient that he or she is welcome. When in the presence of a patient, always involve the patient in your conversations with other staff. Never ignore or exclude the patient as such behav-

TABLE 7-2 Communication Messages Conveying Impatience

- Interrupting people when they are speaking
- Answering telephone calls curtly
- Finishing another person's sentence
- Rushing the patient
- Eating lunch at your desk
- Looking at your watch or the clock
- Doing two things at one time
- Not looking up from your work when someone approaches
- Rushing around the office

ior is disrespectful (Figure 7-3). If the conversation is of a business or confidential nature, then the conversation should be held elsewhere.

Effective medical assistants are able to demonstrate empathy but should be cautious about using sympathy for their patients. Empathy is the willingness or the ability to understand what the patient is feeling without necessarily experiencing the same thing. Sympathy, on the other hand, is feeling sorry for or pitying the patient. Patients react much better to an empathetic listener than to a sympathetic one. You can acquire the skill of empathic listening using these simple nonverbal techniques: nodding, leaning toward the patient or positioning yourself so you are at their eye level, and indicating by your facial expression that you understand what they are saying (Figure 7-4).

Med Tip: Since we all share the same human emotions, there will be times when you become distressed over a patient's situation. It is not possible to be a concerned health care provider and remain totally unemotional at all times. If you become upset over a patient's situation, you can simply excuse yourself for a few moments. Realize that your emotions and concern are another indication that you have chosen the correct field.

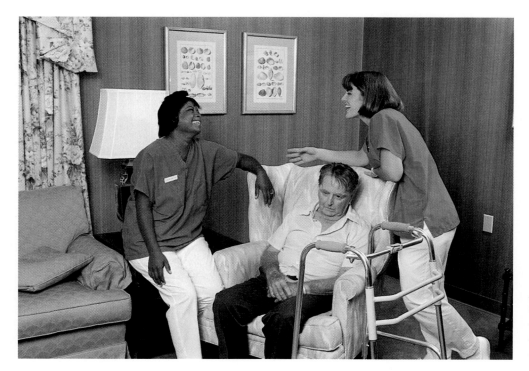

Figure 7-3
Conversations held in the presence of the patient should include the patient.

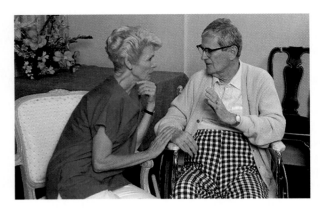

Figure 7-4 Empathy draws a more positive response from the patient since it is based on the willingness of the medical assistant to understand what the patient is experiencing.

Communication Techniques

The ability to encourage a patient to communicate effectively is critical when you wish to perform a patient assessment, or evaluation, to determine what the patient's problems are. But, how do you stop a patient who is talking about seemingly irrelevant issues? First of all, it is important to understand that the patient is probably nervous. Many people talk when they experience this feeling. You may have to direct the communication in order to gain feedback from the patient. Feedback refers to any response to a communication.

Directive Communication Techniques

The medical assistant can often assist the communication process by directing the patient's comments, using specific communication techniques, so that the sharing between the patient and medical assistant is productive. Open-ended questions, or questions that require more than yes or no responses, can be most useful in gaining feedback or drawing out patient information. Using such questions or directive methods, you will be able to obtain the information the physician will require to treat the patient. See Table 7-3 for a list of directive communication techniques with a description and an example of each technique.

TABLE 7-3   **Directive Communication Techniques**

Technique	Description	Example
Open statement	Encourage the patient to discuss freely.	"Please describe your pain for me."
Closed statement	Direct the patient to make a yes/no or simple response.	"Are you having pain?"
Reflecting	Direct the conversation back to the patient by repeating the patient's words.	Patient: "I'm afraid of what the doctor will find." MA: "You're afraid of what the doctor will find?"
Acknowledgement	Indicate understanding.	"I understand what you are saying."
Restating	State what the patient has said but in different terms.	Patient: "I can't sleep." MA: "You say you're having trouble getting to sleep at night?"
Add to an implied statement	Verbalize implied information.	Patient: "I'm usually relaxed." MA: "And today you're not relaxed?"
Seek clarification	Request more information in order to better understand.	Patient: "I don't feel good." MA: "Tell me what your symptoms are."
Silence	Remain silent or make no gesture in response to a statement.	Patient: "I don't know what's wrong but something is."

Feedback

Feedback is critically important when working with patients since you must determine if they really understand what they have heard. This can be either verbal or nonverbal. Sometimes the verbal message and the nonverbal message patients send do not agree. For instance, when you ask a patient, "How are you feeling" and the patient states, "Fine," but, since, the patient is walking with a painful looking limp, you doubt the verbal statement. Always try to ask specific questions such as, "Do you have any pain," "Tell me about your reaction to the medication" or "Tell me what you need to see the doctor about."

Assertive Versus Aggressive Behavior

Most instances of communication within the work setting involve convincing someone else to cooperate with you. Whether patient or staff communication is your goal, the methods to achieve cooperation are the same. As a medical assistant there are occasions when you will have to convince both patients and staff to listen to you. Using assertive behavior techniques can make this easier.

Being assertive means that you make a point in a positive manner. Being aggressive, on the other hand, is considered a negative behavior and indicates a type of pushiness when trying to convince others. In fact, aggressiveness has been compared to making a verbal attack against another. Many people resort to aggressive behavior without meaning to.

Acquiring the ability to use assertive behavior means that you will learn to offer new ideas or even unwanted ideas to people in such a fashion that they will not feel threatened. For instance, when calling a patient regarding nonpayment of a bill you will need to gain the patient's acceptance. If the patient becomes angry at the beginning of the conversation in response to an aggressive comment, such as "Are you aware that your bill is now two months overdue? When are you going to pay it," the patient could become defensive and hang up. Since most patients know when they have not paid a bill, it is not necessary to use threatening language. A better approach would be to state who you are and indicate that you are helping Dr. Thompson with his billings. In a calm but assertive manner, you would then ask questions that could prompt a positive response from the patient. These questions might include, "How can I help you in clearing up these payments? Perhaps we can discuss your making a small payment on your account twice a month. What would be an amount that you could afford?"

> **Med Tip:** Always consider a patient's feelings when asking questions within hearing distance of other patients. Asking questions such as "What is your birth date," "When was your last menstrual period," and "Why are you here to see the doctor," can be embarrassing for many people and breaches patient confidentiality.

Some of the most difficult communication problems occur with other staff members (Figure 7-5). Good staff communication depends on positive, respectful interactions. When thoughtless or condescending comments are made, permanent damage to relationships can occur. Condescending means taking a superior attitude and acting as though you are better than someone else. Withdrawing from the group, feeling angry and hurt, and discussing other staff members behind their backs, causes office morale to suffer. Using assertive behavior with fellow staff members means that you assert your own needs without threatening theirs. For instance, if it is your turn to have a holiday off and you have been scheduled to work, it is better to state, "I'm sorry I can't work that day. Since I worked overtime on the last holiday, I have made plans for this one." An aggressive statement, such as "It's not fair. I always have to work on holidays and the others don't" would imply favoritism or special treatment of some

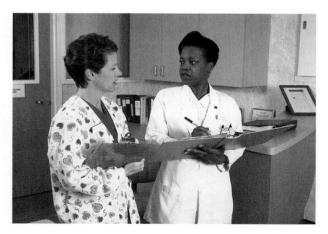

Figure 7-5 Staff members often find it difficult to communicate with other staff members.

staff and might cause a supervisor to become defensive.

Table 7-4 has other examples of assertive and aggressive reactions. In some examples, you are turning a negative statement into a positive statement.

Greeting Patients

A patient should be greeted within one minute of entering the office. If you are speaking on the telephone when the patient comes in, be sure to acknowledge the patient's presence with a smile and nod. Give your full attention to the patient as soon as you complete the telephone conversation.

Discussing Sensitive Issues with Patients

Discussing issues involving money such as a patient's bill and personal financial responsibility can be very sensitive. Patients should be advised before the first visit of physician's charges for specific services or treatment. Inquiries regarding the patient's medical insurance and procedure for payment of fees should also be reviewed prior to the first visit so that there is no confusion over payment at the time services are rendered.

Loyalty to Your Employer

You represent your employer or physician every time you speak to a patient or caller. You must support the physician and his or her reputation in every instance. In your position, you may become privileged to personal information about your employer. Under no circumstances, whether inside or outside of the office, should that information be discussed. It's perfectly acceptable to state, "I really can't answer that" or "I'm sorry, but I don't know" in response to patient's or other staff member's questions.

A loyal employee protects and defends an employer when other employees engage in negative conversation. See Table 7-5 for examples of loyal responses to questions or comments about your employer's personal life.

TABLE 7-4   **Comparison of Assertive and Aggressive Behavior**

Assertive Behavior	Aggressive Behavior
"This medication works best when it is taken on a regular daily basis."	"You know you can't expect this medication to work when you're not taking it every day."
"Let me find someone who can answer that question for you."	"That's not my job."
"Your behavior is inappropriate."	"Why did you do that? It was stupid."
Knocking on door and then coming into an exam room to say: "Excuse me Dr. Thompson, you are needed on the telephone."	Rushing into an exam room to say: "Doctor, you've got a telephone call."

TABLE 7-5   **Responses That Communicate Loyalty**

Question/Comment	Sample Response
"I guess Doctor Thompson can't see me on Wednesday because he's playing golf."	"Dr. Thompson's day off is Wednesday, but he could see you on Saturday."
"I hear Dr. Thompson and his wife are divorcing?"	"I really have no information about Dr. Thompson's personal life."
"I've been waiting 1 hour to see Dr. Thompson. Why is he so slow?"	"I'm sorry you've had a long wait. Dr. Thompson has had many very ill patients today. May I reschedule your appointment?"

Listening

You might think that some people are born with effective listening skills and others are not. Whether this is actually the case doesn't matter. The important thing is that effective listening can be learned and developed just like other skills. Here are some guidelines you can follow to promote effective listening.

Guidelines: Effective Listening

1. Stop talking! You cannot listen if you are talking.
2. Let the speaker know you want to listen. Paraphrase what has been said to show that you understand.
3. Remove all distractions. This includes radio, telephone, computer, and other interruptions.
4. Try to see the other person's viewpoint.
5. Do not argue with or criticize the speaker. This puts people on the defensive and may make them "clam up" or even become angry.
6. Before each person leaves, confirm what has been said.
7. Stop talking!

Effective listening involves more than just the sense of hearing. You must almost be able to feel what the person is trying to communicate to you. There are three types of listening: passive, active, and evaluative.

- *Passive listening* means that you are listening without offering any response. This is a very effective listening style to use when people are troubled, angry, and just need to talk to someone.

- *Active listening* involves your participation by offering feedback to the speaker by asking questions or giving a response.

- *Evaluative listening* is a vital skill for the medical assistant. This type of listening requires that you be able to make a judgment about what you are hearing and to respond quickly. Evaluative listening is used daily when answering the telephone or talking to a patient who has come in for assessment and examination.

Barriers to Communication

Some of the more obvious barriers to effective communication, such as the distraction of loud background noise, can be eliminated by the medical assistant. However, there are other barriers that we are not even aware of that result in either no communication or a distorted message being received. In order to understand the patient, you must overcome the barriers to effective communication (Figure 7-6).

Giving the patient false reassurance that "everything will be all right," can result in the patient's reluctance to talk to you about personal or health related fears. Such comments can also lead to liability issues for the physician if the patient believes that a promise for recovery has been made.

The medical assistant may also put up other barriers to communication without meaning to. These include not looking at the patient when the patient is speaking, interrupting the patient, abruptly changing the subject, and using mean-

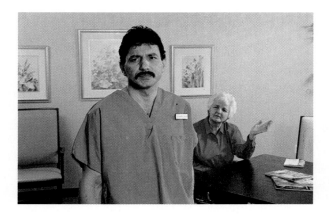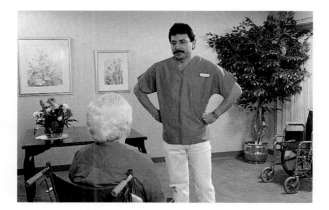

Figure 7-6   The medical assistant's body language may present a barrier to communication.

ingless statements to soothe the patient just to name a few.

> **Med Tip:** Remember that patients come in to see the physician because they have a problem. Never treat them in a condescending manner.

Defensive Behaviors

Patients will also put up barriers to effective communication when they are under the stress of an illness. These barriers are called defensive behaviors. A defensive behavior is a reaction to a perceived threat that is usually unconscious. Defensive behaviors are also referred to as coping behaviors. Some defensive behaviors are discussed in Table 7-6.

TABLE 7-6 Defensive Behaviors

Behavior	Description	Example
Compensation	Substitution of an attitude, feeling, or behavior with its opposite.	Mrs. Matthews believes the lump in her breast is cancer. However, she smiles and laughs whenever you talk to her about it.
Denial	Unconsciously avoiding an unwanted feeling or situation.	Mr. Morgan cancels an appointment to have a PSA (blood) test for prostate cancer in spite of having symptoms associated with prostate trouble.
Displaced Anger	Expressing angry feelings toward persons or objects which are unrelated to the problem.	Mrs. Matthews is angry at being diagnosed with cancer. She takes this anger out on her family members.
Disassociation	Not connecting one event with another.	Mary Sims is a nurse who works with alcoholic patients. In her free time she drinks to excess.
Introjection	Adopting the feelings of someone else.	Mr. Morgan's friends have said that the PSA test is reliable and could relieve his anxiety about having prostate cancer. He believes them and has the test.
Projection	Placing your own feelings onto another person.	Mr. Morgan becomes irritated when the medical assistant calls to remind him of his appointment. He wrongly decides that she is irritated with him or dislikes him. In reality, he is upset with himself.
Rationalization	Justifying thoughts or behavior to avoid the truth.	Mary Sims believes that the appetite suppressant benefit of smoking offsets the risk of developing cancer.
Regression	Turning back to former behavior patterns in times of stress.	Jimmy, who is toilet-trained, reverts to bed-wetting during hospitalization.
Repression	Keeping unpleasant thoughts or feelings out of one's mind.	Mr. Morgan denies any urinary frequency when questioned by the physician.
Sublimation	Directing or changing unacceptable drives for security, affection and/or power into socially or culturally acceptable channels.	Mrs. Matthews is worried about having cancer and uses up energy cleaning her house.

Use of Medical Terminology

You will become adept at understanding the language of medicine. The abbreviations that are used in medicine are a form of communication for people working in the health care field. However, your patients have little understanding of medical terminology. You may wish to teach patients a few simple terms so that they can better understand the physician's instructions on items such as prescriptions. However, you must make an effort to avoid using the "shorthand" or abbreviations of medical terminology with the patients.

Patients may be reluctant to admit they do not understand. You will then assume that they have been properly instructed which is not the case.

Med Tip: Abbreviations such as "NPO," meaning nothing by mouth, are not readily recognized or understood by patients. Always write out clear instructions regarding preparations for tests and taking medications.

Handling the Angry Patient

One of the most difficult communication problems involves the angry patient. It can be a difficult task for the medical assistant to refrain from taking the patient's comments personally. People have different styles and coping behaviors when they are frightened (Figure 7-7). Many patients who enter the physician's office are fearful of the diagnosis they may hear. Some patients become frightened of the equipment in the office or have an unwarranted fear of pain.

The job of the medical assistant is to remain calm and use professional techniques to direct the patient's anger into a positive channel. For instance, many patients will gain control over their anger when the medical assistant offers a comment such as, "I'm really sorry you feel this way. Let's see if we can solve the problem."

You may have to take the patient into a private office if you cannot calm the patient immediately. Disruptive patients can upset others waiting to see the physician. While it is not necessary to give in to the unreasonable demands of a patient, realize that an upset patient is often expressing the need for you to listen carefully, without judging, and assist in solving the problem. Whenever possible, try to gently direct the patient's comments to the solution of the problem.

In the case of an angry caller, you must remember that no matter how angry a patient becomes, you cannot respond in anger. The role of the medical assistant is to assess or evaluate the situation. Remain calm and speak to the patient in a quiet, calm tone of voice, projecting your concern for the patient in the present situation. Often, this will be enough to calm the patient down. If it does not work, however, ask your supervisor or office manager for assistance. Otherwise, ask the patient if you may return the call after you have been able to gather more information to be of help.

Communicating with Fellow Staff

A positive attitude can make the difference between keeping and losing a job. A positive attitude is easier to project if you are happy in your work. The work group you are a part of is an important factor in your attitude.

Work groups need to become a cohesive team. In order to do this, many work groups also become social groups. It is beneficial to talk about hobbies, travels, sports, family, and friends with other staff members to bring about an atmosphere of trust and understanding. The social aspect of staff communication should not interfere with work productivity, but it is a necessary step in establishing an effective work team.

Technical language is necessary for the practice of medicine. It should not be used to gain status or to show off. Using language in this way can confuse issues rather than inform people and it creates bar-

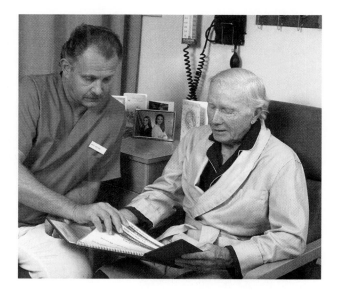

Figure 7-7 The medical assistant often has to reassure and comfort the patient before effective communication can take place.

riers to effective communication among team members. Everyone on the health care team must be able to understand the medical or technical terminology used. In some cases, staff may be reluctant to discuss issues or provide feedback. You will find yourself recognizing in staff some of the same barriers to communication or defense mechanisms that have already been discussed. You will want to use some of the techniques presented to draw out fellow staff members and promote effective communication. To assess your own attitude, you might ask yourself the following questions:

- Do I complain unnecessarily?
- Do I give everyone the impression that I really enjoy my work?
- Do I try to remain cheerful at all times?
- Do I perform all my work without complaint?
- Am I cooperative?
- Do I treat patients and coworkers the way I like to be treated?

Telephone Techniques

If you work in the "front office" area, much of your day will be spent on the telephone (Figure 7-8). The telephone techniques used when speaking on home telephones are generally more informal and chatty than the style of conversation that is expected in a professional medical office. For example, slang such as "hi" is not used.

Answering the Telephone

Your manner of answering the telephone frequently determines how the conversation will flow. A clear, pleasant voice conveys the message to the caller that the call is welcome. The proper way to answer the telephone is to pick it up by the second ring and begin with a greeting such as "Good morning" or "Good afternoon." An example of a correct telephone greeting would be:

> "Good afternoon, Drs. Thompson and Williams. This is Mary. How may I help you?"

It is most important to clearly state the name of the physician or the medical practice. The greeting should be consistent among all staff members. This information is usually part of the orientation/training for staff who will be answering the telephone.

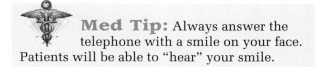

Med Tip: Always answer the telephone with a smile on your face. Patients will be able to "hear" your smile.

Using the Hold Function

One of the most sensitive issues relating to telephone courtesy is use of the "hold" function (Figure 7-9). The "hold" function refers to the ability to keep more than one call on the line at a time. Holding a call is permissible when the person being called will come onto the line within a short period of time or when you are already speaking to a caller on another line. However, the "hold" function is abused when callers are left "on hold" for indefinite periods of time.

If you are already speaking with a caller when a second call comes in, it is proper to ask the first caller if you may place him or her on hold for a moment in order to answer the second call. It is discourteous to handle the second caller before returning to the first call. An example of a typical conversation follows:

> First caller: "Mrs. Mendez, may I place you on hold for a moment? I have another call."

> Second caller: "Good afternoon, Drs. Thompson and Williams. Would you please hold?"

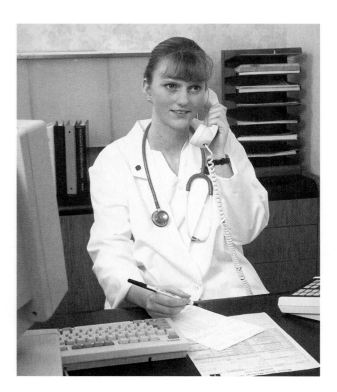

Figure 7-8 The medical assistant spends many hours on the telephone assisting patients.

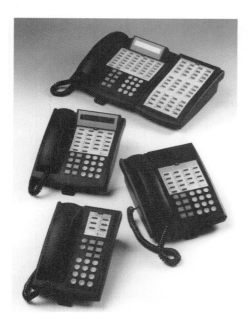

Figure 7-9 Choose the telephone unit that offers the features needed in your office.

It is important to allow the second caller time to say they will allow you to place them on hold. If this second call is an emergency, you would handle it immediately. It is never appropriate to simply state, "please hold" or "hold" to either of your callers and then cut the line off without hearing each caller's response. This type of rude behavior, which might even be dangerous in the case of an emergency, is one of the most frequent causes of complaints among patients.

When placing a caller on hold, until the physician or person the caller wishes to talk with can pick up the line, the medical assistant should explain that there may be a few minutes delay. You may also ask if you may take a number and have the

Med Tip: Research has found that patients who have established a good relationship with their physicians and office staff are less willing to bring a lawsuit against them. It goes without saying that patients must always be provided quality medical care. However, courteous treatment of patients does pay extra dividends.

physician return the call. In some cases, the caller will ask to remain on hold. Regularly check back with the caller or callers "on hold" each in turn to let the caller(s) know you have not forgotten him or her. An example of this type of conversation is:

"Dr. Williams is with a patient. May I take your number and have her return your call?" When you check back every 30 seconds on the holding caller, you will ask if they still wish to hold. For example, "Mrs. Mendez, Dr. Williams is still with a patient. Do you wish to continue holding or should I give her your telephone number and message?"

It is your responsibility to try to keep the telephone lines clear for incoming calls. Therefore, it is not a good idea to have patients "on hold" for very long. See Table 7-7 for a list of things to avoid when using the "hold" function.

Screening Telephone Calls

One of your most important functions to keep the office running smoothly is to effectively screen telephone calls. This means that you must be able to determine which calls will go directly into the physician, which calls you can handle either with scheduling or instructions, or which calls need to have a message taken (Figure 7-10).

TABLE 7-7 **Placing a Caller on Hold: Things to Avoid**

When placing a caller on hold always avoid:

• Switching the caller to "hold" before he or she states the reason for the call.

• Placing several callers on hold at the same time.

• Going back to the "hold" call and asking, "Who are you waiting for?"

• Cutting off calls by careless use of the hold button.

• Leaving a caller "on hold" for several minutes without checking back on the caller.

• Playing loud music on the telephone line while the patient is "on hold."

• Stating rudely "Hold" or "Hold please" without giving any explanation.

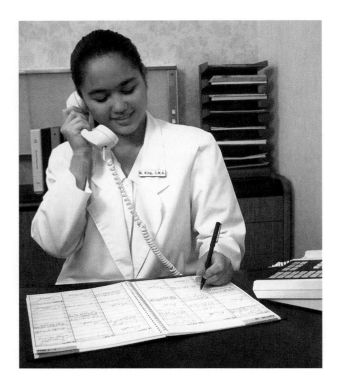

Figure 7-10 Scheduling appointments over the telephone is very common.

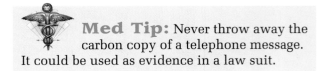

Whenever you answer the telephone, you will ask the person the reason for the call. Some callers will be reluctant to tell you. In those cases, you will still handle the call as a message. If the caller refuses to give his or her name, you will generally not take a message in to the physician.

It is more time efficient for physicians to set aside a time period to return all telephone calls and most physicians do this. Patient callers generally understand that a physician cannot be interrupted during a patient examination or conference.

If the physician is out of the office or otherwise unavailable, you may ask the patient if someone else can be of help. Sometimes, the nurse may be able to handle the problem. If you work in a joint practice, one of the physicians is usually assigned to handle telephone calls on a particular day.

Pharmaceutical representatives who wish to speak to the physician about a new product or drug are not usually put through to the physician unless otherwise instructed. You would simply take a message, including the representative's name, company, and telephone number.

Always follow the procedure Taking a Telephone Message to be sure you have taken all the necessary information when you take a telephone message.

Personal Calls to the Physician

The physician will also receive personal calls in the office. Physicians work long hours and often encourage family members to call them at the office. Most physicians will instruct you on how they wish their personal calls to be handled. In some cases, they will want you to knock on the exam room door and simply state, "Doctor, you are wanted on the telephone." In other cases, physicians may ask you to give them telephone messages as soon as they come out of the exam room. Generally, family members do not wish to interrupt the physician during a patient examination.

Personal calls from other physicians are handled in the same manner. Physicians wish to talk

---

PROCEDURE: Taking a Telephone Message

1. Give the correct greeting.
2. Use a message form or pad with a carbon copy to keep a record of the message.
3. Print the date and time of the call.
4. Print the full name and telephone number of the caller. (Always ask to have the name spelled.)
5. Write the name of the person being called.
6. Write down the complete message. Avoid using abbreviations other than accepted medical abbreviations. Include symptoms such as temperature, rash, emesis, and duration of symptoms.
7. Write your initials to indicate that you took the message.

to other physicians as soon as the call comes in whenever possible. These calls may relate to a patient consultation question that needs to be answered immediately.

Prescription Refill Requests

Telephone requests to have prescriptions refilled are frequent. As a medical assistant, you are not able to call in this order without the physician's direct order. Therefore, all these messages must go directly to the physician. In some offices, this can be done with voice mail via a separate line for pharmacies. Refill messages are then typically taken off two times a day. Always follow the procedure taking a Prescription Refill Message when a caller gives you a message for a prescription refill.

Local Calls

Some telephone systems are set up so the caller is required to dial "9" to get an outside line for local calls—telephone calls within your own area code. In this case, after dialing "9" you then dial the number without using the area code (9-555-7777).

Many offices have strict rules on the use of the telephone by staff. Usually, a pay telephone is provided for use by patients and staff to avoid tying up the office line(s) which should be available at all times for patient emergencies and the running of the office. It is important to follow these rules and to advise staff of them.

Long Distance Calls

You will be asked to place long-distance calls—telephone calls outside your area code—for the physician (Figure 7-11). You may also need to make travel arrangements or call other medical facilities for information. Long distance calls can be costly and are based on the type of call made and the length of time spent on the telephone line. If you accidentally reach an incorrect long-distance number, dial "O" immediately, and explain that you dialed an incorrect number to the operator who will credit the call for you.

Telephone Logs

In many offices, a telephone log is maintained to keep track of all long distance calls. This log is compared with the telephone bill when it arrives. Your office may have a policy of charging the patient for long-distance calls. The billing charge from the telephone bill can then be added to the patient's bill. The telephone log also makes it possible to catch any abuses such as excessive personal calls.

A typical log will include: name of the person called, telephone number called, name of person placing the call, date and time of the call, city and

---

PROCEDURE: Taking a Prescription Refill Message

1. Print the name of the patient. (This name may be different from the name of the caller.)
2. Write down the patient's telephone number.
3. Write down the name of the medication. Ask the caller to spell the medication if you are unclear about what the caller is saying.
4. Write down how long the patient has been on the medication.
5. Write down the patient's symptoms (why prescription is still needed).
6. Take the patient's age and weight (if a child).
7. Ask for the name and telephone number of the pharmacy and the prescription number.
8. Tell the caller you will give the message to the physician.
9. Tell the caller that you will call back if the prescription cannot be refilled.
10. Pull out the patient's chart for the physician to review and attach the telephone message to it.

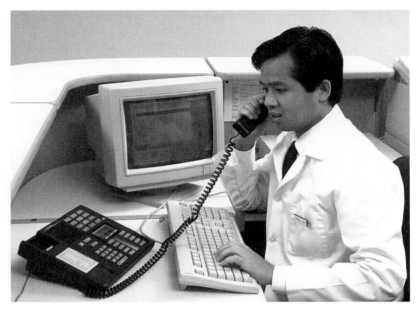

Figure 7-11   Typical telephone system in physician's office.

state called, length of call, and the purpose of the call. You may also indicate who is to be charged for the call. For example, bill patient, bill Dr. Williams, or bill office.

Direct Distance Dialing (DDD)

Direct Distance Dialing (DDD) refers to calls made outside your area code without the assistance of an operator. To place a long distance call using DDD, dial "1," then the area code followed by the number (1-312-555-7777). If you know the number you are calling but do not have an area code, you can find the listing of area codes at the front of the telephone directory. If you do not know the number of the person you are calling, dial Directory Assistance—555-1212—using the correct area code preceded by "1." For example, 1-312-555-1212 would connect you to Chicago information.

Operator-Assisted Calls

Operator-Assisted Calls are used when you place a collect call in which the receiver pays for the call, calls charged to a third number, person-to-person calls, station-to-station calls, and some credit card calls. This type of telephone call is more expensive than DDD. To request operator assistance dial "O" before the number (0-555-7777). The operator will then come onto the line.

Collect Calls

Collect Calls are calls for which the charges are reversed. In other words, the person receiving the

call pays the charges rather than the caller. Your office should have a policy on whether or not to accept collect calls. The physician may reverse charges if he or she is calling from out-of-state. If a patient calls the physician collect, always explain that the call will be placed on the patient's bill. You would generally not accept a collect call from a pharmaceutical company or an unknown person.

Conference Calls

When several people from different locations wish to have a telephone discussion, you would place a conference call. This means, for example, that two physicians at a distance from each other may speak with a patient at a third location at the same time. While these calls are more expensive than regular long-distance calls, they can save money in the long run, since you do not have to make several long-distance calls to relay the same information. The procedure for placing a conference call follows. *Note:* To make the best use of such telephone calls be aware of any telephone systems variations in your office.

Time Zones

You must be aware of time zones within the United States and foreign countries when placing long distance calls. The continental United States and parts of Canada are divided into four time zones based on parts of the country: Eastern, Central, Mountain, and Pacific. As you move from East to West across the United States, there is a one hour difference (earlier) in each time

1. Gather the telephone numbers of all participants before beginning the call.
2. Determine the time that everyone will be available for the conference call. (You may have to call people ahead of time to determine a convenient time.) Be aware of time zone differences when arranging conference calls.
3. Dial "O" for operator. Give the operator the name and telephone number (area code first) for each person to be called.
4. The operator will then place a call to each of the parties. When all the other participants are on the line, the operator will come back to the original caller (you) and the conversation can then begin. If you are placing this call for your physician, he or she will then pick up on your line.
5. If you are setting the conference call up ahead of time, tell the operator when you wish the conference call to begin.

zone. So, while it is 10:00 a.m. in New York (Eastern), it is 9:00 a.m. in Illinois (Central), 8:00 a.m. in Arizona (Mountain), and 7:00 a.m. in California (Pacific).

It is generally a good idea to post a copy of the time zones near the telephone (Figure 7-12). This way you can plan long-distance calls based on "office hours" in each time zone. A call placed at 3:00 p.m. in California will be received in New York at 6:00 p.m. when the office you are calling may be closed.

Using an Answering Service

Many medical offices use an answering service for times when there is no one in the office. This service can be in effect 24-hours a day or just at designated times, for example during the night, over lunch, or during peak hours of the day to relieve staff. The answering service personnel take calls from a location other than the office; then they either call or page the physician directly. In some cases, a list of non-emergency messages are

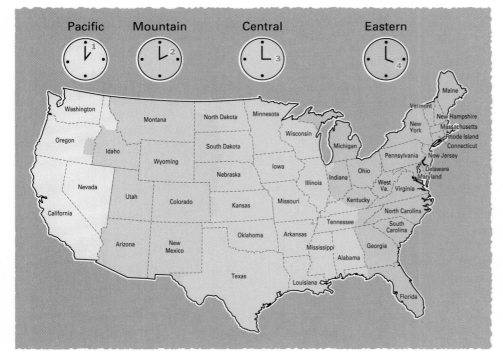

Figure 7-12   Have a time zone map located near the telephone to assist you with long distance calls outside your time zone.

kept until morning when staff arrives in the office. Messages taken during the lunch hour can be faxed to the office. An answering service is ideal for emergencies since the physician can be reached at all times. There is a monthly charge for this service.

Many offices will use an answering machine which contains a recorded message when no one is available to take the call. The medical assistant takes all the messages off the machine upon returning to the office. This is not as costly as an answering service, but, in this case, callers cannot have their problems handled immediately. *Note: The message machine should give callers a number to call if it is an emergency.*

Handling an Emergency Telephone Call

Since you cannot see the telephone caller, it can be difficult to determine a true emergency by talking to someone over the telephone. It is critical to get the caller's name and telephone number immediately in case you are disconnected. If an emergency is taking place during the telephone call, then alert the physician immediately.

In some cases, the patient may be hysterical or crying. If your voice remains calm and reassuring, you may be able to calm the patient. If the caller is extremely upset, ask if there is someone else who can come onto the telephone. Your role is to gain as much information from the caller as possible so that the emergency can be handled quickly. Try to keep the caller on the line. Table 7-8 lists some sample questions to ask when handling a telephone emergency.

Never take an emergency call lightly. Emergencies can become life-threatening if no treatment is provided. If you have any questions about whether the call is actually an emergency, you must assume it is and alert the physician. Malpractice suits have been brought against medical assistants who have failed to correctly handle an emergency.

List of Medical Emergencies

- Allergic reactions (anaphylactic shock)
- Asthma
- Broken bone
- Burns that blister
- Drug overdose
- Eye injury/foreign body
- Gunshot/stabbing wound
- Heart attack
- Inability to breathe (or difficult breathing)
- Loss of consciousness
- Premature labor
- Profuse bleeding
- Severe pain, including chest pain
- Severe vomiting and/or diarrhea
- Suicide attempt or suicide threats
- High temperature

If the physician is not in the office, then ask your supervisor or the office manager to assess the nature and seriousness of the emergency. If you are alone in the office, keep the caller on the tele-

TABLE 7-8 Questions to Ask When Handling a Telephone Emergency

1. Name of the patient and the relationship of the caller (parent, spouse, friend, passerby).

2. What is the emergency?

3. When did the emergency occur?

4. How severe is the emergency?

5. What are the patient's symptoms? (Problems breathing? bleeding? extreme pain? other symptoms?)

6. What has been done for the patient?

7. Has anyone called an ambulance?

8. Who is the patient's primary physician?

9. Where is the emergency?

Note: Some specialists, such as obstetricians and cardiologists, may have additional questions they wish to have you ask the caller.

phone while you call *911* on another line. Tell the caller what you are doing and have the appropriate identifying information: patient name, location/address, telephone number and what the emergency is. Or, tell the patient or relative making the call to call *911* directly, and, in this case, you would notify the physician and the emergency room (if known) of the situation.

Med Tip: Remember that only the physician is qualified to determine what is an emergency. It is considered "practicing medicine without a license" for a medical assistant to make this determination.

LEGAL AND ETHICAL ISSUES

Medical assistants must use caution when communicating with patients. Providing false hopes for recovery or implying that the physician may be able to cure a patient is not only unethical but can result in liability for the physician and the medical assistant.

Placing incidents in writing also involves careful thought and caution. It is important to chart exactly what occurred and what the patient stated rather than the medical assistant's feelings about the situation. Recording the patient's comment, "I have an overwhelming feeling of hopelessness," is a better indication of the patient's emotional state than the comment, "I think the patient is depressed," This last comment reflects the medical assistant's judgment of the patient's appearance or what the patient said, not what the patient has said about himself or herself.

PATIENT EDUCATION

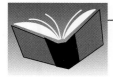

Patient education must be presented in a manner suited to the patient. In most cases, direct contact between the learner (patient) and the instructor (medical assistant) provides the best atmosphere for learning. As a medical assistant, it will be a great advantage if you are able to use the communication techniques discussed in this chapter effectively.

Lifestyle changes can greatly affect the ability to acquire new information and some patients may use several barriers to block communication such as, rationalization and denial. A patient concerned over a life-threatening diagnosis, may not be in a receptive mood for education or instruction. If you sense that a patient's uncooperativeness comes from defensive or anxious behavior, you may be able to draw the person out using open-ended questions. With a mutual trust established, it is more likely that needed instruction can be given.

Brochures and pamphlets can also be helpful for explaining health care issues. Material should be clearly and simply written. The patient with a language barrier will need an interpreter when an explanation regarding treatment or medication is given. Free brochures are available to physicians through organizations such as the American Diabetes Association.

Summary

Communication is a necessary requirement for everyday living. In the health care field, the ability to communicate effectively is essential for success—to call and request that a prescription be renewed, to share symptoms and be diagnosed properly, to provide patient education, or to arrange travel plans for the physician. The concern you have for any of these individuals will come through in your words, actions, gestures and/or your tone of voice. You can become an effective communicator by practicing some of the basic techniques presented in this chapter.

Competency Review

1. Define and spell the glossary terms for this chapter.
2. Explain what you would say to a patient who says that the medications Dr. Thompson gave her last week have made her sick.
3. Using your local telephone directory find the area codes for Pittsburgh, PA; St. Paul, MN; Los Angeles, CA; and Miami, FL.
4. When it is 9:00 in New York what time will it be in the cities listed in question #3?

5. Write a telephone message for a patient who calls for a refill of Estrace 1 mg. daily.

6. How would you handle the following call: "Help me. I'm having trouble breathing and I'm having chest pains."

7. Explain what you would say to the patient who complains to you about Dr. Thompson.

8. Explain what you would say to the patient who is angry at the delay in the waiting room.

PREPARING FOR THE CERTIFICATION EXAM

Test Taking Tip — Remember that when taking a multiple choice test, the answer is always there! Don't try to second-guess the teacher and worry about another response that is not given.

Examination Review Questions

1. The basic units of the communication process are
   (A) source of a message, for example the patient
   (B) message, for example written words
   (C) channel for communicating a message, for example the telephone
   (D) receiver of a message, for example the physician
   (E) all of the above

2. A nonverbal form of communication would include
   (A) doing more than one thing at a time
   (B) folding one's arms across one's chest
   (C) finishing a sentence for a patient for the purpose of expediting the taking of the patient's history
   (D) B and C
   (E) A, B, and C

3. Consider the following statement a medical assistant might make to a patient: "You say you are still in pain from your hysterectomy. On a scale of 1 to 10, with 1 being very little pain and 10 being the worst you could imagine, how would you rank your pain level at this moment?" What directive communication technique is this statement an example of?
   (A) open statement
   (B) closed statement
   (C) reflective statement
   (D) acknowledgment
   (E) seeking clarification

4. Which of the following statements regarding assertive versus aggressive behavior is FALSE?
   (A) assertiveness is generally considered a very positive form of communication
   (B) aggressiveness is generally considered a very negative form of communication
   (C) assertiveness can be compared to a verbal attack against another person
   (D) all of the above
   (E) none of the above

5. Placing your own feelings onto another person is an example of which of the following defensive behaviors?
   (A) rationalization
   (B) projection
   (C) compensation
   (D) displaced anger
   (E) disassociation

6. When dealing with a very angry patient, which of the following statements would BEST diffuse the situation?
   (A) "I am very sorry there was an error on your billing statement. Let me see if our billing clerk can fix it while you are here."
   (B) "Please come back when you are less angry. It will be easier to talk to you then."
   (C) "I will not listen to you while you are expressing your anger, but I will listen as soon as you calm down."
   (D) "I think you are feeling angry because, without a medical background like mine, you simply do not understand the situation."
   (E) "I am going to refer you to my supervisor."

7. Which of the following statements regarding proper telephone techniques is TRUE?
   (A) using any slang words, including "hi," is generally unacceptable
   (B) the manner in which a medical assistant answers the telephone often determines the flow of the conversation

(C) a proper telephone greeting would include identifying yourself by name

(D) A and B

(E) A, B, and C

8. The correct procedure to follow when taking a prescription refill message from a patient includes writing down the

(A) patient's name and telephone number

(B) name of the medication and the length of time the patient has been taking the medication

(C) patient's symptoms

(D) pharmacy's prescription number, name, and telephone number

(E) all of the above

9. The type of long distance call that might be used to facilitate the consultation of one physician with another is called a/an

(A) operator-assisted call

(B) conference call

(C) DDD

(D) collect call

(E) station-to-station call

10. When handling an emergency telephone call from a patient, the FIRST thing a medical assistant should do is

(A) get the caller's name and telephone number

(B) ascertain whether or not, it is in fact, an emergency

(C) gather as much information as possible about the emergency in the shortest amount of time

(D) ask to speak with someone other than the patient if the patient/caller is too hysterical to communicate the details of the situation

(E) ask if an ambulance has been summoned

ON THE JOB

For over 2 years, Linda Lewis, a medical assistant, has been employed by Drs. Norek and Klein who specialize in gerontology. Also on staff are 2 registered nurses, a medical laboratory technician, and a medical social worker.

The daughter of one of the doctor's patients has just called the office. She is very distraught at the seemingly diminished capacity of her mother and insists on speaking to the doctor.

Linda explains that both of the physicians only take emergency calls during patient appointment hours, but that she will take a detailed message. The caller, however suggests that not only should her call be considered an emergency, but that she will sue the doctor if the call is not handled accordingly.

What is your response?

1. What should Linda do to immediately diffuse the situation?

2. Is this clearly a case where the call should be passed on to one of the registered nurses or even the medical social worker?

3. Is this a case where, because of the threat of an impending suit, the physician should be called to the telephone?

4. How could Linda ascertain whether or not this, indeed, is an emergency? Is it even up to her as a medical assistant to make such a determination?

5. Since this is the patient's daughter, rather than the patient herself, does Linda have any reason to even enter into a conversation with the caller? Could Linda be ethically bound by confidentiality to not even admit the woman's mother is a patient?

References

Cohen, A., Fink, S., Gadon, H., and Willits, R. *Effective Behavior in Organizations.* Homewood, IL: Irwin, 1992.

Covey, S. *The Seven Habits of Highly Effective People.* New York, NY: Simon and Schuster, 1989.

Gudykunst, W. *Bridging Differences: Effective Intergroup Communication.* London: Sage Publications, 1994.

Hellriegel, D. and Slocum, J. *Management.* Cincinnati: South-Western Publishing, 1996.

MEDICAL ASSISTANT ROLE DELINEATION CHART

Highlight indicates material covered in this chapter

ADMINISTRATIVE

ADMINISTRATIVE PROCEDURES

- Perform basic clerical functions
- Schedule, coordinate, and monitor appointments
- Schedule inpatient/outpatient admissions and procedures
- Understand and apply third party guidelines
- Obtain reimbursement through accurate claims submission
- Monitor third-party reimbursement
- Perform medical transcription
- Understand and adhere to managed care policies and procedures
- *Negotiate managed care contracts (adv)*

PRACTICE FINANCES

- Perform procedural and diagnostic coding
- Apply bookkeeping principles
- Document and maintain accounting and banking records
- Manage accounts receivable
- Manage accounts payable
- Process payroll
- *Develop and maintain fee schedules (adv)*
- *Manage renewals of business and professional insurance policies (adv)*
- *Manage personal benefits and maintain records (adv)*

CLINICAL

FUNDAMENTAL PRINCIPLES

- Apply principles of aseptic technique and infection control
- Comply with quality assurance practices
- Screen and follow up patient test results

DIAGNOSTIC ORDERS

- Collect and process specimens
- Perform diagnostic tests

PATIENT CARE

- Adhere to established triage procedures
- Obtain patient history and vital signs
- Prepare and maintain examination and treatment areas

- Prepare patient for examinations, procedures, and treatments
- Assist with examinations, procedures, and treatments
- Prepare and administer medications and immunizations
- Maintain medication and immunization records
- Recognize and respond to emergencies
- Coordinate patient care information with other health care providers

GENERAL (TRANSDISCIPLINARY)

PROFESSIONALISM

- Project a professional manner and image
- Adhere to ethical principles
- Demonstrate initiative and responsibility
- Work as a team member
- Manage time efficiently
- Prioritize and perform multiple tasks
- Adapt to change
- Promote the CMA credential
- Enhance skills through continuing education

COMMUNICATION SKILLS

- Treat all patients with compassion and empathy
- Recognize and respect cultural diversity
- Adapt communications to individual's ability to understand
- Use professional telephone technique
- Use effective and correct verbal and written communications
- Recognize and respond to verbal and non-verbal communications
- Use medical terminology appropriately
- Receive, organize, prioritize, and transmit information
- Serve as liaison
- Promote the practice through positive public relations

LEGAL CONCEPTS

- Maintain confidentiality
- Practice within the scope of education, training, and personal capabilities
- Prepare and maintain medical records
- Document accurately
- Use appropriate guidelines when releasing information
- Follow employer's established policies dealing with the health care contract
- Follow federal, state, and local legal guidelines
- Maintain awareness of federal and state health care legislation and regulations
- Maintain and dispose of regulated substances in compliance with government guidelines
- Comply with established risk management and safety procedures
- Recognize professional credentialing criteria
- Participate in the development and maintenance of personnel, policy, and procedure manuals
- *Develop and maintain personnel, policy, and procedure manuals (adv)*

INSTRUCTION

- Instruct individuals according to their needs
- Explain office policies and procedures
- Teach methods of health promotion and disease prevention
- Locate community resources and disseminate information
- *Orient and train personnel (adv)*
- *Develop educational materials (adv)*
- *Conduct continuing education activities (adv)*

OPERATIONAL FUNCTIONS

- Maintain supply inventory
- Evaluate and recommend equipment and supplies
- Apply computer techniques to support office operations
- *Supervise personnel (adv)*
- *Interview and recommend job applicants (adv)*
- *Negotiate leases and prices for equipment and supply contracts (adv)*

SOURCE: Reprinted by permission of the American Association of Medical Assistants from the *AAMA Role Delineation Study: Occupational Analysis of the Medical Assisting Profession.*

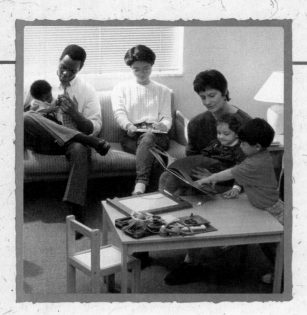

8

Patient Reception

LEARNING OBJECTIVES

After completing this chapter, you should:
1. Define and spell the glossary terms for this chapter.
2. List the receptionist's responsibilities.
3. Explain the procedure for opening the office.
4. List the information to be obtained from the new patient.
5. Describe how to handle the angry patient.
6. Describe how to handle a waiting room emergency.
7. Explain the procedure for closing the office.
8. Explain the legal and ethical issues related to the duties of the receptionist.
9. Describe the look of a professional.

ADMINISTRATIVE PERFORMANCE COMPETENCIES

After completing this chapter, you should perform the following tasks:
1. Prepare a medical office for the day's patients.
2. Correctly collate and review a patient's record to prepare for the next day's appointments.
3. Assist a new patient (or role playing partner) to correctly complete a registration form.
4. Explain an assignment of benefits form to a patient (or role playing partner).
5. Identify equipment/furniture placement that would allow for efficiency and comfort in the office.

Glossary

collating Collect in one file all materials pertaining to a patient, and group this information by category, for example, progress notes and laboratory reports.

co-pay A medical insurance plan which requires the patient pay a designated amount or percentage (for example $10 or 20%) of a bill for medical services or medication. This amount is usually collected at time of service. The rest of the bill (in this example 80%) is paid by the insurance company.

demographic Data relating to descriptive information such as age, gender, ethnic background, and education.

facsimile (fax) An electronically transmitted document containing print and/or graphic information.

medical emergency A patient condition which may be life-threatening if not treated.

no-show Patient's failure to keep an appointment without notifying the physician's office personnel.

overbooking The practice of scheduling more than one patient in the same time slot. This practice is not recommended. This is also referred to as double or triple booking.

receptionist A physician's staff employee, often a medical assistant, who greets and assists patients as they come into the office. The receptionist usually sits in an area where the waiting patients can be observed.

scheduling system A method that is used in a particular physician's practice to provide efficient services.

Patient reception requires a multi-skilled individual whose manner, physical appearance, and tone of voice projects a professional, confident, and caring manner. A small office will have fewer employees, than one with several physicians, therefore, the medical assistant in a small office will perform many of the tasks described in this chapter. In the role of receptionist, the medical assistant performs many important duties which make the office run smoothly and efficiently. Some of these duties are quiet and behind the scenes; others require constant interaction with patients. The medical assis-

tant who functions as a receptionist must do everything possible to ensure patient safety and confidentiality at all times during the office visit.

Duties of the Receptionist

The number of patients as well as the nature of the medical practice, for example, whether it is a solo practice or a corporation of several physicians, will determine what duties or tasks the medical assistant performs in the role of receptionist—the person who greets and assists incoming patients (Figure 8-1).

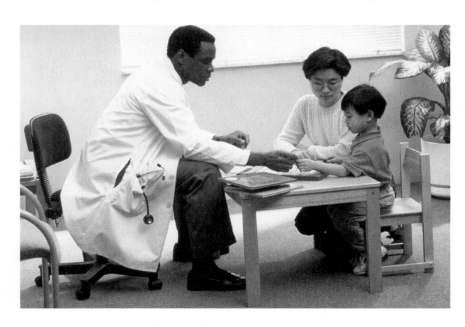

Figure 8-1 A pediatrician's pleasant waiting room.

The duties of a receptionist may include opening the office, greeting patients upon arrival, assisting a new patient with completion of the proper forms, maintaining a clean and safe environment in the waiting room, managing any disturbance in the waiting room, and handling a medical emergency. In addition, the receptionist may also handle incoming telephone calls for the office, schedule returning appointments, and make reminder calls for upcoming appointments.

Med Tip: The terms waiting room and reception room are used interchangeably. In some facilities, especially the larger clinics, a reception area for registering patients is separate from the waiting area.

Personal Characteristics and Physical Appearance

The receptionist is the first person a patient will see upon entering the office. Presenting a positive public image is important since your appearance reflects on the entire staff. Careful grooming, good hygiene, and the correct dress need to be observed. Office policy will dictate the preferred clothing. In general, uniforms may consist of white dresses or pantsuits for women and white slacks with a white jacket or white pullover top for men. If street clothes are worn, then a tailored white knee-length laboratory coat may be worn to protect clothing.

Hygiene, at a minimum, consists of daily bathing, use of a deodorant, good oral care, and clean clothing. Makeup, hair styles, and jewelry worn by male and female medical assistants should reflect professionalism. Accessories should be conservative and minimal—generally limited to one finger ring, a watch with a second hand, name tag and a professional association pin. Long hair is best worn tied back and off the shoulders so that it does not cover one's eyes when bending over a patient to provide care. Nails should be well-trimmed and only clear polish should be used.

Name pins/tags should be visible at all times. Many offices use only first names in capital letters or fairly large print with your title printed below in slightly smaller print. So if your name is JANICE, the words *Medical Assistant* will be printed under your name.

Professionalism displayed by the use of discreet language, behavior, and grooming is a key characteristic of a receptionist.

Med Tip: Misunderstandings about your title or role in patient reception can cause serious problems for the patient, the physician, and yourself. Remember: Women in white tend to be referred to as "nurse" by patients, while males in white are often called "doctor." When patients mistakenly refer to you as "nurse" or "doctor," gently remind them you are a medical assistant.

Opening the Office

The medical assistant or receptionist whose responsibility it is to open the office arrives 15-20 minutes before office hours begin. In addition to the receptionist's welcoming greeting, a well-lighted, clean, and inviting environment do much to cheer patients. After checking that the reception area is ready for patients and that there is a record for each patient who will be seen that day, the patient examination rooms should be checked in the event that something was missed in the overnight cleaning. A procedure for opening the office follows.

Collating Records

Collating records refers to collecting all records, test results, and information pertaining to the patient who is scheduled to be seen by the physician. Collating also refers to organizing the sub-group information (for example laboratory and x-rays results) in records for the days appointments as well as when filing. This should be part of "pulling records."

Collating records is usually done the day before patients are seen. The records of patients scheduled for Monday are pulled and collated on the previous Friday. These records are then

Med Tip: The terms record, file, and chart can be confusing in the discussion of patient documents. A record or chart refers to a medical record containing information such as laboratory and x-ray results, physical history, a record of vital signs and physician's orders. A file is generally a bookkeeping record. A patient's file may contain information about billing, payments, and insurance forms that have been processed and it is kept separate from the medical record.

PROCEDURE: Opening the Office

1. Turn on the lights in the patient waiting area before the first patient arrives.
2. Check that the heating or air conditioning and computer are working properly.
3. Observe overall waiting room for safety hazards such as frayed electric cords, slippery floor, or torn carpeting. Place a warning sign near any safety hazard and report it immediately to the office manager.
4. Check magazines and recycle or discard any that are torn, damaged, or outdated.
5. Check for level of cleanliness per housekeeping services and report inadequate services. *Note:* Since housekeeping services and hazardous waste removal are separate and frequently performed after office hours in larger facilities, the "checking" referred to in *a* and *b* below are really a double check that services were completed the day or evening before.
   a. Check that examination rooms are cleaned and well-stocked. Hazardous waste containers need to be emptied daily and sharps containers must be changed when they are 3/4 full.
   b. Check patient restrooms to determine cleanliness and supplies.
6. Unlock file cabinets in which records are kept.
7. Take calls from the answering machine or answering service. Handle any that need immediate attention.
8. Unlock the outer office door.
9. Compare the master list of all patients who will be seen during the day against the records that were pulled during the previous office hours. A patient may have been added to the schedule after the records were pulled. This patient's record must be pulled, reviewed, and added to the other records. Make phone calls to gather any laboratory test information that is missing from the record. Provide the physician(s) and nurse(s) with a copy of the list of any laboratory test information that you have called for but has not yet been received.
10. Type and place a list of all patients who will be seen that day on the physician's desk.

locked in a file cabinet for overnight storage. The number of patients seen in some medical offices with several physicians may require collating of records earlier than the day before the patient's visit. Always follow the policy of your office.

The physician's orders and notations from the previous visit must be reviewed to make sure that all necessary information has been received and is in the record. If laboratory test or x-ray results are not present in the record, then you will have to call the laboratory to obtain an oral report. This telephone report is written into the patient's record, however, when the report is received, it is placed in the patient's record also.

This is quite often done by the clinical medical assistant. In some offices and laboratories, the facsimile (fax) machine can be used to send reports between facilities. A facsimile, or fax, is an electronically transmitted document containing print and/or graphic information.

In some offices, the records are to be placed in the order in which the patients will be seen. A printed appointment list is placed on top of the collated records. This list serves as a checklist to keep track of patients who have been seen by the physician. As a patient is seen, his or her name is checked off the list. A copy of this same list is placed on the physician's desk on the morning of the patient's visit.

Greeting the Patient upon Arrival

In the role of receptionist, the impression the medical assistant makes on the patient is often the patient's first impression of the physician and the medical office staff. The impression you make—good or bad—tends to flavor the patient's opinion of everyone. Therefore, that first impression is very, very important.

Emergency patients or those with a contagious disease should enter the office through a private office entrance if there is one and be escorted directly into an exam room. This is done in order not to alarm the other patients and to limit exposure to contagious germs.

In some offices, the receptionist sits behind a glass window which slides open easily, allowing the receptionist to personally greet each patient entering the office (Figure 8-2). If the receptionist is on the telephone when a patient enters, then looking up and smiling is a good way to acknowledge the patient's presence.

Patients must always take precedence over other visitors to the office, for example a pharmaceutical or drug company representative who has come to explain how some new equipment works or describe a new drug. Scheduling such a visit when there are few or no patients in the office might be a better solution. Non-emergency conversations with other staff persons should always be interrupted to respond to a patient.

Use caution and speak in a low voice when mentioning another patient's name over the telephone or to another staff member within hearing distance of any patients in the waiting room. This is a violation of confidentiality and can be grounds for a lawsuit. The reason for the glass enclosure is to protect the confidentiality of patients. Always close the partition when you are speaking on the telephone.

Quickly pick up ringing phones by the second ring if possible, and always take a message if you are busy with another call or a patient in the office. It is better to call the patient back if you are unable to answer a question or have to look up information than to leave the patient on hold. Callers should not be left on hold for longer than one minute.

Med Tip: Remember the caller is unaware of what is happening in the office. If you are checking a patient "out," the patient (in the office) will understand the telephone interruption.

Signing-in

A sign-in sheet or patient register is maintained at the reception desk. The sign-in sheet, which will differ from office to office, usually has space for the patient's name, address, time of arrival, and the name of the physician the patient will see. The sign-in sheet allows the receptionist to maintain a continuous record of all patients who come into the office.

It is important to have every patient sign the register and include their address since patients frequently forget to notify the physician's office of changes. The receptionist should verbally relate

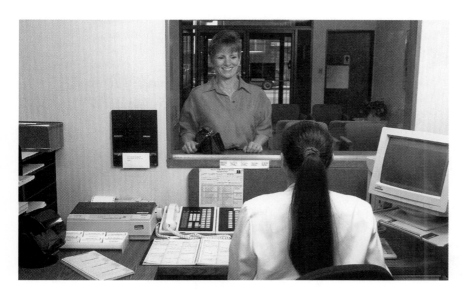

Figure 8-2 A typical reception area.

address and telephone information to the patient, for example "Mrs. Jones, do you still live at 43 Home Avenue? Is your telephone number still . . . ?" The sheet should be checked for accuracy and completeness. This can be critical for billing purposes. As each patient is taken into the examination room, a check mark is placed next to the patient's name. It is not recommended to draw a black line through the names since this can obliterate the address. This is only one way of patients signing in, each office develops a system that works for its flow of patients.

In some offices, the sign-in sheet is filed in a designated folder at the end of the day to provide another record of the patients seen during that day. If the policy is to destroy the sign-in sheet, then maintain confidentiality. *Note:* Some offices are starting to move away from sign-in sheets due to confidentiality concerns.

Registering New Patients

New patients will need to fill out a complete patient registration form containing demographic information such as DOB and Social Security number (Figure 8-3). Place the form on a clipboard with a pen attached and have the patient complete the form while he or she is waiting to be seen by the physician. Some offices send forms to patients to be completed at home and submitted at the time of the first visit; others request new pa-

Med Tip: Patients can be embarrassed to admit they cannot read or write. If you suspect this is the case, quietly move them to a private setting in which you can help them complete the new patient questionnaire.

tients arrive 15-30 minutes early to complete the necessary forms. Give precise instructions and indicate what portion of the form the patient must complete, if there are two sides to be completed, and where the patient's signature is required. Assist patients who are unable to read and write either because they are illiterate or due to a physical disability.

With computer assisted registration, you can input dictation directly onto the computer terminal. Refer to Chapter 12 for more information on computer assisted office functions.

Request to see the patient's insurance card including Medicare and Medicaid cards if applicable. Medicare is the federal health care insurance program for older adults over 65 and disabled persons who qualify; Medicaid is the federal program which provides medical care for qualified low income families. The program is jointly funded by state and federal governments.

It is a good rule to ask the patient politely if any insurance information has changed. This

---

PROCEDURE: Registering a New Patient

1. If you were occupied when the new patient signed the patient register, call the patient to the desk as soon as you are free.

2. Give the patient a pen and the patient information form attached to a clip board. Instruct the patient to complete both sides of the form, and then sign and date it. If the patient is not able to read the questions then read them to the patient in a private setting. *Note:* Observe the patient periodically to see if the patient is having difficulty reading and/or understanding the instructions on the form.

3. Explain the billing and payment policy. This should be done

verbally but can be reinforced by giving the patient an informational brochure that includes the office hours, emergency phone numbers and other relevant policies.

4. Have patient sign an assignment of benefits form so that the patient's insurance company can make payments directly to the physician. Figure 8-4 is an example of an assignment of benefits form.

5. Check the completed form to determine if the information is complete and legible.

6. Ask the patient to have a seat until the physician is ready.

PATIENT REGISTRATION FORM
(Please Print)

Date: _____

Patient's
Name: _____   DOB: _____ / _____ / _____
      First   Middle   Last   Month Day Year

Address: _____   Phone: _____ / _____ - _____
        Street   City   State   Zip   (Area code)

Patient's SS#: _____ - _____ - _____   Driver's License #: _____   Occupation: _____

Method of payment (circle):   cash   check   credit card   insurance co-payment

Primary Insurance Co.: _____   Policy/Group #: _____

Medicare #: _____   Medicaid #: _____

Person
Responsible
For Payment: _____   _____
         First   Middle   Last   Relationship

Address: _____   Phone: _____ / _____ - _____
        Street   City   State   Zip   (Area code)

Employer Name: _____   Dept: _____
            First   Middle   Last

Address: _____   Phone: _____ / _____ - _____
        Street   City   State   Zip   (Area code)

Spouse or
Nearest Relative: _____   _____
          First   Middle   Last   Relationship

Address: _____   Phone: _____ / _____ - _____
        Street   City   State   Zip   (Area code)

How were you referred to this office? _____

_____

Statement of Financial Responsibility: I, _____ ,
do hereby agree to pay all medical charges incurred by the above listed patient. I further understand
that these charges are my responsibility regardless of insurance coverage.

Responsible Person's Signature: _____

Figure 8-3   Patient Registration Form.

AUTHORIZATION TO PAY BENEFITS TO PHYSICIAN

I hereby authorize that payment of any insurance benefits covering medical charges be made directly to the physician/surgeon.

Signature of insured patient: _____

Date: _____

Figure 8-4   Assignment of Benefits Form.

can decrease the chances of lapsed coverage. Photocopy both sides of the card(s) and be sure that the copy is legible. Insurance billing cannot be completed without complete information. Check on the insurance card to see if there is a patient co-pay which requires the patient pay a certain amount/percentage of the total bill. Indicate the co-pay in the appropriate place on the patient's record so the amount can be collected by the cashier at the end of the visit.

Follow the procedure for registering a new patient: 1) to assist the patient to complete the forms accurately and 2) to be sure you have all the information required.

Charge Slips

The charge slip (also referred to as encounter form or superbill) used in most medical offices is a part of the billing process. Some offices use a charge plate system or computer program which will imprint the patient's name and identification number on all forms used including the charge slip. The appropriate charge slip is attached to the medical record of each patient who is to be seen by the physician on that day. At the end of the visit the physician indicates what treatment was given and what the charge is. The charge slip is then given to the receptionist or the cashier by the patient. Payment or arrangements for payment are made before the patient leaves the office.

All patients must be issued a charge slip before they leave the office. In a case in which there is no charge for the visit, as in a follow-up visit after surgery, the physician will write "no charge" or N/C on the slip. For accounting purposes there should be a charge slip number for each patient. The patient is entitled to and should receive a copy of the charges. The charge slip will contain a list of the most common CPT (current procedural terminology) and ICD-9 (International Classification of Diseases) Codes identifying diagnosis related charges. See Chapter 14 for detailed information on charge slips and Chapter 17 for a discussion of medical insurance.

Consideration for the Patient's Time

One of the most common complaints heard from patients is the excessive amount of time they have to spend in the waiting room before being seen by a physician. Patients are generally understanding when they are told the physician has an emergency which has resulted in a schedule delay. However, in most cases, the physician is running behind schedule through human errors with the scheduling system, such as overbooking. Delays are also caused by not allowing enough time on the schedule due to failure to get accurate information concerning the reason a patient wishes to see the doctor.

In general, a 20 minute wait is accepted by most patients. If the wait is going to be longer, then you should approach each patient and ask if the patient prefers to wait or wishes to reschedule the appointment. Patients generally respond well to a quiet explanation from the receptionist regarding how long the wait will be. Unfortunately patients are sometimes forgotten by the receptionist after they sign in. Since the patient's only contact in the office is the receptionist, it is critical that a concerned approach be used. Always check on your waiting patients periodically. Know the office policy regarding which type of complaint is seen immediately without waiting.

Make every effort to calm an angry patient so that he or she is no longer angry when going in to see the physician. When a patient complains of a long delay in seeing the physician, never become angry in return or tell the patient, "It's not my fault." An empathetic medical assistant can imagine how the nervous and ill patient must feel.

Escorting the Patient into the Examination Room

All patients should be personally escorted into the examination room (Figure 8-5). In most instances, this is done by a medical assistant assigned to patient care rather than by the receptionist. Select the correct record and clearly call the patient's name. If there is doubt that you have the correct patient, ask the patient to give you his or her name. Verify the name with the record you have requesting additional information, such as senior (Sr.) or junior (Jr.), if necessary. Walk at the patient's rate of speed and offer special assistance to patients using a wheelchair, crutches, walker, or cane. You may wish to make pleasant conversation to make the patient feel at ease.

Place the patient's record in the proper location. Do not leave the chart in the room with the patient. Often there is a slot on the outside of the examination room door for the record. Enter the room with the patient. Clearly explain exactly what items of clothing the patient should remove. Point out the gown or sheet to be used after the patient has undressed. Assist any patient who is unable to remove his or her clothing. Always protect the patient's modesty as you help the patient undress. Efforts made by medical staff to protect a patient's modesty are important to the patient.

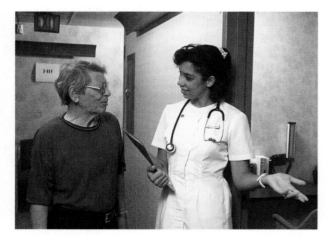

Figure 8-5 Medical assistant escorting patient from reception area to examination room.

Med Tip: It is necessary to specifically tell the patient exactly what articles of clothing to remove so the physician can perform a physical examination without being hampered by articles of clothing.

After the examination has been completed, return to the exam room and knock before entering. Give the patient instructions about what to do next. For example, you might say to the patient, "You may dress now. The doctor will come back to talk to you shortly" or "Stop at the reception desk (or other designated area) after you have dressed, and I'll explain the test the doctor has ordered."

Make it a point to speak with patients before they leave. In some cases the patient may need to make a payment, talk to the cashier, make another appointment, or have a specific test or procedure explained. A simple "good-bye" brings closure to each patient's office visit.

If discussion is needed, it should be done in a private area out of the hearing range and view of the other patients.

Med Tip: Inquire from the patient how he or she wants to be addressed. Never use the patient's first name until you have done this. Some patients are offended by such familiarity.

Managing Disturbances

If a patient becomes angry or starts speaking in a loud voice try to handle the situation immediately. It is always advisable to ask the patient to come into a quiet office where the problem can be discussed and handled.

If a private office is not available, the problem must be handled quickly and quietly in another area. Generally, people will respond to a sincere statement such as, "I'm sorry there's a problem. Let's see how we can solve it." Ask the patient to identify what he or she perceives the problem to be and then discuss the possible solutions. Frequently, the angry patient will respond well if the medical assistant uses a very quiet, calm manner. With practice a medical assistant can become adept at calming the angry patient. If the patient is drunk or disorderly, follow the office policy regarding when to call the police.

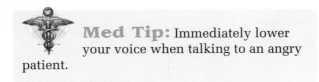

Med Tip: Immediately lower your voice when talking to an angry patient.

Children

Children pose a special problem. Usually, children go into the exam room with the adult and then are removed only if private areas are to be examined on the parent. If a child is left alone in the office while the parent is seen by the physician then the medical assistant must observe that the child remains safe at all times. It is advisable to explain to the parent before he or she leaves the office that children cannot be left unattended.

On rare occasions, a physician treats a child without the parent being present. In such a case, a medical assistant or other staff person will stay with the child during the examination or procedure. Teenagers often have things to ask the doctor that they may not want their parents to hear.

Medical Emergencies in the Waiting Room

There will be occasions when a **medical emergency** occurs in the physician's office (Figure 8-6). Ill patients may come directly to the physician's office instead of first calling the physician or 911. In this case, you must stop whatever you are doing to immediately give assistance. Ask another staff member to alert the physician. Tell available staff to give you assistance or to call 911 if emergency transport to a hospital is necessary. If all the rooms are full, you can ask the other waiting patients to step into the hall to avoid these patients becoming anxious during the emergency.

If cardiopulmonary resuscitation (CPR) is necessary, begin immediately without moving the patient from the waiting room. Follow the CPR procedure presented in Chapter 34.

If a patient's condition requires emergency treatment and equipment which your physician is able to provide in the office setting then immediately take the patient into an examination room. Assist the patient onto an examination table if possible. This patient should not be left unattended. Another staff member should alert the physician that the patient requires immediate attention. Many offices have an intercom system that allows communication from the reception area to all rooms in the office so that medical personnel can be summoned quickly.

If a family member who is present wishes to accompany the patient into the examination room, allow the person to do so unless prohibited by office policy. When treatment begins, a staff member will ask the family member to step out of the room.

No-Shows

Accounting for "no-shows," the patients who did not keep their appointments, is done at the end of the day. Some offices have a standard practice to call the patient to determine why the appointment was not kept and to reschedule another appointment. There is sometimes a policy to charge for no-show appointments. It is important that the receptionist learn and use the procedure to be followed for "no-shows" as stated in the policy manual in the office in which he or she works.

One person, usually the office manager, is responsible for alerting the physician to the patient "no-shows." Physicians are notified immediately about a patient whose condition warrants attention. Calling patients the day before their visits to remind them of the appointments may lower the number of no-shows.

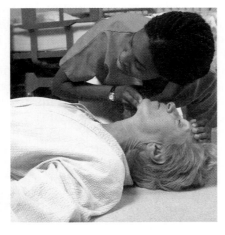

Figure 8-6 Medical assistant handling an emergency.

Med Tip: Documentation of all "no-shows" is important to protect the physician in the event of a patient's lawsuit which charges the physician with abandonment or withdrawal of the physician's services.

After the patient has been re-scheduled, place a notation on the patient's record about the failed appointment, the date, action taken, the result, and initials of the person performing the documentation.

If the patient fails to keep two or more appointments the physician needs to be informed. The physician may wish to send a letter declining to continue treating the patient or dismissing the patient from the practice.

Closing the Office

Closing the office at the end of the day and opening the office in the morning are two major functions of the medical assistant. These functions are key to operating a well run office. A procedure for closing the office at the end of the day is presented here.

Office Environment: Physical Appearance

The reception area consists of the waiting room and the reception desk. A counter top or ledge to hold a sign-in sheet for patients is useful. Figure 8-7 illustrates the design of a typical waiting room and reception/appointment desk. Ideally, the desk will be enclosed with a glass partition that can be closed for privacy when the receptionist is handling a telephone call.

The file room or storage area for records is usually close to the receptionist's area for quick accessibility during telephone calls and the scheduling process. See Figure 8-8 for an example of a typical file room.

The desk surface should be neat and not contain confidential information regarding patients such as records, open appointment book, and billing

---

PROCEDURE: Closing the office

1. Leave at least 30 minutes at the end of the day to close the office.

2. Check all records used during the day for any orders that may have been missed. In addition, make sure that every visit is posted to be billed.

3. Records for patients who will be seen during the next day should be pulled, reviewed, and collated during the day. Place the collated records with charge tickets attached and the master list of the next day's scheduled patients in a locked file cabinet overnight. Also, make a copy of this master list of patients for each physician. Locking this file protects the confidentiality of the patients. This is your responsibility as receptionist.

4. All money received from patient payments must either be deposited in a bank or locked in the office safe. It is wise to have a person designated to make a daily bank deposit, varying the time of deposit regularly. Many offices now use a courier for this task. For purposes of quality control, the person completing the bank deposit and the person making the deposit should not be the same. Both people should be bonded. Completing a bank deposit is discussed in Chapter 16.

5. Turn off electrical equipment and appliances. *Note:* Some equipment such as an incubator, fax machine, and computers, may require 24 hour operation. Check with your supervisor regarding the special requirements of your office.

6. Check all examination rooms to make sure they are clean and supplied for the next day.

7. Straighten the reception room.

8. The answering service must be activated before leaving. Know the name of the physician who is accepting emergency calls, or on call, until morning. Remind the physician who is on call.

9. Activate the security system if there is one.

10. Always double-check to make sure the door is locked.

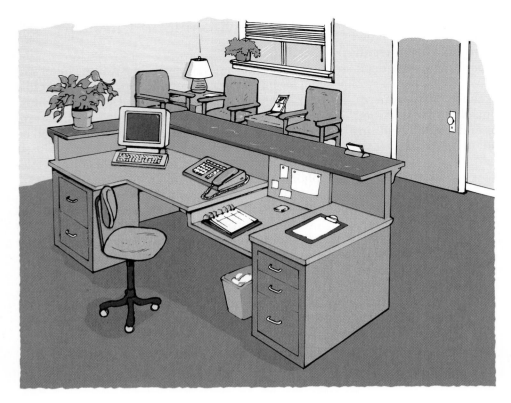

Figure 8-7 Typical waiting room and reception/appointment desk.

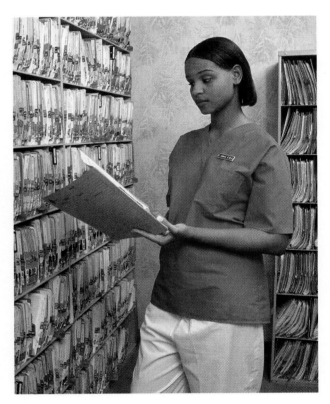

Figure 8-8 A typical file room.

information. Periodically, the receptionist or another staff member assigned may need to straighten up the reception area and the waiting room, especially magazines and brochures.

Reading material in the reception room should be selected that is suitable for male and female patients of all ages. For sanitary reasons, it is a good idea to place magazines in a plastic binder which can be washed periodically.

Med Tip: Patients often judge a medical practice by the quality of reading material in the reception room. Every effort must be made to have current literature in excellent condition placed in neat containers throughout the office. Old magazines can be recycled.

Comfortable seating that provides good support and is easily cleaned is most suitable. Over stuffed chairs and couches should be avoided. Such furniture cannot be moved easily by housekeeping during daily cleaning and most people prefer individual seating in public areas.

All materials placed for patient reading must be screened to make sure they meet the standards of your office and would not upset the patients. Medical journals are generally not a good choice and fund raising materials are inappropriate.

Television is not usually provided since it is difficult to provide entertainment that is suitable for all your patients. Ill patients may not want the distraction or noise of television. Soft background music can be used effectively in waiting rooms to muffle conversations between staff or patients. Video tapes for teaching are available and provide an excellent source of information to waiting patients.

Children's toys and books should be washable and not have small removable parts. Small blocks, balls, and stuffed toys are not good toys for a reception room. Large building blocks, stiff covered books, and large plastic toys which are washable can be placed on a small sized table for children. These toys should be disinfected regularly with bleach water to prevent cross-contamination or the spread of disease from one patient to another through contact with the toys.

Green plants can soften the institutional feeling in a medical office. Many offices contract with a plant service since live plants can be difficult to maintain. If the office in which you work does not have a plant maintenance service then carefully observe for any plants that need replacement or use artificial plants.

Smoking is not allowed in medical offices. No smoking signs can be obtained by calling the American Cancer Society. Remind patients who complain about this restriction that patients with respiratory conditions have difficulty in smoke-filled rooms.

If a patient with a communicable disease visits the office, he or she should be placed in a designated area to minimize spreading disease. After the visit is over, the office should be disinfected immediately. Refer to Chapter 19 for information on asepsis or infection control. Every office should have a hazardous control manual regarding OSHA guidelines.

Housekeeping

Ideally, a housekeeping or medical office cleaning service will thoroughly clean the front office area and the examination rooms every night. Regular housekeeping services are usually not responsible for handling hazardous waste containers. Instead, hazardous waste including sharps, should be disposed of in designated containers and removed from the office or facility properly. There are specific Occupational Safety and Health Administration (OSHA) and Environmental Protection Agency regulations controlling the disposal of hazardous waste.

Med Tip: A simple thing like a torn carpet edge may be a real safety hazard and should be reported immediately. The patient's safety should be your priority. Always protect the patient, particularly the handicapped or ill patient, in any situation where there is a possibility of injury. Maintain a phone list of heating, air conditioning, maintenance and security personnel along with the building manager's number. Remember: Your employer is liable for such injuries.

LEGAL AND ETHICAL ISSUES

The receptionist must protect the safety of the patients at all times during the office visit. Be sure to eliminate safety hazards, make sure exits are clearly marked, and place warning signs to identify wet floors. The receptionist must know how to evacuate the waiting room in the event of fire. A map should be placed on the wall indicating where the patient waiting area is in relation to the nearest exits.

Current CPR certification is necessary for the receptionist and all medical office staff. The receptionist must be familiar with the policies of the office regarding emergency treatment of patients and respond quickly to waiting room emergencies. Training in handling telephone emergencies must be included in the receptionist's orientation to the job.

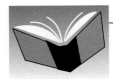

PATIENT EDUCATION

Patient education often begins with the patient's call for an appointment. Two other important sites for patient education are at the reception desk and in the waiting room. For example, education regarding office hours, policies, insurance form submissions, and emergency telephone numbers can be handled at the reception desk. The receptionist may give instructions regarding tests and procedures such as fasting before a particular blood test. In smaller offices where the receptionist handles insurance processing, education can take place regarding the patient's responsibility in the process.

Patient education is supported through the use of descriptive informational office practice brochures, literature from the American Cancer Society, American Diabetic Association, and American Heart Association, and bulletin displays on various aspects of health. Some offices provide a brief video presentation about selected procedures or health concerns.

Summary

The receptionist's role can be one of the most demanding and most interesting positions in the medical office. While attending to the general running of the office, the medical assistant, as receptionist must greet all patients, assist new patients in registering being sure to get necessary health and insurance information, answer calls, schedule patients as well as open and close the office, contact and document "no-shows," and more. All this requires a calm, caring, and organized individual who can keep patient information confidential and protect the safety of the patient during the office visit. The patient is most important.

Competency Review

1. Explain the steps you would take if you are the first person to arrive and must open the medical office.
2. Describe how a professionally groomed receptionist would appear.
3. Explain what you would do if a patient suddenly collapsed in the reception room.
4. Discuss steps a medical assistant would take to assist in preventing a claim of abandonment against a physician.
5. Describe the important characteristics of a typical waiting area.

PREPARING FOR THE CERTIFICATION EXAM

Test Taking Tip — Computer grading cards have a space for you to print your name as well as bubble spaces for the correct answers. Always double check that you have printed your name on the exam or computer grading card before handing in the test.

Examination Review Questions

1. This is Mrs. Mendez' first appointment to see Dr. Williams. Upon her arrival, you would have all of the following forms for her to read and/or sign EXCEPT
   (A) patient information sheet
   (B) physician's emergency phone numbers
   (C) authorization to pay physician form
   (D) sign-in sheet
   (E) all of the above are correct

2. When a patient enters the office and you are on the telephone, what is the correct procedure to follow?
   (A) continue speaking with the patient on the telephone, and after you have completed the telephone conversation look up and handle the walk-in patient
   (B) place the telephone patient "on-hold" and tell the walk-in patient to sign in

(C) smile at the walk-in patient to indicate that you see him or her and finish talking with the patient on the telephone

(D) tell the patient on the telephone you will call back later, then handle the walk-in patient

(E) none of the above

3. When handling the angry patient, it is best to

(A) ask the patient to have a seat in the reception room

(B) calmly tell the patient you are sorry he or she is angry and take the patient to an empty exam room

(C) tell the patient that you have to cancel his appointment since you cannot have loud, angry patients in the office

(D) let the patient continue to talk until the patient's anger is gone

(E) have someone else handle this patient

4. "No-show" appointments are documented

(A) when the staff person assigned to document "no-shows" comes in for work

(B) at the beginning of the next day

(C) at the end of the day of the failed appointment

(D) only on the sign-in sheet

(E) do not have to be documented

5. Suitable toys for the children's area of the reception room would include all EXCEPT

(A) large plastic toys

(B) tiny blocks

(C) hard cover books

(D) cloth washable books

(E) all the above are suitable

6. Mr. James has walked into the office and collapsed. Dr. Williams is not there. Which of the following would a medical assistant do?

(A) alert a staff member to help Mr. James while you call 911

(B) assist Mr. James and call out or ask another staff member to call 911 for help

(C) call 911 immediately and wait by the door to direct the emergency team

(D) if Mr. James is alert, advise him to go to the hospital to meet Dr. Williams, then call Dr. Williams to alert her that

an emergency patient is on his way to the hospital

(E) none of the above are correct

7. Which of the following statements, regarding the collation of patient records, are FALSE?

(A) patient records for the day's appointments are usually pulled and collated 2 days before the appointment

(B) patient records are usually pulled and collated for an appointment immediately after the reminder call

(C) only a written report of test results is entered into a patient's records not the actual laboratory report

(D) all of the above

(E) none of the above

8. What is the name of the billing document that most medical offices use where the physician indicates a patient's treatment and the charges?

(A) assignment of benefits form

(B) authorization to pay form

(C) charge slip

(D) insurance slip

(E) billing slip

9. What, in general, is the maximum number of minutes that should be an acceptable amount of time for a patient to wait on the day of a scheduled appointment?

(A) 10

(B) 15

(C) 20

(D) 25

(E) 30

10. Which of the following should NOT be considered a medical emergency in an office waiting room?

(A) a potentially contagious patient's incessant coughing

(B) a crying child with a very upset stomach

(C) a patient, whose chief complaint is nausea over the past several days, who has just vomited

(D) a disgruntled patient

(E) all of the above

ON THE JOB

Dr. Morrison, a child psychiatrist, who is in solo practice, employs one medical assistant in her office. This medical assistant is multi-skilled, like all medical assistants, and, essentially, handles all of the administrative and clinical tasks in the office.

It is 3:00 P.M. and a parent has just arrived for a 3:30 P.M. appointment with her 10 year old daughter. The child is a new patient of Dr. Morrison's that was referred by her attending physician. She has a relatively long history of combative and destructive behavior and the referring pediatrician is seeking a psychological evaluation from Dr. Morrison. Psychotropic medication of some sort may be a viable treatment option.

The medical assistant has asked the mother and daughter to please be seated and to fill out some registration forms. The child is acting out—pulling cushions off of the waiting room couch, wildly ripping the pages of the magazines, whining and kicking at her mother. The behavior seems to be escalating as the mother tries to frantically control her child while, at the same time, follow the instructions of the medical assistant and fill out the registration forms.

What is your response?

1. What if anything, should the medical assistant do?
2. Would it be appropriate, for example, for the MA to interrupt Dr. Morrison's current session?
3. Might this be considered a medical emergency?

References

Badasch, S. and Chesebro, D. *Introduction to Health Occupations.* Upper Saddle River, NJ: Brady/Prentice Hall, 1997.

Becklin, K. and Sunnarborg, E. *Medical Office Procedures.* New York: Glencoe, 1996.

Black, H. *Black's Law Dictionary.* St. Paul: West Publishing Co., 1991.

Taber's Cyclopedic Medical Dictionary, 18th ed. Philadelphia: F.A. Davis, 1997.

The New American Desk Encyclopedia. A Signet Book: NY, 1989.

Strategies for Success

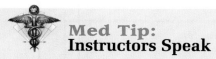

Med Tip:
Instructors Speak

Think of the first day of your medical assisting program as if it were the first day of your career as a medical assistant! Dress, think, and conduct yourself as if you are actually working in a medical office. Then, when it is time for the *first day of your first job,* you will have developed the professionalism to succeed.

Use a calendar or date book to record your assignments, quiz dates, and examination dates.

Linda Ramge, MT (ASCP), CMA
Matthews, North Carolina

Read! Become informed! For example, learn about new procedures, new research, and new equipment in the medical assisting field.

Linda Bednar, CMA
Cedar Brook, New Jersey

Show initiative and enthusiasm. Be excited about what you're doing and what you're learning.

Lynn Augenstern, CMA, MA
Endwell, New York

Show resourcefulness—the key to being a good Medical Assistant is not in knowing all the answers but in knowing how to find them.

Nina Theirer, CMA
Fort Wayne, Indiana

Think and practice professionalism; be prepared, expect to learn, and dress for success.

Dee A. Stout, BA, MA
Kansas City, Missouri

Learn from change. Each time a schedule change is announced, or a rule is revised, use this change as an opportunity to practice being flexible. Flexibility is one of the keys to becoming a successful medical professional.

Ursula Backner, CMA
Debra Hampton, BSPH, LPN, CPC
Catherine Schoen, CMA
Indianapolis, Indiana

MEDICAL ASSISTANT ROLE DELINEATION CHART

Highlight indicates material covered in this chapter

ADMINISTRATIVE

ADMINISTRATIVE PROCEDURES

- Perform basic clerical functions
- Schedule, coordinate, and monitor appointments
- Schedule inpatient/outpatient admissions and procedures
- Understand and apply third party guidelines
- Obtain reimbursement through accurate claims submission
- Monitor third-party reimbursement
- Perform medical transcription
- Understand and adhere to managed care policies and procedures
- *Negotiate managed care contracts (adv)*

PRACTICE FINANCES

- Perform procedural and diagnostic coding
- Apply bookkeeping principles
- Document and maintain accounting and banking records
- Manage accounts receivable
- Manage accounts payable
- Process payroll
- *Develop and maintain fee schedules (adv)*
- *Manage renewals of business and professional insurance policies (adv)*
- *Manage personal benefits and maintain records (adv)*

CLINICAL

FUNDAMENTAL PRINCIPLES

- Apply principles of aseptic technique and infection control
- Comply with quality assurance practices
- Screen and follow up patient test results

DIAGNOSTIC ORDERS

- Collect and process specimens
- Perform diagnostic tests

PATIENT CARE

- Adhere to established triage procedures
- Obtain patient history and vital signs
- Prepare and maintain examination and treatment areas

- Prepare patient for examinations, procedures, and treatments
- Assist with examinations, procedures, and treatments
- Prepare and administer medications and immunizations
- Maintain medication and immunization records
- Recognize and respond to emergencies
- Coordinate patient care information with other health care providers

GENERAL (TRANSDISCIPLINARY)

PROFESSIONALISM

- Project a professional manner and image
- Adhere to ethical principles
- Demonstrate initiative and responsibility
- Work as a team member
- Manage time efficiently
- Prioritize and perform multiple tasks
- Adapt to change
- Promote the CMA credential
- Enhance skills through continuing education

COMMUNICATION SKILLS

- Treat all patients with compassion and empathy
- Recognize and respect cultural diversity
- Adapt communications to individual's ability to understand
- Use professional telephone technique
- Use effective and correct verbal and written communications
- Recognize and respond to verbal and nonverbal communications
- Use medical terminology appropriately
- Receive, organize, prioritize, and transmit information
- Serve as liaison
- Promote the practice through positive public relations

LEGAL CONCEPTS

- Maintain confidentiality
- Practice within the scope of education, training, and personal capabilities
- Prepare and maintain medical records
- Document accurately
- Use appropriate guidelines when releasing information
- Follow employer's established policies dealing with the health care contract
- Follow federal, state, and local legal guidelines
- Maintain awareness of federal and state health care legislation and regulations
- Maintain and dispose of regulated substances in compliance with government guidelines
- Comply with established risk management and safety procedures
- Recognize professional credentialing criteria
- Participate in the development and maintenance of personnel, policy, and procedure manuals
- *Develop and maintain personnel, policy, and procedure manuals (adv)*

INSTRUCTION

- Instruct individuals according to their needs
- Explain office policies and procedures
- Teach methods of health promotion and disease prevention
- Locate community resources and disseminate information
- *Orient and train personnel (adv)*
- *Develop educational materials (adv)*
- *Conduct continuing education activities (adv)*

OPERATIONAL FUNCTIONS

- Maintain supply inventory
- Evaluate and recommend equipment and supplies
- Apply computer techniques to support office operations
- *Supervise personnel (adv)*
- *Interview and recommend job applicants (adv)*
- *Negotiate leases and prices for equipment and supply contracts (adv)*

SOURCE: Reprinted by permission of the American Association of Medical Assistants from the *AAMA Role Delineation Study: Occupational Analysis of the Medical Assisting Profession*.

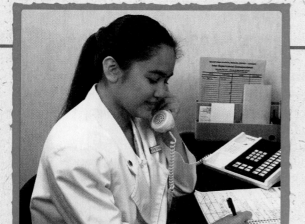

9

Appointment Scheduling

LEARNING OBJECTIVES

After completing this chapter, you should:
1. Define and spell the glossary terms for this chapter.
2. Name and describe 4 scheduling systems.
3. List and describe 4 pieces of equipment used in the scheduling process.
4. Identify 10 conditions that qualify as emergencies.
5. Explain the importance of correct documentation when a patient does not keep an appointment.
6. State the process for handling a patient referral.
7. Describe the process for scheduling a hospital admission and surgery.
8. Summarize the ethical implications related to scheduling.

ADMINISTRATIVE PERFORMANCE COMPETENCIES

After completing this chapter, you should perform the following tasks:
1. Prepare a new schedule book.
2. Form a matrix to integrate the physician's schedule with patient services/appointments and holidays.
3. Schedule patients using all methods of scheduling described in this chapter.
4. Schedule a patient for surgery.
5. Rearrange a schedule for a physician who is late in arriving in the office due to an emergency.
6. Arrange for a patient's admission to the hospital.
7. Correctly document a "no-show" appointment.

Office hours are usually determined by the physician or group of physicians in a practice. The scheduling system used in each office is dependent on a variety of factors including the physician's preference, type and size of practice, and amount of flexibility required by the physician(s). The two basic types of appointment scheduling systems are (1) scheduled appointments and (2) open office hours.

There are some medical facilities such as free-standing urgent care centers which offer extended evening hours and may be open 24-hours a day. Free-standing urgent care centers are facilities that are prepared to handle situations requiring immediate but not life-threatening medical care. These facilities are not always attached to a hospital or other large treatment center. The patients arrive without an appointment and are generally seen in the order of arrival. A medical office or facility using such a system is said to have "open" office hours.

Appointment Scheduling Systems

Physicians, especially in metropolitan areas and large medical practices, prefer to see patients according to a set schedule. As soon as a day's schedule of time slots is filled then that day is closed to any new appointments. In this way, the physician is better able to spend an appropriate amount of time with each patient in an unhurried manner.

There are several variations used for scheduling. These scheduling variations are:

- Specified time scheduling
- Wave scheduling and modified wave scheduling
- Procedure grouping
- Double booking

All of these scheduling variations are described here along with the benefits and limitations of each type.

Specified Time Scheduling

With this method of scheduling each patient is given a specific time slot. The time allocated to each patient will depend upon the reason for the office visit—the type of examination or testing that is to be done. For example, a complete physical examination may require 1 1/2 hours. In an office based on 15 minute increments, or time slots, this patient would be given 6 time slots in a row equaling the 1 1/2 hours needed. This method prevents a large backlog of waiting patients.

The drawback to specified time scheduling is that some patients may not provide enough information about their medical problems at the time the appointment is scheduled, in spite of careful questioning by the medical assistant. For instance, consider the case of a patient who is given a thirty minute appointment but who really needs to have

1 or 1 1/2 hours for a thorough physical examination. Since not enough time was allocated for the visits, the schedule will back up.

Some patients will discuss topics that are unrelated to the complaint that brought them into the office. This can be time consuming, frustrating for the physician, and not beneficial to the patient. It is the medical assistant's responsibility to get accurate information when scheduling patients so that the correct amount of time on the schedule is reserved for them. If the patient is going to require more time than was originally scheduled the physician may have to ask the patient to make another appointment. The following chart is an example of specified time scheduling for a family practitioner.

Specified Time	
1:00	John Matthews—ear irrigation
1:15	Jacob Ives—well-baby checkup with vaccines
1:30	Laurie Steck—PAP smear
1:45	↓ ↓ ↓
2:00	Amy Morgan—well-baby checkup with vaccines
2:15	Whitney Gall—BP check
2:30	Mario Lopez—skin rash (poss. contagious)

All the above appointments will require 15 minutes with the exception of the PAP smear which is a 30 minute appointment. Many offices will build in time—known as "catch up" time—in either the morning or afternoon for emergencies.

Wave Scheduling

Wave scheduling provides built-in flexibility to accommodate unforeseen situations such as patients who require more time with the physician, a late arriving patient, or the patient who fails to keep an appointment (no-show). Wave scheduling can also be helpful in handling the patient who needs to be seen by the physician but does not have an appointment.

The purpose of wave scheduling is to begin and end each hour on time. Each hour is divided into equal segments of time depending on how many patients can be seen within an hour. For example, a dermatologist may only require 10 minutes with

each patient which would mean that 6 patients could be scheduled in any hour. However, most physicians require 15 or 20 minute time slots in which to see patients.

For appointments averaging 20 minutes, three 20-minute appointments would be scheduled within each hour period of time and for appointments averaging 15 minutes, four appointments would be scheduled during the entire hour.

Using wave scheduling all the patients are told to come in at the beginning of the hour in which they are to be seen. These patients are then seen in the order in which they arrive. Since some of the patients require more time, some may not come in at all, and some may be late, wave scheduling allows for the actual time used by patient appointments to average out over the hour.

Med Tip: It is a good policy under wave scheduling to put the patient's chart on top of the charts as the patient arrives regardless of the time of the patient's appointment.

The chart that follows provides an example of wave scheduling compared with specified time appointments.

Wave Scheduling		Specified Time	
1:00	John Matthews	1:00	John Matthews
	Jacob Ives	1:20	Jacob Ives
	Laurie Steck	1:40	Laurie Steck
2:00	Amy Morgan	2:00	Amy Morgan
	Whitney Gall	2:20	Whitney Gall
	Mario Lopez	2:40	Mario Lopez

Using wave scheduling (left column), if John Matthews arrives 15 minutes late, Jacob Ives arrives ten minutes early, and Laurie Steck arrives thirty minutes late all patients could still be seen within the hour (1:00–2:00) time frame. If Whitney Gall failed to keep her 2:00 p.m. appointment, the other two appointments, Amy Morgan and Mario Lopez, could be seen without a gap in the physician's schedule since they would have arrived at 2:00 p.m.

The drawback to wave scheduling is that when all the patients arrive exactly on time and each patient appointment takes 20 minutes, then the last patient will have to wait 40 minutes to be seen. Patients do not like to know that other patients have been scheduled in the same time slot that they have. However, wave scheduling is a useful method when a medical practice requires flexibility.

Modified Wave Scheduling

Wave scheduling can be modified to avoid the possibility that any patient would have to wait 40 minutes to be seen by the physician. This system is also built on the hour as the base of each block of time. There are many variations of **modified wave** scheduling.

One example would be to have three patients scheduled at intervals during the first half hour with none scheduled for the second half hour. All three patients would be actually seen during the entire hour period, but the physician would not be waiting for a late arriving patient. With this system the physician can still spend 20 minutes with each patient without having to wait for any patients to arrive. See the modified wave chart for one example of this type of scheduling.

Modified Wave	
1:00	John Matthews
1:10	Jacob Ives
1:20	Laurie Steck
1:30	↓ ↓
1:40	↓ ↓
2:00	Amy Morgan
2:10	Whitney Gall
2:20	Mario Lopez
2:30	↓ ↓
2:40	↓ ↓

Scheduling by Grouping Procedures

Many physicians prefer to have similar procedures and examinations scheduled during a particular block of time. For example, a obstetrician may prefer to have all new patients scheduled together on two mornings a week since they will require a longer physical examination. An allergist may group all skin testing together on three afternoons a week. A pediatrician may do well-baby check-ups during particular hours each day.

Double Booking Patients

Double booking, which is the practice of scheduling two patients to be seen during the same time slot without allowing for any additional time in the schedule, is considered to be a very poor practice. If each patient will need a 20 minute appointment, and both are scheduled from 1:00 p.m. to 1:20 p.m., then the entire afternoon's schedule will be late by 20 minutes at least. Using a modified form of wave scheduling will eliminate this problem since enough time is actually allowed in the schedule for all the patients.

Open Office Hours System

An open office hours system is the least structured of all the systems. The hours in which the office is open are posted and patients may arrive at any time during those hours. The patients are seen in the order of their arrival.

Some physicians prefer this method since the schedule is not disrupted by patients who miss an appointment. The physician and office staff may be able to leave the office on time at the end of the day since the danger of running behind schedule is gone. This method is more common in rural areas and in free standing emergency centers.

The disadvantages to this method include having too many patients arrive at the same time which frequently results in long delays—waiting time—for the patient. The physician and staff can be overworked during peak times of the day and may have no patients during other times. Most physicians in busy metropolitan areas do not use this system.

Patient Scheduling Process

Each office will have its own method for appointment scheduling. The appointment is usually entered into an appointment book or on computer. Figure 9-1 depicts a sample page of an appointment book.

When scheduling a patient appointment always begin by asking the purpose of the visit. You will then know how much time to allow. Refer to

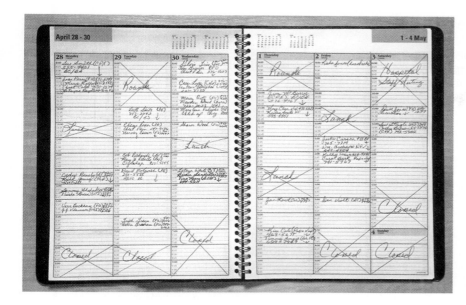

Figure 9-1 An appointment schedule book to be used for a single physician.

Table 9-1 for estimates of the amount of time to be allotted for specific office procedures.

Ask if there are any dates/days and times of day the patient would not be available. Once you have narrowed down the dates the patient is available then offer one or two choices of dates and times. Be sure to state the date, day and time. Using pencil enter the appointment the patient selected into the schedule book, repeating the day, date and time to the patient. If the patient is making the appointment in person write the date and time on an appointment card for the patient. Use the following guidelines when scheduling patients.

Forming a Matrix

Forming a **matrix,** or blocking-out the schedule book, refers to crossing out periods of time on the daily schedule when the physician will not be available to see patients. Some of these blocked-out segments include times when the physician is seeing patients in the hospital, surgery, lunch and break times, segments of time for returning telephone calls, meetings, and out of town trips (Figure 9-2).

Several weeks of the schedule book are blocked-out or prepared at one time. It is not good practice to block out the entire schedule book for the year since there may be unexpected changes in the physician's schedule. All blocking-out and scheduling is done in pencil. Actually cross out the blocks of time when the physician is unavailable and write the reason across the line.

Scheduling Free Time for the Physician

Ideally, there should be a few minutes built into the schedule between the end of one patient visit and the beginning of another patient's visit. However, most schedule systems do not allow for time between patients. Therefore it is important to build in small blocks of time during the day when the physician can return telephone calls, catch up on charting, read mail and journals, or just rest. The best time for this is at the end of the morning's schedule and again at the end of the day. Some physician's prefer to return all morning telephone calls when they return from lunch.

Building this free time block into the office daily schedule at the same time each day, is very important and every effort should be made not to schedule last minute appointments during this time. These "buffer" periods are excellent backup times for emergencies that may have to be seen that day.

Cancellations and Missed Appointments

Appointments are canceled for any number of reasons. Sometimes the patient experiences an unforeseen emergency, is too ill or too fatigued to get to the office, or actually forgets the appointment. On the other hand, the physician may have

TABLE 9-1 Time Estimates for Specific Office Procedures

Procedure	Time in Minutes
Allergy testing	30–60
Cast check	10
Cast change	30
Complete physical with EKG	60
Blood pressure check	15
Dressing change	15
Minor surgery procedure	30–45
Office visit : Established patient	
Low complexity	5–10
Medium complexity	15–20
High complexity	20–30
Office visit: New Patient	
Low complexity	10–15
Medium complexity	15–30
Complete physical	30–45
Pelvic examination with PAP test	30
Patient education	30–45
Post-operative check-up	15–20
Prenatal examination (first visit)	30–60
Prenatal checkup	15
Prostate examination	30
School physical	15–30
Suture removal	10
Well-baby checkup	15

Guidelines: Scheduling Patients

1. Understand the scheduling system used in your office.
2. Use a pencil so that appointments can be erased to make changes as needed.
3. Set up a matrix by blocking out all time periods when the physician is not available (hospital rounds, vacation) for appointments before scheduling patients. Ideally, setting up a matrix or appointment blocking done on the computer is done three months ahead of time.
4. Schedule appointments by beginning with the first empty appointment in the morning or early in the afternoon, and then fill in the day. Do not schedule appointments at the end of the day with large open gaps in between.
5. Print the patient's full first and last name next to the appropriate time on the schedule. Add Jr. for junior and Sr. for senior if there are two patients with the same name in a family.
6. Ask the patient for a current work and home telephone number with the area code. Write these numbers next to the patient's name.
7. Write the reason for the visit on the schedule using accepted medical abbreviations (Example: PAP test).
8. Allow the correct amount of time for the appointment. If an appointment will take more than the minimum time allotted on the schedule (for example 15 minutes), then use an arrow to indicate that the patient will be using 2 or 3 blocks of time. In some offices, a line is drawn across the time blocks.

Note: In offices where scheduling is done by computer, enter the patient information as directed by the on-screen prompts.

to cancel the appointment due to an emergency at the hospital or even a patient emergency in the office. In all but the case of the forgotten or missed appointment, the medical assistant is usually able to adjust the schedule so as not to inconvenience the physician or the patients who do come to the office on time. Missed appointments happen with no warning, so the medical assistant has less opportunity to make satisfactory adjustments. Make every attempt to reschedule and document these attempts in the patient record.

Patient Cancellations

Make every attempt to fill up a void in the schedule caused by a patient cancellation. One method is to call the patient who has the last appointment for the day and ask the patient if it is possible to

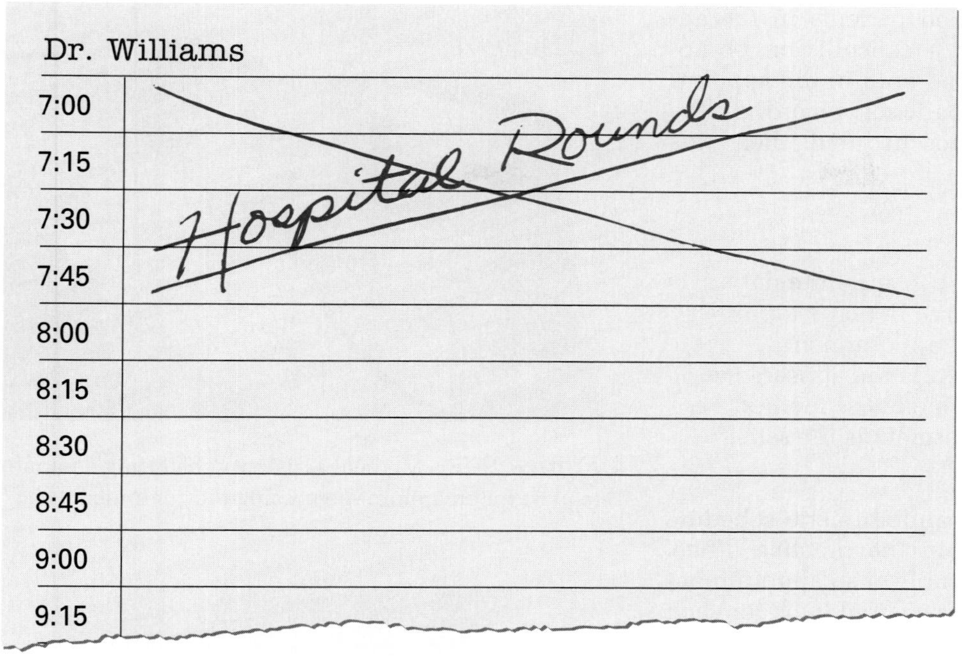

Dr. Williams

7:00	
7:15	
7:30	*Hospital Rounds*
7:45	
8:00	
8:15	
8:30	
8:45	
9:00	
9:15	

Figure 9-2 Forming a matrix or blocking-out the schedule is done to reserve time for hospital rounds and other times when the physician is not available for office visits.

come in earlier. This will allow for some free time at the end of the day for the physician. In the event that a long appointment, such as a one and a half hour appointment for a complete physical, has been canceled you will have to attempt to move up an entire group of patients. Many offices maintain a list of patients who wish to be called if there is an appointment open at the last minute. This practice is good in that it is beneficial to both the patient and the physician.

No-shows

No-shows or failed appointments occur when a patient does not show up to keep an appointment. If a patient misses an appointment write "no-show," N/S, or cancellation above the scheduled appointment. Also record the missed appointment (along with the reason such as cancellation) in the patient's record.

Every effort must be made to reschedule the missed appointment. The patient must be contacted by telephone to attempt to determine the reason for the "no-show." If the patient does not reschedule, then note in the patient record the time and date that you spoke with the patient.

This careful documentation is required to protect the physician from a claim of patient abandonment. See Chapter 5 for more information on abandonment. If the patient has rescheduled the appointment, write the new appointment date in the patient's record and in the schedule book.

Med Tip: It is not good practice to reprimand the patient for missing an appointment. Make every effort in the future to give the patient either a written reminder or a telephone reminder call of an appointment.

Physician Called away from Office

If the physician is called away to handle an emergency at the hospital or an office emergency puts the schedule behind, it is expected that patients who have not yet arrived be called to reschedule their appointments. Patients who arrive at the office to discover their appointment has been canceled should receive an apology.

Be sure to document the cancellation in the patient's record noting the reason for the cancellation. Every attempt must be made to reschedule the appointment.

The Appointment Book

The appointment book is a legal document that can be subpoenaed by the court. It is a record of the physician's day and time spent in contact with patients. Appointment books should be kept for several years in case of a court case. If there are any changes from the scheduled patients in the appointment book, such as a cancellation or no-show, these should be noted both in the appointment book and in the patient's record. If the appointment has been rescheduled then this should be noted also.

> **Med Tip:** The appointment book is referred to in many terms including schedule book, appointment calendar, or date book. While the appearance of these documents is different the method used to record the appointment is the same.

There should be an appointment schedule book for each physician in the practice office. Refer to Figure 9-1 for a sample of an appointment book. Setting up a different colored book for each physician helps to eliminate mistakes. Writing each physician's name in bold letters also helps eliminate confusion. Maintain patient confidentiality during the scheduling process. The appointment book should never be left in an area that is visible to visitors at the reception desk.

Also, the appointment book should be archived for future reference with a hard copy or back up tape for computer scheduling. Files are archived by placing them in a storage container or facility and keeping them for several years as back-up documentation.

Computer-assisted Scheduling

Many offices keep all records in a computerized system (Figures 9-3 and 9-4). Only the times when the physician is available appear on the computer screen. Prompts will direct you to necessary information. You will need to backup computerized schedule information frequently to prevent loss. A computerized system provides a print-out of the schedule.

Advance Booking

Ideally, before leaving the office, the patient will schedule his or her next appointment. This practice is known as advance booking. It is possible to book patients far in advance because most medical offices prepare their schedule books from 3 to 6 months ahead of time. However, it is not recommended that appointments be scheduled more than 3 months in advance. Refer to the section on Forming a Matrix earlier in this chapter for infor-

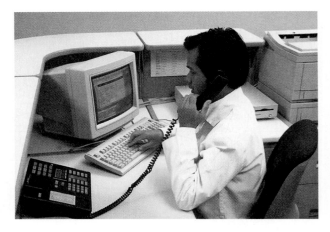

Figure 9-3   Medical assistant scheduling a phone request for an appointment using the computer.

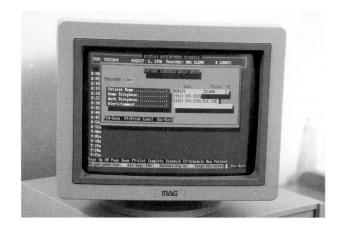

Figure 9-4   Many larger medical offices have switched to computer scheduling.

mation on blocking-out or preparing the appointment book. Advance booking is done for regularly scheduled checkups or required follow-up appointments, for example after surgery.

Appointment Cards

Appointment cards with the name, address, and telephone number of the physician's practice have space to write in the date and time of the next appointment. A card should be given to each patient at the time the next appointment is made (Figure 9-5).

A follow-up reminder card with the same information can be sent to arrive a week before the scheduled appointment. Some offices have the patient complete a self-addressed postcard type of reminder which is then filed in a small file box (tickler file) under the date the postcard should be

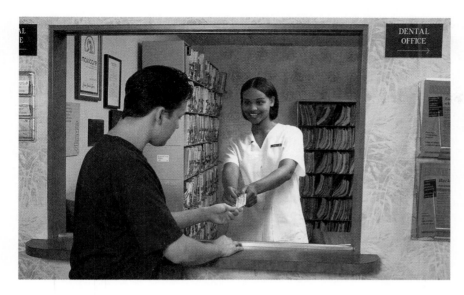

Figure 9-5 Medical assistant gives the patient an appointment card.

mailed. Such reminders are used for annual PAP tests.

When appointments are made over the telephone the reminder card is completed by the medical assistant and filed under the correct date to be mailed. Some medical offices place a reminder phone call the day before a scheduled appointment.

Follow-up

A follow-up appointment, if needed, should be scheduled before the patient leaves the office. Always write down the date and time of the next appointment on an appointment card. Include the patient's first name since families may have more than one person seeing the same physician. This is considered good office management since the only follow-up needed from the medical assistant is an appointment reminder call a day or two before the appointment.

Follow-up Calls

Making follow-up calls to check on a patient's progress addresses quality of care. A "tickler file" is maintained for this purpose. Patients are grateful that their physician and staff are concerned about their welfare even after they leave the office. By using the follow-up call system, it is possible to have a patient come back in for immediate care in the event that he or she is having difficulty after a procedure or office visit. This is especially important if you feel the patient may still be unclear about directions for care prior to leaving the office.

Patient Referrals

The physician may refer the patient to another facility or physician for further testing and treatment. Ideally these arrangements are made by the medical assistant while the patient is present.

The patient must be consulted about any preferences for date and time. When scheduling an admission to a hospital or other facility, the medical assistant must provide pertinent information either over the telephone or on an admissions form.

Health maintenance organizations (HMOs) and Medicare require pre-certification (approval) before allowing for payment for referrals. Pre-certification is obtained by calling the insurer (HMO, Medicare), giving patient information, and requesting approval.

Scheduling Admission to the Hospital

The medical assistant is responsible for scheduling all patient admissions to the hospital or other facility for diagnostic testing. Patients do not schedule their own admissions. When scheduling a direct admit to the hospital, be sure to contact the patient's insurance company for pre-admissions approval. Table 9-2 provides a description of the patient information supplied when scheduling hospital admissions.

Provide the patient with a detailed explanation of the time, date, and preparation needed for the admission. It is always better to place detailed information in writing. Many offices have preprinted information to hand to the patient.

TABLE 9-2 Patient Information Supplied when Scheduling Hospital Admissions

Information	Explanation
1. Patient's full name	Verify spelling of first and last name.
2. Address	Ask the patient to state current address.
3. Social security number	May be taken from the patient record.
4. Age/Date of birth	Check birth date in patient record.
5. Telephone number	Ask patient for current number and area code.
6. Requirement	Type of room or special requirement such as no smoking.
7. Admitting diagnosis	Take this from the physician's statement in the patient record.
8. Recent prior admission	Ask the patient for last admission date.
9. Physician's name	Give physician's name.
10. Insurance information	May fax copy of insurance card.
11. Person's name at insurance company who gave pre-approval.	Forms are also available from insurance company.

This should, however, be personalized with the patient's name. Even when preprinted materials are used, a complete, concise, verbal explanation of the important points should be given by the medical assistant.

Scheduling Surgery

The patient is not usually present when the surgery is actually scheduled. Surgery may fall into several categories: routine, elective, or urgent. Routine surgery refers to a surgical procedure that the physician believes is necessary but not an emergency. Procedures such as hysterectomy, prostatectomy, tonsillectomy, and cataract removal all fall in this category.

Elective surgery is a surgical procedure that has the approval of the physician but one which is not necessary to treat an acute health problem. A patient may request an elective procedure such as plastic surgery, vasectomy, or tubal ligation. You must call the patient's insurance company for authorization of coverage for all elective surgery. A form can also be sent to the company and kept on file.

An emergency procedure requires immediate surgery to prevent severe damage or death to the patient. Emergency surgical procedures include appendectomy, cholecystectomy for acute gall bladder attack, tracheotomy, and surgery to stop internal bleeding.

Once you have determined the category of the surgery from the physician then call the surgery department and talk to the scheduler. If the surgery is urgent, arrangements will have to be made to prepare a surgical room immediately. If a non-urgent admission is scheduled, the time and date will be established according to the first opening on the surgical schedule. You may also have to place a call to the assistant surgeon to notify him or her of the scheduled surgery. Table 9-3 describes the information the surgical scheduler will need.

The medical assistant will make arrangements for an anesthetic (for the surgery) at the same time the surgery scheduling is done. Arrangements are made for the anesthesiologist to speak with the patient.

Patient Instructions for Surgery

Patients should be told what to expect before undergoing surgery or diagnostic procedures. It is the physician's responsibility to explain the procedure and the risks involved to the patient.

The medical assistant is responsible for explaining the preparation that is necessary. This preparation may include laboratory tests, fasting, medicated preparations inserted into the rectum such as enemas to expel fecal material, skin preparations such as showers with germicidal soap, and any other special instructions. It is good practice

TABLE 9-3   Information Needed to Schedule Surgery

The following information is required when scheduling surgery.

1. Day and time the surgeon wishes to perform the surgery.

2. Physician's current diagnosis of the patient's condition.

3. Type of surgery that is to be performed.

4. Amount of time the surgeon will require to perform the procedure.

5. Names of the surgeon and assisting surgeon(s).

6. Patient's full name, age, and sex.

7. Patient's telephone number with area code.

8. Any special instructions (for example will the patient require blood reserved in case of transfusion)

9. Pre-authorization from patient's insurance company if required.

to provide written instructions. Some offices have patient instructions for how to prepare for various procedures printed ahead of time and available for distribution to patients after the medical assistant has verbally reviewed the instructions with the patient.

Med Tip: Careful written or verbal instruction by the medical assistant can do much to reduce natural fear that patients have before surgical procedures. Never discuss the procedure in such a way as to instill fear in the patient.

Exceptions to the Appointment System

Special problems may arise which mean that the schedule cannot be maintained. These include patient emergencies and handling patients with acute conditions. Acute conditions are illnesses or injuries that come upon the patient suddenly and require treatment.

The medical assistant must listen carefully to all the patient's complaints to be able to accurately assess the seriousness of the patient's condition. Acute illnesses which require medical attention, but are not life threatening, must be distinguished from life-threatening emergencies. In general, sudden onset of pain must be considered an emergency until otherwise determined. The medical assistant will ask questions regarding where the pain is located, when it first appeared, the strength

and duration of pain, and if the patient has experienced the same pain before. The physician should *always* be asked if there is *any* question regarding a potential emergency.

If an emergency exists, such as in severe chest pain, then the physician is informed of the call immediately. If a physician is not available then the medical assistant refers the patient to the nearest emergency center. If the patient is not able to make his or her own arrangements for transportation then the medical assistant will do this by arranging for taxi or med-van service. Table 9-4 lists emergency (life-threatening) conditions, while Table 9-5 lists acute illnesses which will require that the patient be seen by a physician as soon a possible.

Triage, which is the process of sorting or grouping patients according to the seriousness of their condition, becomes necessary when there is more than one seriously ill patient waiting to see the physician.

Salespersons and Other Non-patient Visitors

Companies that manufacture drugs are referred to as pharmaceutical companies. Their salespersons, also called representatives (reps) visit physicians to explain the latest drugs on the market. They have information relating to the expected effects and recommended dosages of these medications.

Physicians try to arrange time in their schedules to meet with selected pharmaceutical representatives. Most offices have a policy for

TABLE 9-4   **Examples of Emergency Conditions**

Emergency Conditions	
Acute allergic reaction	Head injury
Allergic reaction with respiratory distress	Laceration
Coma	Loss of consciousness
Convulsions	Pain and/or numbness after the application of a cast for fracture
Diabetic reaction	Poisoning
Difficulty breathing	Severe bleeding
Drowning/near-drowning	Severe dizziness
Drug overdose	Severe nausea, vomiting, and diarrhea lasting more than 24 hours
Foreign object in the eye	Severe pain (especially chest pain)
Fracture	Sudden acute illness
Gunshot wounds	Sudden paralysis of part or all of the body

TABLE 9-5   **Examples of Acute Conditions**

Acute Conditions	
Earache	Pain in abdomen that is not severe
Eye infection	Skin rash
Fever lasting more than 24 hours	Sore throat and/or swollen glands
Infection that is visible to patient (for example: a red, swollen area after an injury)	Unusual discharge (for example: blood in urine)
Pain or burning upon urination	Vomiting

working with the drug reps. If the physician is to meet with the pharmaceutical rep, then the medical assistant will escort the representative into the physician's private office (Figure 9-6).

If the physician is interested in a new drug product the rep may leave samples of this product. The medical assistant has a responsibility to place all drugs into a secured storage area.

All visitors to the physicians office should be treated with courtesy. Not all visitors are allowed in to see the physician. In general physicians will see their family members or other physicians if they come unannounced into the office. Take in a written note to the physician with the names of the visitors. If the physician is able to talk with them you can escort them into his or her private office.

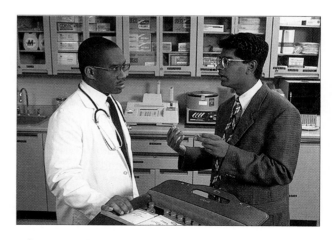

Figure 9-6   The medical assistant talking with a pharmaceutical representative.

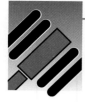

LEGAL AND ETHICAL ISSUES

There are many ethical concerns relating to the scheduling process. The appointment book is a legal document which records the physician's time spent with patients. This record can validate actual services provided and billed for Internal Revenue Service (IRS) verification. Documentation of canceled appointments and no-shows is critical. Keep in mind that a physician may be liable for a lawsuit on the grounds of abandonment and negligence, if a patient who requests to see the physician, is not seen by the physician through some fault of the physician or the physician's staff. The patient may claim that the physician did not offer treatment or provide follow-up care. If a patient cancels an appointment or does not show up for an appointment, the physician is not at fault. Hence the need for correct documentation.

The medical assistant has a great responsibility to correctly screen and assess the patient's need for immediate treatment. The physician has a legal responsibility to see patients who are acutely ill or need emergency care. The severity of the patient's health problem should be related to the physician objectively. Factors such as like or dislike of a patient are inappropriate and should not enter into the decision-making process. It is unethical for the medical assistant to decide that a patient is lying about his or her need to see the physician. All patients have the right to be seen by their physician.

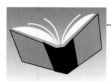

PATIENT EDUCATION

Patients will need a detailed explanation of what they need to do to prepare for the appointment. Laboratory tests or procedures which require preparations such as enemas or taking nothing by mouth (NPO) after midnight need to be explained carefully.

If pre-registration is required before the patient arrives for an appointment the extra time needed must be explained to the patient. Prior approval from insurance companies for payment is paramount. Patients must be taught to know what their insurance policy covers.

Summary

An efficiently managed medical office requires careful attention to the scheduling function. The medical assistant is responsible for carefully assessing the patient's need for an appointment. Providing the correct amount of time on the schedule for the patient visit works to ensure that the needs of patient and physician are met. However, the medical assistant must remain flexible in scheduling since patients with emergencies and acute illnesses must be seen immediately.

Most offices maintain an open time in the schedule to handle daily acute illnesses.

A calm manner is the best approach to handling a schedule that has fallen behind. Quick thinking and planning by rescheduling patients can alleviate stress for the physician who falls behind. Careful documentation of all patients who fail to keep appointments, either through cancellation or "no-show," can assist the physician in avoiding a lawsuit for abandonment of the patient.

Competency Review

1. Define and spell the glossary terms for this chapter.
2. Write an office policy for handling emergency telephone calls.
3. Role play instructing a patient regarding admission to the hospital for a surgical procedure. Use another student as the patient.
4. Correctly document a patient appointment cancellation.
5. Use a computerized scheduling system to integrate patient information and appointment scheduling.

Test Taking Tips — Concentrate intensely when taking an exam. If you find your mind wandering, stop briefly and recoup your concentration.

Examination Review Questions

1. Mark Adams is scheduled to have a post-operative check-up. He has been given a 15 minute appointment at 1:00 p.m. His wife, Maria, has an appointment on the same day at 1:15 p.m. What type of scheduling system is the physician using?

   (A) wave scheduling

   (B) specified time scheduling

   (C) modified wave scheduling

   (D) double booking

   (E) open office hours

2. How far ahead of time should an appointment book be "blocked-out?"

   (A) 1 year

   (B) 6 months

   (C) 3 months

   (D) to be done when you make an appointment

   (E) not to be done at all

3. What is the best method to use when a patient cancels an early afternoon one-hour appointment?

   (A) move up the last appointment (15 minute exam) for the day into that slot

   (B) leave the time free for the physician to get caught up with paper work

   (C) do nothing since the physician is always running late

   (D) call several patients who have asked to be placed on a waiting list and try to fill the entire hour

   (E) try to change all of the rest of the afternoon appointments to one hour earlier

4. When the patient requires surgery the medical assistant would

   (A) give all the information to the patient so that the patient can schedule the surgery at a convenient time

   (B) ask the surgeon who will be performing the surgery to schedule it

   (C) call the surgery scheduler where the surgery will be performed and schedule the time

   (D) place the surgery request in writing and send it to the surgical center

   (E) none of the above

5. All the following are either medical emergencies or acute conditions which require an appointment as soon as possible EXCEPT

   (A) earache

   (B) severe pain

   (C) eye infection

   (D) pain with urination

   (E) fever of 99.8° F for past two weeks

6. To assist the physician in avoiding a claim by a patient for abandonment the medical assistant would

   (A) tell the patient that he or she will have to find another physician for treatment

   (B) screen out all patients who really do not need to be seen by the physician

   (C) call the patient to attempt to re-schedule the appointment and document the telephone call

   (D) nothing special needs to be done

   (E) all of the above

7. Double booking patients:

   (A) is one of the most acceptable ways of patient scheduling in terms of practice time management

   (B) generally considered poor practice

   (C) involves scheduling two members of the same family at the same time

   (D) always forces the physician to utilize less time per patient

   (E) none of the above

8. What procedure for appointment scheduling refers to crossing out periods of time when the physician is unavailable?

(A) double booking

(B) wave scheduling

(C) forming a matrix

(D) modified wave scheduling

(E) archiving

9. When a patient does not show up for an appointment:

(A) the medical assistant should write "N/S" above the scheduled appointment

(B) record the missed appointment in the patient's record

(C) record the reason for the missed appointment in the patient's record

(D) all of the above

(E) none of the above

10. Which of the following is applicable to appointment cards?

(A) include the name, address and telephone number of the practice

(B) should be given to each patient whether the patient wants one or not

(C) includes all of the same information as the follow-up reminder card

(D) are generally only used for past "No-Shows"

(E) are preprinted with the patient's name prior to the day's appointment

ON THE JOB

A pharmaceutical representative, has just arrived at the office of Dr. Joseph Henderson, a board certified orthopaedic surgeon. The waiting room is literally swarming with patients waiting to see Dr. Henderson because he was delayed with an unexpectedly complicated lumbar spinal fusion and laminectomy.

The representative is very insistent, almost belligerent, about seeing the physician immediately even though she did not have an appointment to see him. In fact, the visit was totally unexpected as the representative had just been in two weeks prior to today.

Last time the representative was in, she gave Dr. Henderson a variety of readily usable and dispensable medication. She has more of the same today—injectable cortisone with Novocain, muscle relaxants, NSAIDs, and even some Tylenol with codeine. Usually, Dr. Henderson is

quite receptive to receiving these samples as they help to ease the financial burden of his patients on whom he uses or to whom he dispenses the samples. The office is, in fact, running quite low on these particular medications because of Dr. Henderson's heavy patient load.

What is your response?

1. What should the medical assistant consider doing in this situation?

2. Should a rep. ever take precedence over scheduled appointments?

3. Does the fact that Dr. Henderson usually is quite anxious to receive any and all samples for his patients enter in as a factor?

4. Does the diminished supply of these samples alter the situation?

5. Can the medical assistant ever accept delivery of any or all of these samples?

References

Becklin, K. and Sunnarborg, E. *Medical Office Procedures.* New York: Glencoe, 1996.

Health Care Law and Ethics. Chicago: American Association of Medical Assistants, 1996.

Humphrey, D. *Contemporary Medical Office Procedures.* Belmont, CA: Wadsworth, 1990.

Lipman, M. *Medical Law & Ethics.* Upper Saddle River, NJ: Brady/Prentice Hall, 1994.

MEDICAL ASSISTANT ROLE DELINEATION CHART

Highlight indicates material covered in this chapter

ADMINISTRATIVE

ADMINISTRATIVE PROCEDURES

- Perform basic clerical functions
- Schedule, coordinate, and monitor appointments
- Schedule inpatient/outpatient admissions and procedures
- Understand and apply third party guidelines
- Obtain reimbursement through accurate claims submission
- Monitor third-party reimbursement
- Perform medical transcription
- Understand and adhere to managed care policies and procedures
- *Negotiate managed care contracts (adv)*

PRACTICE FINANCES

- Perform procedural and diagnostic coding
- Apply bookkeeping principles
- Document and maintain accounting and banking records
- Manage accounts receivable
- Manage accounts payable
- Process payroll
- *Develop and maintain fee schedules (adv)*
- *Manage renewals of business and professional insurance policies (adv)*
- *Manage personal benefits and maintain records (adv)*

CLINICAL

FUNDAMENTAL PRINCIPLES

- Apply principles of aseptic technique and infection control
- Comply with quality assurance practices
- Screen and follow up patient test results

DIAGNOSTIC ORDERS

- Collect and process specimens
- Perform diagnostic tests

PATIENT CARE

- Adhere to established triage procedures
- Obtain patient history and vital signs
- Prepare and maintain examination and treatment areas

- Prepare patient for examinations, procedures, and treatments
- Assist with examinations, procedures, and treatments
- Prepare and administer medications and immunizations
- Maintain medication and immunization records
- Recognize and respond to emergencies
- Coordinate patient care information with other health care providers

GENERAL (TRANSDISCIPLINARY)

PROFESSIONALISM

- Project a professional manner and image
- Adhere to ethical principles
- Demonstrate initiative and responsibility
- Work as a team member
- Manage time efficiently
- Prioritize and perform multiple tasks
- Adapt to change
- Promote the CMA credential
- Enhance skills through continuing education

COMMUNICATION SKILLS

- Treat all patients with compassion and empathy
- Recognize and respect cultural diversity
- Adapt communications to individual's ability to understand
- Use professional telephone technique
- Use effective and correct verbal and written communications
- Recognize and respond to verbal and non-verbal communications
- Use medical terminology appropriately
- Receive, organize, prioritize, and transmit information
- Serve as liaison
- Promote the practice through positive public relations

LEGAL CONCEPTS

- Maintain confidentiality
- Practice within the scope of education, training, and personal capabilities
- Prepare and maintain medical records
- Document accurately
- Use appropriate guidelines when releasing information
- Follow employer's established policies dealing with the health care contract
- Follow federal, state, and local legal guidelines
- Maintain awareness of federal and state health care legislation and regulations
- Maintain and dispose of regulated substances in compliance with government guidelines
- Comply with established risk management and safety procedures
- Recognize professional credentialing criteria
- Participate in the development and maintenance of personnel, policy, and procedure manuals
- *Develop and maintain personnel, policy, and procedure manuals (adv)*

INSTRUCTION

- Instruct individuals according to their needs
- Explain office policies and procedures
- Teach methods of health promotion and disease prevention
- Locate community resources and disseminate information
- *Orient and train personnel (adv)*
- *Develop educational materials (adv)*
- *Conduct continuing education activities (adv)*

OPERATIONAL FUNCTIONS

- Maintain supply inventory
- Evaluate and recommend equipment and supplies
- Apply comptuer techniques to support office operations
- *Supervise personnel (adv)*
- *Interview and recommend job applicants (adv)*
- *Negotiate leases and prices for equipment and supply contracts (adv)*

SOURCE: Reprinted by permission of the American Association of Medical Assistants from the *AAMA Role Delineation Study: Occupational Analysis of the Medical Assisting Profession.*

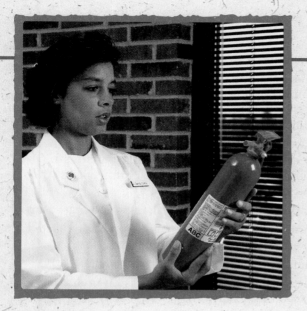

10

Office Safety, Facilities, and Equipment

LEARNING OBJECTIVES

At the completion of this chapter, you should:
1. Define and spell the glossary terms for this chapter.
2. Identify 6 general safety measures.
3. Define the RACE formula and discuss its use.
4. Discuss 6 disaster rules.
5. Describe electrical, radiation, mechanical, and chemical safety hazards.
6. List and describe 4 types of medical waste.
7. Define OSHA Bloodborne Pathogens Standards.
8. Describe the three points that must be included in an Exposure Plan.
9. List and discuss 5 guidelines for using protective measures as indicated by OSHA.
10. Discuss the importance of Universal Precautions for the medical assistant.
11. List and describe 6 rules for proper body mechanics.
12. State the difference between capital equipment and expendable equipment.
13. State the proper procedure for handling drug samples.
14. List 15 items commonly found in a physician's bag.

ADMINISTRATIVE PERFORMANCE COMPETENCIES

After completing this chapter, you should perform these tasks:
1. Correctly adhere to OSHA Bloodborne Pathogens Standards.
2. Demonstrate the correct sequence of events, using the RACE formula, if a fire occurs.
3. Demonstrate proper body mechanics for moving equipment from the floor to the counter.
4. Complete an incident report.
5. Assemble equipment for a physician's bag.

Glossary

bloodborne pathogens Disease producing microorganisms transmitted by means of blood and body fluids containing blood.

body mechanics Methods of standing and lifting objects in order to avoid injury and fatigue.

caustic Capable of burning or eating away tissue.

fire extinguisher Canister containing material capable of putting out many types of fires including paper, electrical, wood, and cloth.

grounded Connected to an electrical current or circuit with the ground through a conductor or other solid connection.

incident report Formal written description of an incident, such as a patient falling, occurring in a medical setting.

inventory A list of articles with a description and quantity of each.

mandate Require.

morale Positive or negative state of mind of employees (as regards a feeling of well being) with relationship to their work or work environment.

parenteral Medication route other than the alimentary canal (oral and rectal). Parenteral routes include subcutaneous, intravenous, and intramuscular.

pathogens Disease producing microorganisms.

terminal disease A disease which is expected to end with death.

vendor A supplier of material goods.

virulent Relating to transmission of disease. Exceedingly harmful.

Just as in any workplace, general safety measures, employee safety, housekeeping safety, proper body mechanics, office security, and measures to insure a clean, pleasant environment are critical to maintaining the safety and comfort of the medical assistant and the patient. In a medical workplace, additional safety issues may arise including biological hazards, bloodborne pathogens, and the handling of drug samples.

General Safety Measures

Since medical assistants work throughout the medical office including the front office, clinical area and laboratory setting there are several general safety rules that should be observed. These guidelines or rules, designed to protect you, your coworkers and the patients, are presented here.

Figure 10-1 shows two common office hazards which should be corrected or removed whenever they are observed.

Disaster Plan

A disaster is anything that can cause injury or damage to a group of people. Disasters in a medical office include: fire, flood, tornado, earthquake, or explosion. The guidelines for disaster contain basic rules to follow when a disaster strikes.

Physical Hazards

Physical hazards in the work place include fires, electrical and radiation hazards, and mechanical failures.

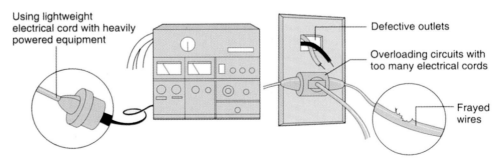

Figure 10-1 Office hazards.

Guidelines: General Safety Measures

1. Walk never run in a medical office. If an emergency situation occurs, move quickly without running.
2. Always walk on the right-hand side of the hallway. Wheelchairs and carts bearing patients use the same hallways as employees and visitors. Some medical facilities have a mirror on the wall or ceiling at hallway junctions so that people do not collide.
3. Use handrails when using stairways.
4. Never carry uncapped syringes or sharp instruments in hallways or between exam rooms.
5. Keep floors clear. Immediately wipe up spills or call housekeeping to assist. Never pick up broken glass with bare hands. Use OSHA standards when cleaning up glass, spilled specimens and liquids.
6. Open doors carefully to avoid injuring someone on the other side.
7. Replace burned out light bulbs immediately, especially over exit signs.
8. Report all unsafe conditions at once.
9. Wear long hair pulled back and tied to prevent it from coming into contact with hazardous materials.
10. Shoes should cover the entire foot. Open-toe, open-heel, or high-heel shoes are not recommended in the medical office due to the danger of slipping and other injuries.
11. No food is ever placed in the same refrigerator with laboratory specimens or refrigerated drugs.
12. There should be no eating, drinking, or smoking in the medical office, except in designated areas.
13. File cabinets should be mounted against the walls to avoid accidental tipping when a heavy top drawer is opened.
14. Floors should be clean but not so highly polished that they cause slipping. All spills must be cleaned immediately. A hazard sign should always be placed near a wet floor. Figure 10-2 illustrates hazard signs for wet floors.
15. All controlled substances (narcotics) must be stored in a locked cabinet. A record of all narcotic administration must be maintained according to the Drug Enforcement Administration (DEA) regulations. Any loss of drugs must be reported to the regional office of the DEA immediately. The local police should also be notified.

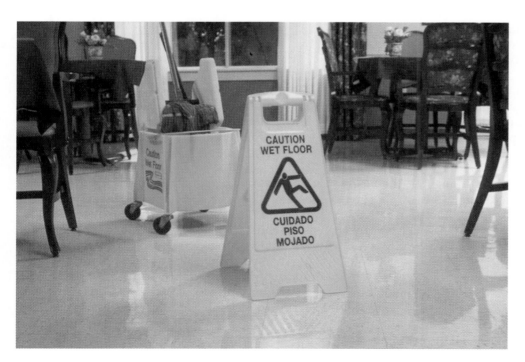

Figure 10-2 Caution signs should always be used to warn people of wet floors.

1. Remain calm. Count to 10 and assess the situation.
2. Make sure that you are not in danger.
3. Remove all others (patients and employees) who are in immediate danger, if it is safe for you to do this.
4. Make sure that the fire department has been called in the event of a fire.
5. Notify others of the emergency according to the policy of the facility.
6. Use stairs, never the elevator.

All medical facilities must have a disaster plan. This plan should include the following:

- The floor plan of the facility
- The nearest exit
- The location of alarms and fire extinguishers.
- How to use fire equipment such as extinguishers and hoses.
- Your role when a disaster strikes.

Fire Safety

Fire extinguishers should be attached on walls where the potential for fire is the greatest, such as in the laboratory areas. Fire extinguishers generally are canisters containing material capable of putting out many types of fires. Each employee should be instructed on the proper use of all fire equipment including extinguishers and fire hoses. Smoke alarms should be placed in strategic areas such as waiting room, laboratory, and hallways. These should be tested periodically.

Large medical clinics and offices will often hold a yearly fire drill in which the local fire department will demonstrate fire equipment and the most effective means for putting out fires. However, even small medical facilities should hold a fire drill periodically throughout the year with mandatory attendance required of all employees. Staff meetings are ideal times in which to hold fire drills since most employees are present at that time. A fire drill prepares each employee to know where the fire exits are and how to act in a calm manner during this emergency.

There are few exceptions to the "No Smoking" policy in medical offices. In addition to the health hazard to the smoking patient there are additional dangers from cigarettes, cigars, and pipes. Some of the chemicals used in a medical office are volatile which means they easily convert into a flammable gas. Also, some patients may be receiving flammable oxygen from portable equipment.

Patients sometimes dispose of ashes and cigarettes in waste baskets and other trash receptacles when they smoke in the office or near the doorway to the office. This can be a serious fire hazard.

Med Tip: Always be on the alert for patients and visitors who use paper cups or other highly flammable containers as ashtrays.

In the event of a fire, the following items should be available:

1. *Telephone numbers* of fire and police departments attached to all telephones, including extensions.
2. *Fire extinguishers,* which are periodically checked on a posted schedule, to assure they are in good working condition. The date and initials of the person responsible for testing the equipment should be legible.
3. *Exits and stairways* should be clearly marked and free of debris at all times. A diagram of all exits should be posted near the fire extinguishers.
4. *Vital records* should be easily identified by staff so they can be saved if possible in an emergency.

Fires need oxygen, heat, and fuel in order to start. These three factors are present in the medical office: flames from matches and cigarette sparks provide the heat; chemicals, papers, and plastics normally present in medical offices can provide the fuel; and air containing oxygen. Oxygen does not burn by itself. However many offices have an oxygen supply or portable oxygen tanks. Extra oxygen in the room can support combustion which means that materials will catch fire if heat and fuel are present also. The medical assistant must be observant in order to prevent these fires from starting.

After notifying the fire department, the most important function during a fire is to see that all patients and employees are safely out of danger. All patients should be told to immediately leave the building. Any patients who need assistance should be helped. Exam rooms and bathrooms need to be inspected in the event a patient is still in the building.

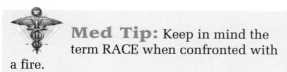

Med Tip: Keep in mind the term RACE when confronted with a fire.

R = remove the patient from vicinity of the fire.

A = activate the alarm and alert other staff members.

C = contain or confine the fire by closing all doors.

E = extinguish the fire if it is safe to do so.

See Figure 10-3 for a summary of fire safety.

Electrical Safety

Electrical shock is a hazard in the medical office, and in particular in the laboratory due to the equipment being used. All equipment should be grounded, or connected to the ground, according to the manufacturer's instructions. All plugs should be three-pronged and not frayed. Extension cords should not be used at all. But, if they are necessary, the extension cords must be able to take the additional load placed on them. They should not be draped across the floor in areas where people can trip.

The circuit breakers in the office should be clearly marked in the event the medical assistant needs to find them during an electrical fire or shock. If an employee or patient is being shocked, he or she should not be touched. The main source of power should be turned off immediately. You may have to administer cardiopulmonary resuscitation (CPR) and call for help if the victim is unresponsive after the power is turned off.

Radiation Safety

In most medical offices the exposure level of radiation is well below the limits which have been established by federal and state regulations. Some specialists, such as orthopedic physicians and surgeons, require frequent x-rays of their patients to determine the level of healing taking place.

Always pay close attention to signs near radiology rooms and equipment indicating that there is danger due to exposure to radiation. Employees who work around x-ray equipment on a regular basis must wear a small radiation badge that indicates the level of radiation the person is receiving. A lead apron and gloves must be worn by medical personnel if they are in close proximity to a patient receiving x-rays.

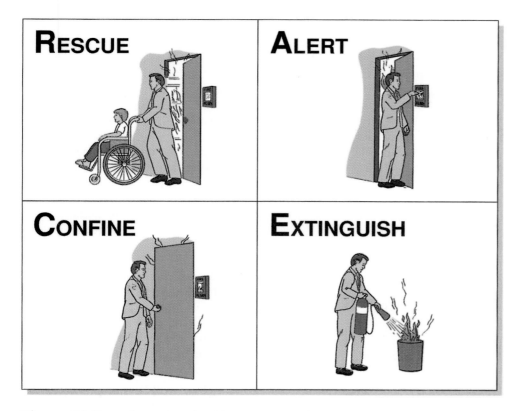

Figure 10-3   A fire safety plan like RACE saves lives.

Exposure to radiation has a cumulative effect. This means that continued exposure and build-up of radiation is the most dangerous. Most medical assistants working in a physician's office will not be exposed to excessive radiation.

Mechanical Safety

Many pieces of equipment in the medical office can cause harm if they are not used properly. Some of these pieces of equipment include the centrifuge, autoclave, sterilizers, and oxygen equipment. All of these pieces of equipment come with detailed instructions. In most cases, the equipment must be grounded with a three-prong plug and will require a particular type of loading technique. This equipment is discussed in later chapters.

Med Tip: Remember to ask for instructions when using unfamiliar equipment. It is better to admit ignorance than to make a disastrous mistake!

Chemical Hazards

Medical offices may contain chemicals, such as hydrochloric acid (HCl), which are highly **caustic** and can cause severe burns. Carefully read all labels for instructions when disposing of chemicals. All chemical spills should be carefully cleaned up, using a spill clean-up kit containing absorbents and neutralizers.

Any caustic chemical or material that comes into contact with the skin or eyes should be washed immediately. The skin should be washed under cold running water for at least five minutes; the eyes should be rinsed for a minimum of fifteen minutes.

Med Tip: When working with an acid, always add the acid to water (instead of water to acid) to avoid a violent chemical reaction that could cause injury. MSDS (Material Safety Data Sheets) are required for all hazardous materials and drugs.

Employee Safety

All employees need the assurance that they work in a safe environment. Following guidelines for the correct handling of waste materials and using

proper **body mechanics** to avoid injury are two areas that all employees should understand.

Biological Hazards

Hospitals, dental practices, veterinary clinics, laboratories, nursing homes, medical offices, and other health care facilities generate 3.2 million tons of hazardous medical waste each year. Much of this waste is dangerous, especially when it is potentially infectious or radioactive. There are four major types of medical waste:

- Solid
- Chemical
- Radioactive
- Infectious

Solid Wastes

Solid waste is generated in every aspect of medicine including administration, cafeterias, patient rooms, and medical offices. It includes trash such as used paper goods, bottles, cardboard, and cans. Solid waste is not considered hazardous, but can cause pollution of the environment. Mandatory recycling programs have assisted in reducing some of the solid waste in the country.

Chemical Wastes

Chemical wastes include substances like germicides, cleaning solvents, and pharmaceuticals. This waste can create a hazardous situation like a fire or explosion. It can also cause harm if ingested, inhaled or absorbed through the skin or mucous membranes. Do not pour toxic, inflammable, foul-smelling, or irritating chemicals down the drain. These chemicals are generally placed in sturdy containers such as buckets. The Materials Safety Data Sheet (MSDS) gives information on handling chemicals safely and should include specific disposal information.

Radioactive Wastes

Radioactive wastes have increased with recent advances in nuclear medicine and include Iodine 123, Iodine 131, and Thallium 201. Radioactive waste is any waste that contains or is contaminated with liquid or solid radioactive material. It is not generated by x-rays or other external beam therapy procedures. Radioactive waste must be clearly labeled as "radioactive", and never placed into an incinerator, down the drain, or in public areas. These waste products must be removed by a licensed facility.

Infectious Waste

Infectious waste identifies any waste material that has the potential to carry disease. Between 10 and 15 percent of all medical waste is considered infectious. Infectious waste, which is handled every day, includes laboratory cultures, blood and blood products from blood banks, operating rooms, emergency rooms, doctor and dentist offices, autopsy suites, and patient rooms.

The three most dangerous types of infectious pathogens (microorganisms) found in medical waste are hepatitis B virus (HBV), hepatitis A virus (HAV), and the human immunodeficiency virus (HIV) which causes acquired immune deficiency syndrome (AIDS).

Hepatitis, a virulent potentially lifethreatening infection of the liver, is transmitted directly or indirectly from blood and feces. AIDS is a virus that attacks the immune system and is considered a **terminal disease**. These diseases are discussed more thoroughly in Chapter 19.

Infectious waste must be separated from other solid and chemical waste at the point of origin (medical office). Infectious waste must be labeled, decontaminated on-site, or removed by a licensed removal facility for decontamination. Methods for treating infectious waste include:

1. Steam sterilization
2. Incineration
3. Thermal inactivation
4. Gas/vapor sterilization
5. Irradiation sterilization
6. Chemical disinfectant

Steam sterilization, which saturates waste with high temperature steam in an autoclave, and incineration are the most commonly recommended treatments for most infectious waste including:

1. Blood cultures
2. Sharps (such as needles and scalpels)
3. Isolation wastes
4. Pathological waste
5. Dialysis unit waste

OSHA Bloodborne Pathogens Standards

Medical office laboratories must follow the Occupational Safety and Health Administration (OSHA) guidelines for handling contaminated materials. These guidelines are available from the US Department of Labor in Washington, DC.

In December of 1991, OSHA released a set of regulations that was designed to reduce the risk of medical employees to infectious diseases. The OSHA standards went into full effect in 1992 and are formally known as OSHA Occupational Exposure to Bloodborne Pathogens Standards. There is a severe penalty of up to $7,000 for each violation of the standards by employers.

OSHA standards must be adhered to by any employee who has occupational exposure. Occupational exposure is defined as a reasonable anticipation that the employee's duties will result in skin, mucous membrane, eye, or parenteral contact with **bloodborne pathogens** or other potential infectious material. Examples of employees who have occupational exposure are medical assistants, physicians, nurses, laboratory workers, and housekeeping personnel. The OSHA standards mandate that each employee with occupational exposure must be offered the hepatitis B vaccination at the expense of the employer. If the employees refuse the vaccine, they must sign a waiver. The potential infectious materials include:

- Body fluid contaminated with blood.
- Saliva in dental procedures.
- Amniotic fluid.
- Cerebrospinal fluid.
- Tissues, cells, or fluids known to be HIV-infected.
- Microbiological waste (kits or inoculated culture media).
- Pathologic waste (human tissue).
- Any unidentified body fluid.

The OSHA standard refers to urine, stool, sputum, nasal secretions, vomitus and sweat only if there is visible evidence of blood present.

OSHA requires that each medical office have a written Exposure Control Plan to assist in minimizing employee exposure to dangerous infectious materials. This exposure plan must be reviewed by all office staff and updated annually. An Exposure Control Plan must include:

1. *Exposure Determination:* listing of job classification within the office and whether there is danger of occupational exposure to infectious waste materials in each job (for example medical assistants, custodians, and housekeeping personnel).
2. *Method of Compliance:* includes specific measures to reduce the risk of exposure.

3. *Post-exposure:* Evaluation and Follow-up: specifies the steps followed when an exposure incident occurs.

An OSHA record for each employee must be kept on file. This includes documentation of the employee's review of the Exposure Control Plan for the facility. In addition records must be maintained on each employee regarding hepatitis B vaccination and an exposure incident report. These report records must be maintained for the duration of employment plus 30 years. Records of all training sessions must be maintained for 3 years.

Personal Protective Equipment

Personal protective equipment refers to clothing and equipment that protects the employee from contact with infectious materials. Protective equipment includes gloves, protective eyewear, masks, gowns, and laboratory coats. Table 10-1 describes what protective clothing is appropriate .

Universal Precautions

Prior to the implementation of OSHA Standards, the US Centers for Disease Control (CDC) in Atlanta issued recommendations that became known as Universal Precautions. According to Universal Precautions, all blood and bodily fluid contact is to be treated as if it contains the HIV, HBV, or other bloodborne pathogens. OSHA Standard states that Universal Precautions must be maintained at all times when there is a potential for contamination by bloodborne pathogens.

Guidelines: Using Protective Equipment and Clothing from OSHA

1. The employer must supply the protective clothing and provide cleaning or disposal of it.
2. The clothing or other equipment must be of a strength to act as a barrier to infectious materials reaching the employee's street clothing, work clothing, eyes, mouth or skin.
3. Disposable gloves may not be reused.
4. Eye protective equipment must have solid sides to prevent infectious material from entering the area.
5. All equipment and clothing must be removed and placed in a designated container before leaving the medical office.

More complete guidelines, known as Standard Precautions, were issued by the CDC in 1996. These guidelines are discussed more fully in Chapter 19.

Housekeeping Safety

All members of the housekeeping department must receive careful instruction regarding OSHA standards. Housekeeping personnel should not empty biohazard waste and sharps containers. They only empty office trash containers. However, since they are around potentially dangerous infectious materials they must receive training.

TABLE 10-1 **Protective Equipment and Clothing**

Clothing/Equipment	When Used
Gloves	Anticipate contact with blood, infectious materials, open wounds or skin is broken on hands. Examples: venipuncture, capillary stick, wound care, injections, minor surgery, cleaning contaminated equipment, such as contaminated surfaces of thermometers.
Mask	Anticipate spray with blood or infectious materials. Often used with eye shields.
Eye/Face Shields	Anticipate spray with infectious materials, droplets of blood, or other infectious matter. Example: performing blood smear.
Gowns, Lab Coats	Anticipate gross contamination of clothing during a procedure. Examples: minor surgery, laboratory procedures.

1. Immediately clean and disinfect contaminated surfaces after exposure to infectious materials. Figure 10-4 shows one type of single-use cleanup kit. All surfaces must be decontaminated on a regular schedule that is posted, signed, and kept with OSHA records.

2. Never pick up broken glass with hands. Use a dust pan or other mechanical device.

3. Properly bag contaminated clothing and laundry in leak-proof labeled bags. Contaminated laundry should not be handled or washed at the medical office or with other non-contaminated clothing.

4. Handle regulated waste (highly infectious material such as contaminated needles and surgical waste) by placing in clearly labeled biohazards waste containers (Figure 10-5). Waste must be removed by a licensed waste disposal service and incinerated or autoclaved before placing in a designated land fill area.

5. Replace a damaged biohazard bag by placing a second bag around the first. Do not remove infectious material from the damaged bag.

6. Use puncture-proof, sealable, biohazard sharps containers for all needles and sharps, such as razors and glass pipettes (Figure 10-6).

   • Place the container close to the work area.
   • Keep sharp container upright.
   • Never reach into the sharps container or push sharps further into the container.
   • Replace sharps container when 2/3 full.
   • Seal and label sharps containers before placing with biohazard waste for removal by disposal service.

7. Wash hands both before and after using gloves.

8. Personal protective equipment (PPE) may not be worn out of the laboratory areas. Failure to observe this precaution may result in an OSHA citation.

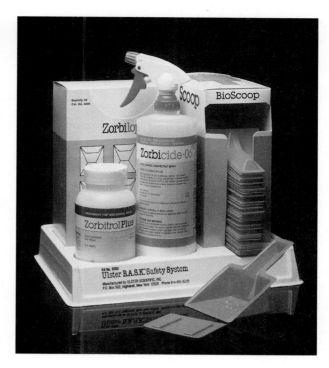

Figure 10-4   One type of single-use cleanup kit.

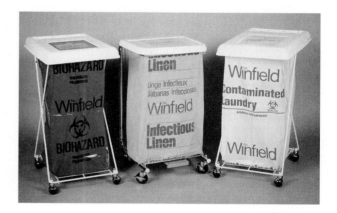

Figure 10-5   Examples of waste and hazard containers.

Cleaning supplies, which are stronger than those used for normal household cleaning, should be stored in a locked room or cabinet when not in use (Figures 10-7 and 10-8).

Proper Body Mechanics

Medical assistants move, lift, and carry many things—equipment, supplies and even patients. Correct body mechanics can prevent muscle strain, permanent injury, and increase efficiency.

Body mechanics is the proper coordination of body alignment, balance, and movement. Table 10-2 describes the principles of body mechanics.

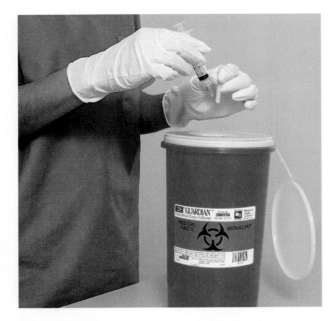

Figure 10-6 Handle needles and syringes carefully.

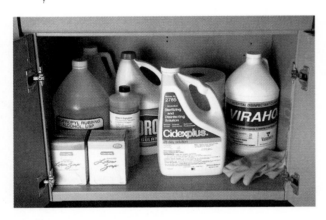

Figure 10-7 Cleaning supplies.

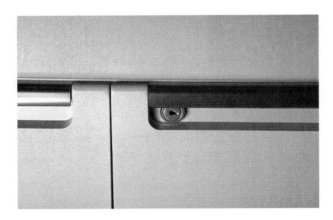

Figure 10-8 Cleaning supplies—locked.

Guidelines: Proper Body Mechanics

1. Keep your back straight.
2. Bend at the hips and knees.
3. Keep feet approximately 6 to 8 inches apart to provide a wide base of support.
4. Use the longest and strongest muscles which are in your legs.
5. Do not twist.
6. Use the weight of your body to help push or pull an object.

Figures 10-9 through 10-11 provide a demonstration of proper lifting techniques.

Office Security

There are unique security issues in a physician's office. Medical offices make an attractive target for a thief or drug addicted person who can sell stolen drugs. Doors and windows need to have secure locks. Only a few authorized personnel should have keys for opening and closing the office. If a key is missing, all locks should be changed. Many offices have electronic security systems that are activated when the last person leaves the office. In order to enter the building a predetermined code has to be entered into the system. If the code is not entered within a specified number of seconds, an alarm will be activated in the local police station.

Prescription pads can be stolen and forged. Therefore, to remove such a temptation, they should be placed out of sight, preferably in a locked cabinet or drawer.

Incident Report

Any unusual occurrence or accident is referred to as an incident in the medical setting. Some examples of incidents are

- A patient falls on wet floor.
- A housekeeping employee is stuck by a needle while emptying a trash container.
- A patient receives the wrong medication.
- A patient misplaces or loses personal property, such as a hearing aid or dentures while in the office.
- Syringes and needles missing from the supply cupboard.
- A patient faints while having blood drawn.
- A medical assistant receives a needle stick from a contaminated needle.
- An employee's purse is missing.
- An abusive patient using vulgar language.
- Missing prescription pads.

TABLE 10-2 Principles of Proper Body Mechanics

Movement	Description
1. Stoop.	• Do not bend from your back. • Stand close to the object you are moving. • Keep feet 6 to 8 inches apart to create a base of support. • Place one foot slightly ahead of the other. • Bend at the hips and knees keeping the back straight, lower the body and hands down to the object. • Use the large leg muscles to assist in returning to a standing position.
2. Lift firmly and smoothly.	• If you think you cannot move a heavy or awkward load get help. • Grasp the load with a firm grip. • Lift the load by using the large leg muscles. • Keep the load close to the body.
3. Use the center of gravity for carrying a load.	• Keep your back as straight as possible. (Hint: You should not be able to feel your clothing touch your back if you are standing straight.) • Keep the weight of the load close to your body and centered over the hips. • Put the load down by bending at the hips and knees. • When two or more people carry the load, have one person give the commands to lift or move the object.
4. Pull or push rather than lift a load.	• Remain close to the object you are moving. • Keep feet apart with one slightly forward. • Have a firm grasp on the object. • Crouch down with feet apart if the object is on the floor. • Bend your elbows and place hands on the load at chest level. • Keep back straight. • Push up with your legs in order to stand up with the load.
5. Avoid reaching.	• Evaluate the distance before reaching too far for an object. • Stand close to the object. • Do not reach to the point of straining. • To change direction, point your feet in the direction you wish to go. • Keep the object close to your body as you lower it.
6. Avoid twisting.	• Do not twist your body.

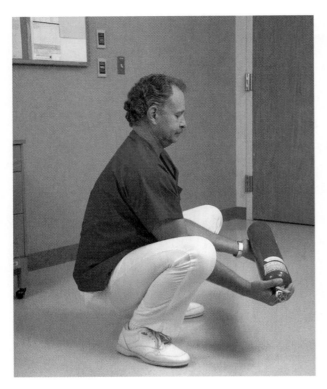

Figure 10-9 Correct position when lifting a heavy object off the floor.

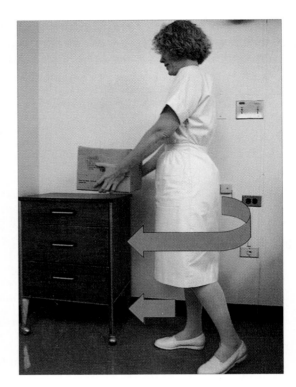

Figure 10-11 When changing direction of the movement, use a pivot turn of the feet.

Whenever any unusual occurrence or incident takes place a written report must be made. This is called the **incident report** and can protect both the employer and the medical assistant against possible lawsuits.

> **Med Tip:** Remember to record any unusual occurrence in writing. Memory of what actually happened can fail over time. A written record of what happened and what corrective action was taken can assist in determining if something was an accident or negligence.

Incident reports should be completed immediately in black or blue ink. The incident should be described as simply as possible. Only objective information is included, such as "Patient fell while getting onto examination table." Do not include subjective comments, such as "Patient was not paying attention to what he was doing."

Your medical office should have its own customized form. However, most incident forms include the following information.

- Names of all persons involved.
- Date and time of the incident.

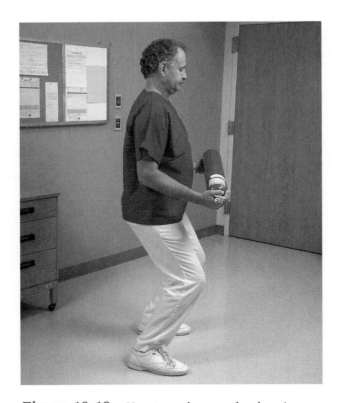

Figure 10-10 Use strong leg muscles, keeping back straight, when lifting.

- Exact location of the incident (including the address of the medical facility and the location of the incident within the facility).
- Name of the person to whom the incident is reported and the time of the report.
- Brief description of what happened.
- Names of all witnesses.
- Name and description of any equipment involved in the incident.

- Action taken at the time of the incident.
- Action taken to prevent a recurrence.
- Signature and title of person completing the report.

A copy of the incident report should be placed in a master incident report file, the patient's file, and the employee's record. Figure 10-12 is one example of an incident report form.

INCIDENT REPORT

Name of injured party _____ Date _____

Address _____ Telephone _____

_____

Was the injured party: ☐ Employee ☐ Patient ☐ Other _____

Date of accident/incident _____ Time of incident _____

Where did incident occur? _____

Names of witnesses (include titles):

_____   _____

_____   _____

What first aid/treatment was given at the time of the incident?

_____

_____

Who administered first aid? _____

Briefly describe the incident. _____

_____

_____

_____

_____

Names of employees present at time of incident/injury:

_____

What, in your opinion, caused the accident? _____

_____

Follow up: What steps have been taken to prevent a similar accident? _____

_____

_____

Date _____   Employee s signature _____

Date _____   Supervisor s signature _____

Figure 10-12   An example of a typical incident report.

Medical Office Facility

The pleasant physical atmosphere created by a cheerful, clean office makes an immediate impression upon patients. It also adds to the general positive morale of the employees. Morale refers to the positive or negative state of mind of employees (as regards a feeling of well being) with relationship to their work or work environment. Things to be considered in setting up and maintaining a medical office include room temperature, office layout, and examination room(s).

Temperature

The temperature throughout the reception area and examination rooms should be maintained at around 74°F. Patients in the exam rooms have frequently disrobed and may be chilled in just a disposable gown.

Facilities Planning

Furnishings should be arranged to create an easy traffic pattern for patients to follow as they enter and leave the office. There should be adequate space in the waiting room for a wheelchair to be maneuvered with ease. See Figure 10-13 for an illustration of a typical office layout.

Medical offices are divided into two areas: administrative and clinical. The administrative area contains the reception area and front desk, waiting room, file storage, insurance and billing area, and office equipment such as computers and telephone system.

The clinical area contains the exam rooms, physician's office and/or consultation room, treatment room for office surgical procedures, supply room, clean and contaminated utility areas, and a laboratory which contains all blood drawing, specimen analyzing, and electrocardiogram (EKG) equipment.

Some medical offices will also have a small recovery room with a bed or cot. This is used while the patient recovers from a minor surgical procedure.

Examination Rooms

Examinations rooms should only contain furnishings and equipment needed to examine a patient. Figure 10-14 illustrates a typical patient exam

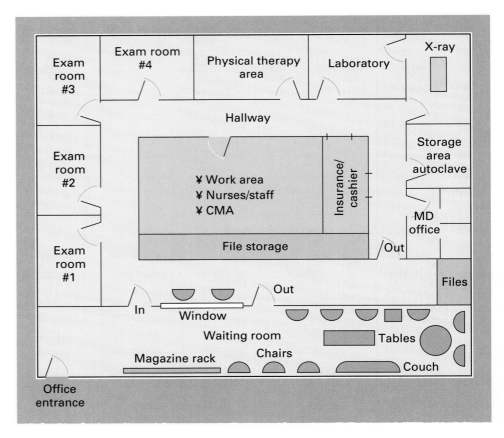

Figure 10-13 A typical office layout.

room. All instruments and supplies, such as disposable gowns, towels, tissues, and sheets, are kept in the exam room supply cabinets, if possible. Medications are never kept in the exam rooms at all but are brought in from the main supply cabinet when needed. A small sink with a foot operated faucet, an adjustable goose-neck lamp, telephone extension, one chair, exam table, and a stool for the physician are the only furnishings necessary.

The exam rooms should be soundproof so that conversations cannot be heard from one room to another. The exam table should be arranged so that the patient is not exposed when the door is opened.

Bathrooms

Separate bathrooms do not have to be maintained for male and female patients. The door should be clearly marked for patients and be wheelchair accessible with handrails around the toilet. Most medical office bathrooms are now built with an alarm button that patients can push if they need help.

Employees should have their own bathroom facilities which are clearly marked for them. Bathrooms and facilities must conform to regulations regarding the handicapped.

Office Equipment

Office equipment that is categorized as capital equipment includes: office furnishings, carpeting, typewriters, word processing equipment, computers, exam tables, refrigerators, and EKG equipment. Some medical specialties, such as ophthal-

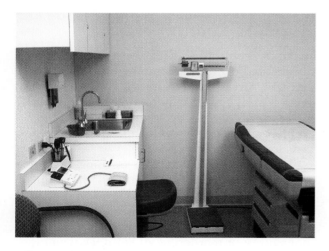

Figure 10-14 A patient exam room should be simply but efficiently designed and furnished.

mology and radiology, require a heavy expenditure in capital equipment.

Capital equipment refers to items that require a large dollar amount to purchase (generally over $500) and have a relatively long life. The distinguishing factor between capital equipment and general office supplies is the life expectancy (useful life) of the product.

Capital equipment also has a financial life which is referred to as depreciation. Depreciation is a loss in value of the product resulting from normal aging, use or deterioration. An allowance is made for this type of loss of value for tax purposes. Therefore the office accountant will account for capital items differently than for general office supplies.

A master list should be maintained of all the physical assets, or capital equipment, in an office. This allows the physician to maintain an **inventory** of assets.

Administrative Equipment

Most medical offices will have the following administrative equipment:

- *Calculator:* Used for mathematical calculation for billing and determining medication dosages.
- *Checkwriter:* Used to mechanically process paychecks. May be used in conjunction with a computer system.
- *Computer:* (discussed in Chapter 12).
- *Word processor:* Used for typing statements and letters.
- *Laser printer:* Used in conjunction with a computer for letter quality printing. Creates images with a laser beam and then transfers the image to paper with pressure and heat.
- *Facsimile (FAX) machine:* Used to send copies from the office via the telephone system (Figure 10-15).
- *Dictation/transcription machine:* (discussed in Chapter 13).
- *Telephone system:* (discussed in Chapter 9).
- *Scanners:* Used to "read" text and graphic files.
- *Copy machine:* Used to copy, reduce, enlarge, collate, and copy in color documents in the medical office (Figure 10-16).

Warranties

A warranty is a guarantee in writing from the manufacturer the product will perform correctly under normal conditions of use. The warranty provides

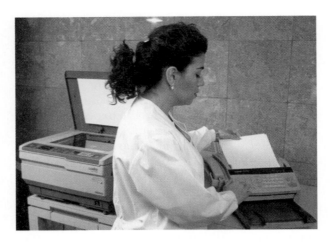

Figure 10-15 FAX machines have become an essential item in all medical offices.

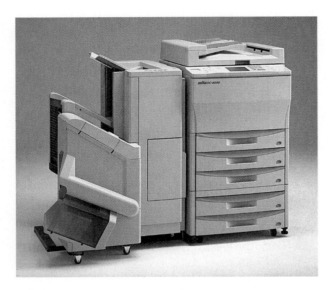

Figure 10-16 A photocopy machine is just one of many kinds of business office equipment.

for a replacement of defective parts at no charge within a certain period of time. An extended warranty can be purchased to cover the period of time after the warranty has expired. For example, a copier may have a one year warranty, but an extended warranty can be purchased to cover parts replacement after the year has expired.

Some office equipment which is heavily used, such as copy machines, carry a service contract for preventive maintenance. This provides maintenance and cleaning of equipment even when it is working properly to avoid a breakdown. A maintenance contract will state in detail what is actually covered by the contract. The dates and frequency of service should be noted carefully.

Literature relating to warranties and preventative maintenance contracts should be kept in a designated file. Since office equipment is expensive these contracts are important.

Equipment Records

Records need to be maintained relating to receipts for major purchases, operating manuals, instructions, guarantees, repair and maintenance instructions. Lists of service people and telephone numbers should be maintained. Many offices maintain a current file of business cards. Ideally, the registration and ID number of each item is maintained in a separate file from the warranty.

Supplies

Vendors, or suppliers, are selected based on several factors including: quality, price, service, and availability. In general, it takes multiple vendors to provide all supplies for a medical practice. Catalog services can provide ease of availability, competitive pricing, and fast delivery.

Many vendors will provide a discount on supplies when they are ordered in large quantities. This results in a unit cost savings. The drawback to this method is that many offices do not have enough storage space to handle a large inventory of supplies. Some suppliers will store excess inventory for you.

Supplies should be rotated on the shelves so that the newer supplies are in the back of the shelf and the older supplies are used first (Figure 10-17).

Expendable supplies and equipment include items that are used up in a short period of time and have a relatively inexpensive unit cost. Examples of expendable office supplies are found in Table 10-3.

Inventory Control

Inventory control requires constant supervision since a medical office cannot afford to run out of supplies. Since many supplies are purchased at lower cost due to unit buying practices, it can be costly to run out and have to suddenly purchase supplies at full price with additional shipping costs for faster service.

Most offices maintain an ongoing inventory system which helps to determine the point at which to reorder supplies. Whenever an item is removed from the supply cabinet it is marked on the inventory sheet. A staff member is assigned the responsibility of reordering all supplies when they get to a certain level so that the supply is never to-

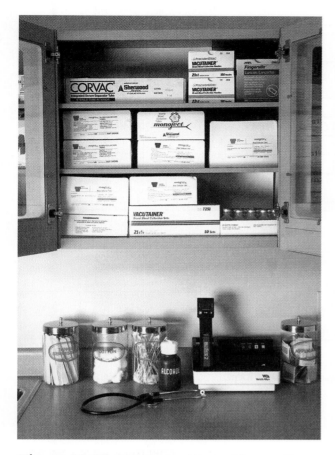

Figure 10-17   Rotate supplies so older supplies are used first.

lating the amount of time it takes to receive a new order, an estimate can be made of when to place an order. For example, if 50 disposable vaginal speculums are used in a gynecologist's office per week and there is a three week reorder period, then a new order must be placed when the supply reaches 150. Since a gynecologist may have seasonal periods when the office is busier, it would be advisable to reorder 200 speculums to prevent running out.

Many offices develop color-coded reorder reminder cards which are inserted into the stack of inventory items. As the color card comes to the top of the stack it is time to reorder. Inventory reminder cards can be maintained with a date for reorder. Some suppliers maintain their own records and will notify the medical office when it is time to reorder.

A list of inventory items should be kept in the procedures manual. Many inventory records are now maintained by using the computer. Table 10-4 provides an example of an office inventory record.

Drug Samples

Pharmaceutical representatives from the drug companies will supply medical offices with samples of medications. These are small packages with one or two doses of a drug. The physician may give these to the patients so they have a day's supply of medicine until they can get a prescription filled.

Drug samples should be kept together in an organized fashion in a cupboard or drawer in the supply room. It is advisable to keep all drugs together by category (for example, sedatives, antibiotics, hypertensives). The expiration dates on drug samples have to be carefully monitored. All samples should be discarded when they have expired. This is done by flushing the medications in the toilet or returning them to the drug company.

tally depleted. The amount of time necessary to have the order processed and delivered needs to be known. See Figure 10-18 for a sample inventory order form.

It takes experience to be able to calculate how long inventory items will last. However, records can be reviewed to determine how many items were used during a three month period. Then, by calcu-

TABLE 10-3   **Expendable Office Supplies**

Type	Example
Paper supplies	Exam table paper, disposable gowns, drapes, paper towels, sterilization bags and tapes, stationary, photocopy paper, insurance and chart forms, laboratory order forms, appointment books, EKG paper, receipt book, appointment cards, current CPT and ICD-9 coding books.
Clinical equipment	Disposable speculums, ear and nose speculum covers, catheters, tongue blades, thermometers, cotton tipped applicators, lubricant, needles, syringes, suture material, dressings, tape, elastic bandages.
Office supplies	Pens, pencils, highlighters, desk blotters, stapler(s).

ORDER	ITEM NAME:	ON ORDER

ORDER QUANTITY: ____________ **REORDER POINT:** ____________

ORDER	QTY	REC D	COST	PREPAID	ON ACCT	ORDER	QTY	REC D	COST	PREPAID	ON ACCT

INVENTORY COUNT:

	JAN	FEB	MAR	APR	MAY	JUN	JUL	AUG	SEP	OCT	NOV	DEC
19 ___												
19 ___												

ORDER SOURCE: **UNIT PRICE:**

The King Company
222 East Maple Avenue
Anytown, IL 60000

Figure 10-18 Sample inventory order form.

TABLE 10-4 **Equipment Inventory Record**

Item	Serial #	Purchase Date	Location
IBM Selectric II Typewriter	XX 12345	2/14/97	Reception
IBM Selectric II Typewriter	XC 54321	2/14/97	Laboratory
IBM G40 Computer	4-190-L1001	9/19/97	Reception
Hewlett-Packard Inkjet Printer	2342VXF	9/19/97	
Xerox Copier	AS 98765	6/2/96	Billing

Doctor's Bag

All physicians have a medical bag with general supplies and also specific supplies that relate to their area of specialization. The medical assistant may be asked to take on the responsibility of making sure there is an ample supply in the bag of anything the physician might need. Since the physician's bag contains medications, it should be locked and kept in a locked closet or office.

The contents of a physician's bag varies depending on the personal preferences and specialty of the physician. Items generally found in a physician's bag include:

- Adhesive tape
- Alcohol or disinfectant
- Ball-point pen
- Culture tubes for throat cultures
- Hypodermic syringes and needles
- Lubricant
- Microscopic slides and fixative
- Ophthalmoscope
- Otoscope
- Pen flashlight
- Percussion hammer
- Portable sphygmomanometer
- Prescription pad
- Probe
- Scissors
- Specimen containers
- Sterile dressings
- Sterile gloves
- Sterile hemostat/forceps
- Sterile scalpel
- Sterile suture set

- Sterile swabs
- Sterile tongue depressors
- Stethoscope
- Sutures
- Thermometer (oral and rectal)
- Tourniquet

Drugs carried in physician's bag may include:

- Adrenaline
- Thorazine
- Demerol
- Antibiotic (for example, penicillin)
- Antihistamine
- Seconal
- Spirits of ammonia

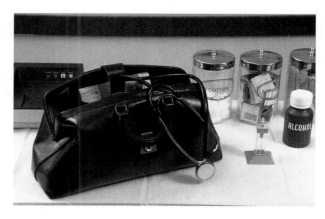

Figure 10-19   Contents of the physician's bag.

These medications are discussed more thoroughly in Chapter 31. Figure 10-19 illustrates the supplies contained in the physician's bag.

A checklist should be prepared of everything the physician wants in the bag. The bag should be checked on a daily basis by the medical assistant.

1. Check all the contents against the checklist and replace all items that are missing.
2. Remove any specimens. Make sure they are labeled and send them on for processing.
3. Remove all used instruments, clean, sterilize, and return them to the bag.
4. Replace all disposable items.
5. Make sure that all instruments are in proper working condition (for example, batteries in flashlight).
6. All sterile instruments should be re-sterilized on a weekly basis even if they were not used.
7. Replace all sterile items when the date has expired.

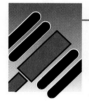

LEGAL AND ETHICAL ISSUES

The employer has the responsibility, according to OSHA guidelines, to protect the employee's health from infectious disease. The medical assistant has a responsibility to correctly follow OSHA guidelines for self-protection and to protect other employees and patients.

The medical assistant has a duty to report any incident such as the accidental administration of a medication to a patient, a patient fall or injury, or theft.

Working with inventory requires integrity. Office and medical supplies must not leave the medical office unless the physician orders them for the patient. Vendors and suppliers must be dealt with in an honest manner.

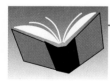

PATIENT EDUCATION

Safety precautions are the responsibility of all medical office personnel. The medical assistant's thorough understanding of medical office policy regarding fire safety, infectious waste, and office security results in better patient education, understanding, and protection.

Some patients are insulted when the person caring for them applies gloves before touching them. The medical assistant may need to explain to patients the rationale for wearing protective clothing by medical personnel.

Summary

Safety measures including general safety, employee safety, emergency plans such as fire, the handling of biological hazards and bloodborne pathogens, housekeeping procedures, proper body mechanics, security, and environment are essential to maintaining a safe and pleasant workplace. The efforts of a medical assistant can be critical in insuring that all of these components are carefully regarded.

Competency Review

1. Define and spell the glossary terms for this chapter.
2. List 6 safety rules to follow in medical offices.
3. Upon arriving for a blood pressure checkup, Jeff Deal slips on the newly washed floor and hits his head on the edge of the front desk. Dr. Williams immediately checks Mr. Deal and determines that, other than a small bruise on his head, he appears to be fine. There is a hazard sign indicating the wet floor. This accident occurred at 9:00 a.m. on December 21st. Complete an incident report using the form in Figure 10-12.
4. List and describe 15 items commonly found in the physician's bag.
5. What do the letters R-A-C-E represent?
6. You have been asked to draft the OSHA Exposure Plan for your office. What three points must you include in this plan?
7. Describe 5 guidelines stated in the OSHA Standard for using protective equipment.

PREPARING FOR THE CERTIFICATION EXAM

Test Taking Tip — When answering multiple choice questions always eliminate the incorrect responses by crossing through them on the exam.

Examination Review Questions

1. Medical waste consists of all of the following except
   (A) radioactive waste
   (B) occupational waste
   (C) infectious waste
   (D) chemical waste
   (E) solid waste

2. To provide protection from HIV or HBV, when carrying a urine specimen wear
   (A) gown
   (B) mask and goggles
   (C) mask and gloves
   (D) gloves
   (E) gloves and eye shield

3. Use Standard Precautions when giving an injection to which type of patient?
   (A) HIV positive patient
   (B) small child
   (C) hypertensive patient
   (D) diabetic patient
   (E) all of the above

4. An incident report would be used for all of the following EXCEPT
   (A) missing syringes
   (B) theft
   (C) employee arriving late for work
   (D) patient fall
   (E) lost dentures

5. Proper body mechanics mainly involves the use of which muscles?
   (A) arm
   (B) back
   (C) leg
   (D) neck
   (E) all of the above

6. OSHA reports for employee Hepatitis B vaccine records must be maintained for at least
   (A) 30 years
   (B) 3 years
   (C) 1 year
   (D) forever
   (E) none of the above is correct

7. Hepatitis B is transmitted through
   (A) blood
   (B) blood and feces
   (C) feces
   (D) mucus membranes
   (E) all of the above

8. Factor(s) required for fire to start?
   (A) oxygen
   (B) fuel
   (C) heat
   (D) spark
   (E) all of the above

9. Capital equipment includes all of the following except
   (A) carpeting
   (B) EKG machine
   (C) pictures
   (D) files
   (E) typewriter

10. When working with vendors you should expect all of the following except
    (A) unit pricing
    (B) inventory count
    (C) competitive pricing
    (D) fast delivery
    (E) quality assurance

ON THE JOB

Gail Rowe, a medical assistant in Dr. Williams's practice, has been asked to take over responsibility for equipment, including acquisitions, and maintaining an inventory of consumable supplies. Gail knows that Dr. Williams was displeased with how the last medical assistant stocked the inventory and that they were 20% over budget. Dr. Williams expects Gail to remedy the situation and to replace one of the older EKG machines.

Gail calls Bob O'Malley, a medical supplier, to discuss the purchase of the new computerized EKG machine. Bob tells Gail that he can get her a deal on the new piece of equipment saying, "If you give me your business, I'll make it worth your while. . . ." He further explains that the machine can be "dirt cheap" as long as Gail agrees to purchase all of the EKG supplies from him like the last medical assistant did. Bob invites Gail out to lunch saying that they can work out the details then.

What is your response?

1. Is it ethical for Gail to let Bob buy her lunch?
2. Is lunch an appropriate venue for discussing the acquisition of new medical equipment?
3. If Bob is alluding to a kickback, is it ethical for Gail to be a party to such a thing?
4. Must Gail keep Dr. Williams appraised of her dealings with Bob? All of them?
5. Should Gail trust that Bob will give her the best deal or should she get other quotes?
6. If Bob brings up the prior medical assistant during conversation, is it ethical for Gail to discuss why she left the practice and Dr. Williams's feelings about her performance?
7. How can Gail approach Bob regarding the cost of the machine and consumables given that her mission is to bring down costs?

References

Badash, S., and Chesebro, D. *Introduction to Health Occupations.* Upper Saddle River, NJ: Brady/Prentice Hall, 1997.

Decker, M. "The OSHA Bloodborne Hazard Standard." *Infection Control and Hospital Epidemiology.* 12:7, 1992.

Gerberding, L. "Reducing Occupational Risk of HIV Infection." *Hospital Practice.* June, 1991.

Handling Medical Waste. Virginia Beach, VA: Coastal Video Communications Corp., 1993.

Kelsay, E. "Understanding OSHA's Bloodbourne Pathogens Standard." *Professional Medical Assistant.* July/August, 1992.

Michels, K. "Final OSHA Bloodbourne Standard Released." *AANA Journal,* 60:1, 1992.

O'Brien, L., Bartlett, K. "TB Plus HIV Spells Trouble." *American Journal of Nursing.* 92:5, 1992.

Richardson, D. "OSHA Releases Final Standard on HIV, Hepatitis B Exposures." *American Nurse,* 24:1, 1992.

Rodriques, P. "Handling and Disposal of Infectious Waste in the Office Setting." *Orthopedic Nursing,* 10:5, 1991.

US Department of Health and Human Services, Centers for Disease Control and Prevention. Draft Guidelines for Isolation Precautions for Hospitals. *Federal Register.* Washington, DC: US Government Printing Office, November 7, 1994.

MEDICAL ASSISTANT ROLE DELINEATION CHART

Highlight indicates material covered in this chapter

ADMINISTRATIVE

ADMINISTRATIVE PROCEDURES

- Perform basic clerical functions
- Schedule, coordinate, and monitor appointments
- Schedule inpatient/outpatient admissions and procedures
- Understand and apply third party guidelines
- Obtain reimbursement through accurate claims submission
- Monitor third-party reimbursement
- Perform medical transcription
- Understand and adhere to managed care policies and procedures
- *Negotiate managed care contracts (adv)*

PRACTICE FINANCES

- Perform procedural and diagnostic coding
- Apply bookkeeping principles
- Document and maintain accounting and banking records
- Manage accounts receivable
- Manage accounts payable
- Process payroll
- *Develop and maintain fee schedules (adv)*
- *Manage renewals of business and professional insurance policies (adv)*
- *Manage personal benefits and maintain records (adv)*

CLINICAL

FUNDAMENTAL PRINCIPLES

- Apply principles of aseptic technique and infection control
- Comply with quality assurance practices
- Screen and follow up patient test results

DIAGNOSTIC ORDERS

- Collect and process specimens
- Perform diagnostic tests

PATIENT CARE

- Adhere to established triage procedures
- Obtain patient history and vital signs
- Prepare and maintain examination and treatment areas

- Prepare patient for examinations, procedures, and treatments
- Assist with examinations, procedures, and treatments
- Prepare and administer medications and immunizations
- Maintain medication and immunization records
- Recognize and respond to emergencies
- Coordinate patient care information with other health care providers

GENERAL (TRANSDISCIPLINARY)

PROFESSIONALISM

- Project a professional manner and image
- Adhere to ethical principles
- Demonstrate initiative and responsibility
- Work as a team member
- Manage time efficiently
- Prioritize and perform multiple tasks
- Adapt to change
- Promote the CMA credential
- Enhance skills through continuing education

COMMUNICATION SKILLS

- Treat all patients with compassion and empathy
- Recognize and respect cultural diversity
- Adapt communications to individual's ability to understand
- Use professional telephone technique
- Use effective and correct verbal and written communications
- Recognize and respond to verbal and non-verbal communications
- Use medical terminology appropriately
- Receive, organize, prioritize, and transmit information
- Serve as liaison
- Promote the practice through positive public relations

LEGAL CONCEPTS

- Maintain confidentiality
- Practice within the scope of education, training, and personal capabilities
- Prepare and maintain medical records
- Document accurately
- Use appropriate guidelines when releasing information
- Follow employer's established policies dealing with the health care contract
- Follow federal, state, and local legal guidelines
- Maintain awareness of federal and state health care legislation and regulations
- Maintain and dispose of regulated substances in compliance with government guidelines
- Comply with established risk management and safety procedures
- Recognize professional credentialing criteria
- Participate in the development and maintenance of personnel, policy, and procedure manuals
- *Develop and maintain personnel, policy, and procedure manuals (adv)*

INSTRUCTION

- Instruct individuals according to their needs
- Explain office policies and procedures
- Teach methods of health promotion and disease prevention
- Locate community resources and disseminate information
- *Orient and train personnel (adv)*
- *Develop educational materials (adv)*
- *Conduct continuing education activities (adv)*

OPERATIONAL FUNCTIONS

- Maintain supply inventory
- Evaluate and recommend equipment and supplies
- Apply computer techniques to support office operations
- *Supervise personnel (adv)*
- *Interview and recommend job applicants (adv)*
- *Negotiate leases and prices for equipment and supply contracts (adv)*

SOURCE: Reprinted by permission of the American Association of Medical Assistants from the *AAMA Role Delineation Study: Occupational Analysis of the Medical Assisting Profession.*

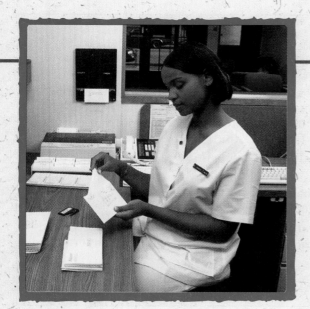

11

Written Communication

LEARNING OBJECTIVES

After completing this chapter, you should:

1. Define and spell the glossary terms for this chapter.
2. Name and describe eight areas to consider when letter writing.
3. Identify the eight parts of speech and use them correctly.
4. Explain the process of proofreading and editing.
5. Describe the process of drafting correspondence using the four methods of letter styles.
6. List and describe how to prepare an envelope to meet the standards of the US Postal Service.
7. State the four classifications of mail service.
8. List and describe six special services offered by the Postal Service.
9. Identify four mail handling tips.
10. Summarize the ethical implications related to written correspondence.

ADMINISTRATIVE PERFORMANCE COMPETENCIES

1. Compose a letter using correct terminology, positive tone, gender neutral language, and correct grammar.
2. Proofread and correct correspondence.
3. Compose a letter using the four main parts for a letter.
4. Type medical office correspondence using the block, modified block, modified block with indented paragraphs, and the simplified letter styles.
5. Identify the three basic sizes of letterhead stationery and envelopes.
6. Correctly fold and insert a letter into an envelope.
7. Process large amounts of mail by separating into the four categories and handling each piece of mail only once.
8. Address an envelope using the correct format to facilitate postal service scanning.
9. Select references from a professional library.

Glossary

active voice   The subject of the sentence performs the action.

block   Style of letter writing in which all lines are flush with the left margin.

gender bias   Indicating either male or female by the type of language used.

gender neutral   Unable to determine which gender is referred to based on the language used.

homophones   Words which sound alike but have different meanings and spellings.

modified block   Style of letter writing in which the date, complimentary close, and signature line begin in the center with all other lines at the left margin.

passive voice   The subject of the sentence receives the action.

proofreading   Reviewing or reading printed, typed, and handwritten material to check for content (grammar, spelling, style) and mechanical (typing, printing) errors.

redundant   Repetitive.

thesaurus   Reference book that lists words alphabetically and gives synonyms for each entry word.

transcription   Listening to dictation of a medical record while typing it into a written record.

Medical assistants draft many types of correspondence to be signed by the physician/employer. These letters must reflect the professionalism of the medical practice and the physician. The physical appearance of letters depends on the selection of quality paper, letterhead design, and the choice of formats for the letters. But, the most professional looking correspondence is quickly and harshly judged when the letter is written in a negative or condescending tone, and is filled with grammatical errors. Correspondence should be positive in tone and well written.

Handling incoming mail requires efficiency in sorting, dating, and reading all correspondence. Correct handling of the mail can save money and time for the medial practice. Initiative in handling mail quickly and accurately is paramount.

Medical transcription, which is the processing of medical records, dictation, requires careful attention to detail, a thorough knowledge of medical terminology, and excellent typing skills. This type of written correspondence is covered fully in Chapter 13.

Letter Writing

Letters from a medical office must be professional, courteous, businesslike, project a positive tone, and protect the confidentiality of the physician and the patient. This requires some diplomacy. For example, when drafting a sensitive letter requesting payment for a long overdue bill or to advise a patient to seek the services of another physician, such letters should be clear and to the point. The situation should be explained and the expected outcome presented—"Please send a check for (amount due)" or "Please call to make payment arrangements." Threats or derogatory comments are never acceptable in professional correspondence and may have legal consequences for the sender. The following letters are examples of positive and negative tones in writing.

Negative Example:

Dear Mrs. Murray:
You have repeatedly failed to take medications as prescribed and follow my recommended treatment. Since you have again failed to keep an appointment, I am forced to withdraw as your physician, and I request that you find another physician immediately.

Positive Example:

Dear Mrs. Murray:
During your last visit, we discussed the necessity of continuing medical treatment for you to recover fully from your recent medical problems. Therefore, I am concerned that you failed to keep your appointment this week and have not called the office to schedule a new appointment. Your health continues to be important to me so I am requesting that you call me as soon as possible to discuss future treatment.

If we are unable to reach a mutual understanding about your medical treatment and appointment schedule, I regret that I will not be able to continue as your physician. In that event, you will receive a letter indicating that you have a month's notice in which to secure the services of another physician.

Word Choice

The use of correct words when writing office correspondence includes avoidance of the use of technical terms, gender bias, long sentences and paragraphs, excessive use of the personal pronoun "I", repetition, and the passive voice.

Technical Terminology

When writing a letter to medical professionals or institutions that employ medically trained staff, the use of correct medical terminology is essential. This terminology is specialized and is easily understood by medically trained professionals. Many patients are not familiar with medical terminology, and, in fact, may not understand or may be intimidated by this style of writing. Table 11-1 lists selected medical terms with corresponding synonyms that may be more easily recognized by patients. The medical terms in the left-hand column are appropriate for medically trained personnel correspondence (physician to physician, physician to the medical record, medical assistant to hospital); the terms in the right-hand column are more easily understood by patients.

Removing Gender Bias

Unfortunately it is quite common in the medical field to assume that every nurse is female and all physicians are male since this was the case many generations ago. Federal legislation is in place to eliminate gender bias in the workplace. This means that, according to the law, either a male or female can be hired for any position.

Gender-neutral terms are preferred to reflect this change in the workplace. This means that any reference to a particular gender (male or female) should be eliminated. For example, a male orderly should be referred to as a medical attendant, cleaning ladies are called housekeeping or cleaning personnel, a stewardess is called a flight attendant and the chairman of a committee is referred to as the chair of the committee.

Written correspondence must also reflect this same neutral bias toward the genders. When writing about physicians, do not refer to them as males or nurses and medical assistants as females. For example, "The patient was referred to a hospital dietitian for diabetic diet instruction. The patient was told to ask *her* about a food exchange list." This wording assumed the dietitian was a female. A better statement would be, "The patient was instructed to ask the dietitian about a food exchange list." In order to write in a gender-neutral style, you may have to rewrite the sentence or change a pronoun from singular to plural. For example, you might say, "The *physicians* were asked to discuss *their* gynecology practices."

Sentence and Paragraph Length

Short, concise sentences and paragraphs are preferred in medical writing. Sentence length should never exceed twenty words. Eliminate all words that are unnecessary. The paragraph should only cover one point. A good paragraph contains from two to six sentences. Your reader may stop reading if the paragraph is too long.

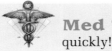 **Med Tip:** Get to the point quickly!

Personal Pronoun

Whenever possible, it is preferable to avoid the use of the personal pronoun "I" in professional writing. It is better to focus writing on the word "you" since this involves the reader. For example, a statement such as, "I am asking that any overdue balance be cleared up immediately. I will have to take steps to send this account to a collection agency if it is not paid immediately," is considered negative. When requesting a patient to pay an overdue bill, it is better to write, "We know that you will want to clear up any overdue account. This overdue balance may have been an oversight on your part. If that is the case, would you kindly remit your payment in the enclosed envelope."

Repetition, Redundancy, and Inflated Phrases

The reader of your correspondence wants to know in concise terms what you are telling them. Avoid

TABLE 11-1 Medical Terms and Corresponding Synonyms

Medical Term	Synonym
carcinoma	Cancer
cardiac	Heart
dermatitis	Skin irritation
diabetes mellitus	Diabetes
gastric	Stomach
gynecology	Study of female diseases
hepatic disease	Liver disease
hyperglycemic	Excessive blood sugar
hypertension	High blood pressure
larynx	Voice box
leukocytes	White blood cells
MI	Heart attack Myocardial infarction
nephroses	Kidney disease
NPO	Nothing by mouth
otolaryngology	Study of ear and throat
para I	First delivery
pc	After meals
thrombus	Blood clot

repeating the same statement over again. **Redundant** expressions include such terms as "each and every, first and foremost, and physician's patient." The above examples can be simplified by stating "each, first, or the patient."

Inflated phrases can usually be eliminated without any loss of meaning. Common examples are introductory word groups such as "in my opinion, I think that, it seems that, one must," and so on. Table 11-2 contains examples of inflated patterns of writing versus concise terms.

Active Versus Passive Voice

The active verbs can make writing more interesting. In the **active voice** the subject of the sentence does the action; in the **passive voice**, the subject receives the action. Although both voices are grammatically correct, the active voice is considered more effective because it is simpler, more direct, and less wordy.

To transform a sentence from the passive to active voice, make the actor the subject of the sentence. Table 11-3 contains examples of statements in both active and passive voice.

Composing Letters

Composing letters can be a simple process when an organized approach is used. The guidelines shown on page 202 may help.

Spelling

There are several words in the English language which have similar pronunciations but very

TABLE 11-2   Inflated Phrases Versus Concise Terms

Inflated	Concise
Along the lines of	Like
As a matter of fact	In fact
At all times	Always
At the present time	Now, currently
At this point in time	Now, currently
Because of the fact that	Because
By means of	By
By virtue of the fact that	Because
Due to the fact that	Because
For the purpose of	For
For the reason that	Because
Have the ability to	Be able to
In light of the fact that	Because
In the nature of	Like
In order to	To
In spite of the fact that	Although, though
In the event that	If
In the final analysis	Finally
In the neighborhood of	About
Until such time as	Until

different meanings and spellings. These words are called **homophones**. They pose problems unless the writer is careful about their usage. Table 11-4 contains some of the most common homophones.

Computer software programs cannot be depended upon to correct word use since they do not "understand" the data input or content of the correspondence. For example, use of the word *effect* or *affect* depends on the content and could not be determined by the software program. Both spellings are correct and only the individual using the word in the sentence would be able to determine if the word is the correct choice.

English grammar books, such as *The Bedford Handbook for Writers,* contain lists of the most fre-

quently misspelled words in the English language. See Table 11-5 for examples of the most commonly misspelled medical terms.

Capitalization

General rules for capitalization are given in Table 11-6.

Plurals

Some basic rules for forming plurals of words are
- Abbreviations are formed into plurals by adding an *s* (EKGs, DRGs)
- Plurals of nouns are formed by adding an *s* or an *es* (physicians, suffixes)

TABLE 11-3 Active Versus Passive Voice

Active voice	Passive voice
The medical assistant took the patient's blood pressure measurement.	The patient's blood pressure measurement was taken by the medical assistant.
The surgeon performed an appendectomy on the patient.	An appendectomy was performed on the patient by the surgeon.
The medical committee reached a decision.	A decision was reached by the medical committee.

Guidelines: Composing Letters

1. Determine the reason for the correspondence. Write down the main purpose for the letter.
2. Make a list of all the points you will cover in the letter. Have any supporting documents, such as the patient's medical record or billing file available. Prepare a rough draft of the letter. Arrange the ideas in a logical manner so the reader will be able to follow them easily.
3. Make sure the letter has a *beginning, middle,* and *end.*
   - The beginning or introduction should catch the interest of the reader.
   - The middle should contain all the supporting facts and details relating to the purpose for the letter.
   - The end should be brief, pleasant, and indicate any action that is to be taken by the reader or the writer.
4. Use a natural style of writing; avoid pretentious language. Avoid medical terms when writing to the lay person. Also avoid inflated phrases (see Table 11-2).
5. Use a positive tone—negative writing should always be avoided.
6. Writing should contain the five "Cs." It should be:
   - Clear
   - Complete
   - Concise
   - Consistent
   - Courteous
7. Pay particular attention to spelling, punctuation, and grammar.

Basic rules for forming plurals of medical terms with specific endings are listed in Table 11-7 along with examples for each.

Numbers

In general, the numbers 1 to 10 are spelled out—one to ten—in correspondence. For numbers greater than ten, it is acceptable to use the number designation, for example 128, 1020, 32. The only exception to this rule is when the number is at the beginning of a sentence. It should then be spelled out. See Table 11-8 for a further description of the use of numbers in correspondence.

Parts of Speech

Traditional grammar recognizes eight parts of speech: noun, pronoun, verb, adjective, adverb, preposition, conjunction, and interjection. Many words are able to function as more than one part of speech. For example, depending on its use in a sentence, the word cut can be a noun—The cut is fresh—or a verb—The surgeon cut into the organ. Table 11-9 provides a quick reference to parts of speech.

Error Correction in Office Correspondence

Word processing has made correspondence correction much easier. Word processing allows the writer to display the document on the screen of the word processor or computer or reenter the document and make changes. This new document is then saved and printed.

Corrections made to typed letters require the use of correction ribbons, tapes, or fluids. Any corrections on correspondence should be inconspicuous. If more than a few words need correction then the entire document needs to be retyped. It is

TABLE 11-4   **Common Homophones**

Word	Meaning	Word	Meaning
accept	to receive	fare	money for transportation, food or drink
except	to take or leave out		
advice	opinion about what to do for a problem	hear	to sense by the ear
		here	this place
advise	to offer advice	hole	hollow place
affect	to exert an influence	whole	entire; unhurt
effect	result; to accomplish	its	of or belonging to it
all ready	prepared	it's	contraction for it is
already	by this time	know	to be aware of
altar	a structure on which religious ceremonies are held	no	opposite of yes
		lessen	to make less
alter	to change	lesson	something learned
always	every time; forever	loose	free; not secured
all ways	every way	lose	to be deprived of
bare	naked	pair	set of two
bear	to carry; to put up with	pare	to trim
brake	something used to stop movement; to stop	pear	fruit
break	to split or smash	patience	calm endurance
buy	to purchase	patients	a doctor's clients
by	near	personal	private; intimate
choose	to select	personnel	a group of employees
chose	past tense of choose	precede	to come before
cite	to quote	proceed	to go forward
sight	vision	quiet	silent; calm
site	position, place	quite	very
complement	to complete	right	proper or just; correct
compliment	praise	rite	a ritual
conscience	sense of right and wrong	write	to put words on paper
conscious	awake; aware	stationary	standing still
elicit	to draw or bring out	stationery	writing paper
illicit	illegal	taught	past tense of teach
fair	lovely; light-colored	taut	tight

(Continued on next page)

TABLE 11-4   Common Homophones (Continued)

Word	Meaning	Word	Meaning
than	besides	waist	midsection
then	at that time; next	waste	to squander
their	belonging to them	weak	feeble
they're	contraction of they are	week	seven days
there	that place or position	weather	state of the atmosphere
through	by means of; finished	whether	indicating a choice between alternatives
threw	past tense of throw	who's	contraction of who is
thorough	careful; complete	whose	possessive of who
to	toward	your	possessive of you
too	also	you're	contraction of you are
two	one or more in number		

TABLE 11-5   Commonly Misspelled Medical Terms

abscess	defibrillator	ischium	perforation	respiratory
additive	ecchymosis	larynx	pericardium	roentgenology
aerosol	effusion	leukemia	perineum	sagittal
agglutination	epididymis	malaise	peristalsis	sciatica
albumin	epistaxis	malleus	peritoneum	serous
anastomosis	eustachian	mellitus	petit mal	sphincter
aneurysm	fissure	menstruation	pharynx	sphygmo-manometer
anteflexion	glaucoma	metastasis	pituitary	squamous
arrhythmia	gonorrhea	neuron	plantar	staphylococcus
bilirubin	hemorrhage	occlusion	pleura	suppuration
bronchial	hemorrhoids	oscilloscope	pleurisy	trochanter
calcaneus	homeostasis	osseous	pneumonia	venous
capillary	humerus	palliative	polyp	wheal
cervical	idiosyncrasy	parasite	prophylaxis	xiphoid
chromosome	ileum	parenteral	prostate	
cirrhosis	ilium	parietal	prosthesis	
clavicle	infarction	paroxysmal	pruritis	
curettage	intussusception	pemphigus	psoriasis	
cyanosis	ischemia	percussion	pyrexia	

considered unprofessional for a document to have a "white-out" type of correction fluid apparent on the document.

Standard Components of the Business Letter

All letters contain the same basic parts starting at the top of a letter and moving down to the end.

TABLE 11-6 Rules for Capitalization

First word of

- Sentences
- Expressions used as sentences
- Each item in a list or outline
- Salutation and closing of a letter

Proper name of person, place, or thing

- John F. Kennedy
- New York City
- Sears Tower

Noun that is part of a proper name

- Professor Mary King
- Dr. Beth Williams
- Michigan Avenue

Med Tip: Note that error correction within a typed correspondence and within the medical record are handled differently. Corrections can be made within typed materials, before they are sent out or filed, to correct such items as typing and grammatical errors. However, corrections made within the patient's medical record must be handled according to the method described in Chapter 21. The use of white-out correction fluid, erasures and other types of document alterations cannot be made on the medical record, which is a legal document.

These include the heading, date, inside address, salutation, body, closing, and reference initials. In some specialized cases, such as with insurance correspondence, there may be special components added for clarification such as the insurer's identification number.

Heading

Medical office letters are usually typed on letterhead stationery bearing the name of the physician (Beth Williams, MD) or practice (Windy City Clinic), address, telephone number, and FAX number. See Figure 11-1 for an illustration of letterhead stationery. If the physician does not use letterhead stationery, the letter should be typed or printed on good quality bond paper with the return address typed above the date on the upper left side of the paper.

TABLE 11-7 Rules for Forming Plurals of Medical Terms (nouns)

Ending	Rule	Example
a	ae	vertebra to vertebrae
ax	aces	thorax to thoraces
ex, ix	ices	apex to apices
is	es	metastasis to metastases
on	a	ganglion to ganglia
um	a	ovum to ova
us	i	nucleus to nuclei
y	ies	biopsy to biopsies
nx	ges	phalanx to phalanges

TABLE 11-8   Use of Numbers in Correspondence

Type	Explanation of When to Use
.Decimals	Write using figures without commas (23.04).
Figures	Only numbers (including 1-10) are used in tables, statistical data, dates, money, percentages, and time.
Measurements	Write out in figures (23 inches).
Percentages	Write out in figures and spell out percent (20 percent).
Tables	When typing numbers or placing them in columns align as follows: • Arabic numerals (1, 2, 3) aligned on the right. • Decimals (1.33) are aligned on the decimal. • Roman numerals (I, II, III) are aligned on the left.
Time	Do not use zeros when writing on-the-hour time. Use AM and PM with the time designation (10 AM, not 10:00 AM).

TABLE 11-9   Eight Parts of Speech

Part of Speech	Definition	Example
noun	Names a person, place, or thing.	Medical assistant, office.
pronoun	Substitutes for a noun.	I, me, you, he, him, she, her, it, we, us, they, them.
verb	Helping verb: comes before main verb. Main verb: asserts action, being, or state of being.	Operate, write, speak, obtain, is, are, am.
adjective	Modifies a noun or pronoun, usually answering the questions: Which one? What kind of? How many?	*Responsible* medical assistant. The articles *a, an,* and *the* are adjectives.
adverb	Modifies a verb, adjective, or adverb usually answering the questions: When? Where? Why? How? Under what conditions? To what degree?	Gently, extremely, nicely, quietly.
preposition	Indicates the relationship between the noun and pronoun that follows it and another word in the sentence.	About, above, across, after.
conjunction	Connects words or word groups.	And, but, nor, for, so, yet, after, although.
interjection	Word used to express strong feeling.	Oh, hurrah, ouch.

Date

Every correspondence must have a current date. The month must not be abbreviated, followed by the day and year (January 1, 1999). The date is usually placed three lines (spaces) below the letterhead or on line 15 if there is no letterhead. Four to six lines (spaces) are left after the date before the inside address.

Inside Address

The inside address contains the name, title, company name (if applicable), and address of the per-

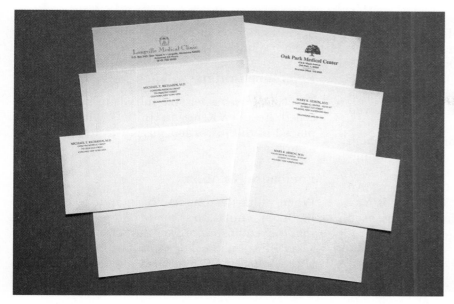

Figure 11-1 Different letter-head stationery and envelopes.

son who is to receive the correspondence. This is typed at the left margin and single spaced. If there is a company name (for example, medical practice, clinic, hospital) it must be typed exactly as shown on their own letterhead.

All words in the inside address (such as street name) are spelled out fully. The city is followed by a comma, the two-letter state abbreviation followed by two spaces, and then the ZIP code. If the inside address contains a long line it may be divided into two lines so that the inside address is in balance. The second of these two lines would be indented two spaces. See the example below.

Marvin Hammer, MD
123 Bonneymeadow
  Plaza in the Park
Chicago, IL 60610

Business courtesy recommends always including a title with the receiver's name on the inside address. For example:

Beth Williams, MD
Ms. Helen Daly
Mrs. Homer Olson
Mr. Thomas Freeman
Miss Jane Merryweather

Salutation

The salutation, a courteous greeting, is typed at the left margin and spaced two lines below the

Guidelines: Using Courtesy Titles

1. *Mr.* is always an appropriate title for men.
2. If there is a professional title, such as *MD* or *PhD*, this is used instead of the courtesy title.
3. *Ms.* is used when the marital status of a woman is unknown.
4. *Mrs.* is appropriate for a married woman if she prefers that title. However it is always safe to use *Ms.*
5. *Miss* is appropriate for unmarried women who prefer that title. It is also used for young girls.
6. Two people at the same address with different last names should be addressed individually. For example: Dr. Beth Williams and Mr. Allan Radde.
7. A professional title, such as *owner*, *president*, *manager*, may be placed next to the name or below it depending on which is a better balance.

Allan Radde, President Dinesh Shey, PhD
Radde and Associates Department Chair

8. If there is no record of the correct spelling of a receiver's name, then call the company or office and ask for the correct spelling.

inside address. The name in the salutation must agree with the name in the inside address. If the letter is going to a physician named Williams, the salutation would read, "Dear Dr. Williams:." A colon is placed after this type of salutation. If the person is well known to the writer, the first name is often used, for example "Dear Beth," followed by a comma.

When sending a letter to a company in which the individual who will receive the letter is unknown, use salutations such as "Dear Sir or Madame" or "Dear Ladies and Gentlemen." An anonymous salutation, such as "To whom it may concern," while generally avoided, may be used when the reader is unknown.

Body

The body contains the purpose of the letter. The body begins two spaces below the salutation and is single spaced, with a double space between each paragraph. The paragraphs of the body are either blocked or indented depending on the style (format) of the letter. A letter may be any length, however, most letters bearing a single message are usually two to three paragraphs in length and contained on a single page.

Med Tip: Remember: due to the large amount of mail that comes into a medical office, the reader may not wish to read long letters. Limit letters to one page whenever possible.

Closing

The letter closing consists of a complimentary close containing a courtesy word(s), such as "Sincerely," "Sincerely yours," or "Yours truly." This appears two spaces below the end of the body of the letter.

The signature line is typed four spaces below the complimentary close and contains the name and title of the writer. If the name and title are on the same line, they are divided with a comma. The personal title of the writer (such as Mr. and Ms.) is not included in the signature line. The exception to this is when the writer may wish to indicate his or her gender if the reader may be confused, for example, Ms. Leslie Lapointe or Mr. Pat Timmons.

The signature of the writer must be placed on the letter directly above the typed signature line before it is sent. A handwritten signature indicates to the reader that the writer has read and approved

the letter. Since a signature can be difficult to read, the full name of the sender is always typed on the signature line.

Reference Initials

The typist uses reference initials to indicate who typed the letter. Reference initials, when used, are placed at the lower left margin in lowercase, for example *bff*.

Enclosure Notation

When other documents are included along with the letter a notation is made on the letter indicating the enclosure. Examples of enclosures are x-ray films, medical records, and brochures. The abbreviation ENC. is used or the word "Enclosures" can be written out.

> Enclosures (2)
> x-ray lumbar spine
> surgical report 12/12/19xx

Copy Notation

A copy of all correspondence is always filed in the office. In some cases a copy of the letter is sent to someone other than the addressee. This is noted at the bottom left of the letter by typing the initials "cc:" before the recipient's name. The title of the recipient is often added.

> For example:
> cc: Jane Paulson, Office Manager

Two-Page Letter

When the letter is too long to fit on one page, a second sheet of plain stationery is used. Letterhead stationery is used only for the top sheet. The plain, bond second sheet should be of the same quality and color as the top letterhead stationery. A margin of one inch is left at the bottom of the first page.

Med Tip: Do not leave a "widow/orphan" at the top of the second page. A "widow/orphan" refers to a lone line. At least two lines of the first page should be carried over to the second page if a paragraph must be divided.

Leave a one inch margin at the top of the second and all subsequent pages. Place a heading, such as the name of the individual the letter is being sent to and the page number, at the top of each subsequent page. This is usually placed in the top right margin.

Form Letters

Form letters can save time for the medical assistant. A form letter is developed when the same letter is sent to several different people. Figure 11-2 illustrates an example of a form letter that can be used as a base when constructing a letter of withdrawal. The letter would be personalized with the patient's name and the signature of the physician.

The use of a computer and/or a word processor with memory individualizes the form letter. The body of the letter, called the constant information, is retained in the computer's memory or on a computer disk. The areas of the letter that require personalization, such as the date, inside address and salutation, are called the variables. The variables can be stored on a separate disk and/or database and then merged into the disk or main drive of the computer which stores the constant information. In this manner a set of data, such as names and addresses of patients for billing purposes, can be used with a form letter enclosed

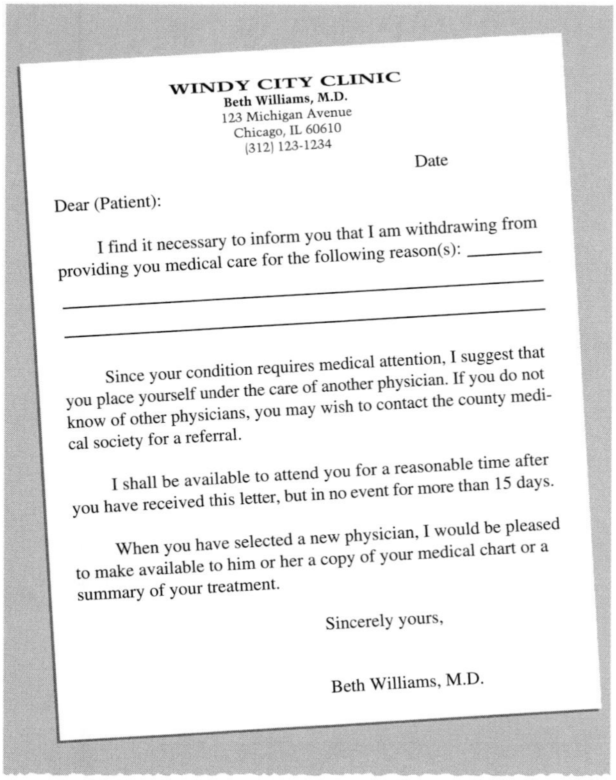

WINDY CITY CLINIC
Beth Williams, M.D.
123 Michigan Avenue
Chicago, IL 60610
(312) 123-1234

Date

Dear (Patient):

I find it necessary to inform you that I am withdrawing from providing you medical care for the following reason(s): _____

_____

Since your condition requires medical attention, I suggest that you place yourself under the care of another physician. If you do not know of other physicians, you may wish to contact the county medical society for a referral.

I shall be available to attend you for a reasonable time after you have received this letter, but in no event for more than 15 days.

When you have selected a new physician, I would be pleased to make available to him or her a copy of your medical chart or a summary of your treatment.

Sincerely yours,

Beth Williams, M.D.

Figure 11-2 A form letter is a type of letter that is sent repeatedly to many patients.

with the monthly bill. Chapter 12 contains more information regarding the use of the computer in the medical office.

Form letters require few changes. A file of frequently used form letters should be maintained in the office files. The physician may review a copy of a form letter and make a few changes which can easily be added by the medical assistant.

Letter Styles

Letter styles vary depending on the purpose. Letter styles include **block**, **modified block** (standard), modified block with indented paragraphs, and a simplified letter style. Block and modified block are the most commonly used in the medical office.

The block letter style format is spaced with all lines, from the date through the signature line, flush with the left margin. There is a space separating each paragraph and between inside address, salutation, body, and close. Since there are no indentations for paragraphs, this format saves typing time.

The modified block (standard) style letter has the date, complimentary closing, and the signature line beginning at the center and moving toward the right margin. All other lines are flush with the left margin. This is often preferred since it has a professional, neat appearance. This format requires more time to type since the typist must set and use tabs. The modified block style letter with indented paragraphs is identical to the modified block except that the paragraphs are indented five spaces.

Med Tip: Tabs are set when typing to automatically indent lines to the same point within the document. For instance, tabs are used when working with columns of figures so that all figures line up evenly.

A simplified letter style format is spaced with all lines flush with the left margin. The salutation line is omitted. In its place is a subject line which appears on the third line below the inside address. This subject line is in capital letters and draws attention of the reader to the purpose of the letter. A complimentary closing is also omitted. The signature is also typed in all capital letters on the fifth line below the body. This format is an abbreviated style of writing letters relating to patients. Figure 11-3 shows sample letter formats: block, modified

(a)

WINDY CITY CLINIC
Beth Williams, M.D.
123 Michigan Avenue, Chicago, IL 60610
(312) 123-1234

August 1, 19xx

Thomas Moore
123 Lee Street
Louisville, KY 40223

Dear Mr. Moore:

With the season for colds and flu fast approaching, it is time once again for flu shots. Supplies have arrived and flu shots will be administered starting October 3. Please call the office to schedule a visit for your flu shot at your earliest convenience.

If you wish to wait to get your flu shot at the time of your next appointment, it is not necessary to call the office. An appointment card with the date and time of your next appointment is enclosed.

Sincerely,

Beth Williams, MD

ENC: Appointment card
cc: B. Reed, Office Manager

(b)

WINDY CITY CLINIC
Beth Williams, M.D.
123 Michigan Avenue, Chicago, IL 60610
(312) 123-1234

August 1, 19xx

Thomas Moore
123 Lee Street
Louisville, KY 40223

Dear Mr. Moore:

With the season for colds and flu fast approaching, it is time once again for flu shots. Supplies have arrived and flu shots will be administered starting October 3. Please call the office to schedule a visit for your flu shot at your earliest convenience.

If you wish to wait to get your flu shot at the time of your next appointment, it is not necessary to call the office. An appointment card with the date and time of your next appointment is enclosed.

Sincerely,

Beth Williams, MD

ENC: Appointment card
cc: B. Reed, Office Manager

(c)

WINDY CITY CLINIC
Beth Williams, M.D.
123 Michigan Avenue, Chicago, IL 60610
(312) 123-1234

August 1, 19xx

Thomas Moore
123 Lee Street
Louisville, KY 40223

Dear Mr. Moore:

With the season for colds and flu fast approaching, it is time once again for flu shots. Supplies have arrived and flu shots will be administered starting October 3. Please call the office to schedule a visit for your flu shot at your earliest convenience.

If you wish to wait to get your flu shot at the time of your next appointment, it is not necessary to call the office. An appointment card with the date and time of your next appointment is enclosed.

Sincerely,

Beth Williams, MD

ENC: Appointment card
cc: B. Reed, Office Manager

(d)

WINDY CITY CLINIC
Beth Williams, M.D.
123 Michigan Avenue, Chicago, IL 60610
(312) 123-1234

August 1, 19xx

Thomas Moore
123 Lee Street
Louisville, KY 40223

RE: FLU SHOT

With the season for colds and flu fast approaching, it is time once again for flu shots. Supplies have arrived and flu shots will be administered starting October 3. Please call the office to schedule a visit for your flu shot at your earliest convenience.

If you wish to wait to get your flu shot at the time of your next appointment, it is not necessary to call the office. An appointment card with the date and time of your next appointment is enclosed.

BETH WILLIAMS, M.D.

ENC: Appointment card
cc: B. Reed, Office Manager

Figure 11-3 Example of four letter formats: a) Block style; b) modified block style; c) modified block style with indented paragraphs; and d) simplified letter style.

block (standard), modified block with indented paragraphs, and simplified letter style.

Interoffice Memoranda

Interoffice memoranda, also called memos, are correspondence sent to people within the office or organization. They are used to inform personnel about meetings, general changes that affect everyone, special projects or news items. The memo is an inexpensive means to communicate with others in the office setting. They do not require postage and are delivered through the interoffice mail route.

Memos are generally written on a short form developed for that purpose. The memo may contain a heading much like the letterhead stationery to indicate the office where they originated. They contain the word MEMORANDUM at the top of the form. Also included are the typed words DATE:, TO:, FROM:, and RE: or SUBJECT:. The memo is most often handwritten. The memo form is meant to be used within the office setting and should never be used to send information outside of the office. An example of a memo form follows.

```
┌─────────────────────────────────────────────┐
│       WINDY CITY MEDICAL CENTER              │
│              MEMORANDUM                      │
│   DATE:                                      │
│                                              │
│     TO:                                      │
│                                              │
│   FROM:                                      │
│                                              │
│   SUBJECT:                                   │
│                                              │
│                                              │
│   cc:                                        │
│                                              │
└─────────────────────────────────────────────┘
```

Proofreading

Proofreading for errors in content and typing is critical. The professionalism of the office is judged, in part, by the appearance of correspondence and documents that come out of that office. Proofreading or reading cannot be overemphasized. Even small omissions, such as commas, are noticed by readers.

Most computer programs contain "spelling and/or grammar check" components. These should always be used before printing the document. You may have to add frequently used medical terms to the program. After printing out the document, there should be a careful reading of all correspondence to catch any content or typing errors. Pay close attention to the spelling of names and procedures. When typing figures always double-check to make sure all decimal points are placed in the correct position. Look for sound-alike terms, such as right and write or anti-and ante-. Proofread for errors both in grammar and in typing.

Med Tip: After first proofreading a document for errors in content, there is another step to take in looking for typing errors. Read the typed material backwards to catch double words, such as "the the" and misplaced letters. By doing this, you will not be reading the content and should only see the typing errors. If possible, have a person who is unfamiliar with the content read and review the material for errors. Take the time to review the proofreading guidelines provided here from time to time.

Guidelines: Proofreading

1. Proofread and correct errors before printing the document, whenever possible.
2. Use a ruler, pencil, or edge of a piece of paper to follow each line as you proofread.
3. Check the content to see if it flows in a logical order.
4. Check for missing and/or repeated words.
5. Check grammar, spelling, and punctuation.
6. Check where the word breaks occur.
7. Verify the spelling of proper names and titles.
8. Verify numbers in dates, figures, and time (hours of the day).
9. Read the opening and closing carefully.
10. Proofread at least twice.
11. Check the general appearance of the letter for spacing and format.

Proofreader's Marks

There are marks that are generally accepted for use when proofreading large documents. These are especially helpful when a second person is proofing the document, such as the physician. See Figure 11-4 for a list of proofreader's marks.

Editing

Editing is similar to proofreading in that you must read the final material to check for accuracy. Editing also involves reading the printed material to determine if it is clear. When editing medical reports, you cannot change the content of the report or alter the meaning in any way. If you believe the meaning is unclear, you must check with the writer of the report before making any editorial changes.

When editing material you have composed, such as an informational form letter to be sent to all patients, changes can be made to increase clarity.

Abbreviations

Only accepted medical abbreviations can be used in medical reports and when filing insurance doc-

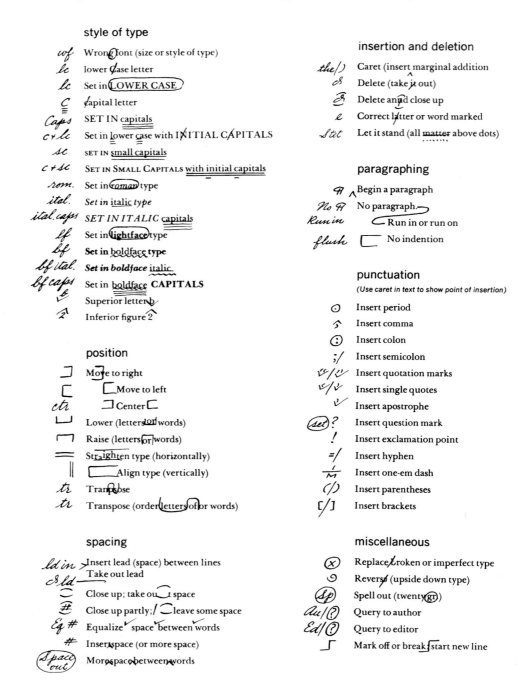

Figure 11-4 Proofreader's marks.

uments. A list of accepted medical abbreviations is included in the appendix of this textbook.

Individual physician offices may use an abbreviation on progress notes that is related to that practice. For example, a urologist may write "L," meaning leaking urine when coughing, on his or her progress notes. While this is not an acceptable abbreviation, it can be used to conserve space and simplify documentation within that particular office.

Reference Materials

Every physician's office contains general reference books—medical dictionaries—as well as textbooks related to the physician's specialization, for example pediatric textbooks in a pediatrician's office. Figure 11-5 illustrates a library reference shelf in a physician's office.

A complete office library should include the following:

- A desk dictionary, such as *The American Heritage Dictionary, The Random House Collegiate Dictionary, Webster's New World Dictionary of the American Language* or *Webster's New Collegiate Dictionary* which all contain current meanings and pronunciations. The dictionary should also be used when in doubt about the correct spelling of a term.
- A medical dictionary, such as *Taber's Cyclopedic Dictionary,* assists with the correct spelling, pronunciation and meaning of medical terms and diagnoses. Other medical dictionaries may include color illustrations to enhance the meaning of terms.
- A *Physician's Desk Reference* (PDR) should

be accessible in all offices to verify the correct spelling and meaning of drugs. The *PDR* is published each year and with supplements during the year to update this reference. The *PDR* is indexed by

1. Manufacturer
2. Brand name (trade name, such as Tylenol)
3. Generic name (common name, such as aspirin)
4. Chemical name (represents a chemical formula, such as acetylsalicylic acid)
5. Drug category
6. Product identification and information
7. Diagnostic information

Med Tip: It is not possible to know the names and correct spelling of all the drugs which are prescribed. Always look up the correct spelling of unfamiliar drugs.

- Use coding books when transcription and insurance forms involve procedural and diagnostic coding. Maintain references of the most recent CPT (Current Procedural Terminology), HCPCS, and the ICD-9-CM (Figure 11-6).
- A **thesaurus**, such as *Roget's International Thesaurus,* provides synonyms (similar meanings) for each entry word. At the back of Roget's thesaurus is an index to the groups of synonyms that make up the bulk

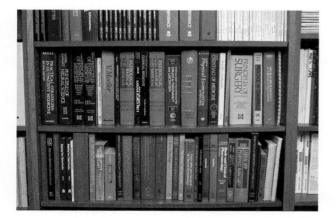

Figure 11-5 Medical reference textbooks are an essential component in the physician's office.

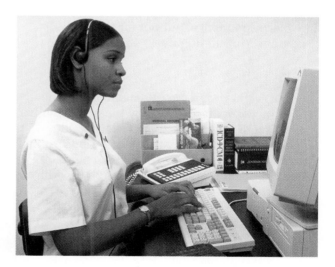

Figure 11-6 Coding books are kept within easy access of the transcriptionist/insurance coder.

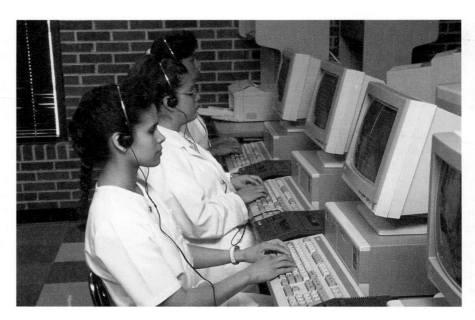

Figure 11-7 Transcriptionists working on medical records.

TABLE 11-10 **Stationery and Envelopes**

Stationery	Dimensions	Envelope Size	Dimensions
Standard	8 1/2″ × 11″	No. 10	9 1/2″ × 4 1/8″
Monarch	7 1/4″ × 10 1/2″	No. 7	7 1/2″ × 3 7/8″
Baronial	5 1/2″ × 8 1/2″	No. 6 3/4	6 1/2″ × 3 5/8″

of the book. For example, look up the adjective 'still,' and you will find references to lists containing the words tranquil, motionless, silent, and dead. Using a thesaurus, helps the writer find exactly the right way to convey the intended meaning. A thesaurus is used for office correspondence, but not for medical transcription (Figure 11-7).

Med Tip: Remember that the exact terms used by the physician in dictation or when writing in the medical record must be used by the person transcribing these notes into a typewritten document. Therefore, a thesaurus would not be used for transcription work.

Preparing Outgoing Mail

Letterhead stationery, which contains the name and address of the sender, comes in three commonly-used sizes. These are: standard, monarch or execu-

tive, and baronial. The more common letter sizes with their matching envelope sizes are shown in Table 11-10.

The standard letterhead is used for most office correspondence. A smaller version of this, the monarch or executive style, is used by some physicians for their social correspondence. The baronial letterhead is a half-sheet of the standard size and is used for brief letters and memoranda. Each size of letterhead stationery has an appropriate size envelope. See Figure 11-8 for an illustration of different letter sizes.

Folding Letters and Inserting into Envelopes

There are recommended methods for folding and inserting letters into envelopes so the contents can remain confidential and be easily removed. See Figure 11-9 for an illustration of folding a letter.

Number 10 Envelope
1. Bring up the bottom third of the letter and fold with a crease.

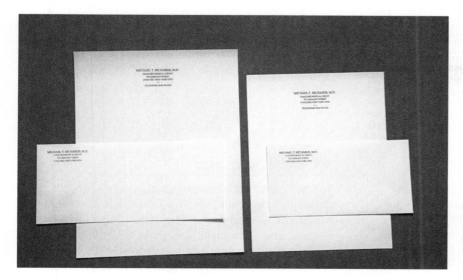

Figure 11-8 Letterhead stationery sizes are varied to suit the needs of the sender. Envelopes are sized to match different letter sizes.

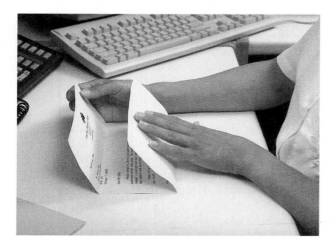

Figure 11-9 A well folded letter fits easily into the envelope and is easily removed by the person who receives it.

2. Fold the top of the letter down to 3/8 inch from the first creased edge.
3. Make a second crease at the fold and place this edge into the envelope first.

Number 6 3/4 Envelope
1. Bring the bottom edge up to 3/8 inch from the top edge.
2. Make a crease at the fold.
3. Fold the right edge one third of the width of the paper, and press a crease at this fold.
4. Fold the left edge to 3/8 inch from the previous crease and insert this edge into the envelope first.

Envelope Formats

The United States Postal Service (USPS) has recommended guidelines when typing envelopes. This is meant to improve the handling and delivery of the mail. Optical Character Recognition (OCR) equipment used by the postal service scans, reads, and sorts the envelope. For optimal efficiency of OCR scanning, the address must be typed on the envelope using single spacing and all capital letters with no punctuation.

The last line in the address must include the city, state two-digit code, and the ZIP code. It cannot exceed 27 characters in length. See Figure 11-10 for a listing of the two digit letter abbreviations for states.

A more traditional style of typing envelopes with the initial letter in capital letters and small letters for the rest of the address is still accepted by the post office.

The bottom margin of the No. 10 envelope (business size) should be 5/8 inch with one inch margins on the left and right sides. The No. 6 3/4 envelope should have a two inch margin on the left side with the address 12 lines from the top of the envelope.

A return address for the sender should always be placed in the upper left hand corner in the event the letter must be returned to the sender. Envelopes can be printed with the address of the sender in this position.

ZIP Codes

The five-digit ZIP code was introduced in the 1960s to increase the post office's efficiency in

TWO-LETTER ABBREVIATIONS

UNITED STATES and TERRITORIES

Alabama	AL	Montana	MT
Alaska	AK	Nebraska	NE
Arizona	AZ	Nevada	NV
Arkansas	AR	New Hampshire	NH
California	CA	New Jersey	NJ
Canal Zone	CZ	New Mexico	NM
Colorado	CO	New York	NY
Connecticut	CT	North Carolina	NC
Delaware	DE	North Dakota	ND
District of Columbia	DC	Ohio	OH
Florida	FL	Oklahoma	OK
Georgia	GA	Oregon	OR
Guam	GU	Pennsylvania	PA
Hawaii	HI	Puerto Rico	PR
Idaho	ID	Rhode Island	RI
Illinois	IL	South Carolina	SC
Indiana	IN	South Dakota	SD
Iowa	IA	Tennessee	TN
Kansas	KS	Texas	TX
Kentucky	KY	Utah	UT
Louisiana	LA	Vermont	VT
Maine	ME	Virgin Islands	VI
Maryland	MD	Virginia	VA
Massachusetts	MA	Washington	WA
Michigan	MI	West Virginia	WV
Minnesota	MN	Wisconsin	WI
Mississippi	MS	Wyoming	WY
Missouri	MO		

Figure 11-10   Every state has a two digit letter abbreviation.

mail handling. ZIP codes begin on the East Coast with the number "0" eventually increasing to the number "9" on the West Coast and Hawaii. The first three numbers of the ZIP code identify the city and all five digits combine to identify the individual post office and zone within the city. Four more digits have recently been added to the ZIP code by the USPS. These four digits follow a hyphen behind the first five and represent the addressee's street location. The 9-digit ZIP code has eliminated many handling steps at the postal service and improved service.

Using a Postage Meter

Many offices use a postage meter that will automatically stamp large mailings. The postage can be printed directly onto an envelope with a meter. Postage can also be printed onto an adhesive backed strip that is placed directly onto a package. Metered mail does not have to be stamped when it arrives at the post office. The meter is taken into the post office for calibrating.

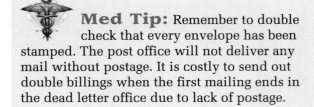

Med Tip: Remember to double check that every envelope has been stamped. The post office will not deliver any mail without postage. It is costly to send out double billings when the first mailing ends in the dead letter office due to lack of postage.

Classifications of Mail

The classifications of mail vary according to weight, type, and destination. Mail is weighed in ounces and pounds. The most common types of mail are: first class, priority, second class, third class, fourth class, and express mail. Table 11-11 describes these classifications of mail.

Size Requirements for Mail

The USPS standardized envelope sizes in order to machine sort mail. Minimum mail sizes have been established. Domestic mail must be at least 0.0007 inch thick. A further restriction on size requires that mail 1/4 inch or less in thickness must be 3 1/2 inches in height and at least 5 inches long. All mail not meeting this requirement is considered nonstandard.

The post office will place a surcharge on mail that is nonstandard. A surcharge will be placed on First Class and Third Class mail weighing 1 ounce or less if the following apply:

- Length exceeds 11 1/2 inches
- Height exceeds 6 1/2 inches
- Thickness exceeds 1/4 inch

Med Tip: Before doing a special mailing, such as promotional materials, it is wise to measure and weigh the final material in the envelope. This assures the correct postage is placed on the mail.

Special Postal Services

Specialized services include Certified Mail, certificate of mailing, special delivery, registered mail and special handling.

Certified Mail

Mail which includes contracts, mortgages, birth certificates, deeds and checks which are not valuable themselves but would be difficult to replace if

TABLE 11-11 **Classifications of Mail**

Type	Description
First Class	Letters, postcards, business reply cards.
	Letters weighing less than 11 ounces.
	Sealed and unsealed handwritten or typed material.
Priority	First class mail weighing more than 11 ounces.
	Maximum weight of 70 pounds.
	Postage calculated based on weight and destination.
Second Class	Newspapers and periodicals which have received second class mail authorization.
	Copies of newspapers and periodicals mailed by the general public are not able to receive the second class rate.
Third Class	Catalogs, books, photographs, flyers, and other printed material. Also called "bulk mail."
	Must be marked "Third Class."
	Must be sealed.
Fourth Class	Printed material, books, and merchandise not included in First and Second Class.
	Must weigh between 16 ounces and 70 pounds.
	There are size limitations also.
Express Mail/ Next Day Service	Available 7 days a week.
	Up to 70 pounds in weight and 108 inches around.
	Expected delivery by noon.
	Shipping containers are supplied.
	Pickup service in some areas.

lost can be mailed as Certified Mail (Figure 11-11). They would need to be mailed at the First Class rate with a special fee added for Certified Mail. Certified Mail assists in tracking and collecting this mail. A receipt verifying delivery can be requested for a fee. Certified Mail can also be sent by Special Delivery if the extra fee is paid. Certified Mail records are maintained at the post office for two years.

Certificate of Mailing

For a small fee, a certificate of mailing can be obtained at the post office. This document will demonstrate

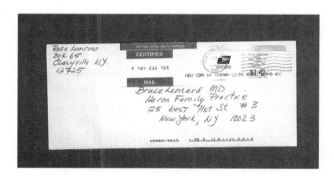

Figure 11-11 Items that would be difficult to re-place or bearing legal significance are sent by Certified Mail.

proof that mail was posted. This is useful for mailing items such as tax returns which need to be received by a certain date.

Special Delivery

When fast delivery of an item is needed, special delivery service can be requested from the postal service. Special delivery is useful for shipping perishables, such as specimens, since the post office will deliver these items beyond the regular delivery service hours (for example, on Sundays and holidays). There is a fee for this service.

Special Handling

Special handling can be requested for third- and fourth-class items. "Special handling" is stamped across the package. The fee for this service is based on the weight of the item.

Insurance

Insurance can be purchased for third-class, fourth-class, and priority mail. The sender will then be reimbursed if this mail is lost or damaged. The sender receives a receipt from the post office at the time of purchase of the insurance. This receipt along with the damaged goods must be presented when reimbursement is necessary.

Registered Mail

Registered mail is the safest way to send first-class or priority mail. A fee is paid for this service and a signed record is kept for each piece of registered mail. Registered mail is tracked as it moves throughout the mail system which helps to reduce loss.

Registered mail is the preferred route to send valuables such as jewelry, currency, stocks and bonds. The sender must declare the value of the items and seal the envelope. The sender receives a receipt which should be kept in the event the item is lost and needs to be traced in the postal system.

Registered mail is insured for the value declared at the time of registration. For an additional fee the sender can request a return receipt indicating the time, place of delivery, and the receiver's signature.

Postal Money Orders

A postal money order can be purchased at the post office. The money order is replaceable if lost or stolen and can be mailed instead of the actual cash. They are available in several denominations and the fee varies according to the amount of the postal money order.

Forwarding Mail

First class is the only type of mail that can be forwarded to another address without paying an additional fee. Cross out the incorrect address and add the new address and return to the mail carrier or post office. The post office will forward mail for up to six months.

Mail Recall

If mail has been placed into the mail box or given to a postal carrier by mistake, it can be recalled by the sender. The sender can call the post office and request the item be held for them. When the sender goes to the post office to reclaim the mail, he or she will be asked to complete a "Sender's Application for Recall of Mail." If the mail is still at the post office, it will be returned to the sender upon completion of this form. If the mail has already left the post office, the postal clerk will call the post office where that mail has been sent and ask that the mail be returned. The sender must pay all the expenses incurred in an attempt to recall the mail, including the phone calls placed by the postal service. If the mail has already been delivered to the addressee, the sender will be notified.

Tracing Lost Mail

All receipts for mailed goods should be retained until receipt of the mail has been acknowledged. If the mail has not arrived after a reasonable period of time, the post office will attempt to trace it for you. First class mail is not easy to trace since there is no receipt for it. The postal service requires a special form to be completed before they will trace mail.

Returned Mail

When mail has been returned and marked "undeliverable," it cannot be re-mailed until new postage is added. It is advisable to place the contents into a new envelope with the correct address, place the proper postage according to weight on the envelope, and re-mail.

Electronic Mail (E-mail)

All written materials that are transmitted electronically are referred to as electronic mail. The documents may include letters, reports, and pictures. These mails may be sent over telephone lines, cables, computers, microwaves, and satellites. Electronic mail allows the medical assistant to edit, correct, and transmit documents very quickly to another location. Electronic mail cannot be used if the *original signature* on the document needs to be sent.

Facsimile (FAX)

Another electronic means of sending a written communication is by using a FAX machine. The FAX is an exact duplication of a document that is then transmitted to another location via a facsimile (FAX) machine. The telephone lines are used to transmit FAX documents. The original document is inserted into the FAX machine, the receiver's phone number is dialed and when the connection is made the document is transmitted over the phone lines resulting in a printed document at the receiver's FAX machine. A cover sheet should be sent first which includes information about the sender (company, name, and telephone and FAX numbers) telephone number of the receiver, date, and number of pages.

Intelpost

INTELPOST is a service offered by the US Postal Service in cooperation with foreign countries. Mail sent by INTELPOST is taken to an INTELPOST mail processing center where it is transmitted by FAX equipment, via satellite, to the destination INTELPOST post office. An image of the document is then printed at this post office. The paper image can be picked up at the destination post office or delivered by the postal service.

Mail Handling Tips

To facilitate time management within the medical office all mail should be handled only once. For ease and efficiency in handling large amounts of mail, the following guidelines should be noted.

Guidelines: Handling Large Amounts of Mail

1. Have all supplies in one place when processing the mail. These include a letter opener, pencil, stapler, time and date stamp and pad, paper clips, and file folders.
2. Sort the mail before opening into first-class, personal/confidential, second-, third- and fourth class.
3. Discard and recyle all third-class mail immediately if it will not be used by the office.
4. Place a current date and time of arrival on each piece of mail as it comes into the office. Purchase a rubber stamp and pad from an office supply store so that the date can be changed each day.
5. Stamp the name of the medical office across all periodicals and newspapers (Second-class) that will be placed in the waiting area for patients' use.
6. Lay all the envelopes flap down to reduce the motions involved in opening a large amount of mail. Many mail handlers open all the envelopes before dealing with individual contents. This saves time but may cause items to fall out of the envelopes.
7. Do not open mail marked "personal" or "confidential". Place it in the physician's box unopened unless otherwise instructed.
8. Attach all enclosures in each envelope with a paper clip. Avoid stapling since these will have to be removed later and may damage sensitive materials such as x-rays. If an enclosure is noted within the correspondence but is not included in the envelope write "no" next to enclosure with your initials to indicate it was not included. Clip the opened envelope to the mail until the mail is completely processed. In some cases a return address is only on the envelope and not on the inside correspondence.
9. Open all the mail and clip together the inside contents before handling the individual correspondence.
10. Annotate the mail as soon as possible after it is opened. An annotation consists of writing a short comment in pencil to indicate the purpose of the letter, and underline the critical portions of the letter. If another document is referred to in the letter, then take initiative by pulling it from the file and attaching it to this correspondence.
11. Route the mail immediately after opening. Another department or physician may be waiting for the document.

LEGAL AND ETHICAL ISSUES

The medical assistant must carefully monitor all dated material to assure that replies are made on a timely basis. Confidential mail and correspondence including checks and payments are handled on a regular basis. This is a grave responsibility. Since the US Postal Services is regulated by the federal government, any tampering or deliberate mishandling of mail is a federal offense.

A non-threatening tone of correspondence can promote the profession of medicine to the reader.

Any attempts to threaten a patient in writing can lead to charges of harassment. Courteous language, presented in a diplomatic manner, can result in compliance and prevent a lawsuit.

An error in correspondence may not be caught by the physician before he or she signs the document. The medical assistant must carefully proofread all correspondence before it leaves the office to protect the physician from legal problems.

PATIENT EDUCATION

Much of the patient education materials used in the medical office is prepared and distributed in printed form. This type of marketing and public relations for the office includes pamphlets, brochures, and letters of instructions. In many cases, the information will have to be interpreted for the patients who have difficulty with vision, reading, or understanding medical information. This is an excellent opportunity to provide additional patient teaching. By asking the patient to repeat some of the material that has been explained, you can test the patient's understanding.

When advising patients about correspondence they should be cautioned about placing cash into the mail. Payments should always be made by check or in person.

Summary

The responsibilities of the medical assistant relating to office correspondence are multifaceted. These include being able to draft correspondence for the physician's signature using correct grammar and style and efficiently handling mail. Effective mail handling includes using the most efficient and cost-saving form of mail service. These responsibilities must be handled in a professional, courteous, and diplomatic manner. Correct handling of written communication allows the medical assistant to demonstrate his or her initiative.

Competency Review

1. Define and spell the glossary terms for this chapter.
2. How would you track a missing piece of mail?
3. Describe how you would sort through 40 pieces of mail containing first-, second-, third-, and fourth-class mail.
4. Address an envelope using the method recommended by the USPS for use with Optical Character Recognition Equipment (OCR).
5. Describe what types of material you would send by certified mail.
6. Type a short letter using both the block and modified-block with indented paragraph style.
7. Why do you think companies (and medical offices) use letterhead stationery?

PREPARING FOR THE CERTIFICATION EXAM

Test Taking Tip — When taking a computer generated exam, be sure to mark all the spaces on the answer sheet. A blank space is automatically wrong. Try to answer every question even if you have to guess. You may be correct.

Examination Review Questions

1. Which of the following is not a method used for classifying mail?
   (A) weight
   (B) date
   (C) destination
   (D) type
   (E) all of the above

2. What is the maximum weight (in pounds) for priority mail?
   (A) 100
   (B) 150
   (C) 17
   (D) 70
   (E) 50

3. What is the term that means "to note the important points or items in a letter or document"?
   (A) annotate
   (B) announce
   (C) notify
   (D) proofread
   (E) classify

4. What is the term that means "to indicate the presence of an error or correction needed on a letter or document"?
   (A) annotate
   (B) sort
   (C) notify
   (D) proofread
   (E) classify

5. What type of mail is used to send valuables, such as currency and jewelry?
   (A) special handling
   (B) priority mail
   (C) registered mail
   (D) special delivery
   (E) all of the above

6. What category of mail can be insured?
   (A) first class
   (B) second class
   (C) third class
   (D) fourth class
   (E) all can be insured

7. The two letter abbreviation for Michigan is
   (A) MH
   (B) MN
   (C) MI
   (D) MG
   (E) MA

8. Which of the following would NOT be used on a memorandum?
   (A) writer's name
   (B) subject
   (C) complimentary close
   (D) date
   (E) all of the above are used

9. Which of the following is NOT found in a thesaurus?
   (A) alphabetical listing
   (B) index
   (C) synonyms
   (D) medical terminology
   (E) all of the above are found

10. The proofreader's mark that means "insert a space" is
    (A) #
    (B) //
    (C) [
    (D) sp
    (E) tr

ON THE JOB

Diane Webb, a medical assistant in Dr. Williams' office, has been asked to proofread a letter that was prepared by a temporary secretary. Follow the rules for proofreading, grammar, capitaliza- tion, and spelling found in this chapter to correct the errors in this letter. Type this letter using the modified block style and prepare it for Dr. Beth Williams' signature.

Dear Docter Stacey:

I right this letter to inform you that I am pleased that you would chose me to present at your conference. Its a great complement.

Their are several cases which I can site. I would like you're recommendation since I no you will be frank with me. We must all ways be discrite and conscience of patience's rights when presenting cases relating to there conditions. We must remain mindful that patients have there legal rites.

I have the following x-ray studies which I can include: xyphoid process, greater trocanter, pere-toneal abcess, left calcanus, fracture of right clavical, and a fractured ileum and ischeum. Let me know which of these rentgeneology studies you would prefer.

Please advise me on how to procede.

Sincerely yours,

Dr. Beth Williams

References

Becklin, K. and Sunnarborg, E. *Medical Office Procedures*. New York: Glencoe, 1996.

Hacker, D. *The Bedford Handbook for Writers*. Boston: Bedford Books of St. Martin's Press, 1991.

McMiller, K. *Being A Medical Records Clerk*. Upper Saddle River, NJ: Brady/Prentice Hall, 1992.

Morrow, N. *Being a Medical Transcriptionist*. Upper Saddle River, NJ: Brady/Prentice Hall, 1992.

Oliverio, J., Pasewark, W., and White, B. *The Office: Procedures and Technology*. Cincinnati, Ohio: South-Western Publishing Co., 1993.

Smith, L., and Grisolia, J. *Communication and English for Careers*. Upper Saddle River, NJ: Brady/Prentice Hall, 1994.

Strategies for Success

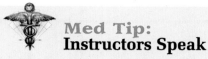

Med Tip:
Instructors Speak

After the externship interview and when you complete an externship, remember to send a thank you note.

John P. Cody, MPH, MBA, CMA
Richfield, Minnesota

Demonstrate the ability to translate what you know to an understandable level for the patient, whether an adult, child, or ESL-adult.

Nina Theirer, CMA
Fort Wayne, Indiana

When presented with a classroom or clinical situation, think through all the alternatives before making a decision. Remember, no two situations will be the same—so think critically.

Eugenia Fulcher, RN, BSN, CMA
Waynesboro, Georgia

Set career goals for yourself, *both* short term and long term goals.

Dee A. Stout, BA, MA
Kansas City, Missouri

Realize that learning is a lifelong process. Learning does not stop once classes have ended, particularly in the medical field, where changes occur constantly. Be prepared to spend some part of your professional life reading journals, attending workshops, and exchanging new information and ideas with other professionals to be sure you are up-to-date on the latest changes and improvements in the field.

Ursula Backner, CMA
Debra Hampton, BSPH, LPN, CPC
Catherine Schoen, CMA
Indianapolis, Indiana

MEDICAL ASSISTANT ROLE DELINEATION CHART

Highlight indicates material covered in this chapter

ADMINISTRATIVE

ADMINISTRATIVE PROCEDURES

- Perform basic clerical functions
- Schedule, coordinate, and monitor appointments
- Schedule inpatient/outpatient admissions and procedures
- Understand and apply third party guidelines
- Obtain reimbursement through accurate claims submission
- Monitor third-party reimbursement
- Perform medical transcription
- Understand and adhere to managed care policies and procedures
- *Negotiate managed care contracts (adv)*

PRACTICE FINANCES

- Perform procedural and diagnostic coding
- Apply bookkeeping principles
- Document and maintain accounting and banking records
- Manage accounts receivable
- Manage accounts payable
- Process payroll
- *Develop and maintain fee schedules (adv)*
- *Manage renewals of business and professional insurance policies (adv)*
- *Manage personal benefits and maintain records (adv)*

CLINICAL

FUNDAMENTAL PRINCIPLES

- Apply principles of aseptic technique and infection control
- Comply with quality assurance practices
- Screen and follow up patient test results

DIAGNOSTIC ORDERS

- Collect and process specimens
- Perform diagnostic tests

PATIENT CARE

- Adhere to established triage procedures
- Obtain patient history and vital signs
- Prepare and maintain examination and treatment areas

- Prepare patient for examinations, procedures, and treatments
- Assist with examinations, procedures, and treatments
- Prepare and administer medications and immunizations
- Maintain medication and immunization records
- Recognize and respond to emergencies
- Coordinate patient care information with other health care providers

GENERAL (TRANSDISCIPLINARY)

PROFESSIONALISM

- Project a professional manner and image
- Adhere to ethical principles
- Demonstrate initiative and responsibility
- Work as a team member
- Manage time efficiently
- Prioritize and perform multiple tasks
- Adapt to change
- Promote the CMA credential
- Enhance skills through continuing education

COMMUNICATION SKILLS

- Treat all patients with compassion and empathy
- Recognize and respect cultural diversity
- Adapt communications to individual's ability to understand
- Use professional telephone technique
- Use effective and correct verbal and written communications
- Recognize and respond to verbal and non-verbal communications
- Use medical terminology appropriately
- Receive, organize, prioritize, and transmit information
- Serve as liaison
- Promote the practice through positive public relations

LEGAL CONCEPTS

- Maintain confidentiality
- Practice within the scope of education, training, and personal capabilities
- Prepare and maintain medical records
- Document accurately
- Use appropriate guidelines when releasing information
- Follow employer's established policies dealing with the health care contract
- Follow federal, state, and local legal guidelines
- Maintain awareness of federal and state health care legislation and regulations
- Maintain and dispose of regulated substances in compliance with government guidelines
- Comply with established risk management and safety procedures
- Recognize professional credentialing criteria
- Participate in the development and maintenance of personnel, policy, and procedure manuals
- *Develop and maintain personnel, policy, and procedure manuals (adv)*

INSTRUCTION

- Instruct individuals according to their needs
- Explain office policies and procedures
- Teach methods of health promotion and disease prevention
- Locate community resources and disseminate information
- *Orient and train personnel (adv)*
- *Develop educational materials (adv)*
- *Conduct continuing education activities (adv)*

OPERATIONAL FUNCTIONS

- Maintain supply inventory
- Evaluate and recommend equipment and supplies
- Apply computer techniques to support office operations
- *Supervise personnel (adv)*
- *Interview and recommend job applicants (adv)*
- *Negotiate leases and prices for equipment and supply contracts (adv)*

SOURCE: Reprinted by permission of the American Association of Medical Assistants from the *AAMA Role Delineation Study: Occupational Analysis of the Medical Assisting Profession.*

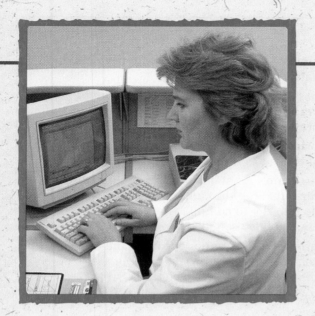

12

Computers in Medicine

LEARNING OBJECTIVES

At the completion of this chapter, you will:
1. Define and spell the glossary terms for this chapter.
2. Explain the difference between hardware and software.
3. List 3 ways to ensure confidentiality of medical records when using a computer.

ADMINISTRATIVE PERFORMANCE COMPETENCIES

After completing this chapter, you should perform the following tasks:
1. Receive, organize, and prioritize information using computers.
2. Perform basic secretarial skills using a word processor.
3. Apply computer concepts for office procedures.
4. Evaluate and recommend equipment for the practice.

Glossary

CPU   Central processing unit.

disk   Storage medium for data and software.

dot matrix printers   Impact printers that produce characters by impacting small dots onto the paper's surface; capable of producing graphic images as well as text material.

floppy disk   Magnetic disks with a magnetic oxide coating over a thin slice of plastic used as a storage medium.

K   See kilobyte.

kilobyte(s) (K)   A measure of storage capacity or memory.

main memory   That part of the central processing unit which stores data and program instructions; it does not perform any of the logical operations, for example computations or sorting.

microcomputer   Small computer systems designed to be portable, including desktop, laptop notebook, and handheld computers.

microprocessor   A small chip that does the work of processing data in a microcomputer.

monitor   Screen which allows the user to see input and output.

mouse   Pointing and selection device to input data.

password   A word or phrase that identifies a person and allows access or entry to a program or records.

printer(s)   An output device for hard copy; classified as impact and nonimpact.

program   A set or sets of programmed instructions that tell the computer hardware what to do in order to complete the required data processing (also called software).

prompt   A reminder or hint to the user that some action must be taken by the user before processing of data can continue.

RAM   Random-access memory.

ROM   Read-only memory.

software   A set or sets of programmed instructions that tell the computer hardware what to do in order to complete the required data processing (also called a program).

terminal   Also called a monitor or dumb terminal; allows the computer operator to see input and output.

The uses of computers in medicine are many and varied. Depending on the size of the practice, some or all of the functions normally performed in the front office may be done with computers and specialized programs. In order to be successful in the administrative, clinical, and lab areas, the medical assistant must be familiar with computers and how they can be used.

Use of Computers in Medicine

As the cost of computers and programs shrinks, and the cost of doing business in any medical office grows, more and more functions of the medical office are being done with computers. Computers give the advantages of speed and often eliminate having to key or enter information more than once. Just as write-it-once revolutionized office bookkeeping, computer programs have adopted the write-it-once principal and given medical practices the flexibility of entering patient information such as name, address, insurance information, and other data one time, then using this information to complete tasks such as appointment scheduling, billing and payment information, generating statements, and preparing insurance forms.

Computers are invaluable in collecting inventory data, for example the number of PAP smears performed. Sophisticated programs allow the medical practice to computerize chart information, obtain laboratory results from remote sites instantly or search through a large quantity of information about the patient's disease or condition, speeding diagnosis and treatment. Figures 12-1 and 12-2 illustrate ways the computers have become invaluable in diagnosing, monitoring, and reporting the patient's progress.

Types of Computers

Computers used in the medical office today are of the microcomputer variety. This means that a small piece of electronic hardware, called a chip, allows the processing of information in a very small amount of space. Computers today fit on a desk, in your lap, or even in a device the size of a hand-held calculator. Before the microchip revolution, computers took up a great deal of room and used a vastly different technology. In the early

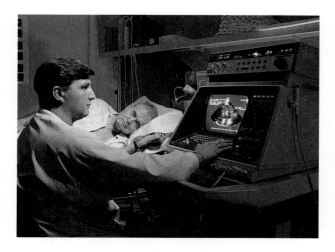

Figure 12-1   Echocardiography examination.

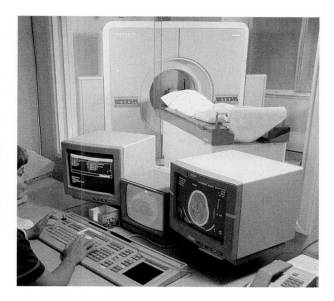

Figure 12-2   CT brain scanning.

days of computers, what now fits on your desk took an entire room and had the same amount of memory.

Early Computers

Minicomputers were the next step in the evolution of computer processors. These computers could fit comfortably into an office and took up approximately the same space as a filing cabinet. Early computers were not particularly easy to use. Normally the operator or user had a blank screen and was required to memorize a language the computer understood in order to use any program. These early computers were very functionally limited.

Minicomputers were manufactured and programmed to do data processing (numbers with few words) or word processing (words with few numbers). Trying to perform both data processing on a word processor or word processing on a data processor was difficult and required many hours of training. As technology became more sophisticated, the programmers added menus, to make using programs easier for the user and cutting the time it took to be able to use a program effectively.

Microcomputers in the Medical Office

Today, the distinction between data processing and word processing has been completely eliminated. Computers process information of all types rapidly and easily. As computers have become more "friendly" and manuals become more readable, computer users are able to learn a program in a much shorter period of time. This technology is now used to save time, eliminate duplication of effort, and decrease errors (Figure 12-3).

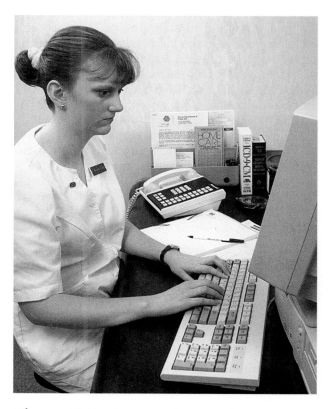

Figure 12-3   Computers have now become essential equipment in today's medical office.

With microchip technology and more sophisticated monitors, programmers were able to add visual elements to computer programs, making the programs even easier for the novice to use. With a mouse (an electronic pointer) some keyboard commands have been completely eliminated. The mouse allows the user to point to a picture (or icon) of the desired program or function, and point-and-click through program features.

Basic Computer Components

Although there are still many different computer manufacturers, every computer works the same way, no matter who makes it. Every computer, old or new, has two basic parts: the hardware and the software. Table 12-1 lists the different types of hardware, software, and storage components needed to run computers. Figure 12-4 illustrates the components of a computer system.

Hardware is the category of all the parts of the computer that you can see or touch. Every computer made has a central processing unit, or CPU. The CPU, often called the "heart," "brains," or main memory of a computer, acts as a traffic policeman, directing the computer's activities and sending electronic signals to the right place at the right time. The time it takes for the electronic signals to come and go is measured in megahertz. The higher the megahertz, the faster the computer can move information from one place to another. At the heart of the CPU is the microprocessor, which has a number indicating its size. For example, if you think of the 286 microchip as a 2-lane highway, it allows information to travel in and out at the same time (2 lanes of traffic). The 386 processor has 3 lanes. The 486 has 4, and so on. The more "lanes," the larger the amount of information which can be moved at one time.

Memory

Computers also have a number for memory. Memory is measured in kilobytes (Kb or K). Each kilobyte is 1,000 bytes (or characters) of information. This memory is further divided into RAM and ROM. RAM, or random-access memory, is the highest number a computer can hold all at once.

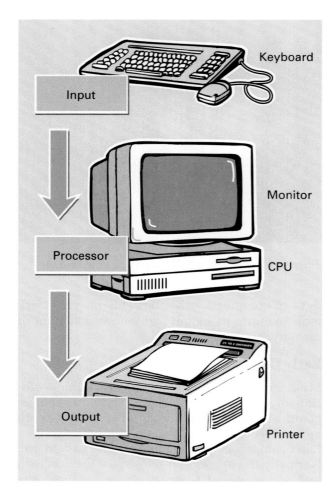

Figure 12-4   Components of a computer system.

For example, a computer with 64K RAM, can "hold" or process 64,000 kilobytes at one time. The ROM, or read-only memory, is used to store information which is not actively being used by the computer at that moment. RAM, however, is only good as long as the computer is not turned off. Once the computer is turned off, or powered down, all information stored in RAM is lost. Storage capacity is also measured in kilobytes. The higher the number of kilobytes, the more information a particular storage media can hold.

TABLE 12-1   **Hardware, Software, and Storage Components**

Hardware	Software	Storage
Central processing unit (CPU)	Systems	Diskettes/floppy disks
Peripherals: monitor, printer, CD ROM, modem, scanner, cables, and other equipment	Applications	Hard disks Magnetic tapes

Hard Drive

Today's computers are based on hard-disk technology. By programming convention, this special magnetic storage media, contained inside the computer, is called the "C drive." This storage area is controlled by the CPU, and information written to this magnetic media is called by the CPU when needed to make the computer run. Both programs and information can be stored on a hard-disk drive. The more visual the software, the larger the amount of storage space required. Today's programs, many of which run with *Windows* technology and are highly visual, require larger amounts of storage space than the simpler, keyboard-command-driven programs used in earlier years.

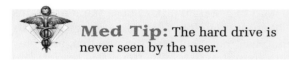 **Med Tip:** The hard drive is never seen by the user.

As programs and computers get even more sophisticated, the required amount of storage space, as well as the size and speed of the processor, have risen, making some computers purchased only a few years before obsolete.

Floppy Disk

Information can also be stored on other media. This media is called a diskette or floppy disk and comes in two sizes, the older 5 1/4 diskettes, and the newer 3 1/2 diskettes. These are placed into openings in the computer called disk or diskette drives. By inserting a diskette, information and programs can be moved or copied from one place to another. This allows the user to move programs and information from one computer to another easily and quickly. These diskette drives also have names. The first diskette drive the computer recognizes is, by programming convention, called the "A" drive. The second is called the "B" drive.

CD-ROM

CD-ROM stands for "Compact Disc Read-Only Memory." It is a data storage system for personal computers using internal or external CD-ROM players with CD-ROM discs. Computer programs, databases, and other large amounts of information on CD-ROM discs are digitally encoded and may not be changed by the user. Stored data may include simple text programs, entire encyclopedia programs, photo and sound libraries, and/or, complex motion pictures or animations. The data is randomly accessed in the same manner as a floppy disk. However, a CD-ROM disc is capable of holding or storing more information than 1,000 floppy disks.

Some computers have multimedia capabilities which allow the user to record and access a variety of sounds and music, photos, animations, and videos. Multimedia functions require the large storage capacity that CD-ROM discs offer.

Monitors

In order to communicate with a computer, the user also needs to see what is happening. The monitor or terminal is the means which allows the user to do this. Monitors can be purchased in black-and-white, or with color options. The clearer the color, the more expensive the monitor. Today's technology takes advantage of the colors and clarity by allowing for pictures to be imported onto a screen.

Printers

To turn the information on the monitor into paper, printers are used. The least expensive of these options are the dot matrix printers. These impact printers use pins against an inked ribbon and the characters they produce are actually a series of dots. The more pins the printer has, the closer the printed output looks to typewritten copy. And as the number of pins increases, the cost of the printer also goes up. Some dot matrix printers can produce documents which are nearly impossible to distinguish from typewritten copy. Some are able to add graphics.

An ink jet printer also works on the dot matrix principle, but with ink that is blown onto the paper. The characters are still made up of dots. Ink jet printers are usually quieter and faster than dot matrix printers, can print graphics, and can print in color if the proper ink cartridge and software have been installed. These printers are more costly than the dot matrix printers.

Laser printers use lasers to burn the ink onto the paper. These nonimpact printers, while most expensive of the three printer options, are the most versatile printers available today. They are faster and quieter than either the dot matrix or ink jet printers, can produce typewritten quality work, and are able to add color to documents with available color print options.

Software

Software or program is the name given to the set or sets of instructions that allow the computer to perform its functions. Contrary to what you might think, computers are not intelligent. Their capabilities are controlled by the humans who write the instructions that tell them what to do. All software is a list of instructions that tells the computer what action to take in a given case.

Every computer starts with an operating system. This is a set of very basic instructions to the CPU to turn on the computer. The most common operating system is called DOS, or disk operating system. If only DOS is loaded on a computer, the user will hear a beep when turning on the computer, and then receive a message called a prompt. Depending on which drive the computer is instructed to look at first by its operating system, the user might see a C>: or an A>: on the screen. At this point, the user must instruct the computer what to do next by typing in a command (written in the DOS language) and pressing the key marked "ENTER" or "RETURN." While using DOS to find a program is not difficult, it requires the user to remember the name of the program wanted, to type it in correctly, and then to press the confirmation key (ENTER or RETURN).

The next layer of programs, which work with the operating system, are called "overlays." These overlay programs allow the user to choose from a menu instead of having to type a command at the opening prompt. By using arrow keys, function keys, or a mouse, the user can choose from words or pictures the desired program, so that even an in-experienced user can choose a task more easily. The overlay programs most users are familiar with is the Microsoft Windows 3.1 (now up to 7.0) program, which lets the user choose a function from pictures, or icons. Using a mouse, the user moves the pointer arrow to the icon of the program and clicks a special key on the mouse. The *Windows* program translates this for the CPU, and the program is called to the screen.

The third layer of programs are called application programs. These programs perform a special function such as accounting, word processing, or data management (Figure 12-5).

Accounting programs for medical offices exist in many forms, from very simple to extremely sophisticated. Most medical office accounting programs allow the user to track charges and payments and to generate bills. These same programs also have instructions for processing accounts payable, writing checks for the practice, and may include an option to handle the office payroll and general ledger.

More sophisticated medical management packages include other functions, such as appointment scheduling, insurance processing, and even coding. Software manufacturers usually update their programs to keep pace with new technology and new regulations. It is not uncommon practice in the software industry to issue an up-

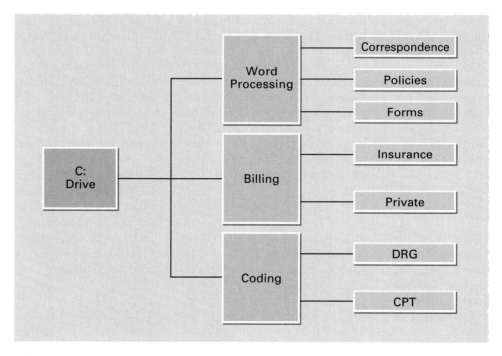

Figure 12-5 Programs are located in directories or folders and subdirectories.

dated version of an older program at one- or two-year intervals. It is important for the successful medical assistant to be aware that new regulations may make some software obsolete, so the program must be changed before it can again be useful to the practice.

The most complex medical management programs include options that allow the practice to keep records for clinical research, maintain patient charts and records, generate letters through a word processing feature (Figures 12-6 and 12-7). As with most computer components, the capability of the program is usually directly proportional to its cost. The more expensive the program, the more it can do.

Advantages of a medical management programs are many (Figure 12-8). After entering patient information only once, the practice is able to schedule an appointment, record charges and payments, generate an insurance form, print a statement (including notices of delinquency accounts or "aged" accounts), track the number of days before payment is received from the insurance company, and write a reminder letter or postcard to the patient about an upcoming appointment.

Most practice management packages do require some training, however. Depending on the user and the difficulty of the program, it may take weeks before the user is completely comfortable with all the functions of the program. It is also very time consuming to convert records from paper to computer, as all patient information must be entered into the computer program's database before it can be used.

However, the advantages of using a computer system to handle routine front office tasks outweigh the disadvantages and, as the cost of doing business for a medical practice goes up, it is to the practice's advantage to use the computer as a tool to hold down the costs of routine tasks.

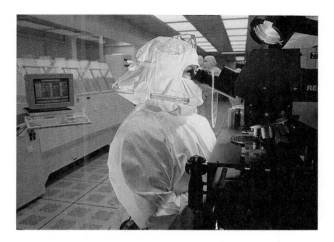

Figure 12-7   Lab results can be entered in a computer system and compared with other samples using a program that analyzes and sorts entries based on predetermined characteristics.

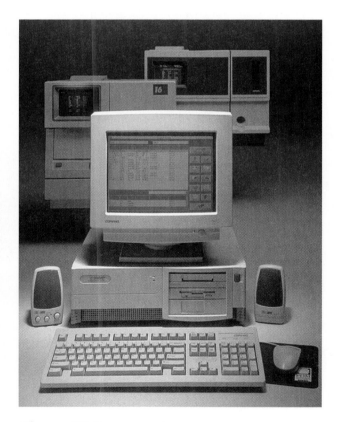

Figure 12-8   Patient data management system.

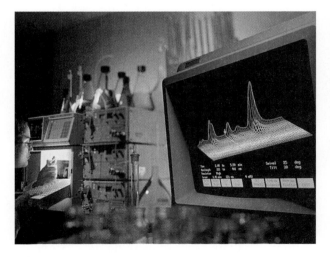

Figure 12-6   Computers are of tremendous benefit to medical researchers who must create, maintain, and update records with test results for large databases.

Security for the Computer System

The same legal standards of confidentiality apply to all patient records, whether on paper or on the computer. It is absolutely essential for the successful medical assistant to understand that other patients should not be able to see computerized records any more easily than paper records. This may require some thought and planning when a computer system is used for record keeping in the front office.

First, the screen should be positioned so that it cannot be easily seen by patients. A privacy screen around the computer work station may be necessary, depending on office layout. Another safeguard available is a screen saver which blanks out the screen without removing any data, but covers up what is on the screen so that no one but the user can see it.

Second, it is imperative that the records are accessible only to those who are authorized to use them. Keeping patient records safe may require using a **password.** Medical management programs often have several tiers of security, allowing one system administrator (the person in charge of the computer program) to limit access to patient records to those who need to see them. For example, the person who does appointment scheduling in a particular practice may not need to see a patient's financial records. The system administrator can "lock" the appointment scheduler out of financial records altogether, or assign a very limited access to the data.

Without a proper password, the user has no access at all to the data and must "log in" or type in his/her password, followed by an acceptance key (ENTER or RETURN) in order to use the program at all. It is important to guard a password carefully. It should not be shared with co-workers or written where someone else will see it. When choosing a password, avoid using the names of children or significant others (these would be too easy for someone else to guess). Use a word or a set of numbers that has significance to you, but is also easily remembered. If you must write your password down, write it in a secure place and do not identify it as a system password.

In order to avoid losing all data in the event of a system failure, fire, or equipment theft, it is also recommended that all data be backed up

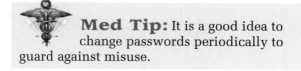

Med Tip: It is a good idea to change passwords periodically to guard against misuse.

(copied onto disks) at regular intervals and that these backups be stored in a secure location outside the office. Again, confidentiality is of the utmost importance, and access to backup files should be carefully guarded.

Med Tip: Recommendations for backup: Do this daily. Keep a separate tape for each workday (Monday through Friday). At the end of the work day, save onto tapes and take one off the premises to ensure data will not be lost.

Selecting a Computer System

The office manager in conference with the physician is usually responsible for selection of the computer system. However, as computer sophistication grows and makes old technology obsolete, it is quite possible that you will be involved in the selection of a computer system for the practice.

Med Tip: Remember: the hardware and the software are two different issues! The hardware without the software is worthless, and the wrong software can make even the most technologically advanced computer system a very expensive desk decoration.

It is important to make the selection of a computer system cautiously. The guidelines presented here offer direction and support to individuals charged with the task of making such a costly purchase.

Electronic Claims

With the advent of remote communications through electronic mail (e-mail) and modems, computers in one location can now "talk" to computers across the street, across the state, and across the country. This technology has allowed many insurance companies to offer electronic claims services or ECT (electronic claims transmission). This service tremendously speeds the path of an insurance claim and puts the dollars for services rendered in the practice's bank account in as few as three working days. Such access can be obtained through a "clearing house" or remote computer with transfer to multiple insurance carriers.

Guidelines: Selecting a Computer System

1. Before beginning the search for a new computer system, it is important to establish

   - How will the computer be used?
   - How many people will be using the computer system?
   - How much storage space is needed now and for several years into the future?

Remember, the more visual the program, the more space it will require to run. The more patients added to a particular database, the more storage space will be needed to keep pace with the size of the practice.

2. The second phase of the computer search should focus on the software currently being used.

   - Is it meeting the needs of the practice?
   - Does everyone who uses it understand how to use it?
   - Will the current programs transfer to a new system?

Changing programs adds to the cost of a new computer system and must be considered carefully in any system change. (WARNING: Some programs may not run correctly or at all when computer hardware has been changed!) Software can also be developed or modified for a specific purpose or office.

3. The third critical element of a computer search is the budget and costs related to budget, for example, monthly billing and insurance claim mailings. Questions that need to be asked are

   - How much can be spent to buy a new system?
   - Must any of the programs be changed in order to work on the new system?
   - How soon is this new system needed?
   - Is delivery/installation time a critical factor?

4. Once the hardware and software analysis has been completed, it is time to look at the products on the market. Some questions that should be asked are

   - Are there manufacturers who have a better service record than others?
   - What happens if the computer system breaks down?
   - Who pays to have it fixed?
   - Who decides what parts (components) of the system are needed—the practice or the computer salesperson?
   - Is some software already loaded on the computer or does the practice need to load all the software?

5. Next, the needs of the practice must again be examined. What things are absolutely essential and which are just "nice-to-haves?" It is always a good idea to narrow the choices down to one or two. Then, just as with buying a car, a "test drive" is in order. Does the system do what the salesperson said it would? Are there problems that can be discovered only by trying out the system?

6. Identify a support system of computer experts who can provide ongoing technical assistance and quick on site service for computer software and hardware problems.

7. Purchasing a service contract to take effect when the warranty covering parts, repair, and service expires is an option that you may wish to consider. Training contracts are available with firms that will provide employer training on new software and hardware.

Computer system selection is a large responsibility and while the final decision usually rests with a financial manager, the system's users can make or break the success of any given installation. Users that are not happy with the selection are not as apt to use the system to its fullest capability, and this will, in the end, cost the practice money. Therefore, it is imperative that as many users as possible be involved in the selection process in order to make sure that the money being spent on a system is well spent.

Table 12-2 provides a list of frequently used computer terms and definitions in addition to the glossary terms for this chapter. It would probably be helpful to have a list such as this available to distribute to staff at training sessions to support new computer users.

TABLE 12-2   List of Frequently Used Computer Terms

Term	Definition
backup	A copy of work or software batch data stored for processing at periodic intervals.
batch	Data stored for processing at periodic intervals.
boot	To start up the computer.
catalog	List of all files stored on a storage device.
characters per second	Speed measurement for printers.
cursor	Flashing bar, or symbol, which indicates where the next character will be placed.
daisy wheel printer	An impact printer that "strikes" characters onto a page, much like a typewriter; unable to produce graphic images, but does produce letter quality output.
database	Computer application which contains records or files.
data debugging	Process of eliminating errors from input data.
disk drive	A container which holds a read/write head, an access arm, and a magnetic disk for storage.
DOS	Disk operating system.
downtime	Time a computer cannot be used because of maintenance or mechanical failure.
electronic mail (e-mail)	Use of a telephone, modem, and appropriate hardware and software to allow transmission of data electronically from computer to computer.
file	A collection of related records.
file maintenance	Data entry operations including additions, deletions, and modifications.
format	Methods for setting margins, tabs, line spacing, and other layout features.
GIGO	"Garbage in, garbage out" which means if you input incorrect information you will receive incorrect output.
hard copy	A printed copy of data in a file.
hardware	The actual physical equipment that is used by a computer to process data.
input	Entering data into the computer system.
interface	Technology that allows two or more non-connected computers to exchange programs and data. Also referred to as a network.
keyboard	An input device, similar to a typewriter keyboard.
menu	A list of options available to the user.
modem	Hardware device which converts digital signals to analog signals for transfer over communication lines or links.
output	Processed data translated into final form or information to be used.

(Continued)

Term	Definition
peripheral	Devices required for the input, output, processing, and storage of data; includes mouse, disk drive, keyboards, printers, and joysticks.
scrolling	Feature which allows the computer operator to control the location of the cursor within a document.
security code	A group of characters that allows an authorized computer operator access to certain programs or features. Password.
write protect	Feature of storage devices which allows the data to be seen, but not changed.

Electronic claims submission requires the same information as a paper copy of an HCFA-1500 form, but instead of sending the claim form by mail, all information is sent directly to the insurance company's computer over telephone lines. This type of submission is referred to as a paperless claim. To send a claim electronically

1. Collect all information needed about the patient, including diagnostic and procedure codes as though you were completing an HCFA-1500 form. However, the claim form on the screen may not be identical to a hard copy of the HCFA form.
2. Connect your computer to the insurance company's computer, using instructions provided by the insurance company. This is normally accomplished by dialing a telephone number and waiting for connection confirmation. Once the connection has been established, type in your unique identification number and password and follow the instructions on the screen.
3. Fill out the claim form as you would the HCFA 1500. When the insurance carrier's computer recognizes the physician's identification number, it will automatically assign a processing number to the claim. Keep track of this number for future reference; it is your confirmation that the claim has been received.

Software programs are available which allow claim processing without the need to re-enter some of the data more than once. Figure 12-9 shows the Azron laptop electronic chart which allows the user to handwrite information on the screen, store the handwritten information, and convert it into a patient chart.

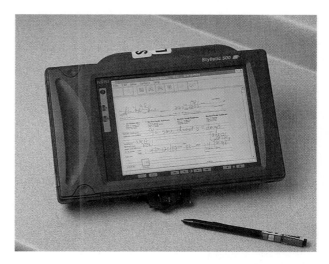

Figure 12-9 Wireless pen based portable computer helps create a paperless office.

Word Processing

Just as there are a myriad of programs for medical management, word processing programs range from very simple to very complicated. Most word processing programs function similarly to the old typewriter technology. The user inputs (types) information on a keyboard that is similar in appearance and basic functions to a typewriter keyboard. From that point forward, however, the differences between typing and word processing are large. With word processing, the user may view the copy prior to printing for modifications. Words, sentences, paragraphs, and even pages can be moved throughout the document. Other features of word processing include: automatic centering, indenting, underlining, bolding, italics, and font style.

More sophisticated word processing programs allow the user to

- Check spelling and grammar
- Create tables, charts, and graphs

- Automatic playback of frequently-used words, phrases, and letters
- Generate form letters to every person or to selected individuals in the database

It is advisable to add a spell check for medical terminology as well as a medical encyclopedia where this is financially feasible.

Word processors are used in medical offices to

- Generate and print letters, postcards, newsletters, patient information booklets, and sheets.
- Generate (type) patient chart records, history and physical exams, operative reports, and discharge reports.

While word processing is still used in some medical offices, computerized systems, and, in particular, computerized charting, is the wave of the future (Figure 12-10).

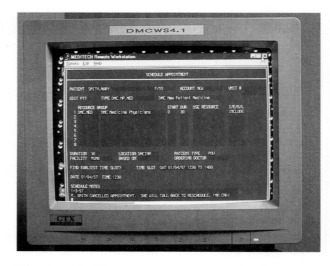

Figure 12-10   Computerized charting.

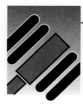

LEGAL AND ETHICAL ISSUES

The same standards of patient confidentiality apply to data stored on computers that apply to any and all patient records. The medical office must guard against unethical and illegal accessing and use of computer equipment for illegal purposes. Information contained within the computer must be protected, as must the computer hardware and software.

Employees of the practice must be educated and trained to understand the importance of security methods and to prevent loss or damage to valuable equipment and programs. Informed employees can follow the proper procedures to report suspicious occurrences within the workplace. The medical assistant must have an understanding of his or her own liability and the physician's liability in the processing of medical records.

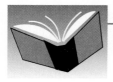

PATIENT EDUCATION

Most patients have now accepted computer technology as a part of conducting any business. Some patients, however, are still fearful that unauthorized persons may have access to their records. By using discretion in the handling of all medical records, the successful medical assistant conveys to the patient, without words, that confidentiality is of the utmost importance to the practice, thus reassuring the patient.

Summary

The use of computers is becoming more commonplace in medical offices today. In medical offices, computer use is especially useful in eliminating some of the more time-consuming tasks associated with appointment scheduling, charting, billing, and insurance processing. The successful medical assistant is a computer literate professional who deals easily with the challenge of finding new and efficient ways to use available technology.

Competency Review

1. Define and spell the glossary terms for this chapter.
2. Using a microcomputer, boot up the computer. Notice what information is displayed on the screen before the computer is "ready" to work. What disk operating system is being used? Does a menu or sub-menu appear when the computer has been booted or is the computer using a version of Windows? Are any security codes required to use the programs listed? If so, what are they?
3. What type of printer is used by the computer system? Is it an impact or a nonimpact printer?
4. Print a list of all the files on the hard drive.
5. Select a word processing program and type a simple letter, reminding a patient that he or she is due for a blood pressure check. Use the spell checking feature before printing the letter.
6. Enter a patient into a medical management software database. Use yourself and your own information as the data.
7. Complete an HCFA-1500 form for your personal insurance.

PREPARING FOR THE CERTIFICATION EXAM

Test Taking Tip — Read every question carefully to the very end. Do not assume you know what the question is until you have read every word. It is sometimes helpful to use your finger as a pointer to make sure you haven't missed a detail.

Examination Review Questions

1. Which of the following is considered a software element of computers?
   (A) hard disk
   (B) central processing unit
   (C) diskette
   (D) kilobyte
   (E) program
2. Which of the following is NOT considered hardware?
   (A) printer
   (B) DOS
   (C) monitor
   (D) keyboard
   (E) central processing unit
3. What type of printer is considered the most versatile?
   (A) laser
   (B) dot matrix
   (C) ink jet
   (D) word processor
   (E) typewriter
4. What is/are the advantages of a medical management program?
   (A) enter patient information only once
   (B) can print statements
   (C) can track days before payment is received from insurer
   (D) can print delinquency notices
   (E) all of the above
5. What is NOT recommended to establish computer security?
   (A) position screen away from patients
   (B) use a password that is unknown to the patient but that you can remember easily
   (C) have tiers of security that limit access to patient information to authorized employees
   (D) use screen savers to blank out the screen
   (E) change password frequently
6. Electronic mail is
   (A) physically entering data into the computer system
   (B) a backup copy of work or software
   (C) a process of eliminating errors from input data

(Continued on next page)

(D) use of a telephone, modem or hardware and software to transmit data from computer to computer

(E) physical equipment used by a computer to process data

7. A prompt is

(A) a set of instructions that tells the computer hardware what to do

(B) a reminder or hint to the user that some action must be taken

(C) processed data translated into final form

(D) methods for setting margins, tabs, and layout features

(E) a measure of storage capacity

8. The computer program that contains all records and files is known as

(A) software

(B) catalog

(C) database

(D) batch

(E) format

9. All of the following office functions can be performed by word processing EXCEPT

(A) user can input information using a typewriter-like keyboard

(B) user can see the copy that will be printed

(C) user can correct errors on the screen before printing takes place

(D) user can generate form letters

(E) all of the above are functions of word processing

10. To protect against a loss of data and information processed by the computer, a medical assistant should

(A) change the password frequently

(B) use electronic mail

(C) use word processing whenever possible

(D) make backup copies on a diskette

(E) handwrite a backup copy for the file

ON THE JOB

Elizabeth Maxwell, a medical assistant for Dr. Casey, is responsible for entering charges and payments into the office's computer system. One of Dr. Casey's patient's, Stephanie Cross, who is recovering from elective cosmetic surgery on her nose (rhinoplasty) has called to ask Elizabeth to submit her surgery bill to the insurance company with the statement that the surgery was necessary due to an auto accident. Stephanie tells Elizabeth that her insurance will not cover elective surgery and she is concerned that she will not be able to pay Dr. Casey unless Elizabeth processes the charges in this manner.

Later the same day, Diana Muldaur, who sits at the desk next to Elizabeth, has forgotten her computer password. She asks to use Elizabeth's password "just for today."

What is your response?

1. What should Elizabeth tell Stephanie Cross? Should she convey the request to Dr. Casey?

2. What should she do if Dr. Casey requests her to process the charges according to Elizabeth's request?

3. What should Elizabeth tell Diana Muldaur?

References

Becklin, K. and Sunnarborg, E. *Medical Office Procedures.* New York: Glencoe, 1996.

Computers in the Medical Office. New York: Glencoe/McGraw-Hill, 1996.

Gylys, B. *Computer Application in the Medical Office.* Philadelphia: F.A. Davis, 1991.

Johnson, J., Witaker, M., and Johnson, M. *Computerized Medical Office Management.* Albany, NY: Delmar Publishers, 1994.

Oliverio, J., Pasewark, W., and White, B. *The Office: Procedures and Technology.* Cincinnati, Ohio: South-Western Publishing Co., 1993.

Workplace Wisdom

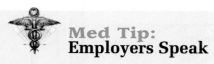

Med Tip:
Employers Speak

Demonstrate good basic skills.

Lynn Bowersfield
Assistant Administrative Director
Department of Medicine
Cooper Health System
Camden, New Jersey

Be willing to learn new skills and tackle new tools such as the computer. Adaptability will get you ahead today.

Opal Howard
Human Resources Specialist
Wendy Krieg
Assistant Director Centra Care
Florida Hospital
Orlando, Florida

Be willing to wear many hats—no longer can employers hire one person for a limited set of tasks.

Linda Davis-Rogers
Recruiter
Sharp Health Care
San Diego, California

Develop computer skills. Although you do not have to be a pro, you may need to register patients or input billing.

Jody Jesson
Principal Staffing Coordinator
UCLA Medical Enterprise
Los Angeles, California

Show a willingness to do whatever needs to be done. Keep an open mind; health care is changing and no one can say any longer, "It's not my job."

Kathy Robson
Human Resources Generalist
The Ohio State University Medical Center
Columbus, Ohio

Be willing to do whatever needs to be done. In today's environment, there is no room for the attitude, "It's not my job."

Lynn Bowersfield
Assistant Administrative Director
Department of Medicine
Cooper Health System
Camden, New Jersey

MEDICAL ASSISTANT ROLE DELINEATION CHART

Highlight indicates material covered in this chapter

ADMINISTRATIVE

ADMINISTRATIVE PROCEDURES

- Perform basic clerical functions
- Schedule, coordinate, and monitor appointments
- Schedule inpatient/outpatient admissions and procedures
- Understand and apply third party guidelines
- Obtain reimbursement through accurate claims submission
- Monitor third-party reimbursement
- Perform medical transcription
- Understand and adhere to managed care policies and procedures
- *Negotiate managed care contracts (adv)*

PRACTICE FINANCES

- Perform procedural and diagnostic coding
- Apply bookkeeping principles
- Document and maintain accounting and banking records
- Manage accounts receivable
- Manage accounts payable
- Process payroll
- *Develop and maintain fee schedules (adv)*
- *Manage renewals of business and professional insurance policies (adv)*
- *Manage personal benefits and maintain records (adv)*

CLINICAL

FUNDAMENTAL PRINCIPLES

- Apply principles of aseptic technique and infection control
- Comply with quality assurance practices
- Screen and follow up patient test results

DIAGNOSTIC ORDERS

- Collect and process specimens
- Perform diagnostic tests

PATIENT CARE

- Adhere to established triage procedures
- Obtain patient history and vital signs
- Prepare and maintain examination and treatment areas

- Prepare patient for examinations, procedures, and treatments
- Assist with examinations, procedures, and treatments
- Prepare and administer medications and immunizations
- Maintain medication and immunization records
- Recognize and respond to emergencies
- Coordinate patient care information with other health care providers

GENERAL (TRANSDISCIPLINARY)

PROFESSIONALISM

- Project a professional manner and image
- Adhere to ethical principles
- Demonstrate initiative and responsibility
- Work as a team member
- Manage time efficiently
- Prioritize and perform multiple tasks
- Adapt to change
- Promote the CMA credential
- Enhance skills through continuing education

COMMUNICATION SKILLS

- Treat all patients with compassion and empathy
- Recognize and respect cultural diversity
- Adapt communications to individual's ability to understand
- Use professional telephone technique
- Use effective and correct verbal and written communications
- Recognize and respond to verbal and non-verbal communications
- Use medical terminology appropriately
- Receive, organize, prioritize, and transmit information
- Serve as liaison
- Promote the practice through positive public relations

LEGAL CONCEPTS

- Maintain confidentiality
- Practice within the scope of education, training, and personal capabilities
- Prepare and maintain medical records
- Document accurately
- Use appropriate guidelines when releasing information
- Follow employer's established policies dealing with the health care contract
- Follow federal, state, and local legal guidelines
- Maintain awareness of federal and state health care legislation and regulations
- Maintain and dispose of regulated substances in compliance with government guidelines
- Comply with established risk management and safety procedures
- Recognize professional credentialing criteria
- Participate in the development and maintenance of personnel, policy, and procedure manuals
- *Develop and maintain personnel, policy, and procedure manuals (adv)*

INSTRUCTION

- Instruct individuals according to their needs
- Explain office policies and procedures
- Teach methods of health promotion and disease prevention
- Locate community resources and disseminate information
- *Orient and train personnel (adv)*
- *Develop educational materials (adv)*
- *Conduct continuing education activities (adv)*

OPERATIONAL FUNCTIONS

- Maintain supply inventory
- Evaluate and recommend equipment and supplies
- Apply computer techniques to support office operations
- *Supervise personnel (adv)*
- *Interview and recommend job applicants (adv)*
- *Negotiate leases and prices for equipment and supply contracts (adv)*

SOURCE: Reprinted by permission of the American Association of Medical Assistants from the *AAMA Role Delineation Study: Occupational Analysis of the Medical Assisting Profession.*

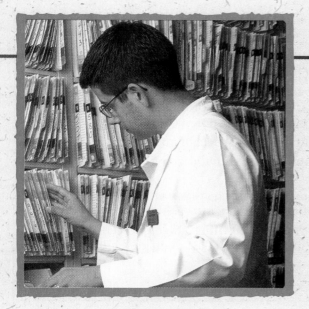

13

Medical Records and Transcription

CHAPTER OUTLINE

LEARNING OBJECTIVES

After completing this chapter, you should:

1. Define and spell the glossary terms for this chapter.
2. Describe three types of file storage units.
3. State the "Rules for Filing."
4. List and discuss 5 types of numerical filing systems.
5. Describe color-coded alphabetic and numerical filing systems.
6. State an effective system used for cross-referencing.
7. Describe how to find a missing file.
8. Define what a tickler file is.
9. Describe 3 pieces of equipment used for medical transcription.
10. State the "Rules of Editing."
11. Discuss the 6 types of reports found which may be dictated and require transcription.
12. Describe the equipment available for the physically challenged individual.

ADMINISTRATIVE PERFORMANCE COMPETENCY

After completing this chapter, you should perform the following tasks:

1. File patient records using both the alphabetic and numerical filing system.
2. File and retrieve patient records using a color-coded system.
3. Establish a "tickler" file.
4. Transcribe the following types of reports:
   a. History and physical
   b. Consultation report
   c. Operative report
   d. Pathology report
   e. Radiology report
   f. Discharge summary
5. Locate a missing file.

Glossary

accession Record of numbers assigned to each new patient name.

active Medical files of patients who are currently being seen by the physician. These may cover from 1 to 5 years, depending on the office policy.

alphabetic Filing system based on the letters of the alphabet.

archives Records that are no longer needed, such as when a patient dies, but must be kept for legal purposes.

closed Medical files of patients who have indicated that they are no longer patients or who have died. These files are kept in storage for legal reasons.

editing Rearrangment or restatement of a word or group of words in a document.

inactive Medical files for patients who have not been seen, according to the time period set up by the office policy (generally 1 to 5 years).

microfiche Sheets of microfilm.

microfilm Miniaturized photographs of records.

numeric Filing system which assigns an identification number to each person's name.

terminal digit filing Medical record filing system based on the last digits of the ID number.

Medical records are the sources of all documentation relating to the patient. They contain past history information, current diagnosis and treatment, and correspondence relating to the patient. Billing materials are often maintained in a separate accounting record. They can be maintained in a variety of ways which include paper (hard copy files), computer database files, and microfilm (miniaturized photographs of records) and microfiche (sheets of microfilm). Medical records management requires careful attention to accuracy, confidentiality, and proper filing and storage.

The Medical Record

The medical record contains all the written documentation that relates to the patient. Each patient's medical record will contain essentially the same categories of material but with information unique to each patient. For example, not every patient will have a consultation report from another physician, or a surgical report. See Figure 13-1 for an example of handwritten documentation in a medical chart. Table 13-1 contains a list of standard reports that can be found in a medical record.

The format for the medical record may also reflect the physician's specialty. For example, an obstetrical practice will use a format that includes questions pertaining to the prenatal (before birth) and postnatal (afterbirth) periods. See Figure 13-2 A and B for a health history summary for a maternal/newborn record system.

Most medical offices and hospitals use SOAP (subjective, objective, assessment, and plan) chart-

ing and the POMR (problem oriented medical record). See Figure 13-3 for an example of SOAP charting. Chapter 21, Assisting with Physical Examinations, contains a detailed description of the SOAP method.

The medical record is a legal document and, as such, should not contain flippant or unprofessional comments, such as "This patient is a very

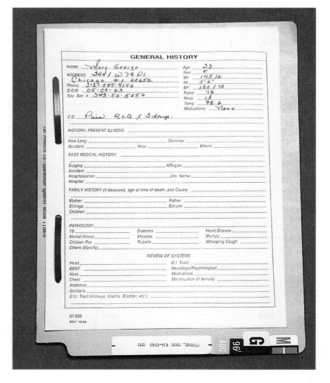

Figure 13-1 Handwritten documentation.

TABLE 13-1 Standard Medical Record

Contents
Patient's past medical history
History of present illness
Review of systems (Assessment of body systems)
Chief complaint (CC)
Progress notes
Family medical history
Personal history
Medication history with notations on refill orders
Treatments
X-ray reports
Laboratory results
Consultation reports (referrals)
Diagnosis
Other patient-related correspondence: • Informed consent documentation, when appropriate • Signature for release of information • Copy of living will

annoying person." However, everything that is done during a patient's medical visit, ordered over the telephone, or discussed with a patient over the telephone, must be documented in the medical record. See Figure 13-4 for an example of a medical assistant writing in a medical record.

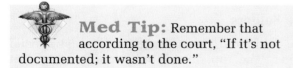

Med Tip: Remember that according to the court, "If it's not documented; it wasn't done."

Supplies and Equipment

Choosing the type of file system, including the file folder coding system, used in the office is an important decision since all files must be maintained within that system. Some large offices hire an office consultant to set up a filing system. While the office staff are generally consulted when setting up a new file system, the decision is made by the physician and the office manager.

Files

There are three categories of files or records in a medical office: active, inactive, and closed.

- **Active** records relate to patients who have been seen in the past few years and are currently being treated. Each medical practice may have its own policy regarding what constitutes an "active" file, but it is usually from 1 to 5 years.
- **Inactive** records relate to patients who have not been seen within the time period determined by office policy. These files are still maintained within the office but they are generally kept in a separate storage file cabinet. These patients have not received a formal notification that the physician has terminated caring for them. They may return when a medical problem develops.
- **Closed** records are those of patients who have actively terminated their contact with the physician. This occurs when they move

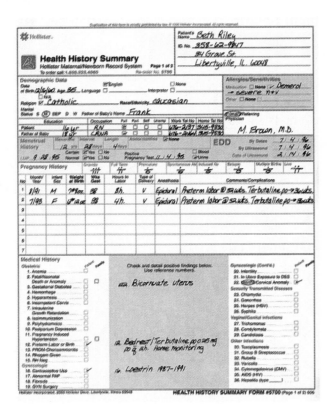
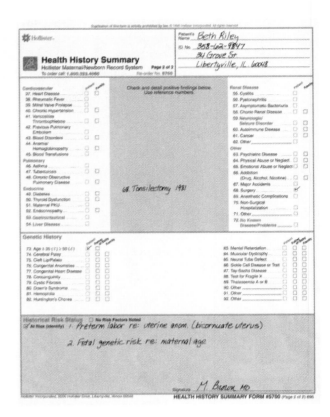

Figure 13-2 A and B Health History Summary for Maternal/Newborn Record System.

away, ask to have their records sent to another physician, or death occurs. These files can be placed in storage boxes and are referred to as **archives,** since they are no longer needed but must be kept for legal reasons.

Fireproof cabinets are used to file documents such as patient records, tax records, insurance policies, and canceled checks.

File Storage

Three types of file storage commonly used in a physician's office are vertical, lateral, and movable.

- Vertical—Set up with two to four stacked pullout drawers holding up to 100 files per drawer. This type of file storage system is heavy and space consuming.
- Lateral—Set up with shelves allowing for easy access to files by pulling them off the shelves. This system often uses a color-coded method for visual recognition of files.

- Movable—Set up with electrically powered or manually controlled file units that move on tracks in the floor. This type of open filing system is space saving since the file units can be moved close together when they are not needed. This system is also useful for books and journals since the floor can be reinforced when the track is installed.

File Folders

File folders are also designed to meet special needs. The top or side edge contains tabs at spaced intervals. These tabs are marked with identification labels. If files are stored with alternating tab cuts, it is easier to read the labels in the file drawer. The identification label is attached to the top tab in a vertical file cabinet or to the side edge of the file in a lateral file cabinet.

The patient's record may be placed within a separate tabbed folder that remains in the filing cabinet. The file folders may be color-coded to indicate the primary care physician. Each physician

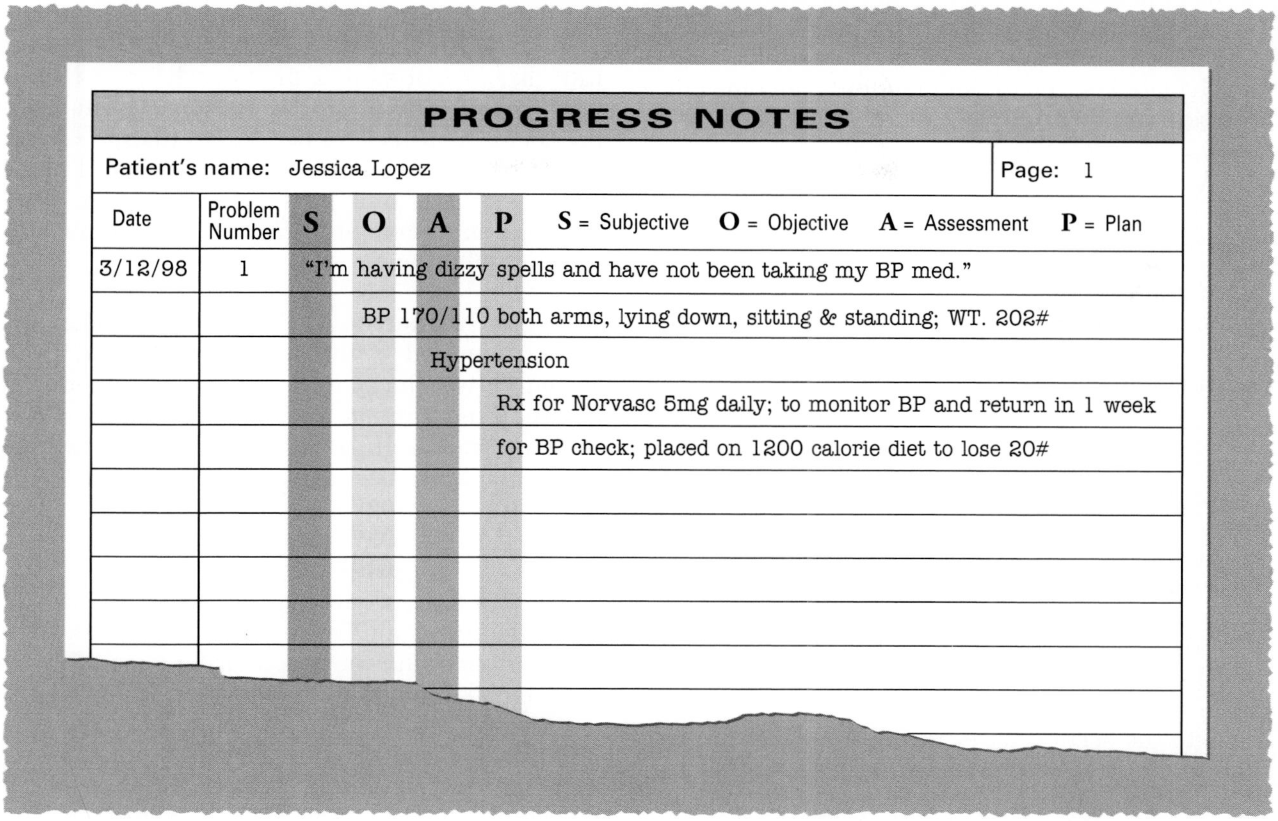

PROGRESS NOTES

Date	Problem Number	S	O	A	P	S = Subjective O = Objective A = Assessment P = Plan

Patient's name: Jessica Lopez   **Page:** 1

Date	Problem Number	S O A P
3/12/98	1	"I'm having dizzy spells and have not been taking my BP med."
		BP 170/110 both arms, lying down, sitting & standing; WT. 202#
		Hypertension
		Rx for Norvasc 5mg daily; to monitor BP and return in 1 week
		for BP check; placed on 1200 calorie diet to lose 20#

Figure 13-3   Example of SOAP charting.

would be assigned a folder color. This helps keep files in order in large clinics.

Guides

Divider guides are used to separate files in the drawer or on the shelf. These guides are of heavy pressboard and should be placed every 1 1/2 to 2 inches to separate the file folders.

The divider guide breaks the files into subsections using a letter (for example A, B, C, or A-B, Invoices) or a numerical system by patient number.

An out-guide is placed in the file when a file is removed to indicate where the file should be returned. The out-guide is usually a distinctive color, such as red, to indicate a file is missing.

Labels

The label on the file folder has a main purpose of identifying what is in the file (patient's name). However, the label can also include a color coding stripe which can be used for other purposes, such as identifying the primary care physician. The label on the file drawer contains the topic and the range of files.

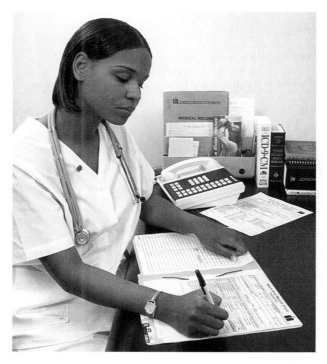

Figure 13-4   Medical assistant documenting patient call in medical record.

For example: **Patient Histories**
A-D

The label on the divider contains the range of files between that divider and the next.

For example: **Aa-Ba**

Rules for Filing

Three commonly used systems for filing are the **alphabetic, numeric,** and subject filing. Alphabetizing is a component of all the methods and will be explained in detail. Color-coding is used in all three systems to assist in locating files, refiling, and prevent misfiling.

Alphabetic System

Alphabetizing is the most common system for filing records in a physician's office. (A hospital generally uses an ID numeric system for filing patient records). In this system Abbott would be filed before Bacon since "A" appears before "B" in the alphabet. If the first letter is the same, then move to the second letter in the name. Abbott is filed before Acker. This does not pose problems when filing a last name since everyone understands the alphabet. However there could be confusion when filing Jacob James Jergens, Jr. and Jacob James Jergens III. Or determining how correspondence from 23rd Avenue Clinic should be filed.

The key to alphabetic filing is to divide the names and titles into units (first, second, and third). The unit is the portion of the name that is used for filing or indexing purposes. For example:

- Unit 1 Jergens
- Unit 2 Jacob
- Unit 3 James

The first letter of each unit is then used to determine where the file is to be placed. When filing a large number of files, use the first letter of the first unit and place all the files from A-Z in order. Then take each group of A files and use the second letter and consecutive letters to place them in order. If the entire first unit is the same, as in Smith, then move onto the second unit, and third unit. For example, Smith, Loren comes before Smith, Michael which comes before Smith, Michelle. Table 13-2 describes basic rules for alphabetic filing.

Numerical Filing Systems

A numerical patient identification system is used in hospitals and many of the larger clinics. A number is assigned to each patient's medical record. This is generally a 6-digit number divided into three sections of 2 digits each (for example 05-72-21). Veterans Administration hospitals use the social security number with 9 digits.

There are several types of numerical filing including straight numerical filing, filing by terminal digit, middle digit filing, unit numbering, and serial numbering.

Straight Numerical Filing The simplest numerical method is the straight numerical filing system in which each record is filed sequentially based on its assigned number. The numbers used in this system begin at 01 and continue upward.

Example:	01	101	886
	02	102	887
	03	103	888
	04	104	889

In this type of system, the file space will become depleted rapidly as new files are added to one section. This requires constant reshifting of files to make room for the new files.

Terminal Digit Filing Terminal Digit filing, based on the last digits of the ID number, evenly distributes the files within the entire filing system which eliminates the need for frequent reshifting of files, providing enough space was designated when the filing system was setup.

Filing using terminal digits requires dividing the files into 100 primary sections, starting with 00 and ending with 99. The three sections of numbers assigned to each file are designated as tertiary, secondary, and primary sections respectively.

Example: 05 72 21
tertiary secondary primary

To file a record using this system, find the file section matching the patient's primary digits (21). Within that section, match up the secondary digits (72), and file the record according to the tertiary digits (05).

Middle Digit Filing Using the same 6-digit numbering system as with the terminal digit system, the middle digit filing system places the middle digits as the primary numbers.

Example: 05 72 21
secondary primary tertiary

In this example, find the section marked 72, within that section find the 05 area, and then file the record according to the tertiary digit, 21.

Unit Numbering This system assigns a number to patients the first time they are seen or admitted to a hospital. All other hospitalizations or hospital

TABLE 13-2   Rules for Alphabetic Filing

Rule and Example

1. Names are filed: last name, first name, middle name (or initial). Each letter in the name is a separate unit.

   Example: Krause, Marvin K. is placed before *Krause, Marvin L.*

2. Initials come before a full name.

   Example: Brown, H. is placed before *Brown, Henry.*

3. Hyphenated names are treated as one unit. This applies to the names of individuals and businesses.

   Example: Amy Freeman-Smith is indexed under *F* for *Freeman.* It is considered *Freemansmith* for indexing purposes.

4. Titles (and initials) are disregarded for filing but placed in parentheses after the name.

   Example: Dr. Beth Ann Williams is indexed as *Williams, Beth Ann, (Dr).*

5. Married women are indexed using their legal name. The husband's name can be used for cross-referencing.

   Example: Mrs. Mary Jane Smith is indexed as *Smith, Mary Jane (Mrs. John).*

6. Seniority units, such as *Jr.* and *Sr.,* are filed in a numerical order from first to last.

   Example: Jacob James Jurgens, Sr. comes before *Jacob James Jurgens, Jr.*

7. Numeric seniority terms are filed before alphabetic terms.

   Example: Jurgens, Jacob James III indexed before *Jurgens, Jacob James, Jr.*

8. Mac and Mc can be either filed alphabetically as they occur or grouped together depending on the preference of the office.

9. Foreign language names are indexed as one unit.

   Example: Mary St. Claire is indexed as *Stclaire, Mary.* Carol van Damm is indexed as *Vandamm, Carol.*

10. If company names are identical, the address, by state, then city, street, may be used in the index. The ZIP code is not used to index files.

    Example: ABC Drugs, 123 Michigan Blvd., Chicago IL is indexed before *ABC Drugs, 1450 N. Ash, Kalispell MT.*

11. If individual's names are identical, use the birth date or mother's maiden name. Avoid using address since that can change.

    Example: Mark Richard Jones is indexed as *Jones, Mark Richard* (5/12/65) and *Jones, Mark Richard* (2/12/89).

12. Disregard apostrophes.

    Example: Megan O'Connor is indexed as *Oconnor, Megan.*

13. Business organizations are indexed as they are written.

    Example: *Lincoln Memorial Hospital* is correct.

(Continued on next page)

TABLE 13-2 *(Continued)*

Rule and Example
14. Disregard small terms, such as *a, and, the,* and *of.*   Example: The Whitefish Drug Store is indexed as *Whitefish Drug Store (The).*
15. Numeric characters are indexed before alpha characters.   Example: 23rd Avenue Clinic would be indexed before the *Nineteenth Street Medical Center.* A separate file is set up for all numeric files.
16. Names with religious titles, such as Sister Mary Murphy would be filed with the last name first, and then with the religious title.   Example: *Murphy, Sister Mary.*
17. Compound words are filed as they are written.   Example: South West Physician Service is filed before *Southwest Physician Service.*

visits use the same number. This method requires that all the records be kept at the same location.

Serial Numbering With a serial numbering system, the patient receives a different medical record number for each hospital visit. The patient acquires multiple records which are stored at different locations. For example, a hospitalization, laboratory work, and a mammogram will all receive different numbers and be filed within their own systems.

The assigned numbers are kept in an **accession** record in which numbers in sequential order (1, 2, 3, 4, 5, 6...) have a name placed next to them as each new name is entered. This record can also be maintained on the computer. Figure 13-5 illustrates a medical assistant filing in a medical records room.

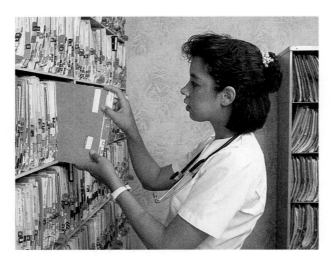

Figure 13-5 Medical records room.

Med Tip: Remember to have a backup for all computer files, such as accession records, in the event of a loss of computer power.

Subject Matter

Filing by subject is used for general files, such as invoices, correspondence, resumes, and personnel records. This method is adequate as long as the files are relatively small. If these files become large, then another method, alphabetic or numerical, will have to be devised.

Color-Coding Systems

To decrease the number of misfiled charts and aid in file retrieval many medical record departments will use a color-coded system on their file folders. This system assigns a color for each number from 0-9. Color bars on the end of each file folder correspond to the medical record number. Usually only the three primary digits are color-coded. When files are in the correct placement, the color bands will all have the same pattern. In this manner any misfiles are easily seen. Filing records is simplified since the correct color band can be located on the file shelf.

Color Bands Two popular color-coding methods using a numerical system are the Ames Color File System and The Smead Manufacturing Company's method. Table 13-3 lists examples of the numerical color-coding systems used by these two systems.

TABLE 13-3   Numerical Color-Coding Systems

Ames Color File System			Smead Corporation System		
0 - red	4 - purple	8 - pink	0 - yellow	4 - orange	8 - red
1 - gray	5 - black	9 - green	1 - blue	5 - brown	9 - black
2 - blue	6 - yellow		2 - pink	6 - green	
3 - orange	7 - brown		3 - purple	7 - gray	

TABLE 13-4   Alpha-Z Alphabetic Color-Coding System

Color	White Letter No Stripe	White Letter White Stripe
Red	A	N
Dark Blue	B	O
Dark Green	C	P
Light Blue	D	Q
Purple	E	R
Orange	F	S
Gray	G	T
Dark Brown	H	U
Pink	I	V
Yellow	J	W
Light Brown	K	X
Lavender	L	Y
Light Green	M	Z

There are also color-coded methods using an alphabetic system. One example is the Alpha-Z system by The Smead Manufacturing Company. This system is based on 13 colors using white letters on a colored background (for example, the letter "A" is on a solid red background) for the first one-half of the alphabet, and the addition of a white stripe on the colored background for the second half of the alphabet (for example, the letter "N" is a red background with a white stripe). This color-coding system is described in Table 13-4.

The Alpha-Z system uses file labels to denote the patient's name, and a color label with the letter of the alphabet to indicate the index unit. For example, Emily Jane Smith would be labeled Smith, Emily Jane with an orange color block containing a white stripe and the letter "S." Two other color blocks would be added to the label for the secondary and tertiary letters of the index unit (in this example, "E" on a solid purple background, and "J" on a solid yellow background.

This system is ideal for the large practice with many patients having the same surnames. It can be adapted to a particular office's needs. For example, only the last name is color-coded (Joseph Evans has only one solid PURPLE color label). After the files are color-coded, they are then alphabetized within their particular "color" category.

In large practices with several physicians, each physician may have a color assigned to him or her. For example, Dr. Williams' patients might all have medical file folders with a yellow label. Figure 13-6 is a photo of a color-coded medical record.

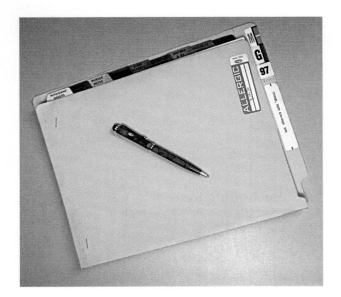

Figure 13-6   Color-coded record.

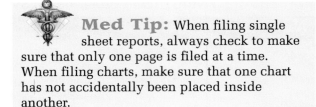

Guidelines: Locating Missing Files

- Look for a file with a "sound-alike" or "look-alike" name. For example, Smith or Smits.
- If using a color-coded system, look for a folder with the same color-coding.
- If using a numeric system, look for a transposing of numbers. For example, 236984 for 263984.
- Look for a transposing of letters.
- Look for an alternative spelling. For example, Keane for Kane.
- Look at the folders that were filed before and after the missing record. For example, pull out the schedule of all patient's who were seen on the same day as the patient whose file is missing.
- Look on the physician's desk, in and out baskets. Also ask other staff, such as the billing clerk, to examine their desks.

Cross-Referencing

Due to the large number of files processed in a busy office and the confusion over surnames (for example, how are step-children's names filed for easy access?), cross-referencing of files is recommended. Cross-referencing refers to alerting the health worker that a file may be found under another name. For example, if Mrs. Henry Watts also uses her maiden name, Farideh Rahman, then a file insert into Henry Watt's file could state, "See Rahman, Farideh for Mrs. Henry Watts. Cross-referencing can be a simple, but useful, tool for finding and avoiding "lost" records.

In some medical practices, a color-coded "year" tab is placed on folders of patients who are seen once a year. This hastens the purging of "inactive" files.

Locating Missing Files

One of the most time consuming and frustrating activities relating to medical records is locating a "missing" file. Ideally, everyone who removes a file from a cabinet should add that file name or number to a master file sheet. In addition, a marker should be placed in the file indicating a file was removed.

If a systematic search takes place, the file can usually be located quickly. In the case of one piece of paper which has been misfiled with other papers, it may not be located. In this case, the medical assistant will need to get another copy of the paper from the original source (for example, a laboratory or radiology report).

The best way to avoid losing a file, is to file all records methodically and carefully.

Tickler Files

A tickler file is used to remind the medical assistant of an event or action that will take place at a future date. The tickler file contains patients' names and telephone numbers, dates when action or activities should occur, and actions to take. The tickler files should be reviewed on a daily basis so that actions are taken on time. For example, tickler files can be used as reminders to call patients to set appointments, to pay certain invoices, or to send fees for the physicians' license renewals. Figure 13-7 is a example of a tickler file using a file drawer. Figure 13-8 illustrates an index card tickler file.

Releasing Medical Records

The physician owns the medical record but the patient has the legal right of "privileged communication" and access to their records. Therefore, the

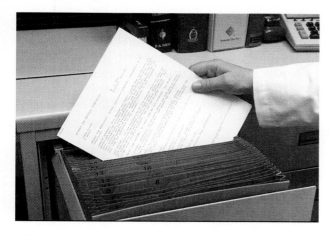

Figure 13-7 Tickler file using a file drawer.

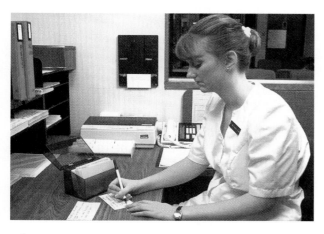

Figure 13-8 Index card tickler file.

patient must authorize release of his or her records and state in writing that the medical records may be released. The patient may have access to his or her records and request a copy of those records. Since some records are large and require excessive duplicating time and expense, the physician may charge to provide this service.

> ✦ **Med Tip:** Never send an original record. Always send a copy. In the case of x-ray film, the physician may allow the original to be sent under the stipulation that it be returned. Never give medical record information over the telephone.

Never release records directly to a patient without the physician's permission. The informa-

tion contained in the record can be upsetting to some patients without the proper explanation.

The Statute of Limitations

Each state varies somewhat on the legal time limits (statute of limitations) to keep records and documents. Legally, all medical records should be stored for 7 years from the time of the last entry. However, most physicians store medical records permanently since malpractice suits can still be filed within 2 years from the date of the knowledge of the occurrence or malpractice event. For example, a minor child can file a malpractice suit relating to a birth injury 2 years from the date he or she reaches the age of maturity and became aware of the injury.

Medical Transcription

Medical transcription involves translating dictated or written medical information and producing a permanent record into a typed format. The information can relate to a patient's office or hospital visit, a specific hospital report such as radiology, pathology or lab, or a manuscript for publication.

There is an absolute need for accuracy to ensure the correct interpretation when editing the physician's dictation. The same professional standard relating to confidentiality is necessary when handling transcription even though the transcriptionist may never see the patient.

Medical records must be professionally prepared following appropriate formats. They should be free of errors and correctly filed. Remember medical records are always subject to possible subpoena by the courts.

Medical Transcriptionists

Medical transcriptionists are men and women who have excellent typing and grammar skills, a knowledge of medical terminology, and a desire for accuracy.

The medical transcriptionists must understand words and how to use them. This includes an understanding of etymology, phonetics, synonyms, acronyms, antonyms, homonyms, and eponyms.

- Etymology is the study of word origins. An understanding of the derivation (for example Latin or Greek) of a medical term helps in understanding the meaning.
- Phonetics are the keys to pronunciation. These are found in all standard

dictionaries and aid in deciding how a combination of letters is pronounced. Correct pronunciation is a key to correct spelling.

- Synonyms are words with like meanings (for example, fever and pyrexia).
- Acronyms are words that are structured by taking the first letter of each word in a group of words (for example, AIDS for acquired immune deficiency syndrome or CPR for cardiopulmonary resuscitation).
- Antonyms are words with opposite meanings (for example, supine and prone).
- Homonyms are words that are spelled alike, pronounced alike, but have different meanings (for example, the word draw as "to draw blood" or to "draw a conclusion").
- Eponyms are names of diseases based on the physician or patient who first documented the disease (for example, Bright's disease).

Sound-Alike Words

Caution must be used when writing words that have the same, or similar, sound. When taking medical dictation off a recording device, such as a Dictaphone, it can be difficult to discern the term based on the physician's pronunciation. To compound the problem, many medical terms actually sound alike when spoken, but have very different meanings.

Transcriptionists must take special precautions when transcribing tapes to make sure they have heard the correct terms. In many cases, the content of the material will determine which is the correct term. For instance, mastitis, meaning an inflammation of a mammary gland, and mastoiditis, an inflammation of the mastoid bone in the middle ear, sound alike in pronunciation. However, the mammary gland in the female breast and the mastoid bone in the ear are located in different body systems and are not generally discussed in the same context.

There are other terms, such as ureter and urethra, which are organs located in close proximity to each other in the urinary system. These two terms must never be confused. When in doubt always ask the dictating physician to clarify the term for you. You may have to look up the exact definition of the word in a medical dictionary. Table 13-5 contains an extensive list of words that sound alike.

Editing

Editing, the rearranging or restatement of a word or group of words in a document, requires skill. It is particularly important that the editor (in this case the transcriptionist) has the ability to know how to edit the text without affecting the intended meaning of the text.

Rules for Editing The medical transcriptionist must understand both when and when not to edit. Editing refers to making sure that grammar, punctuation, spelling, and word usage are all correct even if the person dictating the material is incorrect. The typed transcription must be clear, concise and easy to understand. However, care must be taken not to change the meaning of the material during the editing process. If the transcriber is unclear about a word or the meaning of a dictated term, the report should be flagged. This means that a colored tag or stick-on is applied to the report when it is submitted to the physician indicating there is a question about something on the report. If the word or words are not decipherable, then a blank line is left on the report where the word should be. Rules for *when* and *when not* to edit are presented in Table 13-6.

The medical assistant must acquire the ability to work closely with the physician in order to understand his or her dictation and editing needs.

Transcription Reminders

Transcriptionists must consider policies of physicians and hospitals when editing, trying not to change dictated material to reflect their own style and/or taste in writing. The dictated material should reflect the personal style of the individual physician.

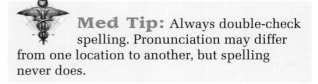
Med Tip: Always double-check spelling. Pronunciation may differ from one location to another, but spelling never does.

The American Association for Medical Transcription (AAMT) publishes *The AAMT Book of Style for Medical Transcription,* which contains useful information about appropriate abbreviations, cancer classifications, and medical terminology.

Just as there are rules for the transcriptionist to follow, there are also guidelines when giving dic-

TABLE 13-5 Sound-Alike Words

Words That Sound Alike					
addiction	adduction	abduction	hypertension	hypotension	
amenorrhea	dysmenorrhea		ileum	ilium	
antidiarrheic	antidiuretic		infection	infestation	
antiseptic	aseptic	asepsis	keratosis	ketosis	
arteritis	arthritis		larynx	pharynx	
aural	oral		lymphangitis	lymphadenitis	
callus	callous		macro	micro	
chronic	chromic		mastitis	mastoiditis	
cirrhosis	serosa		menorrhea	menorrhagia	metorrhagia
contusion	concussion	convulsion	mucous	mucus	
corneal	cranial		nephrosis	neurosis	
cocci	coxa		palpation	palpitation	
cystostomy	cystotomy	syctoscopy	precardiac	pericardium	
diaphysis	diastasis	diathesis	perineal	peroneal	
epigastric	epispastic		perineum	peritoneum	
embolus	thrombus		stasis	staxis	
facial	fascial		sycosis	psychosis	
foci	fossae		ureter	urethra	
gavage	lavage		vesical	vesicle	

tation. Some of these guidelines are presented in this chapter.

Transcription Equipment

The equipment required for medical transcription includes dictation equipment including transcribers, typewriters, word processing equipment and reference materials. Newer methods of transcription include computerized voice recognition technology (VRT). Explanations of each follow.

Transcribers

Medical transcribers are machines that allow the transcriptionist to take oral dictation and turn this into written material and documents. These typically have an audiocassette tape (onto which the physician or other health care worker has dictated information); headphones for private listening, a speed, volume, and tone control; and a footpedal to free the hands for typing.

The cassette mechanism of transcription equipment has the ability to play, stop, rewind and fast forward the tape. However, the footpedal is used for most playing and rewinding since it is faster.

A standard cassette transcriber uses a standard size audio tape (3 15/16″ × 2 1/2″). The microcassette transcriber uses micro-sized tapes (2″ × 1 1/4″). A mini-cassette transcriber, used almost exclusively as transcription equipment, requires a slightly larger tape (2 3/16″ × 1 3/8″) than the microcassette. The correct tape must be used with the appropriate medical transcriber.

TABLE 13-6   Editing Guidelines

Edit	Examples
Grammatically incorrect dictation	Incorrect: "There was no scars, adhesions, masses." Correct: "There were no scars, adhesions, or masses noted."
Ambiguous and/or unclear dictation	Incorrect: "Dr. William's, the primary care physician, was contacted after she had the cerebrovascular accident." Correct: "Dr. Williams, the patient's primary care physician, was contacted after the patient had the cerebrovascular accident."
Inaccurate or inconsistent dictation	Incorrect: "The patient's SMACK-7 values were within normal limits." Correct: "The patient's SMAC-7 values were within normal limits."

Do not edit	Examples
When unsure of the meaning	Incorrect: "Upon exam of right eye, cataract found in left eye."
(Flag report for physician to make correction.)	Correct: "Upon exam of _____ eye, cataract found in _____ eye."
When the meaning would change	Incorrect: "Fracture of ileum."
(Flag report for physician to make the correction.)	Correct: "Fracture of _____ (ilium or ileum)."

Guidelines: Giving Dictation

1. State what is being dictated and any special requirements such as size, type of paper, and number of copies.
2. Spell out the full names of all persons named in the report or correspondence. Provide a full address including ZIP code if the correspondence is to be mailed.
3. Speak clearly directly into the dictating equipment or microphone of the tape recorder. Do not eat or drink while dictating.
4. Alert the transcriber to a new paragraph by saying, "Period paragraph."
5. Indicate punctuation when appropriate, such as commas, quotation marks, and question marks.
6. Turn off the recorder when thinking rather than using fillers such as "um."

Med Tip: It is important to coordinate the type of dictation equipment the physician uses with the type of equipment the transcriber uses for medical transcription. Some newer models of transcription equipment can accommodate different sizes of tapes (dual capacity transcribers).

Word Processing

Word processing has made medical transcription more efficient. The word processor has the ability to create and maneuver text without having to cut and paste a paper document. The word processor also is able to save the document. This allows the typist to work on a document, save it, retrieve it at a later time, and work on it again. Corrections during the typing process can easily be made. For example, if a dictated word is not clear on the tape, the transcriptionist can leave a blank for that word with a question mark, and add the correct word before finishing the document by speaking to the dictator (physician).

Another advantage of the word processor over the typewriter is the ability to make multiple original copies of the document.

Voice Recognition Technology (VRT)

This new technology allows the physician to speak into a microphone connected to a computer program which translates the dictation into a typed report. VRT requires the physician to provide several samples of speech by reading manufacturer-provided scripts to activate the program. Since this is a time consuming process, not too many physicians have adopted this system in their offices. However, it is used in some hospital medical records departments and as the equipment becomes more user-friendly, it will become more accessible.

Transcription Equipment for the Physically Challenged

There are many adaptations for persons with a physical impairment, such as lower limb paralysis, blindness, and deafness. Foot pedals can be replaced with hand or voice activated equipment for a person in a wheelchair or with lower limb impairment.

The blind and visually impaired can use video magnifiers which use high-powered lenses to enlarge copy. A device called a TActile CONverter allows the blind person to read printed material by placing one hand inside the converter holding a printed document and "reading" the material with the index finger resting on the transmitter plate.

Blind transcriptionists are able to proofread their material through the use of a voice synthesizer. A Braille-Edit program allows blind and sighted persons to work together using a microcomputer.

The deaf or hearing impaired are able to use a telecommunications device for the deaf (TDD) which will place sound onto paper. They can then type it into the correct format for a medical record.

Use of Computers in Medical Transcription

The office computer is generally of the microcomputer variety, which takes up little space and can perform a variety of functions, including word processing. This office computer may also be used for a variety of other functions including billing and scheduling. The microcomputer has a larger storage capacity than the word processor. In addition, programs to aid in medical transcription, such as a thesaurus, medical dictionary, spell checker, and various word processing programs can easily be installed on the computer.

Types of Reports

Several types of medical reports require transcribing. These all use the same medical terminology and abbreviations; however, each uses a particular format. Six types of reports are described in this chapter: history and physical, consultation report, operative note, pathology, radiology, and discharge summary.

History and Physical

The history and physical report originates with the physician during the patient's first office visit or with the admitting physician or resident during the admitting process in the hospital. This report is a composite of the patient's past history that led up to the present illness (PI); the past social and family history; a review of all symptoms; and the physical findings as a result of the current examination. The history and physical report is typed based on these categories.

The patient will provide an oral past history including hospitalizations, allergies, chronic illnesses, and immunizations. The social and family history presents any precipitating factors such as a history of smoking, and a family history of diseases/disorders such as cancer, heart disease, and mental illness. A review of all symptoms is the physician's evaluation as a result of the physical exam. A history and physical report will include:

- Patient's name and medical record number
- Medical transcriber's name
- Date of examination
- Chief complaint (CC)
- Details of present illness
- Relevant past family and social history
- Allergies and medication history
- Inventory of body systems: HEENT, GI, Cardiovascular, GU, Respiratory, MS, and Endocrine, for example.

The comprehensive physical exam includes:

- General appearance
- Nutrition

- B/P
- Head-EENT, mouth, and scalp
- Neck, thyroid
- Thorax, breasts
- Lymphadenopathy
- Heart and lungs
- Abdomen
- Pelvic/Genital area, Rectal
- Neurologic including reflexes
- Skin
- Impression and plan

Consultation Report

There are many situations in which a physician would ask another physician to provide a second opinion on a patient's case. The patient generally would be examined by the second physician and then a report dictated. The report is sent to the attending physician (the requesting physician). The consultation report will include:

- Patient's name and medical record number.
- Date of consultation.
- Medical transcriptionist's name.
- Referring physician.
- Reason for the consultation.
- Physical and laboratory evaluations.
- Consulting physician's impression and recommendations.

It is appropriate to close this report, which is supplied in letter format, with a complimentary close such as, "Thank you for this referral."

Operative Note

The operative report describes a surgical procedure. The surgeon is expected to dictate this report as soon as possible, preferably immediately after, the procedure is completed. The surgeon's name, date of procedure, preoperative and postoperative diagnosis, and the actual findings during the procedure are included in this report.

This report includes a description of the actual procedure which will include location and length of the incision, the layers of skin and tissue that were incised, types of instruments used (in some cases), which organs and tissues were removed, and all materials that were used in closing the wound. The estimated amount of blood loss, and a sponge count are included. The condition of the patient at the end of the procedure is stated, such as "Patient tolerated procedure well,"

"Patient awake and responding," or "Patient taken to recovery room."

Pathology Report

The pathology report is generated by the pathologist as the result of examining tissue and organs removed during a surgical procedure (such as a biopsy) or at an autopsy. An autopsy report is generated after a patient's death to determine the cause of death. A pathology report focuses on microscopic (histology and cytology) findings as well as a gross (overall) description of the tissues or organs. This report is related to disease findings and not laboratory findings, which are conducted on body fluids.

Radiology Report

A radiology report is completed by the radiologist to document results of diagnostic procedures such as x-rays, CT (computerized tomography) scans, MRI (magnetic resonance imaging) scans, nuclear medicine procedures (bone and thyroid scans) and other fluoroscopic examinations.

Discharge Summary

The discharge summary is completed on every hospitalized patient and summarizes the hospitalization. It explains why the patient was admitted, a summary of the patient's history and a review of what occurred during the hospitalization. A discharge diagnosis is included in this report. The patient's condition upon leaving the hospital is noted.

Additional Reports

Other reports may be dictated concerning a patient, such as an emergency room report, psychiatric note, special procedures, for example a cardiac catheterization, and autopsy reports.

Reference Materials

Reference materials should be kept near the medical transcriptionist's work station. These references include standard dictionary, medical dictionary, *Physician's Desk Reference (PDR)*, grammar reference book, drug index, and a transcription style book for correct use of abbreviations, capitalizations, and punctuation. Reference materials are discussed further in Chapter 11, Written Communications.

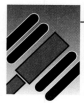

LEGAL AND ETHICAL ISSUES

Confidentiality of medical records must be maintained at all times. The medical record is the legal property of the physician. However, the physicians and their staff have a responsibility to treat the medical record with care since it contains a documentation of the patient's medical history. Physicians must arrange for storage facilities to keep records of inactive or closed files since they could be needed at a future date for patient care, unless the patient is deceased, or be subpoenaed into court.

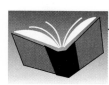

PATIENT EDUCATION

Many patients believe that the medical record is their property since it is a history of their medical care. The medical assistant must be able to explain that the physician owns all the equipment and files in his or her office but, patients have a right to see and have a copy of their medical records. Patients can be confused and distressed if they receive their medical record without any explanation. The physician has the responsibility of explaining the record to the patient and the medical assistant can reinforce this explanation.

Summary

Handling a patient's medical record requires an efficient system which results in few missing or misfiled records. As a medical practice grows, it may be necessary to replace a simple system based on an alphabetic system with a numerical or even a color-coded system. Every medical practice needs a method for alerting staff when a file has been removed from the record area. A "tickler" system that is used faithfully can reduce the number of omissions such as forgetting to remind the physician to renew a medical license. Medical transcription work can be a rewarding career for a skilled typist and there are opportunities available for the physically challenged individual, as well.

Competency Review

1. Define and spell the glossary terms for this chapter.
2. Describe where you would find Emma Helme's file. She has not been seen by Dr. Williams for 2 years and has had no communication with her. Is this an active, inactive, or closed file?
3. Set up a tickler file system for your school assignments during this semester.
4. Jane Wallace, who is visually impaired, has asked your advice regarding a career in medical transcription. What would you tell her?
5. You are missing a file for Sean Roy. Discuss what process you would use to find this file.
6. Mr. Crosby is angry and demanding that you give him his medical chart so that he can take it to another physician. How do you handle Mr. Crosby's anger and his request for his medical file?

PREPARING FOR THE CERTIFICATION EXAM

Test Taking Tip — Arrive early at the examination site so that you can become comfortable with the surroundings before you begin the test.

Examination Review Questions

1. In filing correspondence for Janelle Louise Daniels (Mrs. Kevin Masters), 123 Valley Drive, Kalispell, MT 59999, which of the following would NOT be used as an indexing unit?
   (A) Carey
   (B) Daniels
   (C) Jerome
   (D) Masters
   (E) ZIP code

2. What is the third indexing unit in the following name: Mr. Richard Allan Richards, Jr.
   (A) Richards
   (B) Richard
   (C) Allan
   (D) Jr.
   (E) all the above are correct

3. The most commonly used filing system is based on what method?
   (A) numerical
   (B) color coding
   (C) alphabetical
   (D) unit numbering
   (E) straight numbering

4. Dr. Gemma Reingold is filed as
   (A) Reingold, Dr. Gemma
   (B) Dr. Gemma Reingold
   (C) Reingold, Gemma
   (D) Reingold, Gemma (Dr.)
   (E) none of the above is correct

5. Maura Fitzpatrick has been assigned the patient ID number 239431. To search for her file you will look under 94, then 23, then 31. What system are you using?
   (A) unit numbering
   (B) middle digit filing
   (C) terminal digit filing
   (D) straight numbering
   (E) service numbering

6. Adrian Washington has been assigned a color using the Alpha-Z color-coding system. Under what color would you find his chart?
   (A) lavender with white stripe
   (B) light brown
   (C) dark brown with white stripe
   (D) yellow
   (E) yellow with white stripe

7. David Jesse Montgomery III's file would be filed in what relation to David Jesse Montgomery, Jr.'s file?
   (A) before
   (B) after
   (C) with David Jesse Montgomery, Jr.'s file
   (D) the designations III and Jr. are ignored when filing
   (E) none of the above is the correct answer

8. VRT is an example of (a/an)
   (A) phonetics
   (B) synonym
   (C) acronym
   (D) antonym
   (E) etymology

9. Transcription equipment includes all of the following EXCEPT
   (A) computer
   (B) typewriter
   (C) transcriber
   (D) word processor
   (E) all of the above are correct

10. A report containing information about the tissue removed during a surgical procedure is called a/an
    (A) consultation report
    (B) operative note
    (C) pathology report
    (D) additional report
    (E) history report

ON THE JOB

Monique Adams, a 73 year old female, has been referred to Dr. Lopez from Dr. Williams for a consultation after having a chest x-ray that indicated a suspicious area in the right main stem bronchus.

Mrs. Adams has complained of retrosternal chest pain and a nonproductive cough. Dr. Lopez admitted Mrs. Adams to Memorial Hospital for a bronchoscopy and another chest x-ray. The bronchoscopy revealed a small cell undifferentiated carcinoma of the right lung. Her SMA profile (blood work) and physical examination findings were unremarkable. Dr. Lopez believes the disease is limited to the right lung.

Dr. Lopez discussed the results of the bronchoscopy and biopsy with the patient. He also discussed her options which include a combination of chemotherapy and radiation, or the option of no treatment at all. The patient was dismissed to consider her options for treatment and then return to Dr. Williams for medical care. Her discharge diagnosis is small cell carcinoma of the right lung.

Compose and type a consultation letter that Dr. Lopez might send to Dr. Williams including the above information.

References

Blake, R. *The Medical Transcriptionist's Handbook.* Cincinnati, Ohio: South-Western Publishing Co., 1993.

Dick, R. and Steen, E. editors. *The Computer Based Record.* Washington, DC: National Academy Press, 1991.

Fremgen, B. *Medical Terminology.* Upper Saddle River, NJ: Brady/Prentice Hall, 1997.

Johnson, J., Whitaker, M., and Johnson, M. *Computerized Medical Office Management.* Albany, NY: Delmar Publishers, 1994.

Kotoski, G. *CPT Coding Made Easy.* Gaithersburg, MD: Aspen Publishing, Inc., 1993.

Leonard, P. *Quick and Easy Medical Terminology.* Philadelphia, PA: W. B. Saunders, 1990.

Marshall, J. and Harris, J. *Being a Medical Clerical Worker.* Upper Saddle River, NJ: Brady/Prentice Hall, 1990.

McMiller, K. *Being a Medical Records Clerk.* Upper Saddle River, NJ: Brady/Prentice Hall, 1992.

Morrow, N. *Being A Medical Transcriptionist.* Upper Saddle River, NJ: Brady/Prentice Hall, 1992.

Spooner, A., ed. *The Oxford Thesaurus.* Oxford, England: Clarendon Press, 1993.

The Merck Manual, 16th ed. Westpointe, PA: Merck, Sharpe and Dohme Research Laboratories, 1990.

MEDICAL ASSISTANT ROLE DELINEATION CHART

Highlight indicates material covered in this chapter

ADMINISTRATIVE

ADMINISTRATIVE PROCEDURES

- Perform basic clerical functions
- Schedule, coordinate, and monitor appointments
- Schedule inpatient/outpatient admissions and procedures
- Understand and apply third party guidelines
- Obtain reimbursement through accurate claims submission
- Monitor third-party reimbursement
- Perform medical transcription
- Understand and adhere to managed care policies and procedures
- *Negotiate managed care contracts (adv)*

PRACTICE FINANCES

- Perform procedural and diagnostic coding
- Apply bookkeeping principles
- Document and maintain accounting and banking records
- Manage accounts receivable
- Manage accounts payable
- Process payroll
- *Develop and maintain fee schedules (adv)*
- *Manage renewals of business and professional insurance policies (adv)*
- *Manage personal benefits and maintain records (adv)*

CLINICAL

FUNDAMENTAL PRINCIPLES

- Apply principles of aseptic technique and infection control
- Comply with quality assurance practices
- Screen and follow up patient test results

DIAGNOSTIC ORDERS

- Collect and process specimens
- Perform diagnostic tests

PATIENT CARE

- Adhere to established triage procedures
- Obtain patient history and vital signs
- Prepare and maintain examination and treatment areas
- Prepare patient for examinations, procedures, and treatments
- Assist with examinations, procedures, and treatments
- Prepare and administer medications and immunizations
- Maintain medication and immunization records
- Recognize and respond to emergencies
- Coordinate patient care information with other health care providers

GENERAL (TRANSDISCIPLINARY)

PROFESSIONALISM

- Project a professional manner and image
- Adhere to ethical principles
- Demonstrate initiative and responsibility
- Work as a team member
- Manage time efficiently
- Prioritize and perform multiple tasks
- Adapt to change
- Promote the CMA credential
- Enhance skills through continuing education

COMMUNICATION SKILLS

- Treat all patients with compassion and empathy
- Recognize and respect cultural diversity
- Adapt communications to individual's ability to understand
- Use professional telephone technique
- Use effective and correct verbal and written communications
- Recognize and respond to verbal and non-verbal communications
- Use medical terminology appropriately
- Receive, organize, prioritize, and transmit information
- Serve as liaison
- Promote the practice through positive public relations

LEGAL CONCEPTS

- Maintain confidentiality
- Practice within the scope of education, training, and personal capabilities
- Prepare and maintain medical records
- Document accurately
- Use appropriate guidelines when releasing information
- Follow employer's established policies dealing with the health care contract
- Follow federal, state, and local legal guidelines
- Maintain awareness of federal and state health care legislation and regulations
- Maintain and dispose of regulated substances in compliance with government guidelines
- Comply with established risk management and safety procedures
- Recognize professional credentialing criteria
- Participate in the development and maintenance of personnel, policy, and procedure manuals
- *Develop and maintain personnel, policy, and procedure manuals (adv)*

INSTRUCTION

- Instruct individuals according to their needs
- Explain office policies and procedures
- Teach methods of health promotion and disease prevention
- Locate community resources and disseminate information
- *Orient and train personnel (adv)*
- *Develop educational materials (adv)*
- *Conduct continuing education activities (adv)*

OPERATIONAL FUNCTIONS

- Maintain supply inventory
- Evaluate and recommend equipment and supplies
- Apply computer techniques to support office operations
- *Supervise personnel (adv)*
- *Interview and recommend job applicants (adv)*
- *Negotiate leases and prices for equipment and supply contracts (adv)*

SOURCE: Reprinted by permission of the American Association of Medical Assistants from the *AAMA Role Delineation Study: Occupational Analysis of the Medical Assisting Profession.*

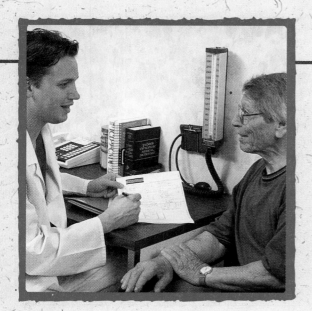

14

Fees, Billing, Collection, and Credit

LEARNING OBJECTIVES

After completing this chapter, you should:
1. Define and spell the glossary terms for this chapter.
2. Discuss how fees are determined and be able to discuss this with patients.
3. Discuss the patient information required at the time of registration and thereafter to maintain the records needed for billing.
4. Discuss credit policy.
5. Describe the various billing methods and preparation of billing statements.
6. Discuss the collection process and the legalities involved.
7. Understand the procedures for aging accounts.

ADMINISTRATIVE PERFORMANCE OBJECTIVES

After completing this chapter, you should perform the following tasks:
1. Collect the patient data necessary to maintain and update accurate records.
2. Establish office billing procedures.
3. Monitor billing processes.
4. Establish collection procedures.
5. Control accounts receivable.
6. Maintain collection control records.
7. Conduct periodic review of collection control.
8. Process accounts for legal collection.

Service to the patient is the primary concern of any medical practice, but revenue is also necessary to maintain a viable business. The process of setting up a fee schedule, extending credit, billing and collection are an important part of the medical practice. The medical assistant must be aware of the importance of a sound billing and collection system to ensure that patients understand their financial responsibility to the doctor and to offer assistance in setting up financial arrangements.

Professional Fees

The fee is determined by the physician, taking into consideration the time and services involved (Figure 14-1) as well as the prevailing rate in the community. The economic level of the community and the average fee charged will determine the prevailing rate.

Usual, customary, and reasonable **(UCR)** refers to:

- The usual fee a physician would charge his or her private patients.
- The customary fee for the same procedure charged by the majority of physicians with similar training in the same geographic and socioeconomic area.
- The reasonable fee that a patient might be expected to pay for similar services.

Government sponsored insurance programs maintain a record of the usual charges submitted for specific services by individual doctors. The physician will make the final determination as to

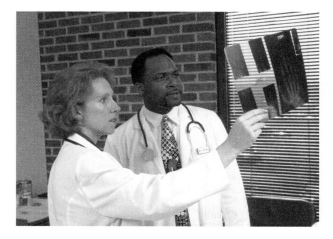

Figure 14-1   A physician's services frequently involve consultation with other staff members.

what the fees for services will be. It is the medical assistant's responsibility to convey this information to the patient in a positive, responsible manner.

It is necessary to initiate a discussion of fees with the patient so that they are informed of costs and can plan for medical expenses. Patients are entitled to an accurate estimate of their obligations. The medical assistant must become comfortable with these discussions. A thorough knowledge of the physician's practice and policies will help to handle any misunderstandings. A thorough understanding by the patient will help to minimize collection problems later.

Some medical offices have a statement displayed addressing the issue of fee policy. For example, a plastic surgeon's statement may include actual fees for services. A typed fee schedule should be available for quick reference. The medical assistant, if instructed by the physician, should be able to quote fees or a range of fees from this schedule. This schedule will have been approved by the physician and will be updated as needed.

Med Tip: Posted information regarding payment policies helps patients become aware of office procedures. It also encourages discussion of such matters.

Computerized offices will maintain a database that includes procedure codes and fees. This database will need to be periodically updated as fees change or at least once a year. Although payment at the time of service is preferred in most cases managed care and contractual agreements are in effect and the payment is made by a third party.

Billing

Payment of medical services can be achieved in one of three ways. First, there is payment at time of services which is the preferred method (Figure 14-2). The second method is billing and extending credit. The third and least desirable is the use of outside collection assistance.

The medical assistant needs to become familiar with health insurance coverage and the various plans. As HMOs, IPAs, and PPOs become a major influence in the office, levels of benefits, co-payments and deductibles are important aspects

of the fee and billing process. Patients can become easily confused about these matters so health care providers and their staff need to be knowledgeable in these areas. (See Chapter 17 for an explanation of HMOs, IPAs, and PPOs.)

Billing Methods

The faster you bill a patient or insurance company the faster you will receive payment. Figure 14-3 shows a hand-held computer that enhances billing capabilities. Billing methods depend on the preferences of the medical office. Billing may be done internally or externally.

Internal billing can include the use of the superbill, or encounter form, ledger card, and follow-up mailed statements. The superbill is commonly used and can serve as charge slip, billing statement, and also as a document for insurance processing. See Chapter 15 for a discussion of the superbill. It will contain all the information required for insurance claims including name and address of patient, name of insurance carrier, insurance ID number, service code numbers, fees, place and date of service, diagnosis codes, doctor's name, address and signature. Since the information on the superbill/encounter form is complete, it can easily be transferred to the insurance claim form.

Statements may be handwritten or typewritten or photocopies of the ledger card may be used. The ledger card is used to record the charges, adjustments, and payments for the patient. The statement must be good quality and large enough to allow itemization of charges. Photocopied statements must be clear and legible and can be sent in a window envelope.

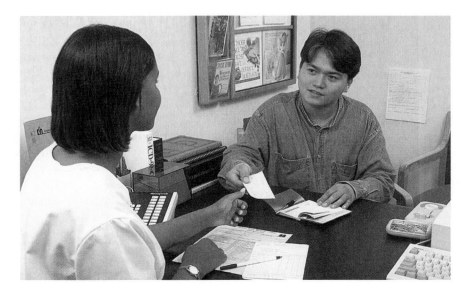

Figure 14-2 Payment at the time of service is the preferred method.

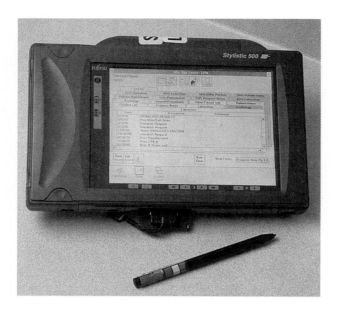

Figure 14-3 A hand-held, electronic, sensitive screen medical chart.

> **Med Tip:** Envelopes should be imprinted with ADDRESS CORRECTION REQUESTED under the return address.

External billing will involve the use of an outside billing service and may be utilized for large volume billing.

Accurate information is absolutely necessary when billing patients. Good records are essential to follow-up with collections. The patient registration form is a good way to establish an information base. The following information is needed to maintain a current billing file for each patient and should be included on the registration form:

- Full name of patient
  (If the patient is a minor, then the full name and address of the parent or guardian is needed)
- Address (residence and mailing address, do not accept post office box only)
- Telephone number (both home and work)
- Occupation (address and telephone of employer)
- Nearest relative (telephone and address)
- Insurance information (company and address, telephone)
- Social Security number
- Driver's license number

If the patient and the subscriber, or the person who holds the insurance policy, plan or contract, are the same, this information is taken only once. If the patient is covered under a policy held by another family member (the subscriber), then the same information relating to home address, tele-

> **Med Tip:** Patient billing information should be updated every 6 months to 1 year by having patients fill out new forms.

phone number, employer's name and address, and so on need to be taken.

Once the account has been set up, the medical assistant must be made aware of any changes to information. Patients should be reminded at each visit of the need to inform the office of any changes to information with particular attention to changes of address, telephone number, employer and insurance information. A notice can be posted at the reception desk as a reminder to patients. The receptionist should also ask at the time the patient checks in.

Superbill/Encounter Form

The superbill is the document generated by the office and used as a charge slip, statement, and insurance reporting form (Figure 14-4). This document provides a comprehensive list of patient services, with respective codes and fees, on which the physician indicates with a check mark the services that have been rendered. The superbill can be used to input computer information for billing.

Computerized Billing

Computer software is available for internal billing purposes, however many offices with regular, monthly, large-volume billing utilize outside computerized billing services. Many different programs exist and can be custom designed for the needs of the office. Databases will include patient information, procedure and diagnosis codes, and insurance companies. Options are available to print statements, ledgers, and receipts.

The Billing Period: Frequency of Billing

Consistency with billing procedures is very important. The medical assistant must have a thorough understanding of office policy with regards

BILLING NAME			NAMES OF OTHER MEMBERS OF THE FAMILY		
PATIENT'S NAME					
HOME PHONE		WORK PHONE			
OCCUPATION			RELATIVE or FRIEND		
EMPLOYED BY			REFERRED BY		
INSURANCE INFO				SOCIAL SECURITY #	

WINDY CITY CLINIC
Beth A. Williams, M.D.
Family Practice
123 Michigan Avenue
Chicago, IL 60610
(312) 123-1234

STATEMENT TO:

TEAR OFF AND RETURN UPPER PORTION WITH PAYMENT

DATE	PROFESSIONAL SERVICE	FEE		PAYMENT		ADJUST-MENT		NEW BALANCE	
8-2-97	85015	40	-					40	-
9-15	90080	95	-					135	-
	87068	34	-					169	-
10-8	Insurance			142	30			26	70

PROFESSIONAL SERVICE CODES:

1. OFFICE VISIT	8. DRUGS/SUPPLIES/MATERIALS	15. CASTS
2. HOME VISIT	9. COLLECTION OF LAB SPEC.	16. LABORATORY
3. HOSPITAL VISIT	10. SPECIAL REPORTS	17. X-RAY
4. EMERGENCY ROOM	11. OTHER SERVICES	18. ALLERGY TEST
5. CONSULTATION	12. SPEC. DIAGNOSTIC SERVICES	19. NO CHARGE
6. IMMUNIZATION	13. SPEC. THERAPEUTIC SERVICES	20. ADJUSTMENTS OR CORRECTIONS
7. INJECTION	14. SURGICAL	21. TOTAL CARE

BETH A. WILLIAMS, M.D.
ILLINOIS LICENSE # G-1234

Figure 14-4   The superbill has multiple uses.

to the timing of billing. When a billing date for an account has been established, it is extremely important not to vary the timing of the mailing statements.

There are two types of billing: once-a-month billing and cycle billing. Once-a-month billing requires that statements leave the office in time to reach the patient no later than the last day of the month. Cycle billing requires that certain portions of the accounts receivable are billed at given times during the month. For example, patients whose names begin with A-F would be billed on the 1st of the month, G-L on the 7th, and so on. The advantages of cycle billing over once-a-month billing are (1) the avoidance of once-a-month work overload and (2) a stable cash flow. The medical assistant can handle routine duties each day with the inclusion of statements, rather than intensive billing responsibilities once a month. By spacing the billing periods, more time can be given to each statement.

Patients must be made aware of the timing of billing statements. If a change is made, patients should be notified. This can be done by enclosing a notice of billing policy changes in each statement, two months prior to the change.

Billing Third-Party Payers and Minors

Third party payers include a party or person other than the patient, such as an insurance company, who assumes responsibility for paying the patient's bill. Patient registration should include information regarding insurance. Patients should be asked to provide all insurance ID cards and copies should be made and kept on file.

A signed assignment of benefits form, which is good for 1 year, can be used by the office to ensure that insurance payments are made directly to the physician. In some offices, a copy of the driver's license and Social Security card is filed.

Bills for minors are addressed to parents or legal guardians (Figure 14-5). Never bill a minor. Minors are not responsible for bills unless they are declared emancipated. (See Chapter 5 for discussion of emancipated minor.) The parent who brings the child for treatment or the subscriber to the primary insurance policy is responsible for payment. Financial agreements between divorced or separated parents are their personal business. However, if documentation exists in the minor's file as to financial responsibility, then that party should be billed.

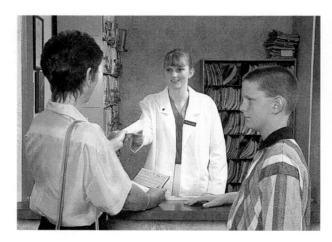

Figure 14-5   Parents or legal guardians are responsible for the medical bills of their minor children.

Credit Policy

Payment at the time of service is the ideal method of collection. The front desk assistants need to overcome any inhibitions regarding discussion of fees and payments. Patients can be informed, when they call to schedule an appointment, of office policies regarding payment. This is the first step in the collections process.

Med Tip: Patients not prepared to pay at the time of service should receive a billing statement when they leave the office with a request to send payment immediately.

The medical assistant must find out the policies the doctor wants administered and consistently and fairly maintain them. A credit policy is an important part of any accounts receivable system.

If payment is collected upon completion of the service, there is no problem. But, if payment is deferred, then credit arrangements must be made. This is best done during the patient's initial visit. All necessary information should be gathered from the patient with regard to demographics, insurance, employment, and signatures.

The medical assistant must have an understanding of the federal laws affecting credit. One of the most important is Regulation Z of the Truth in Lending Act (formerly the Consumer Protection Act of 1968), which was enacted to protect the consumer. This is an agreement between doctor and patient to accept payment in more than four installments. Under this act the physician must provide disclosure of information regarding finance charges. If there are to be no finance charges, the form should be completed stating this fact. The original form is given to the patient and a copy is retained by the doctor. The disclosure must be very specific and the patient must sign it in the medical assistant's presence.

Credit Bureaus operate as sources of credit data on individuals. Many of them specialize in medical-dental collections. They may supply data verifying a patient's employment, residence and payment history. The medical office needs to be sure that it is working with a reputable credit bureau.

Collections

Every medical office should have a collection policy in place, as it is not advantageous to the office to have a haphazard method for collecting overdue accounts. The medical assistant must understand the collection policy of the medical practice and must administer it consistently and fairly according to the physician's directives. Most practices have a collection process in place that allows for timely and effective collections. These guidelines for collections will be useful in creating and maintaining positive collection procedures.

Guidelines: Collections

1. Seek immediate payment.
2. Use charge slips or superbills.
3. Secure accurate patient information and update as needed.
4. Inform patient at the time of the appointment of possible fees and responsibility .
5. Outline all fees and finance charges for the patient.
6. Confirm third party responsibility.
7. Bill consistently following office policy.
8. Institute collection procedures as needed with personal interview, telephone calls, and letters.
9. Follow-up on all commitments by the patient.

Collection Process

Accounts that are seriously overdue become very difficult and costly to collect. Patients need to be educated on billing and collection procedures so that there is a clear understanding of expectations. The patient information booklet given to new patients should have a section outlining office policy regarding billing and collection. Patients need to be encouraged to openly discuss problems or questions they might have with respect to their bills.

The reasons a bill is not paid vary. Some reasons are

- Patient does not feel that the bill is important.
- Patient is unable to pay (for whatever reason).
- Misunderstanding about the fee.

The medical assistant must determine in a timely manner what the problem is so that it can be addressed, and the office can continue with the collection process. Occasionally, when there is no hope of recovering this money from the patient, the physician will "write-off" or cancel an unpaid debt. He or she will try to avoid doing this if it is at all possible.

Delinquent Accounts

Failure to collect delinquent accounts affects the medical practice in many ways. Patients who owe money may stay away from the office out of embarrassment due to their financial situation and failure to collect delinquent accounts may imply guilt on the part of the physician as to the quality of care. Ultimately, failure to collect delinquent accounts burdens the entire practice due to lost revenue.

Aging Accounts Receivable

It is extremely important to age all accounts receivable. Age analysis refers to the process of determining how long an account has been past due, and then instituting the necessary collection procedures. Computerized systems will allow the medical assistant to print out an aging report with a 30, 60, and 90 day and over analysis. This can be used to determine what the next collection step should be. Manual systems may use a coding system to age accounts with various colors or flags to indicate the different ages. These may be attached directly to the patient's ledger card.

Collection Techniques

The medical office may employ several methods of collection. Reminder notices, telephone calls, collection letters, and finally a collection agency may be used. The physician decides office policy regarding collection of overdue payments; the medical assistant has the responsibility to carry out the policy consistently and fairly.

A personal interview can be a very effective collection method. The patient who is seen in the office for an appointment and has an outstanding account is readily available for discussion with the office staff. This is the time to tactfully bring attention to the overdue account and to make arrangements with the patient for payment.

Reminder notices can be placed on bills when mailed to patients asking for their prompt attention to a past due bill. Other reminder notices may ask a patient to contact the office if there is a question about the past due bill. If no payment or contact is made then a reminder letter is sent. It should not be a form letter but rather an individual letter that lets the patient know that their account is being reviewed and there is concern as to the unpaid debt. Tactful, professional telephone calls may also become part of the collection process and sometimes can be more effective than the letter. The last option may be the use of a collection agency when all other attempts at collection have failed.

Regulations

There are some general rules to follow when attempting to collect overdue accounts and there are laws that govern issues regarding collection. One is the Fair Debt Collection Practices Act. Office staff involved with billing and collections need to be familiar with the laws of their particular state when applying collection techniques. Basic rules or guidelines are provided here to assist you in the task of making collections.

As stated above, violation of these rules could be an offense under the Fair Debt Collection Practices Act, which is a federal law that protects debtors from harassment.

In summary, do not make threatening statements that will not be acted upon. Collection telephone calls must be between the hours of 8 AM and 9 PM (Figure 14-6). Avoid calling debtors at their place of employment. Never use a postcard or put an overdue notice on the outside of an envelope.

Telephone Collections

A telephone call at the right time and in the right manner can be more effective than a letter. The medical assistant must be sure to make the call tactful, brief, and to the point. Make sure that all conversation is with the debtor. If the debtor is not

Guidelines: Making Collections

1. Never threaten an action that you do not intend to take. For example, do not tell the patient that his or her account will be handed over to a collection agency if full payment is not received by this afternoon.
2. Do not make a collection telephone call before 8 AM or after 9 PM, and do not call on Sundays and holidays.
3. Do not make a collection call to the patient's workplace.
4. Carefully identify the person accepting the telephone call. Do not discuss a delinquent account with anyone except the debtor.
5. Never raise your voice, use profane language, or show anger in any way.
6. Do not misrepresent yourself, by implying you are someone other than who you are.
7. Do not charge interest unless the debtor has agreed to make 4 (or more) installment payments at a particular rate of interest.
8. Do not harass or intimidate the debtor.

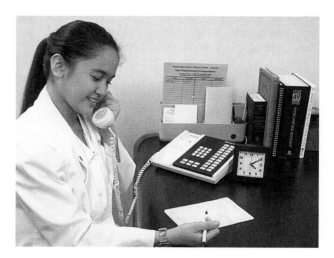

Figure 14-6 Collection calls are made between 8 AM and 9 PM.

available, only a message should be left stating the individual needs to contact the office. A firm commitment to make payment is obtained before ending the conversation. If there is no result by the date mutually agreed upon then the next step in the collection process must be instituted.

WINDY CITY CLINIC
Beth Williams, M.D.
123 Michigan Avenue, Chicago, IL 60610
(312) 123-1234

Date

Patient Name
Street Address
City, State and ZIP Code

Dear Patient:

   Your balance of $400.00 has been on our books for 18 months. Normally at this time, because your payment is long past due, your account would be handed over to our collection agency. However, we prefer to hear from you regarding your preference in this matter.

   Please check one of the following options, and return this letter to our office:

☐   I would prefer to settle this account. Payment in full is enclosed.

☐   I would like to make regular weekly/monthly payments of $ _____ until this account is paid in full. My first payment is enclosed.

☐   I don't believe that I owe this amount for the following reasons(s):

_____

_____

_____

_____
patient's signature

   Failure to return this letter will result in turning this account over to a collection agency.

Sincerely Yours,

Beth A. Williams, M.D.

Figure 14-7   Reminder letter.

Collection Letters

The personalized letter has many advantages over the form letter. Patients who receive the personalized letter will feel that their account has been reviewed individually rather than just another form letter that has been sent to every patient with an overdue balance. The letter may be inserted with the statement. The letter should include an inquiry as to why the bill has not been paid. There should be an offer to assist the patient with making payment arrangements. The letter must convey the message that something needs to be done. Figure 14-7 provides an example of a reminder letter.

Special Problems

Even with the best billing and collection system problems arise. There will be some accounts that the medical assistant will find challenging to collect. An example of such a challenge or collection problem is a "skip". This requires immediate action as this individual has a balance and has moved without leaving a forwarding address. The greater the amount of time it takes to locate the "skip" the less likely you are to receive payment. "Skips" can be traced by checking the registration form to confirm addresses, calling telephone numbers, and calling references without divulging the nature of the call. "Address Correction Requested" on the statement envelope may help to get the statement delivered.

Med Tip: The Post Office may charge a fee for "Address Correction Requested," but it is a sound investment nonetheless.

Bankruptcy

A patient who files for bankruptcy is protected by the court. When notice is received of a patient's bankruptcy all collection attempts must cease and the medical office must file a claim for payment.

Claims Against Estates

When a patient dies a bill should be sent to the estate of the deceased. Contacting next of kin will provide information regarding who is the administrator of the estate. It is important to follow-up with the collection of bills to prevent the impression of any physician fault with the care of the deceased.

Statutes of Limitations

Statute of limitations refers to the amount of time a legal collection suit may be brought against a debtor. This will vary state to state and should be checked with state agencies. If you have aging accounts that are more than 3 years old, you should investigate the statute of limitations in your state before spending time, effort, and money to collect the debt.

Using a Collection Agency

Professional collection agencies are available to use when all other collection attempts fail. Be sure to review the account with the physician before turning it over for collection.

The collection agency should be chosen carefully. Reputable agencies will have references that can be checked and will be happy to discuss

their collection methods. Further checks can be done with the Better Business Bureau and national credit agencies.

Med Tip: Visit the collection agency office before choosing one. It should be professional and willing to discuss collection procedures with you.

Collection agencies charge for their services either by a flat fee per account or a percentage of the amount collected. In either case the physician's office needs to be aware of the costs involved when using this method to collect fees. Do not include the diagnosis when sending financial information to the collection agency.

Once the patient is told the account is going to a collection agency it must, by law, go. After the account has been turned over no further collection attempts can be made by the physician's office. The collection agency will need copies of patient information and itemized statements showing the dates and amounts of all transactions. If the patient should contact the office after the account has been turned over for collection, the patient should be referred to the collection agency.

Accounts Receivable Insurance

Accounts receivable insurance may be purchased to protect against accounts receivable loss. The accounts receivable balance is reported each month and ledgers are kept in a secure place within the office.

Public Relations

Working with fees, billing, collections, and credit presents one of the most effective opportunities for projecting a positive image of the medical practice. The medical assistant must project a professional, but caring approach when working in the area of collections.

Asking the patient, "How can we help you to work out a suitable payment plan?" is much more effective then asking, "When are you going to pay your bill?"

Information about the compassionate treatment given your patients quickly spreads throughout the community by word of mouth. Such free positive publicity can have a great effect at promoting the medical practice.

LEGAL AND ETHICAL ISSUES

Financial information regarding the patient is confidential. All discussions whether in person or on the telephone should be conducted in an area out of view and hearing of other patients. Credit information about a patient is also confidential and may not be released without the patient's expressed permission.

Statements outlining credit arrangements and interest charges must be in writing. If the responsibility for payment is to be handled by a person other than the patient, a signed statement by the third party is necessary to verify this obligation.

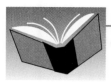

PATIENT EDUCATION

The patient must have a thorough understanding of office policy with regards to financial matters. The initial visit to the office should include information on fees, payment, and financial arrangements. This can be addressed in a patient information booklet or pamphlet given to the patient. Patients who will require surgical or other medical procedures should be made aware of fees, insurance allowances and methods of payment. The patient must understand that he or she has the ultimate responsibility for all charges.

The informed patient will have a clear understanding of all obligations to the office and will be more likely to discuss financial arrangements. This mutual understanding helps to minimize the problems of collection of delinquent accounts.

Summary

The professional health care facility will have in place office policy regarding fee setting, billing and collection. The medical assistant has the responsibility to carry out such policy with a professional, courteous attitude. Informed patients will have a better understanding of office expectations. This helps to lessen the problems encountered with accounts receivable. When an account does become a collection dilemma, a series of steps can be instituted to quickly and efficiently address any problems. The goal of such policy is to protect the financial well being and goodwill of the practice.

Competency Review

1. Define and spell the glossary terms for this chapter.
2. With a fellow student, role play a telephone conversation you would have to collect an overdue bill of 60 days for $225 from Samuel Jones, who is unemployed.
3. What statements can you make to a patient to encourage payment at the time of service?
4. Write a sample collection letter from Dr. Beth Williams to Samuel Jones identified in question number 2 above.
5. Discuss the ethical considerations involved when making collections.

PREPARATION FOR THE CERTIFICATION EXAM

Test Taking Tip — When studying for the examination, be sure to review the items you found most difficult to learn first, then review the topics you found easier to learn. In other words, tackle the difficult content first when you are most alert.

Examination Review Questions

1. The detailed record maintained by the medical office of a patient's financial transactions is called a/an
   - (A) ledger
   - (B) accounts payable record
   - (C) register
   - (D) reconciliation
   - (E) medical record

2. Once an account has been referred for collection the office should
   - (A) discuss payment with the patient
   - (B) not attempt to collect
   - (C) call the patient's employer
   - (D) cancel the balance
   - (E) send a reminder letter

3. The form which serves as the documentation of services, as a billing statement and an insurance processing form is a/an
   - (A) receipt
   - (B) ledger
   - (C) account
   - (D) superbill
   - (E) credit memo

4. A "skip" has/is
   - (A) forgotten to pay
   - (B) lost his or her job
   - (C) moved with no forwarding address
   - (D) not a collection problem
   - (E) none of the above

5. Which of the following is a last resort in the collection process?
   - (A) collection agency
   - (B) telephone call
   - (C) personal interview
   - (D) collection letter
   - (E) none of the above

6. Regulation Z of the Truth in Lending Act requires physicians to outline costs, including finance charges when payment arrangements are made in
   - (A) two or more installments
   - (B) four or more installments
   - (C) eight or more installments
   - (D) three or more installments
   - (E) five or more installments

7. Effective collection letters are
   - (A) brief, simple, and encourage the patient to take action
   - (B) preprinted form letters
   - (C) unsigned
   - (D) impersonal and demand cash
   - (E) all of the above

8. Claims against estates should be
   - (A) canceled
   - (B) sent to collection
   - (C) discounted
   - (D) sent to the administrator of the estate
   - (E) addressed to the next of kin

9. The BEST way to convey billing and collection information to the patient is to
   - (A) include it in a patient information booklet
   - (B) discuss it over the phone
   - (C) discuss it when the visit is over
   - (D) include it on the registration form
   - (E) all of the above can be effective

10. The final decision to send an account to collection is made by
    - (A) the medical assistant
    - (B) the physician
    - (C) the patient
    - (D) the lawyer
    - (E) the collection agency

ON THE JOB

Services were rendered to Jeffrey Boylan on October 1, 1996. It is now 45 days since Mr. Boylan received care, and he has not yet made a payment on his outstanding balance of $150.00. At this point the office's policy requires that a letter be sent to him reminding him of his indebtedness. Using the proper guidelines for composing a collection letter, prepare correspondence to be sent to Mr. Boylan.

Address:

Mr. Jeffrey Boylan
14 Meadow Road
Anytown, State 12345

References

Backstrom, I. *Medical Office Management.* Chicago: American Association of Medical Assistants, 1991.

Becklin, K. and Sunnarborg, E. *Medical Office Procedures.* New York: Glencoe, 1996.

Cohen, A., Fink, S., Gadon, H., Willits, R. *Effective Behavior in Organizations.* Homewood, IL: Irwin, 1992.

Hellriegel, D., and Slocum, J. *Management.* Cincinnati: South-Western Publishing, 1996.

Johnson, J., Whitaker, M., and Johnson, M. *Computerized Medical Office Management.* Albany, NY: Delmar Publishers, 1994.

Larson, K., and Miller, P. *Fundamental Accounting Principles.* Homewood, IL: Orwin, 1993.

Meigs, R., and Meugs, W. *Accounting: The Basis for Business Decisions.* New York: McGraw-Hill, Inc., 1993.

Oliverio, J., Pasewark, W., and White, B. *The Office: Procedures and Technology.* Cincinnati, Ohio: South-Western Publishing Co., 1993.

Seelig, J. *Accounts Receivable and Collections for the Medical Practice.* Chicago: AAMA, 1992.

MEDICAL ASSISTANT ROLE DELINEATION CHART

Highlight indicates material covered in this chapter

ADMINISTRATIVE

ADMINISTRATIVE PROCEDURES

- Perform basic clerical functions
- Schedule, coordinate, and monitor appointments
- Schedule inpatient/outpatient admissions and procedures
- Understand and apply third party guidelines
- Obtain reimbursement through accurate claims submission
- Monitor third-party reimbursement
- Perform medical transcription
- Understand and adhere to managed care policies and procedures
- *Negotiate managed care contracts (adv)*

PRACTICE FINANCES

- Perform procedural and diagnostic coding
- Apply bookkeeping principles
- Document and maintain accounting and banking records
- Manage accounts receivable
- Manage accounts payable
- Process payroll
- *Develop and maintain fee schedules (adv)*
- *Manage renewals of business and professional insurance policies (adv)*
- *Manage personal benefits and maintain records (adv)*

CLINICAL

FUNDAMENTAL PRINCIPLES

- Apply principles of aseptic technique and infection control
- Comply with quality assurance practices
- Screen and follow up patient test results

DIAGNOSTIC ORDERS

- Collect and process specimens
- Perform diagnostic tests

PATIENT CARE

- Adhere to established triage procedures
- Obtain patient history and vital signs
- Prepare and maintain examination and treatment areas

- Prepare patient for examinations, procedures, and treatments
- Assist with examinations, procedures, and treatments
- Prepare and administer medications and immunizations
- Maintain medication and immunization records
- Recognize and respond to emergencies
- Coordinate patient care information with other health care providers

GENERAL (TRANSDISCIPLINARY)

PROFESSIONALISM

- Project a professional manner and image
- Adhere to ethical principles
- Demonstrate initiative and responsibility
- Work as a team member
- Manage time efficiently
- Prioritize and perform multiple tasks
- Adapt to change
- Promote the CMA credential
- Enhance skills through continuing education

COMMUNICATION SKILLS

- Treat all patients with compassion and empathy
- Recognize and respect cultural diversity
- Adapt communications to individual's ability to understand
- Use professional telephone technique
- Use effective and correct verbal and written communications
- Recognize and respond to verbal and nonverbal communications
- Use medical terminology appropriately
- Receive, organize, prioritize, and transmit information
- Serve as liaison
- Promote the practice through positive public relations

LEGAL CONCEPTS

- Maintain confidentiality
- Practice within the scope of education, training, and personal capabilities
- Prepare and maintain medical records
- Document accurately
- Use appropriate guidelines when releasing information
- Follow employer's established policies dealing with the health care contract
- Follow federal, state, and local legal guidelines
- Maintain awareness of federal and state health care legislation and regulations
- Maintain and dispose of regulated substances in compliance with government guidelines
- Comply with established risk management and safety procedures
- Recognize professional credentialing criteria
- Participate in the development and maintenance of personnel, policy, and procedure manuals
- *Develop and maintain personnel, policy, and procedure manuals (adv)*

INSTRUCTION

- Instruct individuals according to their needs
- Explain office policies and procedures
- Teach methods of health promotion and disease prevention
- Locate community resources and disseminate information
- *Orient and train personnel (adv)*
- *Develop educational materials (adv)*
- *Conduct continuing education activities (adv)*

OPERATIONAL FUNCTIONS

- Maintain supply inventory
- Evaluate and recommend equipment and supplies
- Apply computer techniques to support office operations
- *Supervise personnel (adv)*
- *Interview and recommend job applicants (adv)*
- *Negotiate leases and prices for equipment and supply contracts (adv)*

SOURCE: Reprinted by permission of the American Association of Medical Assistants from the *AAMA Role Delineation Study: Occupational Analysis of the Medical Assisting Profession.*

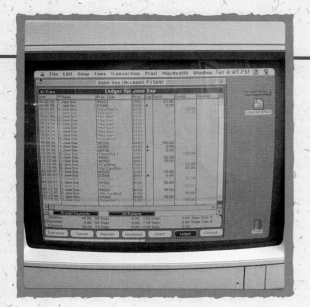

15

Financial Management

LEARNING OBJECTIVES

After completing this chapter, you should:
1. Define and spell the glossary terms for this chapter.
2. Describe the manual, pegboard, and computerized systems for record keeping.
3. State the advantages of the pegboard system.
4. Describe the difference between accounting and bookkeeping.
5. Describe which taxes are withheld from the employee's paycheck.
6. Discuss the types of payroll records.
7. Differentiate between a credit and a debit balance.
8. State the accounting equation.
9. List the rules of bookkeeping.
10. State the five sections of the pegboard day sheet.

ADMINISTRATIVE PERFORMANCE COMPETENCIES

After completing this chapter, you should perform the following tasks:
1. Prepare a daily posting proof using the pegboard system.
2. Balance a day sheet.
3. Calculate a payroll check.
4. Demonstrate proficiency in using the write-it-once (pegboard) system of accounting.

Financial management, in the medical office setting, involves setting up an efficient and effective method of bookkeeping (maintaining accounts) for billing patients as well as careful attention to employee payroll and withholding requirements.

Accounting Systems

Accounting is the art or science of reporting the financial results of a business. The basis of accounting is the ability to make an analysis, statement, or summary about financial matters. Many physicians hire an accountant or accounting service to prepare tax returns and prepare financial statements that are used to obtain bank financing. If the physician is in a partnership with other physicians, the accountant's financial statements will assist in dividing the earnings among the partners. Providing accurate financial records to the accountant is one of the medical assistant's responsibilities (Figure 15-1).

Bookkeeping is the process of keeping the accounts for a business. Bookkeeping is a continual process and should be done daily. The medical assistant or office manager may assume this duty, or the medical practice could hire a bookkeeper. All receipts and charges should be entered immediately into a daily journal, day sheet, or record. Receipts, in duplicate, must be written for all money received. One copy is given to the patient and one copy stays in the office file.

Bookkeeping is a precise skill requiring great attention to detail. Most offices use the computer for bookkeeping records. However, the manual method is still used in some smaller offices. Guidelines for manual bookkeeping provided here or those followed in your office offer sound, basic rules for the beginning or practiced bookkeeper.

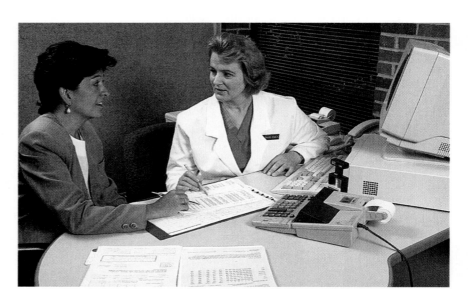

Figure 15-1 The office manager or an assigned medical assistant may work closely with the accountant.

Guidelines: Manual Bookkeeping

1. Use a black pen and clear penmanship. Do not use pencil.
2. Keep the columns straight with decimal points lined up.
3. Check all arithmetic carefully for errors, such as misplaced decimal points or errors in adding and/or subtracting.
4. Do not erase, write over, or use opaque correction fluid. Make all corrections by drawing a straight line through the incorrect figure and writing the correct figure above it.
5. Try to work in a quiet place each day without interruptions. Bookkeeping should not be done at the front desk while answering the telephone and greeting patients.
6. Pay close attention to detail.
7. Form all numbers carefully to avoid errors in calculations. Use care to avoid transposing numbers (for example 79 instead of 97).
8. Always find errors as soon as they appear. Do not carry the error forward in the account books.
9. Double check every entry.
10. Do not discuss patient financial records with other staff members. They are confidential.

Patient Accounts

The medical office is a unique business in that the services are not always paid for at the time of delivery, as they are in a business such as retailing. Patient accounts require careful bookkeeping to assure that insurance payments are correctly posted, or recorded, when received, patient's statements are accurate, and that the physician receives payments for services rendered. Most medical offices are run on a "cash" basis which means that the charge for a medical service is entered in the financial records as income only when the payment is received. The accrual basis of accounting for income, which is used by retailers and merchants, enters income when the service is rendered, even if a payment has not been received.

For an example of the components of a patient billing system, see Figure 15-2.

Accounts Receivable

Money owed to the physician is called accounts receivable. The accounts receivable ledger is a journal containing a record of all the patient's accounts. Terms that relate to accounts receivable are

1. Credit—Indicates when a payment has been received on an account. To credit an account means to record a payment to the account. A patient has a credit balance when a payment exceeds a charge.

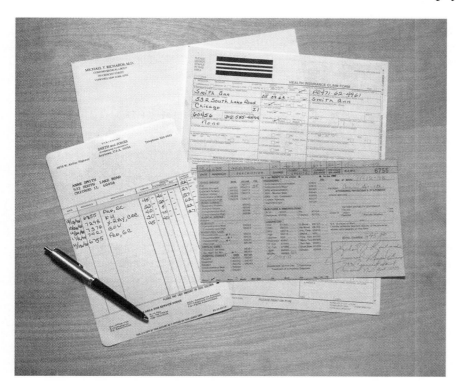

Figure 15-2 Components of a patient billing system.

2. Debit—Indicates when a charge has been entered into the account. To debit an account means to subtract from that account. In some methods of bookkeeping, debits are entered in red. If the balance of the account is negative (a debit balance), this can be indicated by placing the total in red ink or in brackets. A physician's practice usually operates with a debit balance since the total charges to patients exceed the amount paid by all the patients due to delays in payment from insurers and others.

3. Adjustment—Entering a change into the account record such as a discount, write-off, or an amount not allowed by an insurance company (disallowance). A discount is entered as a credit since this amount will be subtracted from the total amount owed.

4. Balance—Is the difference between the debit (money owed) and the credit (money paid).

> **Med Tip:** Accountants use the terms "debit" and "credit" as technical descriptions of the two sides of a journal entry—a part of the "double entry" system used in accounting. The term "credit" is also used to describe payments made by a patient or any adjustment which reduces a patient's balance. The term "charge" is frequently used interchangeably with the term "debit." Do not let these differing terms and differing uses of the same term confuse you.

Accounts Payable

Accounts payable are the amounts the physician owes to others for equipment and services which have not yet been paid. Examples of accounts payable expenditures in a medical office are

1. Office supplies, such as paper goods, day sheets, appointment cards, scheduling books.
2. Medical supplies and equipment.
3. Equipment repair and maintenance including housekeeping.
4. Utilities such as telephone and electric.
5. Taxes.
6. Payroll.
7. Rent.

Records relating to accounts payable include the purchase orders, packing slips which come with the delivered goods, and the invoice requesting payment. The medical assistant, or bookkeeper, who is handling accounts payable payments must carefully document the payment made on the check stub and place the check number onto the retained invoice copy.

Bookkeeping Systems

Medical practices use two basic types of bookkeeping systems: single-and double-entry.

Single-Entry Bookkeeping

In a single-entry system, the bookkeeper, or medical assistant assigned to this task, records all financial transactions into the bookkeeping system just once. She or he makes a single-entry. This is a simple system to learn, inexpensive, and requires only three key records:

- Journal, or day sheet, which is also called the daily journal or log.
- The cash payment journal. (See Figure 15-3 for illustration of one type of cash payment record—the checkbook and stubs.)
- The accounts receivable ledger which contains a record of the money owed to the physician.

Some offices will also have a journal for payroll records and petty cash (Figure 15-4). Petty cash vouchers are used to identify petty cash expenses (Figure 15-5).

Double-Entry Bookkeeping

In double-entry bookkeeping, a financial transaction is recorded in two different places. Therefore, a double-entry is required. This system is inexpensive but requires a trained bookkeeper.

The "double-entry" forces a balance since all accounting procedures require two entries which keep the accounting records in balance. For example, when a patient pays an outstanding bill, cash is recorded as an asset, and the receivable, which was the money owed or an asset, is eliminated.

Accounting is based on the premise that the assets of the business less the liabilities of the business equals the net worth of that business. This is expressed by the standard accounting formula: Assets = Liabilities + Net Worth. It uses

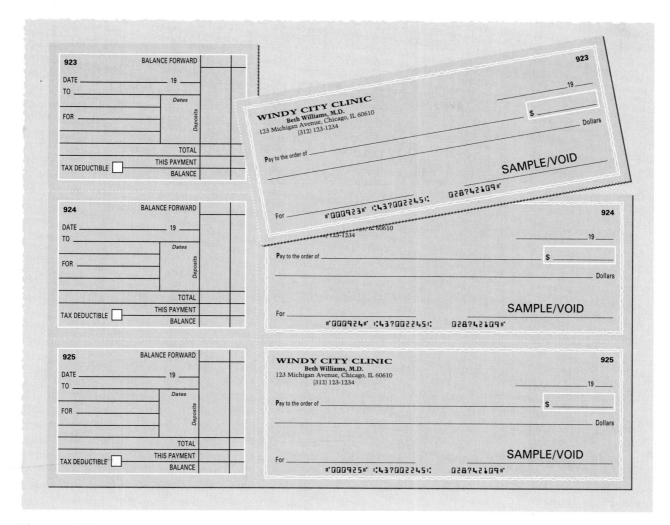

Figure 15-3   Cashbook and stubs—cash payment record.

Number	Date	Description	Amount	Office Expenses	Car	Misc.	Balance
	6-1	Fund established					75.00
1	6-2	Postage due	1.42	1.42			73.58
2	6-8	Taxi — (2)	8.00		8.00		65.58
3	6-10	Delivery charge	3.98			3.98	61.60
4	6-25	Supplies	11.62	11.62			49.98
		Total	25.02	13.04	8.00	3.98	
	7-1	Balance 49.98					
ck #	790	25.02					
		75.00					

Figure 15-4   Petty cash record.

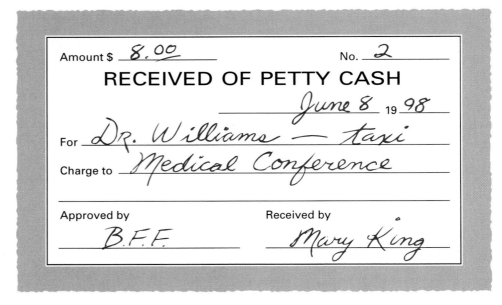

Figure 15-5 Petty cash voucher.

the double-entry system which assures that the accounts are in balance.

Assets include everything owned by the medical practice such as cash, bank accounts, money owed to the physician, equipment and real estate. Liabilities are money the medical practice owes to its creditors. An example of this would be money owed to their medical supplies **vendor** (supplier).

The Pegboard System (Write-It-Once System)

The pegboard system is used to document patient bills and payments. This system is also called the write-it-once method since a system of interrelated forms are placed onto the pegboard and used with the same master day sheet. It is an efficient system since the same data is entered on all the forms at one time. The pegboard system is inexpensive as long as all employees are trained in its use. The forms manufactured by one company are usually not compatible with forms from another company.

The actual pegboard is a firm-backed board that contains pegs along the left-hand side. These pegs hold the perforated edges of a day sheet (same as a daily journal) firmly onto the pegboard. Other forms can be held firmly by the pegs so that when posting is done the form, such as a superbill, will not slip.

Required Pegboard System Forms

There are four components of the pegboard system. These are

- Day sheets
- Ledger cards
- Superbill (Charge/encounter slips)
- Receipt forms

These forms have a carbon ribbon attached or are on special paper which will permit entering charges, payments, and adjustments onto the master day sheet, the charge slip (superbill), and the patient's ledger card at the same time. See Figure 15-6 for examples of pegboard system components.

Day Sheets The day sheet component of the pegboard system is used to list or post each day's financial transactions: charges, payments, adjust-

Med Tip: The disadvantages to the pegboard system are that one cannot erase using this system since it is carbonized. Therefore, corrections must be made carefully by drawing a line through each error. However, if an error is made on one document, such as the ledger card, it is made on all the documents. This makes the error consistent and more easy to find.

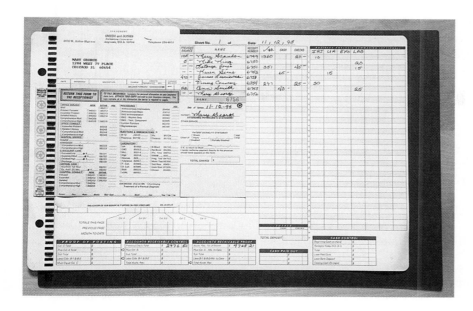

Figure 15-6   Components of the pegboard system

ments, and credits. The day sheet, one for each day of the month must be balanced at the end of each day. The balance from the previous day is carried over to the present day's day sheet as part of the balancing process. In a large or busy practice, there may be more than one day sheet generated per day. The day sheet contains five basic sections which are described in Table 15-1.

> **Med Tip:** The day sheet is also referred to by other names in some offices, for example, the day journal.

See Figure 15-7 for an example of the accounting pegboard system. Remember that the pegboard system, using the double entry system based on the accounting equation, requires that each side of the equation must be balanced.

See Figure 15-8 for a cash control proof and Figure 15-9 for a posting proof.

Ledger Cards

Ledger cards are maintained for each patient or for a family as a whole. These provide a record of all services and charges provided for that patient and his or her family and can also be used as statements. Refer to Figure 15-10 for examples of ledger cards.

The ledger card will contain all the charges for the entire family being seen by the physician. The correct charge for each individual family member must be placed next to the appropriate name so that insurance billings can be made correctly. The front of the ledger card will contain:

- Name of patient
- Mailing address
- Description of the activity (office visit, post-op visit, prenatal visit)
- Amount of the charge and/or payment
- Adjustment(s), if there are any
- Total balance due by that patient or family

The back of the ledger card includes space for information regarding the collection process. This includes the name, address, and telephone number of the employer of the person responsible for the bill, the spouse's employer's name, address and telephone number, the name and address of the nearest relative, and insurance information. There is also a space for additional comments such as the name of a secondary insurer.

When using the pegboard system, the ledger card is placed under the superbill (charge slip) and directly over the day sheet making sure to line up the entry line on the ledger card with the next available space on the day sheet. It is important not to miss any lines when entering information onto the day sheet.

Ledger cards can be copied and used as a statement which is sent to the patient. In offices using a computerized billing system, the bill is

TABLE 15-1 Day Sheet Sections

Section	Description
Section 1	The individual transaction, such as patient charges are posted in this column. The ledger card, charge slip and receipt forms are used when posting in this column. Included in this column are • Patient name • Description of transaction • Charges and credits • Previous and current balances
Section 2	This is the deposit portion of the day sheet. Some forms actually include a detachable slip that can be used as a deposit slip into a bank account. A payment made by the patient would also be listed under the appropriate right-hand column (cash, check, insurance).
Section 3	This is the column that is optional, and may or may not be used depending on the needs of the practice. For example, it can be used to break down the type of service that was provided (office visit, office surgery, hospital visit).
Section 4	This is the totals column/row. Each of the columns feeding into this bottom section is totaled at the end of the day.
Section 5	This section is critical in checking that the accounts balance. It also keeps track of the cumulative accounts receivable figure owed by all the patients. This column is useful in determining how much money is still outstanding or owed to the physician by looking at just one number.

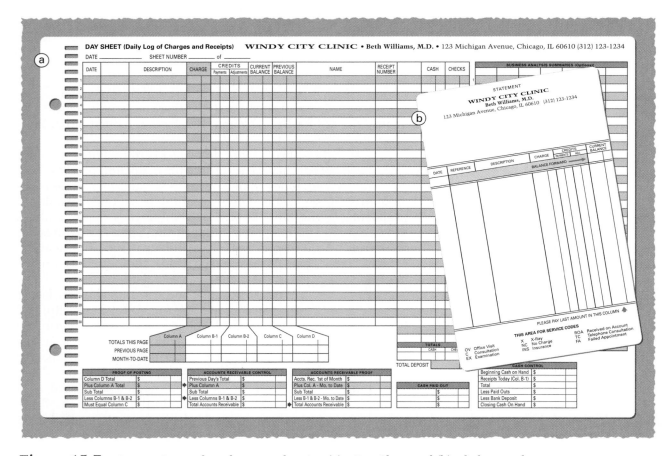

Figure 15-7   Accounting pegboard system showing (a) a Day Sheet and (b) a ledger card.

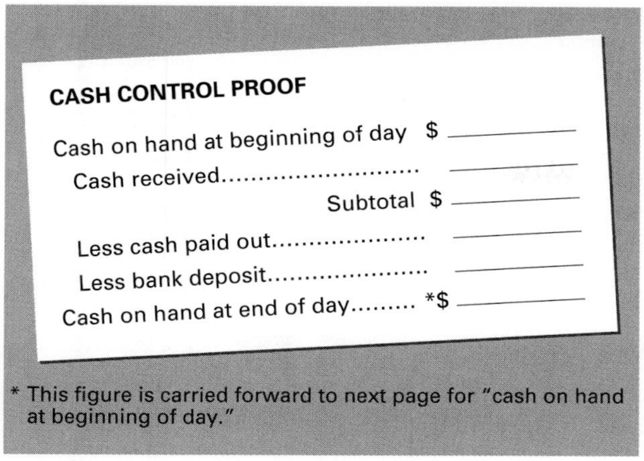

Figure 15-8 Cash control proof.

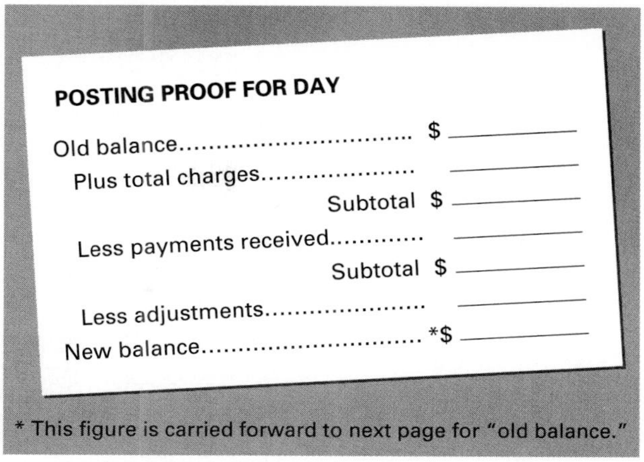

Figures 15-9 Posting proof.

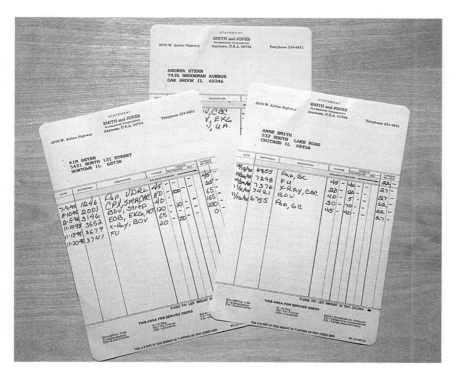

Figure 15-10 Examples of ledger cards.

generated by the computer. Ledger cards are kept in a separate file container that is sized to fit them. This container is usually kept in an accessible spot close to the receptionist or person responsible for handling charges and billing.

Superbill (Charge/Encounter Slip) A superbill, or charge slip, is a two- or three-part carbonized form that has several functions. It gives the patient a record of the account activity (charges, payments, adjustments) for the day and, thus, can

be used as a receipt. It also provides a record which can be used for insurance purposes. The third copy can be kept in the patient's file.

The superbill contains the most commonly performed procedures/services and diagnoses in that physician's practice along with the appropriate insurance code. There is a blank space provided in the event the physician performs a procedure/service not listed on the superbill. Figure 15-11 A–B are examples of a superbill form and a computer-generated superbill.

WINDY CITY CLINIC

UROLOGIC GYNECOLOGY
GENERAL GYNECOLOGY
OBSTETRICS

WINDY CITY CLINIC
Beth Williams, M.D.
123 Michigan Avenue, Chicago, IL 60610
(312) 123-1234

ID.# 20-1342846

No. 4815

☐ PRIVATE ☐ BLUE CROSS ☐ BLUE SHIELD ☐ INDEPENDENT ☐ MEDICARE ☐ GOVERNMENT ☐ MEDI-CAL or MEDICAID

PATIENT INFORMATION

PATIENT'S LAST NAME		FIRST		INITIAL	BIRTHDATE	SEX ☐ MALE ☐ FEMALE	TODAY'S DATE / /
ADDRESS	CITY	STATE		ZIP	RELATION TO SUBSCRIBER	REFERRING PHYSICIAN	
SUBSCRIBER or POLICY HOLDER					INSURANCE		
ADDRESS	CITY	STATE		ZIP	INSURANCE ID.#	COVERAGE CODE	GROUP

OTHER HEALTH COVERAGE?
☐ NO
☐ YES   IDENTIFY _____

DISABILITY RELATED TO:
☐ ACCIDENT   ☐ PREGNANCY
☐ INDEPENDENT   ☐ OTHER

DATE SYMPTOMS APPEARED, INCEPTION OF PREGNANCY, OR
ACCIDENT OCCURED: / /

ASSIGNMENT and RELEASE: *I hereby assign my insurance benefits to be paid directly to the undersigned physician. I am financially responsible for noncovered services. I also authorize the physician to release any information required to process this claim.*

SIGNATURE OF PATIENT (or Parent, if Minor) _____   DATE / /

✓	PROCEDURES	CPT-Mod	AMOUNT	✓	PROCEDURES	CPT-Mod	AMOUNT	✓	PROCEDURES	CPT-Mod	AMOUNT
	A. OFFICE VISITS			31	Post-Partum	59430		60	PG Test, Urine	86006	
1	New GYN, Limited	90010			**F. GYN PROCEDURES**			61	Antigen Test	86006	
2	New GYN, Intermediate	90015		32	Irrigation of Vagina	57150*		62	Cytopathology Smear	88155	
3	New GYN, Extensive	90017		33	Insert Pessary	57160*		63	Specimen Handling	99000	
4	New GYN, Comprehensive	90020		34	Pessary Supplies	99070			**I. MISCELLANEOUS**		
5	Return GYN, Minimal	90030		35	Colposcopy	57452		64	Surgical Tray	99070	
6	Return GYN, Brief	90040		36	Biopsy, Cervix	57500		65	Therapeutic Injection	90782	
7	Return GYN, Limited	90050		37	Biopsy, Vagina	57100		66	Injection, Kenalog	J1870	
8	Return GYN, Intermediate	90060		38	Biopsy, Vulva	56600		67	Injection, Xylocaine	J3480	
9	Return GYN, Extended	90070		39	Biopsy, Endometrium	58100		68	Injection, Estrogen	J2655	
10	Return GYN, Comprehensive	90080		40	Biopsy, Skin			69	Injection, Progesterone	J2675	
11	Return GYN, Post-Operative	99024			0.5 cm.	11420		70	Injection, Vitamin B12	P4320	
	B. CONSULTATION				0.6 to 1.0 cm.	11421		71	Special Reports	99080	
12	GYN Consultation, Limited	90600			1.1 to 2.0 cm.	11423					
13	GYN Consultation, Intermed.	90605		41	Cryotherapy, Cervix	57511					
14	GYN Consultation, Compreh.	90620		42	Destruct. Condyloma	56501					
15	GYN Consultation, Complex	90630		43	Diaphragm Fitting	57170					
16	Second Opinion Surgery	90653		44	Diaphragm Supplies	99070					
	C. TELEPHONE CONSULTATION			45	IUD Insertion	58300					
17	Telephone Consult., Simple	99013		46	IUD Supplies	99070					
18	Telephone Consult., Intermed.	99014		47	IUD Removal	58301					
19	Telephone Consult., Compreh.	99015			**G. UROLOGIC PROCEDURES**						
	D. SPECIAL SERVICES			48	Urethral Dilation	53660					
20	ER Service after Office Hrs.	99064		49	Urethral Dilation, Repeat	53661					
21	ER Service during Office Hrs.	99065		50	Bladder Instillation	51700					
22	Night Call before 10 pm	99050		51	Periurethral Injection	53665					
23	Night Call after 10 pm	99052		52	Simple Catheterization	53670					
24	Sunday or Holiday Service	99054		53	Manual Electric Stimulation	97118					
25	Office Non-Schedule	99058			**H. LAB**						
	E. OB CARE			54	Urine Analysis	81000					
26	Prenatal Dx, Consultation	90620		55	Urine Culture	87068					
27	Initial OB, NOrmal	59400		56	Hematocrit	85015					
28	Initial OB, High Risk	59400.22		57	Hemogram	85021			**TODAY'S TOTAL FEE**	$	
29	Return OB, Normal	59420		58	Commercial-Lat.	87087					
30	Return OB, High Risk	59420.22		59	Wet Mount	87210					

✓	DIAGNOSIS	CODE	✓	DIAGNOSIS	CODE	✓	DIAGNOSIS	CODE	✓	DIAGNOSIS	CODE
	Abortion:			Breasts	216.5		Galactorrhea	676.6		Pregnancy Postpartum	V24.2
	Threatened	640.0		Vulva	221.2		Hemorrhoids	455.0		Rectocele	618.0
	Incomplete	637.1		Breast Disorder (Mass)	611.72		Hypertension	401		Retention of Urine	788.2
	Habitual	646.3		Bronchitis	491		Incontinence of Urine	788.3		Stress Incontinence	625.6
	Abnormal Urination	788.6		Carcinoma In Situ:			Interstitial Cystitis	595.1		Urethral Stricture	598
	Abnormal PAP Smear	795.0		Cervix	233.1		Irritable Colon	564.1		Urethral Syndrome	597.81
	Adenomyosis	617.0		Uterus	233.2		Irregular Menstrual Cycle	626.4		Uterine Leiomyoma	218
	Adnexal MAss	625.8		Female Genital Organs	233.3		Malignant Neoplasm:			Uterine Prolapse:	
	Amenorrhera	626.0		Cervical Dysplasia	622.1		Cervix	180.9		Incomplete	618.2
	Anemia	285.9		Cervicitis	616.0		Uterus	182.0		Complete	618.3
	Arthritis	716.9		Contraceptive Management	V25.0		Ovary	183.0		Vaginal Discharge-Non Specific	623.5
	Artificial Menopause	627.4		Cystocele	618.0		Vagina	184.0		Vaginal Enterocele	618.6
	Asthma-Hayfever	493.0		Cystourethritis	595.0		Vulva	184.4		Vaginal Prolapse	618.0
	Atrophic Vaginitis	627.3		Diabetes Melliuts	250.0		Menopausal Syndrome	627.2		Vaginal Vault Prolapse Post	
	Bartholin Abscess	616.3		Thyroid Disorder	246.9		Menometrorrhagia	626.2		Hysterectomy	618.5
	Benign Neoplasm:			Dysmenorrhea	625.3		Oligomenorrhea	626.1		Vulvovaginitis:	
	Cervix	219.0		Dyspareunia	625.0		Obesity	278.0		Non Specific	616.1
	Uterus	219.1		Dysuria	788.1		Ovarian Cyst	620.2		Candida	112.1
	Ovary	220		Ectopic Pregnancy	617.0		Pelvic Inflammatory Disease	614.9		Trichomonas	131.01
	Vagina	221.1		Endometriosis	617.9		Pelvic Peritoneal Adhesions	614.6			
	Vulva	221.2		Enuresis-Unstable Bladder	788.3		Polycystic Ovaries	256.4			
	Benign Neoplasm of Skin:			Frequency of Urination	788.4		Postmenopausal Bleeding	627.1			
	Buttocks	216.5		Functional Disorder:			Post-Op Wound Infection	998.5			
	Abdomen	216.5		Bladder Instability	596.5		Pregnancy Prenatal	V22			

MISCELLANEOUS DIAGNOSIS	DOCTOR'S SIGNATURE
	_____ DATE / /

SERVICES PERFORMED AT: ☐ Office ☐ Emergency Room
☐ **WINDY CITY CLINIC**
123 Michigan Avenue, Chicago, IL 60610
(312) 123-1234
☐ Hospital Calls at $ _____ per Visit

ADMITTED _____ / /
DISCHARGED _____ / /

RETURN VISIT INFORMATION
15 • 30 • 45 • 60
_____DAYS _____WEEKS _____MONTHS ☐ WILL CALL
Procedure: _____

ACCEPT ASSIGNMENT
☐ YES
☐ NO

INSTRUCTIONS TO PATIENT FOR FILING INSURANCE CLAIMS		
1. Complete patient information portion of this form.	TODAY'S FEE....................	$
2. Sign and date.	OLD BALANCE.....................	$
3. Mail this form directly to your insurance company with your own insurance company's form.	ADJUSTMENTS....................	$
4. Patients with health care insurance please remember:	TOTAL DUE......................	$
A. Professional services are charged to the patient, and not to the insurance company.	AMOUNT RECEIVED TODAY.....	$
B. Insured patients are expected to take care of their fees as services are rendered.	☐ CASH ☐ CHECK ☐ C.C.	
C. This office cannot accept responsibility for collecting your insurance claim or for negotiating a settlement on a disputed claim.		
D. You are responsible for payment of your account.	NEW BALANCE....................	$

(A)

Figure 15-11 A–B (a) Example of a superbill or charge slip form.

(continued on next page)

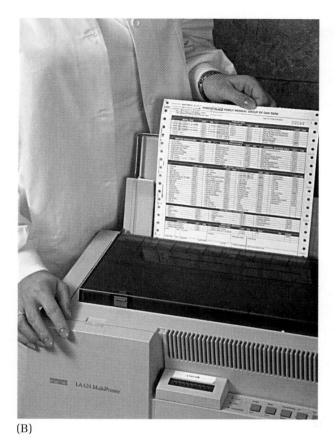

(B)

Figure 15-11   (b) Computer-generated superbill.

Receipt Form   A receipt form is used when a patient payment is made but no service is provided on that day. For example, a patient may come into the office or mail in a check to pay a bill. In some offices, this amount is entered onto the day sheet and ledger card at the same time the receipt form is completed for the patient. If the patient pays the bill with cash, a receipt is given. If the payment is made by check, the patient can use the canceled check as a receipt.

Using the Pegboard System

Every financial transaction, except the use of petty cash, is recorded on the day sheet. Each patient will have a ledger card on which individual financial activity is recorded. When the pegboard system is used, the patient's name, receipt number (the next chronological number on the day sheet), and previous balance are entered on the day sheet with a superbill attached when the patient arrives in the office. The superbill is then removed and attached to the patient's chart. After the patient is seen by the physician, the superbill is put back on

the same line of the day sheet where it was originally written after placing the charge amounts next to the service rendered. See the procedure for using the pegboard system.

If the patient makes a payment in person, then issue a receipt by placing a receipt form on the pegboard in place of the superbill. Place the patient's ledger card onto the day sheet. Enter the previous balance owed on the day sheet, and calculate the new balance after this payment. Post onto the ledger card the date, patient name, a description of the transaction, such as ROA (received on account), and the amount of the payment.

If a payment is made through the mail, a receipt is not sent. The amount credited to the account will appear on the next bill sent to the patient.

Adjustments

Adjustments are any changes made that affect the patient's balance. They can occur when the physician reduces a fee, or agrees to write-off a portion of the charge and accept the insurance payment as

> **Med Tip:** Remember that there must be a balance, based on the accounting equation, when working with financial statements. For every addition in one area, there must be a subtraction in another area in order for the balance to occur.

full payment. For example, if the physician has charged $1500 for a surgical procedure and agrees to accept the insurance payment of $1200, then an adjustment is made for $300. The $300 appears in the adjustment column, and is subtracted from the previous balance to indicate that $1200 is now currently owed. If the $300 was not added to the adjustment column, the totals in section 4 on the balance sheet would not balance. An adjustment or correction also has to be made if there is an error in posting.

Balancing the Day Sheets

To make sure that the accounts and entries are correct, the day sheet(s) need to be balanced at the end of the day. Use a calculator to balance day sheets and always double-check each total. When balancing the day sheet use a calculator with paper tapes, if possible. This will allow a review of

PROCEDURE: Pegboard System

Terminal Performance
Competency: Student will be able to process patient accounts using the write-it-once system without error in posting or mathematics.

Equipment and Supplies
Pegboard
Superbills (Charge Slips)
New day sheet
Ledger cards for each patient scheduled during the day
Calculator

Procedural Steps
1. Place a new day sheet and a strip of superbills (charge slips) onto the pegboard making sure they are fastened securely into the pegs.
2. Complete all the information required at the top of the day sheet (date and page number).
3. Carry balances forward from the previous day sheet and enter it into section 4. These include "Previous Page" columns A–D, "Previous Day's Total," and "Accounts Rec. 1st of Month" which are entered into the Accounts receivable Control and Accounts receivable Proof boxes. This 3rd step is necessary before the day sheet is ready to use.
4. Remove the superbill (charge slip) from the pegboard and clip it to the front of the patient's chart. The physician will enter the procedure performed that day on the appropriate line of the superbill, fill in the diagnosis, and sign the form after he or she sees the patient. The insurance code number is included on the superbill for ease of processing. The superbill is then given to the receptionist by the medical assistant or the patient so that arrangements can be made for payment.
5. To record charges: Place the ledger card under the next superbill (charge slip) and turn back the top two pages of the superbill. Turn back these pages to correctly line up the space for the amount to be posted on the charge slip, and through to the ledger card and day sheet. Write the amount charged pressing firmly and evenly so that this will come through the forms and onto the day sheet.
6. To record payments: When the superbill is received at the front desk, the medical assistant/receptionist will enter the correct charge next to every procedure/service and place this total on the front of the superbill. The superbill is then again placed back on the pegboard, using care to line it up on top of the correct patient's name. The ledger card is then placed UNDER the last page of the charge slip aligning the first blank line of the ledger card with the carbonized entry strip on the superbill. On some types of superbills you will turn back the first two pages of the superbill and enter the total charge and payment into the correct columns. Complete recording this transaction by filling in all the information that the office requires in the far right-hand columns (for example, method of payment such as cash or check).

Med Tip: Try to catch any errors at each step in the balancing process. It is much more difficult to detect an error after all the calculations have been made and the totals are not in balance (equal to each other).

the tape for calculation errors if the figures do not balance.

When errors in posting are corrected, the corrections should be made in the same column as the original posting (Table 15-2).

The steps for balancing the day sheets are presented in Table 15-3.

TABLE 15-2 Correcting Posting Errors

Date	Description	Debit	Credit Payments	Credit Adjustments	Balance
6/19/XX	OV	25.00			25.00
6/19/XX	error in pstg	(25.00)			0

TABLE 15-3 Balancing the Day Sheets

1. Total columns A, B1, B2, C, and D and place the total for each column in the boxes marked "Totals This Page." These column totals then need to be added to numbers brought forward and entered into the "Previous Page" column. This will provide the "Month to Date" total. The "Month to Date" totals are important since they indicate all the credits, charges, and transactions that have occurred from the first day of the month to the present day.

2. The Proof of Posting box is used to make sure that all entries and the totals columns are correct. The numbers used to calculate this figure are taken from the "Totals This Page" column box.

   a. Enter the amount from today's column D total which is the sum of the previous balances into the appropriate box.

   b. Place the total for column A, which represents all the charges for this day, in the appropriate box ("Plus Col. A Total") and create a subtotal by adding Col. D and Col. A totals.

   c. Add column B1 and B2, which are both credit columns (payments and adjustments), together and then enter this amount in the box "Less Col. B1 and B2." This amount will then be subtracted (less) from the subtotal of column D and column A.

   d. If the calculations have been correct, this new subtotal obtained after subtracting column B1 and B2 should be equal to column C, which is the current balance.

      Note that when doing a proof of posting, column D is added to column A minus the sum of columns B1 and B2 and this must equal column C. Therefore, a proof of posting formula is

      $$D + A - (B1 + B2) = C$$

      This means the previous balance (D) plus the charge (A) minus the sum of the payments and adjustments (B1 and B2) is equal to the current balance (C).

Accounts Receivable Control

It is important to keep a running record of all money owed to the physician (accounts receivable). To make sure this number is accurate, an "Accounts Receivable Control" column and an "Accounts Receivable Proof" column are maintained at the bottom of the day sheet.

The day sheet being used on the first day of the month, will have a zero placed in the box marked "Previous Page" if there is no previous page.

If this day sheet page is for the second of the month through the end of the month, there will be a "previous Page" number to place there which is brought forward from the accounts receivable total on the previous page (day before).

The column A and B totals are brought straight across from the Proof of Posting boxes into the correct spaces in the Accounts Receivable Control section. These two figures are added together for a subtotal and then the sum of columns B1 and B2 are subtracted from this amount. This number is the new total accounts receivable figure.

The Accounts Receivable Proof is calculated in the same manner with the last box matching the last box on the Accounts Receivable Control for proof of posting. See Figure 15-12 for an illustration of accounts receivable control.

Accounts Receivable Ratio　An accounts receivable ratio provides a measurement of how fast the outstanding accounts are being paid. The accounts receivable ratio = Current Accounts Receivable Balance ÷ Average Gross Monthly Charges.

For example, if the current accounts receivable balance is $20,000 and the annual gross charges are $120,000, then the average monthly charges are $10,000 ($120,000 ÷ 12). The accounts receivable ratio would = $20,000 ÷ $10,000 = 2 months.

Since a desirable accounts receivable ratio, or the amount of time it takes to have the uncollected debts paid, is 2 months or less, this example is a the high end of the limit. The medical assistant will have to work hard to get collections under 2 months.

Locating Errors

The key to error control is to prevent them in the first place. If there is a difference in the balances of the day sheet, there are several steps that can be taken to locate the error.

1. If the columns on the day sheet do not balance (using the proof of posting box at bottom of day sheet), check all calculations. Ideally you will have saved the calculator tape. Find the difference in the balances and search for that identical amount on the ledger cards and superbill.
2. If an error is divisible by 9, it may be a transposition error. For example, if the difference in the balance is $63, you may find that you wrote $329 instead of $392.
3. Check all the columns, in particular the "previous balance" column to make sure you did not post the amount incorrectly.
4. Check the alignment of all digits to make sure a zero was not misaligned, for example in writing 200 instead of 20. One bookkeeping method for avoiding this type of error, is to use a dash in the cents column instead of two zeros. Thus $45.00 would be written as $45.—.

Computerized Systems

Many offices either perform the accounting function using a computer program, or will be converting to this system in the future. The computer system and program selected will depend on the needs of the office. In some cases a computer consultant is hired to advise on the purchase of the appropriate system based on the size and needs of the practice.

When using a computerized system always back-up data and information on a separate disk which is then stored separately. Some systems also keep the information on the main drive. It is

ACCOUNTS RECEIVABLE CONTROL

Month of __March__, 19 _ _

Accounts receivable at end of preceding month:
$22,500

	Services Rendered	Received from Patients	Adjustments Increase/ (Decrease)	Accounts Receivable Balance
1	$ 800	$ 1000		$22,300
2	$ 700	$ 400		$22,600
3	$ 900	$ 1100	($100)	$22,300
4	$ 1000	$ 700		$22,600

Figure 15-12　Accounts Receivable Control.

advisable to have one hard copy printed of material to be kept on file in the event the computer is not functioning.

Payroll

Payroll responsibilities include making payroll checks for all the staff. This may or may not include the physician depending on how the payment system is set up. Payroll checks are generally issued weekly, biweekly, or monthly. These result in the following pay periods for a year:

- Weekly—52 pay periods a year
- Biweekly—26 pay periods a year
- Monthly—12 pay periods a year

The physician/employer determines the type of pay period the office will use. All employees will then be paid at the same time. See Figure 15-13 for example of payroll.

The employee's payroll check is calculated by first calculating the **gross annual wage**, before taxes and any withholdings are taken out. Use the formula:

(Hourly wage × Number of hours worked per week) × 52 Weeks in a year = Gross pay (or Hourly wage × 2080 Full-time hours in a year = Annual pay)

The annual gross wage for an employee earning $9.00 per hour working a 40 hour week would be:

$$\$9.00 \times 40 \times 52 = \$18,720$$
annual gross wage

To determine the amount the employee earns per day, use the following formula:

(annual gross pay ÷ 52) ÷ 5 = Day's pay

For the example above: ($18,720 ÷ 52) = $360

$360 ÷ 5 = $72

NAME ___Joyce Walker___ SOCIAL SECURITY NO. _123-12-1234_

ADDRESS _22 W. Elm Avenue, Apt 3C_ DATE OF EMPLOYMENT ___6-30-93___

___Goram City, MI 55555___ TELEPHONE ___(010)123-4567___

EXEMPTIONS ___1___ HOURLY RATE _$10.00_

HOURS		GROSS SALARY	DEDUCTIONS					NET SALARY	DATE	CHECK NO.
REG.	O.T.		FWT	SWT	FICA					
80		800 –	72 –	14 –	61⁶⁰			652⁴⁰	7/14	276
80		800 –	72 –	14 –	61⁶⁰			652⁴⁰	7/28	414
72		720 –	64⁸⁰	12⁶⁰	55⁴⁵			587¹⁵	8/11	565
80	4	860 –	77⁴⁰	15⁰⁵	66²⁰			701³⁵	8/25	697
QUARTERLY TOTAL										
YEAR TO DATE										

Figure 15-13 Payroll.

Therefore, if this employee missed a day of work, $72 would be deducted to arrive at the adjusted gross pay ($360 − $72 = $288). Occasionally, an employee will be requested to work overtime or to work more hours than normal for that pay period (a 40 hour week = normal hours). To calculate the overtime pay for an employee who worked 1 day of overtime at the hourly wage of $9.00 simply, divide $9.00 in half ($4.50) and add that amount to the regular $9.00 hourly wage ($9.00 + $4.50 = $13.50). The payment for 1 hour of overtime for this employee would be $13.50 instead of the regular $9.00 payment.

Money is withheld from the employee's paycheck depending on the taxes that must be paid by the employee and employer. This is referred to as **tax withholding**. For example, if the withholding tax is 4% then this amount is calculated based on the employee's gross pay. The taxes are then subtracted from the gross or an adjusted gross pay. This amount is what appears on the employee's paycheck.

Government regulations require that records must be maintained for each employee relating to the following payroll items:

- Amount of gross pay
- Social security number of employee
- Number of exemptions of each employee (taken from W-4 form completed by employee at time of hire)
- Deductions for Social Security, federal, state, and city taxes
- State disability insurance and unemployment tax, where applicable

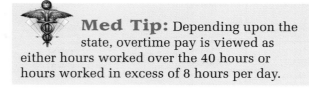

Med Tip: Depending upon the state, overtime pay is viewed as either hours worked over the 40 hours or hours worked in excess of 8 hours per day.

Income Tax Withholding

Federal, state, and city taxes are withheld from the payment to the employee. These tax payments are made directly to the government. Employers have an obligation by law to withhold a portion of their employee's earnings for tax purposes, and report and forward this amount to the government. To determine the amount of money to be withheld from each paycheck, the employee must complete a W-4 form when they are hired (Figure 15-14). The W-4 form must include:

- Employee's name and current address
- Social Security number
- Marital status
- The number of exemptions the employee claims that should be used when calculating the withheld tax money

Tables used to determine the amount of withholding are provided in the Federal Employer's Tax Guide. See Figure 15-15 for a sample federal tax-withholding table. Tables are available for married persons, single persons, and unmarried heads of households and cover weekly, biweekly, monthly, semimonthly, and daily periods.

Social Security, Medicare, and Income Tax Withholding

The federal government **mandates**, or requires, the following taxes be paid: Social Security (Federal Insurance Contribution Act or FICA), Medicare, and federal income tax. These taxes are based on a percentage of the employee's total gross income (see calculation above for determining gross income). The number of exemptions claimed on the W-4 form and the marital status of the employee are taken into account when calculating the tax. The employer has an obligation to match the employee's payment for Social Security and Medicare. This means that if the employee has $100 withheld for Social Security and Medicare, the employer must match the $100 and make a total payment to the government for that employee of $200 ($100 as the employee contribution and $100 as the employer's contribution). The employer does not have to match the federal, state, and local taxes.

Deposit Requirements

The federal tax money withheld and the FICA payment is placed into a federal deposit account in a Federal Reserve Bank or into an authorized banking institution, either at the end of each period or at the end of the month. The Internal Revenue Service (IRS) has a severe penalty for failure to deposit this money.

Employers must file a quarterly report (Form 941—Employer's Quarterly Federal Tax Return) before the last day of the first month after the end of the quarter. These dates are April 30, July 31, October 31, and January 31.

Form W-4 (1997)

Want More Money In Your Paycheck?
If you expect to be able to take the earned income credit for 1997 and a child lives with you, you may be able to have part of the credit added to your take-home pay. For details, get Form W-5 from your employer.

Purpose. Complete Form W-4 so that your employer can withhold the correct amount of Federal income tax from your pay. Form W-4 may be completed electronically, if your employer has an electronic system. Because your tax situation may change, you may want to refigure your withholding each year.

Exemption From Withholding. Read line 7 of the certificate below to see if you can claim exempt status. *If exempt, only complete lines 1, 2, 3, 4, 7, and sign the form to validate it.* No Federal income tax will be withheld from your pay. Your exemption expires February 17, 1998.

Note: *You cannot claim exemption from withholding if (1) your income exceeds $650 and includes unearned income (e.g., interest and dividends) and (2) another person can claim you as a dependent on their tax return.*
Basic Instructions. If you are not exempt, complete the Personal Allowances Worksheet. Additional worksheets are on page 2 so you can adjust your withholding allowances based on itemized deductions, adjustments to income, or two-earner/two-job situations. Complete all worksheets that apply to your situation. The worksheets will help you figure the number of withholding allowances you are entitled to claim. However, you may claim fewer allowances than this.

Head of Household. Generally, you may claim head of household filing status on your tax return only if you are unmarried and pay more than 50% of the costs of keeping up a home for yourself and your dependent(s) or other qualifying individuals.

Nonwage Income. If you have a large amount of nonwage income, such as interest or dividends, you should consider making

estimated tax payments using Form 1040-ES. Otherwise, you may find that you owe additional tax at the end of the year.

Two Earners/Two Jobs. If you have a working spouse or more than one job, figure the total number of allowances you are entitled to claim on all jobs using worksheets from only one W4. This total should be divided among all jobs. Your withholding will usually be most accurate when all allowances are claimed on the W-4 filed for the highest paying job and zero allowances are claimed for the others.

Check Your Withholding. After your W-4 takes affect, use **Pub. 919**, Is My Withholding Correct for 1997?, to see how the dollar amount you are having withheld compares to your estimated total annual tax. Get Pub. 919 especially if you used the Two-Earner/Two-Job Worksheet and your earnings exceed $150,000 (Single) or $200,000 (Married). To order Pub. 919, call 1-800-829-3676. Check your telephone directory for the IRS assistance number for further help.

Sign This Form. Form W-4 is not considered valid unless you sign it.

Personal Allowances Worksheet

A Enter "1" for **yourself** if no one else can claim you as a dependent . . . . **A** _____

B Enter "1" if:
- You are single and have only one job; or
- You are married, have only one job, and your spouse does not work; or
- Your wages from a second job or your spouse's wages (or the total of both) are $1,000 or less.

. **B** _____

C Enter "1" for your **spouse.** But, you may choose to enter -0- if you are married and have either a working spouse or more than one job (this may help you avoid having too little tax withheld) . . . . **C** _____

D Enter number of **dependents** (other than your spouse or yourself) you will claim on your tax return . . . . . . **D** _____

E Enter "1" if you will file as **head of household** on your tax return (see conditions under **Head of Household** above) . **E** _____

F Enter "1" if you have at least $1,500 of **child or dependent care expenses** for which you plan to claim a credit . **F** _____

G Add lines A through F and enter total here. **Note:** This amount may be different from the number of exemptions you claim on your return ▶ **G** _____

For accuracy, complete all worksheets that apply.
- If you plan to **itemize or claim adjustments to income** and want to reduce your withholding, see the Deductions and Adjustments Worksheet on page 2.
- If you are **single** and have **more than one job** and your combined earnings from all jobs exceed $32,000 OR if you are **married** and have a **working spouse or more than one job,** and the combined earnings from all jobs exceed $55,000, see the Two-Earner/Two-Job Worksheet on page 2 if you want to avoid having too little tax withheld.
- If **neither** of the above situations applies, **stop here** and enter the number from line G on line 5 of Form W-4 below.

- - - - - - - - - - - - - - - - - - - **Cut here and give the certificate to your employer. Keep the top portion for your records.** - - - - - - - - - - - - - - - - - - -

Form **W-4**	**Employee's Withholding Allowance Certificate**	OMB No. 1545-0010
Department of the Treasury Internal Revenue Service	▶ **For Privacy Act and Paperwork Reduction Act Notice, see reverse.**	**1997**

1 Type or print your first name and middle initial	Last name	**2** Your social security number

Home address (number and street or rural route)	**3** ☐ Single ☐ Married ☐ Married, but withhold at higher Single rate.
City or town, state, and ZIP code	**Note:** *If married, but legally separated, or spouse is a nonresident alien, check the Single box.* **4** If your last name differs from that on your social security card, check here and call 1-800-772-1213 for a new card . . . . ▶ ☐

5 Total number of allowances you are claiming (from line G above or from the worksheets on page 2 if they apply) . **5** _____

6 Additional amount, if any, you want withheld from each paycheck . . . . **6** $ _____

7 I claim exemption from withholding for 1997, and I certify that I meet **BOTH** of the following conditions for exemption:
- Last year I had a right to a refund of **ALL** Federal income tax withheld because I had **NO** tax liability; **AND**
- This year I expect a refund of **ALL** Federal income tax withheld because I expect to have **NO** tax liability.

If you meet both conditions, enter "EXEMPT" here . . . . ▶ **7** _____

Under penalties of perjury, I certify that I am entitled to the number of withholding allowances claimed on this certificate or entitled to claim exempt status.

Employee's signature ▶ _____ Date ▶ _____ , 19 ____

8 Employer's name and address (Employer: Complete 8 and 10 only if sending to the IRS)	**9** Office code (optional)	**10** Employer identification number

Cat. No. 10220Q

Figure 15-14 W-4 form required by the IRS. *(Continued on next page)*

Deductions and Adjustments Worksheet

Note: *Use this worksheet only if you plan to itemize deductions or claim adjustments to income on your 1997 tax return.*

1	Enter an estimate of your 1997 itemized deductions. These include qualifying home mortgage interest, charitable contributions, state and local taxes (but not sales taxes), medical expenses in excess of 7.5% of your income, and miscellaneous deductions. (For 1997, you may have to reduce your itemized deductions if your income is over $121,200 ($60,600 if married filing separately). Get Pub. 919 for details.)	**1** $ _____
2	Enter: { $6,900 if married filing jointly or qualifying widow(er) $6,050 if head of household $4,150 if single $3,450 if married filing separately }	**2** $ _____
3	**Subtract** line 2 from line 1. If line 2 is greater than line 1, enter -0-	**3** $ _____
4	Enter an estimate of your 1997 adjustments to income. These include alimony paid and deductible IRA contributions	**4** $ _____
5	**Add** lines 3 and 4 and enter the total	**5** $ _____
6	Enter an estimate of your 1997 nonwage income (such as dividends or interest)	**6** $ _____
7	**Subtract** line 6 from line 5. Enter the result, but not less than -0-	**7** $ _____
8	**Divide** the amount on line 7 by $2,500 and enter the result here. Drop any fraction	**8** _____
9	Enter the number from Personal Allowances Worksheet, line G, on page 1	**9** _____
10	**Add** lines 8 and 9 and enter the total here. If you plan to use the Two-Earner/Two-Job Worksheet, also enter this total on line 1 below. Otherwise, **stop here** and enter this total on Form W-4, line 5, on page 1	**10** _____

Two-Earner/Two-Job Worksheet

Note: *Use this worksheet only if the instructions for line G on page 1 direct you here.*

1	Enter the number from line G on page 1 (or from line 10 above if you used the Deductions and Adjustments Worksheet)	**1** _____
2	Find the number in **Table 1** below that applies to the **LOWEST** paying job and enter it here	**2** _____
3	If line 1 is **GREATER THAN OR EQUAL TO** line 2, subtract line 2 from line 1. Enter the result here (if zero, enter -0-) and on Form W-4, line 5, on page 1. **DO NOT** use the rest of this worksheet	**3** _____

Note: *If line 1 is **LESS THAN** line 2, enter -0- on Form W-4, line 5, on page 1. Complete lines 4–9 to calculate the additional withholding amount necessary to avoid a year end tax bill.*

4	Enter the number from line 2 of this worksheet	**4** _____
5	Enter the number from line 1 of this worksheet	**5** _____
6	**Subtract** line 5 from line 4	**6** _____
7	Find the amount in **Table 2** below that applies to the **HIGHEST** paying job and enter it here	**7** $ _____
8	**Multiply** line 7 by line 6 and enter the result here. This is the additional annual withholding amount needed	**8** $ _____
9	Divide line 8 by the number of pay periods remaining in 1997. (For example, divide by 26 if you are paid every other week and you complete this form in December 1996.) Enter the result here and on Form W-4, line 6, page 1. This is the additional amount to be withheld from each paycheck	**9** $ _____

Table 1: Two-Earner/Two-Job Worksheet

Married Filing Jointly				All Others			
If wages from **LOWEST** paying job are–	Enter on line 2 above	If wages from **LOWEST** paying job are–	Enter on line 2 above	If wages from **LOWEST** paying job are–	Enter on line 2 above	If wages from **LOWEST** paying job are–	Enter on line 2 above
0 - $4,000	0	35,001 - 40,000	8	0 - $5,000	0	75,001 - 90,000	8
4,001 - 7,000	1	40,001 - 50,000	9	5,001 - 11,000	1	90,001 - 110,000	9
7,001 - 12,000	2	50,001 - 60,000	10	11,001 - 15,000	2	110,001 and over	10
12,001 - 17,000	3	60,001 - 70,000	11	15,001 - 20,000	3		
17,001 - 22,000	4	70,001 - 80,000	12	20,001 - 24,000	4		
22,001 - 28,000	5	80,001 - 100,000	13	24,001 - 45,000	5		
28,001 - 32,000	6	100,001 - 110,000	14	45,001 - 60,000	6		
32,001 - 35,000	7	110,001 and over	15	60,001 - 75,000	7		

Table 2: Two-Earner/Two-Job Worksheet

Married Filing Jointly		All Others	
If wages from **HIGHEST** paying job are–	Enter on line 7 above	If wages from **HIGHEST** paying job are–	Enter on line 7 above
0 - $50,000	$400	0 - $30,000	$400
50,001 - 100,000	740	30,001 - 60,000	740
100,001 - 130,000	820	60,001 - 120,000	820
130,001 - 240,000	950	120,001 - 250,000	950
240,001 and over	1,050	250,001 and over	1,050

Privacy Act and Paperwork Reduction Act Notice.– We ask for the information on this form to carry out the Internal Revenue laws of the United States. The Internal Revenue Code requires this information under sections 3402(f)(2)(A) and 6109 and their regulations. Failure to provide a completed form will result in your being treated as a single person who claims no withholding allowances. Routine uses of this information include giving it to the Department of Justice for civil and criminal litigation and to cities, states, and the District of Columbia for use in administering their tax laws.

You are not required to provide the information requested on a form that is subject to the Paperwork Reduction Act unless the form displays a valid OMB control number. Books or records relating to a form or its instructions must be retained as long as their contents may become material in the administration of any Internal Revenue Law. Generally, tax returns and return information are confidential, as required by Code section 6103.

The time needed to complete this form will vary depending on individual circumstances. The estimated average time is: **Recordkeeping** 46 min., **Learning about the law or the form** 10 min., **Preparing the form** 69 min. If you have comments concerning the accuracy of these time estimates or suggestions for making this form simpler, we would be happy to hear from you. You can write to the Tax Forms Committee, Western Area Distribution Center, Rancho Cordova, CA 95743-0001. **DO NOT** send the tax form to this address. Instead, give it to your employer.

Figure 15-14   W-4 form required by the IRS. *(Continued)*

WAGE WITHOLDING TABLE

Biweekly Payroll Period—Single Persons
For Wages Paid After December 1996

And the wages are—		And the number of withholding allowances claimed is —										
At least	But less than	0	1	2	3	4	5	6	7	8	9	10
		The amount of income tax to be withheld shall be —										
$580	$600	$118.14	$104.14	$89.14	$74.14	$60.14	$45.14	$45.14	$45.14	$45.14	$45.14	$45.14
600	620	122.67	106.67	93.67	75.87	64.67	49.67	46.67	46.67	46.67	46.67	46.67
620	640	127.20	113.20	98.20	83.20	69.20	54.20	48.20	48.20	48.20	48.20	48.20
640	660	131.73	117.73	102.73	87.73	73.73	58.73	49.73	49.73	49.73	49.73	49.73
660	680	136.26	122.26	107.26	92.26	78.26	63.26	51.26	51.26	51.26	51.26	51.26
680	700	140.79	126.79	111.79	96.79	82.79	67.79	52.79	52.79	52.79	52.79	52.79
700	720	145.32	131.32	116.32	101.32	87.32	72.32	57.32	54.32	54.32	54.32	54.32
720	740	149.85	135.85	120.85	105.85	91.85	76.85	61.85	55.85	55.85	55.85	55.85
740	760	154.38	140.38	125.38	110.38	96.38	81.38	66.38	57.38	57.38	57.38	57.38
760	780	158.91	144.91	129.91	114.91	100.91	85.91	70.91	58.91	58.91	58.91	58.91
780	800	163.44	149.44	134.44	119.44	105.44	90.44	75.44	60.44	60.44	60.44	60.44
800	820	167.97	153.97	138.97	123.97	109.97	94.97	79.97	64.97	61.97	61.97	61.97
820	840	172.50	158.50	143.50	128.50	114.50	96.50	84.50	69.50	63.50	63.50	63.50
840	860	177.03	163.03	148.03	133.03	119.03	104.03	89.03	74.03	65.03	65.03	65.03
860	880	181.56	167.56	152.56	137.56	123.56	108.56	93.56	78.56	66.56	66.56	66.56
880	900	186.09	172.09	157.09	142.09	128.09	113.09	98.09	83.09	69.09	68.09	68.09
900	920	190.82	176.62	161.62	146.62	132.62	117.62	102.62	87.62	73.62	68.02	68.02
920	940	196.15	181.15	166.15	151.15	137.15	122.15	107.15	92.15	78.15	71.15	71.15
940	960	199.68	185.68	170.68	155.68	141.68	126.68	111.68	96.68	82.68	72.68	72.68
960	980	204.21	190.21	175.21	160.21	146.21	131.21	116.21	101.21	87.21	74.21	74.21
980	1,000	210.74	194.74	179.74	164.74	150.74	135.74	120.74	105.74	91.74	78.74	75.74
1,000	1,020	217.27	199.27	184.27	169.27	155.27	140.27	125.27	110.27	96.27	91.27	77.27
1,020	1,040	224.80	203.80	188.80	173.80	159.80	144.80	129.80	114.80	100.80	85.80	78.80
1,040	1,060	232.33	208.33	193.33	178.33	164.33	149.33	134.33	119.33	105.33	90.33	80.33
1,060	1,080	238.86	212.86	197.86	182.86	168.86	153.86	138.86	123.86	109.86	94.86	81.86
1,080	1,100	246.39	218.39	202.39	187.39	173.39	158.39	143.39	128.39	114.39	99.39	84.39
1,100	1,120	252.92	225.92	208.92	191.92	177.92	162.92	147.92	132.92	118.92	103.92	88.92
1,120	1,140	260.45	233.45	211.45	196.45	182.45	167.45	152.45	137.45	123.45	108.45	93.45
1,140	1,160	267.98	239.98	215.98	200.98	186.98	171.98	156.98	141.98	127.98	112.98	97.98
1,160	1,180	274.51	247.51	220.51	205.51	191.51	176.51	161.51	146.51	132.51	117.51	102.51

Figure 15-15 Example of a federal tax-withholding table.

Federal Unemployment Tax

Every employer must contribute to the unemployment tax act. This is mandated under the Federal Unemployment Tax Act (FUTA). If the employer is making payments into a state unemployment fund, this can generally be applied as credit against the FUTA tax amount.

FUTA is the sole responsibility of the employer. It is based on the employee's gross income, but must not be deducted from the employee's wage.

FUTA deposits are calculated quarterly and the amount due must be paid by the last day of the first month after the quarter ends. Therefore, for the first quarter of the year ending on March 31st, the payment must be made by April 30th. An an-

nual FUTA report must be filed to the federal government using Form 940 each year.

State Unemployment Tax

All states have unemployment compensation laws. Most states require only the employer to make payments toward this fund. However, a few states require both the employer and employee to make a payment. In this case, the employer would withhold a certain calculated amount from the employee's pay check.

In some states, the employer does not have to make a payment to unemployment compensation if there are very few employees (4 or less). Each state's regulation concerning tax requirements should be checked carefully before preparing the payroll.

State Disability Insurance

Some states require a certain amount of money be withheld from the employee's check to cover a disability insurance plan. This insurance coverage assists employees in the event they become injured or disabled and unable to work. Money may also be withheld, as requested by the employee, for health, life, and disability insurance, and pension plan contributions.

Annual Tax Returns

W-2 forms must be completed at the end of each year and given to each employee. The amount of wages that were taxable under Social Security and Medicare must be listed separately on the W-2 form. The employer must provide three copies of the W-2 form to each employee from whom these taxes were withheld (one each for federal and state filing and one for the employee's file). This form must be received by the employee by January 31, according to the law. The W-2 form lists the total gross income, total federal, state, and local taxes which were withheld, taxable fringe benefits, such as tips, and the employee's total net income (Figure 15-16).

The preparation of reports to the federal government and the W-2 forms for the employees can be time-consuming and requires some training. Many offices which do not have a bookkeeper, or medical assistant assigned to this duty, use the services of an accountant. The records and reports the accountant will use need to be prepared ahead of time. The pegboard system, if used, can provide summaries of the income, expenses, and payroll for the office. If a manual system is used, the totals for all the tax payment periods should be calculated for the accountant. The accountant will then audit or reexamine all the financial statements for accuracy.

Methods for Calculating Payroll Checks

There are several systems for calculating and issuing payroll checks, which include: manual, pegboard, and computer.

Manual

Meticulous recordkeeping is necessary when performing any payroll function. Separate records are needed for documentation of the gross income, tax withholdings, and each of the checks issued for all employees. This can mean that the records for payroll are kept in more than one record book or log book. For example, the check stub will indicate the name, date, and amount of payroll check, while a log book is needed to track the gross income and withholdings which are totaled monthly, quarterly, and annually.

Pegboard

The advantage of using a pegboard (write-it-once) method is that all or most of the payroll record is in one record.

Computer

There are several software packages available that are used to calculate payroll and tax withholdings,

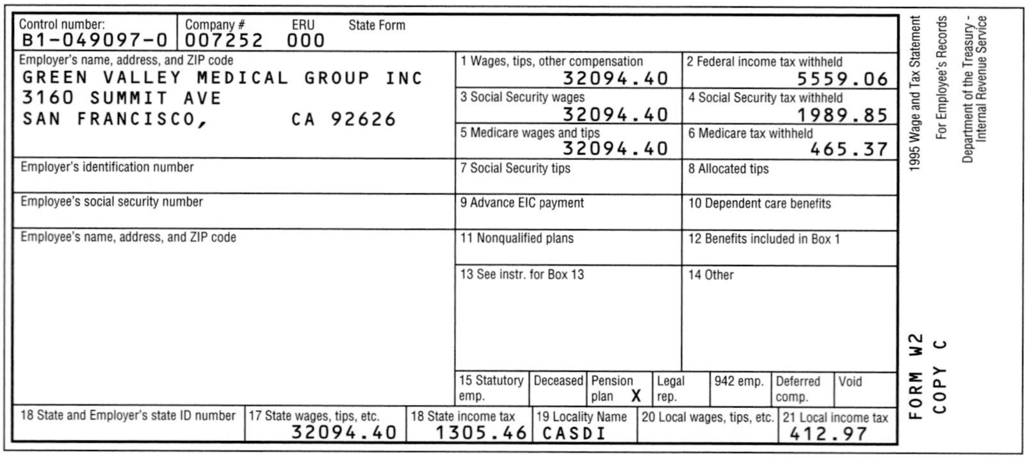

Control number: B1-049097-0 | Company # 007252 | ERU 000 | State Form

Employer's name, address, and ZIP code: GREEN VALLEY MEDICAL GROUP INC, 3160 SUMMIT AVE, SAN FRANCISCO, CA 92626

1 Wages, tips, other compensation 32094.40	2 Federal income tax withheld 5559.06
3 Social Security wages 32094.40	4 Social Security tax withheld 1989.85
5 Medicare wages and tips 32094.40	6 Medicare tax withheld 465.37
7 Social Security tips	8 Allocated tips
9 Advance EIC payment	10 Dependent care benefits
11 Nonqualified plans	12 Benefits included in Box 1
13 See instr. for Box 13	14 Other

Employer's identification number

Employee's social security number

Employee's name, address, and ZIP code

15 Statutory emp. | Deceased | Pension plan X | Legal rep. | 942 emp. | Deferred comp. | Void

18 State and Employer's state ID number	17 State wages, tips, etc.	18 State income tax	19 Locality Name	20 Local wages, tips, etc.	21 Local income tax
	32094.40	1305.46	CASDI		412.97

1995 Wage and Tax Statement | For Employee's Records | Department of the Treasury - Internal Revenue Service | FORM W2 COPY C

Figure 15-16 An example of a W-2 form required by the IRS.

and print payroll checks. Such software programs can provide time savings for office staff over the more traditional manual method. In addition, the amounts calculated for withholding can be more accurately performed with the computer than with the manual method.

In some offices, an outside payroll service is hired to process all payroll checks, withholding payments, and keep records.

LEGAL AND ETHICAL ISSUES

The employer (physician) has a legal responsibility to correctly withhold certain portions of the employee's salary as required for tax and other purposes. In addition the employer must make contributions on behalf of the employee to certain funds, such as unemployment, on a timely basis or receive a penalty. When the responsibility for calculating payroll withholding is delegated to the medical assistant, it is a serious and confidential responsibility.

PATIENT EDUCATION

The patients will call the medical office with questions concerning their bills. The medical assistant needs to be familiar with the accounting system used in the practice, for example, the pegboard system, in order to be able to explain the detailed bill to the patient.

Occasionally a patient makes an overpayment on a bill. This occurs either through error or when the insurance company pays the physician after the patient has already paid for the service. The medical practice has a legal and ethical responsibility to return the overpayment to the patient.

Summary

Whether working with a manual, pegboard, or computerized accounting system, attention to accuracy in bookkeeping is necessary. Handling the payroll for a medical practice requires skill, attention to detail, accuracy, and punctual filing of all forms. In addition, confidentiality relating to employees' salaries is necessary.

Competency Review

1. Define and spell the glossary terms for this chapter.
2. State the difference between a debit and credit adjustment.
3. List the five sections on a pegboard day sheet.
4. Balance a pegboard day sheet.
5. Prepare a payroll check.
6. Prepare a
   a. New day sheet.
   b. Ledger account for a new patient.
   c. Patient charge slip.
   d. Daily posting proof.

Test Taking Tip — Everybody takes tests at their own pace and speed. Keep that in mind when others around you are finishing before you do. Watch the clock and pace yourself.

Examination Review Questions

1. When using the pegboard system, the accounts receivable amount(s) is/are
   (A) the amount of the physician's charge
   (B) the amount received from the patients
   (C) the adjustments made to the fee
   (D) the amount owed to the physician
   (E) the amount the physician owes for purchases

2. The pegboard system is the same as the
   (A) single-entry bookkeeping system
   (B) write-it-once system
   (C) computerized system
   (D) write-it-now system
   (E) none of the above

3. The accounts receivable record tells you
   (A) the effectiveness of the billing system
   (B) total collections divided by gross charges
   (C) how much money is still owed the physician
   (D) how fast outstanding accounts are being paid
   (E) total collections divided by net charges

4. The formula for the accounts receivable ledger is
   (A) $D - A + (B1 + B2) = C$
   (B) $D + A - (B1 + B2) = C$
   (C) $A + C - (B1 - B2) = D$
   (D) $A + (B1 - B2) = C$
   (E) $A - (B1 - B1) = C$

5. Good bookkeeping habits include
   (A) using blue ink to clearly indicate a deficit
   (B) using pencil so that changes can be easily made
   (C) making corrections using opaque correction fluid
   (D) checking each entry once
   (E) aligning columns using decimal point

6. By law, the employer must match employee contributions on what tax?
   (A) disability insurance
   (B) workman's compensation
   (C) state
   (D) social security
   (E) self-employment tax

7. What information is NOT listed on an employee's W-4 form?
   (A) marital status
   (B) number of exemptions
   (C) employee's social security number
   (D) salary
   (E) current address

8. The pegboard allows you to do all of the following with just one writing EXCEPT
   (A) provide a receipt to the patient
   (B) give a notice of the patient's next appointment
   (C) erase errors
   (D) update the patient's account
   (E) provide a copy for insurance purposes

9. Computer data should be recorded in all of the following ways EXCEPT
   (A) printed-out onto a paper (hard) copy
   (B) on the computer's hard drive
   (C) as a back up disk
   (D) manually
   (E) all of the above

10. A trial balance is a/an
    (A) listing of every account column
    (B) listing of accounts receivable
    (C) cash receipts record
    (D) journal entry
    (E) income statement

ON THE JOB

Sally Harris, a medical assistant, has just been hired to work in the front office of Dr. Williams's practice. She is a recent graduate of an accredited school and will be taking her CMA examination in January. Sally has studied the accounting procedure in school but has not had any opportunity to use either the pegboard system or a computerized system for accounting and payroll. Dr. Williams has asked you to mentor Sally and train her in the use of the pegboard system which is currently used in the office.

What is your response?

1. Write a brief description of the system for Sally and explain what equipment is necessary, and how to set up the day sheet, ledger cards, and superbill for each patient.
2. Describe how an error can be found.
3. Create a day sheet for October 1, using five fictitious patient's names, charges, adjustments, and payments. Balance the sheets completing the proof of posting, accounts receivable control and the accounts receivable proof.
4. Explain the proof of posting equation.

References

Andress, A. *Manual of Medical Office Management.* Philadelphia: W.B. Saunders Company, 1996.

Becklin, K. and Sunnaborg, E. *Medical Office Procedures.* New York: Glencoe/McGraw-Hill, 1992.

Humphrey, D. *Contemporary Medical Office Procedures.* Albany, NY: Delmar Publications, 1996.

Larson, K. and Miller, P. *Fundamental Accounting Principles.* Homewood, IL: Orwin, 1993.

McConnell, T. *Moral Issues in Health Care.* New York: Wadsworth Publishing Company, 1997.

MEDICAL ASSISTANT ROLE DELINEATION CHART

Highlight indicates material covered in this chapter

ADMINISTRATIVE

ADMINISTRATIVE PROCEDURES

- Perform basic clerical functions
- Schedule, coordinate, and monitor appointments
- Schedule inpatient/outpatient admissions and procedures
- Understand and apply third party guidelines
- Obtain reimbursement through accurate claims submission
- Monitor third-party reimbursement
- Perform medical transcription
- Understand and adhere to managed care policies and procedures
- *Negotiate managed care contracts (adv)*

PRACTICE FINANCES

- Perform procedural and diagnostic coding
- Apply bookkeeping principles
- Document and maintain accounting and banking records
- Manage accounts receivable
- Manage accounts payable
- Process payroll
- *Develop and maintain fee schedules (adv)*
- *Manage renewals of business and professional insurance policies (adv)*
- *Manage personal benefits and maintain records (adv)*

CLINICAL

FUNDAMENTAL PRINCIPLES

- Apply principles of aseptic technique and infection control
- Comply with quality assurance practices
- Screen and follow up patient test results

DIAGNOSTIC ORDERS

- Collect and process specimens
- Perform diagnostic tests

PATIENT CARE

- Adhere to established triage procedures
- Obtain patient history and vital signs
- Prepare and maintain examination and treatment areas

- Prepare patient for examinations, procedures, and treatments
- Assist with examinations, procedures, and treatments
- Prepare and administer medications and immunizations
- Maintain medication and immunization records
- Recognize and respond to emergencies
- Coordinate patient care information with other health care providers

GENERAL (TRANSDISCIPLINARY)

PROFESSIONALISM

- Project a professional manner and image
- Adhere to ethical principles
- Demonstrate initiative and responsibility
- Work as a team member
- Manage time efficiently
- Prioritize and perform multiple tasks
- Adapt to change
- Promote the CMA credential
- Enhance skills through continuing education

COMMUNICATION SKILLS

- Treat all patients with compassion and empathy
- Recognize and respect cultural diversity
- Adapt communications to individual's ability to understand
- Use professional telephone technique
- Use effective and correct verbal and written communications
- Recognize and respond to verbal and nonverbal communications
- Use medical terminology appropriately
- Receive, organize, prioritize, and transmit information
- Serve as liaison
- Promote the practice through positive public relations

LEGAL CONCEPTS

- Maintain confidentiality
- Practice within the scope of education, training, and personal capabilities
- Prepare and maintain medical records
- Document accurately
- Use appropriate guidelines when releasing information
- Follow employer's established policies dealing with the health care contract
- Follow federal, state, and local legal guidelines
- Maintain awareness of federal and state health care legislation and regulations
- Maintain and dispose of regulated substances in compliance with government guidelines
- Comply with established risk management and safety procedures
- Recognize professional credentialing criteria
- Participate in the development and maintenance of personnel, policy, and procedure manuals
- *Develop and maintain personnel, policy, and procedure manuals (adv)*

INSTRUCTION

- Instruct individuals according to their needs
- Explain office policies and procedures
- Teach methods of health promotion and disease prevention
- Locate community resources and disseminate information
- *Orient and train personnel (adv)*
- *Develop educational materials (adv)*
- *Conduct continuing education activities (adv)*

OPERATIONAL FUNCTIONS

- Maintain supply inventory
- Evaluate and recommend equipment and supplies
- Apply computer techniques to support office operations
- *Supervise personnel (adv)*
- *Interview and recommend job applicants (adv)*
- *Negotiate leases and prices for equipment and supply contracts (adv)*

SOURCE: Reprinted by permission of the American Association of Medical Assistants from the *AAMA Role Delineation Study: Occupational Analysis of the Medical Assisting Profession.*

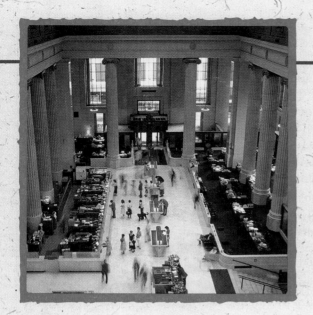

16

Banking Procedures

LEARNING OBJECTIVES

After completing this chapter, you should:
1. Define and spell the glossary terms for this chapter.
2. State the correct procedure for writing a check and check stub.
3. Describe the write-it-once check writing system.
4. State the correct method for endorsing a check based on the guidelines issued by the federal government.
5. Discuss 5 advantages of using checks.
6. List 7 types of checks.
7. Differentiate between the ABA number and the MICR on a check.
8. List and describe 6 steps in the check writing process.
9. State 5 general guidelines when writing checks.
10. Discuss how to correct an error on a check.
11. State the risks associated with accepting a third-party check, cash or check from an out-of-state bank.
12. List the criteria for a negotiable instrument.
13. State and describe 3 types of endorsements.
14. Discuss the reason for not paying bills early.
15. List 6 recurring monthly expenses.
16. Describe the 5 steps to follow when making a deposit.
17. List and discuss 9 steps for reconciling a bank statement.

ADMINISTRATIVE PERFORMANCE COMPETENCIES

After completing this chapter, you should perform the following tasks:
1. Prepare a check and check stub correctly.
2. Prepare a deposit slip.
3. Reconcile a bank statement.

Glossary

ABA number   Code number on right upper corner of printed check to identify bank.

accounts receivable   Money owed to the physician/medical practice.

canceled checks   Deposited checks that have been processed by the bank.

certified   Guaranteed.

credit(s)   Funds added to an account.

currency   Paper money.

debit(s)   Charges against an account.

deposit(s)   To place money (cash and/or checks) into a bank account.

disbursement   Payment of funds (money).

embezzlement   To take money by breach of trust.

fiscal   Relating to financial matters.

Magnetic Ink Character Recognition (MICR) Characters and letters printed on the bottom of the check used as routing information to identify the bank and number of the individual account.

maker (of check)   Person who signs the check (or corporation who pays it). This is the same as the payer.

negotiable   To transfer money to another person (for example, through an endorsement on a check).

outstanding deposits   Checks that have been deposited to one's account but not yet processed by the bank.

payee   Person or company named as the receiving party to whom the amount on the check is payable.

payer   Person signing a check to release money.

postdate   To write a future date on a check and then sign it.

reconciliation (of bank statement)   To adjust one's banking records against a bank statement so that both are in agreement.

signee   Person who signs a check or document.

stop payment   Procedure in which the maker of a check instructs the bank (in writing) not to honor the payment of a check. There is a charge for this service.

third-party check   Check written to the payment of another payee but presented to you as payment (the third payee).

warrant   Written non-negotiable evidence that a debt (money) is due to a person. The warrant can then be used to collect the money.

The medical assistant's responsibility for maintaining control of the medical office's banking procedures is two-fold. First, absolute accuracy is necessary when working with bank deposits, reconciliation of funds, and all related bookkeeping activities. The second responsibility relates to the trust the physician has placed on the employee for handling cash, checks, and accounts. The medical assistant acts as the agent for the physician.

Function of Banking

The basic banking functions are depositing funds, writing checks, transferring funds between bank accounts, withdrawing funds, reconciling statements, and using banking services. Most of the funds that come into a medical office are from the collection of accounts receivable.

Money may need to be withdrawn from a checking or savings account to pay business-related expenses. Every time funds (money) are moved from one account to another or used as cash, it must be handled in a systematic manner and carefully documented. Monthly statements for both checking and savings accounts must be reconciled or balanced to determine what money or funds are available for use.

Bank records are subject to government examination since the federal government regulates banking practices. In addition, the accountant for the medical practice will need accurate records for preparation of federal tax returns.

Types of Bank Accounts

Banks maintain both checking and savings accounts for their customers (Figure 16–1). A checking account allows the owner of the account to write checks to withdraw money from the account to be used as payment for outstanding debts (bills). Cash can also be withdrawn from a checking ac-

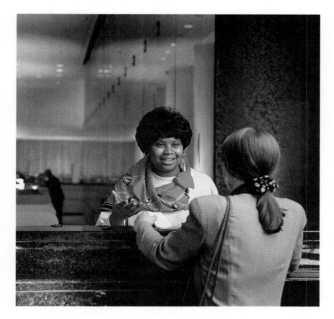

Figure 16–1 Bank teller assisting with customer service.

count. Checking accounts are not usually interest-bearing accounts. Some accounts earn interest only if there is a minimum balance in the account. Generally, the bank charges a fee, or service charge, (for example $5.00 per month) to maintain the account.

A savings account is an interest-bearing account in which funds not needed for daily expenses can be placed. Interest is earned monthly or quarterly. This means the bank will calculate a certain percentage (such as 3%) based on the average balance during a month and pay that amount to the account. Cash can be withdrawn from a savings account or transferred into a checking account. There is usually a limit to the number of monthly withdrawals without paying a fee.

Checks

A check is a written order to a bank to pay or transfer money. A check, which is payable on demand, is considered a negotiable instrument. A negotiable instrument is one which actualizes or permits the transfer of money to another person. In order to have a negotiable instrument it must be:

1. Written and signed by the maker (payer) of the check
2. State a sum of money to be paid
3. Payable on demand or at a fixed date in the future
4. Payable to the holder (payee) of the check

Checks are supplied, for a slight charge, by the bank where the money is held. These are referred to as blank checks since they contain only basic information: the account number, the name, and the address of account owner.

Large medical offices which require a large supply of checks can request a business office checkbook which has several checks per page in a large bound checkbook.

There is standard information included on all checks regardless of the bank which issues them. This preprinted information includes:

- Name and address of payer (person signing the check to release the money)
- Telephone number of payer (in some cases)
- Preprinted sequential number on the corner of each check
- Space for full date
- American Bank Association (ABA) number
- "Pay to the order of" space in which to enter the name of the payee (the person or company to receive the money)
- Space to enter the amount of the check in writing
- Small box or space to enter the amount of the check in numbers
- Space for the signature of payer
- Preprinted name and address of bank
- Magnetic ink character recognition (MICR) figures used for bank processing of the check

The blank spaces must be completed before a bank will honor and cash the check.

Advantages of Checks

Checks are recommended for a variety of reasons including:

1. Safety.
2. Convenience.
3. Ease of maintaining a record or documentation of money transfer.
4. Reliability of records for tax purposes.
5. Summary of deposits from receipts.
6. Protection—Money is protected while in the bank account (banks carry insurance to cover loss).
7. Stop-payment orders which can be issued by the payer to protect any lost or stolen checks.

Types of Checks

The various types of checks include cashier's check, certified check, bank draft, limited check, money order, traveler's check, voucher check, and a warrant.

- *Cashier's checks* are written using the bank's own check or form and are issued by the bank. A cashier's check guarantees the money is available since the bank checks the payer's account before issuing the check. The purchaser can also pay cash to have a cashier's check issued. The funds to pay the check are debited against the payer's account when the check is issued by the bank. Cashier's checks can be requested of a bank by savings account holders who do not have a checking account. There is usually a charge for this service.

- *Certified checks* are similar to a cashier's check since the bank guarantees the money is available. A certified check is actually written on the payer's own check form. The teller/banker will verify this check by placing an official stamp directly on the check. The bank actually withdraws the money from the payer's account when it certifies the check.

- A *bank draft* is a check that is drawn up by a bank against funds (money) that are deposited to its account in another bank.

- *Limited checks* are issued on special check forms that contain a preprinted maximum dollar amount for which the check can be written. There may also be a time limit during which the check is valid or must be cashed. Limited checks are used for payroll checks and insurance payments.

- A *money order* is purchased for the cash value typed on the check. Money orders can be purchased from banks, the United States Postal Service, and other authorized agents. International money orders can be purchased to be cashed in foreign countries. A money order is purchased with cash and there is a charge for this service. Money orders are frequently used by individuals who do not have bank accounts since it is recommended that cash not be sent through the mail. Money orders are considered safe to accept as payment since they are redeemable at the value typed on the front.

- *Traveler's checks* are familiar to most people who travel. These checks are preprinted in certain dollar amounts ($10, $20, $50, $100, $500 and $1000) and are prepaid. Considered a safe means for carrying money when traveling, travelers checks are also convenient since most places will accept a traveler's check and only the payer can cash it. There is a space for two signatures of the payer: one at the time of purchase and another when the check is cashed. The payee is able to check the two signatures, thus protecting the payer in the event the check is stolen or lost. People purchasing traveler's checks are advised to always sign the checks at the time of purchase before leaving the bank.

- *Voucher checks* contain three detachable sections for transaction information. This type of check is frequently used for payroll checks since additional information can be supplied to the payee. The upper portion of the check contains the actual check; the lower portion provides details about the transaction such as any payroll deductions, account to which the check is to be credited, or reason for issuing the check; the third portion is a carbon that remains with the payer as a record of the transaction. This copy can then be filed with any additional information that is available such as invoices or receipts.

Warrant

A **warrant** is not actually a negotiable check. It is a statement issued to indicate that a debt should be paid. For example, an insurance adjuster may issue a warrant indicating that a fire insurance claim should be paid. This warrant then becomes authorization to the insurance company to issue a check as payment.

ABA Number

The **ABA number** is always located in the upper right-hand corner of a printed check. It is printed as a fraction on a business check or as a straight series of numbers (1–109/210) on a personal check. The American Banker's Association (ABA) originated this number to identify the area where the bank on which the check is written is located and to identify the individual bank.

MICR

Magnetic Ink Character Recognition (MICR) is a system of combining characters and numbers located at the bottom left side of checks and deposit slips. The MICR is read by high speed machinery, increasing the speed and accuracy of processing bank statements and check sorting. It also facilitates the bookkeeping process within the bank.

Printed on each check, the MICR forms an identification for the bank and the account. The first series of numbers identifies the bank and the area it's located in. The second series of numbers identifies the individual account. During bank processing, additional numbers are printed across the bottom of the check to indicate the amount of the check.

Check Writing

The check writing process needs to be handled carefully to avoid errors. Methods for check-writing will vary from office to office depending upon the preferences of the physician and/or the accountant. Your office may use a traditional checkbook with individual checks on each page, a business office checkbook, a write-it-once system, or a computer generated check processing system.

Write-it-once System

The write-it-once system is based on the use of a check with a carbon strip on the back that allows a record to be kept of the date, check number, payee, and net amount of the check. A pegboard system (see Chapter 15), check register sheet, and checks with a carbonized writing strip on the back are used for this method. The check register sheet is placed over the pegs of a pegboard. Checks with the carbonized strip on the back edge are then placed on top of the check register, lining up the first line of the check register with the writing line of the first check. Any information that is written on the check (for example: payee, dollar amounts) will then appear on the check register sheet as a permanent record.

The user must press hard when writing on this type of check so that the impression will go through to the check register underneath. The check register has space for 25 checks to be recorded on one page.

Table 16–1 describes the check writing process using a write-it-once system.

Checks must be handwritten in ink or typewritten so they cannot be altered. Pencil is not used for check writing. The signature cannot be typewritten. Correctly written checks require legible handwriting. No blank space should be left before the name of the payee, the written dollar amount, and the numbered dollar amount. This is to prevent another person from altering any of these items. See Figure 16–2 for a sample of correctly written checks.

In some cases, the net amount of the check is imprinted by machine. All the other information is entered by hand. Checks have to be handwritten when using the write-it-once method. Checks with stubs will have to be detached from the stub for typing. However, the stub must be completed immediately.

Checks can be prepared ahead of time by the medical assistant and given to the physician to sign. Attach all materials, such as invoices and statements, to the check for the physician to sign. Writing a check payable to cash ("cash" checks) is not advised. These checks are easily cashed since they have no payee designated and have been signed by the payer. Banks will usually require that the person cashing this type of check endorse the check while in front of the teller. Review the guidelines for check writing to assure checks are written properly.

Errors in Writing Checks

Errors in writing checks can be handled in several ways. Do not erase on checks. They are printed on sensitive paper and erasures may not process correctly. In addition, banks are suspicious of all alterations on checks.

If there is a major error, such as writing out a different dollar amount than appears in the boxed

TABLE 16-1 **Check Writing Process**

1. Move all the checks in the pad to the left so that the smallest numbered check will lay across the check register.

2. Write the name of the payee on the "Pay to the order of" line.

3. Write out the full amount of the check on the "Pay" line.

4. Write the full date and check number in the designated boxes.

5. Write the amount of the check using numbers in the designated area.

6. Finally subtract the amount of this check from the "Balance Brought Forward" line. Write this amount as the new balance forward.

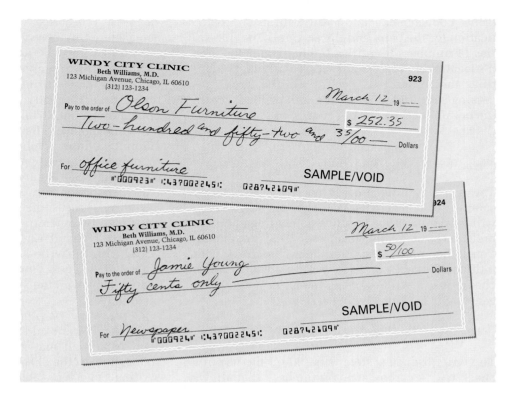

Figure 16–2 Correctly written checks.

space for the numerical amount or the payee name is written in the space meant for the handwritten dollar amount, the check is not valid. In this case, draw a line through the check and write VOID in ink in large letters on the face of the check. Keep the VOID check so that it is not considered missing when the reconciliation of the bank statement is done. If the check has already been signed, many people will tear off and discard just the signature and keep the remainder of the check for a record.

Not all errors will result in voiding the check. If the error is minor, such as writing the number 4 instead of 5 you may change the 4 to a 5 if it is still readable; the signee, the person signing the check, must then initial this change.

Accepting Checks

An office policy should be in place to guide staff about accepting checks from patients. It is acceptable for patients to pay for services with a personal check. Most of the accounts receivable, the outstanding bills, in a medical office are paid by checks written against the bank accounts of patients.

There are some checks that most medical offices consider risky and avoid cashing. These include third-party checks, checks drawn on an out-of-town bank, overpayment of account checks, and "paid in full" checks.

Third-party payer checks refer to a check written by a party unknown to you. You are considered the third party in this process. The patient (the second party), the payee, has received a check from another person which the patient now wishes to use to pay their medical bill. The person who wrote the check is considered the first party. You are at risk in accepting this check since you do not know the payer who has signed the check and, thus, may have trouble collecting the money for which the check is issued. Government checks (for example tax refunds) and payroll checks are examples of third-party checks which are considered to be reliable.

In most cases, these checks will be for an amount greater than the amount of the bill and you would have to issue a refund in cash. This would require maintaining extra cash in the office, additional staff work, and may result in financial loss if the payroll check turns out to be invalid. It is not a good idea to accept these checks.

Checks drawn on out-of-town banks are generally not accepted for payment unless identification is sought from the payee. It is difficult to collect payment if a check is not good, and it may not be easy to reach an out-of-town bank,

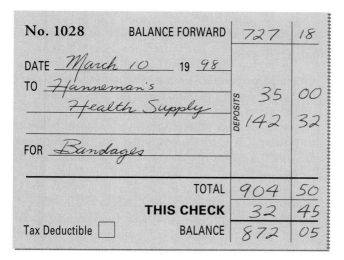

No. 1028 BALANCE FORWARD 727 | 18

DATE *March 10* 19 *98*

TO ~~*Hanneman's*~~

~~*Health Supply*~~

DEPOSITS 35 | 00

142 | 32

FOR *Bandages*

TOTAL 904 | 50

THIS CHECK 32 | 45

Tax Deductible ☐ BALANCE 872 | 05

Figure 16–3 Correctly completed check stub.

Guidelines: Check Writing

1. Fill in the check stub or check record before writing the check.
2. Use ink or typewriter to complete check and stub.
3. Fill in all blank spaces and leave no room for anyone to add anything. Always begin writing or figures at the extreme left of the space.
4. Date the check on the day it is written. Never **postdate** a check. Postdating a check means writing a future date on a check.
5. Use care when spelling the name of the payee. Do not use abbreviations or titles such as MD. Leave no space either before or after the payee's name. If space remains after the name, draw a straight line from the name to the end of the space.
6. Make sure the dollar amount written on the second line agrees with numerical dollar amount entered in the space on the first line.
7. Use care when writing a check for less than one dollar. Write out the amount with the word "only" indicating to the reader that the amount should be noted as less than one dollar. Do not cross out the word dollars. It is not advisable to write checks for less than one dollar. In addition to the time spent bookkeeping such a small amount, many banks place a service charge for each check written. This is a costly practice.

concerning the validity of a check, prior to accepting it.

Occasionally, a patient writes a check for an overpayment of an account. This can happen accidentally if a patient has not maintained adequate records or if the patient's insurance company has also made a payment to the patient's account in the medical office. In this case, a refund needs to be made to the patient. This can be handled by issuing a refund check for the amount of overpayment or returning the incorrect check to the patient if it has not been deposited.

Checks written with the statement added "paid in full" are to be avoided. Patients sometimes write this on their check when they believe they no longer owe any money to the physician. If you deposit the check you acknowledge that this is correct. Therefore, if the patient still owes money on the bill and you deposit the check, you may have difficulty collecting any further payments.

Completing the Check Stub

A check stub can be used as a permanent record of the date, amount, payee of the check, and purpose of the check. The check stub has room to place the new balance which is obtained by subtracting the current check from the previous balance. See Figure 16–3 for an illustration of a correctly completed check stub.

Endorsement of Checks

In order to transfer money from one person to another, the check must be endorsed. According to federal banking regulations, an endorsement is placed on the back of the check within the top 1 and 1/2 inches on the left side of the check as it is turned over. This upper left hand corner is referred to as the "trailing edge" of a check. If the endorsement is not placed within this designated area or extends beyond the 1 and 1/2 inch mark, it can be refused by a bank. An endorsement can either be a written signature of the payee or rubber-stamped. To prevent theft, checks should be endorsed "for deposit only" as soon as they arrive in the mail.

It is common procedure in a medical office to endorse checks at the time they are received. This is often done with an endorsement stamp that contains the doctor's name, account number, and the name of the bank.

Endorsements are regulated by the Uniform Negotiable Instrument Act. A check that has been transferred to more than one person (third-party payer) would have more than one endorsement on the back. Types of endorsements are discussed in Table 16–2.

Mailing Checks

Care should be used when mailing checks so that the check is not visible through the envelope. Special envelopes can be purchased which are non-transparent. Other methods are to place the check in a piece of folded paper or to actually fold the check in half.

Returned Checks

A check may be returned by the bank for a variety of reasons. When this occurs a returned item notice is also included with the check detailing the reason for the return. Checks are returned for example, when the payee name, date, or signature of payer is missing. If a check is returned with the payee's name or date missing, it is acceptable for the medical assistant to fill in the date and physician's name. If the payer signature is missing then the check will have to be returned to the payer. All checks should be reviewed for either a written or stamped endorsement before depositing. It is always wise to place a telephone call to a patient with the reasons for returning their check.

More serious reasons for the return of checks include not sufficient funds (NSF) in the payer's account or a stop-payment order issued by the payer. In the case of NSF, the payer's account does not have enough money to cover the amount of the check. You will need to contact the writer of the check and ask how he or she wishes to make the payment. If funds have been added to the account, the patient (payer) may ask that the check be resubmitted. To resubmit a check, call the payer's bank to determine if there are sufficient funds, write the word resubmit on both the face and the back of the check, make out another deposit slip, and resubmit.

If a **stop-payment** order has been issued by the payer then the bank will not allow the funds to be disbursed. The bank will indicate that you should contact the payer with the terms "refer to maker" on the item notice. This procedure is used when a check has been lost or stolen.

Some medical offices have a policy that if a check is returned for NSF, they will not resubmit the check. They request the payment be made immediately with either cash, a cashier's check, or money order. The returned check should be held

TABLE 16-2 **Endorsements**

Endorsement	Description	Example
Blank	Signature of the payee. Check can be cashed by anyone. This is not used in the business office.	Beth Williams
Full	Indicates person's name, company, account number, bank name, payee's name.	Pay to the order of First Town Bank Beth Williams, M.D. 123-123456
Restrictive	Specifies to whom money should be paid, money's purpose such as "For Deposit Only." Can rubber-stamp the physician's signature. Considered safest endorsement.	Pay to the order of First Town Bank For Deposit Only Beth Williams, M.D. 123-123456

until payment has been made. If the patient has not taken care of the bill, after notification and a sufficient time have elapsed, then advise the patient in writing that the bill will be turned over to a collection agency. Some offices also charge for returned checks.

Paying Bills

All bills should be paid by check for documentation and control purposes. The only exception to this policy would be very small payments, such as daily newspaper delivery and public transportation costs. In these instances, the payments could be made from petty cash. However, it is advisable that all payments, even the daily newspaper, be paid from accounts established with appropriate vendors.

An office policy must be established regarding how often checks are written, for example weekly, biweekly, semimonthly, or monthly. This bill paying schedule must match a schedule of when funds are available for payment of the office expenses. For instance, your office policy may be to send all invoices to patients at the end of the month for payment which is due on the first of the next month. In this case, you would not want to write checks against your account to pay office expenses during the last week of the month since the payments from patients will not have arrived to cover your check writing.

The office banking policy should indicate who is responsible for writing and signing all checks. For good control one person (the medical assistant) should write the checks and another person should be authorized to sign them (office manager or physician). In some medical offices, it requires two authorized signatures in order to transfer funds from one account to another or to write checks over a certain dollar amount, such as $1000.

It is not recommended to pay bills on the day they arrive since they are generally not due for 30 days. During that 30 day period, the money that is used to pay bills can remain in an interest-bearing account. The exception to paying bills as they arrive is when a supplier (vendor) offers a discount if payment is included with the order or paid within 10 days. Since this discount could be as much as 10–20%, it is wise to take advantage of it. Examples of recurring monthly expenses may include:

- Insurance premium(s)
- Rent or mortgage
- Waste removal
- Utilities including telephone charges
- Housekeeping and maintenance expenses
- Laundry
- Equipment rental such as a copy machine
- Taxes
- Maintenance contracts for equipment
- Medical and office supplies
- Postage

A schedule for paying these expenses should be kept on a master calendar or in a tickler (reminder) file. If all checks for expenses are written on a particular day of the month, a planned transfer of funds can be made from a savings account to a checking account to cover these checks.

Hiring an Accountant or Bookkeeping Firm

Larger medical practices may hire an accountant or bookkeeping firm to process all checks. This is an accurate means of handling banking procedures. However, these services can be too costly for smaller medical offices. In some firms, a computerized check-writing service system is used.

Deposits

Deposits of payments can be made to either checking or savings accounts. Deposits refer to money (cash and/or checks) placed into a bank account. Offices will vary somewhat on specific methods of handling deposits, but the following procedures are usually followed:

1. Prepare and make deposits daily.
2. Maintain all records of daily receipts (for checks and cash) together in a safe location.
3. Compare the total on the deposit slip against the total on the day sheet.
4. Keep a duplicate copy of all deposits on file in the office. Photocopy a deposit slip before submitting it to the bank. Some offices copy checks for later references.
5. Keep bank receipts of all deposits on file in the office.
6. Immediately note all deposits in the checkbook.

All deposits should be made to the bank as soon as possible. Until cash and checks can be deposited, they should be stored in a secure location that is not accessible to patients.

Always compare the total credited to the accounts receivable with the total on the deposit slip. Occasionally, a check is omitted from the accounts receivable record. Numbers may be transposed when completing the deposit slip or the accounts receivable total. Using the pegboard, or write-it-once system, results in a duplicate deposit slip. Maintain an accurate balance of all accounts on a daily basis.

Completing the Deposit Slip

A deposit slip is completed every time a deposit is made into a bank account. The slip indicates the total dollar amounts of cash and checks being deposited. Entries on the slip should be printed in black ink. Coins and bills (currency) are totaled separately. Each check must be entered on a separate line. If there are more checks than lines provided, the excessive checks can be entered on the back of the deposit slip. The currency and coins totals and check totals are added together. Then this amount, the total for the deposit, is entered on the bottom line of the deposit slip. See Figure 16–4 for an example of a deposit slip.

Check all deposits on the deposit slip against the day sheet totals. If the two figures do not match, check for the error in several ways:

- Recheck addition.
- Check each item on the deposit slip.
- Check for transposed numbers.
- If the error is still not found, subtract the difference between the deposit slip and the day sheet, then search for an item with that number.
- Check for errors of omission.

Correct order for listing money on a bank deposit is: currency, coins, checks, and money orders.

Deposit to Savings Accounts

All cash and checks can also be deposited into a savings account. When the amount in a checking account becomes greater than the amount needed to

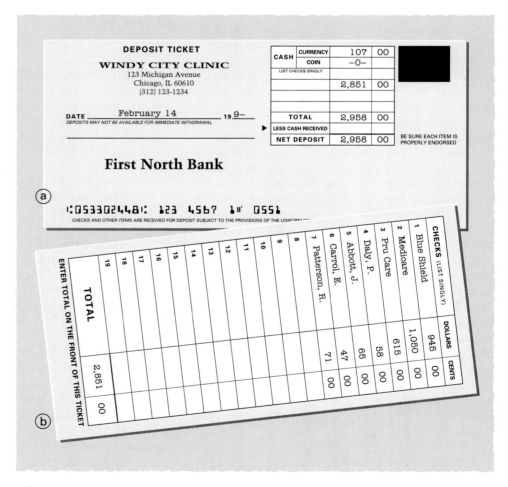

Figure 16–4   A deposit slip.

cover the checks written on the account, deposits can be made into a savings account which will have a greater interest return on the money than a checking account. When transferring funds from a checking account to a savings account, it is advisable to do so by check. This provides a record of the transaction.

A passbook, for maintaining a record of deposits, withdrawals, interest earned, and account balance, is issued with a savings account. The passbook should be kept in a safe place designated for banking materials in the office.

Making the Deposit

Deposits can be made to both the checking and savings accounts in person, by mail, or by night depository. If a deposit is made in person there will be an immediate receipt of deposit. A deposit by mail will result with a receipt by mail. However, cash should not be sent in the mail.

The night depository method can be set up for a business by obtaining a night depository key and depository bags with security locks. The deposit slip, cash, and checks are placed in the bag and then dropped off at the end of the day when the bank may be closed.

It is preferable that only one person be responsible for the deposits and another person be responsible for the receivable records . This separation of responsibilities is a critical method of fiscal or financial control.

Accepting Cash

Cash can be accepted as a form of payment, but this is not encouraged. Receipts must be given for all cash payments. Having large amounts of cash in an office poses a security risk and also holds the potential for the embezzlement of funds. Embezzlement is the taking of funds and involves a breach of trust. Large cash amounts may necessitate making bank deposits more than once a day.

Cash Disbursement

Cash disbursement refers to payments made to your creditors. The term "cash" is misleading, since, in most cases, the disbursement is made by check and not cash. Payment by check provides a permanent record as documentation for taxes and proof of payment.

Bank Hold on Accounts

Occasionally, a bank will place a "hold" on a checking account. A statement may appear indicating "Hold for Uncollected Funds (HCF)." This is usually due to a deposit which needs to "clear" so that the bank can make sure the funds (money) are present before allowing anyone to write a check on that account. This is called a "hold." The bank will not actually credit the account in which the money was deposited until the check has been processed and the funds paid to the payer's bank. These funds cannot be used by the depositor until the check or funds have cleared and the "hold" is removed. The bank will notify the depositor of the length of time for the hold.

Bank Statement

The purpose of a statement from the bank is to confirm the amount of funds that are in each account. The bank statement can uncover errors that have been made in either the office bookkeeping system or the banking bookkeeping system.

A monthly bank statement includes all debits and credits that have been processed. Debits are charges against an account; credits are additions to an account. The statement will include canceled checks. These are checks that have been processed and paid out to the medical practice's creditors by the bank. Many banks no longer return canceled checks which indicates a further need to maintain excellent record keeping on the check stub when the check is written. Figure 16–5 is an example of a typical bank statement.

Reconciliation of Bank Statements

Reconciliation of bank statements refers to the comparison of the figures on the bank statements with the records maintained in the medical office and the adjustment of banking records so that both are in agreement. The purpose of the reconciliation of bank statements is to match the account activity and totals against the medical office records. Bank statements include the following information:

- Account number
- Average collected balance
- Minimum balance
- Tax ID number (usually a social security number of the physician/owner)
- Beginning balance
- Deposit history
- Interest/credits
- Checks/debits
- Service charges
- Ending balance

Bank statements should be reconciled as soon as they are received, and errors that are found

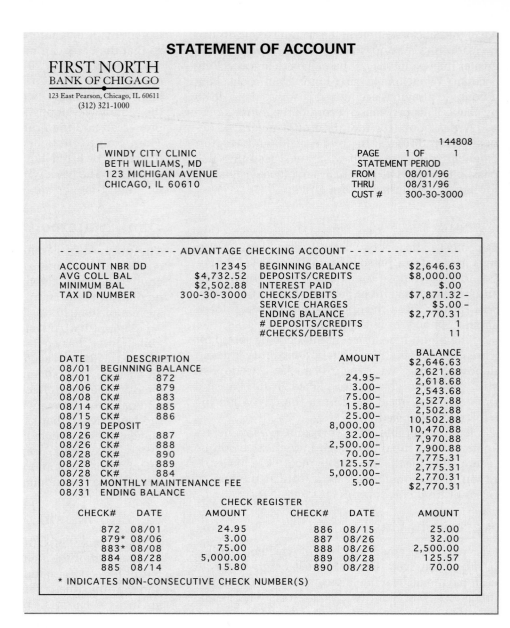

STATEMENT OF ACCOUNT

FIRST NORTH
BANK OF CHIGAGO
123 East Pearson, Chicago, IL 60611
(312) 321-1000

144808

WINDY CITY CLINIC
BETH WILLIAMS, MD
123 MICHIGAN AVENUE
CHICAGO, IL 60610

PAGE   1 OF   1
STATEMENT PERIOD
FROM   08/01/96
THRU   08/31/96
CUST #   300-30-3000

```
- - - - - - - - - - - - - - - - ADVANTAGE CHECKING ACCOUNT - - - - - - - - - - - - - - - -

ACCOUNT NBR DD          12345      BEGINNING BALANCE        $2,646.63
AVG COLL BAL       $4,732.52       DEPOSITS/CREDITS         $8,000.00
MINIMUM BAL        $2,502.88       INTEREST PAID                 $.00
TAX ID NUMBER    300-30-3000       CHECKS/DEBITS          $7,871.32 -
                                   SERVICE CHARGES            $5.00 -
                                   ENDING BALANCE         $2,770.31
                                   # DEPOSITS/CREDITS              1
                                   #CHECKS/DEBITS                 11

                                                           BALANCE
DATE         DESCRIPTION                      AMOUNT      $2,646.63
08/01   BEGINNING BALANCE                                  2,621.68
08/01   CK#        872                         24.95-      2,618.68
08/06   CK#        879                          3.00-      2,543.68
08/08   CK#        883                         75.00-      2,527.88
08/14   CK#        885                         15.80-      2,502.88
08/15   CK#        886                         25.00-     10,502.88
08/19   DEPOSIT                             8,000.00      10,470.88
08/26   CK#        887                         32.00-      7,970.88
08/26   CK#        888                      2,500.00-      7,900.88
08/28   CK#        890                         70.00-      7,775.31
08/28   CK#        889                        125.57-      2,775.31
08/28   CK#        884                      5,000.00-      2,770.31
08/31   MONTHLY MAINTENANCE FEE                 5.00-     $2,770.31
08/31   ENDING BALANCE
                              CHECK REGISTER
   CHECK#    DATE      AMOUNT       CHECK#    DATE      AMOUNT

     872   08/01        24.95        886   08/15        25.00
     879*  08/06         3.00        887   08/26        32.00
     883*  08/08        75.00        888   08/26     2,500.00
     884   08/28     5,000.00        889   08/28       125.57
     885   08/14        15.80        890   08/28        70.00

* INDICATES NON-CONSECUTIVE CHECK NUMBER(S)
```

Figure 16–5   A typical bank statement.

should be corrected immediately. Office policy may indicate an exact date when reconciliation should take place. For better fiscal control, the person reconciling the bank statement should be someone other than the person who prepares the checks and makes the deposits. This can prevent the embezzlement of funds.

If it is an interest-bearing account, the average collected balance is the amount on which the interest will be earned. It is the average amount of money in that account during the period covered by the statement. Any interest credited to the account and/or any service fees charged to the ac-

count, as shown on the bank statement, should be recorded in the checking account records before beginning the reconciliation.

The processed checks will be listed by number. Any checks that are listed in non-consecutive order may be indicated with an asterisk (*).

The reverse side of the bank statement includes information on how to handle errors or questions about the statement, and a form to assist in reconciling the bank statement. The guidelines for reconciling a bank statement provide step-by-step instructions for handling this task.

1. Organize all materials needed: current and previous bank statements, canceled checks (if returned by the bank), and checkbook stubs. If canceled checks are returned by the bank, sort them in numerical order to make reconciling easier.
2. Compare the beginning balance of the current statement with the ending balance of the previous statement. These should be the same.
3. Write the current ending balance in the appropriate space on the reverse side of the bank statement.
4. Compare deposits noted on the statement against your records or receipts by making a check mark next to each correct number.
5. List separately all outstanding deposits. These are deposits made toward the end of the month that have not been included in the current statement. Add these together and place the total on the reverse side of the statement in the space provided.
6. Add the ending balance to the total of deposits not already included and write this amount on the TOTAL line.
7. Compare the value of the checks listed on the statement with the value listed in the checkbook or check stubs.
8. Note all numbers missing from the sequential list of check numbers; these are the checks that have not yet cleared your bank ("outstanding checks"). List all outstanding checks. Add the total for outstanding checks and place that figure on the line indicated on the back of the statement.
9. Subtract the total figure for checks outstanding from the previous total on the back of the statement to determine the current balance. This amount should agree with the amount in your checking account.

Example:

1. Bank balance shown on this
   statement: $_____
       ADD (+)
2. Deposits not credited in this statement,
       (if any) $_____
3. TOTAL $_____
       SUBTRACT (−)
4. Checks outstanding $_____
5. BALANCE $_____

Summary of RULES:

#1 Note ending statement balance.

#2 Add all deposits not yet credited.

#3 Determine subtotal of step **#1** and **#2**.

#4 Subtract total outstanding checks.

#5 Determine balance or final total.

Saving Documentation

Documents relating to banking procedures should be saved in an organized manner. In addition to banking documents, such as copies of deposit slips and check stubs, your records must include the following for verification of business expenses:

1. Receipts
2. Vouchers for expenses and salaries
3. Invoices
4. Statements from suppliers
5. Proof of payments

These supporting documents should be saved in a file with check numbers of payments written on the document. After the bank statement has been reconciled each month, it should be stored with the canceled checks as further documentation of business activity. Remember that business expenses are subject to auditing by the Internal Revenue Service (IRS). Good recordkeeping is essential when providing documentation to the IRS.

LEGAL AND ETHICAL ISSUES

The medical assistant acts as the physician's agent when performing the banking procedures for the medical office. In this capacity, the medical assistant must exercise great care and integrity to protect all cash and check receipts that come into the office. Similarly, all disbursements made by the medical assistant, on behalf of the physician and the medical office, must be handled responsibly. Information relating to the banking practices or the total assets of the physician, or the medical practice, is confidential and should never be discussed outside of the office.

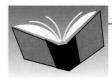

PATIENT EDUCATION

The role of the medical assistant in educating the patient is two-fold: to instruct the patient on the banking practices of the office and to safeguard the patient and the physician from loss of money through carelessness. The patient may be given an informational pamphlet prepared specifically for your office with guidelines and options for payment of services. Patients should be instructed not to send cash through the mail.

Summary

Banking is one of the critical office procedures since it requires careful handling of money and records. This requires a thorough understanding of banking procedures and terminology. Great trust is placed upon the medical assistant by the physician in handling his or her banking needs.

Competency Review

1. Define and spell the glossary terms for the chapter.
2. Using your own bank statement, reconcile it to your checkbook records.
3. Create and complete a check and check stub in the amount of 65 cents drafted to Bill Jay.
4. Call a local bank and request information regarding the various options for checking and savings accounts.
5. Create a bank deposit slip for $23.10 in cash and checks for $54.00, $21.25, $110.00, $29.00, and $9.25.

PREPARING FOR THE CERTIFICATION EXAM

Test Taking Tip — Always have a pair and a spare pencil—three pencils—when preparing to take an exam that requires you to use a computer-generated answer sheet.

Examination Review Questions

1. A check that will become void if written over a certain amount is
   (A) certified check
   (B) limited check
   (C) cashier's check
   (D) warrant
   (E) A and B correct
2. The person who signs the check is the
   (A) maker
   (B) payee
   (C) payer
   (D) teller
   (E) depositor
3. The code number found in the upper right hand corner of a printed check is the
   (A) MICR
   (B) withdrawal number
   (C) registration number
   (D) ABA number
   (E) Social Security number
4. Future-dated checks are referred to as
   (A) postdated
   (B) old
   (C) traveler's
   (D) voucher
   (E) predated

5. Endorsements must be within what measurement of the "trailing edge" according to federal regulations?
   (A) 2 inches
   (B) 1 1/2 inches
   (C) 1 inch
   (D) 1/2 inch
   (E) 3 inches

6. Which of the following is a FALSE statement about check stubs?
   (A) stub should have the purpose of check
   (B) stub should have the name of payee
   (C) stub should have the name of payer
   (D) stub should be filled out after removing from checkbook
   (E) stub should be retained

7. Third-party checks safe to accept are
   (A) patients'
   (B) insurance companies'
   (C) vendors'
   (D) should never be accepted
   (E) out-of-town patients'

8. Reconcile the bank statement and checkbook balance for the following: bank statement $1200, checkbook balance $1350, bank fees $20, outstanding checks $150 and $200. What is the correct checkbook balance?
   (A) $1200
   (B) $1310
   (C) $1330
   (D) $1350
   (E) $1530

9. A legal term for the person who signs the back of a check to transfer the ownership of the money on the check to another is
   (A) restricter
   (B) maker
   (C) endorser
   (D) depositor
   (E) banker

10. "For deposit only to the account of Dr. Williams" is what type of endorsement?
    (A) special
    (B) blank
    (C) full
    (D) restrictive
    (E) A and D

ON THE JOB

During the day Paquita Daley, a medical assistant responsible for handling banking for Dr. Williams, receives 37 checks as payment for patient services. Paquita has (1) endorsed the back of each check, indicating "for deposit only," (2) prepared the deposit slip, and (3) is ready to bundle the checks and place them in a deposit envelope for deposit on her way home. She counts them once more and realizes there are only 36 checks.

What is your response?
1. How should Paquita go about finding her error with the deposit?
2. Would referring to the day sheet help Paquita resolve the problem?
3. Would any other document help reconcile the deposits? If so, which one(s) and how?
4. Given that the bank is now closed, how should Paquita go about making a deposit?
5. If Paquita cannot make a deposit, must the deposit slip be changed? If so, how?
6. What should Paquita do with the checks if she does not deposit them today?

References

Donnelly, J., Gibson, J., and Ivancevich, J. *Fundamentals of Management.* Chicago: Irwin, 1995.

Hellriegel, D. and Slocum, J. *Management.* Cincinnati: South-Western Publishing, 1996.

Johnson, J., Whitaker, M., and Johnson, M. *Computerized Medical Office Management.* Albany, NY: Delmar Publishers, 1994.

MEDICAL ASSISTANT ROLE DELINEATION CHART

Highlight indicates material covered in this chapter

ADMINISTRATIVE

ADMINISTRATIVE PROCEDURES

- Perform basic clerical functions
- Schedule, coordinate, and monitor appointments
- Schedule inpatient/outpatient admissions and procedures
- Understand and apply third party guidelines
- Obtain reimbursement through accurate claims submission
- Monitor third-party reimbursement
- Perform medical transcription
- Understand and adhere to managed care policies and procedures
- *Negotiate managed care contracts (adv)*

PRACTICE FINANCES

- Perform procedural and diagnostic coding
- Apply bookkeeping principles
- Document and maintain accounting and banking records
- Manage accounts receivable
- Manage accounts payable
- Process payroll
- *Develop and maintain fee schedules (adv)*
- *Manage renewals of business and professional insurance policies (adv)*
- *Manage personal benefits and maintain records (adv)*

CLINICAL

FUNDAMENTAL PRINCIPLES

- Apply principles of aseptic technique and infection control
- Comply with quality assurance practices
- Screen and follow up patient test results

DIAGNOSTIC ORDERS

- Collect and process specimens
- Perform diagnostic tests

PATIENT CARE

- Adhere to established triage procedures
- Obtain patient history and vital signs
- Prepare and maintain examination and treatment areas

- Prepare patient for examinations, procedures, and treatments
- Assist with examinations, procedures, and treatments
- Prepare and administer medications and immunizations
- Maintain medication and immunization records
- Recognize and respond to emergencies
- Coordinate patient care information with other health care providers

GENERAL (TRANSDISCIPLINARY)

PROFESSIONALISM

- Project a professional manner and image
- Adhere to ethical principles
- Demonstrate initiative and responsibility
- Work as a team member
- Manage time efficiently
- Prioritize and perform multiple tasks
- Adapt to change
- Promote the CMA credential
- Enhance skills through continuing education

COMMUNICATION SKILLS

- Treat all patients with compassion and empathy
- Recognize and respect cultural diversity
- Adapt communications to individual's ability to understand
- Use professional telephone technique
- Use effective and correct verbal and written communications
- Recognize and respond to verbal and non-verbal communications
- Use medical terminology appropriately
- Receive, organize, prioritize, and transmit information
- Serve as liaison
- Promote the practice through positive public relations

LEGAL CONCEPTS

- Maintain confidentiality
- Practice within the scope of education, training, and personal capabilities
- Prepare and maintain medical records
- Document accurately
- Use appropriate guidelines when releasing information
- Follow employer's established policies dealing with the health care contract
- Follow federal, state, and local legal guidelines
- Maintain awareness of federal and state health care legislation and regulations
- Maintain and dispose of regulated substances in compliance with government guidelines
- Comply with established risk management and safety procedures
- Recognize professional credentialing criteria
- Participate in the development and maintenance of personnel, policy, and procedure manuals
- *Develop and maintain personnel, policy, and procedure manuals (adv)*

INSTRUCTION

- Instruct individuals according to their needs
- Explain office policies and procedures
- Teach methods of health promotion and disease prevention
- Locate community resources and disseminate information
- *Orient and train personnel (adv)*
- *Develop educational materials (adv)*
- *Conduct continuing education activities (adv)*

OPERATIONAL FUNCTIONS

- Maintain supply inventory
- Evaluate and recommend equipment and supplies
- Apply computer techniques to support office operations
- *Supervise personnel (adv)*
- *Interview and recommend job applicants (adv)*
- *Negotiate leases and prices for equipment and supply contracts (adv)*

SOURCE: Reprinted by permission of the American Association of Medical Assistants from the *AAMA Role Delineation Study: Occupational Analysis of the Medical Assisting Profession.*

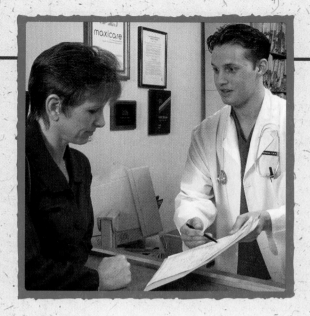

17

Insurance

CHAPTER OUTLINE

LEARNING OBJECTIVES

After completing this chapter, you should:
1. Define and spell the glossary terms for this chapter.
2. Describe group, individual, and government-sponsored (public) health benefits and explain the differences between them.
3. List the information required on a medical claim form and explain why each piece of information is needed.
4. Discuss legal issues affecting claims submission.
5. Explain the differences between health maintenance organizations (HMOs), preferred provider organizations (PPOs), and traditional insurance programs.

ADMINISTRATIVE PERFORMANCE COMPETENCIES

After completing this chapter, you should perform the following tasks:
1. Correctly apply the principles of ICD-9 coding.
2. Correctly apply the principles of CPT coding.
3. Fill out an HCFA-1500 claim form.

Glossary

assignment of benefits   Patient's written authorization giving the insurance company the right to pay the physician directly for billed charges.

benefit period   Period of time for which payments for Medicare inpatient hospital benefits are available.

claim   Written and documented request for reimbursement of an eligible expense under an insurance plan.

coding   Transferring narrative description of diseases and procedures into a number.

coinsurance   A cost-sharing provision requires the insured to assume a portion of the cost of covered services.

copayment (copay)   Amount specified by an insurance plan that the patient must pay before the plan pays (commonly used in managed care plans).

crossover claim   Patient is eligible for both Medicare and Medicaid (also called Medi/Medi).

deductible   Amount of eligible charges each patient must pay each calendar year before the plan begins to pay benefits.

fee schedule   Schedule of the amount paid by a specific insurance company for each procedure or service. Amounts are determined by a claims administrator and applied to claims subject to the fee schedule of a provider's managed care contract.

indemnity schedule   List of determined amounts to be paid for specific services by the insurance carrier on behalf of the insured.

insured   Individual(s) who is covered under an insurance plan.

medically indigent   Person without insurance coverage and with no funds.

nonparticipating provider   Provider who decides not to accept an allowable charge as the full fee for care.

participating provider   One who accepts assignment and is paid directly by the plan.

preauthorization   A requirement of Medicare and insurance companies to obtain prior approval for surgery and other procedures in order to receive reimbursement.

premium   Amount paid for insurance coverage.

prepaid plan   A group of physicians or other health care providers who have a contractual agreement to provide services to subscribers on a negotiated fee-for-service or capitated basis (also called managed care plan).

rider   A written exception to an insurance contract, expanding, decreasing, or modifying coverage of an insurance policy.

subscriber   Person who holds a health benefit plan/contract. This plan, contract, or policy may include other family members.

Health insurance was originally designed to help patients with catastrophic medical expenses, not to cover all costs associated with health care. Health benefits have always existed as a contract between the subscriber (insured) and the carrier (insurance company). As the cost of medical care has escalated, new and different types of health care plans and many regulations have also come into being. In today's medical practices, as much as 85% of a physician's income is paid by some form of medical insurance.

The successful medical assistant understands the importance of insurance to both the patient and the practice. He or she keeps current with regulations governing the health insurance industry and how these regulations affect the practice's reimbursements as well as the patients who are insured under the various policies available. This means the medical assistant must be able to process a written and documented request for reimbursement, or claim, for an eligible expense in a correct and timely manner.

Purpose of Health Insurance

Insurance provides protection against risk, loss, or ruin by contract in which an insurance company or agency agrees to pay a sum of money to the insured in the event of some contingency such as death, accident, or illness, in return for the payment of a premium by the insured. Insurance was not designed to cover all costs associated with health care, but to assist the patient with expenses incurred for medical treatment.

Availability of Health Insurance

Today's insurance is available in three options:

1. Government sponsored programs, which are financed and regulated by federal or state governments for specific groups of people. Some examples of government-sponsored insurance include Medicare, Medicaid, workers' compensation, and CHAMPUS.
2. Group-sponsored or individual policies purchased through commercial insurance companies.
3. Fixed, prepaid-fee plans with contracted health care providers obtained either independently or as a group.

Any of these plans will help with the cost of health care, but they do not cover all expenses. For any of the insurance options, the insured pays a monthly fee, or premium, for specific coverage. Often, the insured also has a deductible, or a sum of money which must be paid before insurance benefits can be paid.

Health Care Cost Containment

The cost of medicine has risen steadily throughout the years. As new treatments to cure disease and prolong life are discovered, these costs are passed on to the consumer or patient. Traditionally, medical care has been rendered on a fee-for-service basis which was a separate charge/fee set up by individual physicians for every service. Insurance carriers set up the policies they offered on this basis, as well. However, as medical care costs rose, the insurers, carriers, the patients, and the medical community began to offer cost-saving alternatives to higher medical costs and the higher costs of medical premiums.

The first cost containment measure initiated was the Peer Review Organization (PRO). This came about when Congress amended the Social Security Act of 1972 and established the Professional Standards Review Organization (PSRO). This was a voluntary group of physicians who monitored the necessity of hospital admissions and reviewed the treatment costs and medical records of hospitals. Unfortunately, the cost of operating this system was more than what the program saved each year. In order to establish stricter

controls over Medicare reimbursement for inpatient costs, Congress created control peer review organizations (PROs). These PROs were intended to determine whether proposed services were reasonable and medically necessary and whether or not the services provided on an inpatient basis could be provided more efficiently on an outpatient basis.

As part of the cost containment process, a patient classification system was developed which provides a means of relating the type of patients a hospital treats to the costs incurred by the hospital. Yale University developed the design of diagnosis-related groups (DRGs) in the late 1960s. The initial idea was to provide a means of monitoring the quality of care and the utilization of services in a hospital setting. Payment rates based on DRGs have now been established as the basis for a hospital's Medicare reimbursements. While DRGs have an effect on hospital reimbursements, they are not used to calculate payments made to outpatient providers. Physicians now have contracts with managed care companies and insurance companies.

Types of Health Insurance Benefits

Many patients (and medical assistants) find the proliferation of health care policies confusing. It is important to understand what type of insurance coverage the patient has and what types of services this insurance covers. Remember, insurance is a contract between the insured (the patient or the patient's family) and the insurance company. Questions about specific coverage should be directed to the insurance carrier, as policies vary widely, even with the same carrier. Many health care providers file insurance forms for patients as a courtesy, but this service is usually not required by the insurance companies.

The most basic insurance policies cover hospital expenses only. For coverage to be effective, the services must be performed on an inpatient basis. There may also be an annual deductible (the portion the patient must pay before the insurance company will pay any benefits). This type of coverage is the least expensive, and is also called hospitalization insurance. Some basic policies also cover limited outpatient services after deductibles have been met.

More extensive coverage, sometimes called major medical, can be obtained for an extra premium. This type of insurance usually begins paying benefits when a large amount of money has been spent on hospitalization. Most major medical coverage becomes effective after the basic policy has reached its limits of coverage.

Surgical insurance is just what its name implies: an insurance policy covering surgical services. These policies are not as common today as they once were; most surgical services are now covered under basic medical coverage.

Disability insurance is a special type of benefit which usually begins paying the patient (not the doctor or the hospital) after the insured has been disabled (unable to work) for a specific period of time. A waiting period of two to four weeks before benefits are paid is not uncommon with these policies. Most disability insurance also requires special forms to be completed by the attending physician before benefits can be paid to the insured.

Medicare supplements are policies which pay benefits on the **copays** and deductibles required and not paid by Medicare. Copays or copayment, also called **coinsurance**, is an amount of money the patient must pay before the insurance plan will pay. This amount can be as little as $10. Some policies require special forms to be filed before benefits can be paid to the insured. It is important for the medical assistant to check coverage with the individual carrier of the supplement policy, as the coverage provided varies widely from carrier to carrier.

Special risk insurance covers a particular illness or injury. For example, there are policies available that will pay benefits only if the patient develops cancer or AIDS. These policies require special forms available from the carrier before payment will be made.

Types of Health Insurance Forms

Cost containment measures have changed the face of insurance in America. Where once there were only commercial insurers, such as Prudential, patients may now choose from a wider variety of health care coverages, many available on a "menu plan" from the insurance carriers. The insured will pay a premium for the insurance coverage. Most insurance providers require **preauthorization,** or prior approval, before the service will be covered.

Commercial Carriers (Insurers)

Commercial carriers are usually for-profit organizations. These insurance companies may offer traditional fee-for-service insurance as well as a managed care option to their subscribers. Generally, the insured pays a premium and receives coverage for specific services. Figure 17-1 A and B shows a repre-

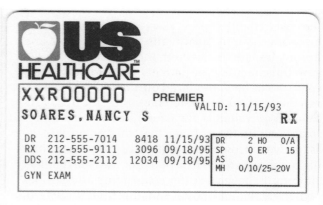

Figure 17-1 A and B   US Healthcare Insurance Card—front and back.

sentative insurance card, listing the name of the insured, the effective date of the coverage, and other information of importance to the health care provider.

> **Med Tip:** Each time a patient is seen in the office, it is a good idea for the medical assistant to verify insurance coverage by making a photocopy of the patient's insurance card and by calling the insurance company.

Blue Cross/Blue Shield

Perhaps the most well known insurance plans are Blue Cross and Blue Shield. These Blue Plans date back to the 1930s when Blue Cross was introduced to provide coverage for hospital costs. Then in 1939, Blue Shield was sponsored by state medical societies in Michigan and California to provide medical and surgical coverage. These services became known as Blue Shield Plans. Today Blue Cross and Blue Shield Plans operate in all states and have become the largest prepayment medical insurance system in the country.

Blue Shield Plans are well known in the medical office since they pay for the physician services. Most Blue Shield Plans are not-for-profit voluntary associations in which subscribers pay in advance for their anticipated health care needs. Become familiar with the Plan representative who serves your area. The representatives are knowledgeable, conduct office seminars, and can answer many questions over the telephone.

Always ask to see your patient's Blue Cross/Blue Shield card. Make a copy of both sides of the card and then return it immediately to the patient. You may also wish to write information regarding the insurance Plan number on the patient's chart in addition to placing a copy of the card in the chart.

If the patient has a card from an out-of-area Blue Cross/Blue Shield Plan, the patient's claim should be processed through the BlueCard Program. Carefully check the card for a three-character alpha prefix to the subscriber identification number. This will identify the Plan to which the member is enrolled. Identification cards with a "PPO in a suitcase" logo in the upper right hand corner indicates that the member is a BlueCard PPO member. For membership and eligibility information, call BlueCard Eligibility at 1-800-676-BLUE (2583) and you will be connected to the subscriber's Blue Cross/Blue Shield Plan. After the patient receives care, send the bill to your local Blue Cross/

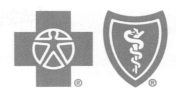

Figure 17-2 Insigna for Blue Cross and Blue Shield.
(The Blue Cross and Blue Shield Names and Symbols are registered marks of the Blue Cross and Blue Shield Association, an association of independent Blue Cross and Blue Shield Plans. Used by Permission.)

Blue Shield Plan. Your local Plan will then electronically send the claim to the subscriber's Plan and you sill receive payment from your Plan.

Refer to Figure 17-2 for an illustration of the Blue Cross and Blue Shield insigna.

Managed Care

Managed care options are available through private insurance carriers and through some government programs. Both Medicare and Medicaid now offer some type of managed care (HMO) arrangements as a choice for participants. In some managed care situations, the patient is assigned a primary care provider (PCP), who is responsible for the overall management of the patient's health. This PCP acts as a gatekeeper, determining the medical necessity of services by specialist providers. At the same time, the managed care organization stresses the concept of wellness, often paying higher benefits for routine health maintenance (physical examinations, routine immunizations, etc.). In this manner, the managed care organization tries to decrease the number of visits a patient needs to make per calendar year for health care services of an acute nature.

This type of plan is referred to as a **prepaid plan** in that a group of physicians will have a contractual agreement to provide services to subscribers on a negotiated fee-for-service basis. A **fee schedule** lists the amount to be paid by the insurance company for each procedure or service, determined by a claims administrator and applied to claims subject to the fee schedule of a provider's managed care contract.

Medicare

Government programs also provide health care benefits. Perhaps the best-known government plan is Medicare. Medicare is actually a two-part health care benefit system. Part A, which covers hospital expenses, provides coverage automatically when an insured becomes eligible for Social

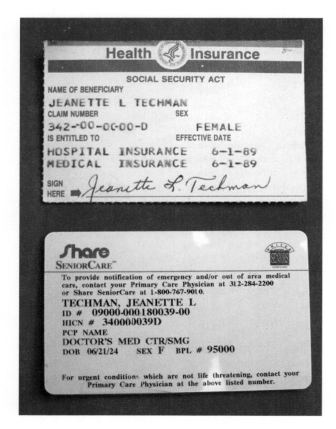

Figure 17-3 Medicare and supplemental private insurance cards.

Security benefits. The patient must apply to receive Medicare benefits from the Social Security Administration. Eligible patients are issued a Medicare card (Figure 17-3).

In order to qualify for Part B Medicare coverage, the insured must pay a monthly premium. This coverage is not automatic, nor does the coverage pay for all services. The patient pays a yearly deductible. After this deductible is met, Medicare will pay for 80% of the approved amount of covered services and the insured is liable for the 20% co-pay. The 80% reimbursement rate of Medicare is based on their Resource-Based Relative Value Scale (RBRVS) which was developed using values for every medical and surgical procedure based on the work, practice, and malpractice expenses and while accounting for regional differences.

Medicare deductibles, covered services, and copays change, so it is important to understand which services are covered under Medicare and which are not. Wise medical assistants maintain their knowledge of Medicare coverages and are knowledgeable regarding the **benefit period**, or period of time for which payments for Medicare hospital benefits are available.

Medicaid

While not directly a federal program, Medicaid also qualifies as a government insurance. Some of the cost of the Medicaid program, designed for the **medically indigent**, or persons without funds, comes from state funds, with some federal money to offset costs. Federal funds may assist by supplying 50-80% of the cost of the state's Medicaid program. Since Medicaid is administered by individual states, the rules for eligibility and for payment vary from state to state. In most instances, however, the patient must qualify for benefits on a monthly basis. Some services require **preauthorization** (prior approval from the Medicaid administrator) or the cost of services will not be paid. When dealing with Medicaid patients, the medical assistant should verify coverage at each and every visit and become familiar with the policies and procedures covering Medicaid in his/her individual state.

Eligibility for Medicare does not automatically confer Medicaid eligibility. In some cases, in which a person is eligible for both Medicare and Medicaid (Medi/Medi) a **crossover claim** is filed.

Military

Military medical benefits are also part of government programs. Active-duty military personnel and their families, as well as retired personnel and their eligible dependents are covered under CHAMPUS (Civilian Health and Medical Program of the Uniformed Services), while spouses and children of veterans with total, permanent, service-connected disabilities or for surviving dependents of veterans who have died as a result of service-connected disabilities are covered under a program called CHAMPVA (Civilian Health and Medical Program of the Veterans Administration).

Providers of service must be approved in order for the patient to receive benefits for services. Special forms are required for claim filing. Certain services require approval from the government agency responsible for administering these programs before payment can be made.

Worker's Compensation

Another type of government mandated insurance is called worker's compensation. This special insurance is for injuries directly related to work. Payment of premiums is the employer's responsibility; the employee pays nothing. In worker's compensation cases, the provider of services must complete a special report called a Surgeon's Report and must submit further reports at predetermined intervals. In addition, if the patient is regularly seen in the practice, any information connected to the injury or illness being treated under worker's compensation must be kept separate from all other patient information. Billing also needs to be done separately and the patient will not be billed for services. Billing statements are sent to the employer or insurer, instead. Because of the special type of documentation required for worker's compensation claims, some providers of service will not see workers' compensation patients. In some states, the patient must see physicians who specialize in these types of cases.

Payment of Benefits

When a covered service has been rendered, the insurance carrier is obligated to pay its portion of the cost. How is this portion calculated? Many insurance carriers use the UCR (usual, customary, reasonable) method. In this model, payment is set by determining

- The usual fee a provider charges the majority of patients for a particular service
- The geographic location of the practice and the provider's specialty
- Any complications or unusual services or procedures

This allows the carrier to establish a payment base for an allowed or covered services.

Indemnity schedules, another means of determining the amount of payment made by an insurance carrier, are based on a maximum amount for a specific service. Payment to the provider of service is based on the lower of either the provider's submitted charge or the fee schedule. This method of payment is very common in managed care situations.

To communicate effectively and efficiently with providers of medical care, insurance companies have adopted several methods of standardizing information received. Many insurance companies, working together and separately, developed a means of calculating pricing factors in reimbursement. The results of these efforts are called Relative Value Studies (RVS). In each instance, the system takes into account the time, skill, and overhead expense of the provider as required for each service. These factors are then turned into unit counts applied to a specific service, allowing for the most efficient and effective method of calculating payment.

Medicare, since 1992, has established payment on a Resource-based Relative Value Scale, which incorporates the Relative Value Studies (RVS), but also allows for increases in charges tied to economic changes and other factors.

Insurance Coding

A last element of payment from insurance carriers is based on a coding system of converting uniform descriptions of medical, surgical, and diagnostic services into numbers. This system, developed by the American Medical Association (AMA) in 1966, allows the providers to communicate more efficiently with insurance carriers about the procedures and services provided to the patient. Reimbursement is then based on the codes submitted. The process of transferring a narrative description of diseases and procedures into numbers is referred to as coding.

In 1983, the Health Care Financing Administration (HCFA) incorporated the CPT coding system into its Common Procedural Coding System (HCPCS). To differentiate between the two, HCFA designated the CPT codes as Level I, and the HCPCS codes as Level II. Level II codes are used to report services, supplies, and equipment provided to Medicare patients for which no CPT code exists.

Procedural Coding

In order to maximize reimbursements for a particular practice, the medical assistant must be familiar with CPT codes and how they are used. The CPT manual is updated yearly and is available for purchase from the AMA in November for use at the beginning of the next calendar year. As codes do change yearly, it is important to code from the most current edition of the CPT manual.

The CPT manual is organized in sections and numerically (Table 17-1). The most commonly-used codes, for evaluation and management services (including office visits), are located in the front of the book. Codes for anesthesia, surgery, radiology, pathology and laboratory, and miscellaneous medical services follow. Several appendices follow, including a complete list of all modifiers used in CPT with descriptions, as well as a quick reference summary of codes that have been added, deleted, or revised.

TABLE 17-1 CPT Manual: Sections and Codes

CPT Section	Code Numbers
Evaluation and Management	99200 - 99499
Anesthesia	00100 - 01999
Surgery	10000 - 69999
Radiology	70000 - 79999
Pathology and Laboratory	80000 - 89999
Medical Services	90700 - 99999

For a beginning coder, the most complex section of the CPT coding system is the Evaluation and Management Services. It is important to understand the difference between a new and established patient, a consultation and a referral, and to be sure the proper place of service (office, hospital, skilled nursing facility, emergency department) is coded. Take a few moments to look through the CPT manual to familiarize yourself with its structure and how codes are presented.

Commonly-accepted descriptions of services or procedures are presented after the code number. There are two types of codes listed. One type stands alone; the other is indented. Only the codes which stand alone have full descriptions. Indented codes include *only that portion of the stand-alone code before the semicolon.* This is an extremely important concept to remember.

Procedures and services are listed by name of service or procedure, anatomic site, condition or disease, synonym, eponym, or abbreviation. In order to code services correctly, locate the desired procedure in the index in the back of the CPT manual. Often a single code is given, although ranges of possible codes (joined with a hyphen) are also a possibility.

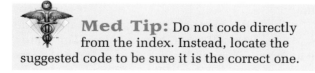

Med Tip: Do not code directly from the index. Instead, locate the suggested code to be sure it is the correct one.

There are times when it is necessary to report a service not contained in the CPT manual. These procedures may be reported using the "unlisted procedure" code for that particular section, or by use of a two-digit modifier. These two-digit codes provide additional information about services provided to a patient.

Diagnostic Coding

Working hand-in-glove with the CPT codes, ICD-9-CM (International Classification of Diseases, Ninth Clinical Modification), provide numeric codes for the patient's diagnoses. In order for an insurance payment to be processed, both codes must appear on a claim form and the diagnosis code must support the medical necessity of the treatment code.

The ICD-9 coding manual is actually three volumes of information. Volume III, which deals with inpatient diagnoses and treatments, and is used to code inpatient procedures, is not used in the medical practice. Therefore, we will concentrate on Volumes I and II. See Table 17-2 for a summary of Volume I and II and Table 17-3 for the steps to take when assigning the proper code.

To understand how to code diagnoses, it is important that the medical assistant understand the organization of the ICD-9 manual. Diagnoses are given a three-digit main code, with fourth and fifth digits when required for certain conditions. To code properly, it is necessary to begin with Volume II, the alphabetic index. Diagnoses and conditions are located alphabetically by condition, not body system. Therefore, when trying to find a code for a closed fracture of the right arm, the coder would begin by looking for the key word "fracture." This term is listed in bold type. The coder would next locate the word "arm." A code number of 818.0 is given. The coder would next turn to the numeric index (Volume 1) and find the code number 818.0. After reading the description, the code 818.0 is determined to be the correct one. Special notes and symbols used in ICD-9-CM coding, such as not otherwise specified (NOS), are listed as reference material in the code books.

TABLE 17-2   Summary of Volume I and Volume II of ICD-9-CM Codes

Volume	Description
Volume I	Tabular List of Diseases (4 sections) 1. Classification of diseases and injuries. 2. Classification of factors influencing health status and contact with health services (V codes). 3. Classification of external causes of injury and poisoning (E codes). 4. Appendices.
Volume II	(3 sections) 1. Index to diseases and injuries. 2. Table of drugs and chemicals. 3. Index to external causes of injuries and poisoning.

Med Tip: The medical assistant must understand that coding must never be done directly from Volume II, and that the numbers given are code numbers not page numbers.

When coding for claim reimbursement, the medical assistant must also understand the significance of a principal diagnosis. The principal diagnosis is the reason the patient sought care on a particular date. Principal diagnosis is used when performing coding in the hospital setting. The primary diagnosis represents the patient's major health problem for that particular claim. This is important when you file a claim for a patient who has more than one diagnosis, for example cancer and a urinary tract infection (UTI). If the UTI is unrelated to the cancer, and the cancer will not affect the treatment or recovery from the UTI, then the code used for that claim would be UTI. Any other diagnoses treated at that time (up to four) must also be listed. For example, if a diabetic patient is seen for an ear infection, the ear infection is the primary diagnosis, while diabetes is a secondary diagnosis.

The ICD-9 coding system also allows for visits (V codes) not directly related to illness or injury. The codes are used to describe a person who is not currently sick, but uses the health care system for some specific purpose such as well baby care or birth control advice. The codes are also used when some circumstance or problem is present that may influence the patient's health, but is not in itself a current illness or problem such as an allergy to penicillin.

E codes are used to describe external causes of injury and poisoning. These codes may not be used as primary or principal diagnoses (they do not stand alone). E codes are used as additional information regarding a particular diagnosis.

The ICD-9 manual also uses tables for certain diseases and conditions. A diagnosis of hypertension, for example, must be coded from the hypertension table. A neoplasm, whether benign or malignant, must be coded from the neoplasm table, and the morphology (behavior) of the neoplasm is coded from a morphology table (M code). Again, the medical assistant should become familiar with the organization of the ICD-9-CM manual in order to code diagnoses properly and correctly.

Claims Processing

Claims are processed at insurance companies by a claims administrator. The claim form is a critical item in claims processing. While there are several forms used for claims processing (Figure 17-4 and Figure 17-5), the most commonly-used form was designed by the Health Care Financing Administration and is called a HCFA-1500. For a claim to be processed, this form must be filled out completely and correctly. The following information is required for all claims:

- The name of the insured's insurance company
- The name of the insured
- The insured's identification number
- The address of the insured
- The telephone number of the insured

TABLE 17-3   Steps for Assigning an ICD-9-CM

Step	Description
Step 1	Locate the condition or diagnosis in Volume II. Conditions may be expressed as: a. Noun (cystitis) b. Adjective (fibrocystic disease) c. Eponym (Addison's disease, Cushing's syndrome) Name of disease or condition includes the name of a person, usually the physician/person associated with identifying, researching, or developing a cure for the disease.
Step 2	Examine the diagnostic statement to determine if the main term specifically describes that disease. If it does not, then look at the modifiers listed under that main term to find a more specific code. Also read any notes or cross references that may apply.
Step 3	Then locate the code in the Tabular Index.
Step 4	Match the code description in the Tabular Index with the diagnosis in the patient's medical record.

Additional guidelines:

A. Any of the codes from 0021.0 through V 82.9 in ICD-9-CM can be used to describe the main reason for the patient visit.

B. First list the ICD-9-CM code for the condition, problem, or diagnosis that is the main reason for the visit. Then list coexisting conditions under additional codes.

C. Use codes at their highest level—5th digit codes first, then 4th digit, 3rd digit, and so on.

D. Do not code questionable or probable or rule-out (R/O) diagnosis. One of the signs or symptoms of the R/O diagnosis will have to be identified by the physician as the reason for the visit (encounter). For example, in R/O cystic fibrosis, the symptom of dyspnea would be coded until a definitive diagnosis of cystic fibrosis is made.

E. V codes describe factors which influence the health status of the patient, such as pregnancy test or vaccination, and are not used to code current illnesses. V codes are located in Volume II.

F. E codes are used for identifying external environmental events or conditions as the cause of injury, some adverse effect, or poisoning. For example, a drug overdose, either accidental or taken as a suicide attempt. The use of E codes (E 930-E 949) is mandatory when coding the use of drugs.

G. M codes, in Appendix A of Volume I relates to the morphology of neoplasms. Morphology codes are not used as the primary diagnosis code; they are listed after the ICD-9 code. Each M code begins with the letter "M." The M codes cannot be used on claims for patient billing.

Data about the patient is also required. In general, the upper portion of the form describes the patient and the lower half of the form (separated by a heavy line) refers to the provider of services, the services provided to the patient and the medical necessity of those services.

As with all patient information, all rules of confidentiality apply. Therefore, the patient must sign a release of information for a claim form to be completed. To make this process simpler, many offices have a standard release form for this purpose. Once the form has been signed and is on file in the patient's record, a notation of "SIGNATURE ON FILE" may be written or typed in box 12 of the HCFA-1500 form. Box 13 deals with payment of benefits. If this box is signed, payment will frequently be made directly to the provider of services. If the box is not signed, or for a contract that cannot be assigned, payment is made to the insured. Many insurance carriers, including Medicare, allow for lifetime assignment of benefits. With a signature on one

WORKER'S COMPENSATION BOARD

ATTENDING PHYSICIAN'S 48-HOUR REPORT

PLEASE PRINT OR TYPE — INCLUDE ZIP CODE IN ALL ADDRESSES — CLAIMANT'S SOCIAL SECURITY NUMBER MUST BE ENTERED BELOW ➡

WCB CASE NUMBER (if known)	CARRIER CASE NUMBER (if known)	DATE OF INURY AND TIME	ADDRESS WHERE INJURY OCCURRED (city, town or village)	SOCIAL SECURITY NUMBER

INJURED PERSON: NAME — AGE — ADDRESS — APT. NO.

EMPLOYER:

INSURANCE CARRIER:

HISTORY

1. State how injury occurred and give source of this information. (If claim is for *occupational disease*, include occupational history and date of onset or related symptoms).

2. Is there a history of unconsciousness? ☐ YES ☐ NO   If YES, for how long?   Were X-Rays taken? ☐ YES ☐ NO

3. Was patient hospitalized? ☐ YES ☐ NO   If YES, state name and address of hospital:

4. Was patient previously under the care of another physician for this injury? ☐ YES ☐ NO   If YES, enter his name and address, and reason for transfer under REMARKS (Item 10).

DIAGNOSIS

5. Describe nature and extent of injury or disease and specify *all* parts of body involved:

TREATMENT

6. Nature of treatment:

Date of first treatment: If treatment is continuing, estimate its duration:

If treatment is not continuing, is this your final report? ☐ YES ☐ NO   If YES, state date of last treatment:

DISABILITY

7. May the injury result in permanent restriction, total or partial loss of function of a part or member, or permanent facial, head or neck disfigurement? ☐ YES ☐ NO

8. Is patient working? ☐ YES ☐ NO   Is patient disabled? ☐ YES ☐ NO   If YES, estimate duration of disability:

CAUSAL RELATION

9. In your opinion, was the occurence described above the competent producing cause of the injury and disability (if any) sustained? ☐ YES ☐ NO

REMARKS

10. Enter here additional information of value, requests for authorization, etc.:

11. Medical testimony is occasionally required. If your testimony should be necessary in this case, please indicate the days of the week (and hours) most convenient to you for this purpose:

Date	Typed or printed name of attending physician	Address

WCB rating code	WCB authorization number	Telephone number	Written signature of attending physician

ANSWER ALL QUESTIONS. AVOID USE OF INDEFINITE TERMS.

Figure 17-4   Health Insurance Claim Form.

PLEASE
DO NOT
STAPLE
IN THIS
AREA

Align by typing an X in box

CARRIER

HEALTH INSURANCE CLAIM FORM

PICA · · PICA

| 1. MEDICARE (Medicare #) | MEDICAID (Medicaid #) | CHAMPUS (Sponor's SSN) | CHAMPVA (VA File #) | GROUP HEALTH PLAN (SSN or ID) | FECA BLK LUNG (SSN) | OTHER (ID) | 1a. INSURED'S I.D. NUMBER (FOR PROGRAM IN ITEM 1) |

2. PATIENT'S NAME (Last Name, First Name, Middle Initial)

3. PATIENT'S BIRTH DATE MM DD YY   SEX M   F

4. INSURED'S NAME (Last Name, First Name, Middle Initial)

5. PATIENT'S ADDRESS (Number, Street)

6. PATIENT RELATIONSHIP TO INSURED Self   Spouse   Child   Other

7. INSURED'S ADDRESS (Number, Street)

CITY   STATE

8. PATIENT STATUS Single   Married   Other
Employed   Full-time Student   Part-time Student

CITY   STATE

ZIP CODE   TELEPHONE (Include Area Code) ( )

ZIP CODE   TELEPHONE (Include Area Code) ( )

9. OTHER INSURED'S NAME (Last Name, First Name, Middle Initial)

10. IS PATIENT'S CONDITION RELATED TO:

11. INSURED'S POLICY GROUP OR FECA NUMBER

a. OTHER INSURED'S POLICY OR GROUP NUMBER

a. EMPLOYMENT? (Current or Previous) YES   NO

a. INSURED'S DATE OF BIRTH MM DD YY   SEX M   F

b. OTHER INSURED'S DATE OF BIRTH MM DD YY   SEX M   F

b. AUTO ACCIDENT?   PLACE (State) YES   NO

b. EMPLOYER'S NAME OR SCHOOL NAME

c. EMPLOYER'S NAME OR SCHOOL NAME

c. OTHER ACCIDENT? YES   NO

c. INSURANCE PLAN NAME OR PROGRAM NAME

d. INSURANCE PLAN NAME OR PROGRAM NAME

10d. RESERVED FOR LOCAL USE

d. IS THERE ANOTHER HEALTH BENEFIT PLAN? YES   NO   If YES, return to and complete items 9a–d.

READ BACK OF FORM BEFORE COMPLETING & SIGNING THIS FORM

12. PATIENT'S OR AUTHORIZED PERSON'S SIGNATURE I authorize the release of any medical or other information necessary to process this claim. I also request payment of government benefits either to myself or to the party who accepts assignment below.

SIGNED _____ DATE _____

13. INSURED'S OR AUTHORIZED PERSON'S SIGNATURE I authorize payment of medical benefits to the undersigned physician or supplier for services described below.

SIGNED _____

PATIENT AND INSURED INFORMATION

14. DATE OF CURRENT: ◄ ILLNESS (First Symptom) or INJURY (Accident) or PREGNANCY (LMP) MM DD YY

15. IF PATIENT HAS HAD SAME OR SIMILAR ILLNESS, GIVE FIRST DATE: MM DD YY

16. DATES PATIENT UNABLE TO WORK IN CURRENT OCCUPATION MM DD YY   From   To   MM DD YY

17. NAME OF REFERRING PHYSICIAN OR OTHER SOURCE

17a. I.D. NUMBER OF REFERRING PHYSICIAN

18. HOSPITALIZATION DATES RELATED TO CURRENT SERVICES MM DD YY   From   To   MM DD YY

19. RESERVED FOR LOCAL USE

20. OUTSIDE LAB? YES   NO $ CHARGES

21. DIAGNOSIS OR NATURE OF ILLNESS OR INJURY. (Relate items 1, 2, 3, or 4 to item 24E by line)

1. |___.___   3. |___.___
2. |___.___   4. |___.___

22. MEDICAID RESUBMISSION CODE   ORIGINAL REFERENCE NUMBER

23. PRIOR AUTHORIZATION NUMBER

24.	A. DATE(S) OF SERVICE						B. PLACE OF SERVICE	C. TYPE OF SERVICE	D. PROCEDURES, SERVICES, OR SUPPLIES (Explain Unusual Circumstances) CPT/HCPCS MODIFIER	E. DIAGNOSIS CODE	F. $ CHARGES	G. DAYS OR UNITS	H. EPSDT FAMILY PLAN	I. EMG	J. COB	K. RESERVED FOR LOCAL USE
	From MM DD YY			To MM DD YY												
1																
2																
3																
4																
5																
6																

25. FEDERAL TAX I.D. NUMBER   SSN EIN

26. PATIENT'S ACCOUNT NUMBER

27. ACCEPT ASSIGNMENT? (For govt. claims, see back) YES   NO

28. TOTAL CHARGE $

29. AMOUNT PAID $

30. BALANCE DUE $

31. SIGNATURE OF PHYSICIAN OR SUPPLIER, INCLUDING DEGREES OR CREDENTIALS (I certify that the statements on the reverse apply to this bill and are made a part thereof.)

SIGNED _____ DATE _____

32. NAME AND ADDRESS OF FACILITY WHERE SERVICES WERE RENDERED (if other than home or office)

33. PHYSICIAN'S, SUPPLIER'S BILLING NAME, ADDRESS, ZIP CODE, AND PHONE #

PIN # _____   GRP # _____

PHYSICIAN OR SUPPLIER INFORMATION

PLEASE PRINT OR TYPE

Figure 17-5   HCFA-1500 form.

Assignment of Lifetime Medicare Benefits

Name of Beneficiary _____

Medicare Number _____

I, the undersigned, request that all authorized Medicare benefits be paid to me or on my

behalf to _____ for all services rendered to me by the
           (Name of Physician or Supplier)

aforementioned provider. I hereby authorize any holder of my medical records to release

to the Health Care Financing Administration and its agents any information necessary to

determine and secure the payment of all benefits.*

Signed _____ Date _____
           (Signature of Beneficiary)

* If you are a patient in a hospital or skilled nursing home, this authorization is in effect for the period of your confinement. Otherwise, this authorization is in effect until you choose to revoke it.

Figure 17-6 A   Health Insurance Claim Form—Assignment of Lifetime Medicare Benefits.

Insurance Benefits Assignment

I hereby declare that I am insured with _____ ,
           (Name of Insurance Company)

and I authorize said insurer to pay and assign directly to _____
           (Name of Doctor)

all surgical and/or medical benefits, if any, otherwise payable to me for services rendered

(as described on attached forms herewith), but not in excess of the recorded charges for

those services. I understand that I am financially responsible for all charges whether or not

paid by said insurer. I hereby authorize said assignee to release any information needed

to secure the payment of all benefits.

Signed _____ Date _____
           (Signature of Beneficiary)

Figure 17-6 B   Health Insurance Claim Form—Assignment of Insurance Benefits.

form, the notation "SIGNATURE ON FILE" can also be made in box 13 (Figure 17-6A and Figure 17-6B). This saves the medical assistant the time required for a patient to sign an insurance claim form during each office visit. The forms, however, must be kept in the patient record and must be available at all times.

One confusing element in insurance processing is the concept of "participating" and "nonparticipating" providers. Most insurance companies will make special incentives available to those who choose to become **participating providers**, which means the physician will accept the insurance company's allowed amount as payment in full (less patient copayments) for services rendered. To become a participating provider, the physician completes a form and is assigned a number which is unique to the physician or practice.

With most insurance plans, payment is made directly to participating providers, while payment is made to the patient in the case for the claims of a **nonparticipating provider**. The nonparticipating provider bills the patient and the patient is expected to pay the charges.

There are advantages to both ways of handling insurance claims. Often, insurance reimburses at a lower rate than the physician bills. In this case, the physician must "write off" or agree to forfeit the amount the insurance company does not authorize. It is an expense of any practice when an associate (medical assistant, insurance claims processing clerk, for example) must be on the payroll to submit and track insurance claims. However, payment is made directly to the physician, often within a few days (especially with electronic claim submission), so that large charges do not accumulate on the physician's accounts receivable. Each practice must weigh the advantages and disadvantages carefully before making a decision to become either a participating or nonparticipating practice.

Many medical offices now use a single sheet to speed the process of reimbursement. This form is called a superbill and lists the patient's name, diagnoses and treatments with additional space to fill in claim information. Some insurance carriers will accept a superbill in lieu of a claim form, although this depends on the specific carrier. Originally, superbills were created to allow patients to file their own claims; however, as insurance rules and regulations have become more complex and coding and documentation requirements more stringent, most medical practices file insurance claims for their patients as a courtesy.

The "birthday rule" is used by insurance claims administrators to determine which parents' benefit plans will pay for the medical bills of a dependent child when the child is covered by the plans of both parents. The plan of the parent whose birthday falls earliest in the year (not the oldest parent) will be the primary plan.

Many medical offices have access to electronic claims filing, a way to send claims over telephone lines, communicating from computer to computer rather than on paper. This process speeds claims processing on both the provider's end and at the insurance carrier's end and many plans allow for direct electronic deposit of payments for insurance claims directly to the provider's bank account.

Occasionally, if a claim is not correct in some way, the insurance company will reject the claim. Some of the most common reasons for claim rejection include:

1. Incorrect or missing patient registration information (name, address, insurance number)
2. Incorrect or missing name of a referring physician
3. Incorrect or missing diagnosis code
4. Overlapping, incorrect, or duplicate dates of service
5. Incorrect place of service
6. Invalid, incorrect, or missing procedure code
7. Incorrect or missing quantity
8. Incorrect or missing modifier

If a claim is rejected for any reason, it must be corrected and resubmitted to the insurance carrier. There are usually time limits for refiling rejected claims, so the medical assistant must be very aware of these deadlines and resubmit the claims before the time has expired. Expired claims will not be processed by the insurance carrier and will ultimately cost the practice money.

As a precaution, the medical assistant should review every claim submitted for accuracy (Figure 17-7). While no one process or procedure can guarantee that a claim will ever be rejected or reviewed, a careful, studious approach to the claims process can ensure greater accuracy.

Continuing Education

The medical assistant who processes the insurance claims should plan to spend at least two to three hours a month on continuing education about insurance. Many insurance companies offer seminars on an annual or semiannual basis to dis-

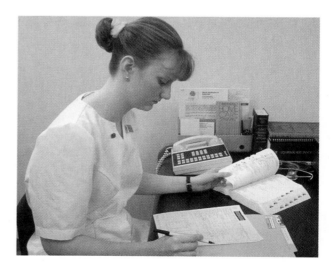

Figure 17-7   Medical assistant reviews forms for accuracy before submitting them.

cuss changes in policies and procedures. Medicare and Medicaid, as well as HCFA, have home pages on the Internet and publish updates and other information of interest on a regular basis. Many carriers have hotlines for specific questions regarding claims and will make information about claims processing available to the practices, including claim tracking, which gives information about the status of a submitted claim.

Billing Requirements

Each insurance carrier has a certain deadline for submitting insurance claims. Claims must be submitted in a timely manner in order to be processed, and if the deadline for filing has passed, no money can be recovered from the insurance carrier. It is extremely important to become familiar with these filing deadlines, which vary from carrier to carrier. It is also important that the appropriate form be used for filing charges. Not all carriers accept the HCFA-1500; some require forms specific to that carrier. Some carriers require supporting documentation (such as reports) which must be submitted in a timely manner.

If a patient has more than one insurance carrier, it is crucial that the primary carrier be determined for proper billing to occur. The claim must be submitted to the primary carrier first for processing, and the claim must be processed and a statement of remittance completed before the information can be sent to any secondary carrier.

As with all aspects of insurance processing, accuracy and attention to detail are the primary concerns. The successful medical assistant keeps abreast of rules, regulations, and changes about insurance claims processing so that the insurance reimbursement for the practice is as high as is allowed for services rendered.

> **Med Tip:** The medical assistant should be on the alert for a **rider** to an insurance contract. The rider is a statement that identifies any exception to insurance coverage. For example, coverage for a pregnancy may not begin until 1 year after the effective date of the insurance.

LEGAL AND ETHICAL ISSUES

When dealing with insurance, confidentiality and honesty are major issues. The patient's right to confidentiality with regard to sensitive medical information must be scrupulously respected. Insurance reimbursement, as it is currently structured, provides a constant temptation to do what is necessary to recover the full amount of charges. As a successful medical assistant, be careful to release only information authorized by the patient, and avoid becoming involved with insurance fraud in any form.

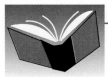

PATIENT EDUCATION

Most patients have difficulty understanding the details of health insurance. Practicing medical assistants often encounter patients who are convinced that, because they have paid premiums to the insurance company, they should pay nothing further to the provider of service. Tact and patience are essential in educating patients about covered and noncovered services.

Summary

Most patients coming into the medical office have some form of health care insurance. These include commercial insurers, Blue Cross/Blue Shield, Medicare, Medicaid, workmen's compensation, and military insurance (CHAMPUS and CHAMPVA). Many patients are members of health care plans, such as health maintenance organizations (HMOs), and preferred provider organizations (PPOs). The medical assistant should have an understanding of working with procedural coding (CPT codes) and diagnostic coding (ICD-9-CM) in order to be able to quickly and accurately process insurance forms.

Competency Review

1. Define and spell the glossary terms for this chapter.
2. Describe what steps you would take to determine if a patient has insurance coverage.
3. What code book is used to code a diagnosis?
4. What code book is used to code an office visit and procedure?
5. Use the health insurance claim forms shown in Figures 17-4 and 17-5 to complete the forms for Jane Doe, 123 Main St., Anywhere, USA 60000; telephone 555-1234, SS# 123-45-6789. She is single and self insured. Jane Doe's insurance number is the same as her SS #.
6. Explain the difference between a primary and secondary diagnosis using the example of stroke and hypertension.

PREPARING FOR THE CERTIFICATION EXAM

Test Taking Tip — Study for an examination by taking notes based on the headings within the chapters of a book. The author believed the items discussed under these topics were important enough to use headings to identify or highlight the content.

Examination Review Questions

1. What is defined as transforming verbal descriptions into numerical designations?
   (A) grouping
   (B) coding
   (C) classifying
   (D) modifying
   (E) rider

2. In ICD-9 coding conventions, E codes
   (A) stand alone
   (B) are required for all diagnoses
   (C) give external causes or factors for illness or injury
   (D) should never be used with V codes
   (E) are the same as CPT codes

3. CPT stands for
   (A) current physician's terminology
   (B) current procedure terminology
   (C) current procedural terminology
   (D) current procedural terms
   (E) none of the above

4. In CPT coding conventions, modifiers are used to
   (A) explain unusual circumstances
   (B) list a patient's treatment options
   (C) frustrate a medical assistant
   (D) communicate with the insurance company via electronic billing
   (E) make the coding statement grammatically correct

5. The HCFA-1500 claim form
   (A) is accepted by every insurance company in the United States
   (B) must be filled out by the patient
   (C) must be filled out by the provider
   (D) is accepted as a standard submission (claim) form by most carriers
   (E) is never used

6. In CPT coding conventions
   (A) both inpatient and outpatient visits use the same code
   (B) inpatient visit codes are different from outpatient visit codes
   (C) use a complicated system to determine whether services were rendered on an inpatient or outpatient basis
   (D) require a call to the insurance company to determine which code to use
   (E) are the same as ICD-9-CM

7. ICD-9 codes
   (A) may require a fifth digit for detail
   (B) never require a fifth digit for detail
   (C) always require a V code to support the diagnosis
   (D) may be coded directly from Volume II
   (E) none of the above

8. When determining payment for a provider, insurance companies consider
   (A) fee schedules

(B) usual, customary, and reasonable charges

(C) relative value studies and resource-based relative value scales

(D) any riders on the contract

(E) all of the above

9. A lifetime assignment of benefits from a Medicare patient

(A) entitles the provider to all the patient's social security and Medicare benefits

(B) may only be given to the patient's family

(C) allows the provider to complete claim forms without the patient's signature on the form

(D) should be sent to the insurance carrier

(E) is also good for Medicaid claims

10. Electronic claim submission

(A) is difficult and costly

(B) is an efficient way to manage accounts receivable relating to insurance claims

(C) is only done on rare occasions in most medical practices

(D) increases the time it takes for an insurance carrier to pay a claim

(E) none of the above

ON THE JOB

Lisa Medina, CMA, processes insurance claims for a large internal medicine practice. You have recently been hired as Lisa's assistant and she has asked you to verify the accuracy of a group of claim forms. As you review the forms, you notice that one of the doctors regularly checks the superbill used in the office at one evaluation/management code level higher than the actual level of service provided. How will you handle this situation?

What is your response?

1. Name some of the options which are possible for handling this situation.

2. Tell which option you would select.

3. Give three reasons for your selection of this particular option.

4. Whose advice might you seek before acting on your choice?

References

Adams, W. *Guide to Coding and Reimbursement.* St. Louis: Mosby Lifeline, 1994.

Buck, C. *Step-by-Step Medical Coding.* Philadelphia: W. B. Saunders, 1996.

Collins, R. *From Patient to Payment.* New York: Glencoe/Macmillan/McGraw-Hill, 1993.

Kotoski, G. *CPT Coding Made Easy.* Gaithersburg, MD: Aspen Publishing, Inc., 1993.

Marrelli, T. *Home Health Standards and Documentation Guidelines for Reimbursement.* St. Louis: Mosby, 1994.

Renfro, J. *Coding Skills for the Medical Assistant.* Chicago: American Association of Medical Assistants, 1993.

MEDICAL ASSISTANT ROLE DELINEATION CHART

Highlight indicates material covered in this chapter

ADMINISTRATIVE

ADMINISTRATIVE PROCEDURES

- Perform basic clerical functions
- Schedule, coordinate, and monitor appointments
- Schedule inpatient/outpatient admissions and procedures
- Understand and apply third party guidelines
- Obtain reimbursement through accurate claims submission
- Monitor third-party reimbursement
- Perform medical transcription
- Understand and adhere to managed care policies and procedures
- *Negotiate managed care contracts (adv)*

PRACTICE FINANCES

- Perform procedural and diagnostic coding
- Apply bookkeeping principles
- Document and maintain accounting and banking records
- Manage accounts receivable
- Manage accounts payable
- Process payroll
- *Develop and maintain fee schedules (adv)*
- *Manage renewals of business and professional insurance policies (adv)*
- *Manage personal benefits and maintain records (adv)*

CLINICAL

FUNDAMENTAL PRINCIPLES

- Apply principles of aseptic technique and infection control
- Comply with quality assurance practices
- Screen and follow up patient test results

DIAGNOSTIC ORDERS

- Collect and process specimens
- Perform diagnostic tests

PATIENT CARE

- Adhere to established triage procedures
- Obtain patient history and vital signs
- Prepare and maintain examination and treatment areas

- Prepare patient for examinations, procedures, and treatments
- Assist with examinations, procedures, and treatments
- Prepare and administer medications and immunizations
- Maintain medication and immunization records
- Recognize and respond to emergencies
- Coordinate patient care information with other health care providers

GENERAL (TRANSDISCIPLINARY)

PROFESSIONALISM

- Project a professional manner and image
- Adhere to ethical principles
- Demonstrate initiative and responsibility
- Work as a team member
- Manage time efficiently
- Prioritize and perform multiple tasks
- Adapt to change
- Promote the CMA credential
- Enhance skills through continuing education

COMMUNICATION SKILLS

- Treat all patients with compassion and empathy
- Recognize and respect cultural diversity
- Adapt communications to individual's ability to understand
- Use professional telephone technique
- Use effective and correct verbal and written communications
- Recognize and respond to verbal and non-verbal communications
- Use medical terminology appropriately
- Receive, organize, prioritize, and transmit information
- Serve as liaison
- Promote the practice through positive public relations

LEGAL CONCEPTS

- Maintain confidentiality
- Practice within the scope of education, training, and personal capabilities
- Prepare and maintain medical records
- Document accurately
- Use appropriate guidelines when releasing information
- Follow employer's established policies dealing with the health care contract
- Follow federal, state, and local legal guidelines
- Maintain awareness of federal and state health care legislation and regulations
- Maintain and dispose of regulated substances in compliance with government guidelines
- Comply with established risk management and safety procedures
- Recognize professional credentialing criteria
- Participate in the development and maintenance of personnel, policy, and procedure manuals
- *Develop and maintain personnel, policy, and procedure manuals (adv)*

INSTRUCTION

- Instruct individuals according to their needs
- Explain office policies and procedures
- Teach methods of health promotion and disease prevention
- Locate community resources and disseminate information
- *Orient and train personnel (adv)*
- *Develop educational materials (adv)*
- *Conduct continuing education activities (adv)*

OPERATIONAL FUNCTIONS

- Maintain supply inventory
- Evaluate and recommend equipment and supplies
- Apply computer techniques to support office operations
- *Supervise personnel (adv)*
- *Interview and recommend job applicants (adv)*
- *Negotiate leases and prices for equipment and supply contracts (adv)*

SOURCE: Reprinted by permission of the American Association of Medical Assistants from the *AAMA Role Delineation Study: Occupational Analysis of the Medical Assisting Profession.*

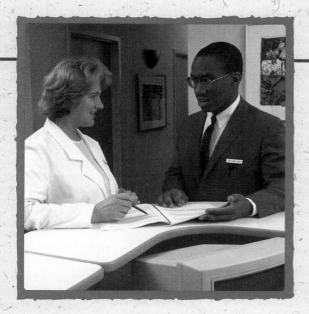

18

Office Management

CHAPTER OUTLINE

LEARNING OBJECTIVES

After completing this chapter, you should:
1. Define and spell the glossary terms for this chapter.
2. Define the systems approach to management.
3. List and discuss the personnel management duties as they relate to the medical office.
4. Discuss the elements of monthly planning including holding staff meetings.
5. Describe time management principles and how a TO DO List would enhance office organization.
6. Differentiate between the employee policy manual and the office procedures manual.
7. Describe 10 responsibilities in assisting the physician to set up a medical meeting.
8. Discuss how to perform basic library research to assist the physician in a medical paper development.
9. List 5 items that belong in a patient information booklet.

ADMINISTRATIVE PERFORMANCE COMPETENCIES

After completing this chapter, you should perform the following tasks:
1. Apply time management techniques to enhance office efficiency.
2. Plan staff meeting and prepare agenda.
3. Orient and train personnel to office procedures.
4. Perform basic secretarial skills for the physician.
5. Design and develop patient information materials.
6. Design and develop a recruitment advertisement for new help.

Glossary

citation To quote an authority.

colleague A fellow member of a profession.

discriminatory To set someone apart or act with prejudice against a group.

draft A preliminary version of a writing.

grievance Real or imaginary wrong regarded as cause for complaint or resentment.

honorarium Small payment for a service (for example, a speaking engagement).

probationary period A trial period during the early months of employment to see if there is a fit between the employee and the position. It is usually 3 months in length. During this period the employee can be dismissed without cause.

protocol The standard (for example, a protocol for behavior).

seniority Refers to the person who has been with the organization longest.

solvent Having sufficient assets (money) to pay debts.

Office management requires special administrative and people skills. Office management cannot be discussed without discussing time management. Careful planning of activities, delegation of tasks, and effective use of all personnel involve careful attention to how time is managed. Several documents are important for a smooth running medical office. These include the personnel policy manual, a procedures manual, and patient information booklets.

Systems Approach to Office Management

Current management philosophy recommends a systems approach when managing a medical office. Under this approach the functions of an office are categorized into systems which must function simultaneously and be integrated into a whole system, the medical office. For example, the administrative component of a medical office can be divided into the following systems:

- Personnel management
- Financial management (including banking, billing, collections, and insurance)
- Scheduling
- Facility and equipment management (including computers)
- Communications (written and oral including patient education)
- Legal concepts

The clinical component of managing an office can be considered a system by itself. A brief description of the various systems that form the medical practice are discussed below.

Personnel Management Responsibilities

These duties include recruitment and selection, probation, performance and salary review, discipline, and maintenance of employee records.

Recruitment and Selection

The recruitment and selection process is used when a medical practice needs to replace a staff member who has left or when more staff is needed for an expanding practice. Recruitment can begin in-house which means that the job vacancy is posted within the medical office before the position is advertised elsewhere. An existing employee may apply for the vacant positions.

If there are no interested or qualified internal candidates, several routes may be used to seek applicants. These include: placement of newspaper and trade journal ads, professional organizations, Internet, formal training programs, and employment agencies. A fee is paid by the employer to the agency if an agency's candidate is hired. Local training programs in colleges are excellent resources also. In most cases, there is a deadline for applications to be accepted.

After all applications have been reviewed, qualified candidates are contacted for personal interviews. A team approach is recommended for interviewing candidates, and staff members participating in the process must be familiar with the fair-employment practice (FEP) laws that affect hiring. Title VII of the Civil Rights Act of 1964, later amended as the Equal Employment Opportunity Act of 1972, (and further amended in 1990), prohibits asking applicants questions—during the interview or on the application—about their race, color, sex, religion, and national origin. For example, asking a female applicant questions such as, "Did you have difficulty finding a baby-sitter today?" or "Do you plan to have children?" is considered discriminatory and is therefore against the law.

The next step in the selection process is to check the references of the applicants. This is done by conducting a brief telephone interview of the reference person. After the references have been checked, the applicants are ranked and the most qualified person is selected as the first choice. If that person does not accept the job offer, the next person on the list can be contacted.

After an applicant has accepted the position, all other applicants should be notified, either by telephone or in writing, that the position is filled. The new employee should receive a written confirmation of the job offer along with the salary. The office manager will usually sign this letter.

The first three months (90 days) is usually a probationary period for all new employees. This time frame allows the supervisor to observe the new employee at work and to determine if the new employee is suited to the position for which he or she was hired. During this probationary period an employee can be terminated without cause. After 90 days, the employer must show just cause, or reason, to dismiss an employee. Absenteeism, poor performance, or violations of OSHA and safety standards are examples of just cause.

Orientation and Training

All new employees are entitled to an orientation to their new position and duties. Large offices and clinics often have formal orientation training sessions that employees attend before beginning their day-to-day assignments. These orientation sessions may include a/an:

- Review and discussion of policy and procedure manuals
- Discussion of employee safety issues
- Explanation of the way the physician prefers to work. If a team approach is used, examples should be provided to help the medical assistant understand his or her role.

Smaller offices with fewer employees may conduct orientation sessions on-the-job as the new employee begins working. This is not ideal but often necessary. Orientation materials and a schedule can be developed to assist in this training process.

Performance and Salary Review

There is generally an annual salary review at which time, if the employee's performance has been acceptable, a merit raise in salary is granted. In some facilities there is a set schedule for salary increases. In most cases, the salary increases are higher than the increase in the cost of living for the year.

The salary increase is often tied to the performance evaluation. However, conducting periodic performance evaluations, to encourage or direct the steady improvement of an employee's performance, is better management policy. The performance evaluation is not meant to find fault with the employee. Often, the evaluation or review provides positive motivation to employees whose performance has been excellent. This is the appropriate time to review office policies and set employee goals for the coming year.

Discipline and Probation

Occasionally it is necessary to discipline an employee. Due to the sensitive nature of medical work there are certain situations which can result in immediate discharge. These include intoxication, drug use, breach of confidentiality, and sleeping on the job. The employee must be sent home on suspension while the incident is investigated. If the facts prove to be true then the employee is dismissed.

For frequent tardiness or absenteeism, an employee may be placed on probation and told that if the situation occurs again the employee will be discharged. In some facilities, both verbal and written warnings are issued before corrective action is taken. Investigating every employee incident prevents someone being falsely fired. For instance, diabetic employees may appear to be on drugs when they are, in fact, having a diabetic reaction.

Any employee incident must be carefully documented with the time, date, and an objective statement about what happened placed into their employee file. Do not trust this type of information to memory. Document immediately. It is always better to have a witness present when dismissing an employee.

Employee Records

There are records that are required by law to be maintained for every employee. These include payroll records. These records include:

- Social security number of employee
- Number of exemptions claimed by the employee (W-4 form)

- Gross (salary before taxes are removed) salary amount
- Deductions for Social Security taxes, federal, state, and city withholding taxes, state disability tax, and state unemployment tax, if applicable.

Payroll is discussed further in Chapter 15.

Financial Management

Financial management includes banking, billing, collections, and insurance collections. This critical area is responsible for generating the income necessary to keep the practice solvent or capable of paying its bills and salaries. Fees, billings, collections, and credit are discussed in Chapter 14. Financial management, including employee record keeping, is discussed in Chapter 15.

Scheduling

The scheduling process involves using a systematic method for patient appointments. This is discussed in Chapter 9. Scheduling also includes managing staff work hours and vacation periods.

Facility and Equipment Management

Facility and equipment management includes facility layout and planning, inventory, maintaining safety and OSHA standards, and equipment replacement. This is discussed in Chapter 10. Computer use in the medical office is presented in Chapter 12.

Communication

Written communication skills are presented in Chapter 11, oral communication, including verbal and nonverbal in Chapter 7, and patient education in Chapter 33.

Legal Concepts

Physicians have their own personal attorney to assist with handling legal documents and issues. However medical assistants must have an understanding of legal terminology. Legal and ethical issues are discussed fully in Chapters 4 and 5.

The Office Manager

The office manager acts as a coordinator for the business activities conducted in the office. Each office varies somewhat, however, the general duties include:

- Acting as liaison between staff and physician/employer
- Conducting performance and salary reviews
- Delegating responsibilities to staff
- Developing and training staff
- Improving office efficiency
- Maintaining employee records
- Maintaining office procedure manual
- Planning and conducting staff meetings
- Preparing patient education materials
- Providing guidelines for patient education
- Recruiting, hiring, and firing
- Supervising cash, banking, and payroll operations
- Supervising employees on a day-to-day basis
- Supervising the purchase/storage of equipment and supplies
- Training new personnel

An office manager needs effective administrative and people skills. Medical assistants who have demonstrated good administrative, clinical, and people skills may seek to be promoted into this position. Other qualities or skills observed in good managers are

- An ability to enforce policy, when necessary
- An ability to organize
- Facility in resolving conflicts
- Creativity
- Diplomacy
- Excellent judgment
- Flexibility
- Leadership/take charge initiative
- Objectivity
- Sense of fairness
- Willingness to continue to learn

The office manager's time is generally spent on administrative and employee issues. The employees, on the other hand, spend most of their time working with patients. A good office manager does not strive to become "the boss," but, rather, to establish and implement a team approach to management by including all staff in the decision-making discussions and process. Ultimately, the manager must make the final decision in conjunction with the physician/employer, but compliance with decisions is much greater when employees have had the opportunity to participate. Table 18-1 describes responsibilities the office manager has to the employees and to the physician.

Many office managers are promoted based on seniority, or promoting the person who has worked

TABLE 18-1   Manager's Responsibilities to Employee and Physician/Employer

Employee	Physician/Employer
Interview	Increase efficiency of office
Hire/Terminate	Meet with doctor to discuss problems/plans
Orientate/Train	Manage calendar for doctor
Arrange work schedules	Assist with meetings
Arrange vacation coverage	Update doctor on insurance changes related to Medicare fee schedules
Conduct performance evaluations	Order CPT and ICD code books and current pharmacology books annually
Consult with doctor regarding salary increases	Renew insurance policies and pay premiums

for the physician the longest. This is not always a wise practice since not everyone is a skilled manager. When no internal candidate is available with the necessary skills or interest for the office manager position, then the physician/employer will have to seek an outside candidate. This is usually handled by placing an advertisement in the medical "help wanted" section of the local newspaper. In some cases, the physician's colleagues will recommend a qualified candidate for the position.

The office manager position is an ideal goal for the medical assistant who (1) enjoys the administrative and the clinical functions of the practice, (2) is looking for more challenge, and (3) wishes to continue learning through further education and/or on-the-job experience.

Monthly Planning

The office manager may wish to develop a system in which the entire month is laid out on a calendar. All physician conferences, staff meetings, vacations, and accountant's and other vendor visits would be noted. This calendar should be placed in an accessible location.

The manager will create and update the physician's own calendar. It is not necessary to include staff vacations on the physician's calendar. However the office manager's vacation schedule and days off should be included.

Staff Meetings

One of the most common complaints in the medical office is the lack of communication between staff and management. Staff members wish to have direct communication with the physician, but this is often

Med Tip: Many physicians carry a personal pocket calendar in which they enter all patient hospital visits and meetings. It is wise to ask the physician to see his or her calendar on a periodic basis so that the master calendar can be updated. If you are asked by the physician to take information from this personal calendar to process billing for the patients seen in the hospital, always make a copy of the pages needed and return the calendar immediately.

not possible in a large practice. The office manager can help resolve this problem by requesting the physician(s) to attend all or part of the regularly scheduled staff meetings, if this is not already being done. Many of the best ideas for office improvement are a result of suggestions made at staff meetings.

Staff meetings should be held on a regular basis. If it is necessary to hold weekly meetings due to the nature of the practice, then the physician(s) may only be invited monthly due to their busy schedules.

The meetings may need to be scheduled during a time period in which there is staff overlap due to shifts or staggered hours. For instance, if the practice is open from 9:00 a.m. to 9:00 p.m. on Thursdays, the meetings could be scheduled for 4:30 p.m. or 5:00 p.m. when all staff would be present. Generally, staff are compensated when they arrive before or remain after working hours to attend a staff meeting.

The office manager usually conducts staff meetings and facilitates team interaction. The office manager determines the time and date for the meeting, and also prepares the agenda, frequently with input from the physician and other staff. The key to a good meeting is a concise agenda that identifies items for discussion, staff responsible, and limits the time allotted. Focusing staff meetings/discussions in this way limits the amount of time wasted. Generally, minutes are recorded for future reference and distributed for review prior to the next meeting. See Table 18-2 for an example of an office staff meeting agenda.

Time Management

One of the greatest attributes of an effective office manager is the ability to effectively manage time. If the manager is organized, the office is usually organized. Time management requires the ability to prioritize what the important tasks are and to complete them on schedule. This is quite different from doing every task as it comes along. The office manager generally has little control over the tasks presented. The control is in how the tasks are handled and delegated.

One of the main responsibilities of the office manager/medical assistant is to manage all the peripheral office functions so that the physician is free to concentrate on practicing medicine. It is possible for the physician to gain an hour each day to devote to administrative and/or patient related tasks that only he or she can do, because tasks such as opening the daily mail, restocking the medical bag, searching for a drug sample to give to a patient, and dealing with pharmaceutical and other sales representatives, are handled by the office manager.

Med Tip: One of the dangers of strictly adhering to time management and goal-setting practices is total concentration on "organizing the office," to the extent that the patient is forgotten in the process. Always take care of a patient who is waiting at the reception desk before concentrating on straightening up the work area.

Before establishing a time management system, it is important to define the office goals with the physician. Physicians' goals vary from complex to simple and from long term to short term. These goals may include: collecting all payments at time of delivery, re-organizing or computerizing billing, limiting the practice, adding a partner or new service, writing a textbook, or plans for early retirement.

TABLE 18-2 **Staff Meeting Agenda**

WINDY CITY CLINIC		
Staff Meeting Agenda		
Date:	December 19, 19xx	
Time:	4:30-5:30 p.m.	
Place:	Staff Conference Room	
Time	**Agenda Item**	**Person Responsible**
4:30	Introduction of new staff	M. King/Office Manager
	Review of last meeting's minutes	
4:35	Discussion of new policies	
4:45	Problems with Insurance	L. Turner/Insurance Coding Clerk
4:55	OSHA protocol for needlesticks	K. Wall/ Lab Tech
5:05	Vacation schedules	M. King
5:10	New office location	Dr. Williams
5:20	New business	Mary King
	Meeting adjourned	

After the goals have been established, priorities can be set. The office manager/medical assistant can establish a priority list of the goals. A priority list is a composite of all the tasks that need to be accomplished to actualize each goal . These can be placed on a TO DO List, as they come to the office manager's attention. Each item is assigned a priority designation of 1, 2, or 3, depending on how critical the item is to complete the task. For example, ordering supplies that are running out is a number 1, while re-arranging a linen cupboard or a file drawer might be a 3. Number 1 priority items must be done first and number 3 last. It is often tempting to do the easier tasks first since they take less time and show an immediate accomplishment. Good use of time management would determine that the inventory order should be placed immediately, and the number 3 priority items be delegated to someone else or completed later, if necessary. It is a good idea to date a TO DO List and to cross off items as they are accomplished. Table 18-3 shows an example of one type of TO DO List.

Make every attempt to do each task, such as handling paper, only once. As mail is opened it needs to be quickly handled and processed. Mail can be quickly sorted according to importance, but it should be handled immediately, if possible.

It is advisable to leave detailed voice mail messages, whenever possible, since they can actually save time. Leaving a detailed message during the first call can prevent having to make another telephone call.

Med Tip: There is an exception to leaving detailed messages. When calling to remind a patient of an upcoming appointment, the patient's confidentiality should be protected. Do not leave a message unless you are certain that only the patient will hear it.

Never trust anything to memory in the medical office. Always write down all instructions from the physician, information from a patient, employee, or supplier. It is better to maintain one small record book and keep all notation in that book rather than have several pieces of paper with information which can be misplaced.

Med Tip: Many medical assistants have learned to carry a small notepad and pen in their pocket at all times.

Some offices require that the in-basket of the day's mail and incoming laboratory reports be emptied before the end of the day. This is a good time management technique to develop.

TABLE 18-3 Medical Office *TO DO List*

Priority	To Do
2	Order paper supplies
1	Arrange Dr.Williams' air transportation to medical convention next week
2	Prepare performance appraisal for J. Jones
3	Reorganize storeroom
1	Type convention speech
1	Place ad for new medical assistant
3	Ask Janet to remove old magazines from reception room
1	Call for PAP test report for Ms. Kohut
2	Block out schedule book for next quarter
3	Ask Mary to take down Christmas decorations
1	Prepare agenda for Thursday's staff meeting

Personnel Policy Manual

The personnel policy manual, also known as the employee handbook, contains information for the employee about the employer-employee relationship, the work environment, and the expectations of the particular medical facility. This manual usually describes the circumstances or grounds for dismissal, such as sleeping, drinking, or swearing on the job. It contains general information about office policies relating to dress and behavior codes, punctuality, office safety, and the role of the employee in an emergency, such as a fire. OSHA guidelines and Standard Precautions are included.

Some issues or benefits about which employees may be given specific information follow.

- Compensation/reimbursement for work-related activities, such as attending conventions and courses (CEU/degree), and parking fees
- Emergency leave
- Complaint/grievance process
- Health benefits
- Holidays
- Jury duty
- Overtime policy
- Pension plan
- Performance review/evaluation
- Probationary period
- Sick leave
- Termination of employment
- Vacation
- Work hours, including flex time

An office manager will find that an updated policy manual can be a useful tool when providing employee counseling. A well-designed policy manual remains flexible enough in design to allow for revision if and when policies change. Small office policy manuals consist of several pages that are copied on-site. In large practices, the manual may be bound and copied at a printing service.

The employee handbook is often the first piece of office literature that the employee is asked to read. Employees should be asked to sign a statement indicating they have read and understand the information contained in it.

Office Procedures Manual

All offices should have a procedures manual describing how to carry out tasks within a particular medical practice. The office procedures manual varies in content from the personnel policy manual. Detailed descriptions, or the standard operating procedure (SOP), of how to perform both administrative and clinical tasks are included in this manual.

The primary functions of a procedures manual are: (1) list the tasks to be performed within the office; (2) standardize the procedure for each task; and (3) describe job responsibilities and titles.

The procedures manual, when properly updated, is an excellent tool for the new employee since it provides guidelines for performing specific tasks. Temporary or substitute employees also find it valuable.

Med Tip: Policy refers to a general statement or course of action, such as "It is office policy that all employees receive hepatitis B (HBV) vaccination." The procedure will describe the steps that need to be performed to carry out the policy. For example, "a series of three injections of HBV will be administered over a 7 month period of time, free of charge to the employee." The terms policy and procedure are used interchangeably in many offices.

Ideally, the procedure manual is contained in a loose-leaf binder which allows for ease of updating with the addition of new pages. Each policy is numbered and dated. As the policy is updated, the number remains the same but the date changes to indicate the revision. The manual should be clearly labeled and available for employees to read.

New policies and procedures are usually distributed or posted for employees in addition to being added to the policy and procedures manuals. In some offices, staff are asked to initial the corner of the policy indicating they have read it.

Table 18-4 contains a list of information that should be included in a procedure manual.

Completing and updating a procedures manual is often a job function of the medical assistant or the office manager. While one person may have responsibility for development of the manual, good manuals are the result of the input from a variety of personnel. The physician/employer should always provide the final review of all policies and procedures.

Medical Meetings and Speaking Engagements

The medical assistant will be asked to assist the physician by making travel arrangements and hotel accommodations and typing any materials

TABLE 18-4   Contents of an Office Procedure Manual

Content	Description
Job Descriptions	Every position including office manager, medical assistant, nurse, technician, housekeeping personnel, and custodian.
Routine Office Tasks	Clinical tasks such as venipuncture, taking vital signs, EKGs, assisting with physical examinations, procedure for assisting with PAP test and other laboratory tests. Administrative tasks such as setting up the schedule book, providing referrals, registering new patients, making bank deposits, completing and filing insurance forms.
Special Procedures	Surgical tray set-ups for individual physicians, assisting with special exams such as proctological exams, using specialized equipment such as ultrasound.
Emergency Procedures	Protocol for handling telephone and office emergencies, description of equipment used for emergency care such as mouth shield for CPR, proper sequence for alerting physician and "911" regarding emergencies.
Quality Assurance	Procedures for maintaining quality control over all laboratory testing and procedures.
OSHA Compliance	Compliance regarding needles, other sharps, specimens, personal protective equipment, regulated waste control, HBV vaccine, laundry disposal, and contaminated equipment.

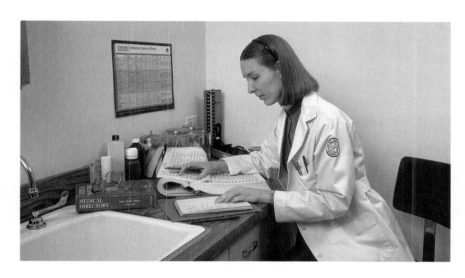

Figure 18-1   Medical assistant preparing a report that the physician will need at a conference.

needed for the trip including an itinerary of the time the physician is away from the office (Figure 18-1). There will be specific duties for the office staff while the physician is away from the office. It is important that the medical assistant and physician have a brief meeting to discuss the plans. A folder with all information relating to this trip should be started. Upon the physician's return, selected materials, such as any speeches and a list of participants, will be filed for future reference.

Travel Arrangements

It is preferable to work with one travel agent or agency that will maintain a profile of the physician's travel preferences, regarding airline(s) (frequent flyer numbers should be on file), seating, special diet, rental car requirements, and hotel accommodations. Always inform the travel agent if convention rates apply, and, if possible, send a copy of convention brochures with details regarding hotel convention rates. For convenience, the physician's credit card number and information regarding senior status will usually be on file.

Reservations should be made as far in advance as possible to obtain the best rates. Provide the agent with all the necessary information, such as dates of departure and return, preferred flight times, city/location of departure and destination, number of travelers, and car, if required. The travel agent will gather information from several airlines unless you state a preference.

Ask the agent for several options regarding times of departure and arrival so the physician has a choice. (The information can be faxed to facilitate review and selection of the best option.) Once the physician has determined the best time for departure, you can make the reservation. At this time, the name(s) of the other traveler(s) accompanying the physician can be given along with any necessary data. In most cases, a travel agent will have the tickets delivered by courier or first class mail per your request.

Hotel Accommodations

After the travel arrangements are finalized, the hotel accommodations can be made. If the hotel is not specified, the travel agent will use information supplied regarding the conference location and travel profile preferences on file to select a hotel. Information regarding room requirements, such as non-smoking or no room above fifth floor and facilities, such as pool, gym, tennis, golf should be part of the travel profile. If the location is not known to the physician, request appropriate brochures and information prior to departure. Arrange for a confirmed reservation in the event that the physician arrives late. Always ask for the hotel reservation confirmation number.

Arrange for transportation between the airport and hotel unless the physician indicates that is not necessary. After all arrangements have been made, prepare an itinerary with the following information:

1. Time(s) and date(s) to and from conference including:
   Name of airline
   Flight number(s)
2. Name, address, telephone number, and confirmation number of hotel.
3. Any necessary information about the conference, such as time to present a paper or attend a conference session or meeting.

Keep a copy of the itinerary in the office file, give one to the physician, and provide a copy for the physician's spouse.

If the conference relates to the physician's office practice, it is tax deductible. All receipts for conference-related expenses must be retained. Upon the physician's return, the expenses can be entered in the accounting record maintained for tax purposes. Collect information about continuing medical education credits.

Setting Up a Medical Conference

Your physician may be involved in a variety of activities, including medical society meetings, that will require making arrangements for large group activities. This can be especially time-consuming if the physician is an officer (president, vice-president, or secretary) of an organization. Some of the activities to prepare for a meeting are listed below.

1. Obtain complete information such as date, number of people attending, and amount of money that can be spent.
2. Select and reserve room(s). Investigate several sites that are large enough to accommodate the meeting. Obtain estimates for food and other services. Select food from sample menus for refreshments, luncheon, or dinner.
3. Obtain a speaker. The program coordinator may perform this function and discuss any **honorarium**, or payment. The speaker should be contacted in writing with all information concerning date, time, and place.
4. Produce a mailing to potential participants with meeting agenda and information about the speakers. Record all reservations as they are returned. Contact by telephone everyone who has not responded by mail.
5. Arrive at the meeting site at least one hour ahead of time to test equipment such as slide projectors and sound system. Greet participants as they arrive.
6. Keep a file of pertinent information for future meetings.

Preparing the Physician's Paper

Physician's are frequently asked to discuss a topic involving their area of expertise or recent research they have conducted. This is referred to as "presenting a paper."

The medical assistant may be asked to assist with conducting a search of the literature (Figure 18-2). This will require going to a library that has medical journals, using the Internet, or the physi-

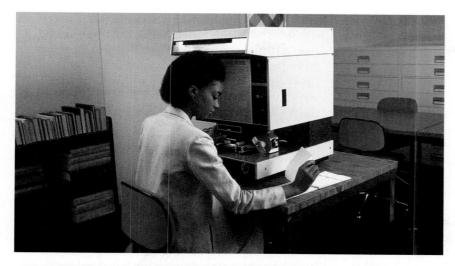

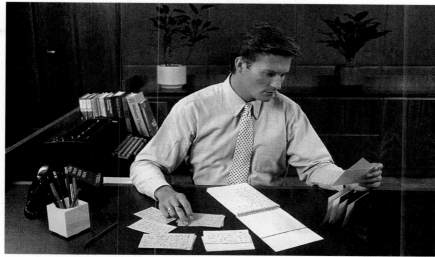

Figure 18-2   The medical assistant's responsibilities may include research from time to time.

cian's own office library. Many physicians subscribe to the *Journal of the American Medical Association* (JAMA) and other specialty journals (Figure 18-3).

The physician may ask you to prepare an abstract which is a summary of a journal article. The abstract must contain a careful notation of the following information:

- Title of article
- Last name and first initial of all authors
- Name of publication
- Publisher's name and city/state location if a book
- Volume number
- Month and year of publication
- Page numbers
- Results of research studies and experiments discussed in article
- Conclusions and recommendations at end of article

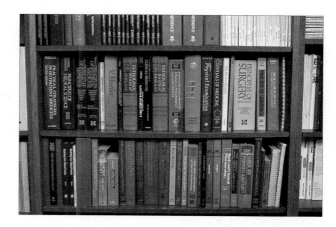

Figure 18-3   Many physicians subscribe to a number of medical journals.

This information is either typed onto index cards or as a one page summary (Figure 18-4). The information is then filed for the physician's use. An example of a book citation is:

Fremgen, B. *Medical Terminology*. Upper Saddle River, NJ: Brady/Prentice Hall, 1997.

Computers or word processing equipment are used to prepare papers and abstracts. The physician may write a draft of the paper. This is a preliminary paper which the medical assistant may be asked to type. The first typed copy should contain wide margins for the physician to add any changes or corrections. All articles and books that are mentioned within the paper must be cited or footnoted to provide credit to the original author. After the physician has made corrections the paper can be typed into its final form.

Patient Information Booklet

Many medical practices use a professional advertising service to develop an informational brochure as a marketing tool. However, a patient information booklet or a variety of patient teaching materials can be developed on-site. They should provide patient information regarding office hours, payment guidelines, appointment and cancellation policy, the telephone answering service, information about the physician(s), a map with directions to the facility, and parking information.

Experience has demonstrated that a good patient information booklet can reduce the number of questions by telephone from patients, enhance the office's image, and reduce the number of patients who fail to follow instructions.

Instruction booklets for patients with special needs or to teach methods of disease prevention can be developed using a format and design similar to the one described in the patient information booklet guidelines.

The patient information booklet should be handed to each new patient at the time of registration or mailed prior to the first appointment. Patient information materials never replace the need for personal instructions to the patient. They augment or reinforce patient teaching.

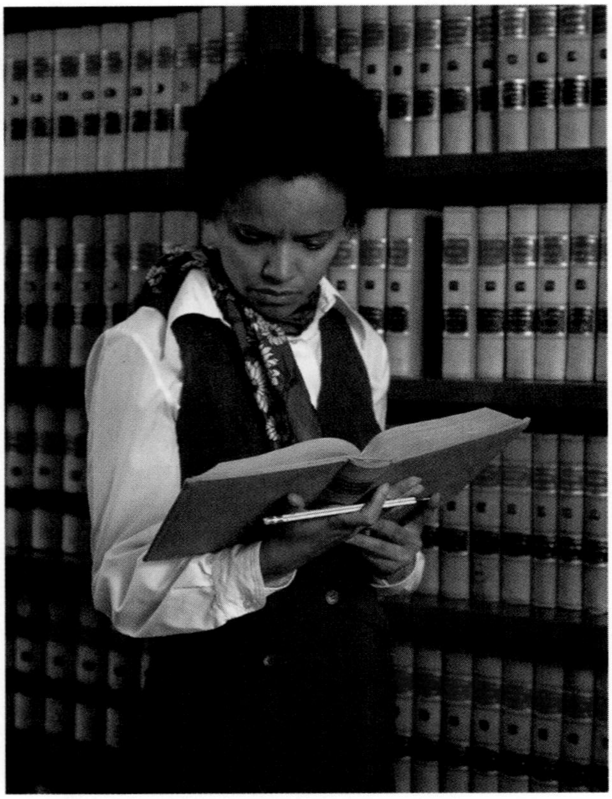

Figure 18-4   Reference librarians can be of great assistance in gathering information for your physician/employer.

Guidelines: Developing a Patient Information Booklet

1. Make the booklet as appealing as possible. Allow white space around all the edges. Use large print for the elderly reader's benefit. The booklet should be small enough that it will easily fit into a pocket or purse.
2. Write the booklet with the reader in mind. Avoid the use of technical medical terms. Never use medical abbreviations in patient literature.
3. Avoid long paragraphs of explanation. Keep the sentences short and concise.
4. Provide a listing of the regular office hours.
5. List any special services offered by the practice or clinic such as patient education classes or blood pressure testing programs.
6. Explain the procedure for having a prescription refilled.
7. Explain the procedure for processing medical insurance forms.
8. Include a general statement about payment of fees, especially if payment is expected at the time of delivery of services. Specific fees are not discussed in patient brochures.

9. Provide information about the physician and the staff. For example, "Dr. Williams is in general practice specializing in family practice. Our pediatrician is Dr. Conway. Our physicians are on staff at two hospitals: Northwestern Memorial Hospital and Children's Memorial Hospital." The name and phone number of the office manager, the person responsible for insurance processing, and the patient educator should be included.

10. State what procedure to follow in case of an emergency. For example, instruct the patients to call "911" if the emergency is life-threatening. Also provide a 24 hour emergency telephone number. Request the patient to keep this number near their telephone.
11. Include a telephone number at the end of the brochure in the event there are additional questions.
12. End the brochure by thanking the patient for taking the time to read the literature.

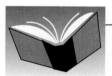

LEGAL AND ETHICAL ISSUES

Confidentiality, as both a legal and ethical concern, is a part of almost every function in the medical office. A good office manager will see that all employees put the patient's needs and confidentiality first. Special care must be taken that only selected office personnel have access to patient records.

The office manager must also protect the confidentiality of all employees by keeping employee records locked. There should never be discussions about one employee's behavior with another employee.

PATIENT EDUCATION

Patients need an introduction to all the caregivers they come into contact within the office. All employees should be taught to identify themselves to patients. Still many patients need further education about the functions that individual employees are able to perform.

Patient information booklets are one of the greatest assists to patient education. While verbal instructions are still necessary, the booklets can enhance learning. Medical assistants need to involve the entire staff in the production of patient literature.

Summary

A smooth running office requires attention to many factors including staff training, good time-management skills, up-to-date policy and proce-dure manuals, and careful attention to detail. A medical office requires the same management skills that any business organization uses.

Competency Review

1. Define and spell the glossary terms for this chapter.
2. Prepare an office procedure for any one of the following tasks: appointment scheduling, patient reception process, taking vital signs, OSHA guidelines.
3. Prepare a monthly calendar for the month of December showing staff vacations and office coverage.

4. Develop a patient information booklet for your own physician's practice.
5. Prepare an employee policy for taking vacation days.

PREPARING FOR THE CERTIFICATION EXAM

Test Taking Tip — Constantly check that you are filling in the correct box when taking a multiple choice exam using a computer-generated answer sheet. If you are off by one line, all the subsequent answers will be incorrect. It is helpful to check the number next to each answer as you enter your selection on the answer sheet.

Examination Review Questions

1. Which of the following would be included in an employee handbook?
   (A) salary amounts
   (B) OSHA guidelines
   (C) protocol for attire
   (D) only A, B, and C
   (E) only B and C

2. Which of the following is a purpose of the procedure manual?
   (A) listing of tasks to perform
   (B) standardization of procedures
   (C) listing of job descriptions
   (D) marketing tool
   (E) only A, B, and C

3. The systems approach to office management is
   (A) performing individual office functions in isolation
   (B) using outside consultants for all financial and business operations
   (C) integrating functions
   (D) not advisable in the office setting
   (E) none of the above

4. Qualities of a good office manager include the following
   (A) flexibility
   (B) authoritativeness
   (C) organization
   (D) creativity
   (E) only A, C, and D

5. Patient instruction booklets should be used
   (A) in place of individual instruction
   (B) to avoid contact with difficult patients
   (C) to prevent lawsuits
   (D) to standardize instruction
   (E) only with hearing impaired patients

6. Employee records must be kept for all of the following EXCEPT
   (A) net salary
   (B) gross salary
   (C) social security number
   (D) number of claimed exemptions
   (E) deductions

7. A *TO DO* List includes
   (A) completed tasks
   (B) non-prioritized items
   (C) daily duties such as emptying trash
   (D) tasks done in the order they appear on the list
   (E) none of the above

8. The HBV is given
   (A) one time only
   (B) three doses over a 3 month period
   (C) three doses over a 7 month period
   (D) to every medical office personnel
   (E) only after exposure to hepatitis

9. The personnel management function includes
   (A) selection
   (B) probation
   (C) firing
   (D) salary review
   (E) all of the above

10. New employee orientations should include
    (A) safety issues
    (B) discussion of the methods one physician uses
    (C) discussion of physician's income level
    (D) explanation of duties
    (E) only A, B, and D

ON THE JOB

Sarah Egan is the office manager in Dr. Williams' practice. Nell Jacobs, who has worked as a medical assistant in the office for one year, has frequently been absent or tardy on Mondays. Sarah suspects that Nell has a drinking problem. However, Nell has never arrived at the office intoxicated—until today. Sarah has just observed Nell stumbling in the parking lot when getting out of her car. Her speech is slurred and her breath has a fruity odor which Sarah thinks could be alcohol. Nell doesn't appear to be understanding anything that Sarah is saying to her.

What is your response?

1. Given the situation, as the office manager, what should Sarah immediately do regarding Nell?
2. If Sarah decides to send Nell home, should she call Nell's husband to come and get her, or, perhaps, insist that Nell go home in a cab?
3. Does Sarah have an obligation to tell Dr. Williams about her suspicions regarding Nell?
4. Should this incident become part of Nell's employment record?
5. Is this incident grounds for firing an employee?
6. Because Nell is a medical assistant and works with patients, is it within Sarah's rights to demand a blood and urine screening for alcohol and drugs?
7. Should the police be notified of the incident?
8. If Nell is indeed intoxicated or under the influence of drugs, is Sarah obligated to provide counseling at an alcohol and drug rehabilitation facility?

References

Backstrom, I. *Medical Office Management.* Chicago: American Association of Medical Assistants, 1991.

Becklin, K. and Sunnarborg, E. *Medical Office Procedures.* New York: Glencoe, 1996.

Cohen, A., Fink, S., Gadon, H., Willits, R. *Effective Behavior in Organizations.* Homewood, IL: Irwin, 1992.

Decker, M. "The OSHA Bloodborne Hazard Standard." *Infection Control and Hospital Epidemiology.* 12:7, 1992.

Donnelly, J., Gibson, J., Ivancevich, J. *Fundamentals of Management.* Chicago: Irwin, 1995.

Hellriegel, D. and Slocum, J. *Management.* Cincinnati: South-Western Publishing, 1996.

Kelsey, E. "Understanding OSHA's Bloodborne Pathogens Standard." *Professional Medical Assistant.* July/August, 1992.

Oliverio, J., Pasewark, W., and White, B. *The Office: Procedures and Technology.* Cincinnati, Ohio: South-Western Publishing Co., 1993.

United States Department of Labor, Occupational Safety and Health Administration. "Occupational Exposure to Bloodborne Pathogens: Final Rule." *Federal Register.* 29 CFR Part 1910.1030. December 6, 1991.

Johnson, J., Whitaker, M., and Johnson, M. *Computerized Medical Office Management.* Albany, NY: Delmar Publishers, 1994.

Workplace Wisdom

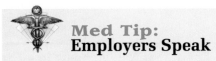

Med Tip:
Employers Speak

Be on time!

Miriam Sanchez, Personnel Officer;
University of Illinois at Chicago
Medical Center;
Chicago, Illinois

Be neat and well-groomed. No gum chewing.

Linda Davis-Rogers
Recruiter
Sharp Health Care
San Diego, California

Implement positive actions and attitudes that provide good customer service to patients and staff members. Go beyond the job description. Exhibit a welcoming attitude; offer reassurance and directions—whatever is needed.

Possess high standards for your own professional performance. If you don't know something, ask someone for help and learn from the experience. Take responsibility for your actions.

Denise Williams
Staffing Specialist (Radnor Office)
University of Pennsylvania
Health System
Philadelphia, Pennsylvania

Show accuracy in following protocols:

- Demonstrate knowledge of and adherence to OSHA standards. For example, Know what to do if blood spills.

- Demonstrate knowledge of laws regarding shipping blood.

Rachael Wallace, RN
Nurse Administrator
Howard Brown Health Center
Chicago, Illinois

Be able to work as a team member. Medical Assistants are an enhancement to the staff and must be able to get along and relate well to everyone. The ability to communicate to the rest of the staff is vital.

Opal Howard
Human Resources Specialist
Wendy Krieg
Assistant Director Centra Care
Florida Hospital
Orlando, Florida

Be able to accept frequent change. These days, procedures are constantly changing. Medical Assistants must be able to adapt to frequent change in order to be valuable to the employer.

Alice Johnson, RN, MA
Director of Nursing
Southern California Region
American Red Cross

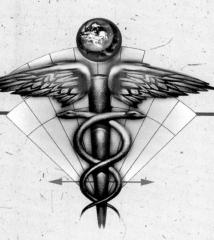

Unit Three

Clinical

MEDICAL ASSISTANT ROLE DELINEATION CHART

Highlight indicates material covered in this chapter

ADMINISTRATIVE

ADMINISTRATIVE PROCEDURES

- Perform basic clerical functions
- Schedule, coordinate, and monitor appointments
- Schedule inpatient/outpatient admissions and procedures
- Understand and apply third party guidelines
- Obtain reimbursement through accurate claims submission
- Monitor third-party reimbursement
- Perform medical transcription
- Understand and adhere to managed care policies and procedures
- *Negotiate managed care contracts (adv)*

PRACTICE FINANCES

- Perform procedural and diagnostic coding
- Apply bookkeeping principles
- Document and maintain accounting and banking records
- Manage accounts receivable
- Manage accounts payable
- Process payroll
- *Develop and maintain fee schedules (adv)*
- *Manage renewals of business and professional insurance policies (adv)*
- *Manage personal benefits and maintain records (adv)*

CLINICAL

FUNDAMENTAL PRINCIPLES

- Apply principles of aseptic technique and infection control
- Comply with quality assurance practices
- Screen and follow up patient test results

DIAGNOSTIC ORDERS

- Collect and process specimens
- Perform diagnostic tests

PATIENT CARE

- Adhere to established triage procedures
- Obtain patient history and vital signs
- Prepare and maintain examination and treatment areas

- Prepare patient for examinations, procedures, and treatments
- Assist with examinations, procedures, and treatments
- Prepare and administer medications and immunizations
- Maintain medication and immunization records
- Recognize and respond to emergencies
- Coordinate patient care information with other health care providers

GENERAL (TRANSDISCIPLINARY)

PROFESSIONALISM

- Project a professional manner and image
- Adhere to ethical principles
- Demonstrate initiative and responsibility
- Work as a team member
- Manage time efficiently
- Prioritize and perform multiple tasks
- Adapt to change
- Promote the CMA credential
- Enhance skills through continuing education

COMMUNICATION SKILLS

- Treat all patients with compassion and empathy
- Recognize and respect cultural diversity
- Adapt communications to individual's ability to understand
- Use professional telephone technique
- Use effective and correct verbal and written communications
- Recognize and respond to verbal and non-verbal communications
- Use medical terminology appropriately
- Receive, organize, prioritize, and transmit information
- Serve as liaison
- Promote the practice through positive public relations

LEGAL CONCEPTS

- Maintain confidentiality
- Practice within the scope of education, training, and personal capabilities
- Prepare and maintain medical records
- Document accurately
- Use appropriate guidelines when releasing information
- Follow employer's established policies dealing with the health care contract
- Follow federal, state, and local legal guidelines
- Maintain awareness of federal and state health care legislation and regulations
- Maintain and dispose of regulated substances in compliance with government guidelines
- Comply with established risk management and safety procedures
- Recognize professional credentialing criteria
- Participate in the development and maintenance of personnel, policy, and procedure manuals
- *Develop and maintain personnel, policy, and procedure manuals (adv)*

INSTRUCTION

- Instruct individuals according to their needs
- Explain office policies and procedures
- Teach methods of health promotion and disease prevention
- Locate community resources and disseminate information
- *Orient and train personnel (adv)*
- *Develop educational materials (adv)*
- *Conduct continuing education activities (adv)*

OPERATIONAL FUNCTIONS

- Maintain supply inventory
- Evaluate and recommend equipment and supplies
- Apply computer techniques to support office operations
- *Supervise personnel (adv)*
- *Interview and recommend job applicants (adv)*
- *Negotiate leases and prices for equipment and supply contracts (adv)*

SOURCE: Reprinted by permission of the American Association of Medical Assistants from the *AAMA Role Delineation Study: Occupational Analysis of the Medical Assisting Profession.*

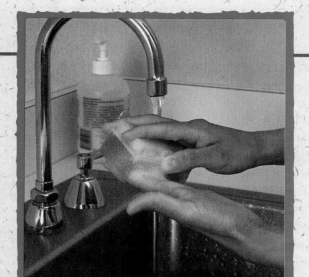

19

Infection Control: Asepsis

LEARNING OBJECTIVES

After completing this chapter, you should:
1. Define and spell the glossary terms for this chapter.
2. Describe the conditions required for the infection process to occur.
3. Discuss the body's defenses against infection.
4. Explain the immune system.
5. Discuss the steps to follow in the infection control systems listed below.
   a. Standard Precautions
   b. OSHA
6. Define medical asepsis.
7. Explain the correct procedure for handwashing.
8. Define surgical asepsis.
9. Explain the difference between sanitization, disinfection, and sterilization.
10. Discuss the five types of hepatitis and their level of contagion.
11. Describe the means of transmission for HIV.

CLINICAL PERFORMANCE COMPETENCIES

After completing this chapter, you should perform the following tasks:
1. Demonstrate the proper handwashing technique for medical asepsis.
2. Demonstrate the procedure for wrapping materials for the autoclave.
3. Demonstrate the correct procedure for disposing of sharps.
4. Disinfect, sanitize, and sterilize materials.
5. Demonstrate procedure for applying nonsterile gloves.
6. Demonstrate procedure for applying and removing isolation gown.

Glossary

aerobic   Microorganism which is able to live only in the presence of oxygen.

anaerobic   Microorganism which thrives best or lives without oxygen.

aseptic   Germ free.

bactericidal   Ability to destroy disease-causing bacteria.

bloodborne pathogens   Disease producing organisms transmitted by means of blood and body fluids containing blood.

carrier(s)   Individual who is unaware he or she has a disease but is capable of transmitting it to someone else (for example "Typhoid Mary" who, legend has it, spread the disease typhoid).

incubation   Period of time during which a disease develops after the person is exposed.

immunity   Resistance to disease.

medical asepsis   Killing organisms after they leave the body.

nosocomial infection   Infection that is acquired after a person has entered the hospital. It is caused by the spread of an infection from one patient or person to another.

opportunistic infections   Infections, such as pneumonia, that occur in a body with a reduced immune system (for example, as seen in AIDS).

pathogens   Disease producing microorganisms.

permeable   Material that allows something to penetrate or pass through.

phagocytosis   Process of engulfing, digesting, and destroying pathogens.

reservoir   Source of the infectious pathogen.

sterile   All microorganisms and spores are killed.

surgical asepsis   A technique practiced to maintain a sterile environment.

syndrome   A set of symptoms or disorders which occur together and indicate the presence of a disease.

WARNING!

For all patient contact, adhere to Standard Precautions
(see pages 342–373). Wear protective equipment as indicated.

Pathogenic, or disease producing organisms, are everywhere. The healthy individual has some resistance to pathogens. However pathogens are especially important to control in the medical office setting since patients who may be already suffering from a disease are more susceptible to infection. The medical assistant must be aware of how easily pathogens can be spread from one person to another or from an inanimate object to a person since lack of knowledge can cause infections to occur.

History of Asepsis

Methods for controlling the spread of infection were used before early man understood the infection process. Religions, such as the Jewish faith, emphasize the careful preparation and cleanliness associated with foods. About 500 years ago, microorganisms known as germs were suspected to be the cause of some diseases. But, it was not until 100 years ago that Semmelweiss, Lister, and Pasteur (discussed in Chapter 2) contributed discoveries to our understanding of germ theory.

Louis Pasteur discovered that many diseases are caused by bacteria and that bacteria can be killed by excess heat. The heat method for killing germs in milk is called pasteurization in his honor. Joseph Lister discovered that germs could be killed using carbolic acid. He was the first to insist on cleaning surgical wounds by spraying the surrounding tissue with carbolic acid. This introduced the principles of *aseptic,* or germ free, technique in surgery. Lister introduced the concept of clean techniques in hospitals which greatly reduced the death rate from amputations from 45 to 15 percent. Semmelweiss taught his medical students to wash their hands before delivering babies. This simple precaution had an immediate effect on reducing the death rate from puerperal sepsis (childbed fever) in new mothers.

Today, we have a better understanding of germs and bacteria thanks to high powered microscopes. Sophisticated equipment can disinfect and sterilize equipment and materials. However, sterilization is meaningless if good aseptic technique is not practiced. With the advent of communicable diseases such as hepatitis, acquired immune deficiency syndrome (AIDS), and tuberculosis (TB) the need for adherence to aseptic technique has become critical.

Microorganisms

Microorganisms are small, living organisms capable of causing disease, which can only be seen with the aid of a microscope. Microorganisms are normally found on the skin, in the urinary and gastrointestinal tract, and in the respiratory tract.

Microorganisms, also called microbes, are bacteria, fungi, protozoa, and viruses. The sizes of microorganisms can be expressed in micrometers. A micrometer is one millionth part of a meter or one thousandth of a millimeter. These microorganisms are listed with descriptions and examples of each in Table 19-1.

See Figure 19-1 for an illustration of pathogens (cocci, bacilli, virus). The study of each of these microorganisms represents a separate science:

- Bacteriology—the study of bacteria.
- Mycology—the study of fungi.
- Protozoonology—the study of protozoa.
- Virology—the study of viruses.

How Microorganisms Grow

Microorganisms occur everywhere in nature and have several requirements to grow: food, moisture, darkness, and a suitable temperature. In addition, some bacteria require oxygen (aerobic) or the absence of oxygen (anaerobic) to live. Table 19-2 presents the four conditions necessary for the growth of bacteria.

Some microorganisms, such as certain types of fungi and bacteria, are necessary for normal body

TABLE 19-1 **Microorganisms**

Microorganism	Description	Example
Bacteria	Most numerous of all microorganisms Unicellular Many are pathogenic to humans Identified by shape and appearance	(See cocci, bacilli, and spirilla below.)
• **Cocci**	3 types of spherical bacteria	
1. **Staphlococci**	Form grape-like clusters of pus producing organisms	Boils, pimples, acne, osteomyelitis
2. **Streptococci**	Form chains of cells	Rheumatic heart disease, scarlet fever, strep throat
3. **Diplococci**	Form pairs of cells	Pneumonia, gonorrhea, and meningitis
• **Bacilli**	Rod shaped bacteria	Gram positive bacilli: tuberculosis, tetanus, diphtheria, gas gangrene
		Gram negative bacilli: *Escherichia coli* (urinary tract infection), *Bordetella pertussis* (whooping cough)
• **Spirilla**	Spiral shaped organisms	Syphilis and cholera
		(Continued on next page)

TABLE 19-1 *(Continued)*

Microorganism	Description	Example
Fungi	Parasitic and some non-parasitic plants and molds Depend on other life forms for their nutrition, such as dead or decaying organic material Reproduction method is budding Yeast is a typical fungus Fungus means "mushroom" in Latin Feed on antibiotics and flourish on antibiotic therapy	*Histoplasma capsulatum* (histoplasmosis), tinea pedis (athlete's foot), candidiasis (yeast infection), and ringworm
Protozoa	One-celled organisms Both parasite and non-parasite Can move with cilia or false-feet Typically 2 to 200 mm in size	Amebic dysentery, malaria, and trichomonas vaginitis
Rickettsia	Visible under a standard microscope Susceptible to antibiotics Transmitted by insects (ticks, fleas)	Rocky Mountain Spotted Fever
Virus	Smallest of microorganisms Can only be seen with electron microscope Can only multiply within a living cell (host) Difficult to kill with chemotherapy since they become resistant to the drug Can be destroyed by heat (autoclave sterilization) but generally not by chemical disinfection More viruses than any other category of microbial agents Feed on antibiotics and flourish on antibiotic therapy	Herpes virus, HIV, ARC, AIDS, common cold, influenza virus, smallpox, hepatitis A, hepatitis B, rabies, mumps, shingles

function. For example, normal flora within the digestive system breaks down food and converts unused food into waste products. In some cases the normal flora will invade areas of the body where they do not belong, and thus, convert to pathogens, which are disease producing microorganisms. For example, *Escherichia coli* (E. coli) is a normal bacteria within the colon where it aids in food digestion. When E. coli moves into the bladder or bloodstream, through improper hygiene habits, such as improper handwashing, it can cause urinary and blood infections.

Those microorganisms which are capable of producing disease (pathogens) grow best at body

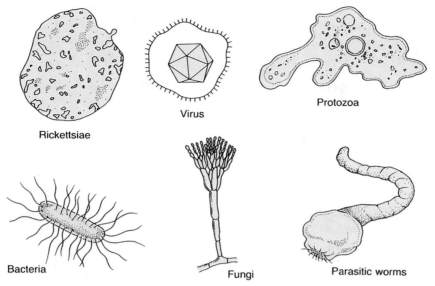

Figure 19-1   Pathogens.

Rickettsiae
Virus
Protozoa
Bacteria
Fungi
Parasitic worms

TABLE 19-2   **Conditions Required for Bacterial Growth**

Condition	Explanation
Moisture	Bacteria grow best in moist areas: skin, mucous membranes, wet dressings, wounds, dirty instruments.
Temperature	Thrive at body temperature (98.6°F). Low temperatures (32°F and below) retard, but do not kill, bacterial growth. Temperatures of 107°F and above will kill most bacteria.
Oxygen	Aerobic bacteria require oxygen supply to live. Anaerobic bacteria can survive without oxygen.
Light	Darkness favors the growth of bacteria. Bacteria will die if exposed to direct sunlight or light.

temperature (98.6°F) destroy and use human tissue as food, and give off waste toxins that are absorbed and poison the body. Table 19-3 lists several disease-causing pathogens as they relate to areas within the human body.

Transmission

Scientists have determined that certain germs can multiply every twelve minutes. If not controlled, germs may spread infection and diseases rapidly from one person to another. The principles of asepsis are applied in the hospital setting to prevent the spread of nosocomial (hospital-acquired) infection. The same emphasis on halting the spread of infection takes place in the medical office setting.

The presence of a pathogenic organism, or microorganism, is not enough to cause an infection to occur. Several factors must be in place for infection to occur. These are

1. The pathogen needs to be present.
2. A reservoir, or source, of disease including individuals who are ill with a disease and human carriers of disease who are unaware they have the disease but can still spread it.
3. A portal of exit, or means of escape, from the reservoir, for example through respiratory tract secretions, intestinal waste products, reproductive tract secretions, blood and blood products, and across the placenta barrier.

4. A means of transmission for the pathogen to pass directly from the reservoir to the new host. That is transmission of the pathogen directly from one person to another or indirect transmission as in the case when an inanimate object, such as milk or water, harbors the pathogen until it is transmitted to a human.

5. A portal of entry, or means of entry, such as the respiratory tract, skin and mucus membranes, reproductive and urinary tracts, blood, and across the placenta, for the pathogen into the new host.

6. A susceptible host which cannot fight off the pathogen.

Microorganisms normally found on the skin may enter the body through a portal of entry and then become pathogens. A portal of entry occurs where the body's defense, such as the skin, has broken down and allows direct access into the body. This can occur when the skin is cut as in a

TABLE 19-3   Disease-Producing Microorganisms

Body Location	Disease
Respiratory system (Nose and throat)	Strep throat (streptococcus)
	Diphtheria
	Scarlet fever
	Influenza (*Haemophilius influenzae* Type b)
	Upper Respiratory Tract Infection (URI)
Cerebrospinal system	Meningitis
Lungs	Pneumonia
	Tuberculosis
Heart and blood	Endocarditis
	Rheumatic fever
Liver	Hepatitis B (Serum hepatitis)
Immune system	AIDS
Intestines	Dysentery
	Typhoid
	Pinworms
	Hepatitis A (Acute infective hepatitis)
Organs of reproduction	Gonorrhea
	Syphilis
Skin	Boils (staphylococcus)
	Impetigo
	Scabies
	Head lice
Tissues	Gas gangrene
	Rheumatic fever (heart tissue)
	Tetanus

surgical incision, an injury causing a skin break, or in any invasive procedure such as the insertion of a needle in venipuncture. Figure 19-2 illustrates a chain of infection. The stages of the infection process are described in Table 19-4.

The Infection Control System

The body has several natural defense mechanisms to prevent the spread of infection. These include:

- Dietary intake of sufficient nutrients to promote health

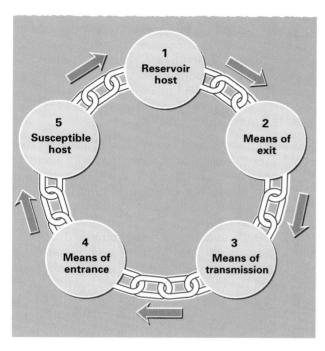

Figure 19-2   Chain of infection.

- Age of the person—the young and aged are more susceptible to diseases of the immune system due to immaturity of the immune system in the young and decrease in effectiveness of the system in the aged
- Adequate amount of rest
  Mechanisms which promote the spread of infection include:
- Presence of other disease processes in the body—diseases such as diabetes and pneumonia can weaken the system
- Genetic inheritance such as diabetes, anemia, cystic fibrosis

The spread of microorganisms can be prevented in two ways: by preventing their spread and by destroying the microorganisms themselves.

Prevention

The human body has several natural barriers to infection. These include the skin, mucous membranes, gastrointestinal tract, lymphoid and blood system. The largest natural barrier to infection is the intact skin. The acid pH of the skin inhibits bacterial action. Mucous membranes lining the body's orifices, respiratory, digestive, reproductive, and urinary tracts also assist in repelling microorganisms. The gastrointestinal tract, containing hydrochloric acid (HCl), causes a **bactericidal** action which destroys disease-producing bacteria.

Lymphoid and Blood System

The lymphoid and blood systems produce antibodies that protect the body from disease. Leukocytes (white blood cells) actively fight pathogenic microorganisms with the process of

TABLE 19-4   **Stages of the Infection Process**

Stage	Description
Invasion	Pathogen enters the body through the portal of entry: respiratory, digestive, reproductive, urinary tracts, and skin.
Multiplication	Reproduction of pathogens.
Incubation period	May vary from several days to months or years during which time the disease is developing but no symptoms appear.
Prodromal period	First mild signs and symptoms appear. A highly contagious period.
Acute period	Signs and symptoms are evident and most severe.
Recovery period	Signs and symptoms begin to subside.

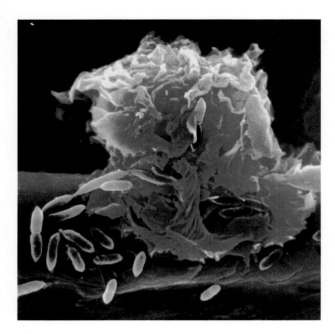

Figure 19-3   Phagocytosis.

phagocytosis. The process of phagocytosis is shown in Figure 19-3. During the process of inflammation, phagocytes engulf, digest, and destroy pathogens. Lymphocytes produce antibodies during the antigen-antibody reaction.

The Antigen-Antibody Reaction

Antibodies, which are protein substances produced by lymphocytes in the spleen, lymph nodes and tissue, and the bone marrow, react in response to antigens (foreign substances). Antibodies have the ability to neutralize antigens or make them more susceptible to phagocytosis. The antibody-antigen reaction occurs in reaction to an invasion of antigens. Immunity, a resistance to disease, is said to have occurred when enough antibodies have been produced to provide protection for weeks, months, or years. The body has a natural protective mechanism called immunity.

Immunity can either be genetic or acquired. Genetic immunity does not involve antibodies. Species immunity protects humans from certain animal diseases such as chicken cholera. It also protects animals from certain human diseases such as measles and influenza.

Acquired immunity, on the other hand, does involve the development of antibodies. This type of immunity may be either natural or artificial and may be acquired either through an active or passive means. Active immunity occurs when antigens are produced by the body. There are two types of active immunity: natural (person is born

with this immunity) and acquired (from an immunization or having had the disease such as with measles). Passive immunity develops when antibodies are artificially introduced into the body.

Active and passive immunity can be produced by both natural and acquired methods. Natural acquired immunity results from having recovered from a disease, such as measles, or being exposed to disease and becoming a carrier, such as in tuberculosis.

Artificial active immunity is the result of receiving vaccinations with inactivated (dead) or attenuated (weakened) organisms. For example, inactivated vaccines include influenza, whooping cough, typhoid, and the polio vaccine (Salk). Examples of attenuated vaccines are measles, polio (Sabin), smallpox, German measles (rubella), and mumps. Artificial passive immunity is produced by injecting a commercially prepared product to produce antibodies. Gamma globulin, used to prevent viral hepatitis, is an example. Acquired immunity is described in Table 19-5.

The Inflammatory Process

The body may react to the invasion of a foreign substance, such as bacteria or a virus, with an acute inflammatory process. This inflammatory process is the result of a tissue invasion of microorganisms from an injury, infection, or an allergy (antigen-antibody reaction).

The inflammatory process produces dilation of blood vessels due to an increased blood flow, production of watery fluids and materials (exudate), and the invasion of monocytes (white blood cells) and neutrophils into the injured tissues to produce phagocytosis. After phagocytosis occurs, the process of repair begins. The signs and symptoms of the inflammatory process are both local and systemic or traveling throughout the body system. See Table 19-6 for a description of this process.

Standard Precautions

The Centers for Disease Control and Prevention (CDC) in 1994 issued new isolation guidelines that emphasize two tiers of approach to infection control. The first and most important tier, or level, contains precautions designed to care for all patients in a health care setting regardless of their diagnosis or risk of infection. This tier contains precautions designed to decrease the risk of transmission of disease through body fluids. It is referred to as "Standard Precautions" and is used regardless of the patient's diagnosis or whether or not the patient has a known infectious disease. It uses the major features of universal precautions and body substance

TABLE 19-5　Acquired Immunity

Type of Immunity	Description
Active acquired natural	By having the disease which results in production of antibodies and "memory cells" which respond when the antigen reappears again.
Active acquired artificial	Administration of a vaccine which stimulates production of antibodies and "memory cells" to prevent that disease from occurring.
Passive acquired natural	Acquired from someone else's antibodies such as from the mother to the fetus through the placenta or through breast milk.
Passive acquired artificial	Temporary protection from gamma globulin (examples tetanus immune globulin, rabies antiserum).

TABLE 19-6　Acute Inflammatory Process

Local	Systemic
Redness	Leukocytosis
Heat	Fever
Swelling/edema	Increased pulse rate
Pain	Increased respiration rate
Stiffness	

isolation, which alerts those in the health care field to handle all materials as if they are contaminated.

Standard Precautions apply to 1) blood, 2) all body fluids (except sweat) regardless of whether they contain blood, 3) non-intact skin, and 4) mucus membranes. Body fluids include:

- Blood
- Body fluids containing visible blood
- Tissue specimens
- Semen
- Vaginal secretions
- Amniotic fluid
- Cerebrospinal fluid
- Pleural fluid
- Pericardial fluid
- Peritoneal fluid
- Interstitial fluid

Also included are feces, nasal secretions, sputum, tears, urine, vomitus, saliva, and breast milk which contain visible blood.

Standard Precautions promote handwashing and the use of gloves, masks, eye protection, or gowns when appropriate for patient contact. Masks, protective eyewear, gowns and gloves are referred to as a barrier type of protection. Standard Precautions are discussed in Table 19-7.

The second tier of the CDC guidelines is focused on the patients who are either suspected of carrying an infectious disease or are already infected. This second tier, which requires extra precautions in addition to the "Standard Precautions," is known as "Transmission-based Precautions." It includes three types of categories: Airborne Precautions, Droplet Precautions, and Contact Precautions.

- *Airborne Precautions* are designed to reduce the transmission of certain diseases, such as tuberculosis (TB), measles, or chickenpox. In addition to practicing Standard Precautions, use Airborne Precautions for patients who are known to be infected with microorganisms which are transmitted via airborne droplet nuclei (smaller than 5 microns) that can remain suspended in the air and widely dispersed throughout a room by air currents. Airborne precautions include isolation of the patient in a private room if hospitalized, with a mask and protective gown used by the health care worker. Hands must be washed before gloving and after gloves are removed. The transport of the patient should be as limited as possible with the patient wearing a mask during transport. All re-usable patient care equipment should be cleaned and disinfected before use on another patient.
- *Droplet Precautions* are used for patients known or suspected to be infected with microorganisms transmitted by droplets generated by a patient during coughing, sneezing, talking or performance of procedures that induce coughing. Examples of these illnesses include: invasive *Haemophilus influenzae* Type b disease (meningitis, pneumonia), invasive Neisseria meningitis disease (meningitis, pneumonia, and sepsis), diptheria, pertussis, streptococcal pneumonia,

TABLE 19-7 Standard Precautions—Equipment and Situations

Precaution	Description
Gloves	Must be worn when in contact with blood, all body fluids, secretions, excretions (except sweat) regardless of whether or not they contain visible blood, mucous membranes, nonintact skin, or contaminated articles.
Gown	Must be worn during procedures (or situations) in which there may be exposure to blood, body fluids, mucous membranes, or draining wounds. Wash hands after removing gown.
Mask/Protective Eyewear (goggles/shield)	Must be worn during procedures that are likely to generate droplets of blood or body fluids (splashes or sprays) as when a patient is coughing excessively.
Handwashing	Hands must be washed both before and after gloves are removed. Hands must be washed immediately if contaminated with blood or body fluids, between patient contact, and when indicated to prevent transfer of microorganisms between other patients and the environment.
Transportation	Precautions must be taken when transporting a patient to minimize the risk of transmitting microorganisms to other patients or environmental surfaces or equipment.
Multiple-use	Common multiple-use equipment, such as blood pressure cuffs or stethoscopes, must be cleaned and disinfected after use or when it becomes soiled with bodily fluids or blood. Single use items are discarded.
Needles and sharp instruments	Must be discarded into a puncture-proof container. Needles should not be recapped.

scarlet fever, mumps, and rubella. Precautions include isolation of the patient in a private room if hospitalized. Hands must be washed before and after gloves are worn. Gloves and gowns must be worn if coming into contact with bodily fluids or blood of the patient. A mask should be worn if the medical assistant is within three feet of the patient and transport of the patient should be limited. All re-usable equipment should be cleaned and disinfected.

- *Contact Precautions* are used for patients known to be infected with a microorganism that is not easily treated with antibiotics and which can be transmitted easily between the patient and health care worker or from patient to patient. Examples of these illnesses include: enteric (intestinal) infections, gastrointestinal, respiratory, skin, or wound infections, diphtheria, herpes simplex virus, impetigo, Hepatitis A, scabies, pediculosis, and zoster. Precautions include isolation of the patient in a private room if hospitalized. Gloves and gowns must be worn if coming

into contact with the patient. A mask and eyewear should be worn if there is potential for exposure to infectious body materials and fluids. When possible do not use patient care equipment on other patients.

Standard Precautions are summarized in Table 19-8.

OSHA

The CDC precautions are required and enforced by OSHA. On December 2, 1991, The Occupational Safety and Health Administration (OSHA) issued

Med Tip: The CDC's "Standard Precautions" are similar to "Universal Precautions" since both are directed at body fluids that are blood, blood-related, or fluids that contain blood. However, "Standard Precautions" are broader since they include precautions for any moist body substance.

TABLE 19-8 **Summary of Standard Precautions**

1. Wear protective barrier equipment (for example, face mask, eye shield, or goggles), when there is any risk of splashing, splattering or aerosolization (becoming airborne in small particles) of potentially infectious body fluids.

2. Wear gloves when there is any potential for exposure to blood or body fluids, secretions, excretions, and contaminated items. This includes performing routine clinical work, touching mucous membranes and the nonintact skin of patients, handling tissue and clinical specimens (Figure 19-4).

3. Wear gloves when drawing blood, including finger and heel sticks on infants, and during preparation of blood smears.

4. Change gloves after each patient. Wash hands before putting on gloves and after removing them.

5. Change gloves if they become contaminated with blood or other body fluids and dispose of properly in biohazardous container.

6. Wash hands or other skin surfaces if they become contaminated with potentially infectious blood or body fluids.

7. Care for linens and equipment that are contaminated with blood, blood products, body fluids, excretions, and secretions in a manner that avoids contact with your skin and mucous membranes or cross-contamination to another person.

8. Wear a gown or other protective clothing when there is a risk of splashing, splattering or other means of exposure to the patient's body fluids.

9. Wear a mask if a patient has an air-borne disease. A special mask is recommended if a patient has an active case of tuberculosis (TB).

10. Use care with needles, scalpels and other sharp instruments to avoid unintentional injury.

11. Dispose of needles and other sharp items in a rigid, puncture-resistance sharps container.

12. Do not recap or handle used needles.

13. Store reusable sharp instruments and needles in a puncture-resistant container.

14. Avoid mouth-to-mouth breathing in all but life threatening situations. Use a mechanical device or mask barrier instead.

15. Use a solution of household bleach (1:10 dilution) to disinfect environmental surfaces and reusable equipment.

16. Use hazardous waste containers for contaminated materials.

Adapted from "Guidelines for Isolation Precaution in Hospitals" developed by the Centers for Disease Control (CDC) and the Hospital Infection Control Practices Advisory Committee (HICPAC), January 1996.

its final standard on Occupational Bloodborne Pathogens which resulted from a concern that healthcare workers face a significant health risk in the occupational exposure to bloodborne pathogens, or disease producing organisms transmitted via the blood. All health care agencies were required to comply with this law by July 6, 1992.

This OSHA directive is aimed at minimizing exposure of health care workers to Hepatitis B virus (HBV) and Human Immunodeficiency Virus (HIV). The OSHA federal standard is now a law which states that Universal Precautions against transmission of bloodborne pathogens cannot just be recommended. They are law and must be observed by employers of health care personnel.

The OSHA guidelines apply to facilities in which the employees could be "reasonably anticipated" to come into contact with potentially infectious materials: body fluids, saliva, and tissues. See Chapter 10 for OSHA guidelines as they apply to all health care workers in a facility.

Physical and Chemical Barriers

Effective physical and chemical barriers are used to maintain infection control. The development of a nosocomial infection, or hospital/medical facility acquired infection, is prevented when careful medical and surgical asepsis is maintained.

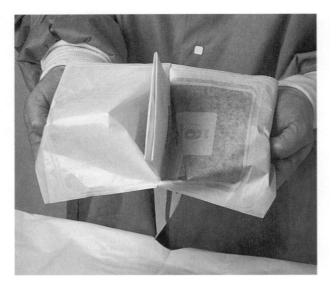

Figure 19-4   Sterile glove packet used for surgery.

Medical Asepsis

Medical asepsis refers to the destruction of organisms after they leave the body. Techniques, such as handwashing, using disposable equipment, and wearing gloves, can help reduce the number and transfer of pathogens. Aseptic technique is a means of reducing the transfer of pathogens in the medical office.

Ordinary hygiene habits of everyday life are a form of medical asepsis. These include handwashing when handling food or after using the bathroom and covering one's mouth during a cough or sneeze. One of the most effective means of reducing pathogenic transmission is through handwashing. This is considered the first stage of infection control since the hands are a primary method for infection to transfer from the host to the receiver. In order to keep the skin free of harmful organisms, there must be frequent handwashing using a disinfectant soap, friction, and warm running water. Jewelry, such as rings, allows germs to hide and grow. See Figure 19-5 for an illustration of hands with jewelry that is likely to catch pathogens.

Medical asepsis is used during "clean" procedures which involve body parts which normally are not sterile. Something is sterile when all microorganisms and spores are dead. Situations involving medical asepsis would include taking oral, aural, and rectal temperatures; obtaining throat or vaginal cultures or smears; obtaining urine, stool, or sputum specimens; administering medications; and cleaning treatment rooms.

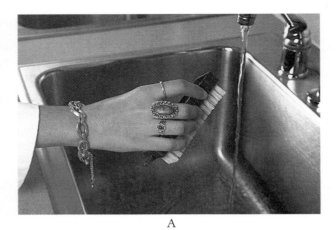

A

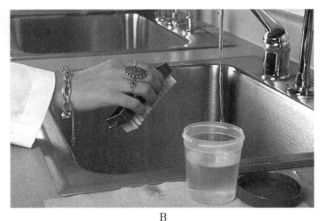

B

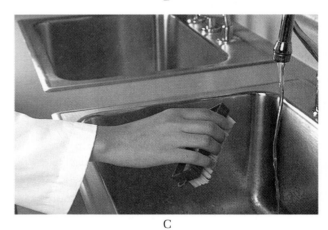

C

Figure 19-5 A-C   Jewelry provides places for pathogens to hide and grow.

Med Tip: Long fingernails should be avoided since a scratch from a nail can break down the body's first line of defense—the skin. In addition, long nails can puncture gloves allowing pathogens to enter.

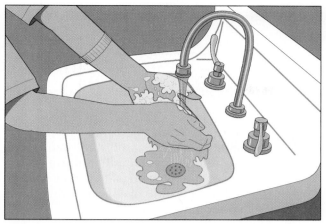

A Hold hands lower than elbows.

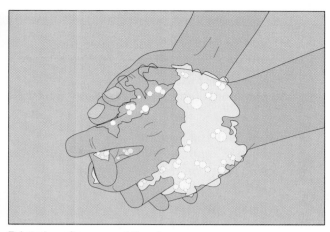

B Interlace fingers and thumbs.

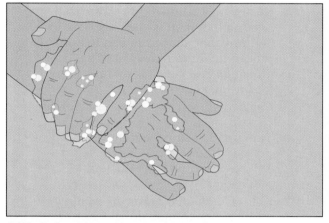

C Wash the wrists with a rotating motion.

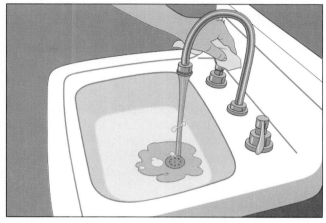

D Turn the water off with a dry paper towel.

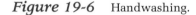

Figure 19-6   Handwashing.

Aseptic techniques which can cause a break in the chain of infection include

- Washing hands before and after any contact with patients or equipment.
- Handling all specimens and materials as though they contain pathogens.
- Using gloves to protect yourself when handling contaminated articles or materials, such as specimens.
- Not wearing jewelry which can attract bacteria.
- Using disposable equipment whenever possible. Dispose of all equipment properly after use.
- Cleaning all nondisposable equipment as soon as possible after patient use.
- Using only clean or sterile supplies for each patient.

- Using a protective covering over your clothes if there is any danger of contaminated materials or supplies coming into contact with your uniform.
- Discarding items that fall on the floor if they cannot be cleaned. All floors are considered contaminated. If in doubt, throw it out!
- Placing all wet or damp dressings and bandages in a waterproof bag to protect persons handling the garbage.

Handwashing

Handwashing provides the first defense against the spread of disease and should be done often. See Figure 19-6 for a demonstration of proper handwashing technique.

PROCEDURE: Handwashing

Terminal Performance
Competency: Student will perform handwashing procedure without error.

Equipment and Supplies
- Soap in liquid soap dispenser
- Nail brush or orange cuticle stick
- Hot running water
- Paper towels
- Waste container

Procedural Steps

1. Remove jewelry (includes rings with the exception of wedding band, watch, bracelets). ***Rationale:*** Jewelry has crevices and grooves which can harbor bacteria and dirt.

2. Stand at sink without allowing clothing to touch sink. Turn water on using paper towel. Discard paper towel. ***Rationale:*** Avoid direct contact with contaminated faucets. Sinks are also considered contaminated. Paper towel is contaminated after touching the faucet(s).

3. Adjust running water to correct lukewarm temperature. Discard paper towel. ***Rationale:*** Hot water may burn skin and cold water will not allow soap lather to form. Improper water temperature can cause chapping and cracking of skin which allows pathogens to enter.

4. Wet hands under running water and place liquid soap (size of a nickel or 1 teaspoon) into palm of hand. If using bar soap, keep the bar in hands and use enough soap to form a lather. Work soap into a lather by moving it over palms, sides, and backs—the entire surface—of both hands for 2 minutes. Use a circular motion and friction. Interlace fingers and move soapy water between them.

Rationale: Friction assists in removing organisms and dirt. If soap bar falls into sink or onto floor during the procedure the medical assistant must start procedure over again. Only use bar soap if liquid soap is unavailable. Soap bars allow the growth of bacteria to occur and must be thoroughly rinsed after each use.

5. Keep hands pointed downward with hands and forearms at elbow level or below during the entire handwashing procedure. ***Rationale:*** Water will run off hands and not back up onto arms for further contamination.

6. Use hand brush and/or orange cuticle stick to clean under fingernails. Thoroughly scrub wedding band if present. ***Rationale:*** Running water and soap may not be sufficient to remove dirt particles under nails.

7. Rinse hands under running water with fingers pointed down using care not to touch the sink or faucets. ***Rationale:*** The sink is not sterile (only clean) and may have contaminants present. Running water will wash away dirt and organisms.

8. Reapply soap and wash wrists and forearms for 1 more minute using circular motions.

9. Rinse hands under running water.

10. Dry hands thoroughly with paper towel. Discard paper towel.

11. Using a dry paper towel turn faucet off. ***Rationale:*** Paper towel will protect clean hands from coming into contact with contaminated faucet handles.

Protective Clothing and Equipment

Protective clothing, such as gowns, gloves, and masks, are worn for two reasons. They are

1. To protect the patient from any microorganisms that might be present on the health care worker's street clothing.
2. To protect the health care worker from carrying microorganisms away from the patient.

In addition, protective devices, such as gloves and masks, assist in protecting the health care worker from contamination with bloodborne pathogens. Nonsterile gowning technique is used for procedures, such as drawing blood, specimen collection, infant handling, and when in contact with a patient who is in isolation. Figure 19-7 A-D illustrates nonsterile gown technique.

Figure 19-8 shows proper technique for putting on an isolation gown and Figure 19-9A-I illustrates how to remove an isolation gown. Proper step-by-step technique for removing gloves is shown in Figure 19-10 A-E.

Surgical Asepsis

Surgical asepsis refers to the techniques practiced to maintain a sterile environment. It is the destruction of organisms before they enter the body.

There are three important steps to take to reach sterility, which is the absence of microorganisms.

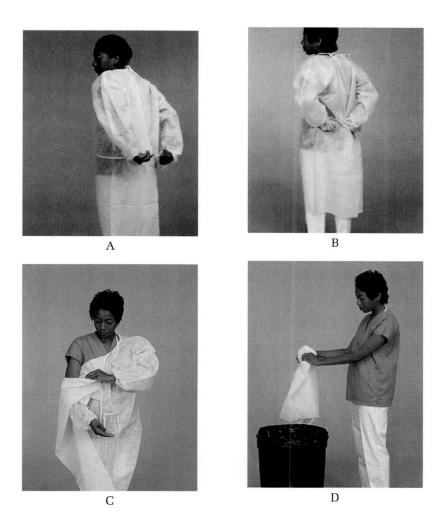

A

B

C

D

Figure 19-7 A-D   (A) Tie the neck piece of the gown and over lap the flaps. (B) Tie the gown securely at the waist. If gloves are to be worn, put them on now. (C) To take off a gown, remove and dispose of gloves properly if you are wearing them. Untie neck and waist. Grasp shoulders. Turn gown inside out as you remove it. (D) Fold up the gown and discard. Do not reuse a gown. Wash your hands.

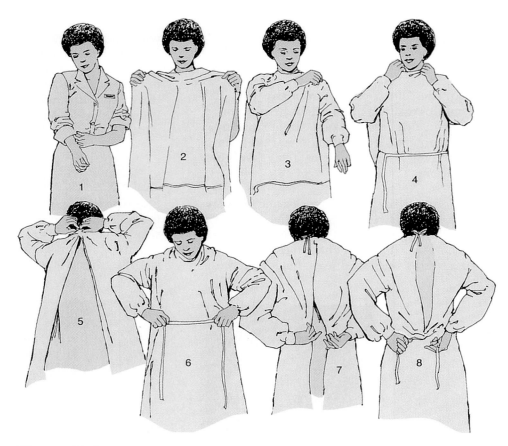

Figure 19-8 Putting on an isolation gown.

These methods for preventing the spread of disease in the medical office are sanitization, disinfection, and sterilization. Sanitization inhibits or inactivates pathogens by means of scrubbing and washing items. Disinfection destroys most or all pathogens on inanimate objects with the use of chemicals such as iodine, chlorine, alcohol and phenol. Sterilization is the destruction of all living organisms and spores with the use of pressurized steam, extreme temperatures, or radiation.

Sanitization

Sanitization includes the careful scrubbing of equipment and instruments using a brush and detergent with a neutral *p*H, such as a soapless soap, rinsing in hot water, and air drying. Sanitization cleans items, but microorganisms and bacteria are not destroyed. Supplies and equipment that do not come into direct contact with the patient or touch only the skin surface must be sanitized. If contaminated material cannot be sanitized immediately, then it should be soaked in detergent and water according to the manufacturer's instructions.

Another means of sanitizing equipment is with the use of ultrasound. In this case the instruments and equipment are placed into a bath tank and sound waves vibrate to break up the contamination. The articles are then rinsed thoroughly. Always follow the instructions of your supervisor regarding the proper procedure for sanitizing instruments or use the procedure provided here.

Disinfection

Disinfection involves a soaking and wiping process. Disinfection destroys or inhibits the activity of disease-causing organisms. Disinfecting agents include chemical germicides, flowing steam, and boiling water. Chemical germicides are used to disinfect heat-perishable objects in the medical office, including some rubber and plastic items, clean floors, and office furniture. Two common disinfectants are zephrin chloride and chlorophenyl.

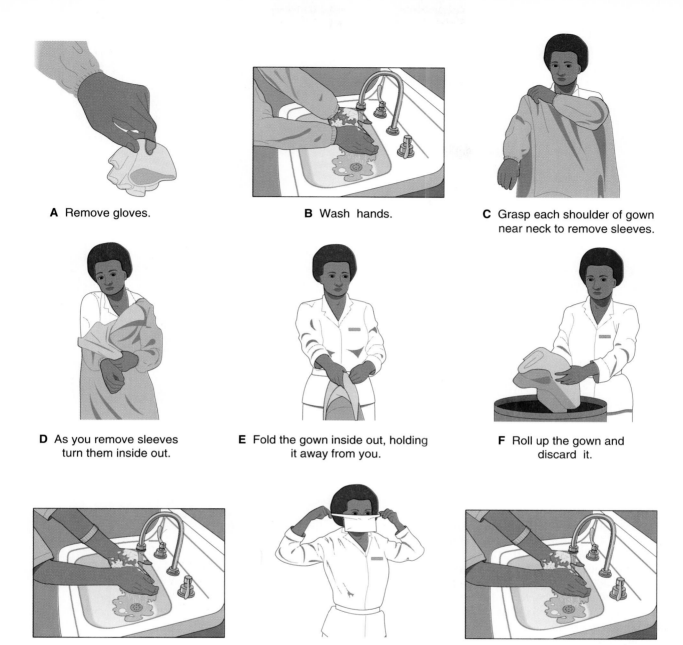

A Remove gloves.

B Wash hands.

C Grasp each shoulder of gown near neck to remove sleeves.

D As you remove sleeves turn them inside out.

E Fold the gown inside out, holding it away from you.

F Roll up the gown and discard it.

G Wash your hands.

H Remove your mask.

I Wash your hands.

Figure 19-9 A-I Removing an isolation gown.

Contaminated instruments and equipment are completely immersed in a germicidal solution according to the manufacturer's instructions from 1 to 10 hours. They are then rinsed in water. (Instruments are rinsed in distilled water to prevent rust and corrosion.) Instruments must be dried after disinfection and rinsing.

Disinfectants can eliminate many organisms, but are not effective against spores (dormant stage of some bacteria), spore-forming bacteria, and some viruses. Some disinfectants, while effective on objects, may be too strong to use on patients (as for example, formaldehyde). The disinfectants, alcohol, and betadine are used when preparing a patient's skin for surgical procedures or injections since antiseptics prevent the growth of some microorganisms.

Objects that come into contact with mucous membranes, such as vaginal speculums, laryngoscopes or thermometers, should be disinfected or even sterilized, if possible. Instruments that cannot

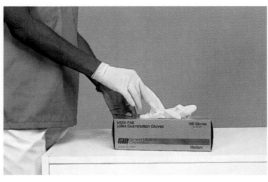

A

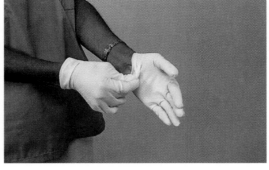

C

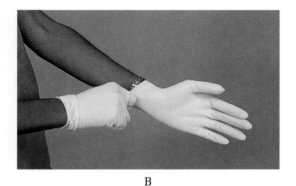

B

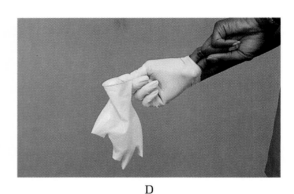

D

Figure 19-10 A-E Removing gloves. (A) Use a clean pair of gloves for each patient contact. (B) Grasp the glove just below the cuff. (C) Pull the glove over your hand while turning the glove inside out. (D) Place the ungloved index finger and middle finger inside cuff of the glove, turning the cuff downward. (E) Pull the cuff and glove inside out as you remove your hand from the glove.

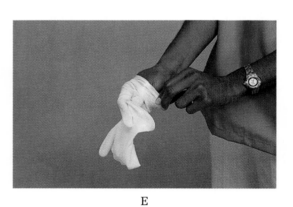

E

be soaked, such as scopes, computers, and electrical instruments) are wiped thoroughly with a germicidal solution. To be effective the entire instrument or item must be fully submersed. Items are generally left in the solution for 15 to 45 minutes. Germicidal solutions must be changed frequently according to the manufacturer's instructions. The chemical disinfection process is referred to as a "cold" process since no heat is used or generated (Figure 19-11).

Chemical disinfectants used for soaking and wiping include soap, alcohol, phenol, acid, alka-

lines (such as bleach), and formaldehyde. Some of these are discussed in Table 19-9.

A means of disinfection that is used in operating rooms is ultra violet rays. Equipment that cannot be soaked is placed under the ultraviolet lamps for a specified period of time. This will kill microorganisms.

Another means of disinfection is the use of boiling water. Moist heat of up to 212°F will kill most forms of pathogens. This is not useful for killing viruses, such as the hepatitis virus or spores which are resistant to other methods of

PROCEDURE: Sanitizing Instruments

**Terminal Performance
Competency:** The student will able to clean and sanitize instruments with no visible contamination remaining.

Equipment and Supplies

Disposable gloves

Rubber (utility) gloves

Plastic Brush

Towel

Sink

Running Water

Container which will hold all the instruments

Low-sudsing (low pH) detergent or germicidal agent

Note: Instruments should be rinsed under warm running water immediately after surgery to remove gross blood, body fluids and tissue. If it is not possible to clean them immediately, instruments should be submerged in water containing a low pH detergent.

Procedural Steps

1. Apply both disposable and rubber gloves. *Rationale:* Instruments have sharp edges which can cut through disposable gloves. Instruments are contaminated with blood and other waste materials.

2. Place low-sudsing (low pH) detergent or germicidal agent in large container with water. Rinse all instruments. *Rationale:* This will clean off gross blood and waste products. A low pH detergent prevents staining on stainless steel surfaces.

3. Rinse instruments in clear water in either sink or container. Delicate and sharp instruments should be separated from general instruments.

4. Scrub each instrument individually with brush and detergent under running water. Open instruments to thoroughly scrub all serrated edges and hinge areas. *Rationale:* Blood and other debris collect in hinges, cracks and on serrated edges.

5. Rinse instrument thoroughly under hot water. *Rationale:* Any detergent left on instrument will prevent the disinfection process.

6. If instruments cannot be cleaned immediately after use then soak them in a solution of water and a blood solvent. When ready to wash instruments begin with step 1. *Rationale:* Soaking instruments prevents blood and other organic material to harden. Hardened blood is difficult to remove.

7. After thoroughly rinsing cleaned instruments, roll them in a towel to dry them. *Rationale:* Drying instruments prevents rust.

8. Check condition of all instruments for defects or remaining soil.

9. Wrap instrument(s) for sterilization.

disinfection. Sterilization cannot occur at this temperature. Stainless-steel, glassware, and instruments can be boiled without damage. The articles are submerged in a container filled with cold water. The water must completely cover the articles to be disinfected. Distilled water should be used when boiling instruments or stainless steel to prevent sediment or deposits from forming. The water is then brought to the boiling point and continues to boil for 20 to 30 minutes for disinfection. When the boiling time has elapsed, the disinfected materials are allowed to cool. To maintain disinfection they must be touched only with sterile forceps.

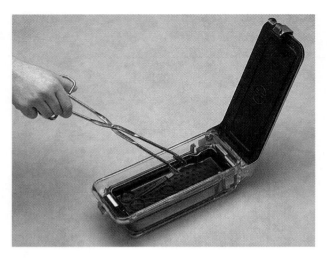

Figure 19-11   Cold chemical sterilizer.

Sterilization

Sterilization results in killing all microorganisms, both pathogenic and nonpathogenic. The use of heat (steam or dry), chemicals, high-velocity electron bombardment, or ultraviolet light radiation are used for this process. Heat sterilization, produced by an autoclave under steam pressure, is able to kill spores, bacteria, and other microorganisms. Dry heat is used for dense ointments such as petroleum jelly.

All supplies including dressings, needles, and instruments that come into contact with internal body tissue or an open wound must be sterile. Once a sterile article is touched by hands or another unsterile object, it is considered contaminated. Sterile gloves must be used when touching sterilized items. See Figure 19-12 A-H for illustration of sterile gloving technique and Figure 19-13A-B for guidelines for removing gloves.

Autoclave

The methods used for sterilization include the autoclave and chemical (cold) sterilization. The autoclave process is an effective means of sterilization in the medical office. Types of autoclaving include: steam under pressure, dry heat (320°F for 1 hour), dry gas, or radiation.

Autoclaving is steam under pressure which destroys the organisms by causing them to explode. This method of sterilization requires 15 pounds of

TABLE 19-9   Disinfection Methods

Method	Description and Use
Alcohol (70% isopropyl)	Used for skin surfaces, equipment such as stethoscopes and thermometers, and table surfaces
	Causes damage to rubber products, lens, and plastic
	Flammable
Chlorine (sodium hypochlorite or bleach)	Use in dilution of 1:10 (one part bleach to 10 parts water)
	Used to eliminate a broad spectrum of microorganisms
	Corrosive effect on instruments, rubber, and plastic products
	Can cause skin irritation
	Inexpensive
Formaldehyde	Used to disinfect and sterilize
	Dangerous product which is regulated by OSHA—must have clearly marked labels
Hydrogen peroxide	Effective disinfectant only for use on non-human surfaces and products
	May damage rubber, plastic, and metals
Glutaraldehyde	Effective against viruses, bacteria, fungi and some spores
	Regulated by OSHA—must have clearly marked labels and use in well ventilated area
	Must wear gloves and masks when using

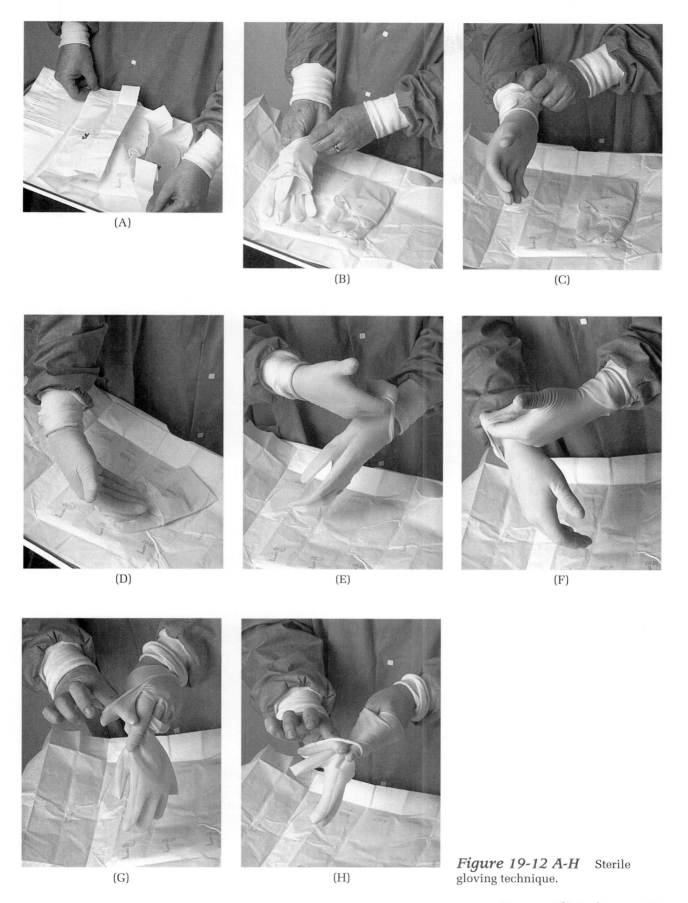

(A)

(B)

(C)

(D)

(E)

(F)

(G)

(H)

Figure 19-12 A-H Sterile gloving technique.

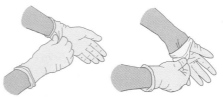

A Grasping the glove just below the cuff with the gloved fingers of the other hand, pull the glove over your hand, while turning it inside out.

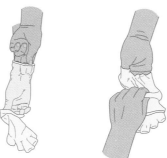

B Place the ungloved index and middle fingers inside the cuff of the glove, turning the cuff downward, pulling it inside out, as you remove it from your hand.

Figure 19-13 A-B   Guidelines for removing gloves.

pressure and a temperature of 250-270°F depending on manufacturer's recommendations. Distilled water must be used in the steam autoclave. The autoclave consists of an outer chamber (jacket), which creates a build-up of steam that is forced into the inner chamber, and an inner chamber in which the materials to be sterilized are placed (Figure 19-14). Depending on the model type there may be three gauges on the autoclave 1) a jacket pressure gauge to indicate pressure in outer chamber; 2) a chamber pressure gauge to indicate the steam pressure in inner chamber; and 3) a temperature gauge to indicate temperature in inner chamber in which items are placed. Some of the newer models have only one gauge. The temperature used in autoclaving (250°F) must be reached before autoclaving the materials. Figure 19-15 displays an ultraclave automatic autoclave/sterilizer.

The microorganisms are killed in autoclaving by the condensation of steam on each of the items, not by the heat produced. Heat is actually transferred to the items by way of the steam condensation. Steam sterilization is not effective if air pockets are present within the packs. A pump within the autoclave will first remove air from the chamber. The pressure level and temperature levels within the autoclave chamber can be built up only after the air is removed. Therefore the gauges indicating pressure and temperature must be monitored by the medical assistant. Table 19-10 describes autoclave sterilization time requirements.

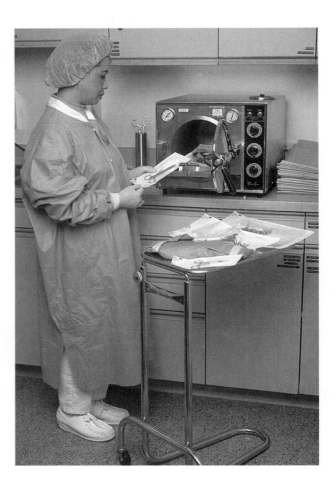

Figure 19-14   Autoclave.

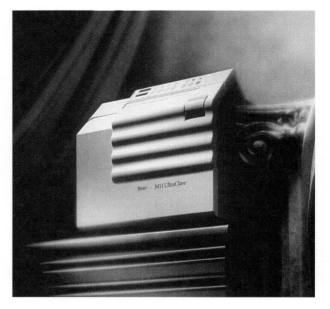

Figure 19-15   Ritter M11 Ultra Clave™ Automatic Sterilizer.

TABLE 19-10 **Sterilization Time Requirements**

Time	Article
15 minutes	Glassware
	Metal Instruments (open tray or individual wrapping with hinges open)
	Syringes (unassembled)
	Needles
20 minutes	Instruments—partial metal in double-thickness wrapper or covered tray
	Rubber products: gloves, tubing, catheters wrapped or unwrapped
	Solutions in a flask (50-100 mL)
30 minutes	Dressings—small packs in paper or muslin
	Solutions in a flask (500-1000 mL)
	Syringes—unassembled individually wrapped in gauze
	Syringes—unassembled individually wrapped in glass tubes
	Needles—individually packaged in paper or glass tubes
	Sutures—wrapped in paper or muslin
	Instrument and treatment trays—wrapped in paper or muslin
	Gauze—loosely packed
60 minutes	Petroleum jelly—in dry heat

Med Tip: Timing for autoclave sterilization cannot begin until both the temperature and pressure gauges are at the recommended manufacturer's reading. These recommendations must be carefully followed.

The autoclave should be thoroughly cleaned (sanitized) and free of any materials or lint before using. If detergent or other cleaner is used for cleaning, it should be completely rinsed before placing objects into the autoclave. The air exhaust valve must be cleaned and free of lint after each use.

The wrapping in which the instruments and materials, such as dressings, to be sterilized are placed must be permeable, or allow steam to pass through and be strong enough to hold together during the steam process. Wrapping materials include heavy paper, muslin, plastic, and stainless steel containers. See Figure 19-16 A-D for an illustration of how to wrap instruments for the autoclave. Instruments with hinges should be open, tubing free of any kinks, and syringes unassembled before wrapping.

The wrapping generally consists of two layers of permeable materials. All items must be completely covered with the wrapping material and fastened with tape which states the date of sterilization and identifies the item. Figure 19-17 displays tapes that have changed color during the sterilization process.

Sterilization pouches or bags are often used for individual instruments. Careful inspection must be made to make sure the bag has not ruptured or been punctured during the autoclave process. Small, lightweight instruments are suitable for pouches. The pouches have sterilization indicators both inside and outside the bag.

Instruments which will be used immediately can be placed in perforated trays and autoclaved unwrapped. Instruments can be sterilized in instrument trays. The lid for the tray is placed next to the open tray of instruments. The lid is immediately placed over the instruments after sterilization. A towel is usually placed under the instruments to absorb moisture during autoclaving.

Items should be wrapped in individual packs which can be handled for storage and use by their outer wrapping without contaminating the inner items. When the autoclaved package is opened, the contents are removed without contaminating them. The autoclave chamber must not be overloaded or the steam will not be able to penetrate the wrapping and sterilize the instruments and materials. Items should be placed on their edges to permit the proper penetration with moisture and heat.

Containers and jars of supplies should be placed on their sides for full sterilization to occur. Solutions should be autoclaved separately since they may boil over during autoclaving. The lid of plastic containers and bags will become sealed upon sterilization.

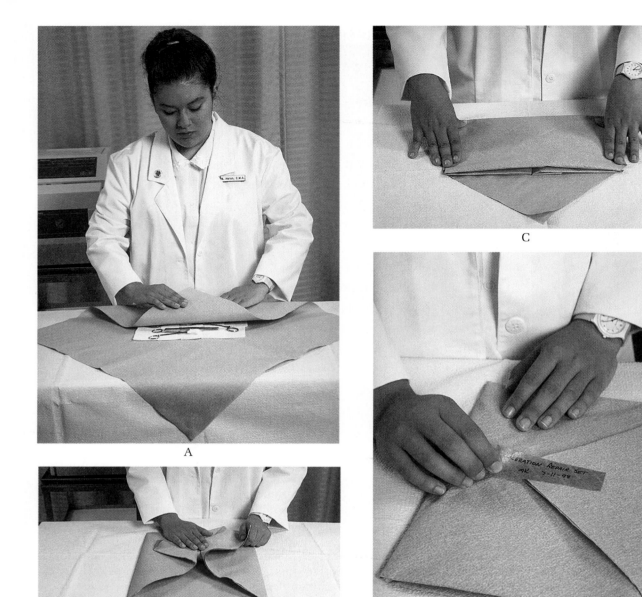

Figure 19-16 A–D Wrapping instruments for the autoclave.

The time or pressure required for autoclaving, according to the manufacturer's recommendations, must never be shortened. If proper timing and pressure is not observed when autoclaving, the items will become warm but not sterile.

Drying Autoclaved Goods

After the process is complete, the drying process is almost as important as the correct temperature and pressure in autoclaving. Wetness on items ("wet packs") can cause a break in sterility since moisture will allow bacteria to grow and be transmitted into the inside of the package. A towel can be placed in the bottom of the autoclave tray to absorb some moisture. "Wet Packs" can be

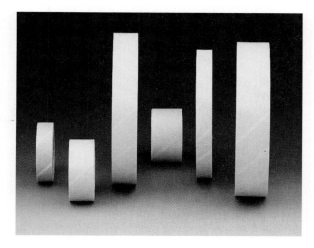

Figure 19-17   Autoclave indicator tape.

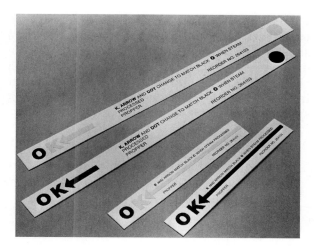

Figure 19-18   Sterility checks.

avoided by allowing for a drying period at the end of autoclaving. To do this open the door of the autoclave 3/4 inch (but no more) just before the drying cycle on the autoclave. Run the dry cycle according to the manufacturer's directions.

Sterilization Indicators

Indicators are used to signify sterilization. Note that the change of color or dots appearing in an indicator strip only indicate that steam has entered the chamber and not that the instruments are sterile. OK strips are placed inside the wrapper or in the chamber. Autoclaving tape turns black after autoclaving. Indicators come in a variety of types including strips and tape. The strips are placed in the center of a pack to indicate that the inner contents have been exposed to the conditions for sterility: correct temperature, correct time, and exposure to moisture. Figure 19-18 illustrates sterility checks.

Shelf-Life

Autoclaved packages are stored with the date visible and the oldest date in front of the stack so that it is used first. Instruments are considered sterile for 21-

Med Tip: Do not open the autoclave door all the way during the drying cycle since the cold air from the room will enter the autoclave and cause condensation to form on the packs and instruments. The rule to follow is that all autoclaved materials should be completely dry when they are removed and remain dry for 1 hour after removal.

30 days (21 days in plastic bags and 30 days in muslin), with a shelf-life of approximately one month. Shelf-life is dependent upon the type of wrapper used. The individual manufacturer's guidelines should be followed concerning when to reclean and resterilize the item. Autoclaved packages cannot be reautoclaved in the same packages without washing, rinsing, drying and rewrapping each item.

Hepatitis and AIDS

Two diseases that require special attention during a discussion of infection control are hepatitis and AIDS since both these diseases affect several million people.

Hepatitis

Hepatitis is a viral disease of the liver resulting in inflammation and infection. Forms of hepatitis are A, B, C, D, and E.

Hepatitis A (Acute Infective Hepatitis)

Hepatitis A is transmitted by fecal waste contamination of food and the water supply. This occurs when food and water become contaminated with fecal waste products of animals or humans. The incubation period, or period of time during which the disease develops after exposure into symptoms, is from 14 to 50 days with a very slow onset of symptoms including fever, loss of appetite, jaundice, nausea, vomiting, malaise, dark urine, and whitish stools.

Hepatitis B (Serum Hepatitis)

Hepatitis B, also called HBV, is transmitted through body fluids including blood, semen, saliva, and breast milk which are contaminated with the virus. This potentially fatal disease can be passed from one drug user to another when sharing a contaminated needle. Hepatitis B is on the increase due to its appearance in persons with HIV and AIDS. The incubation period for this liver infection is 60 to 90 days with a rapid onset of symptoms. HBV symptoms include

- Fever
- Chills
- Diarrhea with clay-colored stools
- Nausea and vomiting
- Orange-brown urine
- Headache
- Anorexia
- Enlarged liver
- Jaundice

The diagnosis of HBV is made through a liver biopsy to identify the virus. Treatment for all forms of hepatitis is a high-protein diet and rest. Treatment for HBV may last for several weeks with the possibility of relapse.

There are two types of vaccine available for HBV: one made from human serum and the other a synthetic product. HBV vaccine is administered in three doses; the second dose one month after the first and the third dose six months later.

Pediatricians and health officials are now recommending that infants and adolescents be vaccinated for hepatitis B due to the rising incidence of this disease. The schedule for infants is for the first dose to be given at time of birth.

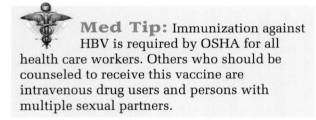 **Med Tip:** Immunization against HBV is required by OSHA for all health care workers. Others who should be counseled to receive this vaccine are intravenous drug users and persons with multiple sexual partners.

Hepatitis C

Hepatitis C, also referred to as non-A and non-B hepatitis, is the most common form of new hepatitis cases every year. The symptoms and treatment are similar to those of hepatitis B.

Hepatitis D

Hepatitis D, also called delta hepatitis, is the most recently identified form of hepatitis. The symptoms of this form of hepatitis can be more severe than with other forms of hepatitis. Hepatitis D is spread through the use of intravenous drugs and intimate contact. There is a

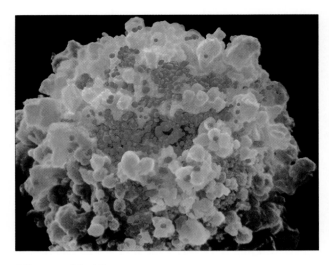

Figure 19-19 The AIDS virus.

rapid growth of this form of hepatitis due to the increased number of HIV and AIDS cases in which it is seen.

Hepatitis E

Hepatitis E is the result of exposure to food contaminated with human feces. It is a major infectious disease in developing countries due to poor sanitary conditions.

HIV/AIDS

Acquired immune deficiency syndrome (AIDS) was first documented in the United States in 1980. This disorder of the immune system was first noted when five homosexual young men were treated for an unusual form of pneumonia, *Pneumocystis carinii,* in Los Angeles. At approximately the same time, doctors were noticing the occurrence of a rare blood vessel malignancy, Kaposi's sarcoma, in homosexual young men in California and New York. The combination of these disorders came to be associated with a syndrome caused by a virus, the human immunodeficiency virus (HIV). Figure 19-19 depicts the AIDS virus.

The Centers for Disease Control in Atlanta reports that about 1.5 million Americans have been infected with HIV and over one-quarter million have AIDS. Globally, the World Health Organization (WHO) suspects there are as many as 15 million cases of HIV and 5 millions cases of AIDS. There is not a cure for HIV or AIDS at this time and people with the disease will have it for the rest of their lives.

This infectious virus causes the immune system, which is the body's shield against infection, to break down and eventually become ineffective by invading the body's macrophages and T-cells, which fight disease. When the T-cells are invaded they render the macrophages useless for fighting off pathogenic invasions.

The various means by which the AIDS virus can enter the body are listed below. They are

- Vaginal, anal, or oral intercourse with a person who has the virus
- Sharing needles or syringes with a person who has the virus
- Receiving transfusions of blood or blood products donated by someone who has the virus
- Receiving organ transplants from a donor who has the virus
- Contaminating open wounds or sores with blood, semen, or vaginal secretions infected with the virus
- Having artificial insemination with the sperm of a man who has the virus

A mother's fetus, or unborn child, may become infected if she contracts the virus before or during her pregnancy. An infant could become infected by being breast fed by a woman with the virus.

The virus can survive well in body fluids such as blood, semen, and vaginal secretions. The virus can stay in cells for months, and even years. During this time the cells will replicate, or reproduce, themselves. The body's defensive T-cells are eventually destroyed by the new viral cells.

Some HIV victims will develop AIDS-related complex (ARC) which has less serious symptoms than AIDS. ARC symptoms include loss of appetite and weight loss, diarrhea, skin rash, fatigue, night sweating, swollen lymph glands, and poor resistance to infection.

Not all HIV patients develop AIDS or any other HIV-related condition. Estimates, according to the CDC, range from 50 percent to 90 percent of patients developing full-blown AIDS. It may take eight to ten years for symptoms of HIV infection to develop and 12 years or more for symptoms of AIDS to develop. The stages of HIV infection are listed below:

- After becoming infected with HIV, it may take a person six weeks to three years to develop antibodies (which means they will not test positive for HIV). Before developing these antibodies, some people with HIV have symptoms that are usually brief but not severe. These might include slight fever, headaches, fatigue, and swollen glands for a few weeks.
- After antibodies develop, the person will test positive for HIV. However, another

period with no symptoms may occur. This "incubation period" can last several years. However, even though there are no symptoms, the immune system becomes increasingly damaged during this time.
- Next, a person with HIV may experience a long period of swelling of the lymph glands in the throat, armpits, and groin. This condition is called "persistent generalized lymphadenopathy" and may last a number of years.
- When HIV has seriously damaged the immune system, a condition called AIDS-related complex (ARC) may occur. These symptoms can include a white coating of the mouth and throat (thrush), similar infections of the skin and mucous membranes of the anus and genital area, and severe viral infections such as herpes.

Med Tip: It is not possible to tell if a person has HIV just by looking at the person. Many people do not know they have HIV because they have no symptoms. In order to be protected, you must use standard precautions as if everyone you come into contact with has HIV or AIDS.

AIDS, the final stage of an HIV infection, includes a variety of viral, fungal, bacterial, parasitic infections, nervous disorders, and cancers. These infections are often present in the healthy body and can be overcome by the immune system. However, in the AIDS patient, the immune system is no longer effective and, hence, the infections become life-threatening. These infections, called opportunistic infections, include:

- *Pneumocystis carinii* pneumonia (PCP)
- Kaposi's sarcoma—a type of skin cancer
- Toxoplasmosis—infestation of parasites that infect the brain and central nervous system

Tuberculosis (TB) is seen with increasing frequency among persons infected with HIV. HIV infection is one of the strongest known risk factors for the progression of TB from infection to disease. However, of the diseases associated with HIV infection, TB is one of the few that is transmissible, treatable, and preventable. An estimated 5% of all AIDS patients have TB according to the CDC.

AIDS is diagnosed based on several factors: functioning ability of the immune system based on tests such as T-cell counts, the presence of one or

Med Tip: Note that testing positive for HIV antibodies does not necessarily mean that a person has, or will develop, AIDS. Positive test results, if leaked to an employer or insurance company, can lead to loss of job, on-the-job harassment, or other serious consequences, even though such actions may be illegal.

more opportunistic infections, and the presence of HIV antibodies. The HIV or AIDS Antibody test, known as ELISA (Enzyme-Linked ImmunoSorbent Assay), is used as a screening test. With a positive ELISA, a patient is said to be HIV positive or HIV antibody positive. The Western Blot test is used to confirm results of the ELISA.

HIV does not survive well outside the human body, and it is not transmitted through air, food, water, pets, or bugs. The virus has been found in tears, saliva, urine, and breast milk. HIV is destroyed by a 1:10 household bleach solution or an application of heat treatment at 132°F (56° C) for 10 minutes. Standard Precautions which include the use of aseptic technique, gloving, careful handling of needles and syringes to avoid puncture wounds, can prevent contracting the virus by health care workers.

HIV and AIDS are no longer considered to be diseases of the homosexual population since they have become increasingly prevalent in women and children.

Med Tip: HIV cannot be obtained from donating blood. The disease is not transmitted through casual contact such as touching.

The symptoms of AIDS are described below:

- T-cell count less than 200 (normal range for T-cells is 500 cells per cubic millimeter of blood).
- Unexplained weight loss of 10-15 pounds in less than 2 months that is not associated with diet or exercise.
- Long-lasting occurrences of diarrhea.
- Unexplained fever, chills, and drenching night sweats for more than 2 weeks.
- Unexplained extreme fatigue.
- Swelling or hardening of lymph glands located in the throat, groin, or armpit.
- Periods of continued, deep, dry coughing that are not due to other illnesses or smoking.
- Increased shortness of breath.
- Appearance of discolored or purplish growths on the skin or inside the mouth.
- Unexplained bleeding from growths on the skin, mucous membranes, or from any opening on the body.
- Severe numbness or pain in the hands and feet, loss of motor control and reflex, paralysis or loss of muscular strength.
- Altered state of consciousness, personality change, or mental deterioration.

There is presently no cure for AIDS. The drugs AZT (zidovudine) and ddC (zalcitabie) have been found effective in boosting the immune system and prolonging life. A combination of these two drugs has resulted in an increase of T-cell counts in some individuals. Supportive measures to improve the quality of life for the AIDS patient include delivery of home meals, nutritional supplements, and hospice care.

The medical assistant may be asked to provide information to a caregiver. Recommendations for caring for someone with AIDS are presented in Table 19-11.

TABLE 19-11 Caring for Someone with AIDS

To protect themselves from infection, caregivers should be reminded to do the following:

- Handle all needles with care. Never replace caps back on needles or remove needles from syringes. Dispose of all needles in puncture-proof containers out of the reach of children.
- Wear latex or rubber gloves if they have any contact with blood, blood-tinged body fluids, urine, feces, or vomit.
- Wash hands after removing gloves.
- Any cut, open sore, or breaks on exposed skin of either the patient or caregiver should be covered with a bandage.
- Flush all liquid waste containing blood down the toilet using care to avoid splashing during pouring. Non-flushable items such as paper towels, sanitary pads and tampons, wound dressings, or items

(Continued on next page)

TABLE 19-11 (Continued)

soiled with blood, semen, or vaginal fluid should be enclosed in a plastic bag and tightly sealed. Check with your local health department or physician to determine trash disposal regulations for your area.

- Use a disinfection solution of one part bleach to 10 parts water to disinfect such items as floors, showers, tubs, sinks. Discard solution in toilet after using.

To protect the person with AIDS from infection:

- If the caregiver has a cold or flu, and there is no one else available to care for the AIDS patient, a surgical-type mask should be worn.
- Wash your hands before touching the AIDS patient.
- Any one with boils, fever blisters (herpes simplex), or shingles (zoster) should avoid close contact with the patient.
- Gloves should be worn if the caregiver has a rash or sores on their hands.
- Persons living with or caring for an AIDS patient should have received all the recommended childhood immunizations and booster shots, including the hepatitis vaccine.
- The AIDS patient should not be in the same room with a person who has, or is recovering from, chickenpox.

The caregiver should:

- Call the local AIDS service organization for support.
- Seek the help of clergy, counselors, and other health care professionals to help cope with feelings of frustration and stress.
- Not be afraid to touch the person with AIDS.
- Encourage the patient to become involved in their own care. Assist them in being active as long as possible.
- Not be afraid to discuss the disease with the patient.

When patients come in for HIV or AIDS testing, they should receive counseling from the physician before and after the test. The counseling should include information on methods for safe sex.

For more information on HIV or AIDS, write to the CDC National AIDS Clearinghouse, P.O. Box 6003, Rockville, MD 20849-6003 or call 1-800-458-5231. The Spanish hotline is 1-800-344-7432. The deaf access hotline is 1-900-AIDS-TTY.

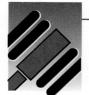

LEGAL AND ETHICAL ISSUES

There is a grave responsibility for the medical assistant to maintain aseptic technique. An ethical concern is that every break in aseptic technique must be reported and corrected immediately. Even when one cannot see a needle puncture in a glove, the wearer of the glove may know there has been a puncture resulting in a break in the barrier to infection. The medical assistant must readily admit if a barrier has been broken so that corrective action can be taken.

The identity of an employee or patient who is HIV positive or has AIDS or hepatitis is confidential and must be respected.

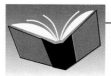

PATIENT EDUCATION

Handwashing must be stressed for all patients. Special emphasis should be placed on washing hands before and after eating, using the toilet, handling contaminated items such as door knobs, or coming into contact with any bodily fluids. Personal hygiene such as daily bathing, oral hygiene, and clean clothes has to be stressed.

Patients truly believe they are carrying out good infection control procedures, when, in fact, there are breaks in the barriers against infection, and as a result infection spreads. The medical assistant must carefully instruct patients concerning the importance of thorough handwashing with soap and warm water before performing such procedures as changing dressings, handling wounds, and colostomy care. Diabetic patients need special instructions on procedures to use to prevent infections developing since they are an at risk population.

Remind the patients that they cannot see germs with the naked eye. Commercial disinfectants are encouraged when cleaning bathrooms and kitchens.

Patients of all ages who are sexually active should be instructed on the proper use of condoms for protection against AIDS, other sexually transmitted diseases, and hepatitis B.

Summary

Good aseptic technique is everybody's business. The medical assistant is often the first barrier against infection in the office. The meticulous attention given to sterilization of all reusable materials and equipment is often the full responsibility of the medical assistant. This is a serious responsibility. All who handle waste products must be trained in safety measures such as Standard Precautions. Document waste removal.

When practicing aseptic technique, know the right way to do something and then never deviate from that method. Never take shortcuts with asepsis.

Competency Review

1. Define and spell the glossary terms for this chapter.
2. Describe the disease transmission process.
3. Develop an infection control plan for a medical office.
4. Wrap and label instruments for autoclave sterilization.
5. Correctly load an autoclave.
6. Correctly follow the step-by-step procedure for sterile gowning and gloving.
7. Call the 800 number of the CDC to request educational brochures that can be used to develop patient teaching materials.

PREPARING FOR THE CERTIFICATION EXAM

Test Taking Tip — Do not look for cues to correct answers by studying the pattern of correct responses. Answers occur in a random pattern.

Examination Review Questions

1. A commonly used disinfectant is
   (A) formaldehyde
   (B) Lysol
   (C) 70% alcohol
   (D) soap
   (E) phenol
2. Most sterilization indicators operate on what principle?
   (A) a color change will revert back when item is contaminated
   (B) original color reappears after 6 weeks
   (C) color change indicates the package has been properly sealed
   (D) color change indicates sterilization is complete
   (E) none of the above
3. Dry heat sterilization is used for
   (A) plastic items
   (B) dressings
   (C) gloves
   (D) surgical instruments
   (E) ointments and powders
4. Steam under pressure, dry heat, and chemical-gas mixtures are used in
   (A) disinfection
   (B) sterilization
   (C) sanitization
   (D) cleaning
   (E) fumigation
5. Before removing sterilized items from the autoclave, they should be allowed to
   (A) change color
   (B) cool
   (C) dry
   (D) depressurize
   (E) all of the above
6. Sterile materials which are wrapped in paper or cloth can be stored for
   (A) one year
   (B) only 10 days
   (C) 6 months
   (D) 21-30 days
   (E) two years
7. Instruments which are being disinfected in boiling water should remain immersed for NOT less than
   (A) 90 minutes
   (B) 60 minutes
   (C) 30 minutes
   (D) 45 minutes
   (E) 15 minutes

8. After the autoclave temperature reaches 250°F, the timer for sterilizing wrapped surgical instruments should be set for
(A) 10 minutes
(B) 15 minutes
(C) 30 minutes
(D) 50 minutes
(E) 60 minutes

9. Which of the following is NOT a cause of incomplete sterilization when using the autoclave?
(A) trapping pockets of air in the autoclave
(B) setting the timer before the correct temperature has been reached
(C) opening the door completely during the drying cycle
(D) placing instruments overlapping one another
(E) placing only one instrument in each packet

10. What conditions are necessary for bacterial growth to occur?
(A) moisture
(B) body temperature
(C) oxygen
(D) light
(E) all of the above

ON THE JOB

Emma Brown, 70 years old, is caring for her 78 year old husband, George. George Brown, a diabetic, has been hospitalized with a recurring leg infection which may lead to amputation of his right leg. George's physical condition may not be able to withstand another massive leg infection. He has been placed on antibiotics and his leg is now healing. Emma Brown will require instruction on irrigating the leg wound and changing her husband's dressing. When the leg wound was cultured, E. coli was present. Emma mentioned to the medical assistant that she is concerned about her own health since she has a colostomy.

What is your response?

1. What patient education is required for Emma regarding the procedure to be used in caring for George?
2. Is it possible that the E. coli was transmitted from Emma's colostomy site to George's leg wound? Explain.
3. Discuss the advantages and disadvantages of the following methods of patient education that you might use:

- Written materials
- Demonstration and return demonstration
- Verbal instructions

References

"CDC Summarizes Final Regulations for Implementing CLIA." *American Family Physician.* 45:6, 1992.

Badash, S. and Chesebro, D. *Introduction to Health Occupations.* Upper Saddle River, NJ: Brady/Prentice Hall, 1997.

Bledsoe, B., Porter, R., and Shade, B. *Paramedic Emergency Care.* Upper Saddle River, NJ: Brady/Prentice Hall, 1994.

Caring for Someone with AIDS. Washington, DC: US Department of Health and Human Services, 1994.

CDC National AIDS Clearinghouse. Rockville, MD: CDC National AIDS Clearinghouse, 1996.

Decker, M. "The OSHA Bloodborne Hazard Standard." *Infection Control and Hospital Epidemiology.* 12:7, 1992.

HIV/AIDS Prevention. Atlanta: Centers for Disease Control, October 1994.

HIV/AIDS Surveillance Reports. Rockville, MD: CDC National AIDS Clearinghouse, 1996.

Kelsey, E. "Understanding OSHA's Bloodbourne Pathogens Standard." *PMA.* July/August, 1992.

Nurse's Pocket Companion. Springhouse, PA: Springhouse Corporation, 1993.

O'Brien, L., Bartlett, K. "TB Plus HIV Spells Trouble." *American Journal of Nursing.* 92:5, 1992.

Taber's Cycolpedic Medical Dictionary, 18th ed. Philadelphia: PA, 1997.

TB/HIV *The Connection: What Health Care Workers Should Know.* Atlanta: Centers for Disease Control, September, 1993.

Technical Guidance on HIV Counseling. *Morbidity and Mortality Weekly Report.* Atlanta: Centers for Disease Control, 42, No.RR-2, 1994.

Wedding, M. and Tolnjes, S. *Medical Laboratory Procedures.* Philadelphia: F.A. Davis, Co., 1992.

Medical Assistant Role Delineation Chart

Highlight indicates material covered in this chapter

ADMINISTRATIVE

Administrative procedures

- Perform basic clerical functions
- Schedule, coordinate, and monitor appointments
- Schedule inpatient/outpatient admissions and procedures
- Understand and apply third party guidelines
- Obtain reimbursement through accurate claims submission
- Monitor third-party reimbursement
- Perform medical transcription
- Understand and adhere to managed care policies and procedures
- *Negotiate managed care contracts (adv)*

Practice Finances

- Perform procedural and diagnostic coding
- Apply bookkeeping principles
- Document and maintain accounting and banking records
- Manage accounts receivable
- Manage accounts payable
- Process payroll
- *Develop and maintain fee schedules (adv)*
- *Manage renewals of business and professional insurance policies (adv)*
- *Manage personal benefits and maintain records (adv)*

CLINICAL

Fundamental principles

- Apply principles of aseptic technique and infection control
- Comply with quality assurance practices
- Screen and follow up patient test results

Diagnostic orders

- Collect and process specimens
- Perform diagnostic tests

Patient care

- Adhere to established triage procedures
- Obtain patient history and vital signs
- Prepare and maintain examination and treatment areas

- Prepare patient for examinations, procedures, and treatments
- Assist with examinations, procedures, and treatments
- Prepare and administer medications and immunizations
- Maintain medication and immunization records
- Recognize and respond to emergencies
- Coordinate patient care information with other health care providers

GENERAL (TRANSDISCIPLINARY)

Professionalism

- Project a professional manner and image
- Adhere to ethical principles
- Demonstrate initiative and responsibility
- Work as a team member
- Manage time efficiently
- Prioritize and perform multiple tasks
- Adapt to change
- Promote the CMA credential
- Enhance skills through continuing education

Communication skills

- Treat all patients with compassion and empathy
- Recognize and respect cultural diversity
- Adapt communications to individual's ability to understand
- Use professional telephone technique
- Use effective and correct verbal and written communications
- Recognize and respond to verbal and non-verbal communications
- Use medical terminology appropriately
- Receive, organize, prioritize, and transmit information
- Serve as liaison
- Promote the practice through positive public relations

Legal concepts

- Maintain confidentiality
- Practice within the scope of education, training, and personal capabilities
- Prepare and maintain medical records
- Document accurately
- Use appropriate guidelines when releasing information
- Follow employer's established policies dealing with the health care contract
- Follow federal, state, and local legal guidelines
- Maintain awareness of federal and state health care legislation and regulations
- Maintain and dispose of regulated substances in compliance with government guidelines
- Comply with established risk management and safety procedures
- Recognize professional credentialing criteria
- Participate in the development and maintenance of personnel, policy, and procedure manuals
- *Develop and maintain personnel, policy, and procedure manuals (adv)*

Instruction

- Instruct individuals according to their needs
- Explain office policies and procedures
- Teach methods of health promotion and disease prevention
- Locate community resources and disseminate information
- *Orient and train personnel (adv)*
- *Develop educational materials (adv)*
- *Conduct continuing education activities (adv)*

Operational functions

- Maintain supply inventory
- Evaluate and recommend equipment and supplies
- Apply computer techniques to support office operations
- *Supervise personnel (adv)*
- *Interview and recommend job applicants (adv)*
- *Negotiate leases and prices for equipment and supply contracts (adv)*

SOURCE: Reprinted by permission of the American Association of Medical Assistants from the *AAMA Role Delineation Study: Occupational Analysis of the Medical Assisting Profession.*

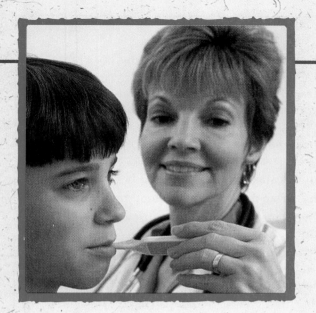

Vital Signs and Measurement

CHAPTER OUTLINE

LEARNING OBJECTIVES

After completing this chapter, you should:
1. Define and spell the glossary terms for this chapter.
2. State the normal values of temperature, pulse, respiratory rates, and blood pressure.
3. List 10 conditions which cause the body temperature to increase or decrease.
4. State 3 situations in which measuring an oral, rectal, and axillary temperature should be avoided.
5. List and describe the 7 pulse sites.
6. State 9 factors that can affect the pulse rate.
7. Describe the respiratory rate range for the various age groups.
8. Discuss the 5 phases of the Korotkoff sounds.
9. Explain the 4 physiological factors that affect blood pressure.
10. Discuss the aneroid and mercury sphygmomanometers.
11. Describe the procedure for measuring temperature, pulse, apical-radial pulse, respiration, blood pressure, height, and weight.
12. Explain 10 causes of errors in blood pressure readings.
13. Convert temperature readings from degrees Fahrenheit (F) to degrees Centigrade (C) (and vice versa).
14. Convert weight in pounds to kilograms (and vice versa).
15. Convert height from inches to centimeters (and vice versa).

CLINICAL PERFORMANCE COMPETENCIES

After completing this chapter, you should perform the following tasks:
1. Demonstrate the correct procedures for measuring oral, tympanic, rectal, and axillary temperature using the correct equipment.
2. Correctly determine pulse rate of the adult.
3. Determine pulse rate of infants and children.
4. Identify Korotkoff sounds.
5. Measure height and weight of infants, children, and adults.
6. Demonstrate the correct procedure for measuring a patient's respiration.
7. Demonstrate the correct procedure for measuring respirations noting the rate, rhythm, and depth.
8. Demonstrate the correct procedure for measuring blood pressure of an adult using both mercury and aneroid equipment.
9. Correctly chart all vital signs.
10. Demonstrate the correct procedure for cleaning and disinfecting a glass thermometer.

Glossary

alveoli Minute air sacs in lungs through which gas exchange takes place between alveolar air and pulmonary capillary blood.

anthropometry Science of measuring the human body as to size of component parts, height, and weight.

antecubital fossa/space Area formed at the inside bend of the elbow.

antipyretic Substance that reduces fever.

arrhythmia Irregular pulse or heart rate.

asymptomatic Without having any symptoms; symptom free.

atypical Unusual; out of the ordinary.

aural Pertaining to the ear or hearing.

auscultatory gap Total loss of sound during phase II of the Korotkoff sounds while taking blood pressure. The sound later reoccurs. This is considered abnormal.

axillary Pertaining to the armpit or area under the arm.

blood stasis Lack of circulation due to a stoppage of blood flow.

cardiac cycle Time from the beginning of one beat of the heart to the beginning of the next beat, including the systole (contraction) and diastole (relaxation).

centigrade or Celsius Scale for measurement of temperature in which 0° C is the freezing point of water and 100° C is the boiling point of water at sea level.

croup An acute viral infection of the upper and lower respiratory tract in children which may result in difficult, noisy breathing.

cyanosis Bluish discoloration of the skin and mucous membranes due to oxygen deprivation.

diaphragm Musculofibrous partition that separates the thoracic and abdominal cavities.

diastole Period in the cardiac cycle during which the heart is relaxed and the heart cavities are being refilled with blood.

emphysema Abnormal pulmonary condition with loss of lung elasticity resulting in overinflation of the lungs and difficulty exhaling—"barrel chest."

Fahrenheit Scale for measurement of temperature in which the boiling point of water is 212° F and the freezing point of water is 32° F at sea level.

frenulum linguae Longitudinal fold of mucous membrane connecting the floor of the mouth to the underside of the tongue.

heart sounds Normal noise produced within the heart during the cardiac cycle.

homeostasis The human body in balance.

hypertension Elevated blood pressure.

hypotension Blood pressure which is below normal.

hypothalamus Portion of brain in the lateral wall of the third ventricle which controls autonomic nervous system functions such as body temperature, sleep, and appetite.

intermittent pulse Skipping an occasional heart beat.

kilograms Metric weight.

lumen Space/cavity within an object or organ.

manometer Device for taking a measurement (for example, pressure).

medulla oblongata Most vital part of the brain which contains the respiratory, cardiac, and vasomotor centers of the brain.

pulse deficit Difference between the rate of the apical pulse and the radial pulse. Normally there is no difference.

palpatory method To determine by using the sense of touch.

pulse pressure Difference between systolic and diastolic readings of blood pressure.

pyrexia Abnormally elevated body temperature; fever.

reading Interpretation of data.

sublingual(ly) Under the tongue.

subnormal Abnormally lowered body temperature.

systole Period during the cardiac cycle when the atria and ventricles contract and eject the blood out of the heart.

thready Pulse rate that is barely perceptible.

tympanic membrane Thin semitransparent membrane separates the outer ear and the middle ear. Also called eardrum.

A healthy human body regulates itself. Vital signs are indicators of the body's ability to maintain homeostasis. Temperature (T), along with pulse (P), respiration (R), and blood pressure (BP) measurements are considered vital signs since they measure some of the body's vital functions and provide necessary information about the patient's physical well being. Vital signs are routinely measured by medical assistants before physical examinations. Care must be taken to be accurate and efficient so the readings or results reflect a true picture of the patient's condition.

Along with the physiology behind body temperature, pulse rate, respirations, blood pressure, and measurement of weight and height, this chapter discusses the normal or average readings for all vital signs at varying ages. Different methods and types of equipment for measuring temperature, pulse rate, respirations, and blood pressure are discussed along with guidelines and ways for choosing the best methods and equipment.

When temperature, pulse, and respirations are measured at the same time it is referred to as TPR. During some office visits only one of the vital signs may be measured, for example blood pressure in a patient with hypertension. Factors influencing readings and procedures with step-by-step instructions for accurately and efficiently measuring vital signs are thoroughly presented.

Note: All health care professionals are required to use Standard Precautions to maintain infection control while measuring vital signs. The details of Standard Precautions will not be repeated for each procedure. The medical assistant is expected to know and continually apply the techniques recommended by the Centers for Disease Control and Prevention as discussed in Chapter 19.

Temperature

An understanding of the way the body maintains a balance between the amount of heat produced and the amount of heat lost is important for the medical assistant. Other factors that inform and assist the medical assistant to measure temperature accurately include knowledge of normal readings, factors that influence readings, how to select and use the proper thermometer, and how to clean and care for equipment.

Physiology of Body Temperature

Since body temperature is regulated through balancing the amount of heat produced in the body with the amount of heat lost from the body, there is normally only a 1-2 degree Fahrenheit (F) variance throughout the day. The hypothalamus, a portion of the brain that controls autonomic nervous system functions, is able to adjust the body temperature as the need for more or less heat production occurs during the day. For example, when a jogger is running on a hot day the body's cooling mechanism reacts to this by creating perspiration which removes some of the excess heat the jogger experiences.

Med Tip: Always be alert for all causes of changes in body temperature. For example, an infant's elevated temperature during an examination may be due to the infant's crying and not due to an illness. Always ask whether the patient has taken aspirin or Tylenol which lower the temperature. Older adults who normally have body temperatures below normal, may be ill even when their temperature is within a normal range for adults.

Temperature Readings

The body temperature of a healthy person is 98.6°F or 37°C, and may vary by 1°F (0.6°C) either up or down during the day. While a slight variance in body temperature is not a cause for alarm, it is important to remember that greater body temperature variations from normal are often the first sign of illness or disease. Table 20-1 describes causes of variations in body temperature.

TABLE 20-1   Variations in Body Temperature

Cause	Description
Time of Day	Body temperature is lower in the morning upon wakening when metabolism is still slow. The lowest body temperature is between 2 a.m. and 6 a.m. The highest body temperature usually occurs in the evening between 5 and 8 p.m. Daily variation in oral temperature can range from 97.6° to 99.6°F (36.4° to 37.3°C).
Age	Infants and children normally have a higher body temperature due to immature heat-regulation. Children often spike a fever late in the day. Older adults usually have a lower than normal body temperature.
Gender	Women may experience a slight increase in body temperature at the time of ovulation.
Physical exercise	Body temperature will rise with exercise due to increased muscle contractions causing an increase in metabolism.
Emotions	Emotions, such as crying and anger, can cause an increase in body temperature.
Pregnancy	An increase in metabolism during pregnancy may cause the body temperature to rise.
Environmental changes	Hot weather can cause serious consequences in older adults whose bodies are unable to regulate body temperature due to a decreased metabolism. Exposure to cold may lower the body temperature.
Infection	An elevated temperature, or fever, may be one of the first signs of an infection. A fever is the body's way of fighting or "killing off" infectious organisms.
Drugs	Drugs may increase muscular activity or metabolism which in turn increases temperature. Antipyretic (fever reducing) drugs, such as aspirin, lower the above-normal temperature.
Food	The process of eating may also raise the body temperature. Fasting decreases metabolism which will cause a lowering of body temperature.

Fever

Fever, or **pyrexia,** is a body temperature above 100.4°F (38°C). At this point it can be stated that the body is producing greater heat than it is losing and is febrile. When the body temperature exceeds 105.8°F (41°C), a serious condition known as hyperpyrexia develops. A body temperature above 109.4°F (43°C) is usually fatal. It can be a result of hyperthermia. Temperatures at this level may result in seizures in infants and small children. See Table 20-2 for a classification of fevers.

Hypothermia

The reverse of a fever is a **subnormal** temperature or hypothermia. This occurs when the temperature falls below 97°F (36°C). At this point, the body is losing more heat than it is producing. This occurs in cases of exposure and near-drowning in cold water. In general a temperature below 93.2°F (34°C) is fatal.

Temperature Taking Sites

Body temperature can be taken in a variety of ways including oral (mouth), aural (ear), axillary (under the arm), and rectal (rectum). The normal temperature—based on statistical averages—for each of these sites is:

- Oral   98.6°F (37°C)
- Rectal   99.6°F (37.6°C)
- Axillary   97.6°F (36.4°C)
- Ear (aural)   98.6°F (37°C)

TABLE 20-2 Classification of Fevers (oral reading)

Fever Level	Fahrenheit (F)	Celsius/Centigrade (C)
Slight	99.6°–100.9°	37.6°–38.3°
Moderate	101.0°–101.9°	38.3°–38.8°
Severe	102.0°–104.0°	38.9°–40.0°
Dangerous	104.1°–105.8°	40.1°–41.0°
Fatal	106.0°–109.4° +	41.1°–43.0° +

As the above figures indicate, the temperature obtained through the rectal method registers 1°F (or 0.6°C) higher than the oral temperature. Axillary temperatures register 1°F (0.6°C) lower than oral temperatures. The medical assistant must document if the temperature was taken rectally by the symbol "R" or axillary by the symbol "AX."

Oral

The oral method of temperature measurement is the most commonly used. There is a potential for error with this method since the patient may not form a tight closure over the thermometer. This allows air to enter the mouth and give a false temperature reading. In recording this measurement, no designation needs to be used to indicate it was taken by the oral route. The thermometer is inserted under the tongue on either side of the frenulum linguae. This is the longitudinal fold of mucous membrane. For an accurate measurement, the patient must be advised not to talk during the procedure.

Aural (eardrum)

One of the newest technologies for accurate temperature measurement involves the aural site. This method uses the area at the end of the external auditory canal for an instantaneous temperature measurement. The tympanic thermometer provides a closed cavity within the easily accessible ear. The aural method is now considered to be the most accurate means of temperature measurement due to the eardrum's proximity to a blood supply and to the hypothalamus. This method also poses the least problems with Standard Precautions.

Axillary (under the arm)

The axillary method has proven to be the least accurate of the four temperature measurement sites.

It is the recommended site for small children unable to understand how to hold an oral thermometer, if a tympanic membrane thermometer is not available. The axillary site is recommended for patients who have had oral surgery, any situation in which the patient may bite the oral thermometer, and mouth-breathing patients. The axillary temperature reading is affected by perspiration. The underarm area should be dry for an accurate reading.

Rectal

The rectal route is considered more reliable than the oral method. The mucous membrane lining of the rectum does not come into contact with air, which could interfere with accuracy, as do the oral and axillary routes. The rectal route is advised for unconscious patients, infants, small children, and mouth-breathing patients. The rectal method is avoided whenever possible due to possible perforation of the rectal wall.

Use the guidelines that follow to determine which method to use when measuring a patient's body temperature.

Fahrenheit/Celsius Conversions

The Fahrenheit (F) scale of temperature measurement is widely used throughout the United States. However, some physicians wish to use the Centigrade (C) or celsius (C) scale. Figure 20-1 shows examples of Fahrenheit and Celsius thermometers. To convert Fahrenheit (F) to Celsius (C), subtract 32, then multiply by 5/9. To convert degrees Celsius (C) to Fahrenheit (F), multiply by 9/5, and then add 32. See Figure 20-2 for a Fahrenheit/centigrade conversion chart and Table 20-3 for temperature scale conversion formulas and examples.

Guidelines: Selecting a Method for Measuring Body Temperature		
Method	**Advisable**	**Inadvisable**
Oral	Most adults and children who are able to follow instructions	Patients who have had oral surgery, mouth sores, dyspnea
		Uncooperative patients
		Patients receiving oxygen
		Infants and small children
		Patients with facial paralysis
		Patients with nasal obstruction
Rectal	Infants, small children	Active children
	Patients who have had oral surgery	Fragile newborns
	Mouth-breathing patients	
	Unconscious patients	
Axillary	Small children	Patients who cannot form an airtight seal around thermometer
Tympanic (aural)	Infants, children, adults	Patient with in-the-ear-canal hearing aids

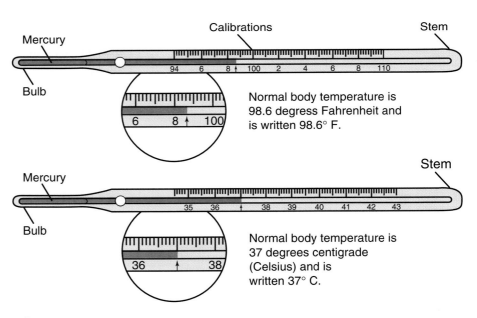

Figure 20-1   Fahrenheit and centigrade thermometers.

Types of Thermometers

Four types of thermometers are available for measuring body temperature: mercury glass thermometers, electronic thermometers, tympanic membrane thermometers, and chemical thermometers (Figure 20-3).

Glass Thermometers

Mercury glass thermometers are available in two shapes to measure temperature using the oral, rectal, and axillary methods. The oral thermometer has a long, slender tip which fits easily under the tongue. A thermometer with a stubby or pear shaped tip is available which can be used for oral, axillary, and rectal temperature taking. On some thermometers there may be a blue dot indicating the thermometer is for oral use or a red dot indicating rectal use.

Mercury Thermometers

The clinical glass mercury thermometer is a glass rod containing a minute amount of the element mercury which is capable of expanding in the tube when it comes into contact with heat. The shaft or stem of the thermometer is calibrated in tenths (0.2, 0.4, 0.6, and so on) of degrees—each short line represents 0.2 of a degree. A whole degree is marked with a long line. The even-numbered degrees are printed on the thermometer. The average normal body temperature (98.6°F) is pointed out with an arrow on the thermometer.

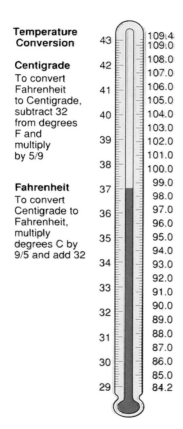

Temperature Conversion

Centigrade
To convert Fahrenheit to Centigrade, subtract 32 from degrees F and multiply by 5/9

Fahrenheit
To convert Centigrade to Fahrenheit, multiply degrees C by 9/5 and add 32

Figure 20-2 Fahrenheit/Centigrade conversion chart.

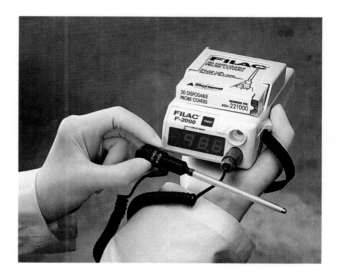

Figure 20-3 Digital electronic thermometer.

TABLE 20-3 **Temperature Scale Conversion Formulas**

Scale	Conversion Formula	Example
Centigrade	$(°F - 32)\ 5/9 = °C$	$101°F - 32 = 69 \times 5/9 = 38.3°C$
Fahrenheit	$(°C \times 9/5) + 32 = °F$	$38.3°C \times 9/5 = 69 + 32 = 101°F$

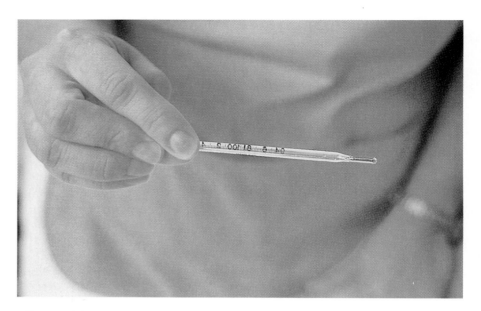

Figure 20-4   Reading a clinical thermometer.

When reading the thermometer, it should be held between the thumb and index finger, at eye level, by the stem end (Figure 20-4). While looking at the edge of the thermometer, keep the lines at the top of the edge and the numbers at the bottom. The stem is then gently rotated until the silver mercury column can be seen in the middle of the lines and numbers. The point where the mercury line stops is read for the body temperature at each two-tenths of a degree. When the mercury appears between two markings it is read at the next higher two-tenths of a degree.

The temperature reading is then recorded. The temperature must be carefully charted with absolute accuracy. Each short line of the thermometer is read as two-tenths of a degree. Always record temperature reading in even numbers when using a mercury thermometer.

Med Tip: Note the difference between a temperature of 100.4 and 104.0. These two temperatures are read as "one hundred and four-tenths" and "one hundred and four point *0.*" Careful attention is needed when recording temperature to avoid a serious mistake.

Plastic Disposable Sheaths

Plastic disposable slip-on sheaths are available to use with both the oral and rectal glass thermometers (Figure 20-5). The sheath comes in a small pa-

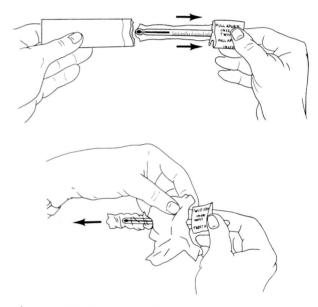

Figure 20-5   Using a thermometer sheath.

per envelope and slips over the tip of the thermometer. The sheath provides a sanitary protective covering and is discarded after use. When using a rectal thermometer, a lubricant is always used over the sheath for ease of insertion into the rectum.

The sheath is removed from the thermometer by pulling on the tear tab which inverts the plastic thus protecting the medical assistant's hands from coming into contact with contamination. Remove and properly dispose of sheath in a hazardous waste container. After the temperature is read,

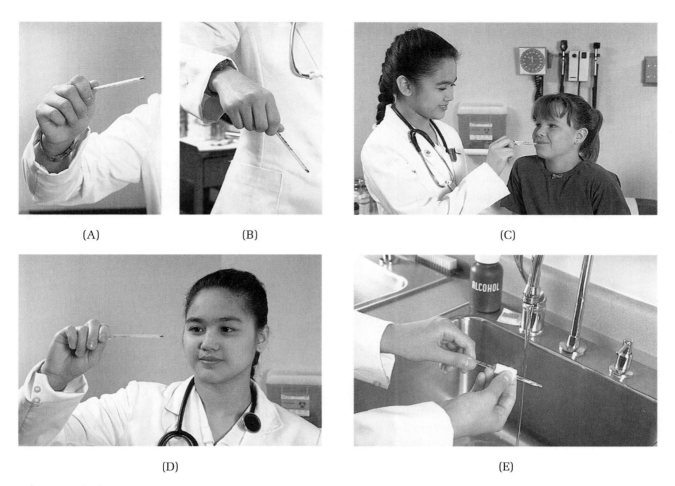

(A) (B) (C)

(D) (E)

Figure 20-6 (A) Taking an oral temperature. (B) Shake down the thermometer. (C) Place the thermometer under the tongue. (D) Medical assistant reads the thermometer. (E) Thermometer is washed with soap and water.

Date	TPR	Initials
9/9/98	100⁶ Ⓡ – 72 – 20	BF

Figure 20-7 Charting temperature.

clean and disinfect the thermometer since mucous membranes may still come into contact with the thermometer.

Figure 20-6 A–E pictures the steps followed in taking an oral temperature.

Figure 20-7 provides an example of how to chart temperature.

A rectal thermometer has a small, round bulb that inserts gently into the rectum. This thermometer may be marked "for rectal use" on its stem and have a red dot indicating the rectal route should be used. It is not safe to use an oral thermometer to take a rectal temperature since the long slender tip may injure tender rectal mucous membranes or can break off in the rectum.

PROCEDURE: Oral Temperature Using a Glass/Mercury Thermometer

Terminal Performance
Competency: Student must be able to accurately perform all steps of procedure and provide a temperature reading within 0.2° of the instructor's reading, unless otherwise instructed.

Equipment and Supplies
Oral mercury thermometer
Disposable plastic thermometer sheath
Watch with second hand
Biohazardous waste container
Patient's record
Paper and pen/pencil

Procedural Steps

1. Wash hands.

2. Apply gloves.

3. Identify patient *Note:* To avoid error call patient by name and check against the name on the patient's record.

4. Ask if patient has recently taken a hot or cold drink or smoked within last 15 minutes. ***Rationale:*** Hot and cold liquids will affect temperature in the mouth. Wait 10 minutes before taking oral temperature.

5. Take thermometer out of container. Do not touch bulb end with fingers. If thermometer is stored in a disinfectant then rinse thoroughly under cool water.

6. Inspect thermometer for any chipped areas or other defects. Discard if damaged.

7. Read the thermometer. If it is not at 95°F, then shake down to that point by firmly holding the end of the glass shaft between the thumb and index finger. Firmly snap the wrist to shake down the mercury within the thermometer.

8. Place plastic sheath on thermometer. Make sure that sheath is tightly in place on thermometer.

9. Place bulb end of thermometer encased in plastic sheath sublingually (under the tongue) in patient's mouth. ***Rationale:*** The space on either side of the frenulum linguae is in close proximity to numerous small blood vessels which will provide an accurate indication of body temperature.

10. Ask the patient to close his or her mouth over the thermometer and hold it in place without biting down. It helps to tell the patient to suck the thermometer rather than to clamp it between their teeth.

11. Leave the thermometer in place for at least 3 minutes. ***Rationale:*** It takes at least 3 minutes for an accurate oral reading to take place. The medical assistant can use this time to take the pulse and respiratory rate.

12. Remove and read the thermometer. If thermometer reads less than 97°F, shake down the thermometer and reinsert for an additional few minutes.

13. Reread the thermometer and write the reading on a piece of paper.

14. Holding tightly by the stem end of the glass shaft pull the plastic sheath off thermometer and discard sheath in biohazardous waste container. ***Rationale:*** The plastic sheath has come into contact with the patient's mucous membranes.

15. Follow the procedure for temporary storage of soiled thermometers.

16. Remove gloves and place in biohazard waste container.

17. Wash hands.

18. Record temperature in patient's record.

19. Follow procedure for cleaning and disinfecting soiled thermometers.

Charting Example
10/23/XX 4:00 p.m. 99°F M. King, CMA

PROCEDURE: Measuring a Rectal Temperature

Terminal Performance
Competency: Student must be able to accurately perform all steps of procedure and provide a temperature reading within 0.2° of the instructor's reading, unless otherwise instructed.

Equipment and Supplies
Rectal mercury glass thermometer
Disposable thermometer sheath
Disposable gloves
Patient's record
Paper and pen/pencil
Tissue
Watch with second hand
Water soluble lubricant
Biohazardous waste container

Procedural Steps

1. Wash hands.
2. Apply gloves.
3. Identify patient. *Note:* To avoid error call the patient by name and check against the name on the patient's record.
4. Explain procedure. If patient is a child, explain the procedure to both parent and child.
5. Place small amount of lubricant on a tissue. ***Rationale:*** Tissue will serve to keep work area clean and also as a temporary receptacle for prepared thermometer.
6. Remove rectal thermometer from container by holding stem end only.
7. Inspect thermometer for any cracks or defects. Discard if damaged.
8. Read the thermometer. If it is not at 95°F, then shake down to that point by firmly holding the end of the glass shaft between the thumb and index finger. Firmly snap the wrist to shake down the mercury within the thermometer.
9. Place plastic sheath on thermometer, making sure that it is tightly in place.
10. Apply lubricant to thermometer by rolling bulb end in lubricant on tissue. Leave thermometer on the tissue. ***Rationale:*** Lubricant allows the thermometer to be inserted easily with reduced chance for injury to mucous membranes. Tissue provides a clean surface for temporary storage of prepared thermometer.

Adult Patient:

a. Instruct patient to remove appropriate clothing so that rectal area can be accessed. Provide privacy for patient.
b. Assist patient onto examining table and cover with sheet/drape. ***Rationale:*** Protect patient's modesty.
c. Instruct patient to lie on left side with top leg bent (Sims position).
d. With one hand raise the upper buttock to expose the anus or anal opening. If unable to see the anal opening, ask the patient to bear down slightly. This will expose the opening.
e. With other hand, gently insert lubricated thermometer 1 1/2 inches into anal canal. Do not force the thermometer into the anal canal. Rotating the thermometer may make insertion easier.

Infant and Child:

a. Ask the parent to prepare the child by removing diaper or underwear.
b. Place the child in a secure position. Place an infant on his or her back. With one hand firmly grasp the ankles and lift them up. This will expose the infant's anus. An older child is more easily controlled when placed on his or her stomach. The parent may assist in holding the child securely. An infant—lying on his or her stomach with legs hanging down—can be placed across the parent's lap.
c. Gently insert the bulb end of a well-lubricated rectal thermometer one inch into the anal canal.

(Continued on next page)

11. Hold the thermometer in place for 5 minutes.
12. Withdraw thermometer.
13. Dispose of the plastic sheath in biohazardous waste container.
14. Read thermometer.
15. Reread thermometer and write the reading on a piece of paper.
16. Place thermometer back on tissue or in a temporary storage container. Never place soiled thermometer on unprotected surface.
17. Wipe anus from front to back removing any excess lubricant.
18. Ask parent to re-diaper and dress infant or child.
19. Assist an adult patient from the examination table. Instruct the patient to dress and assist the patient if necessary.
20. Follow the procedure for temporary storage of soiled thermometers.
21. Remove gloves and place in biohazardous waste container.
22. Wash hands
23. Record temperature in patient's record using (R) to indicate a rectal reading.
24. Follow procedure for cleaning and disinfecting soiled thermometers.

Charting Example

2/14/XX   4:00 p.m.   Temp. 99.6°R
                           M. King, CMA

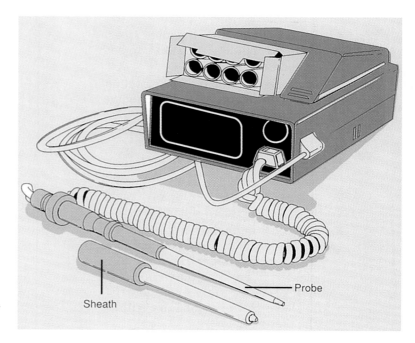

Figure 20-8 Battery-operated electronic thermometers have large digital windows making it easy to read.

Sheath

Probe

Cleaning and Storing Glass Thermometers

The glass mercury thermometer must be cleaned and soaked in a disinfectant after each use. The thermometer is then stored in a proper container. See the following procedure for cleaning and storing glass thermometers.

Electronic Thermometers

The electronic thermometer is becoming very popular. It is considered accurate, easy to read, sanitary, fast, and requires no cleaning or disinfection. These electronic thermometers are battery-operated with digital windows for easy viewing and reading (Figure 20-8). They can ac-

PROCEDURE: Cleaning and Storing Mercury Thermometers

**Terminal Performance
Competency:** Student must correctly clean, inspect, disinfect and store mercury thermometers with 100% accuracy, observing aseptic and safety precautions as prescribed by Standard Precautions.

Equipment and Supplies

70% isopropyl alcohol or other disinfectant for thermometer use

Container with soiled thermometer(s)

Cotton Balls

Soap

Utility or disposable gloves

Water

Biohazardous waste container

Procedural Steps

1. Wash hands.
2. Apply gloves according to office policy. *Rationale:* universal precautions are used to provide protection from contaminated mucous membrane products on soiled thermometer.
3. Take soiled thermometer(s) to sink.
4. Liberally apply soap and water to cotton balls. Holding thermometer by stem, wipe from stem end to bulb by applying friction and rotating the glass stem. *Rationale:* Friction will assist in dislodging contamination from calibrated markings.
5. Discard cotton balls into container.
6. Hold stem of thermometer while rinsing under cool running water. *Rationale:* Hot water will cause mercury to expand and may break thermometer.
7. Inspect thermometer for cleanliness. Note condition of thermometer and

discard if damaged. If soil remains, repeat steps 4 through 6.

8. Holding the stem tightly between thumb and index finger shake mercury down to at least 95.0°F by a quick snapping motion of the wrist. *Rationale:* Wet thermometer may slip out of hand while shaking down. Thermometer needs to be prepared for next use
9. Place thermometer in a container filled with disinfectant. *Rationale:* Thermometer must be completely covered with disinfectant and allowed to remain in solution for at least 20 minutes to be considered disinfected. *Note:* Disinfection in liquid cannot take place without thorough soap and water cleaning first.
10. When all thermometers have been cleaned and placed in disinfectant, then clean soiled thermometer container using soap, water, and disinfectant.
11. Using correct procedure, remove and discard gloves into waste container.
12. Wash hands.
13. Set timer for 20 minutes. *Rationale:* Timer should not be touched until hands have been washed to avoid contamination of timer.
14. After 20 minutes has elapsed, wash hands, rinse thermometers under cool water, and place in sterile storage container.

curately register body temperature within a few seconds.

The electronic thermometer consists of a metal probe which is color-coded: blue for oral and red for rectal. The probe is attached to the battery unit by a flexible cording. A non-flexible plastic disposable cover fits over the probe to provide each patient with a sanitary thermometer (Figure 20-9). This plastic covered probe is inserted under

the patient's tongue or rectally like a mercury thermometer.

The medical assistant will hold the thermometer in place since the reading is performed quickly. The unit will emit a signal when the temperature has registered. The plastic probe shield is then popped into a biohazardous waste container and the probe is replaced into the battery-powered storage unit (Figure 20-10).

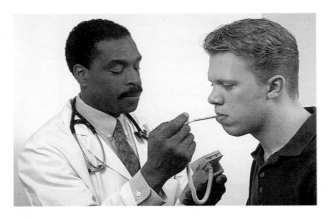

Figure 20-9 The disposable cover, also referred to as a sheath, provides sanitary benefits for the patient.

The electronic thermometer can be used for oral, rectal, and axillary body temperature readings. The blue oral probe is generally used for taking oral and axillary temperatures. Rectal temperatures, taken using the red probe, require lubrication onto the tip of the probe. The rectal probe is inserted 1/2 inch into the adult rectum and 1/4 inch into the child's. The probe may have to be angled slightly to ensure contact with the rectal mucosa.

These units are time-saving but expensive. They are used in medical offices, hospitals, and clinics but rarely by patients in their homes due to cost. The battery-operated unit must be readjusted at intervals to maintain accuracy. The unit should always be returned to the charging stand after each use to maintain the battery.

Tympanic Membrane Thermometers

The tympanic membrane thermometer is used for an aural temperature. The tympanic membrane or aural thermometer is so named because it is able to detect heat waves within the ear canal and near the tympanic membrane. The thermometer calculates the body temperature from the energy generated by these heat waves. Figures 20-11 and 20-12 are examples of tympanic membrane thermometers.

Pulse

Pulse rate is a measurement of the number of times the heart beats in a minute (BPM). Normally the heart beats around 70 times per minute. An increase in circulation will result in a faster heart beat and, thus, a faster pulse rate. A rate above 100 BPM is tachycardia; a rate below 60 BPM is referred to as bradycardia.

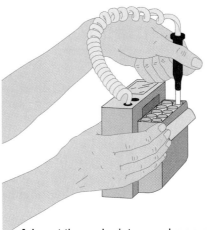

A Insert the probe into a probe cover.

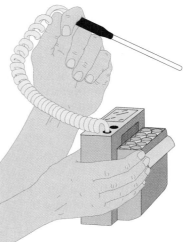

B After measuring the temperature, press to eject the probe cover.

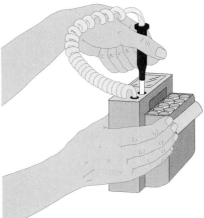

C Replace the probe into the holder.

Figure 20-10 Using the electronic thermometer.

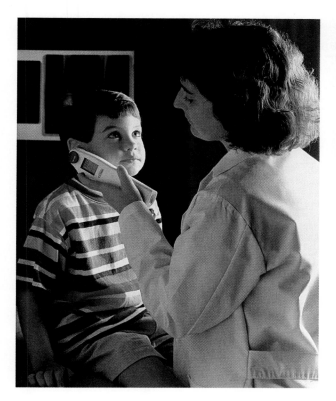

Figure 20-11 Tympanic membrane thermometers are particularly helpful when measuring the temperature of a child.

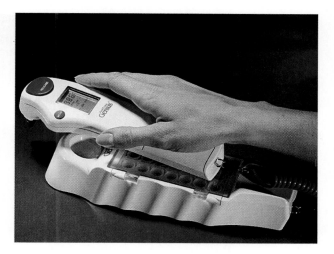

Figure 20-12 Filac tympanic thermometer.

PROCEDURE: Using an Aural (Tympanic Membrane) Thermometer

Terminal Performance
Competency: Student must accurately perform all steps of the procedure and provide a temperature reading with 100% accuracy.

Equipment and Supplies
Tympanic membrane thermometer
Disposable protective probe cover
Paper and pen/pencil
Patient record
Biohazardous waste container

Procedural Steps
1. Wash hands.
2. Identify patient. *Note:* To avoid error call patient by name and check against the name on the patient's record.
3. Explain procedure to patient.
4. Remove thermometer from its base. The display will read "ready."

5. Attach disposable probe cover to the ear piece. ***Rationale:*** The probe cover will assist in keeping probe contamination-free.
6. With one hand gently pull upward on the patient's outer ear if an adult or pull downward if an infant or child. ***Rationale:*** This pulling mechanism will straighten the ear canal for ease of insertion.
7. Gently insert the plastic-covered tip of the probe into ear canal. ***Rationale:*** The ear canal opening is then sealed so that air will not enter and affect the temperature reading.

(Continued on next page)

8. Press scan button which activates the thermometer. ***Rationale:*** An infrared beam is activated which measures the heat waves in one to two seconds.
9. Observe the temperature reading in the display window.
10. Gently withdraw the thermometer.
11. Eject the used probe cover into a biohazardous waste container by pressing the eject button. ***Rationale:*** The medical assistant's hands should not come in contact with the contaminated probe cover.
12. Record temperature using the designation (T) indicating a tympanic temperature. *Note:* Tympanic thermometers can be set to correlate with either an oral or rectal reading. Generally, the oral mode in which 98.6°F is considered normal is used.
13. Return tympanic thermometer to its base.

Charting Example
10/23/XX   4:00 p.m.   Temp. 99.2°F
                          M. King, CMA

PROCEDURE: Measuring Axillary Temperature

Terminal Performance Competency: Student must be able to accurately perform all steps of procedure and provide a temperature reading within 0.2° of the instructor's reading, unless otherwise instructed.

Equipment and Supplies
Oral mercury glass thermometer
Paper and pen/pencil
Patient's record
Tissue
Watch with second hand
Biohazardous waste container

Procedural Steps
1. Wash hands.
2. Identify patient. *Note:* To avoid error call patient by name and check against the name on the patient's record.
3. Explain procedure. If patient is a child then explain procedure to both parent and child.
4. Take thermometer out of container. Do not touch bulb end with fingers. If thermometer is stored in a disinfectant then rinse thoroughly under cool water.
5. Inspect thermometer for any chipped areas or other defects. Discard if damaged.
6. Read the thermometer. If it is not at 95°F, then shake down to that point by firmly holding the end of the glass shaft between the thumb and index finger. Firmly snap the wrist to shake down the mercury within the thermometer.
7. Ask patient to expose axilla. If patient is an infant or child, ask parent to take child's arm out of clothing to expose axilla.
8. Using tissue pat axilla dry of perspiration. ***Rationale:*** Perspiration will interfere with thermometer coming into tight contact with skin.
9. Place bulb end of thermometer into the axillary space. Make sure the bulb comes into contact with patient's skin. ***Rationale:*** Temperature cannot register unless patient's skin touches thermometer.
10. Ask patient to remain still and hold the arm tightly next to the body while the temperature registers. Caution patient not to apply so much pressure that the thermometer breaks.

PROCEDURE: Measuring Axillary Temperature *(Continued)*

11. Leave thermometer in place for 8-10 minutes. Children need to be carefully monitored during this time. Do not leave any patient unattended.
12. Medical assistant can take pulse and respirations while patient is holding thermometer under axilla.
13. Remove thermometer after ten minutes have elapsed and wipe dry with tissue. *Note:* If thermometer reads less than 96°F, shake down the mercury and reinsert for an additional few minutes.

14. Read thermometer.
15. Reread thermometer and write the reading on a piece of paper.
16. Follow the procedure for temporary storage of soiled thermometers.
17. Wash hands.
18. Record temperature in patient's record.
19. Follow procedure for cleaning and disinfecting soiled thermometers.

Charting Example
2/14/XX   4:00 p.m.   Temp. 97.0° AX
                                 M. King, CMA

TABLE 20-4 Factors Influencing Pulse Rate

Factor	Effect on Pulse Rate
Exercise	Activity increases body's requirements. Rate may increase 20-30 beats per minute.
Age	As age increases, pulse rate decreases. Infants and children have a faster pulse rate than adults.
Gender	Female pulse rate is around 10 BPM higher than a male of the same age.
Size	Pulse rate is proportionate to the size of the body. Heat loss is greater in a small body resulting in the heart pumping faster to compensate. Larger males will have slower pulse rates than smaller males.
Physical condition	Athletes and people in good physical condition have lower pulse rate. Lower rate is due to more efficient circulatory system. Pulse rate of 60 or below can be normal for athletes. During sleep and rest the pulse rate may drop to 50–60 BPM.
Disease conditions	Increased pulse rate in thyroid disease, fever, and shock due to increased metabolism.
Medications	Many medications can either raise or lower the pulse rate. Medications such as digoxin are given to regulate the heart beat. Caffeine and nicotine can increase the heart rate in certain people.
Depression	May lower the pulse rate.
Fear, anxiety, anger	May raise the pulse rate.

The pulse rate is influenced by several factors including exercise, age, gender, size, physical conditions, disease states, medications and feelings such as depression, fear, anxiety, and anger. See Table 20-4 for a description of factors influencing pulse rate and Table 20-5 for a list of average pulse rates for different age groups.

TABLE 20-5 Average Pulse Rates by Age

Age	Pulse Rate
Less than 1 year	120–160
2–6 years	80–120
6–10 years	80–100
11–16 years	70–90
Adult	60–80
Older adult	50–65

Characteristics of Pulse

Three characteristics need to be noted and recorded when observing pulse rate: volume, rhythm and condition of arterial wall.

1. *Volume* is the force or strength of the pulse. This is noted as full, strong, normal, bounding, weak, feeble, or thready (barely perceptible). Volume is influenced by the forcefulness of the heart beat, the condition of the arterial walls, and dehydration. A variance in intensity of the pulse may indicate heart disease.

2. *Rhythm* refers to the regularity, or equal spacing of all the beats, of the pulse. Normally, the intervals between each heart beat are the same duration. It is not considered abnormal if the heart occasionally skips a beat. This is referred to as intermittent pulse. Exercise or drinking a caffeine rich beverage may cause this to occur. An arrhythmia is a pulse lacking in regularity. When this occurs on a consistent basis it may indicate heart disease and should be brought to the attention of the physician.

3. The *condition of the arterial wall* should be felt as elastic and soft. A pulse taken in a blood vessel that feels hard and rope-like is considered abnormal and may indicate heart disease such as arteriosclerosis.

Pulse Sites

There are several areas in the body in which the pulse can be easily measured since the artery is located close to the surface of the skin. These pulse sites are: radial, brachial, carotid, temporal, femoral, popliteal, and dorsalis pedis (Figure 20-13). Table 20-6 describes the 7 common pulse sites.

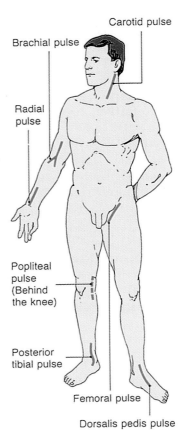

Figure 20-13   Pulse sites.

Figure 20-14 shows a medical assistant measuring a patient's radial pulse as described in the procedure measuring radial pulse rate.

Apical Heart Rate

The apical heart rate is the heart rate counted at the apex of the heart. It can only be heard with a stethoscope placed over the apex. This is considered to be a very accurate heart rate. The apical rate is taken in infants and young children. The physician may also request an apical rate taken when a patient is on heart medications.

An apical-radial pulse rate may be taken to determine if there is a difference between the pulse rate taken at the two sites. An apical-radial pulse must be taken for a full minute. The difference between the two readings is called the pulse deficit. The procedure for taking an apical-radial pulse follows. This measurement requires two people: one to take the radial pulse and one to take the apical pulse. When only one person is doing the procedure, the apical pulse is taken first and then the radial pulse rate.

TABLE 20-6 Location of Common Pulse Sites

Pulse Site	Location
Radial	Thumb side of the wrist approximately one inch below base of the thumb. This is the most frequently used site for counting pulse rate.
Brachial	Inner (antecubital fossa/space) aspect of the elbow. This is the pulse heard and felt when taking blood pressure.
Carotid	Between larynx and the sternocleidomastoid muscle in the side of the neck. This is the pulse used during cardiopulmonary resuscitation (CPR). It can be felt by pushing the muscle to one side and pressing gently against the larynx.
Temporal	At the side of the head just above the ear.
Femoral	Near the groin where the femoral artery is located.
Popliteal	Behind the knee. This pulse is located deeply behind the knee and can be felt when the knee is slightly bent.
Dorsalis pedis	On the top of the foot slightly lateral to midline. This pulse can be an indication of adequate circulation to the feet.

PROCEDURE: Measuring Radial Pulse Rate

Terminal Performance Competency: Student must be able to accurately perform the procedure and provide a radial pulse reading with 100% accuracy, unless otherwise instructed.

Equipment and Supplies
Paper and pen/pencil
Patient's record
Watch with second hand

Procedural Steps

1. Wash hands.
2. Identify patient. *Note:* To avoid error call patient by name and check against the name on the patient's record.
3. Explain procedure.
4. Ask the patient about any recent physical activity or smoking. *Rationale:* Exertion can increase pulse rate. Wait 10 minutes after physical exertion of patient to take pulse.
5. Ask patient to sit down and place arm in a comfortable, supported position. The hand should be at chest level with the palm down.
6. Place finger tips on radial artery on thumb side of wrist. *Note:* Do not use thumb when taking pulse since pulse in thumb may be felt in addition to patient's pulse in wrist.
7. Check quality of pulse.
8. Start counting pulse beats when second hand on watch is at 3, 6, 9, or 12. *Rationale:* One minute is easier to observe at these points.
9. Count the pulse for one full minute. The number will always be an even number.
10. Write the pulse beats per minute immediately on a piece of paper.
11. Wash hands.
12. Record the pulse beats per minute in patient's record, describing any abnormalities in pulse rate.

Charting Example
2/14/XX   4:00 p.m.   pulse = 72
Regular and strong   M. King, CMA

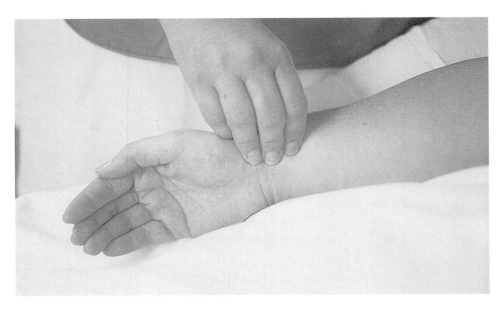

Figure 20-14 Measuring a patient's radial pulse.

Respiration

Respiration, or the act of breathing, is the exchange of oxygen and carbon dioxide (CO_2) between the atmosphere and the body cells. It consists of one expiration or exhalation and one inspiration or inhalation. This is called the respiratory cycle.

Physiology of Respiration

During the process of inspiration, oxygen, which is necessary for body cells and life, is taken into the lungs. The **diaphragm** moves downward, intercostal muscles move outward, and the lungs expand in order to take oxygen into the lungs. During expiration air containing carbon dioxide is expelled from the lungs as a waste product. The diaphragm moves upward and the lungs deflate.

The respiratory process is both external and internal. The external respiratory process is an exchange of oxygen and carbon dioxide between the **alveoli**, the minute air sacs of the lungs, and the blood. The internal repiratory process takes place when blood in the capillaries comes into contact with the alveoli where it picks up oxygen and carries it to cells throughout the body. Carbon dioxide is thrown off as a waste product, carried back to the lungs where it is exhaled. The process then begins all over again with inhalation.

The **medulla oblongata** located in the base of the brain contains the respiratory, cardiac, and vasomotor centers. When the medulla oblongata receives a message indicating there is a buildup of carbon dioxide, this message is translated by the brain into a need for increased respiration to occur. Breathing is actually controlled by the involuntary nervous system. However, breathing is also under some control of the voluntary nervous system.

PROCEDURE: Apical-Radial Pulse (Two-person)

**Terminal Performance
Competency:** Student must be able to accurately perform all steps of the procedure and provide an apical heart rate within 1 point difference of the instructor's reading, unless otherwise instructed.

Equipment and Supplies

Stethoscope

Alcohol wipe/cotton balls with Isopropyl alcohol 70%

Paper and pen/pencil

Patient's record

Watch with second hand

Procedural Steps

1. Wash hands.
2. Prepare stethoscope using alcohol wipe or cotton balls with alcohol on ear pieces and diaphragm of scope. **Rationale:** To prevent carrying organisms into ear canal of medical assistant or between patients.
3. Identify patient. *Note:* To avoid error call patient by name and check against the name on the patient's record.
4. Explain procedure. If patient is a child, explain procedure to both parent and child.
5. Uncover left side of patient's chest. Provide privacy with a drape, if necessary.
6. First person places earpieces of stethoscope in ears with opening in tips forward.
7. Locate apex of patient's heart by palpating to left fifth intercostal space (between fifth and sixth ribs) at the midclavicular line. This is found just below the nipple.
8. Warm chestpiece by holding in the palm of hand before placing onto patient's chest. **Rationale:** This is a comfort measure for the patient. A cold stethoscope can be startling to the patient and may cause a faster heart beat.
9. Second person locates radial pulse in the thumb side of wrist one inch below base of thumb.
10. First person places the chestpiece of stethoscope at apex of heart. When heart beat is heard, a nod is made to the second person and counting begins. Ideally, the count should begin when the second hand is at the 3, 6, 9, or 12.
11. Count for one full minute. *Note:* Both systole and diastole (or lubb/dubb) count as one beat.
12. Remove stethoscope and earpieces.
13. Record the rate and quality of heart beats. Include both apical and radial rates using designation "AP." Calculate the pulse deficit by subtracting the radial pulse rate from the apical pulse rate. *Note:* A pulse deficit may indicate that the heart contractions are not strong enough to produce a palpable radial pulse.
14. Assist the patient with replacement of clothing, if necessary. Assist patient from the examining table.
15. Wipe earpieces and chestpiece of stethoscope with alcohol wipes or cotton balls and alcohol. **Rationale:** Prevent cross-contamination.
16. Wash hands.

Charting Example

2/14/XX	4:00 p.m.	82/78 AP
Pulse deficit = 4		
Quality of beat strong.		M. King, CMA

Characteristics of Respiration

When observing a patient's respirations, three characteristics should be noted: rate, rhythm, and depth.

Rate

Rate refers to the number of respirations per minute and can be described as normal, rapid, or slow. The adult normal range of respirations is 14 to 20 cycles per minute. A respiratory rate, below 12 (bradypnea) or above 40 (tachypnea) in an adult, should be considered a serious symptom. Rapid respirations are usually shallow in depth.

Children have a much more rapid rate of breathing than adults with an average of 30 to 50 cycles per minute. See Table 20-7 for the ranges of respiratory rates of various age groups.

The respiratory rate is usually at a 1:4 proportion of the pulse rate. Many factors affect the respiratory rate. Some of these include an elevated temperature, age, pain, and medical conditions such as asthma. An elevated temperature in both

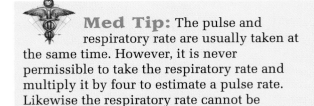

Med Tip: The pulse and respiratory rate are usually taken at the same time. However, it is never permissible to take the respiratory rate and multiply it by four to estimate a pulse rate. Likewise the respiratory rate cannot be determined by dividing the pulse rate by four.

adults and children can result in an elevated respiratory rate. Extreme pain may also cause the respirations to increase.

There are several terms relating to rate used to describe the respirations. Each term is specific to a breathing condition and should be used when observing the patient. A description of these terms is in Table 20-8.

The respiratory rate is affected by both emotional and physical conditions. Table 20-9 lists situations which may cause an alteration in the respiratory rate.

Rhythm

Rhythm is the breathing pattern which occurs at either regular or irregular intervals. In a regular rhythm, inspirations and expirations should be the same in rate and depth. In an irregular breathing pattern, the amount of air inhaled and exhaled and the rate of respiration per minute will vary.

If the breathing rhythm appears irregular after one minute of observation then respirations should be observed for several more minutes for comparison purposes. Patients with emphysema, an abnormal pulmonary condition, may experience no difficulty with inhalation but may struggle to fully exhale. Asthma may also cause an irregularity in breathing rhythm.

TABLE 20-7 Respiratory Rate Ranges of Various Age Groups

Age Group	Average Number Per Minute
Newborn	30–50
1 year old	20–40
2–10 years	20–30
11–18 years	18–24
Adult	14–20

TABLE 20-8 Respiratory Terms Relating to Rate

Term	Meaning	Example
Apnea	Temporary cessation of breathing	Sleep apnea
Bradypnea	Abnormally slow breathing (an adult below 10 per minute)	Near death
Dyspnea	Difficulty breathing	Asthma, pneumonia
Orthopnea	Difficulty breathing when lying down	Emphysema, congestive heart failure
Tachypnea (or hyperpnea)	Rapid respirations	High fever, pneumonia

Depth

The depth of respiration refers to the volume of air being inhaled and exhaled. It is described as either shallow or deep. Shallow respirations with a rapid rate occur in some disease conditions such as high fever, shock, and severe pain.

When a patient is unable to take in enough oxygen during inhalation, the skin and nail beds may appear bluish in color. This is called cyanosis and is due to the increase of carbon dioxide (CO_2) in the blood. In this situation, both the depth of respiration and cyanosis must be noted in the patient's record.

Breath Sounds

Normal respirations have no noticeable sound. Breath sounds occur in some disease conditions. Terms for describing breath sounds are stridor, stertorous, crackles (rales), rhonchi, and wheezes.

1. *Stridor,* a shrill, harsh sound is heard more clearly during inspiration. This sound may be heard in children with croup and patients with laryngeal obstruction.
2. *Stertorous sounds* are noisy breathing sounds such as heard in snoring.
3. *Crackles* or *rales* consist of crackling sounds resembling crushing tissue paper. They are caused by fluid accumulation in the airways and are heard with some types of pneumonia.
4. *Rhonchi,* which are also called gurgles, are rattling, whistling sounds made in the throat. This sound may be heard in a patient with a tracheostomy who requires suctioning of mucous.
5. *Wheezes* are high-pitched, whistling sounds made when airways become obstructed or severely narrowed, as in asthma or chronic obstructive pulmonary disease (COPD).

Med Tip: Chronic obstructive pulmonary disease (COPD) is one of the leading causes of disability and affects approximately 17 million Americans. Cigarette smoking, air pollution, and occupational exposure to dust and fumes are some of the leading causes of this disease. COPD is the result of chronic bronchitis, asthma, emphysema, and heart disease.

TABLE 20-9   **Situations Causing Changes in Respiratory Rate**

Increased Rate	Decreased Rate
Allergic reactions	Certain drugs (for example, morphine)
Certain drugs (for example, epinephrine)	Decrease of CO_2 in blood
Disease (asthma, heart disease)	Disease (stroke, coma)
Exercise	
Excitement/Anger	
Fever	
Hemorrhage	
High altitudes	
Nervousness	
Obstruction of air passage	
Pain	
Shock	

1. Do not explain the procedure to the patient. Attempt to keep the patient unaware that respirations are being measured since the patient may alter the breathing pattern. Appear to be taking the pulse.
2. The temperature and pulse may be taken at this same time if desired.
3. Do not take respiration measurements immediately after the patient has experienced exertion, such as climbing stairs, unless so ordered.
4. Count each inhalation and expiration as one respiration (breathing cycle).

Blood Pressure (BP)

The measurement of blood pressure (BP) is an important vital sign to aid in diagnosis and treatment and is therefore taken routinely. Many medical conditions can be indicated by either a rise or fall in blood pressure. The condition of high blood pressure known as hypertension is often asymptomatic or without any symptoms. An abnormal blood pressure reading can be the first indication of this condition.

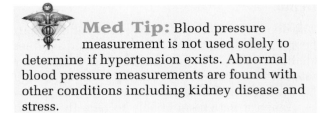

Med Tip: Blood pressure measurement is not used solely to determine if hypertension exists. Abnormal blood pressure measurements are found with other conditions including kidney disease and stress.

Physiology of Blood Pressure

The blood pressure is actually caused by the action of the blood moving against the walls of the arteries. Blood is pushed out of the heart and into the aorta and pulmonary arteries as the ventricles contract. (See Figure 20-15). This, in turn, exerts continuous pressure on the walls of the arteries.

Blood Pressure Readings

Blood pressure levels are taken at two different points called "readings." The two blood pressure readings are systolic pressure, or the highest pressure that occurs as the heart is contracting, and diastolic pressure, which is at the lowest pressure level that occurs when the heart is relaxed (the ventricle is at rest). The pulse beat is felt at the systolic pressure level and is absent at the diastolic pressure level.

PROCEDURE: Measuring Respirations

Terminal Performance Competency: Student must be able to accurately perform all steps of procedure and provide a respiration measurement with 100% accuracy.

Equipment and Supplies
Watch with sweep second hand.

Procedural Steps
1. Wash hands.
2. Identify patient.
3. Assist patient into a comfortable position.
4. Place your hand on the patient's wrist in position to take the pulse.
5. Count each breathing cycle by observing and/or feeling the rise and fall of the chest or upper abdomen.
6. Count for one full minute using a watch with a sweep second hand. If the rate is atypical, or unusual, in any way take it for another minute.
7. Record respiratory rate in patient's record noting date, time, any abnormality in rate, rhythm, and depth, and your signature.

Charting Example
2/14/XX   4:00 p.m.   Resp. 20 and regular
                        M. King, CMA

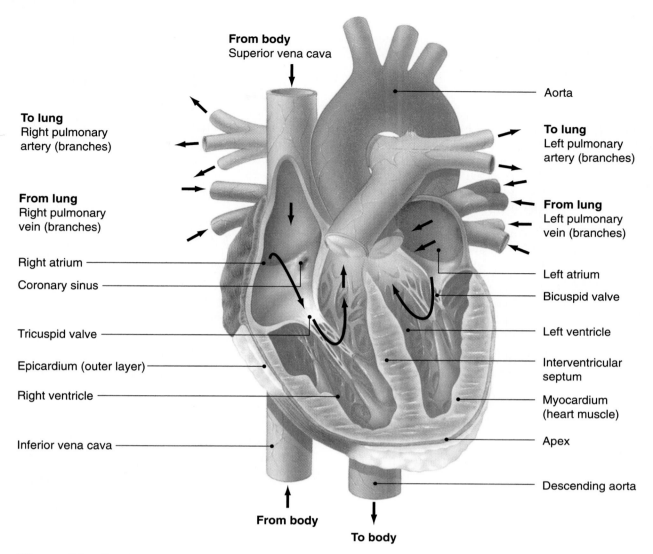

From body
Superior vena cava

Aorta

To lung
Right pulmonary
artery (branches)

To lung
Left pulmonary
artery (branches)

From lung
Right pulmonary
vein (branches)

From lung
Left pulmonary
vein (branches)

Right atrium

Left atrium

Coronary sinus

Bicuspid valve

Tricuspid valve

Left ventricle

Epicardium (outer layer)

Interventricular
septum

Right ventricle

Myocardium
(heart muscle)

Inferior vena cava

Apex

Descending aorta

From body

To body

Figure 20-15   Circulation of blood through the heart.

These two phases of heart activity—contraction and relaxation—are referred to as the **cardiac cycle.** The two **heart sounds** (lubb and dubb) occurring during the cardiac cycle are **systole** at contraction and **diastole** at relaxation.

Korotkoff Sounds

Korotkoff sounds are the sounds actually heard as the arterial wall distends during the compression of the blood pressure cuff. The sounds were first classified into five different phases by the Russian neurologist, Nicolai Korotkoff.

When the blood pressure cuff is first inflated no sound can be heard since the brachial artery is compressed. As air is slowly removed from the cuff during deflation, the Korotkoff sounds become audible. The deflation of air should be at the rate of

2-3 mm Hg per heart beat. The medical assistant should practice taking blood pressure readings slowly in order to be able to identify each phase. Korotkoff sounds are described in Table 20-10.

Pulse pressure is the difference between the systolic and diastolic readings. This is found by subtracting the diastolic reading from the systolic reading. A pulse pressure which is greater than 50 mm Hg or less than 30 mm Hg is considered to be abnormal. For instance, if the blood pressure is 130/82 the pulse pressure would be 48 which is still within the range considered normal. Extremes of pulse pressure can result in stroke or shock.

Readings of blood pressure are in millimeters (mm) of mercury (Hg). The abbreviations, mm and Hg, are not necessary when recording the blood pressure readings. The actual blood pressure is recorded using just the systolic, or highest pressure

TABLE 20-10 Five Phases of Korotkoff Sounds

Phase	Description
Phase I	This is the first faint sound heard as the cuff is deflated. Record this reading as the systolic pressure reading. The cuff must be inflated to a high enough level to hear this first sound during relaxation.
Phase II	The second phase occurs as the cuff continues to be deflated and blood flows through the artery. This sound has a swishing quality. The cuff has to be slowly deflated in order to hear this soft sound. An auscultatory gap is said to have occurred if there is a total loss of sound at this stage which then reoccurs later. An auscultatory gap can occur in certain cases of heart disease and hypertension. An auscultatory gap should be reported to the physician.
Phase III	During this phase the sound will become less muffled and develop a crisp tapping sound as the blood flow moves easily through the artery. If the BP cuff was not inflated enough to hear the Phase I sound, then the Phase III sound may be heard and incorrectly stated as the systolic reading.
Phase IV	The sound will now begin to fade and become muffled. The American Heart Association, which believes Phase IV is the best indicator of the diastolic pressure, recommends the reading at this phase be recorded as the diastolic pressure for a child.
Phase V	Sound will disappear at this phase. Some physicians want both phase IV and phase V recorded for the diastolic pressure reading (for example, 120/78/74 rather than 120/74).

Med Tip: Blood pressure readings, as with all vital signs, should be interpreted using the patient's baseline measurement. This means that a previously-taken blood pressure reading, when the patient was not ill, is used as that patient's "normal" measurement. All subsequent readings are then compared to that patient's "normal" baseline reading.

reading, over the diastolic, or lowest reading. For example, 120/80 would be considered a normal blood pressure reading for an adult. Generally, a *range of normal* is used for blood pressure readings since slight variations can occur between normal healthy adults. A deviation, either rise or fall, from the patient's baseline measurement of 20-30 mm Hg can be significant for that patient.

Blood pressure readings should routinely be started at age five as part of the school physical or earlier if medically necessary. Recommendations are that an elevated blood pressure reading should be found on at least two occasions before the patient is placed on medication, unless the diastolic reading is over 120 mm Hg. Patients should have a complete physical to see why their blood pressure is elevated. Patients with a sustained high

TABLE 20-11 Average Normal Blood Pressure Readings

Age Group	Average Blood Pressure (mm Hg)
Newborn	50/25
6–9 years of age	95/65
10–15 years of age	100/65
16 years to adulthood	118/76
Adult	120/80
Older adult	138/86
Normal adult range	90/60 to 140/90

blood pressure measurement may require further diagnostic evaluation for the presence of other disease conditions, as well as medication to lower the blood pressure. Controlling blood pressure can lower the incidence of stroke and heart attack.

If a patient's blood pressure deviates from the normal range, he or she should be tested again. Ideally, blood pressure is taken while the patient is lying down, sitting, and standing. Average normal blood pressure readings are listed in Table 20-11.

TABLE 20-12 Physiologic Factors Affecting Blood Pressure (BP)

Factor	Result
1. Volume of blood	Increase of blood volume increases the BP. Decrease of blood volume decreases BP. Example: Polycytopenia increases BP, hemorrhage causes volume and BP to drop.
2. Peripheral resistance	Relates to the size of the lumen, the cavity or space, within blood vessels and amount of blood flowing through it. Example: The smaller the size of the lumen, the greater the resistance to blood flow. Fatty cholesterol deposits result in high BP due to narrowing of the lumen.
3. Condition of heart muscle	Strength of heart muscle affects volume of blood flow. The pumping action of the heart and how efficiently it does the job affects the BP. Example: A weak heart muscle can cause an increase or decrease in BP.
4. Elasticity of vessels	The ability of blood vessels to expand and contract decreases with age. Example: Nonelastic blood vessels, as in arteriosclerosis, cause an elevated BP.

While an average blood pressure is listed for a newborn, blood pressure readings are not generally taken on infants. Monitors are used on the very young.

Factors Affecting Blood Pressure

Physiological factors affecting blood pressure include volume or amount of blood in the arteries, peripheral resistance of the vessels, condition of the heart muscle, and the elasticity of vessels. These four factors are discussed in Table 20-12.

Many other factors may affect blood pressure. Two of these are gender and age. Women generally have a lower pressure than men. Blood pressure is lowest at birth and tends to increase as people age. The time of day can also cause blood pressure variations. For example, blood pressure is usually at its lowest point early in the morning just before awakening.

Activities such as standing, sitting, or lying down can affect blood pressure. When blood pressure is measured while the patient is in an erect position it is referred to as an orthostatic blood pressure reading. Orthostatic hypotension refers to a lowered blood pressure occurring when a patient moves from a lying down to an erect position. Sudden movement, or a sudden change in position, with a resulting fall in blood pressure is referred to as postural hypotension.

The pressure reading in the right arm is usually 3 to 4 mm Hg higher than in the left arm. Numerous situations that cause changes in blood pressure readings are listed in Table 20-13. Terms relating to abnormal blood pressure readings are described in Table 20-14.

Blood pressure is a routinely taken vital sign. It is especially important for patients with the following characteristics or conditions:

1. Patients on antihypertensive drugs
2. Patient with a history of heart disease, kidney disease, stroke or hypertension
3. Patients receiving a complete physical examination, including children
4. Pregnant women
5. Preoperative and postoperative patients
6. Patients who are bleeding or in shock
7. Patients with symptoms of a neurological disorder
8. Patient experiencing an allergic reaction

Equipment for Measuring Blood Pressure

There are two pieces of equipment necessary for measuring blood pressure: a sphygmomanometer and a stethoscope. The sphygmomanometer is the instrument used for measuring the pressure the blood exerts against the walls of the artery (Figure 20-16). The stethoscope is a diagnostic instrument that amplifies sound. It is used to detect sounds produced by blood pressure as well as the heart and other internal organs such as the stomach.

Sphygmomanometers

The components of a sphygmomanometer are: manometer, inflatable rubber bladder, cuff, and bulb. The manometer is a scale which registers the actual pressure reading.

TABLE 20-13 Causes of Blood Pressure (BP) Variations

Elevated (Increased) BP	Lowered (Decreased) BP
Anger	Anemia
Certain drug therapies (nicotine, caffeine)	Approaching death
Endocrine disorders, such as hyperthyroidism	Cancer
Exercise	Certain drug therapies (antihypertensives, narcotics, analgesics, diuretics)
Fear, excitement	Decreased arterial blood volume (hemorrhage)
Heart and liver disease	
Increased arterial blood volume	Dehydration
Increased intracranial pressure	Infection and fever
Late pregnancy	Left arm
Lying down position with legs elevated	Massive heart attack
Obesity	Middle pregnancy
Pain	Pain
Renal disease	Starvation
Right arm	Shock
Rigidity of blood vessels (in old age)	Sudden postural changes such as standing
Smoking	Thyroid and adrenal gland disorders: nerve disorders
Stress, anxiety	
Time of day (late afternoon and early evening)	Time of day (during sleep and early morning)
Vasoconstriction or narrowing of peripheral blood vessels	Weak heart

The core of the blood pressure cuff is the rubber bladder which, when inflated, distends to temporarily constrict blood circulation in the arm. A soft material cuff covers the bladder and is placed next to the skin of the patient. The pressure bulb has a thumbscrew attached to a control valve which allows for inflation and deflation of the cuff.

The size of the blood pressure cuff is important. There are three additional sizes available: pediatric, large arm adult, and thigh. A small pediatric cuff is available for children. Blood pressure cuffs are not generally used on infants. The pediatric cuff can also be used on small-limbed adults. A thigh cuff is available when an adult arm is too large for the large arm cuff. When using a thigh cuff, the popliteal artery is palpated for a pulse.

The two types of sphygmomanometers are mercury and aneroid. A discussion follows with illustrations of portable and wall-mounted versions of each type.

Mercury Sphygmomanometer The mercury sphygmomanometer is considered to be the most accurate and is found on the walls in many physicians offices (Figure 20-17). It contains a column of mercury which will rise as the pressure bulb is pressed and the rubber bladder inflated. A calibrated scale runs down both sides of the mercury column. The reading is taken at eye level at the top of the mercury line next to a calibrated scale. This type of instrument must be placed vertically on the wall or on a flat, level surface so that the mercury will rise in a vertical position. Periodic

TABLE 20-14   Abnormal Blood Pressure Readings

Condition	Description
Hypertension	A condition in which the patient's blood pressure is consistently above the norm for his or her age group. Also called high blood pressure. 140/90 is the baseline.
benign	Slow onset elevated blood pressure without symptoms.
essential	This is a primary hypertension of unknown cause. It may be genetically determined.
secondary	Elevated blood pressure associated with other conditions such as renal disease, pregnancy, arteriosclerosis, atherosclerosis, and obesity.
malignant	Rapidly developing elevated blood pressure which may become fatal if not treated immediately.
renal	Elevated blood pressure as a result of kidney disease.
Hypotension	Condition of abnormally low blood pressure which may be caused by shock, hemorrhage, and central nervous system (CNS) disorders.
orthostatic	A temporary fall in blood pressure that occurs when a patient rapidly moves from a lying to a standing position. Dizziness and blurred vision can also be present.
postural	A temporary fall in blood pressure from standing motionless for extended periods of time.

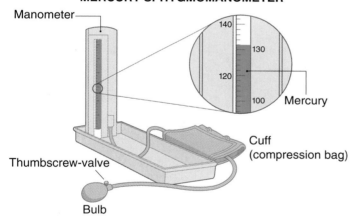

MERCURY SPHYGMOMANOMETER

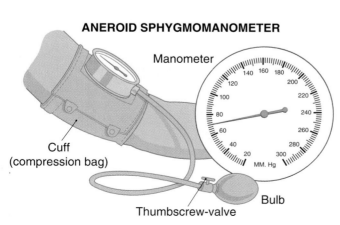

ANEROID SPHYGMOMANOMETER

Figure 20-16   A sphygmomanometer is the blood pressure instrument.

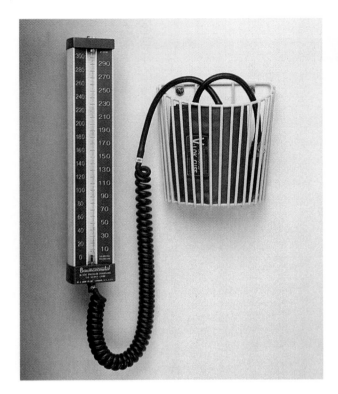

Figure 20-17   Wall mounted mercury sphygmo-manometer.

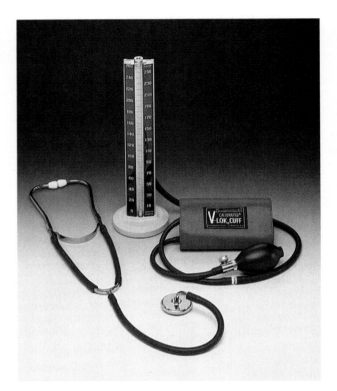

Figure 20-18   Portable mercury sphygmo-manometer.

re-calculation is necessary for accuracy. See Figure 20-18 for an example of a portable mercury sphygmonanometer.

Aneroid Sphygmomanometer The aneroid sphygmomanometer has a round dial that contains a scale calibrated in millimeters (mm) and a needle to register the reading (Figure 20-19). The needle must be at zero before starting the procedure. The aneroid sphygmomanometer should be re-calibrated for accuracy every year by using a mercury manometer as the model. This instrument is easily portable (Figure 20-20).

Diaphragm and Bell Stethoscopes

The stethoscope is used to detect sounds produced by blood pressure. This instrument consists of a chestpiece containing a diaphragm and/or bell, flexible tubing, binaurals, a spring mechanism, and earpieces. The key components of the stethoscope are described in Table 20-15 and shown in Figure 20-21.

Measuring Blood Pressure

After selecting the appropriate equipment, use the following guidelines and the procedure for measuring blood pressure (Figure 20-22).

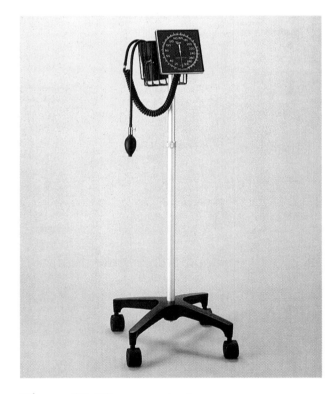

Figure 20-19   Aneroid sphygmomanometer.

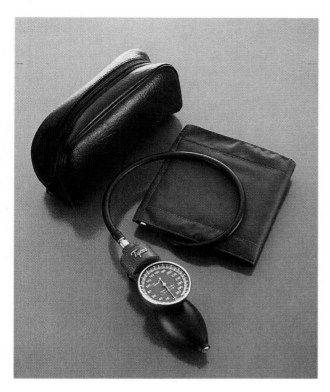

Figure 20-20   Portable aneroid sphygmo-manometer.

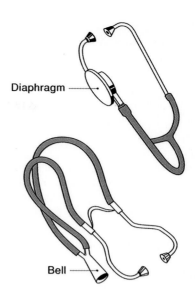

Diaphragm

Bell

Figure 20-21   Diaphragm and bell stethoscopes.

TABLE 20-15   **Components of the Stethoscope**

Key Part	Description
Chestpiece	Portion of the instrument that is placed over the site where the sound is to be heard. May consist of a diaphragm or a bell or both.
Diaphragm	A disc-like sound sensor which picks up both low and high-pitched sound frequencies. More useful for high sounds such as bowel and lung sounds.
Bell	A hollow, curved—bell or cup shaped—sound sensor which may have one, two, or three "heads" which are useful in picking up sounds of the cardio-vascular system.
Flexible tubing	Rubber or plastic tubing to carry the sound from the patient to the binaurals. The usual length of tubing is 12 to 14 inches. You may prefer using longer tubing up to 22 inches. However, some of the sound clarity is lost as the tubing becomes longer.
Binaurals	Rigid small metal tubes that connect the tubing to the earpieces.
Spring mechanism	Flexible external metal spring that holds the binaural steady so that the earpiece will remain in the ear.
Earpieces	Molded plastic tips which attach to the end of the binaurals and are placed in the medical assistant's ears.

Guidelines: Measuring Blood Pressure

1. Attempt to relax the patient by explaining in a calm, quiet manner that the procedure is not painful.
2. Ask if the patient knows what his or her last blood pressure reading was and if the patient has any history of high blood pressure.
3. When taking blood pressure for the first time on a new patient, take a reading in both arms. Usually the BP is higher in the right arm than in the left if the patient is right handed.
4. If you hear the systolic beat immediately, then you have not inflated the cuff enough. However, do not add more pressure to the cuff without deflating it first. Always deflate the cuff completely before attempting to do another pressure reading.
5. Give the patient his or her blood pressure results only if the physician has instructed you to do so. Do not make any statement about the blood pressure being high or low. Let the physician explain the results.

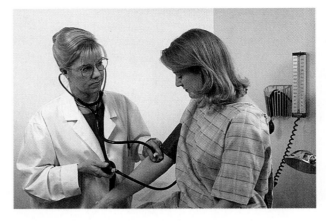

Figure 20-22 Measuring a patient's blood pressure.

PROCEDURE: Taking Blood Pressure

**Terminal Performance
Competency:** Student is expected to obtain a systolic and diastolic reading within 2 mm Hg of the instructor's observance, unless otherwise instructed.

Equipment and Supplies
  Sphygmomanometer
  Stethoscope
  70% Isopropyl alcohol
  Alcohol sponges or cotton balls
  Paper and pen/pencil
  Patient record

Procedural Steps
1. Wash hands
2. Assemble equipment. Thoroughly cleanse the earpieces, bell, and diaphram pieces of the stethoscope. Use an alcohol sponge or cotton ball with 70% Isopropyl alcohol. Allow alcohol to dry.
3. Identify patient verbally and explain the procedure.
4. Assist the patient into a comfortable position. BP is usually taken with patient in sitting position. However, the patient may be lying down, sitting, or standing. If taken while the patient is lying down or standing, note this in the chart. Inform the doctor since the pressure changes in different positions. The patient's arms should not be higher than heart level.
5. Place the mercury sphygmomanometer on a solid surface with the gauge within 3 feet for easy viewing. The sphygmomanometer should be able to be read by the MA but not the patient.

6. Uncover the patient's arm by asking patient to roll back sleeve 5 inches above the elbow. If the sleeve becomes constricting when rolled back, ask patient to slip the arm out of the sleeve. Never take a blood pressure reading through clothing.

7. Have patient straighten arm with palms up. Apply the cuff of the sphygmomanometer over the brachial artery (see Figure 20-22) 1 to 2 inches above the antecubital space (bend in the elbow). Many cuffs are marked with arrows or circles to be placed over the artery. Hold the edge of the cuff in place as you wrap the remainder of the cuff tightly around the arm. If the cuff has a Velcro closure, press it into place at the end of the cuff.

8. Palpate with your finger tips to locate the brachial artery in the antecubital space.

9. Place earpieces in your ears and the diaphragm (or bell) of the stethoscope over the area where you feel the brachial artery pulsing. Hold the diaphragm in place with one hand on the chestpiece without placing your thumb over the diaphragm. The stethoscope tubing should hang freely and not touch any object or the patient during the reading.

10. Close the thumbscrew on the hand bulb by turning clockwise with your dominant hand. Close the thumbscrew just enough so that no air can leak out. Do not close so tightly that you will have difficulty re-opening with one hand.

11. Pump air into the cuff quickly and evenly, until the level of mercury is 20-30 mm Hg above the previously measured BP or the approximated method. Some physicians prefer inflating the cuff to 180 mm Hg as a starting point.

12. Slowly turn the thumbscrew counter-clockwise with your dominant hand.

Allow the pressure reading to fall only 2-3 mm Hg at a time.

13. Listen for the point at which the first clear sound is heard (Phase I of the Korotkoff sounds). Note where this occurred on the mercury column (or spring gauge scale on an aneroid manometer). This is the systolic pressure.

14. Slowly continue to allow the cuff to deflate. The sounds will change from loud to murmur and then fade away. (Phases I, II, III, IV of Korotkoff sounds). Read the mercury column (or spring gauge scale) at the point where the sound is muffled or dull. This is the diastolic pressure (Phase IV of Korotkoff sounds).

15. Continue to deflate the cuff and read the mercury column (or spring gauge scale on aneroid manometer) until the sound is gone. This is Phase V of the Korotkoff sounds. Many physicians will want both Phase IV and Phase V reported for the diastolic reading.

16. Quickly open the thumbscrew all the way to release the air and deflate the cuff.

17. If you are unsure about the BP reading wait at least a minute or two before taking a second reading. Never take more than two readings in one arm since blood stasis may have occurred resulting in an inaccurate reading.

18. Immediately write the BP as a fraction on paper. You may inform the patient of the reading if this is the policy in your office.

19. Remove the cuff.

20. Clean the earpieces of the stethoscope with an alcohol sponge.

21. Wash hands.

22. Chart the results including the date, time, BP reading and your name.

Charting Example

2/14/XX   9:00 am B/P 134/88 left arm, sitting.   M. King, CMA

Estimated Systolic Pressure

The **palpatory method** of feeling the radial pulse while the blood pressure cuff is deflating can be used to determine systolic pressure. This method cannot be used to determine the diastolic pressure or to hear the Korotkoff sounds. However it is useful when a student is learning to take blood pressure readings. The level of inflation necessary to hear the first sound in Phase I can be determined by using the palpatory method. See procedure for using this method.

Note: Follow the general guidelines for taking blood pressure and steps 1 through 10 in the procedure for taking blood pressure. See Figure 20-22 for illustration of measuring blood pressure.

Causes of Errors in Blood Pressure Readings

Table 20-16 describes causes of errors in taking blood pressure readings.

Measuring Height and Weight

Height and weight are two important measurements even though they are not considered vital signs in the true sense of the term. These measurements are called anthropometric measurements since they relate to **anthropometry,** the science of size, proportion, weight, and height.

Height and weight can provide indications of the general health of the patient. Infants who fail to gain weight or "fail to thrive" need close supervision of weight gains and losses. The diagnosis of hormonal imbalances in children resulting in abnormal growth patterns can be picked up through routine comparisons of the child's height and weight against national growth charts. Diabetic patients, pregnant women, cardiac patients, patients with fluid retention, and patients suffering from eating disorders such as bulimia and obesity need to have frequent weight monitoring. Patients prefer privacy when having their body measurements taken. They can remain fully

---

PROCEDURE: Estimating Systolic BP Using Palpatory (Approximated) Method

Terminal Performance
Competency: Student is expected to obtain a systolic reading that is within 2 mm Hg of the instructor's, unless otherwise instructed.

Equipment and Supplies
Sphygmomanometer
Stethoscope
70% Isopropyl alcohol
Alcohol sponges or cotton balls
Paper and pen
Patient record

Note: American Heart Association recommends that approximate systolic BP be determined first by palpatating radial pulse, then pumping up cuff until pulse in no longer felt. This is standard procedure in many cases.

Procedural Steps
1. Place the blood pressure cuff in the usual position on the upper arm.
2. Locate the radial pulse on the thumb side of the wrist.
3. Inflate the blood pressure cuff until the pulse disappears and note the reading on the manometer.
4. Re-inflate the cuff until the pulse once again disappears and inflate another 30 mm Hg to get above the systolic pressure.
5. Slowly deflate the cuff while keeping fingers on the pulse. The point at which the pulse is felt is the systolic pressure.
6. Remember this number if you are going to take a brachial artery blood pressure reading immediately. Write the number on paper if there will be a delay before you can take the complete blood pressure.

Charting Example
Note: This number is not usually charted since it is only used to estimate the systolic BP.

clothed for this procedure. Indicate on the medical record if measurements were taken with clothes on or off.

Scales may be calibrated in either kilograms (metric weight) or pounds (Figure 20-23). In some cases, a scale will have a ruled panel which can be flipped up to reveal both pounds and kilograms. However, the medical assistant must know how to do conversions from pounds into kilograms and vice versa. Table 20-17 contains conversion charts to be used when converting a weight from pounds to kilograms or from kilograms to pounds.

TABLE 20-16   Causes of Errors in Blood Pressure Readings

Source/Cause	Problem
Equipment	Cuff is improper size. The cuff bladder should be 20% wider than the diameter of the extremity where cuff is placed. Large cuffs for obese arms and small cuffs for children should be available in all offices.
	Air leaks around the valve may cause mercury to drop suddenly.
	Air leak in the bladder of cuff delays the inflation rate and could give a false high reading. Air leaks may also occur along the tubing if it is old or worn.
	Mercury column is not calibrated to the zero point.
	Velcro may be worn and does not hold.
Procedure	Patient's arm is not uncovered.
	Medical assistant is too far away from manometer to accurately read gauge.
	Cuff is improperly applied (too loose or too small).
	Cuff is not centered over the brachial artery, 1-2 inches above bend in the elbow.
	End of the cuff is not secured tightly.
	Part of stethoscope tubing or chestpiece touches the blood pressure cuff while taking the pressure reading.
	Failure to locate brachial pulse before placing stethoscope in position.
	The rubber bladder in the cuff was not deflated completely before beginning the procedure.
	Valve on bulb is not completely closed before beginning to pump air into cuff.
	Cuff was not inflated to a level 20–30 mm Hg above the palpated or previously measured systolic pressure or 200 mm Hg.
	Deflation occurs too rapidly to accurately determine the sounds.
	The arm used for the reading is not at the same level as the heart. The arm cannot be held above the level of the heart.
	Failed to wait 1-2 minutes before taking second reading.
	Failed to notice the auscultatory gap.
Patient	Patient is nervous or anxious resulting in a false high reading.
	Patient's arm is too large for accurate reading with available equipment.

TABLE 20-17 Conversion Chart for Pounds and Kilograms

To convert kilograms to pounds (kg to lb):
l kilogram (kg) = 2.2 pounds (lbs)
Multiply the number of kilograms by 2.2
Example: If a patient weighs 64 kilograms, multiply 64 by 2.2.
64 × 2.2 = 140.8 or 141 pounds

To convert pounds to kilograms (lb to kg):
1 pound = 0.45 kilograms
Multiply the number of pounds by 0.45
Example: If a patient weighs 130 pounds, multiply 130 by 0.45.
130 × 0.45 = 58.5 or 59 kilograms

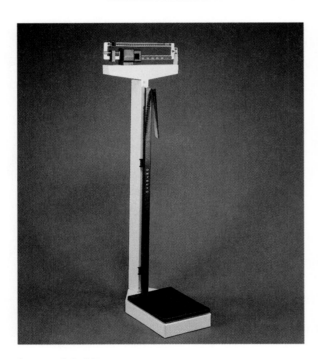

Figure 20-23   Upright scale.

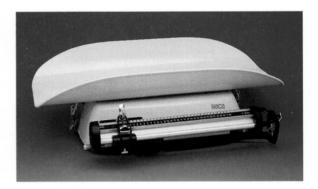

Figure 20-24   Baby scale.

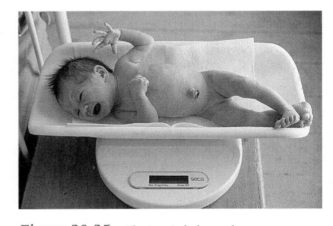

Figure 20-25   Electronic baby scale.

Infant Height and Weight

Figures 20-24 and 20-25 show baby scales used to measure an infant's weight. See the Procedure for Measuring Infant Height and Weight.

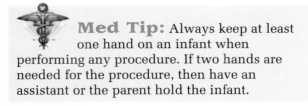

Med Tip: Always keep at least one hand on an infant when performing any procedure. If two hands are needed for the procedure, then have an assistant or the parent hold the infant.

Circumference of the Infant's Head

Some physicians wish to have a measurement taken of the circumference or area around the infant's head. This is performed periodically during infancy to observe for any abnormal enlargement.

PROCEDURE: Measuring Adult Height and Weight

Terminal Performance Competency: Student is expected to obtain a height and weight that is equal to the instructor's observance, unless otherwise instructed, and to perform math conversions.

Equipment and Supplies

Balance scale with bar to measure height
Paper towel
Pen
Patient record

Procedural Steps

1. Wash hands
2. Identify the patient.
3. Explain procedure to the patient.
4. For patients who wish to remove shoes, place a paper towel on the scale. Heavy objects such as keys should be removed and female patients should set their purses aside.
5. Set all the weights to zero. Balance the scale by adjusting the small knob at one end until the balance bar pointer floats in the center of the frame. (A coin can be used to make this adjustment.)
6. Assist the patient onto the scale.
7. Ask the patient to stand still.
8. First move the large weight into the groove closest to the weight you estimate for the patient. If the balance bar pointer touches the bottom of the bar then move the large weight back one notch. Move the small weight by tapping it gently until it reaches a point in which the pointer floats in the center of the frame.
9. Leave the weights in place.

Continue with Height:

10. Ask the patient to place his or her back to the scale, stand erect, and look straight ahead.
11. Raise the height bar in a collapsed position making sure the tip is over the patient's head.
12. Open the bar into the horizontal position and bring it down gently to touch the top of the patient's head. Leave this setting in place.
13. Assist the patient in stepping off the scale.
14. Read the weight scale by adding the number at the large weight to the number behind the small weight to the nearest 1/4 pound. For example, 150 pounds at the large weight and 23 1/2 at the small weight = 173 1/2 pounds.
15. Record this measurement on the patient's record.
16. Read the height as marked behind the movable level of the ruled bar. Record this measurement to the nearest 1/4 inch on the patient's record. (Convert inches to feet by dividing by 12. Chart height in feet and inches.)
17. Return the weights to zero and the height bar to the normal position.
18. Discard paper towel.
19. Wash hands.

Charting Example

2/14/XX   wt. = 140 1/4 lbs with shoes; ht. = 5′ 7″ (67 inches)   M. King, CMA

This is generally performed during each check-up visit until the age of 36 months.

Using a flexible (soft) measuring tape, wrap it once around the baby's head at the forehead level. The circumference is then charted to the nearest 0.1 cm or 1/4 inch along with the height and weight.

The physician may also request to have the infant's chest measurement taken until the age of 12 months. This is used to monitor abnormal growth patterns. A flexible tape measure is held by the medical assistant's thumb at the infant's midsternal level. The tape is wrapped once around the chest above the nipple line and under the axilla. The measurement should be taken while the child is breathing normally and not during crying.

PROCEDURE: Measuring Infant Height and Weight

**Terminal Performance
Competency:** Student is expected to obtain a height and weight that is equal to the instructor's observance, unless otherwise instructed and convert to metric readings.

Equipment and Supplies
Baby scale
Patient record
Pen
Small towel or protector for scale
Tape measure

Procedural Steps

1. Wash hands.

2. Identify infant by stating the infant's name to the parent. Have infant remain with parent while the equipment is being prepared.

3. Place a towel/protector on the baby scale.

4. Balance the scale by placing all the weights to the far left side. Turn the bolt at the right edge of the scale until the balance bar pointer is at the middle of the balance bar.

5. Undress infant (or ask parent to undress infant). Gently lay infant on the scale. Always keep one hand on the infant until the weights are adjusted. Do not leave the infant unattended at any time.

6. Keeping one hand over the infant's body as a safety precaution, move the large pound weight into the groove closest to the weight estimated for the baby. Then move the smaller ounce weight by tapping it gently until it reaches a point in which the pointer floats in the center of the frame.

7. Keep the weights in place while the infant is moved to the examination table for height measurement.

Continue with Height:

8. Holding the tape measure with one hand, place the tape at the top of the side of the infant's head. Stretch the infant out full length as you pull the tape measure down to the bottom of the feet. If you are using a table with a measure bar, place the infant's head at one end of the table with the soles of his or her feet touching the foot board. *Note:* It is preferred to have two people measure the length of an infant. The parent can assist by holding the infant's head still. To measure an active child, make pencil marks at the top of the child's head and at the bottom of the feet on the exam table paper. Then measure the area between the marks.

9. Note the height in inches and fractions of an inch and write it on the paper covering the exam table. Do not take your hands off the infant.

10. Ask the parent to hold the infant while the height and weight are charted in the infant's record.

11. Tell the measurements to the parent.

12. Discard paper towel.

13. Wash hands.

Charting Example
2/14/XX   weight 16 lb. 3 oz., length 30 inches
M. King, CMA

Skin-fold Fat Measurement

In some medical practices body fat is calculated using skin-fold calipers. Areas of fat tissue at the under side of the upper arm are measured by gently grasping the skin (but not the muscle) between the calipers. The measurement is read from the scale on the caliper and charted as "taken by skin-fold caliper."

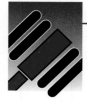

LEGAL AND ETHICAL ISSUES

The medical assistant has an ethical responsibility to use careful, proper technique when performing procedures to measure vital signs since an incorrect reading could lead to misdiagnosis and result in serious consequences for the patient. Proper technique includes: allowing enough time for the temperature to register; using a watch with a second hand when taking pulse and respiration; and never guessing the time when measuring pulse and respirations, just to name a few. Incorrect documentation of vital signs can lead to serious complications for the patient and legal consequences for the physician and the medical assistant.

PATIENT EDUCATION

The medical assistant acts as the resource person for instructing the patient on the correct use of equipment, such as the thermometer, to ensure accuracy in reporting temperatures to the physician.

Teaching methods, include verbal instructions, demonstration and return demonstration, educational pamphlets, and drawings, when necessary, depending on what you are teaching and the patient's educational and motivational level.

Patients must be cautioned that an abnormal vital sign, such as an elevated temperature, should not be ignored with a "wait and see" attitude since a prolonged high fever can result in brain damage and even death.

Patient education will vary. For example, patients suffering from cardiovascular disease should be taught to take their own pulse and to detect abnormalities in pulse rate, rhythm, and volume. Hypertensive patients should be taught the symptoms and causes of high blood pressure and how to monitor their own blood pressure. In addition, patient education is needed to alert the patient to risk prevention, dietary control, the role of exercise, lifestyle choices, and compliance with drug therapy.

Summary

Vital signs are an important objective indication of the patient's overall physical condition. One vital measurement taken alone does not necessarily provide a complete picture. The medical assistant must be able to skillfully take all vital measurements and be able to assess what she or he is observing such as the rate, rhythm, and depth of respirations. Other factors such as age, gender, nervousness and physical condition of the patient may effect vital sign readings.

The accuracy of obtaining and recording vital sign measurements is critical for the ultimate diagnosis and treatment of the patient. Communication skills, while important in all aspects of medical assisting work, are essential when obtaining vital measurements. A positive and sincere approach in interacting with the patient may be enough to put the patient at ease and result in obtaining more valid vital sign measurements.

Competency Review

1. Define and spell the glossary terms for this chapter.
2. Take and record 10 oral temperatures using an oral thermometer within 0.2° of instructor's reading.
3. Take and record an axillary temperature using an oral thermometer within 0.2° of instructor's reading.
4. Take and record 5 aural temperatures using a tympanic membrane thermometer within 0.2° of instructor's reading.
5. Take and record 10 patients' pulse rates within 1 pulse beat per minute of instructor.
6. Count and chart 10 patients' respirations within 1 respiration of instructor's count.
7. Take 10 blood pressure readings within 2 mm Hg of instructor's reading.
8. Measure and record height and weight of 5 patients within 1/4 inch and 1/4 pound of instructor's measurement with conversion to metric included in charting.

PREPARING FOR THE CERTIFICATION EXAM

Test Taking Tip — Circle any key word in the question, such as always or never, to focus on that concept when answering a multiple choice question.

Examination Review Questions

1. Dinesha Reynolds has an oral temperature of 100.4°F. The medical term for this is
   - (A) pyuria
   - (B) purulent
   - (C) hyperpyrexia
   - (D) pyrexia
   - (E) none of the above

2. Which of the following is NOT considered a vital sign?
   - (A) body temperature
   - (B) weight
   - (C) blood pressure
   - (D) respiration
   - (E) all of these are vital signs

3. What is considered the least accurate indicator of temperature?
   - (A) axilla
   - (B) oral
   - (C) eardrum
   - (D) rectum
   - (E) all are equally accurate

4. The ratio of pulse to respirations is usually
   - (A) 1:5
   - (B) 4:1
   - (C) 1:3
   - (D) 1:2
   - (E) none of the above

5. During which phase of the Korotkoff sounds will the sound fade and become muffled?
   - (A) Phase I
   - (B) Phase II
   - (C) Phase III
   - (D) Phase IV
   - (E) Phase V

6. Blood pressure that becomes low when a patient assumes an erect position is called
   - (A) postural hypertension
   - (B) orthostatic hypertension
   - (C) essential hypertension
   - (D) orthostatic hypotension
   - (E) none of the above is correct

7. Mr. Daniels weighs 83.92 Kg. How many pounds does he weigh?
   - (A) 185 lb
   - (B) 195 lb
   - (C) 180 lb
   - (D) 200 lb
   - (E) 210 lb

8. The normal pulse rate (beats per minute) for adults is
   - (A) 40–60
   - (B) 60–80
   - (C) 80–100
   - (D) 100–120
   - (E) 120–160

9. When taking an oral temperature, the thermometer should be left in the mouth for at least how many minutes?
   - (A) 3 minutes
   - (B) 5 minutes
   - (C) 10 minutes
   - (D) 12 minutes
   - (E) 15 minutes

10. When taking a rectal temperature, the thermometer should be left in the rectum for how many minutes?
    - (A) 3 minutes
    - (B) 5 minutes
    - (C) 10 minutes
    - (D) 12 minutes
    - (E) 15 minutes

ON THE JOB

Lakisha is working in an OB/GYN clinic affiliated with a major teaching hospital. Her general responsibilities include registering patients, handling phone calls when the receptionist is on a break, escorting patients into the examination room, taking vital signs, running selected laboratory tests, setting up the clinic examination rooms for gynecological examinations, and providing patient education.

The morning's schedule of patients/visitors follows:

9:00 Adele Bishop	New mother check-up
9:15 Amy Campbell	First OB visit
9:30	↓ ↓ ↓
9:45 Maria Lopez	OB patient in last month of pregnancy
10:00 Meg Rivers	Regular OB check-up
10:15 Vanessa Brown	New gyn patient w/ovarian cyst
10:30	↓ ↓ ↓
10:45 Tiffany Baker	Regular OB check-up
11:00 Vern Simmons	Pelvic inflammatory disease
11:15 Latonya Pike	1st visit after miscarriage
11:30 Emma Thompson	Yearly checkup-gyn patient
11:30	↓ ↓ ↓
12:00 Lunch Break	

Note: During the morning the following occurs:
- When Maria Lopez arrives, she tells Lakisha that she has been bleeding since the weekend.
- A pharmaceutical representative comes in at 10:00 a.m. and is asking to see the doctor.
- Supplies are delivered that must be signed for.
- Dr. Williams is called away to perform a delivery at 11:00 a.m.
- Vital signs including TPR, BP and weight are taken for all OB patients.
- Urinalysis is performed by another medical assistant assigned to the clinic laboratory.

What is Your Response?

1. How should Lakisha handle each of the morning's patients and occurrences?
2. Should Maria Lopez's bleeding be considered an emergency? If so, what is Lakisha's responsibility?
3. Should the representative take precedence over scheduled patients? If so, which ones? If not, what should be said to the rep.?
4. What is the correct procedure for signing for and checking in medical supplies?
5. Since Dr. Williams was called away for a delivery, how should the patients be rescheduled? What about the patients that are already in the waiting room?

References

Anderson, K., and Anderson, L. *Mosby's Pocket Dictionary of Medicine, Nursing, & Allied Health.* Chicago: Mosby, 1994.

Badasch, S. and Chesbro, D. *Introduction to Health Occupations.* Upper Saddle River, NJ: Brady/Prentice Hall, 1997.

Bledsoe, B., Porter, R., and Shade, B. *Paramedic Emergency Care.* Upper Saddle River, NJ: Brady/Prentice Hall, 1997.

Fischbach, F. *A Manual of Laboratory and Diagnostic Tests.* Philadelphia: Lippincott, 1996.

Fremgen, B. *Medical Terminology.* Upper Saddle River, NJ: Brady/Prentice Hall, 1997.

Martine, F. *Fundamentals of Anatomy and Physiology.* Upper Saddle River, NJ: Brady/Prentice Hall, 1995.

Nurse's Pocket Companion. Springhouse, PA: Springhouse Corporation, 1993.

Potter, P., Perry, P. *Fundamentals of Nursing— Concepts, Process and Practice,* 3rd ed. St. Louis: Mosby Year Book, 1993.

Taber's Cyclopedic Medical Dictionary, 18th ed. Philadelphia: F.A. Davis Company, 1997.

MEDICAL ASSISTANT ROLE DELINEATION CHART

Highlight indicates material covered in this chapter

ADMINISTRATIVE

ADMINISTRATIVE PROCEDURES

- Perform basic clerical functions
- Schedule, coordinate, and monitor appointments
- Schedule inpatient/outpatient admissions and procedures
- Understand and apply third party guidelines
- Obtain reimbursement through accurate claims submission
- Monitor third-party reimbursement
- Perform medical transcription
- Understand and adhere to managed care policies and procedures
- *Negotiate managed care contracts (adv)*

PRACTICE FINANCES

- Perform procedural and diagnostic coding
- Apply bookkeeping principles
- Document and maintain accounting and banking records
- Manage accounts receivable
- Manage accounts payable
- Process payroll
- *Develop and maintain fee schedules (adv)*
- *Manage renewals of business and professional insurance policies (adv)*
- *Manage personal benefits and maintain records (adv)*

CLINICAL

FUNDAMENTAL PRINCIPLES

- Apply principles of aseptic technique and infection control
- Comply with quality assurance practices
- Screen and follow up patient test results

DIAGNOSTIC ORDERS

- Collect and process specimens
- Perform diagnostic tests

PATIENT CARE

- Adhere to established triage procedures
- Obtain patient history and vital signs
- Prepare and maintain examination and treatment areas

- Prepare patient for examinations, procedures, and treatments
- Assist with examinations, procedures, and treatments
- Prepare and administer medications and immunizations
- Maintain medication and immunization records
- Recognize and respond to emergencies
- Coordinate patient care information with other health care providers

GENERAL (TRANSDISCIPLINARY)

PROFESSIONALISM

- Project a professional manner and image
- Adhere to ethical principles
- Demonstrate initiative and responsibility
- Work as a team member
- Manage time efficiently
- Prioritize and perform multiple tasks
- Adapt to change
- Promote the CMA credential
- Enhance skills through continuing education

COMMUNICATION SKILLS

- Treat all patients with compassion and empathy
- Recognize and respect cultural diversity
- Adapt communications to individual's ability to understand
- Use professional telephone technique
- Use effective and correct verbal and written communications
- Recognize and respond to verbal and non-verbal communications
- Use medical terminology appropriately
- Receive, organize, prioritize, and transmit information
- Serve as liaison
- Promote the practice through positive public relations

LEGAL CONCEPTS

- Maintain confidentiality
- Practice within the scope of education, training, and personal capabilities
- Prepare and maintain medical records
- Document accurately
- Use appropriate guidelines when releasing information
- Follow employer's established policies dealing with the health care contract
- Follow federal, state, and local legal guidelines
- Maintain awareness of federal and state health care legislation and regulations
- Maintain and dispose of regulated substances in compliance with government guidelines
- Comply with established risk management and safety procedures
- Recognize professional credentialing criteria
- Participate in the development and maintenance of personnel, policy, and procedure manuals
- *Develop and maintain personnel, policy, and procedure manuals (adv)*

INSTRUCTION

- Instruct individuals according to their needs
- Explain office policies and procedures
- Teach methods of health promotion and disease prevention
- Locate community resources and disseminate information
- *Orient and train personnel (adv)*
- *Develop educational materials (adv)*
- *Conduct continuing education activities (adv)*

OPERATIONAL FUNCTIONS

- Maintain supply inventory
- Evaluate and recommend equipment and supplies
- Apply computer techniques to support office operations
- *Supervise personnel (adv)*
- *Interview and recommend job applicants (adv)*
- *Negotiate leases and prices for equipment and supply contracts (adv)*

SOURCE: Reprinted by permission of the American Association of Medical Assistants from the *AAMA Role Delineation Study: Occupational Analysis of the Medical Assisting Profession.*

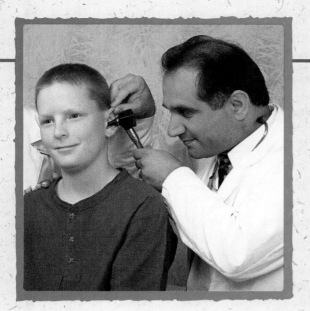

21
Assisting with Physical Examinations

CHAPTER OUTLINE

LEARNING OBJECTIVES

After completing this chapter, you should:
1. Define and spell the glossary terms for this chapter.
2. List and describe the 7 components of the patient history.
3. Discuss the problem oriented medical record.
4. Describe the 4 components of SOAP charting.
5. List the 4 Cs of charting.
6. State 10 guidelines for charting.
7. Discuss the steps to take in preparing a patient for a physical examination.
8. List and describe 8 patient examination positions that are used during a physical examination.
9. Describe 5 examination methods used by physicians.
10. Recognize 6 pieces of equipment commonly used during a physical examination.
11. List laboratory and diagnostic tests that may be ordered as part of a complete physical examination.

CLINICAL PERFORMANCE COMPETENCIES

After completing this chapter, you should perform the following tasks:
1. Obtain and record a past medical history from the patient.
2. Prepare examining room for physical examination.
3. Identify instruments and equipment used by physician when completing physical examination.
4. Prepare patient for a physical examination.
5. Demonstrate knowledge of positions used for physical examinations.
6. Correctly document a patient office visit using both chronological and the problem oriented medical record.

Glossary

acuity   Clearness, sharpness (as of vision).

amplify   To make more powerful, increase sound.

anorexia   Loss of appetite.

anthropometric   Refers to measurements of the human body such as height and weight.

axilla   The armpit.

blood relative   Related to another person by direct birth lineage.

borderline hypertension   Blood pressure which becomes gradually elevated over a period of time until it borders the edge of high blood pressure. A blood pressure of approximately 140/88 is considered borderline hypertension.

bulimia   Eating disorder characterized by recurrent binge eating and then purging the food with laxatives and vomiting.

cyanosis   Bluish coloration to the skin or mucous membranes due to insufficient oxygen getting to the lungs. This may be caused by heart or respiratory disease.

diagnose   To determine the cause and nature of a pathological condition.

differential diagnosis   A distinction between two or more alternative diagnoses.

dyspnea   Difficult or labored breathing.

dysuria   Painful urination.

fixative   Substance that serves to make firm, fixed, or preserved. Used for lab specimens to maintain stability during transport.

halo effect   A white halo appearing around lights which may be an indication of an eye disorder such as glaucoma.

hematuria   Blood in the urine.

hemoptysis   Coughing up blood.

hernia   The protrusion of an organ through the wall of a cavity in which it is usually located.

inguinal   The area of flexion in the groin area between the hips and legs.

jaundice   Yellowish cast to the skin and eye sclera. Usually caused by liver disease or damage, dehydration of the newborn, and bile duct obstruction.

laryngitis   Inflammation of the larynx (voice box) causing temporary loss of voice.

leukoplakia   White patches on mucous membranes which may become cancerous.

leukorrhea   White discharge.

mammogram   X-ray of breasts in women to detect early cancer.

menstrual   Relating to menstruation or monthly uterine blood flow in women.

mensuration   Measurement.

oliguria   Reduced production of urine.

orifice   Opening of a part of the body, such as the mouth.

orthopnea   Difficulty breathing when lying down. Breathing is easier in a straight sitting position.

PAP smear   Also called Papanicolaou test. Used for cytology testing including early detection of cervical and vaginal cancer cells.

peripheral edema   Swelling of the extremities (especially the legs) due to fluid retention.

photophobia   Sensitivity to light.

renal colic   Pain in kidney area usually due to kidney stones.

rheumatoid arthritis   Form of arthritis with inflammation of the joints, stiffness, swelling, and pain. Called crippling, deforming arthritis.

rosacea   Chronic disease of the skin of the face in middle aged and older patients. Resembles butterfly rash of lupus erythematosis.

salivation   Production of fluid (saliva) in the mouth.

speculum   Instrument used to examine canals and body orifices.

symptom(s)   An objective (observable) or subjective (perceived or felt by the patient) change in the body, for example vomiting or muscle soreness, that indicates disease or a phase of a disease.

systemic lupus erythematosis (SLE)   Chronic, progressive inflammatory disease of the connective tissue and skin which resembles rheumatoid arthritis. The characteristic butterfly rash resembles rosacea.

tinnitus   Ringing in the ears.

tympanic membrane   Eardrum.

urticaria   Itchy skin rash, commonly called "hives."

WARNING!

For all patient contact, adhere to Standard Precautions
(see pages 342–373). Wear protective equipment as indicated.

Assisting the physician with the patient's physical examination is a key responsibility of the medical assistant. Along with responsibilities related to obtaining complete patient histories, the medical assistant must prepare the examining room before and after the patient is seen. This includes preparing the instruments required during the examination of the patient. Medical assistants provide patient education before, during, and after the physical examination.

A medical record is prepared for all new patients and requires the completion of a medical history form. The components of the medical history are described in this chapter along with several ways to obtain a medical history. Methods of documenting and updating patient medical records on a regular basis include detailed charting of the current diagnoses, medications, tests, treatments, and findings.

Patient History

Before the physician can adequately assess the patient's condition a past medical history is obtained from the patient. This history assists the physician in assessing the patient's general health status and helps determine a diagnosis of the patient's present problem or condition. The term diagnosis refers to the disease or syndrome a patient has or is believed to have.

Many medical offices give new patients the medical history form to complete when the patient arrives for the first visit with the physician (Figure 21-1). If the patient is expected to complete a history form, then the medical assistant is responsible for making sure that the patient understands the terminology and how to answer the questions.

Some medical offices send the medical history form to the patient's residence with a request that the form be completed and submitted when the patient comes for the first visit. This allows patients the opportunity to check their own records for important dates and the names and dosages of medications the patient may be taking. Even when the form is sent to the patient ahead of time, many offices request patients come to the office a half hour before the actual examination by the physician. This permits the medical assistant to verify that the form is complete, get information required

for billing/insurance, or to help patients who require assistance completing the form.

Some physicians prefer to take all the components of the medical history directly from the patient. On some medical history forms, there are specific questions geared to the physician's specialty. A cardiologist, for example, may require a more extensive history relating to the cardiovascular system.

Whether the patient completes the form at home or in the office, it is important to mark any sections the patient is to skip. Particular care should be taken to assist patients who may be embarrassed that they are unable to complete the form themselves due to frailty, disability, or because they are unable to read. The medical assistant must stress the importance of filling out the form completely. The patient history should include the following six areas.

1. Chief Complaint
2. Present Illness
3. Past Medical History
4. Family Medical History
5. Personal History
6. Assessment of Body Systems (Review of Symptoms)

Med Tip: In an emergency, a physician will have to see the patient before the complete history can be obtained. If the emergency occurs in the office, have a fellow staff member locate the patient's record. Information regarding allergies, prior medical conditions, and current treatment or medications is very important.

Chief Complaint (CC)

The chief complaint is also referred to as the presenting problem. The chief complaint is the reason for the office visit. This is usually stated in the patient's own words such as, "I'm having trouble sleeping," or "I'm out of breath after climbing only 2 or 3 stairs." Duration of symptoms and what the patient has been doing about them must also be documented.

WINDY CITY CLINIC
Beth Williams, M.D.
123 Michigan Avenue
Chicago, IL 60610
(312) 123-1234

Name _____   Date:

Social Security No. _____   Date of Birth _____

Occupation _____

Date of Last Physical _____

Weight Today _____   1 Year Ago _____

Military Services ☐ Yes ☐ No; When and Where _____

☐ Single   ☐ Married
☐ Divorced   ☐ Widowed

Please answer the following questions. Where boxes are provided to check, place a check mark in the box in front of the disease or condition which you have had. *THIS FORM MUST BE COMPLETED AND RETURNED TO THE CLINIC AT LEAST 1 WEEK PRIOR TO YOUR APPOINTMENT.*

FAMILY HISTORY:

Relative	If Living, Give Present Age.	If Deceased, At What Age?	Cause of Death
Father			
Mother			
Siblings ☐M ☐F			
☐M ☐F			
☐M ☐F			
☐M ☐F			
☐M ☐F			
☐M ☐F			

HAS ANY RELATIVE EVER HAD? (Check boxes that apply)

Relationship   Relationship

☐ Asthma _____   ☐ Hay fever _____
☐ Cancer _____   ☐ Ulcers _____
☐ Tumor _____   ☐ Kidney disease _____
☐ Leukemia _____   ☐ Kidney stones _____
☐ Bleeding problems _____   ☐ Gall stones _____
☐ Anemia _____   ☐ Lung disease _____
☐ Diabetes _____   ☐ Mental disorders _____
☐ Gout _____   ☐ Suicide _____
☐ Rheumatism or arthritis _____   ☐ Typhoid disease _____
☐ High blood pressure _____   ☐ Migraine _____
☐ Heart disease _____   ☐ Tuberculosis _____
☐ Strokes _____   ☐ Asthma _____
☐ Epilepsy _____   ☐ Allergies _____
☐ Emphysema _____   ☐ Other _____

HAVE YOU HAD A FAMILY HISTORY OF? (Check boxes that apply)

☐ Heart disease   ☐ Cancer   ☐ Stroke   ☐ Allergies

Figure 21-1   Patient's medical history.

Since only the physician is able to diagnose patient's problems, the medical assistant does not use diagnostic terms when recording the chief complaint. The symptoms would be used for descriptions.

- **Incorrect documentation:**
  10/23/XX Pt. experiencing excessive thirst and unusual weight loss indicative of diabetes.
- **Correct documentation:**
  10/23/XX Pt. c/o excessive thirst and unusual weight loss of 15# during past month.

Present Illness (PI)

The present illness describes the subjective, as well as objective, **symptoms** the patient is experiencing related to the chief complaint. Symptoms refer to the body changes associated with illness or disease such as the vomiting or muscle soreness that often accompanies the flu. The present illness (PI) component of the health history must contain a detailed description of the symptom(s), including the onset, duration, and intensity of each. Each symptom should be documented as to its relationship to the chief complaint (CC).

Past Medical History

This part of the medical history includes all diseases and medical problems the patient has experienced in the past. Dates of major illnesses, hospitalizations, and surgeries are noted whenever possible. A complete past medical history will include information for the following items.

- Childhood diseases
- Major illnesses
- Injuries
- Hospitalization
- Surgeries
- Allergies
- Immunizations
- Current Medications

Family Medical History

Dates of major illnesses, hospitalizations, and surgeries should be included. The family history is a record of the health problems of the patient's **blood relatives**. Blood relatives include the patient's mother, father, sisters, brothers, grandparents, aunts, and uncles related by birth. Family medical histories focus on diseases that may be inherited

such as diabetes mellitus (DM), seizures, heart disease, hypertension, and some types of cancer.

Personal History

Personal histories include lifestyle patterns that could affect the health status of the patient, for example smoking and drinking. The patient's occupation, marital status, sexual preferences are also noted along with the patient's type of diet, choices and frequency of exercise, sleep habits and other health habits. Information about the patient's previous occupation(s) (if the patient has had several occupations) and lifelong hobbies, or interests, often provide helpful information. Table 21-1 provides a list of questions that are included on the patient history form or might be asked to gain a good personal history from a patient.

> **Med Tip:** Patients are often reluctant to offer personal information such as alcohol consumption. The medical assistant may need to ask direct questions to gain necessary information about negative health habits. For example, "How much alcohol do you drink in a day?" or "How many packs of cigarettes do you smoke in a day?" The physician may prefer to ask these questions.

Assessment of Body Systems

The physician conducts this assessment immediately prior to or during the physical examination. This review of systems (ROS) consists of a systematic review of all body systems, beginning with the head and neck area and working downward to the feet through all the body systems.

> **Med Tip:** Document patient comments such as "I'm all alone" or "I just feel that I can't go on." Relay any comments of this nature to the physician since they may indicate an emotional problem in addition to the physical reason the patient is in the office.

Refer to Table 21-2 for a list of conditions that the physician will question the patient about while doing a ROS. See Figure 21-1 earlier in this chapter for an example of a patient history record.

TABLE 21-1 Personal History Questions

Questions to be asked to obtain personal history information:

1. What was the last grade you attended in school?

2. What is your occupation?

3. How long have you done that type of work?

4. Have you been exposed to any toxic or harmful substances such as dust, chemicals, cleaning fluids/fumes, smoke, radiation, pesticides, or paint at work? at home?

5. What do you usually eat for breakfast?

6. Have you gained or lost 10 or more pounds during the past year? Is there a reason?

7. Do you follow a low-fat diet? low salt?

8. What do you do for exercise? how often?

9. How much alcohol do you drink a day? a month? preferred drink?

10. Do you smoke cigarettes? If yes, how many packs a day? filtered?

11. Do you smoke a pipe, cigars, or chew tobacco? If yes, how much?

12. How many cups of coffee do you drink a day? tea? soft drinks w/caffeine?

13. Have you ever used heroin, cocaine, or LSD? OTC drugs? laxatives? How often?

14. Do you have unusual stress at home or work?

15. What are your hobbies?

The physician will also want to know if the patient is currently taking any medications for treatment of any of the conditions.

Med Tip: Patients often forget to tell the physician how much aspirin or other over-the-counter (OTC) drugs they take. Remind patients that aspirin is considered a drug even though it may be purchased over-the-counter. Aspirin can duplicate other medication the physician may prescribe or interfere with the treatment of conditions such as gastric ulcers.

Documentation of Patient Medical Information

There are a variety of formats used for medical charting. One is the chronological record which consists of a blank form with the patient's name stamped or written on each page. The date of each visit, vital signs, and the physician's comments are added at the time of each visit. This type of docu-

mentation may span a period of several years in the patient's record.

With the chronological method of documentation a problem such as borderline hypertension may not be caught unless one reads through all the previous documentation. One would more easily spot a patient's history of hypertension by using the problem oriented medical record (POMR) method of documentation.

Problem Oriented Medical Record (POMR)

The problem oriented medical record (POMR), first developed by Dr. Lawrence L. Weed in 1970, is a popular method of documentation. POMR is based on the patient's problems. Every office employee who comes into contact with the patient or the patient's record, charts information in the same manner.

Problems are diverse and can include any condition or behavior that interferes with normal functions, for example, pain in the upper right quadrant, decreased appetite, fear of crowds, or the inability to pay medical bills. A numbered problem list is developed which appears in the patient's record and

TABLE 21-2   Review of Systems (ROS)

System	Conditions
Head	Headaches, sinus pain, masses, alopecia (unusual hair loss), dizziness, injury or trauma
Eyes	Visual acuity, blurred vision, burning, halo effect, tearing, photophobia (sensitivity to light), discharge, redness, jaundice (yellowing of skin and sclera), known eye diseases, date of last eye exam, prescription glasses, contact lenses
Ears	Tinnitus or ringing in the ears, dizziness, hearing loss, discharge, ear infections, exposure to loud noise on a regular basis
Nose	Allergies, obstruction, sense of smell, pain, discharge
Mouth	Dental work, dentures, gums, sense of taste, teeth, salivation (producing saliva), dryness of mouth, tongue, leukoplakia (white patches, possibly cancerous), gingivitis
Throat	Hoarseness, laryngitis (loss of voice), redness, speech defect, masses, pain
Neck	Tenderness, pain, swelling, difficulty swallowing, enlarged nodes
Respiratory	Dyspnea (labored breathing), cough, asthma, wheezing, allergies, hemoptysis (coughing up blood), chest pain, night sweats, orthopnea (difficulty breathing while lying down), shortness of breath (SOB)
Cardiovascular (CV)	Chest pain, hypertension, peripheral edema, cyanosis, fainting, dizziness
Gastrointestinal (GI)	Nausea, vomiting, anorexia (loss of appetite), bulimia (eating disorder—binge eating followed by purging), indigestion, diarrhea, constipation, hemorrhoids, presence of blood in stool, number of bowel movements daily, hematemesis (vomit blood)
Genitourinary (GU)	History of urinary tract infection, frequency, hesitation, oliguria (reduced urine), hematuria (blood in urine), dysuria (difficult or painful urination), renal colic (kidney pain), stones, discharge, nocturia (urination during the night)
Female Reproductive	Menstrual history, obstetric history, leukorrhea (white discharge), itching, pain, discharge, date of last PAP test, breast self-exam history, sexual habits, menopause symptoms, last mammogram (breast exam)
Male Reproductive	Prostate problems, testicular self-exam, discharge, sexual habits, frequency of urination, decreased stream, nocturia
Endocrine	Growth & development, goiter, excessive thirst, intolerance to temperature change, hormone therapy, diabetes symptoms, irregular menses, symptoms of thyroid disorders
Skin	Rash, urticaria (hives), texture, moles, infection, redness, jaundice, cyanosis, allergies, dry/oily
Musculoskeletal (MS)	Joint pain, swelling, weakness, stiffness, numbness, muscle pain, fractures, discoloration, edema
Neurologic	Fainting, loss of consciousness, headaches, tremor, nervousness, paralysis, pain, memory loss
Psychiatric	Mental health history, emotional stability, depression, stress
General	Weight gain or loss, sleep habits, fatigue

can be tracked to assist in determining the patient's progress. Whenever the patient is seen, the POMR is updated so that the last available information on each numbered problem regarding the patient's condition or problem is dated and identified as the most current data.

SOAP Charting

This method of documentation actually uses a SOAP (subjective, objective, assessment, and plan) approach for documenting each patient problem. Once a problem is identified, it is then SOAPed. The medical assistant documents the subjective statements of the patient and records the objective data such as laboratory results and vital signs. The physician may add objective data and determine the assessment or diagnosis and the plan of treatment. The SOAP method of documenting a medical record is described in Table 21-3.

A problem list for the patient in the example given in Table 21-3 might appear as:

- *Problem List*

    2/14/XX

    Problem No. 1: Diabetes

    Problem No. 2: Hypertension, essential
- *Plan*

    2/14/XX

    Problem No. 1: Diabetic exchange diet

    Regular Insulin, 20 units SC q AM

    Monitor blood sugar levels during day

    Problem No. 2: Norvasc 2.5 mg. daily

    Monitor blood pressure weekly

- *Progress Notes*

    2/14/XX

    Problem No 1: Diabetes

    S - Pt. states thirst has diminished and hunger lessened.

    O - Urine 2+, FBS positive, Gained 4# in past 3 weeks skin turgor good

    A - Diet and medication effective

    P - Continue medication, monitoring blood sugar level daily, adjust insulin levels per instruction, return visit in 2 weeks

    Problem No 2: Hypertension

    S - Pt. states no complaints related to high blood pressure

    O - B/P 148/86 Down 10 points in past 3 weeks

    A - Medication effective

    P - Continue with medication and pt. monitor of B/P weekly. Come in for re-check in 2 weeks

TABLE 21-3   SOAP Charting for 1/24/XX

SOAP	Meaning	Example
S	Subjective symptoms provided by the patient and/or family. The actual patient's words are recorded.	"I'm thirsty and eating all the time but I'm not gaining any weight. I feel tired all the time."
O	Objective findings from vital signs, physical examination, laboratory and diagnostic tests.	B/P 158/96 T = 98°F P = 76 R = 16 Skin turgor (resiliency) poor. Wt. 10# less than 6 weeks ago. Urine 4+ sugar, FBS positive.
A	Assessment including the physician's diagnosis.	Uncontrolled diabetes.
P	Plan including recommended treatments, further tests, medications, consultation, surgery, physical therapy.	Dx: Lab tests for diabetes Tx: Begin diabetic diet & insulin. Instruct on diet and exercise follow-up.

Use the following guidelines when charting.

Med Tip: The 4 Cs of charting are: Concise, clear, complete, and chronological order.

Adult Examination

Patients come to the physician's office for a variety of reasons—illness, emergency, or routine checkup. In all of these instances, the patient is generally given a physical examination. The length and extent of the exam will vary depending on the reason for the visit and the length of time since the last visit.

Purpose of the Physical Examination

The patient's general state of health is assessed during the physical examination. As much as possible in an office setting, the patient's entire body is examined. This means that every **orifice** (opening), major organs, and all body systems are examined. Even if the patient comes into the office with a specific complaint, such as indigestion, the entire body should be examined.

In conjunction with a complete physical examination, laboratory and diagnostic tests may be ordered. This would include a complete blood count, urinalysis, and diagnostic x-rays.

Patient Preparation

Patient preparation includes completing the patient's medical history, determining the reason for this visit, obtaining the patient's height and weight and measuring vital signs—temperature, pulse, respirations, blood pressure. Refer to Chapter 20 for a thorough discussion of vital signs. The vital signs, height, and weight should be placed in the patient's record before the physician sees the patient.

The patient should be requested to empty his or her bladder before undressing. The medical assistant should show the patient where the bathroom is located and give any instructions regarding collecting a urine sample. Supply a urine container that is labeled with the patient's name.

For a complete examination the patient will remove all clothing including underwear and stockings, unless instructed otherwise. A patient gown and drape sheet are left on the exam table for the patient. Instructions on whether the gown is to be worn with the opening in the front or back should be given. If the patient requires help with undressing the medical assistant will remain in the room.

The patient may need to be assisted onto the exam table by holding an arm as they step on a foot stool. Use care when having the patient move onto

Med Tip: Patients may request to use the bathroom when they arrive in the physician's office. Always check to see if a urine sample is required. If a urine sample is not saved at that time it may mean that the patient has to make a return visit with a urine specimen.

the exam table since accidental falls are possible at this point.

The patient's level of anxiety should be assessed. If the patient seems extremely nervous or ill at ease then the medical assistant must attempt to allow the patient to express these feelings. Unusual nervousness should be reported to the physician.

Elderly, frail patients, and children should not be left unattended. If the medical assistant is unable to remain in the room, a family member should be asked to sit with the patient until the doctor begins the examination.

> **Med Tip:** Exam room etiquette requires that one always knock before entering the exam room. Close the door after leaving so that no staff or other patients can see into the patient's exam room. Enter the exam room only if you have a specific reason to do so.

Draping

Small drape sheets are used during the examination to protect the privacy of the patient. An additional benefit of a drape is to provide some warmth to the patient. During the examination, the drape is pulled back to expose only the area being examined.

Sterile drapes are used during surgical procedures to avoid contaminating sterile instruments, suture materials, and dressings. The drape protects the rest of the patient's body from blood or drainage that occurs during surgery. The drapes will be placed in a manner to expose only the site of incision using sterile surgical technique.

Positioning the Patient

The medical assistant will assist the patient into the correct position for the examination. Always explain why you are placing the patient in a particular position. During the examination, the physician may request the patient to change position several times. Since some positions can become uncomfortable, never leave the patient in these positions any longer than is absolutely necessary. Do not leave the patient unattended if there is any danger of injury to the patient due to dizziness or falling.

The more standard positions are discussed in Table 21-4 and illustrated in Figures 21-2 through 21-6.

Assisting the Physician

Medical assistants do not perform physical examinations of patients with the exception of performing measurements of vital signs, height and weight and possibly visual/hearing acuity. The medical assistant may help the physician in the following ways.

1. Position the patient for examination. If the patient is elderly, disabled or a child, the medical assistant may have to help the patient maintain the correct position.
2. Hand instruments, equipment, and other medical supplies to the physician.
3. Document and label specimens.
4. Offer reassurance to the patient.
5. Act as a witness to the behavior of the physician and the patient.
6. Carry out treatment plans such as providing patient instruction, applying dressings, and administering medications.
7. Scheduling further diagnostic tests the physician has ordered.

Diagnosis

Many patients have an annual complete physical examination to assist in maintaining their good health. They may have no chief complaint (CC) or physical problems. The physician will compare the physical condition found during the current examination against the last examination. This is why it is so important to have a current medical record available when the physical examination takes place. In some cases there may be a weight gain, elevated blood pressure or other condition which requires more frequent evaluation, patient education, and even medication.

Other physical examinations are conducted to **diagnose** a problem. The physician analyzes information gathered during the physical examination along with patient's symptoms, vital signs, laboratory findings, and other diagnostic test results. Based on all of this data the physician makes a judgment and comes to a conclusion on the diagnosis. Only the physician is qualified to perform a diagnosis of the patient's condition. The medical assistant must have a thorough understanding of the process in order to assist the physician or type reports or referrals.

Differential Diagnosis

In many situations the symptoms a patient demonstrates can point to more than one condition.

TABLE 21-4 Standard Body Positions

Position	Description	Application
Anatomic	Standing straight with arms at sides and palms forward.	Examine musculoskeletal development, skin color.
Dorsal Recumbent	Patient lies on back with knees bent, feet flat on table.	Vaginal examination when lithotomy position is not advisable, abdominal pain. Rectal examination.
Fowler's	Sitting up with back rest at 90° angle.	When patients have difficulty breathing.
Knee-chest	Patient kneels on table with buttocks raised, head and chest on exam table. Head is turned to side with knees slightly apart.	Rectal examinations.
Left lateral recumbent (Figure 21-5)	Lying horizontal on left side.	Position for surgery (for example right kidney).
Lithotomy	Dorsal-recumbent position with feet on corner of exam table or in stirrups.	Pelvic examinations.
Proctologic (Jack-knife)	Similar to knee-chest but with a greater bend at hips. Special exam table may then be tipped. Patients will lie face down with hips at hinge of table.	Proctologic examination with sigmoidoscope.
Prone (Figure 21-3)	On abdomen with head to one side.	Examine back, spine, or legs.
Right lateral recumbent (Figure 21-4)	Lying horizontal on right side.	Position for surgery (for example left kidney).
Semi-Fowler's	Similar to Fowler's position but with back rest at 45° angle. Semi-sitting position.	Patients with difficulty in breathing.
Sims' (Figure 21-6)	Patient lies on left side, left arm behind body for support, left leg bent slightly and right leg bent sharply.	Rectal examination. Vaginal examination.
Sitting	Patient sits upright with legs over side of the examination table.	Examine head and chest (anterior and posterior).
Supine (Figure 21-2)	Patient lies flat on back.	Examine abdomen, chest, legs.
Trendelenburg Position	Supine position with head lower than feet.	Treat shock, abdominal surgery.

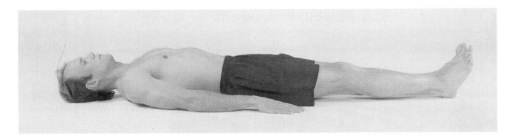

Figure 21-2 Supine position.

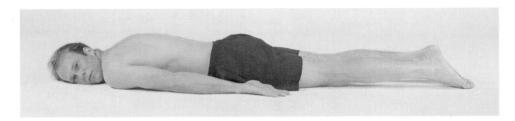

Figure 21-3 Prone position.

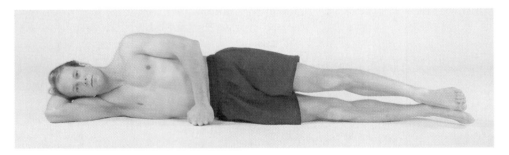

Figure 21-4 Right lateral recumbent position.

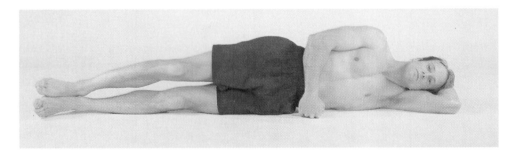

Figure 21-5 Left lateral recumbent position.

The physician will have to make a differential diagnosis. This means that the physician will attempt to rule out (R/O) other diagnoses in favor of the one right diagnosis. A differential diagnosis is indicated in the following manner.

1. R/O rosacea
2. R/O rheumatoid arthritis
3. R/O systemic lupus erythematosis

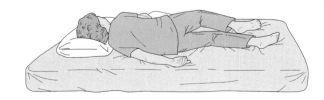

Figure 21-6 Sims' Position.

In the above example, after the laboratory and diagnostic tests have been analyzed the final diagnosis may be systemic lupus erythematosis (SLE).

> **Med Tip:** Note that an R/O diagnosis cannot be used when coding for insurance purposes. The actual diagnosis must be used to determine the correct code number (see Chapter 17).

Examination Methods Used by the Physician

Physicians use five standard examination methods when conducting a physical examination: inspection, palpation, percussion, and auscultation. A fifth method, called mensuration, may occasionally be used. This method involves using calipers or a tape measure to evaluate growth of certain body parts or to determine the size of an abnormality, for example height and weight and head circumference of a baby.

Inspection

Physical inspection requires the physician to visually examine and inspect all exterior surfaces of the body. In addition, a visual inspection is made of interior portions of the body such as the throat, ears, eyes, vaginal wall, cervix, and rectum using an instrument. Any abnormal conditions such as unusual color, size, shape, position or asymmetry are noted (Figure 21-7).

Palpation

Palpation is performed by applying the hands or fingers to the external surface of the body for the purpose of detecting any abnormality or evidence of disease. The physician will palpate all accessible body organs, extremities, and lymph nodes in the neck, axilla, or armpit, and chest. The purpose of this portion of the examination is to determine any unusual tenderness, shape, texture, size, or temperature. Abnormalities and masses in pelvic and abdominal organs can often be discovered through palpation. (Figure 21-8).

Percussion

Percussion refers to using the fingertips to tap the body lightly but sharply so as to gain information about the position and size of the underlying body parts. To do this, two fingers of one hand are placed on the patient's skin and then struck with the index and middle fingers of the other hand. The physician uses his or her fingers to percuss the chest wall and abdomen by a gentle thumping or tapping which produces a standard sound. An alteration of this sound aids in determining the presence or absence of fluid or pus in a cavity (Figure 21-9).

A percussion hammer is used to test the reflexes of the body. As part of a neurological test, the physician gently taps the percussion hammer once against the tendon reflex at the bottom of the patellar (kneecap) bone.

Auscultation

Auscultation means to listen to sounds that are found within the body. Sounds made by the heart, lungs, stomach, and bowel are assessed for strength, presence or absence, and rhythm. These sounds can be heard by using the auscultation method of examination (Figure 21-10). A stethoscope is usually used to amplify body sounds, however, auscultation can also be performed by placing the ear directly over the body surface.

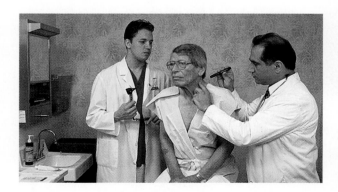

Figure 21-7 Physical examination—inspection.

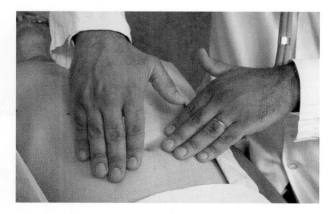

Figure 21-8 Physical examination—palpation.

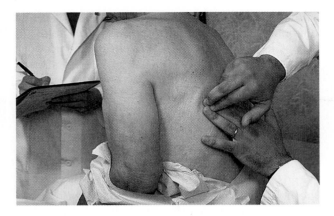

Figure 21-9 Physical examination—percussion.

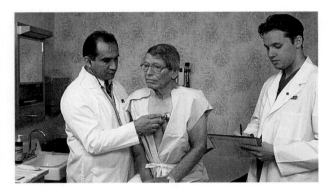

Figure 21-10 Physical examination—auscultation.

Equipment Used for the Physical Examination

In addition to the use of the physician's hands, special instruments and equipment are also used during a physical examination. These include the ophthalmoscope, otoscope, scale, urine cup, stethoscope, laryngeal mirror, reflex hammer, tuning fork, tongue depressor, tape measure, and pocket flashlight (Figure 21-11).

Ophthalmoscope

The ophthalmoscope is used to examine the interior of the eye, especially the retina. External light is focused through the magnifying lens of the ophthalmoscope onto the inner surfaces of the eye to check for abnormalities. The patient needs to be in a sitting position and look straight ahead during this examination.

Otoscope

This instrument allows the physician to inspect the outer ear and tympanic membrane (eardrum). Light is focused through the lens into the ear canal. A protective plastic cover is placed over the speculum to protect against cross-infection between patients.

The otoscope is used with a long and narrow speculum to examine the ear. This speculum can be replaced with a short, wide speculum to examine the nose.

Percussion or Reflex Hammer/Pinwheel

The hammer has a hard rubber, triangular-shaped head for testing neurological reflexes such as found in the tendons of the knee. The pinwheel is

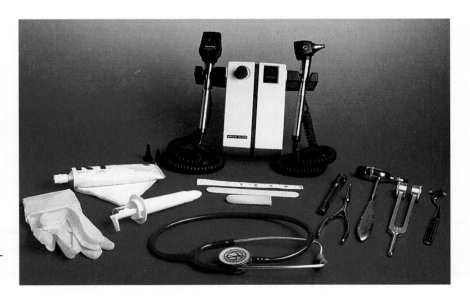

Figure 21-11 Examples of instruments used for the physical examination.

used as part of the neurological examination to test for sensation.

Stethoscope

This instrument is used to amplify sounds (heart, lungs, bowel) heard within the body. It consists of two ear pieces, connecting rubber or plastic tubing, and a chest piece with a bell or diaphragm to amplify the sound.

Tuning fork

The tuning fork consists of two prongs extending from the handle. This instrument is used to test the patient's hearing ability. The tuning fork makes a humming sound which can be heard and felt when vibrated.

Laryngeal Mirror

A small mirror attached to a long handle used for visualizing the larynx. It should to be warmed using warm water to prevent fogging from the patient's breath on use.

Table 21-5 lists the methods and equipment used to examine the areas/parts of the body during a complete physical examination.

Examining Room Supplies

Other supplies such as a sphygmomanometer for taking blood pressure, thermometer(s), cotton tipped applicators, vaginal speculum, **Pap smear** slides and fixative, and tissues should be available in each examining room. Table 21-6 describes some typical supplies and equipment available in an examining room.

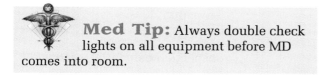
Med Tip: Always double check lights on all equipment before MD comes into room.

Laboratory and Diagnostic Tests

In addition to the physical examination conducted by the physician, a variety of laboratory and diagnostic tests may be ordered. If a test, such as a urinalysis or electrocardiogram, is conducted in the office on the day of the examination, then the results will be available immediately. However, most tests are scheduled by appointment with a separate laboratory or diagnostic facility. Table 21-7 presents an example of tests that might be ordered as part of a complete examination.

Sequence of Examination Procedures

Each physician may have his or her own procedures that are required for each patient. In addition, each physician will specify the order in which they wish these procedures to be conducted. Table 21-8 illustrates an example of a typical sequence of procedures and the person(s) responsible for completing the procedure.

Preparing the Examining Room

The standard furnishings in most examining rooms consist of an examination table with stirrups, a pillow, a footstool, a sink, a small supply cupboard, hazardous waste and sharps containers, a chair, a writing surface, and a telephone for the physician. Physicians in specialized practices, such as ophthalmology, will require specialized furniture and equipment. Figure 21-12 illustrates an examination table with stirrups.

The medical assistant's responsibility is to prepare the room for each patient. All instruments and equipment needed for the examination should be ready for the physician. This equipment should not be left within reach of the patient.

A gooseneck examination light is usually placed near the examination table and moved as needed. The medical assistant is responsible for adjusting the position of any portable lighting for an examination. Due to a danger of tipping over, the portable light should never be placed directly over the patient if the patient will be left alone.

The used gown, examination table paper, and pillow cover are disposed of using universal precautions immediately after the patient leaves the room. Disposable equipment used during the examination is discarded in the proper waste containers. Reusable equipment is taken to a designated area to be cleaned, disinfected, or sterilized. The counter area and sink in the examining room should be decontaminated. Any foul smelling, bloodstained or otherwise potentially infectious materials are placed in the red biohazardous waste

Med Tip: Remove all evidence of the last patient's visit, such as soiled paper on the examination table, before taking the next patient into an examining room. A clean, tidy examining room reflects professionalism and expresses sensitivity.

TABLE 21-5 Equipment and Positions Used During the General Physical Examination

Sitting Position

Area	Body Part	Method/Equipment
Head	Skull, hair, scalp	Inspection and palpation
Ears	Ear canals, ear drum	Inspection with otoscope
Eyes	Visual acuity	Vision chart, Snellen eye chart
	Retina	Inspection with ophthalmoscope
Nose	Nasal passage	Inspection with otoscope and nasal speculum
Mouth and throat (pharynx)	Mucous membranes, lips, gums, teeth, tongue, pharynx	Inspection with laryngeal mirror, flashlight, tongue blade
Neck	Thyroid gland, trachea, and cervical lymph nodes	Palpation and inspection
	Carotid artery	Auscultation
Back and spine	Muscles, spinal cord	Palpation and inspection
Chest and lungs	Chest wall, lungs	Inspection, palpation, percussion, and auscultation

Supine Position

Area	Body Part	Method/Equipment
Breasts	Breast tissue, nipples	Palpation
Heart	Heart sounds, apical pulse	Auscultation with stethoscope
Abdomen	Bowel sounds	Auscultation
	Symmetry	Inspection
	Presence of air masses, enlargement	Percussion Palpation
	Uterus	Palpation
Inguinal Area	Inguinal nodes hernia	Palpation
Genitalia	Female: cervix and vagina	Inspection using vaginal speculum
	Male: penis, scrotum, prostate gland	Palpation
Rectal	Anus	Inspection
	Rectum	Inspection using proctoscope
Legs	Circulation	Inspection
	Pulse sites	Palpation

Standing Position

Area	Body Part	Method/Equipment
Musculoskeletal system	Muscle strength	Inspection
	Gait abnormalities	Palpation
Neurological examination	Reflexes	Percussion

TABLE 21-6 Typical Examining Room Supplies

Equipment	Function
Alcohol	Disinfect instruments.
Alcohol wipes	Disinfect and cleanse skin before injections and phlebotomy.
Balance scale	Take patient's weight and height.
Bandages (small)	Applied after taking blood sample and some injections.
Batteries and light bulbs	Extra batteries and light bulbs are required for lighted equipment.
Betadine (or other topical antiseptic)	Used to disinfect skin before minor surgery.
Biohazard waste container	Closed rigid container with biohazardous labeling and appropriate red waste bags.
Cotton balls (sterile and nonsterile)	Used to apply antiseptic or to clean the skin.
Cotton-tipped swabs (sterile and nonsterile)	Used to clean recessed areas, to apply medications and lubricant, and to obtain specimens from the throat and other orifices.
Drapes	Disposable paper or cloth sheet used to cover patient during examination.
Emesis basin	Kidney-shaped receptacle for body drainage, such as sputum, and for used instruments.
Fixative spray	Use to preserve slides.
Gauze dressings (4 × 4 or 3 × 4)	Applied to dress small wounds.
Gloves (nonsterile disposable)	Worn by all staff to protect against microorganisms and blood borne pathogens.
Gloves (sterile disposable)	Worn when performing minor surgery and handling sterile materials.
Gooseneck lamp	Movable light used to focus on a body area for increased visibility.
Hydrogen peroxide (H_2O_2)	Used to clean open wounds.
Irrigation syringe	Used to wash cerumen (earwax) out of ear canal or to irrigate wounds.
Lubricant	Water soluble gel applied to physician's glove, speculum, or rectal thermometer to reduce friction during insertion. Prevents damage to delicate mucous membranes.
Soap dispenser	Used to dispense germicidal soap for handwashing between each patient.
Sphygmomanometer	Machine used to measure blood pressure.
Tape	Used to secure dressings.
Tape measure	Measure lesions, head circumference, body measurements.
Thermometer	Measure temperature.
Tissues	Wipe body secretions.
Tongue depressor	Wooden blade used to hold patient's tongue down while examining mouth and throat.
Vaginal speculum	Instrument used to expand vaginal opening to view cervix.

TABLE 21-7 Laboratory and Diagnostic Tests

Test	Description
Blood chemistry profile	Package (or panel) of chemistry tests provides overview of patient's body chemistries. Less expensive than performing individual tests.
SMA-12 (or Chem 12)	Panel of 12 chemistry tests.
SMAC (or Chem 20)	Panel of 20 tests.
Complete blood count (CBC) including a differential count	Includes red blood count (RBC), white blood count (WBC), hemoglobin (Hg), hematocrit (Hct), RBC indices, platelets, and differential. The differential count indicates abnormalities of RBCs, platelets, and types of WBCs.
Electrocardiogram (ECG/EKG)	Record of electrical activity of the heart. Useful in diagnosis of heart muscle damage causing disruption of electrical activity of the heart and abnormal cardiac rhythm.
Pulmonary function test (PFT)	Breathing equipment used to determine respiratory function and measure lung volume and gas exchange.
Sedimentation rate (Sed rate)	Measures the rate at which erythrocytes (RBCs) settle out of blood in 1 hour. Inflammatory conditions will cause RBCs to settle faster since they are heavier and the SED rate will be higher than normal.
Visual acuity	Sharpness of vision.
Vital signs	Measurements of signs of life which include temperature, pulse, respirations and blood pressure.
Weight and height	Anthropometric measurements of the human body.
X-rays	Radiology studies of body parts (for example chest and spinal).

TABLE 21-8 Sequence of Complete Physical Examination Procedures

Procedure	Responsible Person
1. Registration	Receptionist/Medical Assistant
2. History	Receptionist/Medical Assistant
3. Urine specimen	Medical Assistant or Laboratory Technician
4. Blood specimen	Medical Assistant or Laboratory Technician
5. Vital signs Weight and height Visual acuity	Medical Assistant
6. X-ray	X-ray Technician (provided x-ray room is available; otherwise x-ray completed before the patient's visit)
7. Preparation of patient	Medical Assistant
8. Physical examination	Physician
9. Prior approvals, scheduling of follow-up tests and appointments, referrals	Receptionist/Medical Assistant

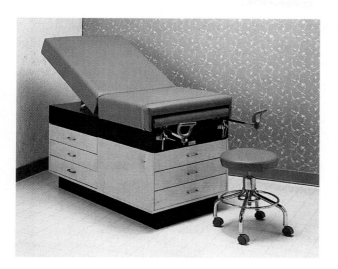

Figure 21-12 Examination table with stirrups.

Med Tip: Prescription pads should be accessible to the physician but out of reach of the patient. Ideally, these are stored in a locked drawer or cabinet. Many physicians carry a pad in their jacket pocket.

container in the examining room. After the patient leaves the room, the bag is removed from the container, sealed, and replaced. Biohazardous waste from all examining room(s), should be stored in a designated area according to OSHA regulations.

The patient's medical record is placed outside the door of the examining room in a wall-mounted rack or in a space designated by the physician. If the patient requests to see the chart, politely inform the patient that you will relay that request to the doctor. The physician must be the one to discuss the record with the patient.

PROCEDURE: Assisting With Complete Physical Examination

Terminal Performance
Competency: Student must be able to perform this procedure with 90% accuracy. (Will correctly perform procedure 9 out of 10 times).

Equipment and Supplies
Equipment and supplies will vary, depending on type and purpose of the examination and personal preferences of the physician.

Alcohol swabs
Drape
Emesis basin
Examination table with clean sheet
Disposable gloves
Laryngeal mirror
Lubricant
Nasal speculum
Ophthalmoscope
Otoscope
Pillow (with clean cover)
Reflex hammer
Scale with height rod
Snellen chart (vision)
Sphygmomanometer
Stethoscope
Tape measure

Thermometer
Tissues
Tongue depressors
Tuning fork
Urine specimen container

Procedural Steps
1. Wash hands.
2. Assemble all equipment in examining room.
3. Identify the patient and explain the procedure. Patients should always be accompanied into the examining room.
4. For comfort and efficiency during the examination, the patient should have an empty bladder. If a urine sample is needed for testing, provide the patient with a urine specimen container and instructions at this time. Otherwise, simply offer the patient the opportunity to use the bathroom now.
5. Take vital signs and measurements (temperature, pulse, respirations,

blood pressure, height, and weight). Document this data in the patient's record or on a complaint slip immediately.

6. Provide the patient with a gown and drape and give instructions on undressing. Have patient wear gown with opening in front if this is appropriate. Allow patient to undress in privacy. ***Rationale:*** Gowns that are open in the front provide easier access to the patient's chest and abdomen.

7. Have patient sit on the side of the examination table with legs hanging over the side. Place a drape sheet over the patient's legs. ***Rationale:*** This position provides easy access to the patient when the physician examines the head, eyes, ears, nose, mouth, neck, throat, breasts, axilla (armpit), chest and heart. *Note:* The physician may prefer to examine the female breasts and axilla when the patient is in a reclining position.

8. Tell the physician that the patient is ready. A female medical assistant should remain in the room if the patient is a female and the physician is a male or if the physician needs assistance.

9. Assist the physician as needed. The patient may require assistance during position changes.

10. Use gloves when handling used equipment which may contain biohazardous materials, such as the laryngeal mirror. The mirror and other contaminated equipment is placed in the emesis basin until it can be carried to the decontamination area.

11. Warm the laryngeal mirror by placing it under warm water. Then dry it with tissue or gauze.

12. As the physician progresses from one section of the body to the next during the assessment of systems, reposition the drape to expose only the portion of the patient's body being examined. Label all specimen slides as soon as possible. Use gloves when handling specimens.

13. When the examination is complete, assist the patient to sit up slowly. *Note:* Some patients experience dizziness if they sit up suddenly. When removing legs from stirrups, take both legs down together to prevent strain on hips and back.

14. Assist the patient off the examination table, as necessary.

15. Ask the patient if he or she requires help dressing. If no help is needed, allow the patient to dress in privacy.

16. Instruct the patient where to go after dressing.

17. After the patient has left the examining room, discard all disposable materials into the appropriate sharps and waste containers. Ideally, sharps should be disposed of as they are used to prevent injury to the patient. Remove soiled linens and place them in the laundry container. Reusable equipment is removed to a decontamination area to be cleaned and disinfected or sterilized.

18. Resupply the examining room.

19. Clean the examination table and replace the soiled linens and gowns.

20. Complete any documentation on the patient's record or the complaint slip.

Charting Example

2/14/XX   3 p.m. CPX by Dr. Williams. Pt. referred to clinic lab for CBC, UA, and mammogram. Pt. to return in 1 week to discuss results. Appointment made for 2/21/XX.   M. King, CMA

Note: The physician will document his or her findings from the CPX on the patient record.

LEGAL AND ETHICAL ISSUES

The physical examination carries with it important legal considerations. There is a contract between the patient and physician. When the patient walks into the office with the expectation of undergoing a physical examination, the patient gives consent—expressed or implied—to be touched by the physician during the examination.

The medical assistant may be required to act as a witness during some examinations such as the gynecological examination. The physician may request that a female medical assistant not be present during a urological examination of a male patient. A female physician may want another person in the room with male patients. The medical assistant will have to be alert to the needs of both the physician and the patient. See Chapter 5 for a discussion of the patient's right to privacy.

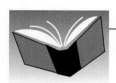

PATIENT EDUCATION

Preparing the patient for the physical examination offers an excellent opportunity for patient education. Additional information can be gathered regarding skin condition and overall hygiene at this time. Instructions on self-examinations such as breast and testicular examinations, dietary suggestions, and general hygiene information can be introduced.

Summary

The patient-physician relationship usually begins the first time a patient is examined by the doctor. Careful preparation of the patient, the examining room, and the medical record is the medical assistant's responsibility. Anticipation of the equipment needed by the physician for the examination process comes through experience. The comfort and safety of the patient during the examination is paramount in that it allows the physician to complete the physical examination efficiently and with the best possibility of obtaining accurate and useful data. Throughout the entire process of the physical examination—before, during, and after—the medical assistant's essential role is to assist the physician by assuring that the medical record, the patient, and the examining room are as completely prepared as possible.

Competency Review

1. What are the omissions in documentation in the following chronological patient record?

   a. 1/23/96 Urticaria T = 98 P = 90 R = 16
      Hydrocortisone cream topical PRN
      B. Williams, MD

   b. 10/23/96   Flu shot, 0.5 ml subq,
      Vaccine Lot #2360   M. King, CMA

   c. 2/20/97   Diet for weight loss given
      Wt. 178, BP 138/72   B. Williams, MD

   d. 5/22/97   Seen in office after treatment of
      fx. of R tibia in ER. Circulation adequate.
      T = 99   B. Williams, MD

   e. 7/12/97   X-ray shows healed tibia. Cast removed from leg. Skin condition noted.
      B. Williams, MD

   f. 10/1/97   Flu shot given   M. King, CMA

   g. 4/5/98   Insurance px BP 146/90 Wt. 182
      T = 97.6; P = 90 R = 20

2. Role play obtaining a patient history with a classmate or family member. Use the sample history form found in this chapter.

3. Take the personal history of a class or family member using questions from Table 21-1.

PREPARING FOR THE CERTIFICATION EXAM

Test Taking Tip — Read quickly through the entire examination before answering the first question. Many times a diagram or another question in the examination will provide some information to help you answer one of the earlier questions.

Examination Review Questions

Select the best answer for each question:

1. For a routine physical examination, the medical assistant will have all of the following equipment ready, EXCEPT
   (A) percussion hammer
   (B) laryngeal mirror
   (C) otoscope
   (D) irrigation syringe
   (E) lubricant

2. Distinguishing between two diseases by contrasting their symptoms is called
   (A) chemical diagnosis
   (B) physical diagnosis
   (C) differential diagnosis
   (D) laboratory diagnosis
   (E) radiologic diagnosis

3. If while taking a patient history, the patient indicates he has chest pain and difficulty breathing, the medical assistant should
   (A) complete taking the history since it will be needed in case of an emergency
   (B) begin administering CPR
   (C) call for assistance
   (D) leave the patient to get the doctor
   (E) wait until the doctor comes in to examine the patient

4. The position the patient is placed in for a pelvic exam is
   (A) semi-Fowler's
   (B) lithotomy
   (C) knee-chest
   (D) prone
   (E) jack-knife

5. Which position is NOT used when a patient is having a sigmoidoscopic examination?
   (A) semi-Fowler's
   (B) dorsal recumbent
   (C) knee-chest

   (D) jack-knife
   (E) none of the above

6. Listening to the sound made when the body is struck is called
   (A) palpation
   (B) auscultation
   (C) inspection
   (D) percussion
   (E) mensuration

7. The patient history that assists the physician to assess the patient's general health and diagnose an existing condition includes: past medical history, personal history, and
   (A) chief complaint
   (B) present illness
   (C) family medical history
   (D) assessment of body systems
   (E) all of the above

8. The actual method of documentation in using the problem oriented medical record (POMR) uses _____ charting
   (A) CC
   (B) PI
   (C) ROS
   (D) SOAP
   (E) ABS

9. Four standard examination methods used when a physician conducts a physical examination are
   (A) inspection, palpation, percussion, and auscultation
   (B) mensuration, palpation, percussion, and auscultation
   (C) inspection, percussion, auscultation, and anthropomorphic
   (D) inspection, anthropomorphic, palpation, and pertussis
   (E) percussion, pertussis, external, and internal

10. The primary reason to position a patient seated on an examination table with legs hanging over the side during a CPX is to

(A) let the patient's legs relax

(B) provide for easy access to the patient for the physician

(C) protect the physician from being kicked during the examination

(D) allow for unencumbered reflex examination

(E) maximize the privacy for the undressed, but draped, patient

ON THE JOB

Jerry Owen, CMA, has been assigned to assist Dr. Williams with Mrs. Lewis's complete physical examination today. Her vital signs were T = 99.6°F, P = 62, R = 14, and BP = 138/90 (borderline hypertension). There was cerumen (earwax) in the left ear which Dr. Williams irrigated. Mrs. Lewis stated she is allergic to penicillin. Blood was drawn for a complete blood count (CBC), a urine specimen was sent to the lab, and a PAP test was done. Mrs. Lewis has also been scheduled for a mammogram at the hospital.

What is your response?

1. How should Jerry prepare the examining room for Mrs. Lewis's CPX?
2. What instruments are needed?
3. How should Mrs. Lewis be positioned?
4. Consider that Jerry is a male medical assistant, what type of assistance should Jerry give Dr. Williams during this CPX?
5. How should this visit be charted? For which part of the documentation is Jerry responsible? Dr. Williams?

References

Anderson, K., and Anderson, L. *Mosby's Pocket Dictionary of Medicine, Nursing, & Allied Health.* Chicago: Mosby, 1994.

DeSando, M. "How Perfect Is 20/20 Vision?" *PMA.* November/December, 1992.

Fiesta, J. "The Physical Exam." *RN.* 54:11, 1991.

Fremgen, B. *Medical Terminology.* Upper Saddle River: Brady/Prentice Hall, 1997.

Lewis, M., and Tamparo, C. *Medical Law, Ethics, and Bioethics in the Medical Office.* Philadelphia: F.A. Davis Company, 1993.

Locher, C. "How to Make the Most of Your Charting." *Journal of Practical Nursing.* 42:2, 1992.

Neubauer, M. "Careful Charting—Your Best Defense." *RN.* 53:11, 1990.

Nurse's Pocket Companion. Springhouse, PA: Springhouse Corporation, 1993.

Taber's Cyclopedic Medical Dictionary, 18th, ed. Philadelphia: F.A. Davis Company, 1997.

MEDICAL ASSISTANT ROLE DELINEATION CHART

Highlight indicates material covered in this chapter

ADMINISTRATIVE

ADMINISTRATIVE PROCEDURES

- Perform basic clerical functions
- Schedule, coordinate, and monitor appointments
- Schedule inpatient/outpatient admissions and procedures
- Understand and apply third party guidelines
- Obtain reimbursement through accurate claims submission
- Monitor third-party reimbursement
- Perform medical transcription
- Understand and adhere to managed care policies and procedures
- *Negotiate managed care contracts (adv)*

PRACTICE FINANCES

- Perform procedural and diagnostic coding
- Apply bookkeeping principles
- Document and maintain accounting and banking records
- Manage accounts receivable
- Manage accounts payable
- Process payroll
- *Develop and maintain fee schedules (adv)*
- *Manage renewals of business and professional insurance policies (adv)*
- *Manage personal benefits and maintain records (adv)*

CLINICAL

FUNDAMENTAL PRINCIPLES

- Apply principles of aseptic technique and infection control
- Comply with quality assurance practices
- Screen and follow up patient test results

DIAGNOSTIC ORDERS

- Collect and process specimens
- Perform diagnostic tests

PATIENT CARE

- Adhere to established triage procedures
- Obtain patient history and vital signs
- Prepare and maintain examination and treatment areas

- Prepare patient for examinations, procedures, and treatments
- Assist with examinations, procedures, and treatments
- Prepare and administer medications and immunizations
- Maintain medication and immunization records
- Recognize and respond to emergencies
- Coordinate patient care information with other health care providers

GENERAL (TRANSDISCIPLINARY)

PROFESSIONALISM

- Project a professional manner and image
- Adhere to ethical principles
- Demonstrate initiative and responsibility
- Work as a team member
- Manage time efficiently
- Prioritize and perform multiple tasks
- Adapt to change
- Promote the CMA credential
- Enhance skills through continuing education

COMMUNICATION SKILLS

- Treat all patients with compassion and empathy
- Recognize and respect cultural diversity
- Adapt communications to individual's ability to understand
- Use professional telephone technique
- Use effective and correct verbal and written communications
- Recognize and respond to verbal and non-verbal communications
- Use medical terminology appropriately
- Receive, organize, prioritize, and transmit information
- Serve as liaison
- Promote the practice through positive public relations

LEGAL CONCEPTS

- Maintain confidentiality
- Practice within the scope of education, training, and personal capabilities
- Prepare and maintain medical records
- Document accurately
- Use appropriate guidelines when releasing information
- Follow employer's established policies dealing with the health care contract
- Follow federal, state, and local legal guidelines
- Maintain awareness of federal and state health care legislation and regulations
- Maintain and dispose of regulated substances in compliance with government guidelines
- Comply with established risk management and safety procedures
- Recognize professional credentialing criteria
- Participate in the development and maintenance of personnel, policy, and procedure manuals
- *Develop and maintain personnel, policy, and procedure manuals (adv)*

INSTRUCTION

- Instruct individuals according to their needs
- Explain office policies and procedures
- Teach methods of health promotion and disease prevention
- Locate community resources and disseminate information
- *Orient and train personnel (adv)*
- *Develop educational materials (adv)*
- *Conduct continuing education activities (adv)*

OPERATIONAL FUNCTIONS

- Maintain supply inventory
- Evaluate and recommend equipment and supplies
- Apply computer techniques to support office operations
- *Supervise personnel (adv)*
- *Interview and recommend job applicants (adv)*
- *Negotiate leases and prices for equipment and supply contracts (adv)*

SOURCE: Reprinted by permission of the American Association of Medical Assistants from the *AAMA Role Delineation Study: Occupational Analysis of the Medical Assisting Profession.*

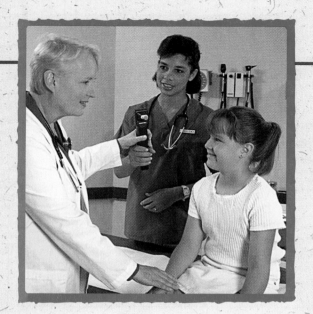

22
Assisting with Medical Specialties

CHAPTER OUTLINE

LEARNING OBJECTIVES

After completing this chapter, you should:
1. Define and spell the glossary terms for this chapter.
2. Prepare patients for examinations and diagnostic procedures.
3. Assist the physician with examinations and treatments.
4. Perform selected diagnostic tests.
5. Instruct patients with special procedures.
6. Follow-up patient's test results.
7. Document special procedures accurately.

CLINICAL PERFORMANCE COMPETENCIES

After completing this chapter, you should perform the following tasks:
1. Prepare a set-up for a PAP test.
2. Explain how to perform a breast self-examination and a testicular self-examination.
3. Assist the physician with a diagnostic examination.
4. Measure color vision using a color chart.
5. Perform a visual acuity test using a Snellen chart.
6. Obtain a wound culture using proper technique.

Glossary

anaphylactic shock   A life-threatening reaction to certain foods, drugs, and insect bites in some people. This can cause respiratory distress, edema, rash, convulsions, and eventually unconsciousness and death if emergency treatment is not given.

benign   Non-threatening, non-cancerous.

contagious   Diseases which can be transmitted from one person to another.

gynecology   The branch of medicine that deals with diseases and disorders of the female reproductive system.

malaise   Discomfort, uneasiness which is often indicative of an infection.

malignant   Cancerous.

metastasize   Cancerous cells or tumors that spread to another location or organ.

pediatrics   The branch of medicine which involves the development, diagnosis, and treatment of diseases and disorders in children.

phenylketonuria (PKU)   A recessive hereditary disease caused by the lack of an enzyme, phenylalanine hydroxylase, which results in severe mental retardation in children if not detected and treated soon after birth.

prognosis   Prediction of the course and outcome of a disease.

visual acuity   Sharpness of vision.

WARNING!

For all patient contact, adhere to Standard Precautions
(see pages 342–373). Wear protective equipment as indicated.

Special examinations and procedures relating to specific body systems are commonly performed in the medical office. The most commonly performed examinations include: pediatric, gynecologic, prenatal, proctoscopic, and sigmoidoscopic. Discussion of these examinations, along with a review of medical conditions related to specific body systems, is presented in this chapter.

The role of the medical assistant is to assist the physician during special examinations and procedures and to instruct the patient before, during, and/or after many of these procedures. Though many of the procedures discussed throughout this chapter are performed in the hospital setting, the medical assistant, as one of the prime educators of the patient, must know and understand a vast amount of medical information regarding these procedures.

To assist their understanding of the systems discussed in this chapter, students should refer to the color anatomical charts in the appendix.

Allergy and Dermatology (Integumentary System)

An allergy is an abnormal response or hypersensitivity to a substance (allergen), such as a medication or pollen, that does not normally cause a reaction in most people. Allergens enter the body through inhalation, injection, swallowing, or contact with the skin. Any substance in the environment can cause an allergy in sensitive persons.

Allergic conditions include eczema, allergic rhinitis, hay fever, bronchial asthma, urticaria (hives), and food allergies. An increase in the blood eosinophil level may occur with allergies.

The symptoms of allergies consist of a local or systemic inflammatory reaction which is characterized by redness, edema and heat. Respiratory symptoms include wheezing, sneezing, coughing, and nasal congestion.

Anaphylactic Shock

In some persons, a life-threatening allergic reaction called anaphylactic shock can occur. Insect stings (for example, bees and wasps) and allergies to drugs, such as penicillin, cause severe reactions. The symptoms include acute respiratory distress, edema, hypotension, rash, tachycardia, pale cool skin, convulsions, and cyanosis. This condition can result in circulatory and respiratory changes and requires emergency treatment consisting of medications (such as, epinephrine to relax smooth muscles in the airways) and, in some cases, endotracheal intubation and mechanical ventilation. If no treatment is received, unconsciousness and death may result.

The treatment for allergies consists of medications, for example benadryl, allergy testing and desensitization. Desensitization, in which minute amounts of the allergen are injected into the patient's system over an extended period of time, is used to develop a tolerance for the allergen. Desensitization is necessary if the allergic reactions significantly interfere with the patient's lifestyle or are life threatening, for example bee stings.

Sensitization

Sensitization is the initial exposure a person has to an allergen, or substance (antigen) recognized as foreign by the body's immune system, which leads to an immune response. On all subsequent exposures to that same substance, such as a pollen allergen, there is a much stronger and faster immune reaction when antibodies develop in response to the antigen. This action is what forms the basis of allergy and other types of hypersensitivity reaction.

Sensitization is deliberately produced during the immunization process when a disease-causing organism, such as smallpox, is injected into the body. The organism is no longer able to become infectious but is still able to cause the body to produce antibodies to fight off the actual disease. Figure 22-1 shows a young patient receiving an allergy injection.

Allergy Testing

Testing is ordered by the physician to determine a patient's sensitivities to allergens. The methods used include scratch or skin testing, intradermal tests, and patch tests.

The scratch method of allergy testing is usually performed on the patient's back or upper

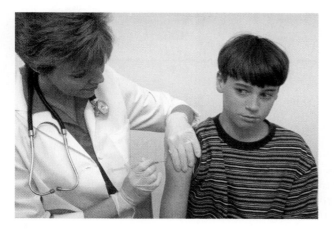

Figure 22-1   Allergy injection.

outer arms. The skin is divided into small squares, which are approximately 1 inch apart, and labeled using a ball point pen to indicate which allergen is used. After scratching the skin with a needle or lancet, a drop of allergen is placed onto the skin at the site of the scratch. Many scratch tests using different allergens can be performed at the same time. If a wheal forms within 15 minutes after placing an allergen on the skin, an allergy is indicated. The patient should be advised to remain in the physician's office for at least 30 minutes after the testing has been completed in the event there is a delayed allergic reaction to the testing.

Intradermal tests for allergy testing are performed by injecting 0.01 to 0.02 mL of the allergen extract into the anterior surface of the forearm. Several tests (10 to 18) can be performed on each arm. A red wheal is a positive sign. An intradermal test is considered more accurate than a scratch test. See Chapter 32 for a more detailed description of intradermal injections.

The patch test consists of placing a small amount of the allergen onto the anterior forearm and then covering this with a plastic covering such as cellophane and tape. Several patch tests can be performed at the same time and these are read after the patches have remained in place for 24-48 hours. Patch tests are used to detect the causative agents in contact dermatitis. Table 22-1* describes common allergies.

> **Med Tip:** "Reading" a skin test means that the test site is observed visually to note any redness and swelling (wheal) which indicates a positive test result. This means the patient is allergic to the allergen.

Dermatology

The skin and its appendages—sweat glands, oil glands, nails, and hair—are known as the integumentary system. The sense organs that respond to changes in temperature, pain, touch, and pressure are located in this system. The skin consists of the epidermis (thin outer membrane), the dermis (middle, fibrous layer), and subcutaneous (innermost layer containing fatty tissue) layers. Medical conditions relating to this system occur in all three layers.

*Tables for Chapter 22 are located in the reference section at the end of the book.

Common Skin Disorders and Treatments

Most skin conditions and diseases are diagnosed, in part, by observing the lesion. Skin lesions can occur whenever the normal surface of the skin is invaded or changed. A skin lesion is not always a sign of disease, such as seen with a non-cancerous nodule. There is generally some discoloration or change from the normal coloration.

Some of the more common lesions are described in Table 22-2 and illustrated in Figure 22-2 (dermatology skin lesions). These terms should be used when charting information relating to any skin lesions.

Bacteria, viruses, and parasites can all invade the skin if its protective barrier is broken down. Some of the more common skin infections are listed in Table 22-3. Table 22-4 describes benign and malignant neoplasms.

Inflammatory skin disorders result in swelling, redness, and often itching over the affected site. These conditions include cellulitis, decubitus ulcers, psoriasis, acne vulgaris and scleroderma.

- Cellulitis is an inflammation of the cellular or connective tissue. Treatment consists of antibiotics.
- Decubitus ulcers, also called bedsores, are open sores caused by pressure over bony prominences on the body due to a lack of blood flow. These can appear in bedridden patients who lie in one position too long. Treatment consists of relieving the pressure through frequent turning and exercise of the patient, thorough cleansing of the wound, and

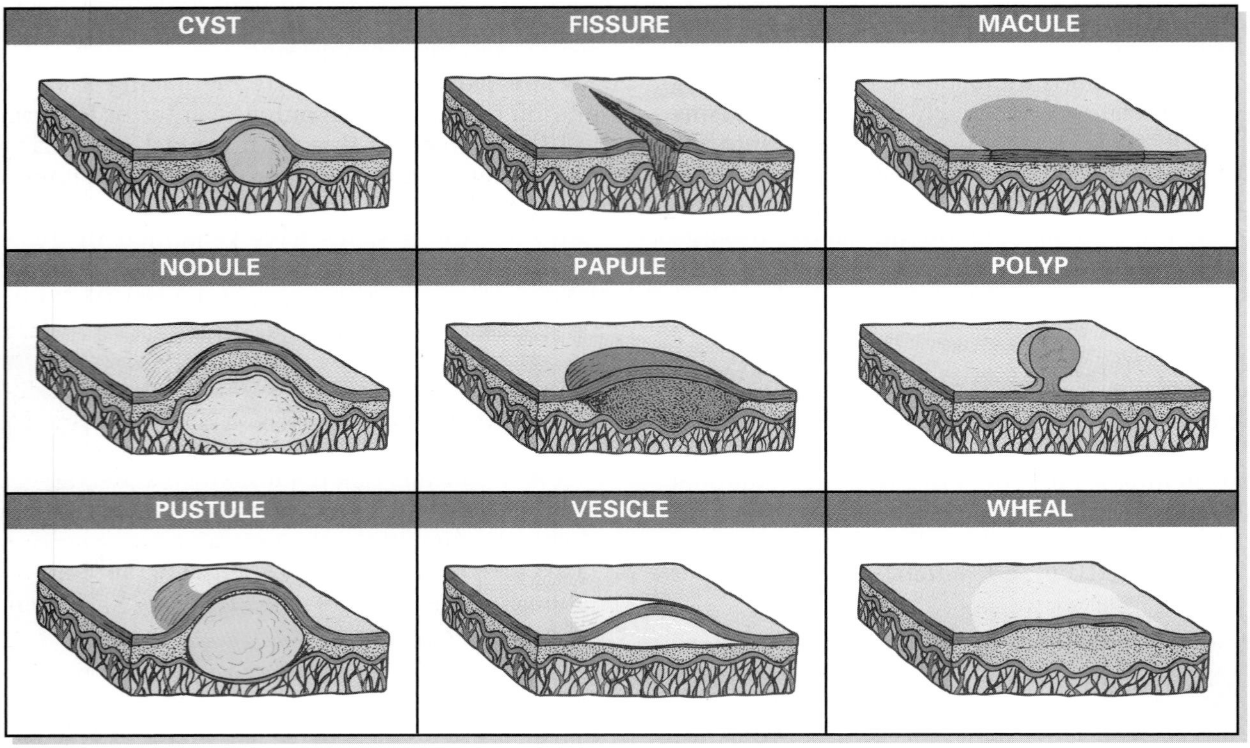

Figure 22-2 Types of skin lesions.
Cyst—A fluid-filled sac or pouch under the skin.
Fissure—Crack-like lesion or groove in the skin.
Macule—Small, flat discolored area that is flush with the skin surface. An example would be a freckle and the flat rash of roseola.
Nodule—Solid, raised group of cells.
Papule—Small, solid, circular raised spot on the surface of the skin.
Polyp—Small tumor with a pedicle or stem attachment. They are commonly found in vascular organs such as the nose, uterus, and rectum.
Pustule—Raised spot on the skin containing pus.
Vesicle—Small fluid-filled raised spot on the skin; blister.
Wheal—Small, round, raised area on the skin that may be accompanied by itching.

topical antibiotics. Deep ulcers may require surgical debridement (removal of dead tissue).

- Psoriasis is a chronic inflammatory condition consisting of crusty papules forming patches with circular borders. Treatment consists of topical ointments, and, in some severe cases, ultraviolet light therapy.
- Acne vulgaris is an inflammatory disease of the sebaceous glands and hair follicles which results in papules and pustules. Treatment consists of thorough cleansing and systemic and topical antibiotics.
- Scleroderma is a disorder in which the skin becomes taut, thick, and leatherlike. There is no treatment unless the skin becomes infected in which case antibiotics may be prescribed.

Med Tip: You need to be aware that whenever your patients hear the term "tumor" they immediately think of cancer. Since a tumor can be either benign or malignant, it is advisable not to use the general term "tumor" when talking to a patient.

Neoplasms

Neoplasms or tumors can be either benign (noncancerous) or malignant (cancerous). Neoplasms are biopsied by surgically removing a small amount of tissue for testing. If the neoplasm is found to be malignant, then the entire tumor is removed.

Oncology is the branch of medicine dealing with tumors. Cancer therapy, consisting of chemotherapy (toxic drugs) and radiation, is used in the treatment of cancer.

Med Tip: Skin cancer has been proven to be directly related to sun exposure. The ultraviolet rays in the sunlight change the DNA structure of skin cells making them receptive to mutations (changes) within the cells which leads to skin cancer. Factor 15 sunscreen is used to prevent sun damage to the skin.

Diagnostic Procedures

A variety of diagnostic tests and procedures are used when treating disorders of the integumentary system. These are described in Table 22-5. These procedures are performed by the physician with the assistance of the medical assistant. See the procedure for taking a wound culture.

Cardiovascular System

A study of the cardiovascular or circulatory system is called cardiology. This system includes the heart and blood vessels. The symptoms of cardiovascular disease and disorders are varied due to the wide variety of precipitating causes (for example, poor circulation, defective heart valves, conduction defect, blood clots in the heart layers or blood vessels). The most common symptoms of cardiovascular disorders are

- Chest pain (crushing type of pain)
- Cyanosis (bluish skin color due to lack of oxygen in the tissues)
- Diaphoresis (excessive sweating)
- Dyspnea (difficult breathing)
- Edema
- Irregular heartbeat

Disorders of the cardiovascular system are described in Table 22-6. Diagnostic procedures and tests related to the cardiovascular system are listed in Table 22-7.

Endocrine System

Endocrinology is the study of the endocrine system. This glandular system secretes hormones directly into the bloodstream. The organs of the endocrine system are of two types of glands: exocrine glands which secrete through a duct or another organ and endocrine glands which produce internal secretions.

The endocrine glands include two adrenal glands, two ovaries in the female, two sets of parathyroid glands, the pancreas (islets of Langerhans), two testes in the male, the pituitary gland, thymus gland, and thyroid gland. The endocrine glands work together as a whole to affect the entire body. Disorders of the endocrine system are discussed in Table 22-8. Table 22-9 lists procedures and tests relating to the endocrine system.

Gastrointestinal System

The gastrointestinal or digestive system includes mouth, esophagus, stomach, small and large intestine and the accessory organs liver, gallbladder, and pancreas. This system stores and digests food, eliminates waste, and utilizes nutrients. Table 22-10 describes common disorders and pathology of the digestive system. Table 22-11 lists procedures and tests relating to the digestive system.

PROCEDURE: Taking a Wound Culture

**Terminal Performance
Competency:** Student will obtain a sample using a swab technique without error.

Equipment and Supplies
Gloves
Culture tube with sterile swab
Tape for dressing
Sterile water for cleansing wound
Sterile 4 × 4 gauze dressing
Hazardous waste container
Bag for soiled dressing
Prepared label for culture tube or pen for labeling tube

Procedural Steps
1. Wash hands.
2. Assemble equipment.
3. Identify patient and explain procedure.
4. Apply gloves.
5. Remove dressing and place in bag.
6. Observe wound for redness, crusting, swelling, odor, and amount of exudate.
7. Using a sterile swab, place it in the wound using a wiping motion. Place the swab in the sterile culture tube. Crush the ampule of preservative that is in the culture tube and seal the tube. Label the culture tube with patient's name, identification number, and date.
8. Clean the wound using sterile water and 4 × 4 gauze squares.
9. Apply sterile dressing over the wound.
10. Remove gloves and dispose of them properly in hazardous waste container.
11. Chart the procedure.

Charting Example
2/14/XX   3:30 PM Small amount of exudate obtained from open wound on L. ankle using sterile swab. Tube labeled and sent to lab. Wound cleaned and dressed. Erythema surrounding wound site. No odor noted. Home care instructions given.

M. King, CMA

Sigmoidoscopy

The sigmoidoscopy, also called proctoscopic or proctosigmoidoscopic examination, is an examination of the interior of the sigmoid colon for diagnostic purposes. This is a useful procedure to assist in the detection of cancer of the colon, polyps, ulcerations, and other disorders of the lower intestinal tract.

The sigmoidoscope, a flexible, metal or plastic instrument with a light source and magnification lens, is used for the sigmoidoscopy. A newer type of flexible sigmoidoscope allows the physician to see further into the colon and view the mucous membranes of the intestines (Figure 22-3). Figure 22-4 pictures a proctoscopic examination table and Figure 22-5 a sigmoidoscope kit.

An obturator is inserted into the sigmoidoscope to guide it into the rectum. The tip of the obturator must be well lubricated to allow for easier insertion. Once into the rectum the physician removes the obturator, or guide, and can then see into the colon through the sigmoidoscope.

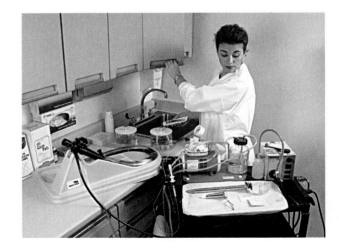

Figure 22-3   Sigmoidoscope in cold chemical sterilizer.

Preparation for this examination is important. Patients should be told to empty their bowel and bladder before coming in for the procedure.

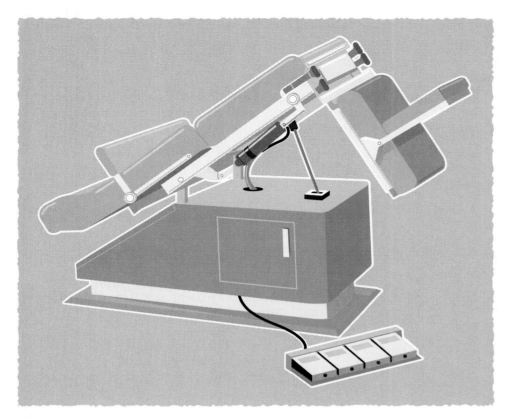

Figure 22-4   Proctoscopic examination table.

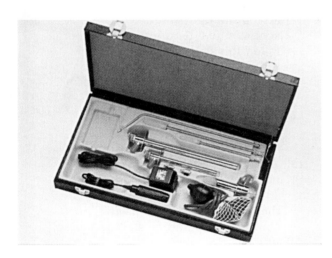

Figure 22-5   Sigmoidoscope kit from Welch-

The physician will usually have the patient take a commercially-prepared enema 2 hours before the examination. They should be advised to drink plenty of clear liquids and eat sparingly the day before the exam. Some physicians will request the patient to refrain from eating raw fruits and vegetables, grains, and dairy products a few days prior to the exam so the colon will be easier to visualize. In some cases a cleansing enema may have to be administered in the physician's office if the patient's bowel is not clear enough. It is critical that every attempt is made to ensure the patient follows the instructions for the bowel preparation since an improperly prepared bowel may result in a reschedule of the procedure.

This procedure can be uncomfortable for patients. The procedure is made easier for patients if they are instructed to concentrate on breathing deeply through the mouth while trying to relax the abdominal muscles. During the procedure the intestinal wall is stretched as the instrument passes through and air may be introduced to distend the wall for easier visualization. This causes the patient to have an urge to defecate and may even be painful for the patient. The procedure only lasts a few minutes, however the patient will need encouragement throughout the procedure.

The physician may take several biopsy samples during the procedure. The patient should sign a consent form for both the procedure and any biopsy of materials.

PROCEDURE: Assisting with a Proctosigmoidoscopy

**Terminal Performance
Competency:** Student will assist the physician during the proctosigmoidoscopic examination by positioning the patient, handling all equipment, biopsy material, and providing support for the patient throughout the procedure without error.

Equipment and Supplies

Sigmoidoscope with obturator, flexible or inflexible (metal or plastic)

Anoscope

Rectal speculum

Insufflator

Suction equipment

Sterile specimen container with preservative

Sterile biopsy forceps

Cotton applicators (long)

Lubricating jelly

Basin of water

Patient drape

Gloves

Patient gown

Patient drape

Small towel or examination table pad

Tissue

Biohazard waste container

Procedural Steps

1. Wash hands.

2. Prepare equipment and supplies. Check all lights and light bulbs in equipment. Prepare a basin of warm water to receive used instruments. Test suction equipment. Place obturator within the sigmoidoscope.

3. Label specimen container with patient's name, address, date, source of specimen, and ID number.

4. Identify patient and explain procedure. Make sure the patient has followed the enema and diet instructions. Check to make sure the consent form has been signed.

5. Ask patient to undress and put on a patient gown.

6. Assist patient into the Sims', lateral, or knee-chest position. Some physicians may use a special proctologic table that will tilt the patient into the correct knee-chest position.

Rationale: In the knee-chest position, the abdominal contents and organs move forward and away from the pelvic area which makes it easier to insert the sigmoidoscope.

7. Drape the patient and place a towel or disposable exam pad under the perineal area.

8. Place lubricant on the physician's gloved fingers for a digital examination.

9. Place metal scope in basin of warm water to warm it before insertion into patient.

10. Lubricate the tip of the scope.

11. Attach the inflation bulb (for air inflation during the procedure) and attach the light source. Turn the scope on just before the physician is ready to use it. *Rationale:* The scope tip becomes warm/hot if turned on too soon and may harm the patient.

12. Remind the patient to take deep breaths and relax the abdominal muscles.

13. Assist the physician by handling instruments and equipment such as suction, cotton tipped applicators, as they are needed. Place used equipment, including suction tubing, into basin of water.

14. Assist with biopsy by holding open specimen containers to receive specimen, while maintaining sterility of container.

(Continued)

15. Clean around patient's anal opening with tissue. Discard in biohazard waste container.
16. Remove gloves and wash hands.
17. Assist patient to slowly sit up.
    Rationale: Sitting up too quickly from the Sims' position can result in dizziness.
18. Ask patient to dress and provide assistance as needed.
19. Apply gloves and clean equipment and room.
20. Remove gloves and document procedure. The physician will document the results of the procedure.

Charting Example
2/14/XX   9:00 AM Assisted patient with sigmoidoscopic examination. Biopsy sent to lab. No dizziness or discomfort noted after procedure.   M. King, CMA

Lymphatic (Immune) System

The lymphatic system, consisting of lymph glands, ducts, and nodes, tonsils, thymus gland, and spleen, are the basis of the body's defense system. This system protects the body against the invasion of foreign microorganisms. It works in conjunction with the circulatory system to purify the blood and drain fluids throughout the body.

In some diseases, such as acquired immune deficiency syndrome (AIDS), the body has lost its natural ability to fight off infection. AIDS is discussed more fully in Chapter 19. Table 22-12 describes common disorders and pathology related to the lymphatic system. Table 22-13 lists procedures and tests related to the lymphatic system.

Musculoskeletal System

The study of the musculoskeletal system of bones and muscles is called orthopedics. Disorders of the musculoskeletal system are discussed in Table 22-14. Table 22-15 lists procedure and diagnostic tests relating to the musculoskeletal system.

Nervous System

The study of the nervous system is neurology. This system consists of the brain, nerves, and spinal cord. Table 22-16 describes disorders and diseases of the nervous system. Table 22-17 discusses procedures and tests relating to the nervous system.

Assisting with Lumbar Puncture

The physician may wish to examine spinal fluid for the presence of bleeding or infection. During this procedure a needle is inserted into the subarachnoid space of the spinal cord. This is usually performed at the level of the 4th intervertebral space. A small gauge needle (22) is passed through the dura. When the stylet, or thin probe, is removed from the needle, cerebrospinal fluid (CSF) will escape which can be collected into tubes for microscopic examination. Patients are prone to headaches after this procedure due to leakage of fluid from the spinal spaces. Headaches can be diminished if the patient is instructed to lie perfectly flat for several hours (6-12) after the procedure. This procedure is more commonly performed in a clinic setting rather than a medical office so the patient can remain flat for the intended time.

A Queckenstedt test may be performed to determine the presence of an obstruction. The medical assistant may assist during this test by pressing the veins in the neck while the physician monitors the pressure using the manometer. First the right side is pressed, then left side, then both together for 10 seconds. Normally the pressure will rise rapidly and then decrease when the pressure is released. In a blockage there will be little or no response to the application of pressure.

PROCEDURE: Assisting With Lumbar Puncture

Terminal Performance Competency: Student will setup equipment, position patient properly, and assist physician during the lumbar puncture without error.

Equipment and Supplies

Sterile glove packets

Personal protective equipment: gowns, masks

Patient gown

3-5 inch lumbar needle (gauge determined by physician)

4 × 4 gauze squares

Sterile test tubes

Local anesthetic, syringe and 25 gauge needle

Sterile drape (fenestrated)

Sterile towel

Antiseptic

Cotton tipped applicators for antiseptic application

Sterile forceps (if sterile skin preparation used by physician)

Spinal fluid manometer with 3-way stopcock

Mayo stand

Adhesive bandage

Biohazard waste container

Biohazard bags

Paper and pen

Procedural Steps

1. Wash hands.

2. Assemble equipment. Prepare the sterile instrument setup (as explained in Chapter 23) and cover with sterile towel.

3. Identify patient and explain procedure. Remind the patient not to move during the procedure. Explain the need to remain flat after the procedure is performed. Take vital signs and record.

4. Make sure consent form is signed and in the patient's record.

5. Ask patient to empty bladder and put on gown with opening in the back.

6. Assist the patient into position.:

   a. Side-lying position: Have patient bring knees up toward chest and move back to edge of table. Place your hands on the patient's legs and shoulder to remind the patient not to move during the procedure.

   b. Forward-leaning position: Have patient sit on the edge of the table and lean forward. Keep your hands on the patient's shoulders to remind the patient not to move during the procedure. ***Rationale:*** These positions allow the space between the vertebra to widen slightly which allows easier insertion of the needle.

7. After gloving, the physician will prepare the skin using antiseptic and sterile forceps. A sterile fenestrated drape is applied to allow a clear view of the puncture site. A local anesthetic is administered before the spinal needle is inserted. Remind the patient that pressure may be felt during the procedure, but that there should be no pain.

8. After the physician has the spinal needle in place, the patient may be allowed to straighten his or her position slightly, as instructed by the physician. The physician will now use the manometer and stopcock to measure the intracranial pressure.

9. If spinal fluid specimens are taken, the medical assistant will apply gloves and hold the test tubes to receive the potentially hazardous fluid. These are labeled in the order they are received (1, 2, 3) with the patient's name and identification number. Place in biohazard bag.

(Continued)

10. Assist the physician, as instructed, if the Queckenstedt test is performed.

11. Monitor the patient during the procedure for signs such as state of mental alertness, cyanosis, dyspnea, and nausea.

12. When the procedure is complete, apply an adhesive bandage over the site. Assist the patient into a flat position. Have the patient remain flat for the required time. Monitor vital signs during this period. If the patient needs to void, a bedpan must be used.

13. Send the specimen to the laboratory for testing.

14. Clean the room and equipment.

15. Chart procedure and your observations. Physician will chart the results.

Charting Example

2/14/XX   9:00 AM   Patient positioned in side-lying position for lumbar puncture performed by Dr. Williams. BP 128/84, P-80, R-16.   M. King, CMA

9:30 AM   LP completed. Pt. tolerated procedure well. BP 122/80, P-78, R-16. CSF sent to lab. Pt. remaining flat.   M. King, CMA

10:00 AM   No discomfort. Dressing dry. Pt. given discharge instructions and verbalized understanding. Spouse remaining with patient. Remaining flat without discomfort.   M. King, CMA

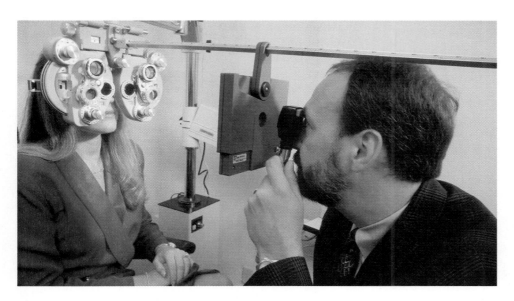

Figure 22-6   Ophthalmologist examining patient.

Special Senses: Eyes and Ears

The study of the eye is ophthalmology. An ophthalmologist treats patients with eye disorders (Figure 22-6). In Figure 22-7 a medical assistant helps a patient with eye care related to contact lenses. Common disorders of the eye, such as glaucoma (Figure 22-8), are described in Table 22-18.

The Ishihara test is printed in either card or booklet form with a single color-dot illustration containing a number on each page or plate. Patients are asked to identify the number they see within the color dots. Patients suffering from color blindness are unable to identify some of the numbers within the allotted time frame (3 seconds). The physician explains the results of this test to the patient. See Figure 22-9 for an example of a chart to test for color-blindness. See the procedure for conducting a color vision test using the Ishihara screening test.

The Snellen chart, and other visual acuity testing charts, are used to test for far vision. This type of chart is hung 20 feet from the patient's eye level in a room with normal lighting.

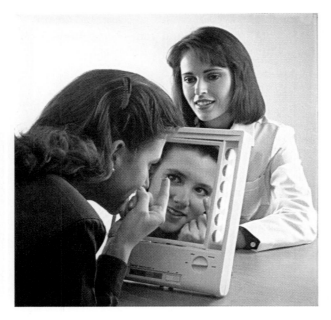

Figure 22-7 Medical assistant helping patient with contact lenses.

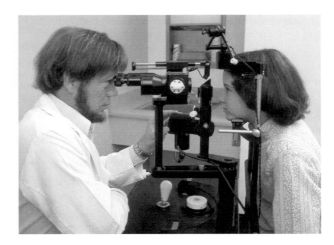

Figure 22-8 Glaucoma test.

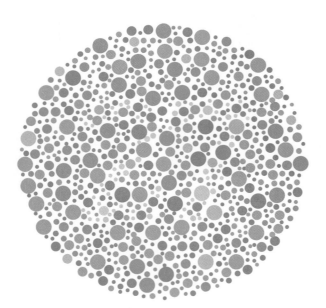

Figure 22-9 Color vision chart.

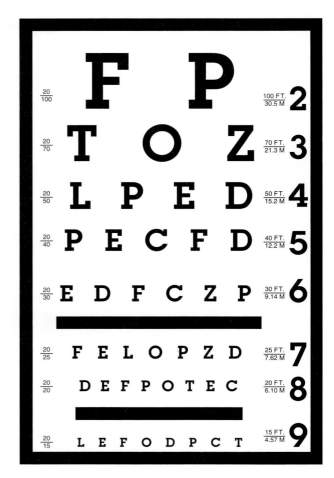

Figure 22-10 Snellen vision chart.

Charts, such as the Snellen chart, contain numbers, pictures, and letters which become progressively smaller. Snellen charts using the letter "E", in gradually diminishing size pointing in different directions, are useful for children or others who are unable to read. Patients are asked to point their finger in the same direction as the "E" is pointing. Figure 22-10 shows the Snellen eye chart. Refer to the procedure for testing vision using a Snellen chart.

PROCEDURE: Color Vision Testing Using the Ishihara Test

**Terminal Performance
Competency:** Student is able to administer color-blindness test to patient without error.

Equipment and Supplies
Ishihara screening booklet/cards
Quiet room with natural lighting, if possible
Paper and pen

Procedural Steps
1. Wash hands.
2. Assemble Ishihara test cards or booklet.
3. Identify patient and explain procedure.
4. Have patient assume a comfortable position, so that he or she can look directly at the booklet/cards, as you hold them 30 inches from the patient's eyes.
   a. Ask patient to identify the number that is formed by the color dots on each card or picture.
   b. The patient will have 3 seconds to identify each number.
5. Ask patient to keep both eyes open during the examination.
6. If the patient is able to identify the number, then write that number after the plate number.
(For example: Plate 1: 7 meaning the patient read the number 7 on plate 1).
7. If the patient is unable to identify any number or the correct number, then indicate with an X.
(For example: Plate 1: X).
8. Chart the results of the procedure including any unusual symptoms such as frequent squinting. If ten or more plates are read correctly, color vision is considered normal.
9. Store booklet/plates out of direct sunlight to prevent fading of color plates.

Charting Example
2/14/XX   3:00 PM   Ishihara test normal.
M. King, CMA

Med Tip: Normal vision is considered to be 20/20 vision. This is based on a patient being able to read material from a distance of 20 feet that a normal eye can see at 20 feet. For example, vision of 20/40 means that the patient can see at 20 feet what the normal eye would be able to see at 40 feet.

Irrigation of the eye is demonstrated in Figure 22-11. Table 22-19 contains procedures and diagnostic tests relating to the eye.

The study of the ear is otology. Otolaryngology refers to the study of the ear and larynx. Otorhinolaryngology refers to that branch of medicine that treats diseases of the ear, nose, and throat.

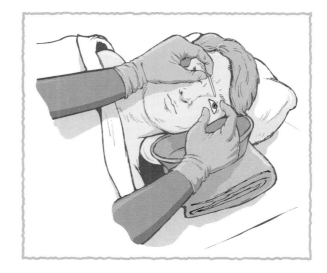

Figure 22-11   Irrigation of the eye.

Terminal Performance
Competency: Student will administer a visual acuity test using the Snellen chart without error.

Equipment and Supplies
Snellen eye chart placed at eye level 20 feet from patient
Eye shield or occluder
Pointer
Paper and pen

Procedural Steps
1. Wash hands.
2. Assemble equipment.
3. Identify patient and explain procedure. Patients may be tested with their glasses (contact lens) on or off, depending on the physician's instructions.
4. Have the patient stand or sit (depending on the height of the Snellen chart) 20 feet from the chart and cover first the left eye with the eye shield. Ask the patient to keep open the eye that is behind the eye shield to prevent squinting.
5. Point to line 3 on the Snellen chart and ask the patient to identify each letter. If the patient is unable to read line 3, then go back to line 1. When the patient can no longer read a line, then record the results as the last line the patient could read.
6. Have the patient place the eye shield over the right eye and test the left vision in the same manner.
7. Also test vision by having the patient read using both eyes.
8. Document findings on patient's record.

Charting Example

2/14/XX	4:00 PM	Snellen eye test
OD 20/30	OS 20/30	OU 20/30
		M. King CMA

The ear is divided into three components: external ear containing the auricle, auditory canal and tympanic membrane, middle ear containing the three bones malleus, incus, and stapes, and the inner ear within the temporal bone. Disorders of the ear generally relate to one of these three divisions. Common disorders of the ear are described in Table 22-20. Table 22-21 describes procedures and diagnostic tests relating to the ear.

Figures 22-12, 22-13, and 22-14 illustrate ear care and assessment techniques.

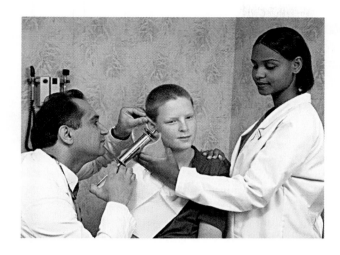

Figure 22-12   Ear irrigation technique.

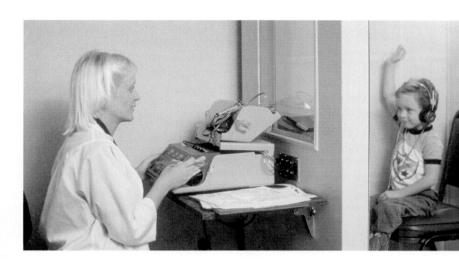

Figure 22-13
Hearing test.

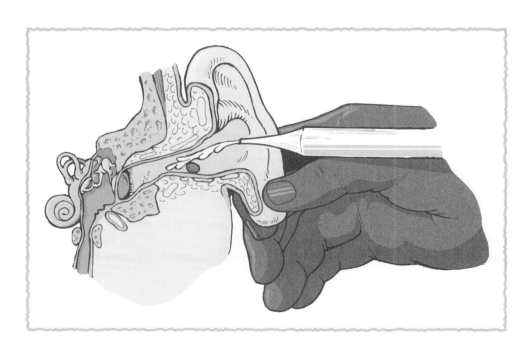

Figure 22-14
Removal of a foreign
body from the ear.

PROCEDURE: Ear Irrigation

**Terminal Performance
Competency:** Student will perform ear irrigation using aseptic technique without error.

Equipment and Supplies

Gloves

Ear syringe and bulb

Emesis basin or ear basin

Basin of warm irrigation solution (per physician order)

Towels

Cotton balls

Biohazard waste container

Procedural Steps

1. Wash hands.
2. Assemble equipment. Check the expiration date of the solution. Check the name of the solution three times. If a solution other than warm tap water is used, warm it slightly by placing the container in a basin of warm water.
3. Identify patient and explain procedure.
4. Apply gloves.
5. Have patient seated with affected ear tilted slightly downward. Place a towel over the patient's shoulder and ask patient to hold the emesis basin directly under the affected ear.
   Rationale: Gravity will assist in the flow of irrigation material into the basin.
6. Clean outer ear with moistened cotton ball.

Rationale: Wash away any gross matter so that it does not enter the ear during the irrigation process.

7. Pour the warmed solution into the basin and fill syringe. Use approximately 50 cc of solution with each irrigation.
8. Perform procedure by pulling up and out on the auricle of adults to straighten the ear canal. After expelling air from the syringe, gently insert the tip of the syringe into the patient's ear. *Rationale:* Gentleness is required to prevent injury to the ear or ear canal with the syringe.

9. Slowly push the solution into the ear without totally occluding the external auditory canal. Try to direct the flow of solution toward the roof of the ear canal. *Rationale:* The solution must have room to flow out of the ear. A buildup of pressure within the ear canal could cause serious damage to the middle ear.

10. Repeat steps 8 and 9 of the procedure until the return is clear.
11. Remove basin.
12. Dry the outer ear and remove the towel.
13. The patient may lie on an examination table on the affected side to allow the water to continue to drain out of the ear.
14. Give the patient cotton balls to wipe away any external drainage. Instruct patient on any home care and remind them not to insert cotton tipped applicators into their ear.
15. Dispose of waste material properly and clean equipment.
16. Wash hands.
17. Document procedure noting the return and any pain or dizziness.

Charting Example

2/14/XX   11:00 AM Ear irrigation to both ears. Cerumen plug removed from Right ear. No pain or dizziness experienced. Patient remained lying on right side for 15 minutes.   M. King, CMA

PROCEDURE: Assisting With Audiometry

**Terminal Performance
Competency:** Student is able to perform audiometric test without error. *Note:* This procedure is performed by the medical assistant only if he or she has been thoroughly trained by the physician.

Equipment and Supplies
Audiometer with headphones
Quiet room or small enclosed cubicle

Procedural Steps

1. Wash hands.
2. Prepare equipment and room. Test equipment or make sure power is on.
3. Identify patient and explain procedure.
   a. Have the patient indicate with a nod or by holding up one finger when the patient first hears a sound.
4. Have patient assume comfortable sitting position and place headphones over one ear.
5. Begin with a low frequency and watch the patient for an indication of when that sound is heard. Plot that on a graph.
6. Gradually increase the frequency until completed with that ear.
7. Have the patient place the headphones over the other ear and perform the same test.
8. Give the graphic results of the test to the physician. The physician will interpret and chart the findings.
9. Clean equipment per manufacturer's directions.
10. Document that the procedure was administered.

Charting Example
2/14/XX   9:00 AM Audiometry test administered in both ears. Results given to Dr. Williams.   M. King, CMA

Pediatrics

Pediatrics is that branch of medicine specializing in the development, diagnosis, and treatment of diseases of children. The physician who specializes in this field is called a pediatrician. There are two categories of pediatric office visits: the well baby visit and the sick child visit.

The well baby visits are for the purpose of establishing and maintaining good health for the infant and child. These visits include immunizations as protection against diseases such as measles, whooping cough, and polio. The well baby office visits are scheduled on a routine basis after birth: 1 month, 2 months, 4 months, 6 months, 9 months, 12 months, 15 months, 18 months, 24 months, and then on a yearly basis.

Children are susceptible to some of the same diseases as adults. These include upper respiratory tract and urinary tract infections. There are other communicable or contagious diseases, which are easily spread from one person to another, which children are especially susceptible to. Some of the childhood diseases can cause permanent damage to susceptible children. For example, a severe case of measles may result in a permanent hearing loss in some children. In addition, measles is dangerous for a pregnant woman to contract during her first three months (trimester) of pregnancy since permanent damage to the unborn fetus can result. Therefore, the Public Health Department requires that all children be immunized against certain diseases.

The Centers for Disease Control and the American Academy of Pediatrics recommend immunization of all babies against hepatitis B. All babies, with parental consent, are given the first dose of hepatitis vaccine while they are still in the nursery. Babies of mothers who tested positive for carrying the hepatitis B virus are given hepatitis immune globulin and hepatitis B vaccine before leaving the hospital. Hepatitis vaccine is given in a series of three injections: 1st dose in the newborn nursery, second dose 1 to 2 months later, and third dose between the ages of 6 and 18 months.

Many contagious diseases are preventable with immunizations. Chapter 32 contains a guide for childhood immunizations. The guide is meant to serve as a quick general reference for an immunization schedule. The report of the Committee on Infectious Diseases (Red Book) of the American Academy of Pediatrics and the Public Health Service Advisory Committee on Immunization Practices should be consulted before developing an office policy. Only the physician can order an immunization schedule or injections for the child. A medical assistant must never give immunizations without the written authorization of a physician. Patients who are ill or have had a fever in the preceding 24 hours should be rescheduled for immunization. Patients who are sensitive to egg protein and antibiotics may have a reaction to immunizations.

During the well baby visits, certain measurements are taken on a routine basis. These include temperature, pulse, respiration, head and chest circumference. These measurements are discussed in Chapter 20. Figure 22-15 shows a baby examination.

The infant's growth is compared against a growth chart which contains the rate of growth against that of other children of the same age. The physician will carefully monitor any significant differences, such as a rapid increase or decrease in the child's growth area. The growth chart is an aid in identifying an abnormal growth or nutritional pattern. As the child advances in age visual acuity, or sharpness of vision, and hearing tests are frequently conducted.

Pediatric Safety

The medical assistant must become skilled at lifting and carrying the baby in a safe position. The cradle position is frequently used for carrying the smaller baby. To use this carry position the medical assistant slips an arm and hand under the baby and grasps the opposite arm. The baby's head is supported by the medical assistant's elbow where the head is "cradled." The other arm of the medical assistant is placed under the baby's buttocks. The baby is then held closely against the chest of the medical assistant.

Med Tip: Always remember to support a baby's head. Even if an older baby is able to hold his or her head upright, the head may suddenly fall backward causing you to lose your grip on the baby. Always keep one hand behind the baby's head to restrain movement.

For some procedures, such as delicate suturing, the physician will ask to have the baby wrapped in a blanket or sheet so their arms and legs are restrained (Figure 22-16 A and B). This safety measure does not hurt the baby and allows the physician to perform a procedure without the baby's sudden movements.

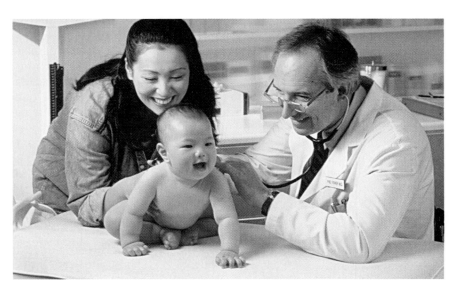

Figure 22-15 Well baby visits involve certain basic examinations.

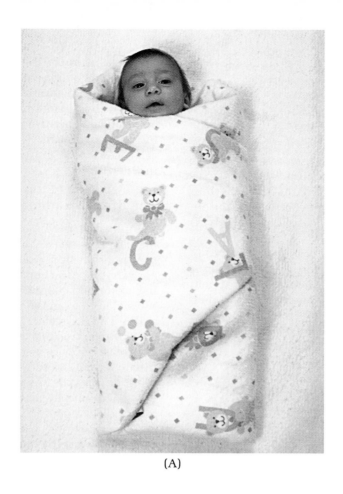

(A)

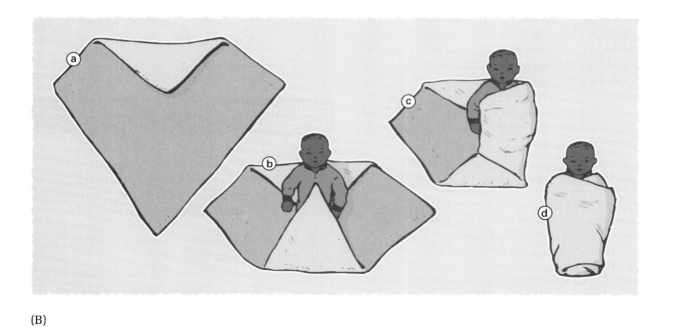

(B)

Figure 22-16 A and B Examples of baby wrap for self containment.

Phenylketonuria (PKU) Screening Test

Phenylketonuria (PKU) is a recessive hereditary disease caused by the lack of an enzyme. This enzyme, phenylalanine hydroxylase, is necessary to convert the amino acid, phenylalanine, into tyrosine which is needed for metabolic function. If this disorder is not treated, severe mental retardation will develop from an accumulation of phenylalanine in the blood. Other conditions such as poor muscle coordination, tremors, hypersensitivity, spasticity, and convulsions may be present.

A screening test for PKU, which is required in many states, is performed at birth. The disorder is seen in both males and females. Treatment consists of a special low-phenylalanine diet. Treatment, with a special diet is usually started around the age of three or four weeks. The **prognosis**, or outcome, of this disorder is excellent with early detection and treatment before three years of age.

Phenylketonuria (PKU) screening is performed on infants between 2 and 7 days after birth. The infant must be on either breast or formula milk for several days before a PKU test can be conducted. Formula-fed babies can be tested earlier than breast-fed babies since formula contains phenylalanine while colostrum, the mother's first breast milk, does not.

PKU testing is done by taking a capillary blood sample from the plantar surface of the baby's foot at either the heel or big toe. The first drop of blood, containing tissue fluid is wiped away, and the second drop of blood is used for the blood sample (specimen). The blood sample is placed onto a circle on a specially treated filter paper which is attached to the PKU test card. The PKU test card is then mailed immediately to a laboratory for testing.

Reproductive Systems

Gynecology is the branch of medicine that deals with disorders and diseases of the female reproductive system. The female reproductive system consists of the uterus, two fallopian tubes, two ovaries, the vagina, and the mammary glands. The practice of gynecology is closely related to the medical specialty of obstetrics, which is the branch of medicine concerned with the management of women during pregnancy, childbirth, and the period of time immediately after childbirth the puerperium (Figures 22-17 A and B). A gynecologist may also be an obstetrician.

Female Reproductive System

An examination of the female reproductive organs will include a breast examination and a pelvic examination to determine the condition of both the external and the internal organs of reproduction. In addition a Papanicolaou (PAP) test may be performed for the early detection of precancerous or early cancer of the cervix and endometrium of the uterus.

The Breast Examination

The physician will generally begin by examining the patient's breasts. The patient lies in the supine position for this examination and is generally asked to place the hand on the side of the breast being examined behind her head. This allows the physician to examine the lymph nodes under that axilla. The physician palpates the breast using his or her finger tips in a circular fashion around all of the breast tissue to search for lumps, tenderness, or inflammation. In addition, any dimpling or puckering of the skin around the breast and nipple is noted. The nipples are checked for cracking, bleeding, or discharge.

The physician will advise the patient to perform a breast self-exam every month, a week after the menstrual period. The medical assistant may have the responsibility of explaining the correct procedure for the breast self-exam. The American Cancer Society also advises a monthly self-exam of both breasts. Women who have reached menopause should examine their breasts on the same day each month. If the woman notes any ab-

---

Guidelines: Performing a Breast Self-Examination

1. Breast examinations should be performed at the same time each month, preferably 7-10 days after the menses.
2. Examine the breasts in three positions: before a mirror, lying down, and in a warm shower.
3. Keeping the fingers flat and using the pads of the three middle fingers, use a circular motion starting at the 12 o'clock position and moving around the breast clockwise. Then use an up and down motion, and then move from the nipple outward covering the entire breast. In this manner all of the breast tissue will be examined.

Hollister™

Initial Pregnancy Profile

Hollister Maternal/Newborn Record System

To order call: **1.800.323.4060** Re-order No **5701**

Patient's Name: Beth Riley

ID. No.: 358-62-9847

34 Grove St.

Libertyville, IL. 60048

History Since LMP

Pregnancy Complications (✓)

1. Vaginal Bleeding ☐
2. Abdominal or Epigastric Pain ☐
3. Headache/Dizziness ☐
4. Change in Vision ☐
5. Hyperemesis ☐
6. Urinary Complaint ☐
7. Febrile Episode ☐
8. Rash with Viral Illness ☐
9. Physical Trauma or Surgery ☐
10. Other ______ ☐

Exposure To Environmental Teratogens

11. HIV, CMV, HSV, Syphilis ☐
12. Rubella, Varicella ☐
13. PKU ☐
14. Encephalitis ☐
15. Occupational Chemicals ☐ (Heavy Metal, Organic Solvent, etc.)
16. Radiation ☐
17. Toxoplasmosis ☐
18. Tuberculosis ☐
19. Other ______ ☐

Check and detail all positive findings below. Use reference numbers.

20. Advised abstention during pregnancy.

Substance Use

20. Alcohol ☑
    type: wine
    amt/day: 5oz/occas.
21. Tobacco ☐
    type ______
    amt/day ______
22. Non-Prescribed Drugs ☐
    type ______
    amt/day ______
23. Prescribed Drugs ☐
    type ______
    amt/day ______
    type ______
    amt/day ______
    type ______
    amt/day ______
24. Street Drugs ☐
    type ______
    amt/day ______
    type ______
    amt/day ______

Physical Assessment

Height	Weight	Pregravid Weight	B.P.	Pulse
5'7"	140	135	114/72	68

System	Normal	Abnormal
25. Skin	☑	☐
26. Neurologic	☑	☐
27. Extremities	☑	☐
28. HEENT/Fundi	☑	☐
29. Mouth/Teeth	☑	☐
30. Neck/Thyroid	☑	☐
31. Breasts/Nipples	☑	☐
32. Cardiovascular	☑	☐
33. Respiratory	☑	☐
34. Abdomen	☑	☐
35. Gastrointestinal	☑	☐
36. Urinary	☑	☐
37. Other ______	☐	☐
Pelvic Examination		
38. Vulva	☑	☐
39. Vagina	☑	☐
40. Cervix	☑	☐
41. Uterus Size 6 Wks	☐	☑
42. Adnexa	☑	☐
43. Rectum	☑	☐

Check and detail abnormal findings below. Use reference numbers.

41. Previously diagnosed

Bicornuate uterus

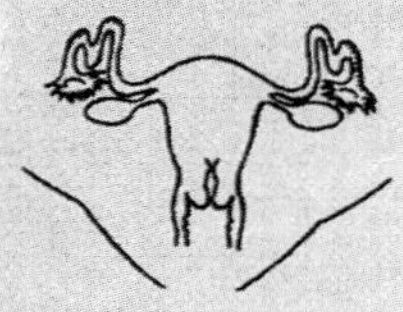

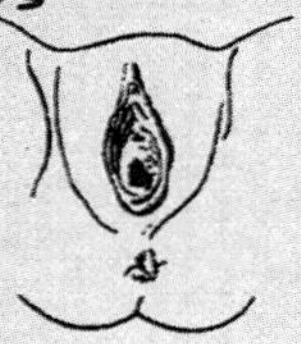

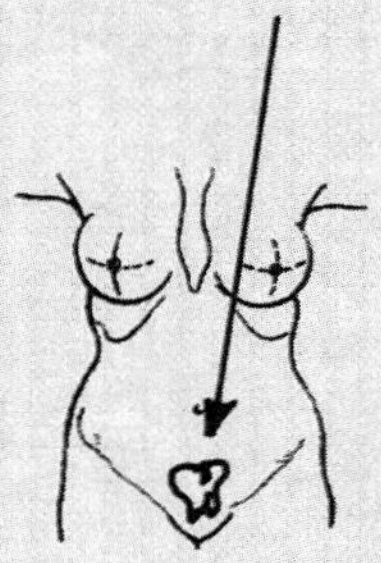

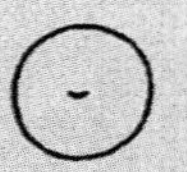

44. Pelvic Type
    ☑ Gynecoid ☐ Anthropoid
    ☐ Android ☐ Platypelloid
45. Measurements
    ☑ Adequate ☐ Inadequate
    ☐ Borderline
46. Diagonal Conjugate Reached
    ☑ Yes ☐ No
    ______ cms
47. Ischial Spines
    ☑ Average ☐ Prominent
    ☐ Blunt
48. Intertuberous Diameter 10 cms
49. Sacrum
    ☑ Concave ☐ Anterior
    ☐ Straight
50. Coccyx
    ☑ Moveable ☐ Malpositioned
    ☐ Fixed
51. Pubic Arch
    ☑ Normal ☐ Narrow
    ☐ Wide

M Brown MD
Examined by

Date 11/8/95

Hollister Incorporated, 2000 Hollister Drive, Libertyville, Illinois 60048

INITIAL PREGNANCY PROFILE FORM #5701 696

Figure 22-17 A and B Initial Pregnancy Profile. *(continued)*

✻ Hollister™

Initial Lifestyle Profile
Hollister Maternal/Newborn Record System
To order call: 1.800.323.4060   Re-order No. **5702**

Patient's Name **_Beth Riley_**
ID. No. **_358-62-9847_**
34 Grove St
Libertyville, IL. 60048

Nutritional Assessment
24 Hour Diet History   **Usual Pattern**

☑ Yes   ☐ No

Nutritional Status   ☑ Well-nourished   ☐ Obese   ☐ Malnourished   ☐ Other____

Eating Disorder ☑ None   ☐ Anorexia   ☐ Bulimia   ☐ Pica

Breakfast	Lunch	Dinner	Snacks
cereal & milk	grilled cheese sand.	spaghetti & meatball	yogurt
banana	fruit	tossed salad	fruit
	veg. soup	garlic toast	nuts
Fluids: coffee 8oz.	Fluids: Milk 8oz	Fluids: Milk 8oz	Fluids: Soft drink & caffeine/H₂O

	No	Yes		No	Yes	Frequency/Amount
Special Diet (i.e. veg, diab...)	☑	☐____	Artificial Sweeteners	☑	☐	____
Food Intolerance/Allergies	☑	☐____	Caffeine	☐	☑	1 coffee/occas. tea
Vitamin/Mineral Supplement	☑	☐____	Excessive Vitamin Intake	☑	☐	____
Other____	☐	☐____	Raw Meat/Fish	☑	☐	____

Activity Assessment
Comments

	No	Yes	
1. Job Outside Home	☐	☑	1. RN, works 12 hr. shifts
2. Work at Home	☐	☑	2. Home maintenance, childcare
3. Frequent Travel	☑	☐	2 + 4 yr. olds.
4. Commute > 2 hrs per day	☑	☐	
5. Exercise	☐	☑	5. Walks 4 mi. 3x/wk
6. Leisure Activities	☐	☑	6. Reading, sewing
7. Other____	☐	☐	

Sexuality Assessment
8. Partners ☐ None ☑ One ☐ Many
9. Physical Changes ☑ None
   Identify____
10. Psychological Changes ☑ None
   Identify____
11. Other____

Psychosocial Assessment
Emotional Status ☑ Happy ☐ Ambivalent ☐ Concerned ☐ Depressed ☐ Angry ☐ Other____

Basic Needs Met	Yes	No	
12. Housing	☑	☐	26. Feels she has adequate experience.
13. Clothing	☑	☐	
14. Food	☑	☐	
15. Finances	☑	☐	
16. Transportation	☑	☐	

Social Support

	Yes	No	
17. Biological Father Involved	☑	☐	
18. Others Available	☑	☐	18. Maternal parents & siblings live in area.

Adaptation to Pregnancy

	Yes	No
19. Planned Pregnancy	☑	☐
20. Lifestyle Modifications	☐	☑

Life Stress

	Yes	No
21. Physical Abuse	☐	☑
22. Emotional Abuse	☐	☑
23. Major Change	☐	☑
24. Serious Illness or Death	☐	☑
25. Other____	☐	☐

Education Assessment

	Yes	No
26. Learning Needs	☐	☑
27. Interest/Motivation	☑	☐
28. Ability to Read/Communicate	☑	☐
29. Access to Information	☑	☐
30. Other____	☐	☐

Preferred Learning Methods

	Yes	No
31. One-on-One Instruction	☑	☐
32. Group Instruction	☐	☑
33. Written Information	☑	☐
34. Audio/Video Information	☐	☑
35. Demonstration/Practice	☑	☐
36. Other____	☐	☐

Personal/Cultural/Religious Customs Affecting Care and/or Learning
☐ None ☑ Identify____

Initial Lifestyle Risk Status ☑ No Risk Factors Noted
☐ At Risk (Identify)

Signature _J. Smith RNC_   Date _12 16 95_

Hollister Incorporated, 2000 Hollister Drive, Libertyville, Illinois 60048

INITIAL LIFESTYLE PROFILE FORM #5702 696

Figure 22-17 A and B

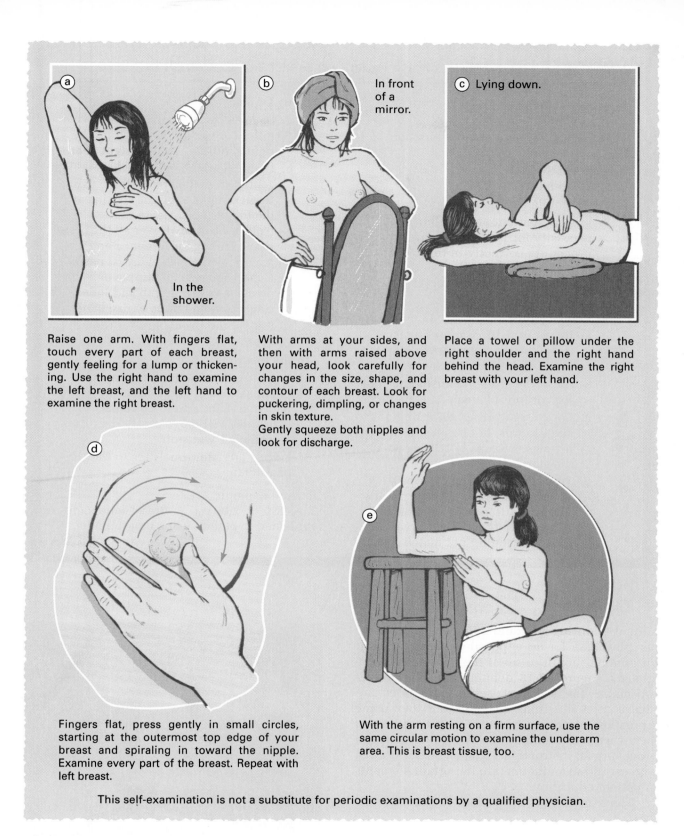

(a) In the shower.

Raise one arm. With fingers flat, touch every part of each breast, gently feeling for a lump or thickening. Use the right hand to examine the left breast, and the left hand to examine the right breast.

(b) In front of a mirror.

With arms at your sides, and then with arms raised above your head, look carefully for changes in the size, shape, and contour of each breast. Look for puckering, dimpling, or changes in skin texture.
Gently squeeze both nipples and look for discharge.

(c) Lying down.

Place a towel or pillow under the right shoulder and the right hand behind the head. Examine the right breast with your left hand.

(d) Fingers flat, press gently in small circles, starting at the outermost top edge of your breast and spiraling in toward the nipple. Examine every part of the breast. Repeat with left breast.

(e) With the arm resting on a firm surface, use the same circular motion to examine the underarm area. This is breast tissue, too.

This self-examination is not a substitute for periodic examinations by a qualified physician.

Figure 22-18   Correct procedure for a breast self-examination.

PROCEDURE: Instructing a Patient on Breast Self-Examination

Equipment and Supplies
Breast Model, if available
Pamphlets on breast self-examination

Procedural Steps
1. Wash hands.
2. Assemble equipment.
3. Identify patient and explain the necessity for performing the procedure correctly in three different positions each month. Use the breast model to explain the correct application of fingertips.
4. **Before a mirror:**
   a. Inspect the breasts for any irregularity in shape while arms are at the side of the body.
   b. Raise the arms overhead and look for contour changes in each breast.
   c. Look for swelling, dimpling of the skin, lumps, or changes in the nipples, such as retracting or discharge.
   d. With palms resting on hips, flex check muscles to observe for any obvious differences in breasts. *Note:* the left and right breasts on most women do not match exactly.

Lying Down:
   a. To examine the right breast place a pillow or rolled towel behind the right shoulder with the right hand.
   b. Using the left hand with fingers flat, gently press the breast tissue using small circular motions starting at the top of the breast in the 12 o'clock position. Cover all the breast tissue feeling for lumps or any abnormal changes in breast tissue. Gently squeeze the nipple of each breast between thumb and index finger to note lumps or discharge.
   c. Repeat the procedure for the left breast.

In the Shower:
   a. Using the flat fingertips check breast tissue and underarm tissue when skin is wet. *Rationale:* Hands will move easily over the softened wet skin.
5. Report any abnormalities to the physician.

Charting Example
2/14/XX   2:00 PM   Breast self-exam explained to patient using breast model.
M. King, CMA

---

normality during an examination she should call her physician for an appointment and not wait for another month to see if the abnormality disappears. Figure 22-18 demonstrates the correct procedure for a breast self-examination and Figure 22-19 illustrates a medical assistant using a prosthetic teaching breast to instruct a patient on breast self-examination. The guidelines and procedure for instructing a woman on performing a breast self-examination are important elements in patient education.

The American Cancer Society recommends that:

1. Women between the ages of 20 and 39 have a breast examination performed by a physician every three years; women over 40 should have one every year.

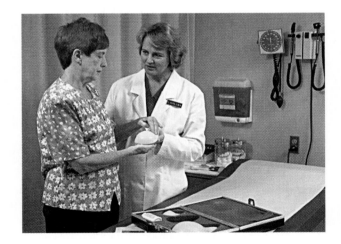

Figure 22-19 Medical assistant using a prosthetic teaching breast to instruct a patient on breast self-examination.

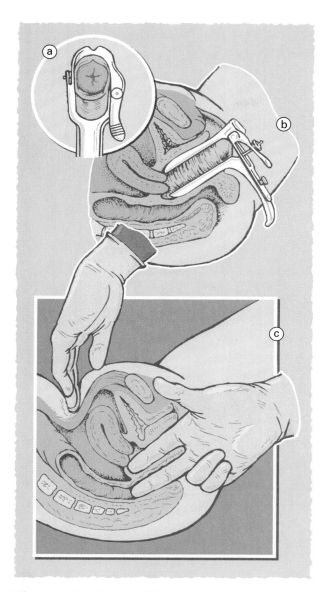

Figure 22-20 a and b Speculum examination and manual examination for woman.

2. Women between 40 and 49 who are without any symptoms of breast cancer should have a mammogram every 1-2 years; women over 50 should have a yearly mammogram.

The Pelvic Examination

The gynecologic examination, or pelvic exam, is generally included as part of a routine physical examination for the female. It may also be conducted alone in order to diagnose a problem relating specifically to the female reproductive organ. The medical assistant is usually present to assist with a gynecologic examination. Figure 22-20 illustrates the speculum and the manual examination for women. The patient may need reassurance that the procedure is painless, especially if it is the first gynecologic examination the woman has had.

Figure 22-21 displays instruments used for a PAP smear and Figure 22-22 A and B a-b] shows an Andwin Safetex One PAP Smear Kit and a PAP smear. The colposcope (gyne) used to ID abnormal tissue is shown in Figure 22-23 See the procedures for assisting with a pelvic examination and a PAP test.

Table 22-22 describes common disorders and pathology of the reproductive system. Procedures and diagnostic tests relating to the female reproductive system are described in Table 22-23.

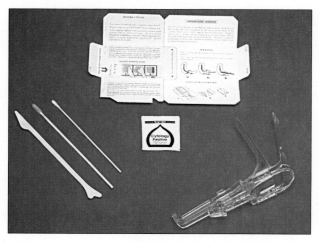

Figure 22-21 Instruments needed for a PAP smear.

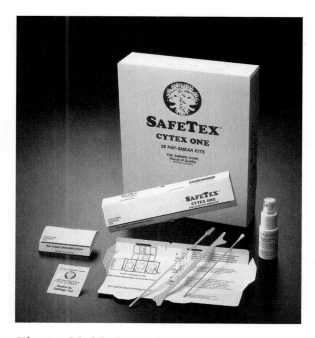

Figure 22-22 A Andwin Safetex One PAP Smear Kit.

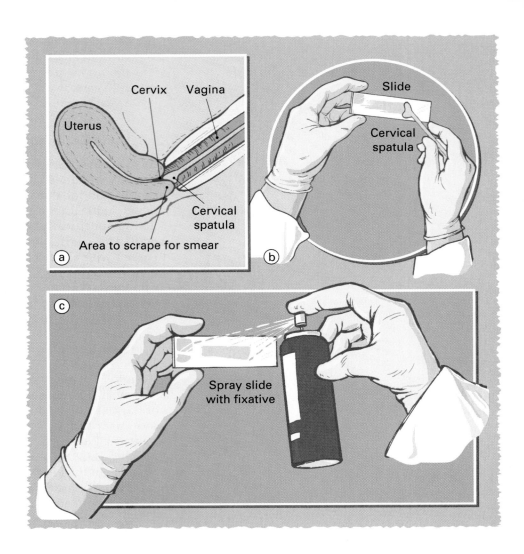

Figure 22-22 B
Preparing PAP smear.

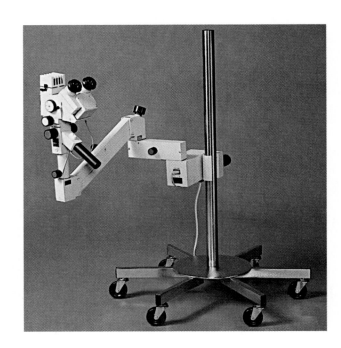

Figure 22-23   Seiler Colposcope 121.

PROCEDURE: Assisting With a Pelvic Examination and PAP Test

**Terminal Performance
Competency:** Student will set-up and assist with a gynecologic examination including collection of PAP smear without error.

Equipment and Supplies
Vaginal speculum

Water-soluble lubricant

Cotton-tipped applicator

Patient drape

PAP smear materials: cervical spatula, glass slides, fixative spray or liquid, identification label

Laboratory request form

Cleansing tissue

Gloves

Container for contaminated vaginal speculum

Goose-neck lamp

Biohazard waste container

Procedural Steps
1. Wash hands.
2. Assemble equipment.
3. Label slides and complete the laboratory form.
4. Identify patient and explain procedure.
5. Direct the patient to the bathroom to empty her bladder.
6. Request patient to remove clothing from the waist down and use drape to cover herself.
7. Position the patient into the dorsal lithotomy position with her buttocks at the edge of the table and feet in the stirrups. Expose the genitalia by moving the drape away from this area while it still covers the legs.
8. Adjust goose-neck lamp and place physician's stool in proper position at end of examination table.
9. Assist the physician with procedure:
   a. Apply gloves.
   b. Hand gloves and equipment to physician as needed. Place lubricant onto the speculum as the physician holds it.
   c. Hold the microscopic slide as the physician places the smear on the slide.
   d. Spray fixative on the slide.
   e. Place the slide into container with label.
10. Hold the receptacle as the physician places the contaminated speculum into it. Set the container into the sink for later cleaning.
11. Apply lubricant to the physician's gloved fingers in preparation for the manual examination.
12. Properly dispose of gloves into hazardous waste container and wash hands.
13. Assist the patient to sit up by (1) helping her move back on the table, (2) taking her feet out of the stirrups, and (3) helping her to a sitting position.

Note: The physician will chart the procedure.

Male Reproductive System

The male reproductive system is a combination of reproduction and urinary systems. The major male organs of reproduction are located outside the body in the scrotum and penis. The scrotum (scrotal sac) contains two testes and the seminal ducts. The penis contains the urethra which carries both urine and sperm to the outside of the body. The internal organs of reproduction are the seminal vesicles, ejaculatory duct, and the prostate gland. Common disorders of the male reproductive system are described in Table 22-24.

The Testicular Examination

Procedures and diagnostic tests relating to the male reproductive system are described in Table 22-25. See Figure 22-24 A-D for an explanation of testicular self-examination for the male patient.

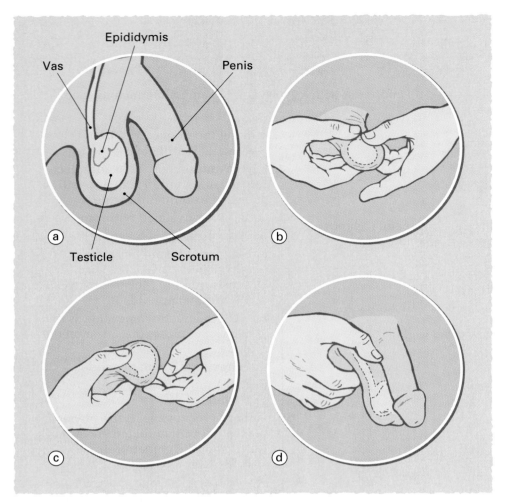

Figure 22-24 (A)–(D)   (a) Male reproductive system. (b) Begin by examining the testicles. Roll the testicle gently between the thumb and fingers while applying very slight pressure while attempting to feel any hard, painless lumps. (c) Next examine the cord behind each testicle (the epididymis). This may be tender and is the location of most non-cancerous conditions. (d) Continue the examination by gently feeling the tube that runs up from the epididymis (the vas). The vas is normally a smooth, firm movable tube.

Sexually Transmitted Diseases

Both genders—male and female—are susceptible to sexually transmitted diseases if they are sexually active. Table 22-26 contains a description of some of the more common diseases.

    There are many genetic disorders that one or both parents can pass on to their child. Table 22-27 contains a description of several.

Respiratory System

The respiratory system consists of the nose, pharynx, larynx (voicebox), trachea, bronchi, and lungs. This branch of medicine is called pulmonary medicine. A description of disorders and pathology of the respiratory system is in Table 22-28. Table 22-29 describes procedures and diagnostic tests relating to the respiratory system.

Urinary System

The organs of the urinary system are the bladder, two kidneys, two ureters which are the tubes that carry urine from the kidneys to the bladder, and one urethra which carries the urine from the bladder to the outside of the body. Table 22-30 describes the disorders and diseases of the urinary system. Procedures and diagnostic tests relating to the urinary system are described in Table 22-31.

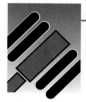

LEGAL AND ETHICAL ISSUES

Many of the procedures and immunizations discussed in this chapter require written consent either from the patient or the parents, if the patient is a child. Careful explanation of the benefits and risks associated with all treatments should be explained by the physician. The medical assistant needs to reinforce the physician's explanation and determine if the patient has understood the explanation.

The patient has a right to privacy and confidentiality during the examination process. Doors should be closed during any examination or procedure and patients, including children, should be draped to protect their modesty. The examination of infants and children carries an additional safety risk since they are unable to protect themselves. The medical assistant must never leave an infant or child unattended.

PATIENT EDUCATION

Many patients are not ready either physically or emotionally to fully understand their medical diagnosis. The medical assistant will need to be able to clearly explain in simple language any terms that are confusing to the patient. All follow-up instructions regarding further treatment, appointments, medications, and mobility need to be explained and documented.

The medical assistant will need to utilize many teaching methods to facilitate the patient's comprehension of their diagnosis and treatment plan. Many patients will not be able to understand the medical terminology relating to their illness. Drawing charts for medication dosages, writing instructions for home care and appointment schedules, and asking the patient to repeat what the physician has told them are all effective learning aids.

Summary

The topics presented in this chapter represent a variety of medical specialty areas. No physician's practice will include all of them. Since the profession of medical assisting is for the multi-skilled individual, he or she is expected to have a general knowledge of medicine.

Much of the clinical role of the medical assistant involves assisting with procedures relating to the body systems including: digestive, musculoskeletal (orthopedics), reproductive, urinary, respiratory, integumentary, endocrine, lymphatic, cardiovascular, and special senses. No matter what the task involves, the trademark of a good medical assistant should be careful, caring attention to detail.

Competency Review

1. Define and spell the glossary terms for this chapter.
2. Develop a teaching plan for a patient with diabetes mellitus.
3. Develop a brochure instructing female patients how to do a breast self-examination and male patients a testicular self-examination.
4. Describe the set-up for a PAP smear. What is the medical assistant's responsibility for assisting with this procedure?
5. What are several steps the medical assistant should take in the medical office to assure the safety of the pediatric patient?

PREPARING FOR THE CERTIFICATION EXAM

Test Taking Tip — Study for an examination by writing sample multiple choice test questions and answers.

Examination Review Questions

1. The round, raised skin lesions with itching, that are a positive sign of reaction to allergic testing
   - (A) nodule
   - (B) vesicle
   - (C) papule
   - (D) wheal
   - (E) macule

2. Fungal infectious skin disease which can be detected through use of a Wood's light
   - (A) herpes zoster
   - (B) herpes simplex
   - (C) tinea
   - (D) impetigo
   - (E) scabies

3. A benign neoplasm which results in enlarged blood vessels
   - (A) melanoma
   - (B) nevus
   - (C) keratosis
   - (D) lipoma
   - (E) hemangioma

4. A cardiovascular condition which results in death of tissue from lack of blood supply
   - (A) angioma
   - (B) infarct
   - (C) aneurysm
   - (D) Reynaud's phenomenon
   - (E) murmur

5. When handling a spinal fluid sample during a lumbar procedure, the medical assistant should
   - (A) number the tubes in the order they are obtained
   - (B) wear PPE
   - (C) place tubes in biohazard bag
   - (D) send the specimen to the lab before cleaning the room and equipment
   - (E) all of the above

6. What disease results in edema, slowed speech with enlarged facial features and tongue, drowsiness, and mental apathy?
   - (A) myxedema
   - (B) von Reckinghausen's disease
   - (C) Graves' disease
   - (D) Cushing's syndrome
   - (E) myasthenia gravis

7. A procedure in which contrast medium is used to visualize the bile ducts
   - (A) peritoneoscopy laparoscopy
   - (B) choledocholithotripsy
   - (C) intravenous cholangiogram
   - (D) endoscopic retrograde cholangiopancreatography (ERCP)
   - (E) cholecystogram

8. An immunoassay test used to test for an antibody to the AIDS virus
   - (A) fluorescein angiography
   - (B) Romberg test
   - (C) falling test
   - (D) ELISA
   - (E) fungal scraping

9. A musculoskeletal disorder in which a softening of bone occurs which may result from a deficiency in vitamin D
   - (A) osteomalacia
   - (B) osteoporosis
   - (C) osteoarthritis
   - (D) scoliosis
   - (E) talipes

10. An ophthalmic condition in which the cornea and conjunctiva are affected by bacteria
    - (A) retinitis pigmentosa
    - (B) macular degeneration
    - (C) glaucoma
    - (D) ectropion
    - (E) trachoma

ON THE JOB

Shelia Meyer, a medical assistant, in Dr. Ryan's large cardiovascular practice, is taking the medical history of Edna Helm, an obese elderly woman with congestive heart disease. Edna states, "I'm always short of breath and I perspire all the time. I guess I'm gaining weight, but the funny thing is that only my legs seem heavier. My heart is pounding when I lie down at night; it even seems to stop sometimes. I've even started to wear red nail polish to hide the funny blue color of my nails."

Edna gives you a copy of her medical history from an out-of-state physician. The medical history indicates that she has had the following conditions, tests, and procedures:

Conditions
Positive Babinski sign
Allergic rhinitis

Aortic insufficiency
Ascites
Gastritis
Osteoarthritis

Tests
Holter monitor testing
Radioimmunoassay test
Protein bound iodine test
Glucose tolerance test

Surgical Procedures
Basal cell carcinoma removed in 1992
Sebaceous cyst removed in 1982
Meniscectomy in 1978
Rhytidectomy in 1970

1. Using correct medical terms chart her presenting symptoms.
2. Define each of the procedures and conditions listed on her medical record.

References

American Cancer Society. *Cancer Facts for Women.* Publication no. 2007, April 1992.

Anderson, K., and Anderson, L. *Mosby's Pocket Dictionary of Medicine, Nursing, & Allied Health.* Chicago: Mosby, 1994.

Andrews, L., Fullerton, J., Holtsman., and Motulsky, M. *Assessing Genetic Risks.* Washington DC: National Academy Press, 1994.

Badash, S., and Chesbro, D. *Introduction to Health Occupations.* Upper Saddle River, NJ: Brady/Prentice Hall, 1997.

Clayman, C., *The Human Body.* New York: Dorling Kindersley, 1995.

DeSando, M. "How Perfect Is Your 20/20 Vision? *PMA.* November/December, 1992.

Fiesta, J. "The Physical Exam." *RN.* 54:11, 1991.

Fremgen, B. *Medical Terminology.* Upper Saddle River, NJ: Brady/Prentice Hall, 1997.

Greenberg, A. editor, *Primer on Kidney Disease.* New York: Academic Press, 1994.

Heller, M., and Krebs, C. *Delmar's Clinical Handbook for Health Care Professionals.* New York: Delmar, 1997.

Potter, P., and Perry, A. *Fundamentals of Nursing—Concepts, Process and Practice,* 3rd ed. St. Louis: Mosby Year Book, 1993.

Seidel, H. *Mosby's Guide to Physical Examination.* St. Louis: Mosby Year Book, 1991.

Straasinger, S. *Urinalysis & Body Fluids.* Philadelphia: F.A. Davis, 1994.

Taber's Cyclopedic Medical Dictionary, 18th ed. Philadelphia: F.A. Davis, 1997.

MEDICAL ASSISTANT ROLE DELINEATION CHART

Highlight indicates material covered in this chapter

ADMINISTRATIVE

ADMINISTRATIVE PROCEDURES

- Perform basic clerical functions
- Schedule, coordinate, and monitor appointments
- Schedule inpatient/outpatient admissions and procedures
- Understand and apply third party guidelines
- Obtain reimbursement through accurate claims submission
- Monitor third-party reimbursement
- Perform medical transcription
- Understand and adhere to managed care policies and procedures
- *Negotiate managed care contracts (adv)*

PRACTICE FINANCES

- Perform procedural and diagnostic coding
- Apply bookkeeping principles
- Document and maintain accounting and banking records
- Manage accounts receivable
- Manage accounts payable
- Process payroll
- *Develop and maintain fee schedules (adv)*
- *Manage renewals of business and professional insurance policies (adv)*
- *Manage personal benefits and maintain records (adv)*

CLINICAL

FUNDAMENTAL PRINCIPLES

- Apply principles of aseptic technique and infection control
- Comply with quality assurance practices
- Screen and follow up patient test results

DIAGNOSTIC ORDERS

- Collect and process specimens
- Perform diagnostic tests

PATIENT CARE

- Adhere to established triage procedures
- Obtain patient history and vital signs
- Prepare and maintain examination and treatment areas

- Prepare patient for examinations, procedures, and treatments
- Assist with examinations, procedures, and treatments
- Prepare and administer medications and immunizations
- Maintain medication and immunization records
- Recognize and respond to emergencies
- Coordinate patient care information with other health care providers

GENERAL (TRANSDISCIPLINARY)

PROFESSIONALISM

- Project a professional manner and image
- Adhere to ethical principles
- Demonstrate initiative and responsibility
- Work as a team member
- Manage time efficiently
- Prioritize and perform multiple tasks
- Adapt to change
- Promote the CMA credential
- Enhance skills through continuing education

COMMUNICATION SKILLS

- Treat all patients with compassion and empathy
- Recognize and respect cultural diversity
- Adapt communications to individual's ability to understand
- Use professional telephone technique
- Use effective and correct verbal and written communications
- Recognize and respond to verbal and nonverbal communications
- Use medical terminology appropriately
- Receive, organize, prioritize, and transmit information
- Serve as liaison
- Promote the practice through positive public relations

LEGAL CONCEPTS

- Maintain confidentiality
- Practice within the scope of education, training, and personal capabilities
- Prepare and maintain medical records
- Document accurately
- Use appropriate guidelines when releasing information
- Follow employer's established policies dealing with the health care contract
- Follow federal, state, and local legal guidelines
- Maintain awareness of federal and state health care legislation and regulations
- Maintain and dispose of regulated substances in compliance with government guidelines
- Comply with established risk management and safety procedures
- Recognize professional credentialing criteria
- Participate in the development and maintenance of personnel, policy, and procedure manuals
- *Develop and maintain personnel, policy, and procedure manuals (adv)*

INSTRUCTION

- Instruct individuals according to their needs
- Explain office policies and procedures
- Teach methods of health promotion and disease prevention
- Locate community resources and disseminate information
- *Orient and train personnel (adv)*
- *Develop educational materials (adv)*
- *Conduct continuing education activities (adv)*

OPERATIONAL FUNCTIONS

- Maintain supply inventory
- Evaluate and recommend equipment and supplies
- Apply computer techniques to support office operations
- *Supervise personnel (adv)*
- *Interview and recommend job applicants (adv)*
- *Negotiate leases and prices for equipment and supply contracts (adv)*

SOURCE: Reprinted by permission of the American Association of Medical Assistants from the *AAMA Role Delineation Study: Occupational Analysis of the Medical Assisting Profession*.

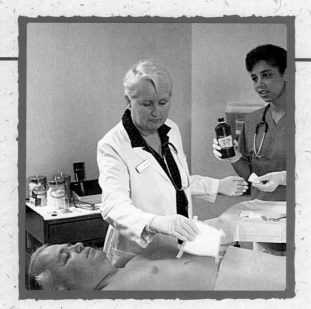

23

Assisting with Minor Surgery

LEARNING OBJECTIVES

After completing this chapter, you should:
1. Define and spell the glossary terms for this chapter.
2. Discuss all 6 guidelines for surgical aseptic technique.
3. List and differentiate between the types of ambulatory surgery.
4. Describe the differences between medical asepsis (clean technique) and surgical asepsis (sterile technique).
5. List and describe instruments for: cutting, dissecting, grasping, clamping, probing and dilating.
6. Explain the rules for handling instruments.
7. Give 5 examples of suture materials, including gauge ranges, with examples of when they may be used.

8. Describe the preparation of the patient for minor surgery.
9. List equipment and supplies used for preparing the patient's skin for surgery.
10. Define "informed consent." Discuss the medical assistant's role in the process.
11. Describe at least 5 surgical procedures that can be performed in the physician's office and indicate the responsibility of the medical assistant for each procedure.

CLINICAL PERFORMANCE COMPETENCIES

After completing this chapter, you should perform the following tasks:
1. Demonstrate proper technique for a surgical scrub and sterile gloving.
2. Demonstrate proper method for opening surgical packs to assure sterility.
3. Demonstrate surgical aseptic technique for preparing the patient's skin for minor surgery.
4. Select, assemble, and prepare equipment for a minor surgical procedure.
5. Identify by name and use the instruments used in minor surgical procedures.
6. Prepare the patient for a minor surgical procedure.
7. Assist the physician during a minor surgical procedure.
8. Remove sutures as directed by a physician.
9. Apply a sterile dressing.

Glossary

ambulatory surgery   A method for performing surgical procedures which allows the patient to walk into and out of the surgical facility on the same day.

anesthesia   Partial or complete loss of sensation.

biopsy   The removal of tissue for purposes of determining the presence of cancerous (malignant) cells.

cryosurgery   Use of freezing temperatures from a probe to destroy abnormal cells.

hyfrecators   Small electrocautery units used to perform minor cautery procedures in the medical office.

incision(s)   Surgical cut into tissue.

invasive   Enters the skin.

Mayo stand   Small portable tray/table used to hold surgical instruments during a procedure.

outpatient surgery   Surgical procedures, which usually require less than 60 minutes, performed in a setting in which the patient is ambulatory and does not stay in the facility overnight.

scrub assistant   A sterile assistant who passes instruments, swabs (sponges) bodily fluids from the operative site, retracts incisions, and cuts sutures.

sterile field   Work area in surgery in which the area is prepared using sterile drapes (cloths) to cover nonsterile areas.

surgical asepsis   A technique practiced to maintain a sterile environment.

WARNING!

For all patient contact, adhere to Standard Precautions (see pages 342–373). Wear protective equipment as indicated.

This chapter discusses surgical aseptic technique, or sterile technique. Procedures requiring sterile technique, such as minor surgical procedures, suture insertion and removal, breast biopsy, incision and drainage, removal of growths, and wound treatment are included. Strict adherence to aseptic technique is necessary when assisting with these procedures. It is important to always remember that an item is either sterile or nonsterile. If there is any doubt about sterility, assume it is nonsterile.

Ambulatory Surgery

Ambulatory surgery is a method for performing surgical procedures in which the patient is able to walk into and out of the surgical facility on the day of surgery. This includes outpatient surgery, surgicenter surgery, and office surgery. Since ambulatory surgery is on the increase, the medical assistant is spending more time assisting the physician with surgical procedures.

Outpatient surgery, with its emphasis on surgical procedures performed outside the hospital setting, has resulted in a cost savings to the consumer and to the insurer. Hospitalization is not required unless there is an unexpected complication. The patient is able to return home after a brief recovery time in the outpatient facility or medical office. The disadvantage to this type of surgery is the short time the health care team has to spend assessing the patient's postoperative condition. It is important for each outpatient facility to develop a consistent follow-up procedure to track the patient's condition after leaving.

Outpatient surgery is generally limited to procedures requiring less than 60 minutes to perform. Terminology relating to surgery are

- *Elective:* Surgery that is considered medically necessary, but can be performed when the patient wishes (for example, removal of benign growths).

- *Emergency:* Surgery that is required immediately to save a life (for example, hemorrhage) or prevent further injury or infection.
- *Optional:* Surgery that may not be medically necessary, but the patient wishes to have performed (for example, cosmetic surgery, vasectomy).
- *Outpatient:* Surgical procedure performed which does not require an overnight stay in a hospital.
- *Surgicenter:* A medical facility that performs ambulatory surgery.
- *Urgent:* Surgery that needs to be performed as soon as possible, but is not an immediate or acute emergency (for example, cancer surgery).

Principle of Surgical Asepsis

Surgical asepsis, or sterile technique, is used when sterility of supplies and the immediate environment is required, as in surgical procedures. Sterile technique results in the killing of all living microorganisms and is necessary during any invasive procedure in which the body is entered such as when administering an injection, making a surgical incision, or working with an open wound.

Open tissues provide an excellent reservoir (host) for infection. Infections can delay the healing process and result in additional medical costs. Sterile technique prevents infection from microorganisms being introduced into the body, thereby decreasing the risk of infection.

Medical asepsis and surgical asepsis are similar in their overall purpose of decreasing the risk of infection. Medical asepsis results in a "clean" approach in which materials can be handled with clean hands or nonsterile gloves. Surgical asepsis requires a sterile hand washing scrub, sterile gloves, and sterile technique when handling materials. See Table 23-1 for a comparison of medical and surgical asepsis.

Med Tip: Remember "clean for clean" and "sterile for sterile". Use clean technique when handling nonsterile items (for example, clean hands when applying a dressing to intact skin). Use sterile procedure when handling sterile materials (for example, must use sterile gloves when touching sterile instruments).

Guidelines for Surgical Asepsis

When practicing surgical asepsis, follow the guidelines presented here or those used in your office as directed by your supervisor.

Med Tip: All personnel should change to street clothes before leaving the medical facility. Nonsterile surgical "scrub suits" should not be worn home. Their purpose is to protect the patient and the health care worker from exposure to pathogenic organisms.

Sterile Scrub and Gloving

Figure 23-1 A-G demonstrates handwashing for surgical asepsis and Figure 23-2 gloving following sterile scrub.

TABLE 23-1 **Surgical Asepsis Versus Medical Asepsis**

Surgical Asepsis	Medical Asepsis
"Sterile" technique used	"Clean" technique used
Absence of microorganisms	Controls microorganisms
Surgical scrub performed	Basic handwashing procedure used
Sterile equipment and supplies required	Clean equipment and supplies
Sterile field	Clean field

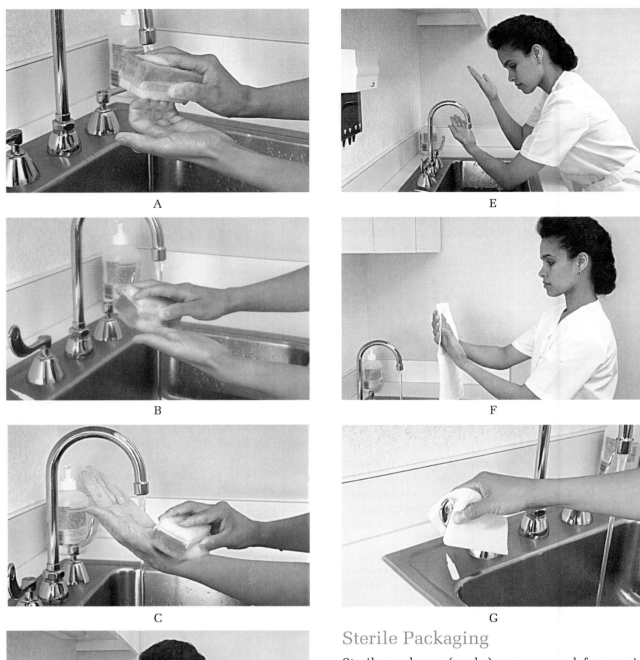

A

B

C

D

E

F

G

Sterile Packaging

Sterile packages (packs) are prepared for use in surgery with either individual pieces of equipment or instruments or several items packed together. These packs are then autoclaved with sterilization indicators and dated. These packs are used for various procedures. For example, all the instruments needed for a procedure, such as a biopsy, are packaged together in a tray and autoclaved. See the procedure for opening a sterile packet. Figure 23-3 A-F demonstrates opening a sterile packet.

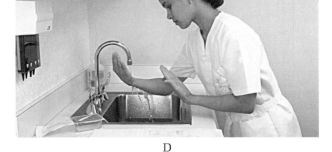

Figure 23-1 A-G   Sterile scrub handwashing.

PROCEDURE: Surgical Handwashing/Sterile Scrub

**Terminal Performance
Competency:** Perform surgical scrub on hands and arms using correct procedure for the appropriate length of time.

Equipment and Supplies

Germicidal Dispenser Soap (not bar soap)

Sterile scrub brush

Sterile towel pack (with 2–3 sterile paper or cloth towels)

Paper towels

Sterile gloves (prepackaged)

Running water (foot pedal preferable)

Nail file

Procedural Steps

1. Remove all jewelry. With nail file remove any gross dirt from beneath fingernails before scrubbing. ***Rationale:*** microorganisms can accumulate in crevices of rings or watch and under fingernails.

2. Assemble equipment.

3. Stand at sink without allowing body to touch it. ***Rationale:*** Sink is considered contaminated with microorganisms.

4. Remove lab coat. Roll sleeves above elbows. Keep hands and arms above waist level at all times. ***Rationale:*** All areas below the waist are considered contaminated.

5. Regulate running water temperature to warm, not hot. ***Rationale:*** Hot water can cause hands to chap and crack which can provide a source of cross-infection.

6. Place hands under running water with hands pointed upward. Allow water to run from fingertips to elbows. ***Rationale:*** If water is running downward from the unscrubbed arm to the hands it would contaminate the scrubbed hands.

7. Apply circle of soap from dispenser and lather well.

8. Vigorously scrub hands and wrists with scrub brush. Wash thoroughly between fingers. Scrub under fingernails. Scrub toward the elbows using 5 minutes on each hand.

9. Raise the hands, bending at the elbow, and place under running water to rinse soap. Allow water to flow from fingertips to elbows.

10. Perform a second lather and scrub if that is the policy in your facility. In this case, use 3 minutes for each scrub.

11. Using a sterile towel (if possible), pat hands dry moving from fingertips to wrists, and then to elbows. The hands should still be held above the elbows.

12. Turn off faucet with fresh towel (if foot lever not available). ***Rationale:*** The faucet and handles are considered unclean. A towel protects the clean hands from contamination.

13. Glove immediately. Keep hands above the waist and folded together until procedure begins.

When assisting the physician/surgeon with the procedure, the medical assistant will "set up" the specific tray or instruments before the procedure begins. The packets are set up on a Mayo stand, which is a small portable table with enough room to hold an instrument tray. For some procedures more than one Mayo stand is used.

Figure 23-4 illustrates dropping a sterile packet onto a sterile field.

Sterile Transfer

Figure 23-5 illustrates how to handle the transfer of sterile equipment from a sterile packet using forceps.

Guidelines: Surgical Asepsis

1. When in doubt about sterility, consider the item nonsterile.
2. All supplies and materials used for sterile procedures must be sterilized at the time of use or prior to use. Check the expiration dates.
3. The human body cannot be sterilized. The patient's skin can be prepared using an antiseptic wash, but will not be sterile. Skin is always considered contaminated (nonsterile).
4. When using sterile gloves:

   - Do not touch the outside of the gloves with bare hands.
   - When wearing sterile gloves, touch only sterile articles.
   - If a sterile glove is punctured by a needle or instrument, remove the instrument from the sterile field, remove and dispose of the damaged glove(s), wash hands, and reglove as soon as possible.

5. Sterile pack (packages):

   - Outer wrappings are considered nonsterile and must not be touched by sterile gloves. Bare hands can only touch the outside wrapper of a pack.
   - Always open sterile packs away from you to avoid touching your clothing, which is considered contaminated.
   - Use sterile packs immediately after opening. Never rewrap them for later use. They must be processed and resterilized.

6. **Sterile field:** A work area which is prepared using sterile drapes (cloth) which hold the sterile supplies during the surgical procedure

   - Never reach or lean across the sterile field. The air above the sterile field is considered part of the field. Contaminated air droplets can fall into the field and cause infection if transferred to the patient.
   - Never talk, sneeze, or cough over the sterile field.
   - Avoid unnecessary movement around the sterile field.
   - Avoid spills on the sterile field. Moisture or wet areas are considered contaminated and must be covered with a sterile drape or towel.
   - Keep all items and gloved hands above waist level or at the level of the sterile field.
   - The sterile field should not be near windows, fans, drafts, or air conditioners since pathogenic microorganisms can be carried through the air currents.
   - A 1-inch perimeter around the outside of the sterile field is considered contaminated since it is in contact with the nonsterile work surface. Therefore place all sterile items in the center of the sterile field.
   - Do not pass anything over a sterile field.
   - Always face the sterile field. If you must turn away or turn your back to the field, cover the sterile field with a sterile towel.

7. All surgical team members (physicians, nurses, medical assistants) wearing sterile clothing must not leave the surgical area unless they rescrub and replace sterile clothing upon reentry.

Handling Surgical Instruments

Surgical instruments have been developed over the past centuries to meet a specific need during an operation such as cutting, suturing, and grasping. In some cases, an instrument developed by a surgeon bears the name of the surgeon, for example Kelly forceps, Halstead mosquito clamp, and the Bozeman uterine forceps.

Instruments Used in Minor Office Surgery

The general classification of instruments is based on their use: cutting, dissecting, grasping, clamping, dilating, probing, visualization and suturing. There are special instruments related to individual specialties such as gynecology, urology, orthopedics, ear, nose, and throat, proctology, obstetrics, and neurology.

PROCEDURE: Surgical Gloving

Terminal Performance
Competency: Apply sterile gloves without a break in sterile technique.

Equipment and Supplies
Double-wrapped sterile glove pack
Note: This procedure follows a surgical hand scrub.

Procedural Steps

1. Assemble equipment and check tape/seal for date and condition of pack.

2. Place the pack on a flat surface at waist height with the cuffed end of the gloves toward you.

3. Open the outside wrapper by touching only the outside of the pack. Leave the opened wrapper in place to provide a sterile work field.

4. Open the inner wrapper without reaching over the pack or touching the inside of the wrapper. Pull inner wrapper edges to each side without touching the inside of the pack. *Rationale:* Nonsterile persons or items contaminate a sterile field by reaching across it.

5. Using the thumb and fingers of your left hand (if you are right-handed) pick up the glove on the right side of the pack by grasping the folded inside edge of the cuff. The glove can be "dangled" slightly off the sterile packing material for easier insertion. *Rationale:* The folded inside edge of the glove will be placed against the skin and thus will be contaminated. The outer portion of the glove must not be touched by an ungloved hand since it must remain sterile.

6. Pull the glove onto the right hand using only the thumb and fingers of left hand. Do not allow fingers to touch the rest of the glove.

7. Place the fingers of the right gloved hand under the cuff of the left glove and pull onto the left hand and up over the left wrist. *Note:* Thumb of right gloved hand should not touch cuff.

8. With gloved left hand, place fingers under the cuff of the right glove and pull up over the right wrist. Thumb should not touch cuff. *Rationale:* The areas under the cuff are considered sterile. Only gloved fingers can touch this area.

9. After the gloves are in place, the fingers can be adjusted, if necessary by using the gloved hands.

10. Removing gloves: Remove the first glove by grasping the edge of that glove (with fingers of the other gloved hand) and pull the first glove over the hand inside out. Discard the first glove into the proper biohazardous waste container. Remove the other glove by grasping edge of the cuff with fingers (of the ungloved hand) and pull the second glove down over hand, inside out. Discard appropriately. *Rationale:* Turning the glove inside out seals in blood and body fluids.

A minor surgical setup will include a standard group of instruments such as scalpel, blades, scissors, hemostat, and suture materials. Instruments are usually made of steel and treated to be rust and heat resistant, stain proof and durable.

Cutting Instruments

Scalpels or knives are used to make incisions, which are surgical cuts into tissue. They are small curved instruments which are made to fit

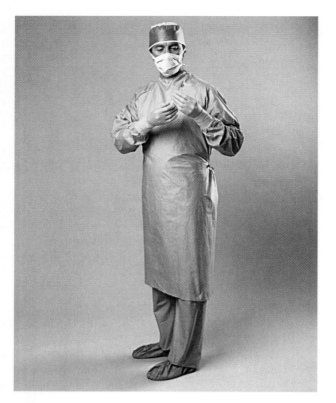

easily into the surgeon's hand. A scalpel blade must be inserted into the scalpel handle. Blades come in various sizes depending on the type of incision and tissue: Number 10 and 12 are curved; Number 11 is used for I & D (incisions and drainage); Number 10 is straight; and Number 10 and 15 are used for foreign body removal. Figure 23-6 illustrates a variety of scalpels and blades.

Figure 23-2   Gloving following sterile scrub.

PROCEDURE: Opening Sterile Packet

**Terminal Performance
Competency:** Open sterile packet (pack) and use it to set up a sterile field without a break in sterile technique.

Equipment and Supplies
　Sterile packet
　Mayo stand
　Waste container
　Sterile forceps

Procedural Steps
1. Wash hands.
2. Assemble equipment. Adjust Mayo stand to correct height.
3. Place packet on Mayo stand so that the folded edge is on top. Place on stand in position so that top flap will fold away from you. ***Rationale:*** You will not have to reach over sterile field to open last flap.
4. Remove tape or fastener and check sterilization indicator and date. Discard in waste container.
5. Pull the corner of pack that is tucked under and lay this flap away from you. It will hang down over the edge of the Mayo stand.
6. With both hands, pull the next two flaps to each side. The packet will still be covered with the last layer of the outer wrapper.
7. Grasp the corner of the last flap, without reaching over the sterile field, and open toward your body without touching.
8. The inside of this outer wrapper is now your sterile field. If you need to arrange items within this field, use sterile forceps. If an inner packet needs to be opened with an instrument setup, then someone wearing sterile gloves must open it.

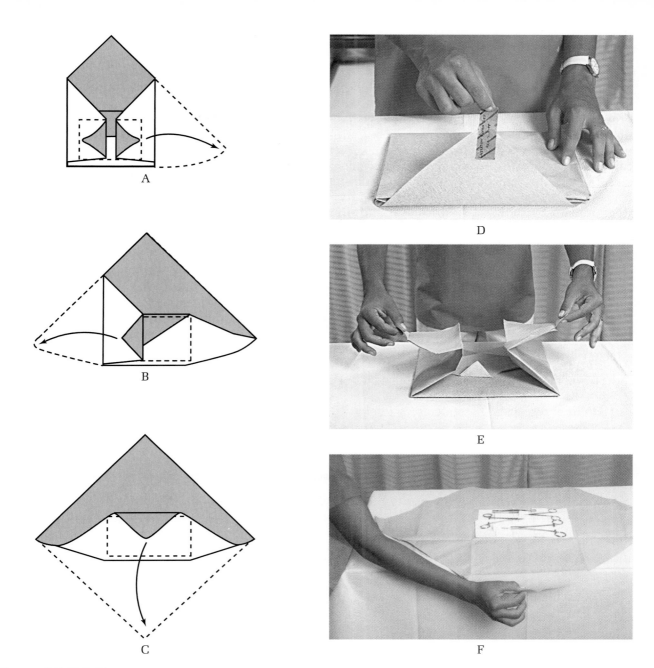

Figure 23-3 A-F   Opening a sterile packet.

Dissecting Instruments

The most common tool for dissecting or cutting tissue is the scissors. Scissors are also used to cut sutures (thread). Scissors have two blades with sharp edges which come together. The tips of scissors vary greatly since a variety of functions can be performed with the tips. Some scissors have blunt tips which can slide under bandages and dressings to cut without damaging the skin.

Operating scissors or suture scissors are used to cut suture material during surgery. They have a hook on one edge that fits under the suture for ease in suture removal. Dissecting scissors are also called straight or Mayo scissors. Metzenbaum scissors are short curved scissors which are used on delicate tissue. The tips of these scissors are blunt to prevent piercing tissue.

Operating scissors are straight or curved with a combination of blades such as sharp/sharp (s/s), blunt/blunt (b/b), and sharp/blunt (s/b); bandage scissors have a blunt tip and a blunt flat edge to allow it to fit easily under a bandage for cutting. Figure 23-7 illustrates a variety of types of scissors.

Grasping and Clamping Instruments

Forceps are used to grasp tissue or objects (Figure 23-8). One type of forceps is a two-pronged instrument which has a spring-type handle that clamps together tightly to prevent slipping. Another type of closure mechanism is called a ratchet closure or clasp. The ratchet clasp allows the forceps to close with differing degrees of tightness. Forceps often have serration, or teeth-like, edges that prevent tissue slipping out of the forceps.

Types of Forceps

- Tissue forceps have teeth and are used to grasp tissue.
- Thumb forceps are two-pronged with serrated tips to hold tissue.
- Sponge forceps are used for holding sponges during surgery.
- Towel clamps are used to hold the edges of sterile drapes together.
- Splinter forceps are used to grasp foreign bodies.

- Needle holder forceps are used to grasp needles during suturing.
- Hemostats are applied to blood vessels to hold vessels until they can be sutured.

Figure 23-8 depicts a variety of types of forceps and Figure 23-9 illustrates hemostats.

Probing and Dilating Instruments

Instruments used to enter body cavities for probing or dilating purposes include:

- *Scope:* An instrument, usually lighted, which is inserted into a body cavity or vessel to visualize the internal structures (Figure 23-10). An obturator is placed inside the scope to guide it into a cavity or canal then removed during visualization of the surgical site. Some obturators have a point which is used to puncture tissue.
- *Speculum:* An unlighted instrument with movable parts which when inserted into a cavity such as the vagina, can be spread apart for ease of visualization and tissue sample removal (Figure 23-11).

PROCEDURE: Dropping Sterile Packet onto Sterile Field

Terminal Performance Competency: Place (drop) sterile item onto a sterile field or into a gloved hand without contaminating the packet or the field.

Equipment and Supplies
Sterile pack (containing for example: prepackaged items such as specimen container or needle and syringe in pull-apart packet)

Procedural Steps
1. Assemble equipment, check date and sealed condition of packet.
2. Locate the edge on the prepackaged item and pull apart by using thumb and forefinger of each hand. Do not let fingers touch the inside of the packet. *Rationale:* The inside of the packet is sterile and the outside is considered contaminated.
3. Pull the packet apart by securely placing remaining three fingers of each

hand against the outside of the packet on each side. The wrapper edges will be pulled back and away from the sterile item.
4. Holding the item securely 8-10 inches from the sterile field, gently drop the contents inside the field. Instead of having you drop the item, the physician may wish to remove the item from the packet by grasping it firmly with his or her gloved hand. *Rationale:* Do not place your unsterile hands and arms over the sterile field.
5. Discard the paper wrapper in waste container.

- *Probe:* An instrument used to explore wounds and cavities usually with a curved, blunt point to facilitate insertion (Figure 23-12).
- *Trocar:* An instrument used to withdraw fluids from cavities. It consists of a cannula (outer tube) and a sharp stylette which is withdrawn after the trocar is inserted. Guide tubing or a wire (Figure 23-13).
- *Punch:* An instrument used to remove tissue for examination and **biopsy** to detect cancerous cells.

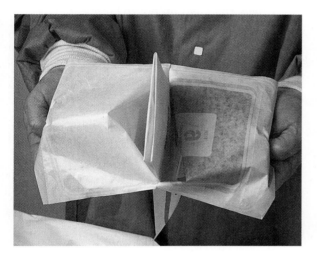

Figure 23-4 Dropping a sterile packet onto a sterile field.

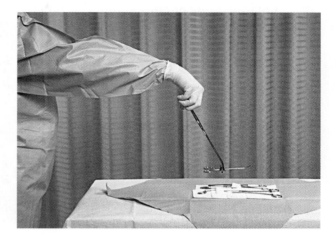

Figure 23-5 Proper way to handle a sterile equipment transfer.

PROCEDURE: Transferring Sterile Objects Using Transfer Forceps

Terminal Performance Competency: Move sterile objects, such as instruments and supplies, within or onto a sterile field or into a gloved hand.

Equipment and Supplies

Sterile transfer forceps in forceps container with sterilant solution such as Cidex

Mayo stand with sterile field setup

Sterile 4 × 4 gauze package, opened

Procedural Steps

1. Grasp forceps handles firmly without separating the tips and remove vertically from the container. *Rationale:* Open forceps tips could touch the sides of the container which are considered contaminated. Remove vertically to avoid dripping solution onto exposed contaminated portion of forceps.

2. Holding forceps vertically with tips down, gently tap tips together to drop excess solution onto a dry sterile 4 × 4 gauze or touch the 4 × 4 gauze to dry the tips.

3. Pick up sterile item to be transferred by holding transfer forceps vertically with tips down. Do not touch the sterile field. Grasp the article to be transferred firmly at its midsection.

4. Place sterile item within the sterile field. *Rationale:* Remember that the outer 1 inch of the sterile field is considered contaminated.

5. Place forceps back into container without touching sides of container.

6. Clean and sterilize the forceps and container in the autoclave once a week. Change solution weekly.

PROCEDURE: Transferring Sterile Solutions onto Sterile Field

**Terminal Performance
Competency:** Pour sterile fluid into a sterile basin on a sterile field without spilling solution or contaminating the field.

Equipment and Supplies
  Sterile saline or other solution as ordered
  Sterile basin
  Mayo stand or side tray
  Waste container

Procedural Steps
1. Wash hands
2. Assemble all equipment. Check expiration dates on solution and sterile basin pack.
3. Set up sterile basin on Mayo tray using inside of wrapper to create a sterile field.
4. Remove cap of solution and place it on a clean surface with outer edge down (inside facing up). Avoid touching the inner surface of cap. *Rationale:* Inside of cap is considered sterile.
5. Check the label on bottle before pouring the solution.
6. Pour a small amount of the liquid into a waste container for discard. *Rationale:* This will dislodge any bacteria that may have collected on the edge of the bottle after opening.
7. Pour the bottle with the label held against the palm. *Rationale:* Protect the label from drips which can destroy the name of solution.
8. Hold the bottle about 6 inches above the basin and pour slowly to avoid splashing.
9. Replace the lid immediately after using.

Specialized instruments are used for disciplines, such as gynecology and obstetrics (Figure 23-14), urology (Figure 23-15), and orthopedics (Figure 23-16).

Guidelines for Handling Instruments

Surgical instruments are expensive and may be delicate. They require special care and attention. In some instances, there might not be a duplicate of an instrument. Even slight damage to an instrument can result in malfunction at a critical time during surgery. The following guidelines can help to prolong the life of instruments.

Suture Materials and Needles

Suture (thread) materials are used to bring together a surgical incision or wound until healing takes place. Suture materials are added to the surgical tray setup when they are needed for a procedure. Sutures come either with or without an attached needle. The package label will indicate type, size, and length of the suture material.

Guidelines: Handling Instruments

1. Instruments should be rinsed, cleaned, and scrubbed with a brush as soon as possible to prevent a hardening of blood and tissue materials.
2. Handle carefully. Do not throw instruments into the basin for cleaning.
3. Avoid allowing large amounts of instruments to become tangled. They are difficult to separate and could result in damaging your protective gloves.
4. Sharp instruments should remain separate from the rest.
5. Delicate instruments, such as those with lenses, should be handled separately.
6. Instruments with ratchets, should be stored open to prolong their life.
7. Check all instruments for defects before sterilizing them. All tips on instruments should close tightly, scissors should cut evenly, and cutting edges should be smooth.

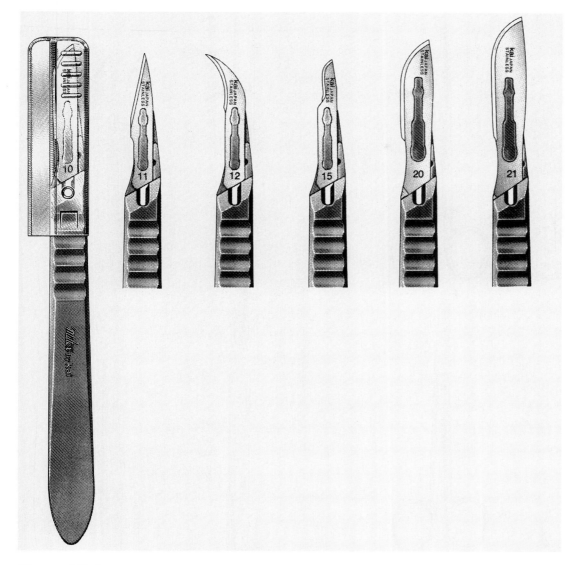

Figure 23-6   A variety of scalpels and blades.

Suture types include absorbable and non-absorbable.

Absorbable Sutures

Absorbable sutures are digested by tissue enzymes and absorbed by the body tissues. They do not have to be removed. Absorption usually occurs 5 to 20 days after insertion. This type of suture, such as surgical catgut (made from sheep's intestinal lining), is used for internal organs such as the bladder and intestines, subcutaneous tissue, and ligating, or tying off, blood vessels. They include plain cat gut, surgical cat gut, and chromic cat gut. Plain cat gut is used in areas where there is rapid healing such as

highly vascular areas of the lips and tongue. Surgical cat gut is used on tissues in which there is fast healing such as the vaginal area. Chromic cat gut has a slower absorption rate and can be used to hold tissue together longer, such as for muscle repair.

Nonabsorbable Sutures

Nonabsorbable sutures are used on skin surfaces in which they can easily be removed after incisional healing takes place. This type of suture material, such as nylon, cotton, silk, dacron, and stainless steel, is not absorbed by the body. Black silk, which can easily be seen, is the most commonly used nonabsorbable suture.

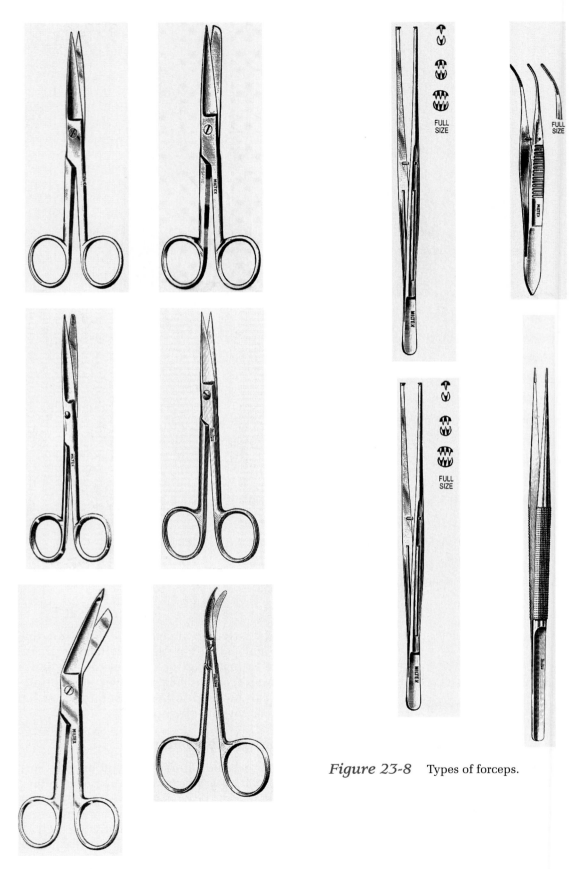

Figure 23-8   Types of forceps.

Figure 23-7   A variety of types of scissors.

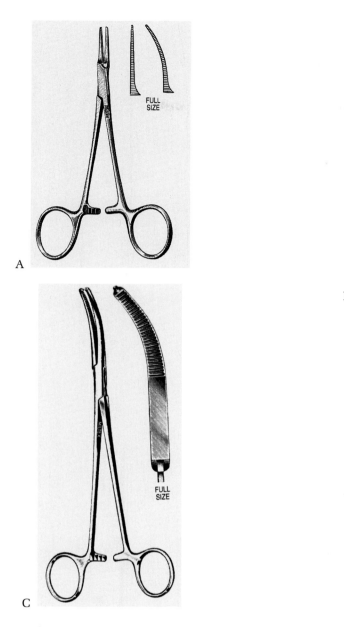
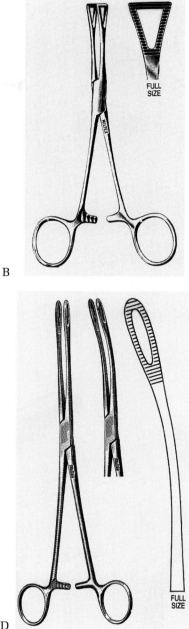

Figure 23-9 Hemostats: a) mosquito forceps; b) Pennington Hemostatic forceps; c) curved forceps; and d) sponge forceps.

Suture Material

Suture material varies and is selected based on the circumstances in which it is used.

- *Silk suture,* while the most expensive, is also considered the most dependable. It is widely used, easy to tie, and used as an all-purpose suture.
- *Nylon suture* has an elasticity and strength that makes it ideal for use in joints and skin

closure. The disadvantage is the difficulty in forming a tight knot.

- *Polyester suture* is considered the strongest of all the standard suture material, with the exception of steel. Polyester is used in ophthalmic, cardiovascular, and facial surgery which all require a strong unbreakable suture since a broken suture could result in permanent damage to the patient.
- *Steel,* such as used in staples, is the most widely used suture material in major

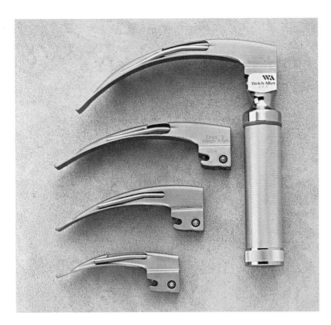

Figure 23-10   Laryngoscope.

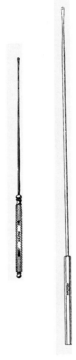

Figure 23-12   Probe.

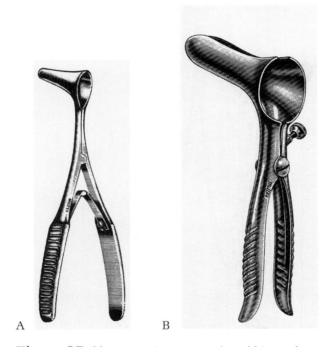

A   B

Figure 23-11   Speculum: a) nasal, and b) rectal.

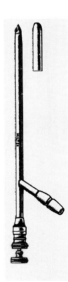

Figure 23-13   Trocar.

surgery. It is the strongest of all staple material.

- *Cotton suture,* with less strength than other suture materials, is no longer widely used.

The size, which is the gauge or diameter of suture material, is stated in terms of 0s, decreas-

ing in size with the number of zeros. For example 6-0 (000000) is the smallest and 0 the thickest. Sizes 2-0 through 6-0 are most commonly used. Delicate tissue on areas such as the face and neck would be sutured with 5-0 to 6-0 suture material. These fine sutures would leave little scarring. Heavier sutures, such as 2-0, would be used for

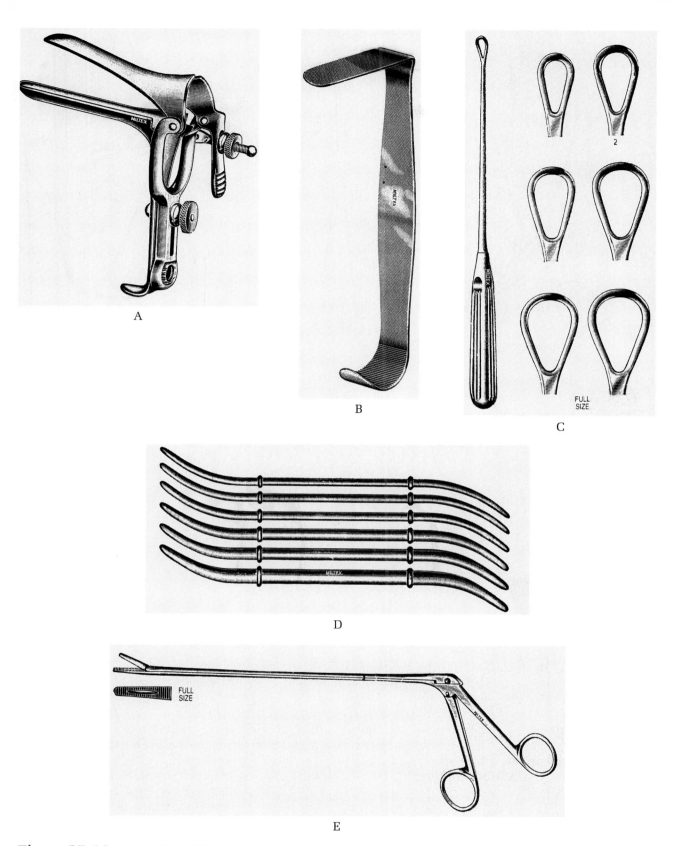

Figure 23-14 Gynecological instruments: a) vaginal speculum;
b) retractor; c) uterine curettes; d) uterine dilators; and e) IUD
removal forceps. *(Continued on next page)*

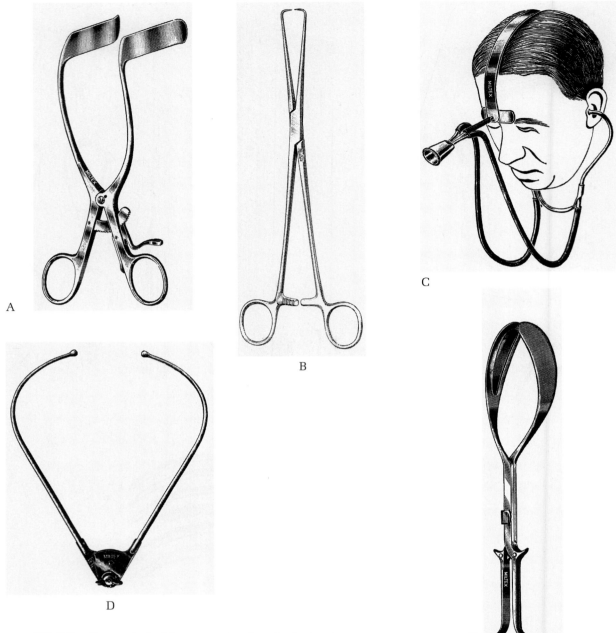

Figure 23-14 Gynecological instruments: a) vaginal retractor; b) uterine tenaculum forceps; c) obstetrical stethoscope; d) pelvimeter; and e) OB forceps. *(Continued)*

the chest or abdomen. The physician determines the type and gauge of sutures to be used. Table 22-2 summarizes suture uses, sizes, and types. Figure 23-17 illustrates different types of suture material.

Suture Needles

Suture needles are available in differing shapes depending on where they will be used. Needles have either a sharp cutting point, used for tissues that provide some resistance such as skin, or a round noncutting point used for more flexible tissue such as peritoneum. They are available in three shapes: straight, curved, or swagged.

The straight needle is used when the needle can be pushed and pulled through the tissue without the use of a needle holder. This type of needle will have an eye that needs to be threaded with the suture material. The suture material will then be double since it will enter the eye from one side and come out the other.

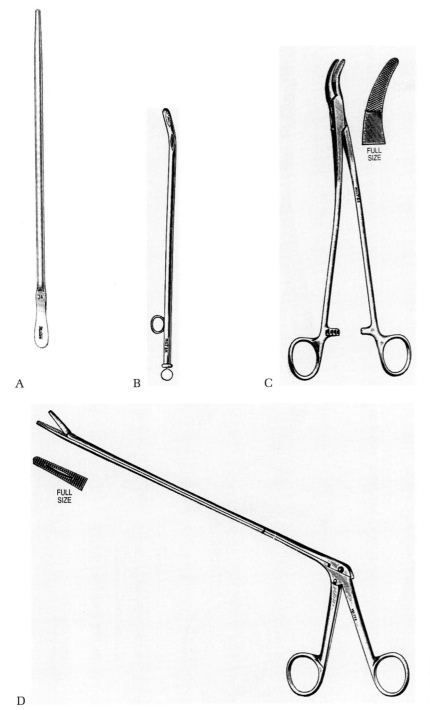

A   B   C

D

Figure 23-15   Urological instruments: a) sound; b) female catheter; c) needle holder; and d) urethral forceps.

Curved needles allow the surgeon to go in and out of a tissue when there is not enough room to maneuver a straight needle. This type of needle requires a needle holder.

A swaged needle is one in which the needle and suture materials are combined in one length. They offer the advantage of not slipping off the needle since they are attached. A swaged needle

pack will contain a label indicating the gauge, type, length of the suture material and the type of needle point (cutting or noncutting).

Other Wound Closure Materials

Other materials used for wound closure include sterile tapes, such as Steri-Strips (Figure 23-18).

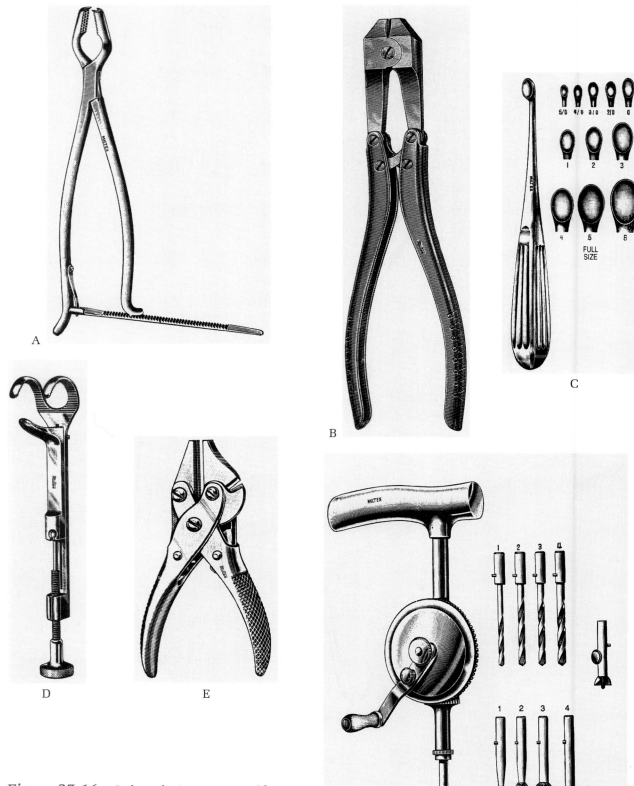

Figure 23-16 Orthopedic instruments: a) bone holding forceps; b) pin cutter; c) bone curettes; d) bone clamp; e) wire cutters; and f) drill set.

TABLE 23-2   **Suture Uses, Sizes, and Types**

Use	Gauge	Type of Material
Blood vessels	3-0 to 0	Chromic gut
	3-0	Cotton
	3-0 to 0	Silk
Eyelid	6-0 to 4-0	Silk
	6-0 to 5-0	Polyester
Skin	6-0 to 2-0	Nylon
	5-0 to 3-0	Polyethylene
	5-0 to 2-0	Stainless steel
Fascia	2-0 to 0	Chromic gut
	2-0 to 0	Silk
	2-0 to 0	Cotton
Muscle	3-0 to 0	Plain gut
	3-0 to 0	Chromic gut
	3-0 to 0	Silk

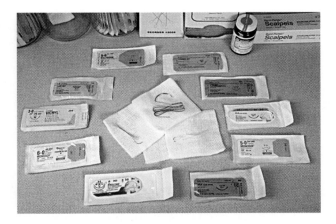

Figure 23-17   Types of suture material.

These sterile, nonallergenic tapes are available in a variety of widths. They are used instead of sutures when not much tension will be applied to a wound, such as on a small facial cut. Sterile tapes must be applied by the physician since only a licensed physician can perform wound closure. The physician may delegate this task to another licensed professional, such as a physician's assistant (PA) or nurse (RN). Staples, made of stainless steel, are applied with a surgical stapler.

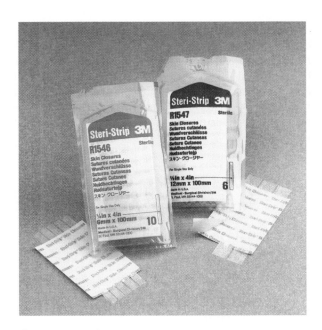

Figure 23-18   Steri-Strips from 3M.

Surgical Assisting

The medical assistant's role in surgical assisting varies depending on the type of office practice and the needs of the physician. For example, an eye surgeon who performs a large number of outpatient cataract operations may employ a full time scrub assistant, scrub tech, or O.R. tech, who will apply sterile gloves and hand instruments to the surgeon. In this case the medical assistant might act as the nonsterile assistant who positions the patient, uses transfer forceps to bring additional supplies as needed, holds the local anesthetic while the surgeon draws up the anesthetic, and applies dressings.

In many practices the medical assistant will scrub, apply sterile gloves, and act as the only assistant for the surgeon. A good assistant can help the procedure flow smoothly. The exact surgical tray setup and sequence of passing instruments will vary depending on the procedure and the surgeon's preferences.

A good assistant will anticipate the needs of the physician, use care in handing instruments, efficiently using care that an injury does not occur, and account for all materials used during the procedure. For example, if absorbent sponges are used to clean out the wound site during surgery, the assistant must maintain an accurate count to ensure that all sponges are removed before the patient's wound is closed.

The two types of assistants in the operating area are designated by the terms scrub and floater. The scrub assistant performs all procedures in sterile protective clothing using sterile technique. Responsibilities include arranging the surgical tray to meet the physician's preferences, handing instruments, swabbing (sponging) bodily fluids away from the operative site, retracting the incision area, and cutting suture materials.

Med Tip: Some physicians will have pictures on cards which demonstrate the setup and instrument packs they prefer.

Figure 23-19 illustrates a medical assistant using proper technique when passing instruments to the physician. See the procedure for assisting the surgeon with a minor surgical procedure.

A float assistant provides the nonsterile needs during a surgical procedure and thus "floats" between the operating table, supplies, and equipment. One of the major roles of the float assistant is to monitor the patient by taking vital signs every 5-10 minutes.

Guidelines: Sterile Technique for Scrub Assistants

1. Always be aware of where your hands are since they should never touch an unsterile area. Immediately reglove if sterility is broken.
2. Arrange the surgical tray for efficiency closing all instruments that were left open during the autoclave process.
3. Close all instruments before passing them. Protect the surgeon from injury by handing needles with the point away from the physician, paying close attention to where scalpel blades and scissors' points are in relation to the physician's hands.
4. Anticipate the physician's needs by memorizing the types of instruments used in a procedure, and the order in which they are most often used. A card index with a list of the preferences for each procedure is useful for this purpose.
5. Do not release your grip on the instrument until you feel the physician take it away. This prevents an instrument falling to the floor and being damaged. In addition you may not have a duplicate of that particular instrument on your tray and it will cause a delay in the procedure.
6. Place the instrument with a firm "slap" into the physician's extended hand. Since he or she may not look up from the surgical site when their hand is extended, do not look away from the instrument until you feel it being taken from you. The handles should be placed into the physician's hands first.
7. If asked to provide retraction to open the incision area for better visualization, follow directions from the surgeon regarding the amount of pull needed. Move slowly and deliberately when retracting. Do not make abrupt, forceful moves.
8. If sutures are used to close the wound, be prepared to cut the suture material. The physician will pull both ends of the suture material together away from the wound. Cut both ends at the same time 1/8 to 1/4 inch above the knot.
9. Many requests for assistance will not be verbalized by the physician. It is important to pay attention and anticipate what instruments or assistance will be required next.

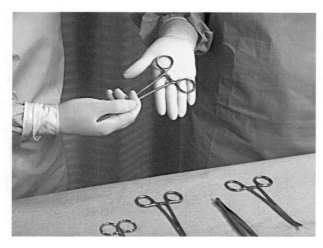

Figure 23-19 Medical assistant using proper technique when passing instruments to the physician.

Med Tip: When practicing to assist as a scrub assistant, practice reaching for an instrument with your eyes closed. This is similar to the conditions under which the physician works since he or she does not look up from the operative site when reaching for instruments.

A surgical setup for a typical minor surgical procedure would include:

- Local anesthetic materials
- 3 cc syringe with needle(s)
- Alcohol sponges to cleanse vial top
- Sterile gloves for surgeon
- 4 × 4 and 2 × 2 gauze sponges
- No. 3 scalpel blades and handle, extra scalpel blades (No. 10, 11, and 15)
- Curved iris scissors
- Tissue forceps
- Straight and curved mosquito forceps
- Straight and curved Kelly forceps
- Towel forceps
- Sterile drape towels
- Needle holder with mounted needle and suture materials
- Sterile specimen container with preservative solution

Figure 23-20 is an illustration of pouring sterile solution into a container and Figure 23-21 shows a sterile instrument setup.

Guidelines: Proper Technique for "Floating" Assistant During Surgical Procedure

1. Immediately report any unusual observations about the patient to the operating physician.
2. Use care not to touch the physician during any assisting since this will contaminate him or her and cause a delay in the procedure while the physician regloves (and regowns if necessary).
3. Provide additional medications such as local anesthetics that are needed during the procedure. This is done by following the correct procedure to identify the medication, clean top of vial/bottle with alcohol, hold vial/bottle upside down so that physician can insert sterile needle into vial without touching the contaminated outer surface, and keep the label in plain view for physician to read. Hold the vial firmly with both hands at your shoulder height for ease of withdrawal by the physician. Do not place the vial in front of your face. Note that the physician will have to use some force to be able to enter the vial with a needle.
4. Since the float assistant is unsterile, this person must perform all light adjustments, patient repositioning, chart notations made during the procedure, requisition forms, and specimen container labeling.
5. The float assistant can place additional sterile materials and instruments onto the sterile field by opening the packet without touching the sterile inside and gently "dropping" them onto the Mayo stand. The sterile scrub assistant or physician may remove them from the inside of the packet as the float holds firmly onto the outside.
6. When holding a container to receive a specimen, tilt the container slightly so the physician can place the specimen inside without touching the rim of the container.

Preparing the Patient for Minor Surgery

For purposes of efficiency some of the preoperative patient preparation can take place before the patient arrives for the procedure. For example, patient education with an explanation of the procedure,

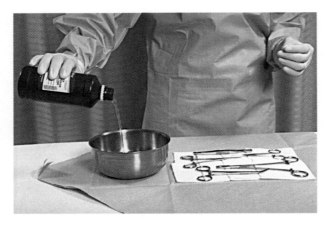

Figure 23-20   Pouring sterile solution into a container.

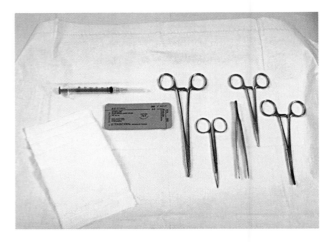

Figure 23-21   Sterile instrument setup.

PROCEDURE: Assisting With Minor Surgery

Terminal Performance
Competency: Prepare all materials and equipment for immediate use in a surgical procedure using sterile technique.

Equipment and Supplies

Mayo stand
Side stand
Transfer forceps and container
Sharps container
Waste container/plastic bag
Biohazard waste container
Anesthetic
Alcohol swab
Sterile specimen container, depending on type of surgery
Sterile pack:

- Sterile gloves (2 pairs)
- Towel pack
- 4 × 4 sponge pack
- Patient drape
- Needle pack and suture materials

Instrument pack(s) including towel clamp pack
Syringe pack
Sterile basin pack (2)

Procedural Steps

1. Wash hands.
2. Open sterile tray packs on Mayo stand and side stand. Use sterile wrapper to create a sterile field. The wrapper will hang over the edges of the tray.
3. Use sterile transfer forceps to move instruments on tray or to place equipment from packets. Materials in peel-away packets should be flipped onto the tray.
4. Open sterile needle and syringe unit and drop gently onto sterile field. Use care not to reach over the sterile field.
5. Open sterile drape packs and towel clamp packs.
6. Open a set of sterile gloves for the physician.
7. After tray is ready with all equipment open and arranged, pull edge of sterile towel across the tray using sterile transfer forceps. *Rationale:* The sterile towel will provide a protective

(Continued)

covering for the sterile tray until the procedure begins. The medical assistant should not leave the room once the tray is set up.

Operative Assist:

8. When the physician has donned the sterile gloves, remove the sterile towel covering the tray of instruments.

9. Remove the towel by standing to one side and grasp the two distal corners. Lift the towel toward you so that you do not reach over the unprotected sterile field.

10. Cleanse the vial of anesthetic with a sterile alcohol swab and hold it upside down in the palm of your hand with the label facing toward the physician. Hold it steady while the physician draws up the anesthetic.

11. Stand to one side of the patient and assist the physician as requested. Supply additional supplies as needed. *Note:* If you assist by handing instruments directly to the physician, you must perform a surgical scrub and wear a sterile gown and gloves.

12. Hold all containers for specimens, drainage, or contaminated 4 × 4s. Wear nonsterile gloves to protect yourself from contact with drainage.

13. Collect and place all soiled instruments in a basin out of the patient's view.

14. Place all soiled gauze sponges (4 × 4s) and dressings in a plastic bag. Do not allow wet items to remain on a sterile field.

15. Immediately label all specimens as they are obtained. Close the specimen container tightly.

16. Periodically reassure the patient by quietly asking how he or she is doing. Do not touch the patient with soiled gloves.

17. When procedure is complete, wash hands before assisting patient.

18. Allow the patient to rest and recover from the anesthetic. Periodically check the patient's vital signs according to office policy.

19. Provide clear oral and written postoperative instructions for the patient. Make sure the patient is stable before he or she leaves the office.

20. Send specimen(s) to the laboratory with requisition slip.

21. Clean, sanitize and sterilize the instruments. Clean and sanitize the room in preparation for the next patient.

22. Wash hands.

Charting Example
The physician will chart the details of the surgical procedure.

preoperative and postoperative instructions, and laboratory testing can take place up to a week before the actual procedure.

Preoperative and postoperative instructions can be presented in a variety of formats including one-on-one discussion, videotapes, brochures, pamphlets, and models. These instructions need to be reinforced either through a telephone reminder, as with notification of the time to arrive for surgery, or through another explanation of the same material. It is especially important to provide postoperative instructions in a variety of formats since the patient may not be fully alert right after the surgery. Family members should be included in these explanations whenever practical.

Preoperative instructions might include an explanation of what laboratory testing is needed and when it is to be done, cleansing enemas, food and fluid restrictions, special bathing/skin cleansing preparations, and bedtime sedative use. At this time the patient can be instructed about when to call the physician postoperatively. The patient should be cautioned to call the medical office if they have any illness, such as a cold or fever, the day of surgery.

Patients should be told orally and in writing to have someone drive them to and from the surgical facility, especially if they will be given a general anesthetic. Questions should be encouraged. However, the medical assistant must refer all

PROCEDURE: Assisting with Suturing

Terminal Performance
Competency: Assist with suture repair of an incision or laceration using sterile technique.

Equipment and Supplies

Mayo stand

Side stand

Anesthetic

Sterile transfer forceps

Sterile saline

Waste container/plastic bag

Biohazardous waste container

Sharps container

Sterile gloves (2 pairs)

Sterile pack(s):

- Patient drape
- Towel pack (four towels)
- 4 × 4 gauze sponge pack

Scalpel blades pack (No. 10 and 15)

Needle and syringe pack

Suture and needle pack (according to physician's preference)

Sterile basin (2)

Suture pack:

- Scalpel handle
- Needle holder
- Thumb forceps
- Two scissors
- Three hemostats

Procedural Steps

1. Use sterile scrub and gloving procedure.
2. Stand across from the physician.
3. Place two sponges ready for the physician near the wound site.
   Rationale: Physician will use sponges to clear drainage during initial inspection of the wound.
4. Assist by using additional sponges to keep wound dry.
5. Pass instruments, such as scissors, to physician using a firm "snap" of the handle into his or her hand.

Rationale: The instrument should be firmly placed in the physician's hand without letting go until the physician has a firm grasp.

6. The blade is placed into the scalpel using a hemostat.
7. Hand the scalpel to the physician with blade edge down to avoid cutting the physician.
8. Continue to use sponges to keep the wound free of drainage.
9. Pass all instruments to the physician as requested. Try to anticipate the need for the next instruments, such as another hemostat or scissors for cutting suture.
10. Pass the toothed forceps to physician if laceration edges need to be grasped.
11. Mount the needle into the needle holder and pass as one unit to the physician using care to keep the suture within the sterile field. Pass the needle holder with the needle pointing outward. Hold the suture with the other hand and do not let go of it until the physician sees it.
12. Using the suture scissors prepare to cut the suture as directed by the physician (usually 1/8 to 1/4 inch from the knot).
13. Sponge the closed wound once with a sponge and discard.
14. Repeat this step with each suture.
15. Handle all soiled instruments after they are used by placing them back onto the sterile field if they will be used again, or discard into the instrument basin.
16. When procedure is complete, remove gloves and wash hands before assisting patient.
17. Allow the patient to rest and recover from the anesthetic. Periodically

(Continued)

check the patient's vital signs according to office policy.

18. Provide clear oral and written postoperative instructions for the patient. Make sure the patient is stable before he or she leaves the office.

19. Clean, sanitize and sterilize the instruments. Clean and sanitize the room in preparation for the next patient.

20. Wash hands.

Charting Example
The physician will chart the details of the surgical procedure.

questions to the physician which relate to the risk of surgery or the possible outcomes.

The patient's vital signs (blood pressure, temperature, pulse, and respirations) should be taken before the procedure.

Med Tip: Ask the patient to restate the instructions if you are concerned that the patient does not understand. You can repeat specific instructions, clarifying the area(s) of confusion for the patient. Then chart, "patient states understanding of the procedure."

Informed Consent

The patient must be provided an honest, thorough explanation of the surgical procedure including the benefits and risks. Informed consent is explained in more detail in Chapter 5, Medicine and the Law. Any invasive procedure in which the body is entered with a scalpel, scissors, or other device requires written permission (consent) from the patient. Procedures in which a body cavity is entered for purposes of visualization, even though no incision is made, such as in bronchoscopy and cystoscopy, also require written consent.

The procedure, with all risks involved, must be explained by the physician. Every attempt must be made to determine if the patient actually understands the explanation given by the physician. The medical assistant can witness the patient's signing the consent form.

Positioning and Draping

Instruct the patient to remove all clothing and put on a patient gown with the ties at the back, unless otherwise instructed. The patient is assisted onto the operating table and placed in the proper position for the procedure by the medical assistant. Every attempt should be made to assure the patient's comfort since the patient may have to remain in one position for an extended period of time. General guidelines for positioning and draping are discussed in Chapter 21, Assisting with Physical Examinations.

Anesthesia

Anesthesia, the partial or complete loss of sensation, is used to block the pain of surgery. Anesthesia can also relax muscles, produce amnesia, calm anxiety, and cause sleep. Medical assistants do not administer anesthetics, but they should be familiar with them and their effects.

The two types of anesthetics are general or local (conduction). A general anesthetic depresses the central nervous system (CNS) to cause unconsciousness. It is generally administered through inhalation or intravenous injection (IV).

Inhalation types of anesthetics are in the form of gases or volatile liquids. In many cases, these are administered after a patient has received a sedative or narcotic to relieve pain or a tranquilizer to relieve anxiety. Sedatives and narcotics are usually administered intramuscularly before surgery. In some cases, they are administered by IV immediately before the general anesthetic is given.

Intravenous anesthetics (IV) are a type of hypnotic sedative that produce anesthesia, or sleep, when given in large doses. Sodium-Pentothal is an example of this type of anesthetic.

Precautions to be taken when administering an general anesthetic include:

- Administering the anesthetic on an empty stomach. This is to prevent vomiting and possible aspiration of vomitus into lungs resulting in pneumonia.

- Cautioning patients not to drive or engage in other activity that could result in harm from an impaired consciousness. General anesthetics can interfere with patient's alertness for 12 to 24 hours after surgery.
- Advising patients to avoid alcohol and depressant drugs 2-3 days before surgery and 1 day after surgery.

Local anesthetics provide loss of sensation in a particular location without overall loss of consciousness. A local anesthetic is also referred to as a conduction anesthetic. The conduction of pain transmission by way of the nervous system is blocked. Examples of this type of anesthetic are

- Topical and local infiltration which act on nerve endings.
- Nerve block which affects pain transmission along a single nerve.
- Regional block, spinal, epidural, or saddle blocks which affect a group of nerves.

A local infiltration anesthetic is injected directly into the tissue that will be operated upon. Examples of a "local" are lidocaine hydrochloride (Xylocaine) and procaine hydrochloride (Novocain). This type of anesthetic is used for such procedures as removal of skin growths, skin suturing and dental surgery. Local anesthesia takes from 5 to 15 minutes to become effective and lasts from 1 to 3 hours. An additional injection of anesthetic may have to be administered when the first has worn off.

Epinephrine, which is a vasoconstrictor causing superficial blood vessels to narrow, is often added to the local anesthetic when the physician is operating on the face and head. The addition of epinephrine allows for better visualization of the surgical site since bleeding is diminished. Epinephrine also causes local anesthetics to be absorbed by the body more slowly. This causes the anesthetic to have a longer lasting effect. Clearly mark anesthetics that have been prepared with the addition of epinephrine. Patients with heart problems could have a reaction to epinephrine causing tachycardia or irregularities.

Nerve blocks are administered by injection into a nerve adjacent to the operative site. This type of anesthetic is used for surgery on hands, fingers, and toes.

Topical anesthetics are local pain control medications that are applied to the skin and produce a numbing effect. These can be applied by drop, spray, or swabbed. They are commonly used in eye procedures. An example of a spray anesthetic is ethyl chloride which produces a "freezing" effect on the skin. Benzocaine (Solarcaine) is another example of a topical anesthetic.

The effects of topical and other local anesthetics occur either immediately or within a few minutes. These effects wear off quickly. Large amounts of local anesthetic, beyond the normal dosages, are not recommended and may result in an adverse reaction in patients. Some patients are allergic to anesthetics and may slip into anaphylactic shock which requires emergency treatment (see Chapter 34, Emergency Care).

Med Tip: An emergency tray or cart containing drugs used to counteract shock and other emergencies should always be available in the medical office.

Patients who receive a local anesthetic in their mouth or throat should be advised not to eat until the effects of the anesthetic wear off to prevent choking on food or burning the mouth. Table 23-3 contains examples of local anesthetics.

TABLE 23-3 **Local Anesthetics**

Anesthetic Agent	Use
Benzocaine	Topical use only
Chloroprocaine	Nerve block, epidural
Lidocaine (Xylocaine)	Infiltration or topical
Mepivacaine	Infiltration nerve block
Procaine (Novocain)	Infiltration; seldom used now
Tetracaine	Infiltration, topical nerve block, spinal

Both the strength and dosage of the anesthetic must be charted. Since only physicians or anesthesiologists can administer an anesthetic, only they can chart the administration. Either the medical assistant or the physician will draw up the local anesthetic. Using the correct procedure for drawing up medication as discussed in Chapter 32, the vial must be correctly identified and then wiped with an alcohol sponge. If the medical assistant draws up the medication then she or he must present both the syringe and the vial to the physician so that the label can be read by the physician. The anesthetic will be injected into the patient's prepared skin by the physician before the physician has donned gloves. This syringe is not placed onto the sterile field since it has been contaminated by the medical assistant's ungloved hands.

If the physician prefers to draw up the anesthetic, it can be done using a sterile syringe after he or she has applied gloves. The medical assistant will hold the vial securely while the physician withdraws the anesthetic without contaminating the needle. The outside of the vial cannot be touched by the physician's sterile gloved hand. This syringe can then be placed onto the sterile field.

Some physicians prefer to change the needle after drawing up the local anesthetic. For example, they may draw up the drug using a 21 gauge needle and then administer the solution using a 23 or 25 gauge needle.

Preparation of Patient's Skin

While skin cannot be sterilized, it can be cleaned using medical aseptic technique. Careful cleansing of skin before performing a surgical procedure will reduce the number of microorganisms on the skin. This will reduce the chance of carrying infection producing microorganisms through the skin during the invasive procedure (incision into skin or entrance of a probe).

In some situations, the physician may order the surgical site to be shaved since bacteria can reside in hair. Care must be taken to avoid scraping or cutting the skin during the shaving process. The physician will order either a dry shave or a wet shave (moistening the skin with soap and water) according to the physician's preference. See procedure for skin preparation. Figure 23-22 illustrates preparation of the patient's skin for surgical procedures. See Figure 23-23 for an example of a dry skin prep tray.

Postoperative Patient Care

Postoperative care includes caring for the patient during recovery from anesthesia, wound care, applying dressings, and patient instructions.

Recovery from Anesthesia

Patients must be observed carefully after surgery for signs of adverse reaction to the anesthetic, bleeding, and circulatory problems. The patient's vital signs (blood pressure, temperature, pulse, and respiration) should be monitored immediately after surgery and then every 15 minutes for the first hour.

Excessive disorientation and inability to arouse within a normal time for recovery should be reported immediately to the physician. The patient should be observed for nausea and/or vomiting. Medications may be ordered by the physician to counteract nausea and vomiting.

Med Tip: Never give fluids to a patient who is not fully alert. This can result in choking. Oral medications for pain, nausea, and vomiting have to be withheld until full recovery from anesthetics. Medications are given by injection until this occurs.

Wound Care

Any break in the skin, whether from an injury or a surgical incision, is referred to as a wound. A surgical procedure requiring an incision through the skin is considered an invasive procedure since the skin is entered and creates a wound. Wounds cause blood vessels to rupture and seep into tissues, which results in skin color changes. Typically, skin coloration during wound healing will change from erythema in a fresh wound to a greenish yellow color, during the healing process involving an oxidation of blood pigments. There are four types of wound classification:

- *Abrasion:* Wound in which outer layers of skin are rubbed away due to scraping. Will generally heal without scarring.
- *Incision:* Smooth cut resulting from a surgical scalpel or sharp material, such as razor or glass. May result in excessive bleeding if deep and scarring.
- *Laceration:* Wound in which the edges are torn in an irregular shape. Can cause profuse bleeding and scarring.
- *Puncture:* Wound made by a sharp pointed instrument such as a bullet, needle, nail, or splinter. External bleeding is usually minimal but infection may occur due to penetration with a contaminated object and there may be scarring.

Wound healing will pass through various stages, including inflammation, as the body starts to fight off potential infection. To prevent infection surgical wounds must be handled carefully. In most situations, a wound or surgical site will require a sterile dressing as protection against bacteria, trauma, to absorb any drainage, and to protect against motion damaging the suture site. The patient should be asked how long it has been since he or she received a tetanus shot. In the event that the shot was not received within the last ten years, the physician should be informed.

The size and shape of the dressing will depend on the size, location and amount of drainage from the wound. Sterile 4 × 4 inch gauze pads (called four by fours) are used for most dressings. If there is drainage expected from the wound, a prepared dressing such as Telfa may be used to prevent the dressing sticking to the wound. See Figure 23-24 for an example of a wound closure

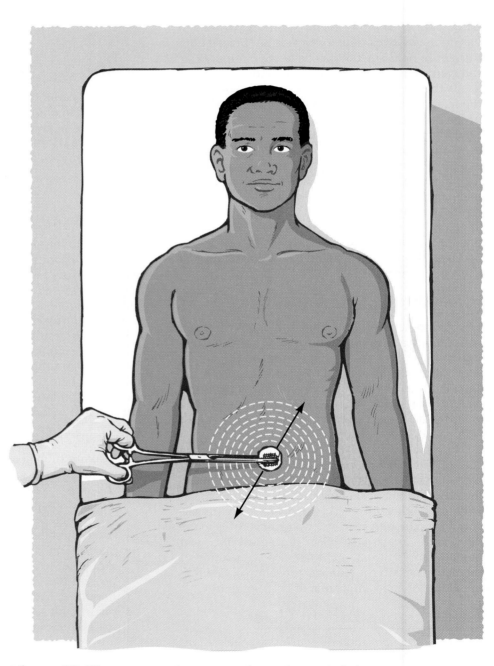

Figure 23-22   Preparing the patient's skin at the surgical site.

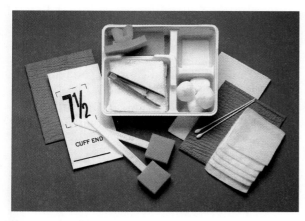

Figure 23-23   Dry skin prep tray.

kit. The procedure for changing a sterile dressing follows.

A dressing is the application of a sterile covering over a surgical site or wound using surgical asepsis. Figure 23-25 illustrates classification of wound healing. A bandage is the application of covering over a nonsterile area using medical asepsis. Figure 23-26 shows various types of bandages.

Suture Removal

Sutures are inserted by the surgeon at the end of a procedure to hold tissues in alignment during the healing process. Sutures generally remain in place from 5-6 days and then have to be removed if they

---

PROCEDURE: Preparing the Patient's Skin for Surgical Procedures

**Terminal Performance
Competency:** To prepare patient's skin for surgical procedure using sterile scrub and shave.

Equipment and Supplies
Antiseptic germicidal soap
Sterile saline
Antiseptic such as betadine
Sterile applicators (8)
Mayo tray or side tray
Waste receptacle (may be included in sterile pack)
Hazardous waste container
Plastic bag for soiled dressings
Sterile Pack:

- Sterile gloves
- Towel pack (3-4 towels)
- Sterile basin pack (3 basins)
- Patient drape
- 4 × 4 gauze sponge pack (12-24 sponges)
- Shave prep kit

Note: This procedure follows a surgical hand scrub.

Procedural Steps
1. Wash hands
2. Assemble equipment by placing packs on Mayo stand or side tray and unwrapping outer wraps from all packs.
3. Identify patient and explain procedure.
4. Have patient remove appropriate clothing and gowning. Ask patient to void, if necessary.

5. Position and drape the patient to provide exposure of the operative site.
6. Unwrap the basin pack. Pour germicidal soap solution into one basin; sterile saline into the second basin; and antiseptic into the third. ***Rationale:*** Liquids are poured by holding the outer nonsterile surface of the containers before applying sterile gloves.
7. Wash using sterile scrub and apply sterile gloves.
8. Drape the skin with two towels placed 3-5 inches above and below the surgical site.
9. With a sterile gauze/sponge apply soapy solution to patient's skin. Use a circular motion starting at the site of proposed incision and move outward. Pass over each skin area only once. Place each used sponge into waste receptacle immediately. *Note:* Some physicians prefer the patient receive a dry shave.
10. Take a fresh sterile gauze/sponge for each cleansing wipe. Repeat this process until the area is completely washed. The last area cleansed will be the outer edges.
11. Rinse using sterile saline on clean gauze/sponge. Pat dry with dry gauze only on the area that has been washed. Avoid touching any other

(Continued on next page)

skin area. ***Rationale:*** The surrounding skin is considered contaminated since it has not been washed.

12. If shaving is ordered, then proceed with the following steps.

13. Apply soap solution to area. Remove razor from shave prep pack. Pull skin taut and shave surgical site in the direction in which the hair is growing. Rinse with saline solution using the single-pass, circular motion as before and pat dry. ***Rationale:*** Shaving against the direction of hair growth can irritate the skin. This skin breakdown will allow bacteria to enter.

14. Reapply soap solution to area and repeat the above process for the time according to office policy (around 5 minutes).

15. Pat dry the entire area with the third sterile towel.

16. Apply the antiseptic solution using two cotton applicators together in the same single-pass, circular motion.

17. Cover the prepared surgical site with the remaining sterile towel.

18. Properly dispose of gloves and soiled materials in biohazard bag/container.

19. To dispose of soiled dressings use the following steps:

    a. Remove gloves.

    b. Place one hand into the empty plastic bag.

    c. Using the hand covered with the plastic bag, pick up all the soiled materials. With other hand pull the outside of the bag over the soiled dressings.

    d. Dispose of this bag in a hazardous waste bag/container.

20. Wash hands and document procedure.

Charting Example

3/12/XX Pt. arrived for removal and biopsy of growth on outer aspect of left forearm. Surgical site prepared using betadine. No cuts or lesions noted.   J. Wall, RMA

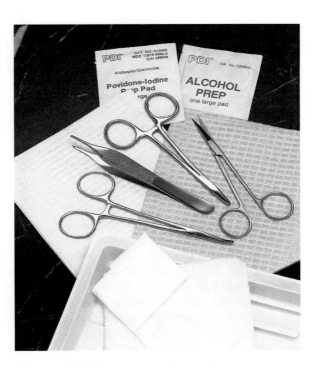

Figure 23-24 Wound closure kit.

are nonabsorbable. If sutures remain in the body too long, they can cause skin irritation and infection. The suture acts as a wick to carry bacteria through the skin and into the subcutaneous tissues. Suture removal times differ depending upon the site:

- Facial sutures may be removed after only 24 to 48 hours to prevent scarring.
- Head and neck sutures remain for 3-5 days.
- Abdominal sutures remain from 5 to 7 days.
- Sutures over weight bearing joints and large bones may remain 7 to 10 days.

The medical assistant prepares the patient for suture removal by removing the dressing, if one is present. Each edge of the dressing is removed by pulling toward the suture line. If the dressing is adhering to the suture line then a small amount of sterile saline or hydrogen peroxide can be used to moisten the dressing for ease in removing.

In some office practices and in some states, the medical assistant is able to remove sutures. The procedure should be explained to the patient re-

PROCEDURE: Changing a Sterile Dressing

**Terminal Performance
Competency:** Change a wound dressing using proper sterile technique.

Equipment and Supplies

Disposable gloves

Antiseptic solution

Solution container

Prepackaged dressing pack

Thumb forceps

Sterile cotton balls

Sterile gloves

Sterile dressing

Adhesive tape

Scissors, if necessary for tape

Waste container/plastic bag

Biohazardous waste container

Mayo stand or side tray

Procedural Steps

1. Wash hands.
2. Assemble equipment using Mayo stand.
3. Prepare the sterile field using aseptic technique using prepackaged dressing packet. Use sterile transfer forceps to place additional sterile items onto the sterile field.
4. Explain procedure to patient.
5. Assist patient into comfortable position with area to be dressed resting on support, such as an examination table.
6. Apply nonsterile gloves.
7. Remove dressing from wound by loosening tape with gloved hands or forceps and pulling it from both sides toward the wound. Without passing the soiled dressing over the sterile field, place it into the soiled waste bag. Do not allow the dressing to touch the outside or edges of the bag.
8. Inspect the wound for signs of infection and inflammation. Note any discharge for type, amount and odor.
9. Discard gloves and contaminated forceps properly. Disposable gloves and forceps are placed in waste container. Reusable forceps are placed in basin for later cleaning.
10. Open sterile gloves and apply properly.
11. Drop antiseptic onto several cotton balls until they are moist but not saturated. Clean the wound by using sterile forceps to hold the cotton. Cleanse the wound moving from top to bottom of the wound once. Use a new cotton ball with antiseptic for each wipe. Move from the inside of the wound to the outside edges.
12. Pick up the sterile dressing with gloved hands and place over the wound.
13. Discard gloves and forceps.
14. Apply adhesive tape to hold dressing in place. Do not apply so tightly as to restrict circulation. The strips of tape should be long enough to hold the dressing in place. Do not wrap the tape entirely around an extremity or completely cover the dressing.
15. Instruct the patient on dressing care and follow-up appointment to see the physician.
16. Chart the procedure including date, time, location and condition of wound and instructions given to the patient.

Charting Example

2/14/XX 11:00 am. Drsg. change on Left anterior forearm. Moderate amt. serous drainage with slight erythema surrounding wound. Incision healing well with edges aligned. Cleansed with betadine. Sterile drsg. applied. Pt. instructed on wound care.   M. King, CMA

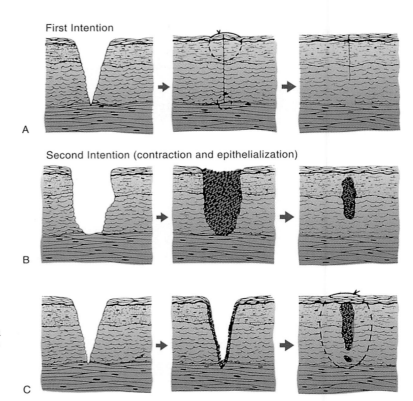

First Intention

A

Second Intention (contraction and epithelialization)

B

C

Figure 23-25 Classification of wound healing: a) First intention: A clean incision is made with primary closure; there is minimal scarring. (B and C) Second intention: The wound is left open so that granulation can occur; a large scar results, b) or the wound is initially left open and later closed when there is no further evidence of infection c).

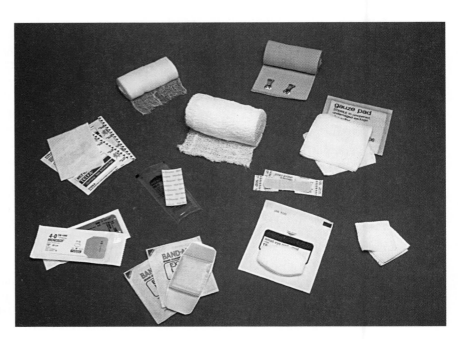

Figure 23-26 Various types of bandages.

minding them that they may feel a pulling sensation. The skin is then thoroughly cleansed with an antiseptic such as alcohol or betadine solution. After opening the sterile suture packet and creating a sterile field with the wrapper, the knot of the suture is gently picked up using a thumb forceps. The suture is then cut with suture scissors below

the knot as close to the skin as possible. The suture is removed by pulling the long remaining suture out. Suture material that is outside of the skin should not be pulled through the skin due to the danger of pulling infection along with it. Very little of the suture is actually pulled through the skin. Suture removal is illustrated in Figure 23-27.

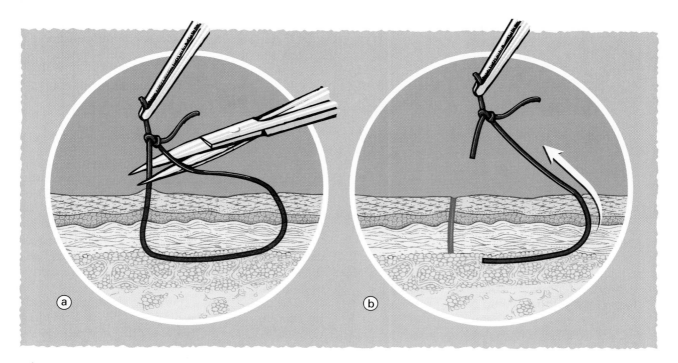

Figure 23-27 Removal of sutures.

A disposable suture removal set is displayed in Figure 23-28.

Surgical Procedures Performed in the Medical Office

Many minor surgical procedures can be performed efficiently in the physician's office. This saves the patient the time and expense of having to go into an ambulatory surgical facility or a hospital. The basic surgical setup is the standard setup with the addition of specific instruments for each procedure. Some of the minor procedures performed in the medical office include biopsy, cautery, colposcopy, cryosurgery, endocervical curettage, suture removal, removal of foreign bodies, incision and drainage, vasectomy, and removal of growths and tumors.

The medical assistant does not administer these procedures but must understand them and their effects so that he or she can assist the physician and the patient. A brief description of some of these procedures follows.

Electrosurgery

Electrocautery, or cautery, is the use of high-frequency, alternating electric current to destroy, cut, or remove tissue. Electrocautery is also used to coagulate small blood vessels. Electrocautery

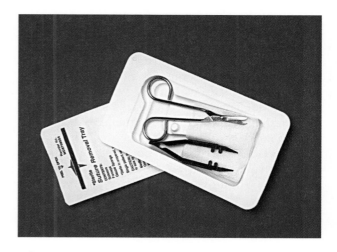

Figure 23-28 Disposable suture removal set.

has the advantage of sealing or cauterizing small blood vessels during a procedure such as small tumor removal, which results in reduced bleeding and cell loss. See Figure 23-29 for photo of a disposable cautery unit. Four types of currents are used in electrosurgery.

- *Electrocoagulation:* Destroys tissues and controls bleeding by coagulation.
- *Electrodessication:* Destroys tissue by creating a spark gap when the probe is inserted into unwanted tissue.

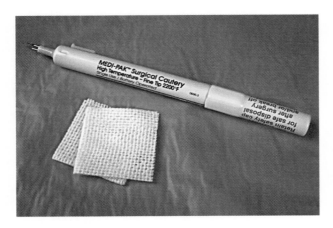

Figure 23-29   Disposable cautery unit.

- *Electrofulguration:*   Destroys tissue with a spark by holding the tip of the probe a short distance away from the unwanted tissue.
- *Electrosection:*   Uses electric current to incise and excise the tissue.

Some physicians have miniature units called **hyfrecators.** The use of electrocautery is being replaced by the electrosurgical unit (ESU) and the ultrasonic surgical unit (USU).

The ESU is able to provide a more controlled, less damaging form of electric current through the use of a variety of attachments. For example, an incision can be made using ESU with a small electrode blade. The blade cauterizes as it cuts thus minimizing bleeding. Other attachments can be used to coagulate and suction.

The USU uses high-frequency sound waves to break apart calcified or sclerosed tissue so they can be removed in small segments. Some models have the ability to suction as they break apart and dissolve body calcifications. In some forms of electrosurgery, a local anesthetic may be administered.

Colposcopy

Colposcopy is an examination of the vagina and cervix performed using a lighted instrument called a colposcope with the patient in the lithotomy position. The colposcope allows the physician to observe the tissues of this area in great detail through light and magnification. Abnormal areas of tissue or cells can then be removed for biopsy, or microscopic examination of cells for cancer. In some cases cryosurgery, using freezing temperatures to destroy cells, is then applied.

Colposcopy is performed

- If abnormal tissue development is observed by the physician during a routine pelvic examination.
- If Papanicoulaou (PAP) smear result is in abnormal range.
- For magnified visualization.
- To obtain a biopsy specimen.

If the physician is unable to visualize the entire cervical canal during the colposcopy, he or she may perform an endocervical curettage (ECC) to scrape endocervical cells from inside the cervical canal. These cells are then sent for further testing to determine any abnormality. (*Note:* Abnormal cell growth can be a sign of a pre-cancerous condition that, if untreated, could lead to the development of cancer.)

The patient may experience slight bleeding after this procedure if a biopsy is taken. Provide a perineal pad for the patient with instructions for home care. The patient should receive instructions to call the physician if there is abnormal pain or bleeding after this procedure.

Cryosurgery

Cryosurgery is used to treat cervical erosion and chronic cervicitis. This procedure is also referred to as cryocautery since the term "cautery" refers to a destruction of tissue. A colposcope is used to magnify the surface of the cervix and then a probe, capable of reaching freezing temperatures, is placed within the colposcope with the patient in the lithotomy position. This produces a freezing effect on tissues which destroys the abnormal cells.

The patient may experience mild cramping and a watery discharge after the procedure. The physician may advise her to take a mild analgesic, such as Tylenol. The patient should be advised against using a tampon which could irritate sensitive tissues for at least a month. Additional instruction should include instructions on reporting any unusual pain or foul discharge, abstaining from sexual intercourse for one month, and the time when she should return for a follow-up visit. The probe used in cryosurgery needs to be sterilized according to manufacturer's instructions immediately after use.

Endometrial Biopsy (EMB)

An endometrial biopsy (EMB) consists of using a curette or suction tool to remove uterine tissue for testing. EMB is performed for a variety of reasons including:

- To detect precancerous and cancerous conditions of the endometrial lining of the uterus.
- To detect inflammatory conditions.
- To determine if polyps are present.
- To assess abnormal uterine bleeding.
- To assess the effects of hormonal therapy.
- To screen for early detection of endometrial cancer (particularly if risk factors are present).

The American Cancer Society considers women with the following factors to be at high risk for endometrial cancer:

- Currently on estrogen therapy
- Obesity
- History of failure to ovulate
- History of infertility
- History of abnormal bleeding

An EMB is performed with the patient in the lithotomy position. The physician performs a bimanual examination of the uterus and administers a local anesthetic. A uterine sound is inserted into the uterus after the anesthetic has taken effect. The specimen is taken by means of a curette or with a suction device to aspirate a specimen. The specimen is sent to the laboratory in a container containing a 10% formalin preservative solution.

Provide a perineal pad for the patient with instructions for home care. The patient should receive instructions to call the physician if there is abnormal pain or bleeding after this procedure. She may experience mild cramping for which the physician may advise her to take a mild analgesic. She should be advised against using a tampon or douching for at least 72 hours.

Incision & Drainage (I & D)

Incision and drainage is performed to relieve the buildup of purulent (pus) material as a result of infection. The purulent discharge may need to be cultured to determine what microorganism is causing the infection, and thus, what antibiotic would be effective. The procedure is performed using sterile surgical technique. It should be remembered that the purulent material may be highly infectious. All soiled dressings and 4 × 4s should immediately be placed in a plastic waste container and then disposed of properly using OSHA guidelines.

A tray setup for an I & D would include:

- Scalpel handle and blades (No. 11)
- Curved iris scissors
- Tissue forceps
- Kelly hemostat
- Retractor
- Thumb dressing forceps
- 4 × 4 gauze squares

Removal of Foreign Bodies and Growths

A foreign body can include a variety of materials from a small splinter or fishhook to a large object, such as an arrow that is imbedded in tissue. Splinter forceps are needed on a tray for foreign body removal.

Growths include tumors, warts, moles, cysts. The most frequent growth removal procedure in the medical office is for cysts which are enclosed fluid-filled sacs. Some growths will be sent to the laboratory for biopsy testing depending upon the physician's instructions. The removal of a foreign body or neoplasm (growth) requires a surgical setup that includes:

- Thumb dressing forceps
- Retractor
- Scalpel handle and blades (No. 10 and 15)
- Curved tissue scissors
- Tissue forceps
- Hemostats
- Blunt probe
- Splinter forceps
- Needle holder
- Suture materials and needles
- Sterile 4 × 4 gauze

Figure 23-30 shows a surgical tray—biopsy removal.

Vasectomy

The vasectomy procedure, tying and cutting of the vas deferens, on the male patient is a surgical procedure that is now commonly performed in the urologist's office. A vasectomy provides a permanent form of birth control for the male. As with any surgical procedure, a consent form needs to be signed and in the patient's record before beginning this irreversible procedure. The patient should be instructed to bring someone with them who can drive them home after the procedure. The patient will be uncomfortable for a short period of time

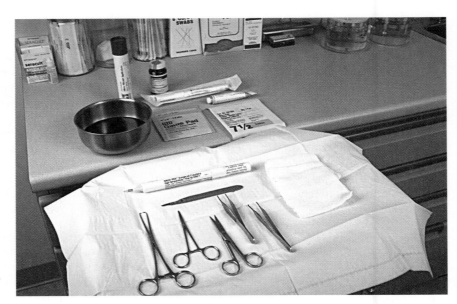

Figure 23-30 Surgical tray— biopsy removal.

(2-3 days). He should be given detailed instructions on home care including activity level and sexual intercourse. The instructions may vary somewhat from one urologist to another. A typical vasectomy tray will include:

- Scalpel handle and No. 15 blade
- Dressing forceps

- Towel clamp
- Straight and Curved Mosquito forceps
- Curved tissue scissors
- Tissue forceps
- Retractor
- Needle holder and suture material
- Suture scissors
- 4 × 4 gauze squares

LEGAL AND ETHICAL ISSUES

All patients must sign an informed consent form before any surgical procedure. This means that it is not enough to just tell the patient what procedure they are having done. The surgeon must also explain the risks, what might occur if nothing is done, and what other options are available. The medical assistant reinforces what the physician has explained and makes sure that there is a patient signature on the consent form before the procedure begins. If there is any doubt about the patient's ability to understand instructions, the medical assistant must bring this to the physician's attention. Preoperative and postoperative instructions should be read to the patient and clarified, if necessary.

Sterility during a surgical procedure cannot be compromised. The medical assistant has an ethical duty to provide the safest surgical environment possible for the patient.

Confidentiality relating to any surgical procedure a patient undergoes must be maintained. It is the physician's role to give the patient information about results of surgical procedures, biopsies, and tests.

Insurance information must be accurately documented. It is considered fraudulent to knowingly provide inaccurate information to an insurance company.

PATIENT EDUCATION

The medical assistant has a prominent role in educating the patient who will have a surgical procedure. Assisting the physician with obtaining the surgical consent is an opportunity to reinforce the physician's instructions. Explanations presented in easy to understand language can assure the patient will follow the correct steps of preparation.

Summary

Assisting with surgery includes maintaining aseptic technique, a thorough knowledge of gowning, gloving, surgical handwashing, setting up sterile instrument trays and passing equipment to the physician, packaging, and preparing the patient for the procedure. Assisting with surgical procedures carries with it a grave responsibility to maintain absolute sterile technique. The medical assistant incorporates a variety of clinical skills when assisting with a surgical procedure.

Competency Review

1. Define and spell the glossary terms for this chapter.
2. Perform handwashing using medical aseptic technique; using surgical aseptic technique.
3. Identify by name the pieces of equipment needed for:
   a. suture removal
   b. incision and drainage
   c. suture of laceration
   d. cervical biopsy
   e. removal of foreign body
   f. dressing change with wound culture
   g. endometrial biopsy
4. You have an open sore on your hand. What procedure should you follow when preparing to assist the surgeon?

ON THE JOB

Victor Krenz is assisting Dr. Connors with the fifth cataract surgical procedure for the day. The patient is Kathy Wall, a diabetic patient, whose condition has been stable enough for her to undergo a surgical procedure. Victor has performed a six minute surgical scrub on his hands before each of the five procedures. Dr. Connors indicates that he is in a hurry to get back to his office for a heavy afternoon schedule of patients. After both Dr. Connors and Victor are scrubbed and gowned and ready to begin the operation, Victor feels a slight prick on the tip of his gloved finger as he moves the sterile syringe and needle on the tray. Dr. Connors, who doesn't notice the accidental needle prick to Victor's glove, states again what a hurry he is in to finish this procedure. Victor knows that if he has to change gloves it will delay the surgery. He also knows that his hands have had a surgical scrub five times that morning and they are clean.

What is your response?

1. Can Victor justify not changing into new gloves?
2. What could happen to Ms. Wall as a result of Victor's needle prick?
3. How should Victor handle this situation?

PREPARING FOR THE CERTIFICATION EXAM

Test Taking Tip — Be sure to eat breakfast or a light meal before taking a major examination, such as the CMA exam.

Examination Review Questions

1. Which of the following should NOT touch a sterile field?
   (A) 4 × 4s
   (B) transfer forceps
   (C) gloved hands
   (D) sterile specimen container
   (E) used instruments

2. The area that is considered sterile on a draped Mayo stand is
   (A) within a 2-inch border
   (B) outside a 2-inch border
   (C) within a 1-inch border
   (D) outside a 1-inch border
   (E) the entire drape is sterile

3. The portion of a hemostat located near the handle that protects it from slipping once it is closed is the
   (A) tooth
   (B) ratchet
   (C) serrated tip
   (D) lock
   (E) clamp

4. An instrument used by an obstetrician to measure an expectant mother's pelvis is the
   (A) curette
   (B) dilator
   (C) pelvimeter
   (D) vaginal speculum
   (E) none of the above

5. What is the correct method for shaving a surgical patient during the skin prep?
   (A) dry shave going with the grain
   (B) wet shave going against the grain
   (C) wet shave before preparing the patient's skin
   (D) wet shave going with the grain
   (E) dry shave after preparing the patient's skin

6. The surgical handwashing is performed
   (A) for 10 minutes using a clean hand brush
   (B) for 10 minutes using a sterile hand brush
   (C) by scrubbing for 2 minutes after removing rings
   (D) with a brush and disinfectant
   (E) using a germicidal soap

7. An example of a small gauge suture used for the skin is
   (A) stainless steel 5-0
   (B) stainless steel 0
   (C) plain gut 3-0
   (D) chromic gut 2-0
   (E) nylon 2-0

8. When applying sterile gloves
   (A) pick up the first glove under the cuff and pull over the other hand slowly
   (B) hold the gloves over the sink while you apply them since the sink is considered "clean"
   (C) place the fingers of the gloved hand under the cuff of the second glove, and then apply
   (D) leave the cuffs turned down after applying since this cuff will catch any spilled fluids
   (E) apply the gloves before setting up the equipment

9. When transferring sterile solutions to a sterile field
   (A) place the cap with outside edge facing up
   (B) place the cap with inside facing up
   (C) place the cap on the Mayo stand
   (D) pour the liquid by stabilizing the bottle on the edge of the basin
   (E) discard the liquid remaining in the bottle

10. A typical surgical setup consists of
    (A) scalpel, blades, trocar, probe, scope
    (B) scalpel, blades, hemostat, probe, scope
    (C) scalpel, blades, hemostat, scissors, suture
    (D) scalpel, blades, hemostat, scissors, suture, scope
    (E) scalpel, blades, scissors, suture, speculum

References

Fremgen, B. *Medical Terminology.* Upper Saddle River, NJ: Brady/Prentice Hall, 1997.

Fry, J., Higton, I., and Stephenson, J., *Colour Atlas of Minor Surgery in General Practice.* Boston: Kluwer Academic Publishers, 1990.

Groah, L. *Operating Room Nursing.* East Norwalk, CT: Appleton and Lange, 1990.

Nurse's Pocket Companion. Springhouse, PA: Springhouse Corporation, 1993.

Potter, P., Perry, P. *Fundamentals of Nursing— Concepts, Process and Practice,* 3rd ed. St. Louis: Mosby Year Book, 1993.

Reichert, M., Young, J. *Sterilization Technology in the Health Care Facility.* Gaithersburg, MD: Aspen, 1993.

Sheldon, H. *Boyd's Introduction to the Study of Disease.* Philadelphia: Lea and Febiger, 1992.

Taber's Cyclopedic Medical Dictionary, 18th edition. Philadelphia: F.A. Davis Company, 1997.

MEDICAL ASSISTANT ROLE DELINEATION CHART

Highlight indicates material covered in this chapter

ADMINISTRATIVE

ADMINISTRATIVE PROCEDURES

- Perform basic clerical functions
- Schedule, coordinate, and monitor appointments
- Schedule inpatient/outpatient admissions and procedures
- Understand and apply third party guidelines
- Obtain reimbursement through accurate claims submission
- Monitor third-party reimbursement
- Perform medical transcription
- Understand and adhere to managed care policies and procedures
- *Negotiate managed care contracts (adv)*

PRACTICE FINANCES

- Perform procedural and diagnostic coding
- Apply bookkeeping principles
- Document and maintain accounting and banking records
- Manage accounts receivable
- Manage accounts payable
- Process payroll
- *Develop and maintain fee schedules (adv)*
- *Manage renewals of business and professional insurance policies (adv)*
- *Manage personal benefits and maintain records (adv)*

CLINICAL

FUNDAMENTAL PRINCIPLES

- Apply principles of aseptic technique and infection control
- Comply with quality assurance practices
- Screen and follow up patient test results

DIAGNOSTIC ORDERS

- Collect and process specimens
- Perform diagnostic tests

PATIENT CARE

- Adhere to established triage procedures
- Obtain patient history and vital signs
- Prepare and maintain examination and treatment areas

- Prepare patient for examinations, procedures, and treatments
- Assist with examinations, procedures, and treatments
- Prepare and administer medications and immunizations
- Maintain medication and immunization records
- Recognize and respond to emergencies
- Coordinate patient care information with other health care providers

GENERAL (TRANSDISCIPLINARY)

PROFESSIONALISM

- Project a professional manner and image
- Adhere to ethical principles
- Demonstrate initiative and responsibility
- Work as a team member
- Manage time efficiently
- Prioritize and perform multiple tasks
- Adapt to change
- Promote the CMA credential
- Enhance skills through continuing education

COMMUNICATION SKILLS

- Treat all patients with compassion and empathy
- Recognize and respect cultural diversity
- Adapt communications to individual's ability to understand
- Use professional telephone technique
- Use effective and correct verbal and written communications
- Recognize and respond to verbal and non-verbal communications
- Use medical terminology appropriately
- Receive, organize, prioritize, and transmit information
- Serve as liaison
- Promote the practice through positive public relations

LEGAL CONCEPTS

- Maintain confidentiality
- Practice within the scope of education, training, and personal capabilities
- Prepare and maintain medical records
- Document accurately
- Use appropriate guidelines when releasing information
- Follow employer's established policies dealing with the health care contract
- Follow federal, state, and local legal guidelines
- Maintain awareness of federal and state health care legislation and regulations
- Maintain and dispose of regulated substances in compliance with government guidelines
- Comply with established risk management and safety procedures
- Recognize professional credentialing criteria
- Participate in the development and maintenance of personnel, policy, and procedure manuals
- *Develop and maintain personnel, policy, and procedure manuals (adv)*

INSTRUCTION

- Instruct individuals according to their needs
- Explain office policies and procedures
- Teach methods of health promotion and disease prevention
- Locate community resources and disseminate information
- *Orient and train personnel (adv)*
- *Develop educational materials (adv)*
- *Conduct continuing education activities (adv)*

OPERATIONAL FUNCTIONS

- Maintain supply inventory
- Evaluate and recommend equipment and supplies
- Apply computer techniques to support office operations
- *Supervise personnel (adv)*
- *Interview and recommend job applicants (adv)*
- *Negotiate leases and prices for equipment and supply contracts (adv)*

SOURCE: Reprinted by permission of the American Association of Medical Assistants from the *AAMA Role Delineation Study: Occupational Analysis of the Medical Assisting Profession.*

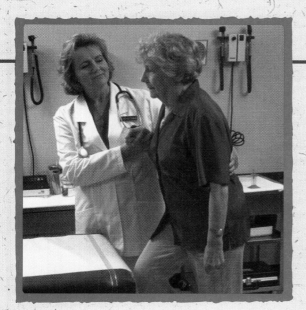

24

Patients with Special Physical and Emotional Needs

LEARNING OBJECTIVES

After completing this chapter, you should:
1. Define and spell all the glossary terms for this chapter.
2. Describe the patient education needs of the colostomy patient.
3. State the mechanism of tube feeding.
4. Discuss intravenous therapy as it relates to the medical assistant.
5. List guidelines when assisting the hearing impaired or the blind patient.
6. Discuss the concerns when assisting the elderly.
7. Describe assisting the terminally ill patient.
8. List and discuss the five stages of dying.
9. List 10 major diagnostic categories of mental disease.
10. State the difference between neurosis and psychosis.
11. Describe 8 health habits to cope with stress.

CLINICAL PERFORMANCE COMPETENCIES

After completing this chapter, you should perform the following tasks:
1. Assist the patient recovering from a stroke.
2. Provide patient education for the ostomy patient.
3. Discuss cast care with a patient.
4. Communicate with the hearing impaired patient.
5. Escort the blind patient into an examination room.
6. Communicate by listening to a patient with a terminal illness.

Glossary

bipolar disorder   Manic-depressive mental disorder.

cerebrovascular accident (CVA)   Hemorrhage within the brain which may result in paralysis and loss of speech.

colostomy   An artificial opening created surgically into the large bowel for the removal of waste (feces).

gerontology   Scientific study of the effects of aging and age-related diseases.

hemiplegia   Paralysis on one side of the body.

holistic   Viewing the human body as a whole organism.

ileostomy   An artificial opening created surgically into the small intestine for the removal of waste.

intravenous   Inserting a medication or fluid into the vein via a needle or tube.

neuroses   Mild emotional disturbances that impair judgment.

psychoses   Severe mental disorders that interfere with a perception of reality.

terminal illness   Illness that is expected to end in death.

Many patients who come into the physician's office or clinic will have physical or emotional problems that are not the main reason for their appointment. The medical assistant must be able to care for the entire person in a holistic fashion.

There are several techniques for assisting patients that are discussed below including providing education for colostomy and feeding tube care. The medical assistant may not be providing direct care for patients who have procedures such as a colostomy, but must understand the procedure to be able to answer questions the patient may have. Medical assistants should not perform procedures outside their scope of practice.

Assisting a Patient Recovering From a Stroke

A cerebrovascular accident (CVA) is a hemorrhagic lesion within the brain which may result in paralysis and the inability to speak. This is commonly referred to as a stroke. The causes of stroke include a cerebral hemorrhage, cerebral embolism, cerebral thrombosis, and compression. A cerebral hemorrhage is the rupture of a blood vessel within the brain. Cerebral embolism results when a clot or foreign body forms in another part of the body and travels to the brain. Cerebral thrombosis is a blood clot forming within a vessel in the brain. Compression as a cause of stroke is the result of a blood clot, or tumor, compressing on a blood vessel with the resulting closure of the vessel.

Occupational therapists and physical therapists assist stroke patients with their recovery. The medical assistant needs to understand the needs of this patient to help with patient education and such techniques as wheelchair transfer.

Many stroke patients recover some use of their limbs as a result of physical therapy and the normal healing process. Speech, in varying degrees, may also return. Assisting the stroke patient requires patience in helping them to communicate their thoughts. See Figure 24-1 for an illustration of assisting a stroke patient.

Patient education is an important component of assisting the disabled patient. There are many assistive devices available for CVA (stroke) and physically challenged patients (Figure 24-2 A and B).

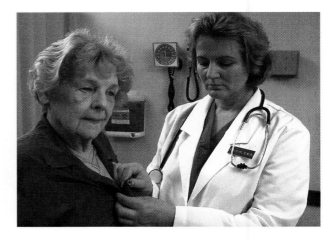

Figure 24-1   Assisting a stroke patient.

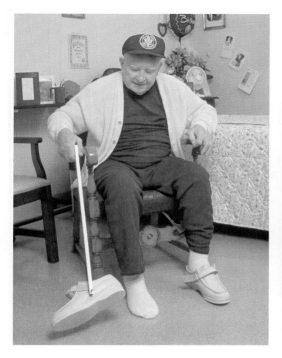
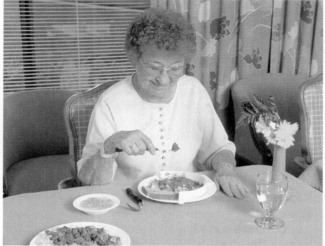

Figure 24-2 A and B   Assistance devices for CVA patients.

The Patient with the Ostomy

The small intestine and large intestine (colon) may become diseased or injured. If large portions of these digestive organs must be surgically removed, it is often necessary to create an artificial opening into the abdomen for the removal of solid body waste. In some cases this is only a temporary mechanism such as might occur while the colon is allowed to heal after an injury.

The creation of this artificial opening into the abdomen is called an ostomy. The actual opening (orifice) is called the stoma. Ostomies are surgically created to treat conditions such as cancer and Crohn's disease. A colostomy is an opening into the large bowel (colon), while an ileostomy is an opening into the ileum of the small intestine. The opening leads directly from the external abdomen into the affected organ (small or large intestine) and resembles a pink rosebud in appearance.

There are several types of colostomies based upon the portion of the intestine that is removed during surgery. There is generally only one opening (single barrel), but in some cases the surgeon will place two openings (double barrel). See an illustration of the various types and placements of ostomies in Figure 24-3.

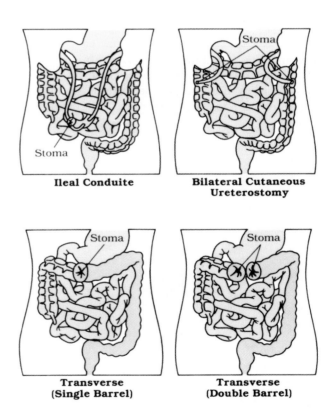

Figure 24-3   Various types and placements of ostomies.

The patient must wear an appliance to collect the waste material as it leaves the body (Figure 24-4). The collection bag is held over the stoma with a special paste, adhesive, adhesive wafer, or a belt (Figure 24-5 A-C). Some collection bags are reusable and need to be cleaned and dried after each use. In this case the patient will need several bags so a fresh one is always available. There are also disposable collection bags available.

Patients should be reminded to change their collection bags when they are full or the seal around the colostomy is broken. In some cases the physician will direct the patient to irrigate their colostomy with a warm water solution to stimulate waste movement. This is similar to an enema.

Patients with a new colostomy will require patient education relating hygiene and handling the colostomy equipment. In most cases the patient will be instructed on home care before leaving the hospital. The medical assistant should be familiar with equipment needs and be able to answer questions the patient may have at the time the patient comes in for an office visit. The procedure for patient teaching of the ostomy patient follows.

Understanding Intravenous Therapy

The medical assistant will not administer intravenous therapy (IV) since only licensed personnel, such as nurses, are permitted to do that. However, the medical assistant will come into

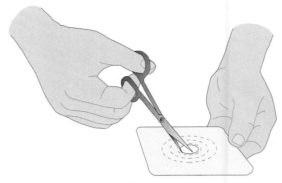

A Cut the hole in the center of the wafer 1/8 inch larger than the stoma.

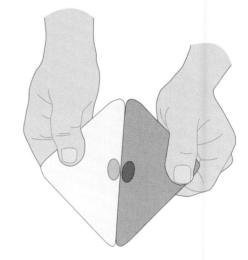

B Peel the backing from the wafer.

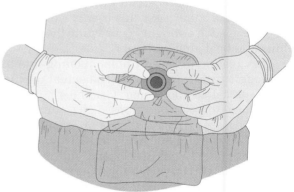

C Place the wafer over the stoma and attach a clean bag.

Figure 24-5   Special paste, an adhesive wafer, or a belt holds the ostomy bag in place over the stoma.

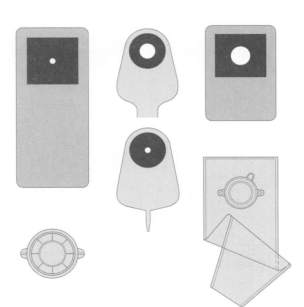

Figure 24-4   Ostomy collection bags.

contact with patients who have intravenous therapy. These include patients in a clinic setting, home-bound patients, or patients who receive chemotherapy on an out-patient basis.

Intravenous therapy is medication or fluid that is administered directly into a patient's vein. Intravenous therapy is prescribed by a physician as either a continuous infusion or drip from a bottle or bag or by single injection (Figure 24-6). A pump may also be used to regulate the flow of the medication into the vein.

Continuous infusion means that the fluid must be running into the vein continuously. If the drip of fluid stops the vein may form a small clot of blood. In this case the IV will have to be restarted by a nurse. To prevent the patient from undergoing this procedure twice, it is wise to report any cessation of dripping immediately.

When the patient receives a single dosage via the intravenous route on a regular basis, a small needle with a port (opening), which is called a Heparin lock, may be inserted into the patient's wrist area. This is sealed with a cap and then taped in place. Each time the patient receives the medication, the cap is removed from the port, and tubing is inserted. Medication is administered through this tubing. In some cases the port opening contains a rubber/plastic stopper and needle can be placed into the port for direct administration of the drug.

If a patient comes into the physician's office with an IV port in place, you should be alert to changes at the IV site and report them to the physician at once. The following should be reported:

- Blood or drainage from the area of insertion
- Redness, pain or swelling in the area
- Blood has backed up into the tubing
- The needle or tube has come loose or been removed by the patient

Understanding Tube Feeding

A patient may come into the office with a feeding tube in place. Tube feedings provide nutritional supplements directly into the patient's upper gastrointestinal tract. The patient receives both liquid food supplements, water, and medication via this route. This method of feeding is used when a patient is unable to swallow due to a surgical procedure such as the removal of the esophagus due to cancer, or the inability to swallow due to paralysis.

The surgeon, after making an incision, inserts a feeding tube in one of several areas: gastrostomy, duodenostomy, and jejunostomy. Figure 24-7 illustrates a gastrostomy tube in place. A plastic bag filled with the fluids is connected to a port of the feeding tube. When the patient is not receiving the feeding, the bag is disconnected, the port sealed and taped to the patient's body, allowing the patient to move around freely.

The patient and his or her family will require support and patient instruction on the need for good hygiene. Remind the patient to discard any feedings that are more than 24 hours old and to warm all solutions to room temperature before placing them into the tube. Tube feedings should be allowed to enter the body slowly using only the force of gravity. The patient should never try to force the contents of the tube feeding bag. Remind the patient to report any symptoms of distress, such as nausea, vomiting, cramps, or diarrhea, to the physician.

Cast Care

Casts are applied for the purpose of immobilizing a broken bone or muscle strain and sprain. A cast may be applied after a surgical procedure on a limb to immobilize the area until healing takes place. Casts are made from a variety of pliable material which the physician will mold to fit the body part. A cast can be considered to be a form of nonflexible bandage. Casts are generally applied using a plaster-type material which is applied wet

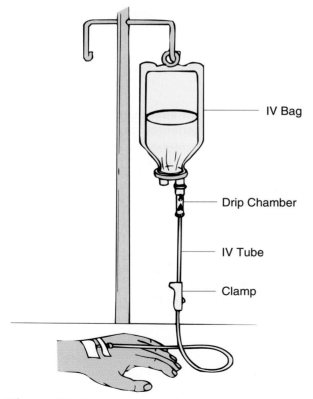

IV Bag

Drip Chamber

IV Tube

Clamp

Figure 24-6   Intravenous therapy.

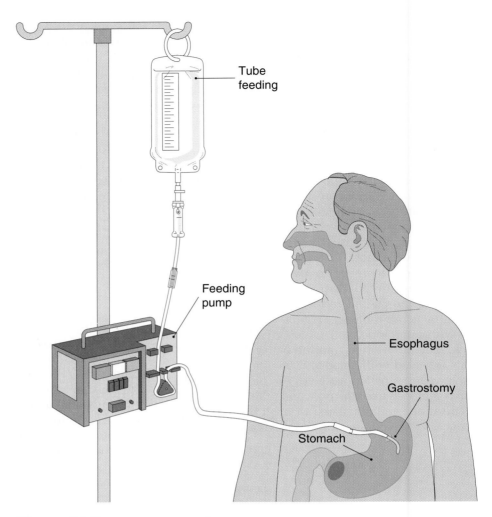

Figure 24-7   A gastrostomy tube.

around a stockinette liner and cotton padding over the limb. As the cast dries it becomes hard. Newer synthetic fiberglass materials are being used to form casts since they are lighter in weight than a plaster cast. The medical assistant should use caution when handling fiberglass materials by wearing protective glasses or eye shield.

The medical assistant may be asked to assist the physician in applying the cast. It may be necessary to hold the limb at the joint areas as the cast is being applied. Remember to handle a damaged limb gently.

After the cast has been applied, it must be left uncovered during the drying process. The limb may need to be supported on a pillow at this time. The patient should be cautioned against moving around until the cast is dry. The cast may become warm or even hot during the drying process. This is normal.

The patient's limb should not become hot or cold once the cast has been applied. Frequent checks of the patient's circulation will alert the

medical assistant to any change in the patient's circulation. The patient should be instructed to call the physician if any of the following problems are observed:

- Circulation restricted by the cast.
- Pain as a result of the cast pinching the skin.
- Excessive itching under the cast.
- Numbness or tingling of fingers or toes.
- Discolored toes or fingers.
- Swelling of the limb around the edge of the cast.
- Discoloration soaking through the cast.
- Loosely fitting cast.
- Foul odor coming from the cast.

The physician should advise the patient on the amount of weight and movement which can be applied to the cast. Remind the patient that nothing should be put into the edges of the cast. The cast should not get wet. The patient may be able to

PROCEDURE: Patient Education for Colostomy Patient

**Terminal Performance
Competency:** Teach patient to care for colostomy using correct medical aseptic technique.

Equipment and Supplies
Ostomy bag
Ostomy belt
Adhesive (if used)
Scissors
Soap
Water
Washcloth
Toilet tissue
Lubricant or skin cream as ordered by physician
Plastic waste bag
Towels
Basin or sink

Procedural Steps

1. Instruct patient to wash hands before starting. The patient does not have to wear gloves, unless he or she wishes to, when performing their own colostomy care. Gloves should be worn by the medical assistant if he or she assists the patient.

2. Assemble equipment in the bathroom on a clean surface. Patient may wish to cover the bathroom counter with a clean towel. If using an adhesive wafer, prepare it by cutting a hole in the center of the wafer 1/8 inch larger than the stoma. Place this on the clean towel.

3. Standing over the open toilet, open the belt holding the appliance in place and remove it. Empty contents into the toilet. It should be placed into a basin or sink for cleaning after the procedure is completed.

4. Remove the soiled plastic stoma bag. If it is disposable, place it into the waste bag. If it is reusable, place it in a basin or sink for cleaning after the procedure is completed.

5. Wipe the area around the ostomy with toilet tissue to remove any loose feces. Dispose of tissue into the toilet.

6. With a wet, soapy washcloth carefully wash the entire area around the ostomy. Rinse with clear water and dry gently.

7. Apply a small amount of lubricant or cream (if ordered) to the skin around the ostomy. Wipe off any excess lubricant so the ostomy bag will adhere securely to the skin.

8. If using an adhesive wafer, peel the backing from the wafer and apply it directly on the skin and with the hole over the stoma opening. If an adhesive is used, place a small amount around the stoma on the skin. Use care in not getting adhesive onto the stoma.

9. Attach a clean bag to the wafer or adhesive.

10. Place the clean adjustable belt around the lower abdomen and loop the stoma bag openings through the belt.

11. Thoroughly clean all reusable equipment in warm, soapy water. Allow the reusable colostomy bag to air dry.

12. Clean bathroom surface thoroughly.

13. Remind the patient that feces contains *E.coli* bacteria which can cause gastrointestinal upsets and disease if not washed thoroughly off surfaces.

Charting Example
2/14/XX   9a.m.   Pt. instructed regarding colostomy care. Pt. stated the procedure correctly. To return for follow-up care.
M. King, CMA

tie a strong plastic bag around the cast in order to take a shower.

> **Med Tip:** Always listen to a patient's complaints about a cast. A limb will frequently become swollen after an injury. When the cast has dried it may constrict circulation due to swelling present. It can be very dangerous to ignore this diminished circulation. The cast will have to be removed immediately if circulation is impaired.

Assisting the Hearing Impaired Patient

Hearing impairment is a problem of the general population for several reasons. First, people are living longer. Since hearing loss accompanies old age, there are a greater number of people over 50 years of age requiring hearing assistance such as a hearing aid. In addition, more people are exposed to loud sounds in the work environment or through the use of earphones when listening to loud music.

Children who are born deaf have several options open to them with the advent of the new amplification (hearing aid) technology and the cochlear implant. Some types of deafness will not benefit from a hearing aid or other technology, however. When this is the case the patient must learn to communicate using sign language, speech reading, or a combination of both.

> **Med Tip:** Deafness is considered the most difficult of all handicaps since it keeps people isolated from communication and social interaction. If a child cannot hear, he or she will have difficulty speaking since learning speech is imitating the speech of others. Basic sign language is not difficult to learn. Simple phrases in sign language should be a part of every medical professional's knowledge base.

Basic hearing tests or screening tests are often performed by the medical assistant in the physician's office. An audiogram may be ordered by the physician when there is a suspicion of moderate to severe hearing loss. This test will illustrate the faintest sounds a patient can hear during audiometric testing. Audiometric testing, con-

Guidelines: Helping the Hearing Impaired Patient

- Never shout. Speak slowly and clearly.
- If the patient does not understand you the first time, rephrase the statement the second time. The patient may not understand again if you use the same phrases and sounds.
- Explain everything carefully before doing any procedure.
- Face the patient when you are speaking. Many hearing impaired have learned some lip reading.
- Have paper and a pen nearby so that you and the patient can communicate in writing. The hearing impaired person is often not able to make all of the speech sounds if he or she has never heard them.
- Allow the patient to listen with your stethoscope earpieces as you speak into the bell.
- Do not speak too loudly or yell at the hearing impaired person.

ducted by an audiologist, tests hearing ability by determining the lowest and highest intensity and frequencies that a person can distinguish (Figure 24-8). The patient may sit in a soundproof booth and receive sounds through earphones as the technician decreases the sound tones or waves.

Assisting the Blind Patient

Blindness can be present at birth or may develop as a result of a disease such as diabetes mellitus. Patients who are blind can remain independent. The medical assistant can communicate and help the blind patient by remembering to follow the guidelines for assisting the blind patient.

Assisting the Elderly Patient

Gerontology is a relatively new area of medical practice. It is the study of the effects of aging on people and the treatment of age-related disorders such as osteoarthritis, congestive heart failure, arthritis, emphysema, cerebrovascular accident (CVA), and Alzheimer's disease.

In general, some of the same conditions that affect a younger population also affect the elderly. The healing time may be longer and elasticity of joints and muscles may be diminished.

Some of the physical problems associated with aging may cause people to lose their independence. These changes include the body's central nervous system slowing down which creates prob-

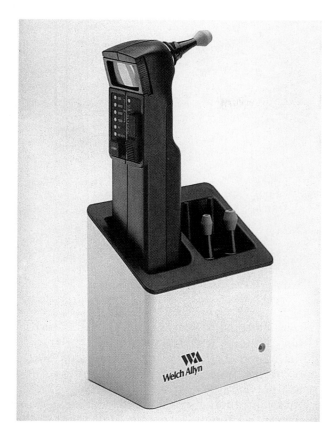

Figure 24-8 Audiometer.

Guidelines: Assisting the Blind Patient

- Always speak to announce your presence when you are near a blind person. In most cases their other senses, such as hearing, will become highly developed. But they may become startled if you touch them without telling them of your presence.
- Offer to guide the patient into an examination room by offering your arm. A blind patient will prefer to hold onto your arm, rather than to have someone grab their arm.
- Try to face the patient and speak clearly. They are unable to read your lips as a normal sighted person can do.
- Describe their surroundings.
- Try not to leave the patient alone for any length of time.
- Explain everything carefully before doing any procedure.

lems in detecting heat, cold, and pain. Thought processes and memory may fail in some people. The senses (hearing, sight, smell, taste, touch) may become diminished. Muscle tone may become

Med Tip: Many people make the mistake of thinking the blind person is also hard of hearing. It is not necessary to speak loudly to this patient.

poor from lack of exercise and muscle atrophy. Bones may become brittle and fracture more easily. Rapid changes in body position may cause the blood pressure to drop with a resulting dizziness and/or fainting called postural hypotension. Circulation may slow down with a resulting effect upon the heart.

Some of these body changes can affect how the elderly will metabolize drugs. Signs of toxicity must be carefully noted so the physician can make dosage adjustments. Many elderly patients remain active and relatively healthy into their late 80's (Figure 24-9).

Alzheimer's Disease

Alzheimer's disease is a progressive disorder of the central nervous system that eventually destroys mental functions. This is a progressive disease which predominantly affects the elderly population. There is no known cause or cure for this disease at the present time. For these reasons, Alzheimer's disease can have a devastating effect on family members as well as on the patient. The medical assistant must be supportive of family members also.

One of the first signs of Alzheimer's disease is loss of memory. While there is a normal loss of some memory as people age (forgetting dates, names, and telephone numbers), the memory loss with Alzheimer's is profound. The patient may not remember where they live and forget who their family members are. The patient with Alzheimer's disease must be kept in safe surroundings with someone observing their movements. The patient cannot be left alone in a waiting or examination room. Other symptoms include agitation, restlessness, irritability, inability to care for oneself, incontinence, and inability to communicate.

Assisting the Patient with Terminal Illness

The medical assistant will come into contact with patients who have a terminal illness. A terminal illness is one that is expected to end in death. This includes conditions and diseases such as cancer, acquired immune deficiency syndrome (AIDS),

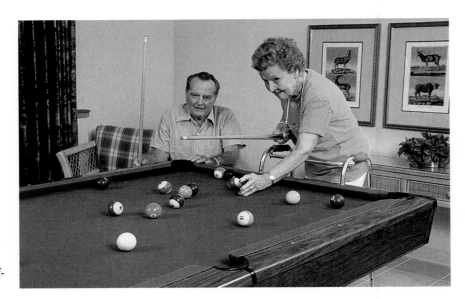

Figure 24-9 Continued activity can have a positive effect on patients.

progressive heart disease, amyotropic lateral sclerosis (Lou Gehrig's Disease), cystic fibrosis, and multiple sclerosis.

In cases in which the dying process is slow for the patient, the medical assistant may have the opportunity to be with the patient on several occasions during office visits. While there is always hope of recovery or finding a cure through research for a disease such as AIDS, it is wise to listen to a patient express his or her fears and concerns rather than to offer false hope for a recovery.

Death is a natural process which everyone must face. People have various ways of coping with their own death based on a variety of influences including culture, religion, personal experience, and age.

Culture

People learn what their own culture expects of them at a very early age by observing family and friends as they handle life events such as births and deaths. In some cultures death is considered a normal end to the life process and accepted with peace. In other cultures death may be feared.

The terminally ill patient and family may have already established a very personal approach or method for handling death and dying. The medical assistant may also have a strong cultural attitude toward death.

Religion

Religious beliefs play an important role in the manner patients handle death and dying. Some patients will have a strong belief in an afterlife. Other patients will follow no particular religious belief. In both cases, the patients' death and dying process can be meaningful and peaceful.

It is considered unacceptable for the medical assistant to attempt to convert the patient to the medical assistant's religious faith. Professionalism mandates that the medical assistant and other staff members recognize and support the patient's right to embrace his or her own religious beliefs.

Personal Experience

The past experiences of the patient and the medical assistant will mold how they approach the topic of death. If the patient has been closely involved with the care of someone who has died a painful death, the patient may fear the same type of death for himself or herself. These patients will need to be able to discuss their fears. In the same manner, if the medical assistant has had past experiences with the death of friends or relatives, it may be easier to assist the patient.

Age

The elderly often have less fear of death than someone younger. In some cases an elderly person may not feel well, have failing eyesight, hearing, and memory, and may look upon death with relief. If the patient wishes to discuss his or her approaching death, the medical assistant should be ready to listen.

TABLE 24-1   Five Stages of Grief

Stage	Description
Denial	A refusal to believe that dying is taking place. This may be a time when the patient (or family member) needs time to adjust to the reality of approaching death. This stage cannot be hurried.
Anger	At this stage the patient may be angry at everyone and may express this intense anger at God, family, and even health care professionals. The patient may take this anger out on the closest person to them. Usually this is a family member. In reality the patient is angry about dying.
Bargaining	The third stage of grief involves attempting to gain time by making promises in return. Bargaining may be done between the patient and God. The patient may indicate a need to talk at this stage.
Depression	This stage is marked with a deep sadness over the loss of health, independence, and eventually life. There is an additional sadness of leaving loved ones behind. The grieving patient may become withdrawn at this time.
Acceptance	The acceptance stage is reached when there is a sense of peace and calm. The patient may make comments such as, "I have no regrets. I'm ready to die." It is better to let the patient talk and not make denial statements such as, "Don't talk like that. You're not going to die."

The Stages of Grief

Doctor Elizabeth Kubler-Ross has spent much of her life devoted to the study of the dying process and working with the dying patient. She has divided the dying process into five stages which she believes all persons go through. It is helpful to understand these stages when attempting to help the dying patient.

According to Kubler-Ross, all those involved with the dying process may go through the five stages. This would include the patient, family members, and caregivers (such as the medical assistant).

The five stages are denial, anger, bargaining, depression, and acceptance. The stages may overlap and may not be experienced by everyone in the stated order but are all present in the dying person, according to Kubler-Ross. The five stages are discussed in Table 24-1.

As the time of death approaches, some of the earlier stages may be repeated. For example, the patient may become angry when they are not able to care for themselves. The critical point to remember when assisting a patient who is dying is that the grieving period is a normal part of the dying process.

Hospice care, which is physical and emotional care provided the dying person, is a growing movement throughout the US. The medical assistant should be acquainted with this option for care of the terminally ill.

Psychology

Psychology is the science of behavior and the human thought process. This behavioral science is primarily concerned with human beings acting alone or in groups. A psychologist is one who is trained in the methods of psychological analysis, therapy, and research.

There is a distinction between normal and abnormal behavior when studying psychology. Abnormal psychology is the study of behavior that deviates from the normal. This includes psychoneuroses, psychoses, psychosomatic disorders, personality and sociopathic disorders, and disturbances occurring in intoxication, brain damage, and brain disease.

All social interactions, such as might occur in the communication process, pose some problems for some people. These problems are not necessarily abnormal. One means of judging if behavior is abnormal is to compare one person's behavior against others in the community. If a person's behavior interferes with the activities of daily living, it is often considered abnormal.

The Mind-Body Connection

Psychologists have discovered that there is a link between stress and illness. There are predisposing factors which create a tendency or susceptibility to become stressed. These include attitudes and feelings (emotions such as optimism or pessimism), health habits (smoking, exercise, drug use and diet), the individual patient's methods for coping, economic and social resources (income, kind of job, security) and the state of the patient's immune system.

Many patients with a major illness go through a period of depression. The disease may cause emotional changes. In turn worry about the disease may cause unhealthy habits such as an increase in smoking or drinking. Patients who have a physical illness such as heart disease, diabetes, or AIDS may become additionally stressed when confronted with the loss of income or a job.

In addition there are personality types in individuals that some psychologists believe may cause the person to become ill. The Type-A behavior pattern individual is considered to be someone who is constantly struggling to achieve, is irritable, hostile, and impatient with anyone who gets in their way, and has a sense of time urgency. It is believed by some psychologists that this type of personality is more prone to some diseases such as cancer and heart disease. Type-B people are considered by the psychologists to be calmer and less intense. Much research has been conducted about the two personality types and not all scientists and psychologists agree about a link between personality and illness.

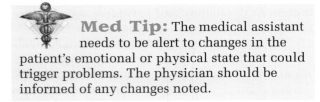

Med Tip: The medical assistant needs to be alert to changes in the patient's emotional or physical state that could trigger problems. The physician should be informed of any changes noted.

Health Habits

Certain major life events such as the death of a loved one, divorce, an unexpected move away from family and friends, unemployment, or illness can trigger stress. Recommendations for coping with stress include:

- Develop a strong support system including family and friends
- Find a balance between perfection and fear of failure
- Eat nutritious meals
- Avoid harmful habits such as smoking and drinking
- Use physical exercise such as walking, jogging, dancing, biking, and swimming

- Look outward to develop a social interest by understanding other people's problems and needs
- Try to see the humor in situations
- Limit the number of activities to a manageable few

Abraham Maslow developed a hierarchy of needs in which he maintained that people had special needs and moved through various levels in achieving satisfaction in life. The hierarchy of needs is based on five elements or levels. These levels are

Level I: Physiological needs such as food, water, and shelter.

Level II: Safety needs which include physical safety as well as security relating to employment.

Level III: Social needs which include having a sense of belonging to a group and the need for social interaction.

Level IV: Self-esteem which includes having a sense of self-worth and pride.

Level V: Self actualization which occurs when the individual achieves all he or she is capable of achieving and has a sense of accomplishment.

Maslow said that he believed a person could not move to a higher level until the basic needs at a lower level were met. An understanding of Maslow's hierarchy of needs is important for the medical assistant since the patients the medical assistant will encounter daily are at different stages or levels of fulfillment of their needs.

For example, one patient may be at Level I and be concerned about how he or she will pay a medical bill. Another patient whose Level II and III needs are met may wish to see the physician about cosmetic surgery as the patient attempts to have his or her self-esteem (Level V) needs met.

Patients who have a life-threatening illness need to have their Level II needs for future security met. For an illustration of Maslow's hierarchy of needs, see Figure 24-10.

Psychological Disorders

Psychiatry is the branch of medicine that deals with the diagnosis, treatment, and prevention of mental disorders. A psychiatrist is a physician specializing in the care of patients with emotional disorders.

Many people will have some type of mental disorder during their life. This is considered normal. A continual state of emotional disorder that disrupts life is considered abnormal. Mental disorders are defined as any behavior or emotional state that causes an individual great suffering or worry, is

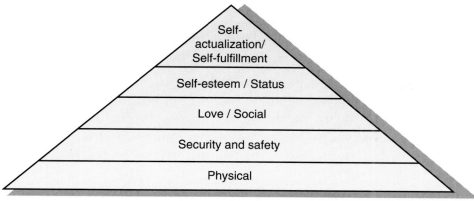

Figure 24-10   Maslow's Hierarchy of Needs.

self-defeating or self-destructive, or disrupts the person's day-to-day relationships. The legal definition of a mental disorder is "impaired judgment and lack of self-control." George Albee, a past president of the American Psychological Association, stated, "Appendicitis, a brain tumor, and chicken pox are the same everywhere, regardless of culture or class; mental conditions, it seems, are not."

The guide for terminology and classifications relating to psychiatric disorders is the *Diagnostic and Statistical Manual of Mental Disorders* (DSM-IV, 1994) which is published by the American Psychiatric Association. Major diagnostic categories of mental disorders in the DSM-IV are described in Table 24-2.

Mental diseases can be divided into three major categories: neuroses, psychoses, and personality disturbances.

Neuroses

Neuroses are mild emotional disturbances that impair judgment. Patients suffering from neuroses are able to tell the difference between fantasy and reality. Neuroses include anxiety, compulsions, hysteria, hypochondria, and obsessions.

- Anxiety is a vague feeling of apprehension, worry, uneasiness, or dread. A certain amount of anxiety is normal.
- Compulsions consist of a repetitive act which is performed by the patient to relieve fear connected with an obsession.
- Hysteria is a lack of control over emotions which may result in an outburst, amnesia, or symptoms such as sleepwalking.
- Hypochondria is an abnormal concern about one's health with the false belief of suffering from a disease despite being assured otherwise by the physician.

- Obsession is a neurotic mental state in which a patient has an uncontrollable desire to dwell on an idea or emotion. The patient is usually aware of the obsession and tries to resist the thoughts.

Psychoses

Psychoses are severe mental disorders that interfere with the patient's perception of reality and their ability to cope with the demands of daily living.

- Delusion is a persistent, strongly held, false belief that is most likely wrong. It is seen in persons with a psychosis who cannot separate delusion from reality. The most serious delusions are those that cause the patient to harm themselves or others.
- Depression is a mental disorder marked by an altered mood. The symptoms may include agitation, loss of energy, feelings of worthlessness, self-reproach, diminished ability to concentrate, and recurrent thoughts of death.
- Hallucination is a false perception which has no relation to reality. It may be visual or auditory. The patient's judgment may be impaired and he or she will not be able to distinguish between the real and the imaginary.
- Manic-depressive state is a mental disorder characterized by mood swings between excessive excitement and depression. This is also referred to as bipolar disorder.
- Schizophrenia is a psychotic disorder marked by a variety of symptoms which can include delusions, hallucinations, disorganized and incoherent speech, severe

TABLE 24-2 Major Diagnostic Categories of Mental Disorders

Category	Example
Anxiety disorder	Phobias, panic attack, compulsive rituals.
Cognitive disorder	Delirium, dementia, amnesia (resulting from brain damage), toxic substances, or drugs, degenerative disorders such as Alzheimer's.
Disorder diagnosed in infancy and childhood	Mental retardation, attention deficit disorders such as hyperactivity or inability to concentrate and developmental problems.
Dissociative disorder	Dissociative amnesia in which important events cannot be remembered after a traumatic event, and dissociative identity disorder (multiple personality disorder) in which two or more personalities or identities are present.
Impulse control disorder	Inability to resist an impulse to perform some act that is harmful to the individual or others such as pathological gambling, stealing (kleptomania), setting fires (pyromania), or having violent rages.
Personality disorder	Inflexible behavior patterns that cause distress or the inability to function. These include paranoid, narcissistic, and antisocial disorders.
Mood disorder	Major depression, bipolar disorder (manic depression), chronic depressive mood.
Schizophrenia and other psychotic disorders	Characterized by delusions, hallucinations, and severe disturbances in thinking and emotion.
Sexual and gender identity disorder	Transsexualism (wanting to be the other gender), sexual performance (lack of orgasm, premature ejaculation, or lack of sexual desire), or unusual or bizarre sexual acts.
Disorder with physical symptoms and no organic cause	Paralysis, heart palpitation, dizziness. Also referred to as hypochondria.
Substance-related disorder	From excessive use of or withdrawal from alcohol, amphetamines, caffeine, cocaine, hallucinogens, nicotine, opiates, and other drugs

emotional abnormalities, and a withdrawal into an inner world.

- Psychopathic behavior occurs when an individual is unconcerned about others to the point of being completely antisocial. These individuals may lack a conscience, and are often manipulative.

Personality Disorders

Personality disorders include antisocial reactions, paranoia, and narcissistic behavior.

- Antisocial reactions are characterized by socially negative actions such as stealing, lying, manipulating others, violence, a lack of social emotions (guilt, shame, empathy), and impulsive behavior. This is also referred to as sociopathic behavior.
- Narcissistic behavior refers to abnormal self-love and self-admiration.
- Paranoia occurs when a patient demonstrates intense feelings of persecution and jealousy. It is also characterized by other symptoms of schizophrenia such as delusions.

With some mental disorders, particularly severe depression, the patient may become so distraught as to threaten or attempt suicide. Often the suicidal person doesn't really want to die, but just wishes to escape an intolerable situation.

> **Med Tip:** The medical assistant must take all threats of suicide from patients as serious. Psychologists tell us that there is no clear "suicidal type" which means that we cannot predict who will actually take his or her own life. Always tell the physician about any discussion a patient has concerning suicide. If you believe a patient is in danger of suicide do not be afraid to ask the patient, "Are you thinking about suicide?"

Treatments

Treatments for mental disorders include a variety of methods including psychotherapy, psychopharmacology, and electroconvulsive therapy (ECT).

Psychotherapy

Psychotherapy is a method for treating mental disorders by mental rather than physical means. This includes psychoanalysis, humanistic therapies, and family and group therapy.

- *Psychoanalysis* is a method of obtaining a detailed account of the past and present emotional and mental experiences from the patient in order to determine the source of the problem and eliminate the effects. It is a system developed by Sigmund Freud which encourages the patient to discuss repressed, painful, or hidden experiences with the hope of eliminating or minimizing the problem.
- *Humanistic therapies* are also called "client-centered" or "nondirective therapy." The therapist does not delve into the patient's past when using these methods. The patient is helped to feel better by building their self-esteem and a feeling that they are respected.
- *Family and group therapy* is solution focused. The therapist places minimal emphasis on the patient's past history and places a strong emphasis on having the patient state their goals and then finding a way to achieve them.

Psychopharmacology

Psychopharmacology relates to the study of the effects of drugs on the mind and particularly the use of drugs in treating mental disorders. The main classes of drugs for the treatment of mental disorders are antipsychotic drugs, antidepressant drugs, "minor" tranquilizers, and lithium.

- Antipsychotic drugs are the major tranquilizers which include chlorpromazine (Thorazine), haloperidol (Haldol), clozapine (Clozaril), and risperidone. These drugs have transformed the treatment of patients with psychoses and schizophrenia. The medications will reduce the patient's agitation and panic and shorten the schizophrenic episode. One of the side effects of these drugs is involuntary muscle movements which approximately one-fourth of all adults who take the drugs develop.
- Antidepressant drugs are classified as stimulants and alter the patient's mood by affecting levels of neurotransmitters in the brain. Antidepressants, such as monoamine oxidase (MAO) inhibitors, are nonaddictive but they can produce unpleasant side effects such as dry mouth, weight gain, blurred vision, and nausea.
- "Minor" tranquilizers include Valium and Xanax. These are also classified as depressants and are prescribed for anxiety. However they are the least effective in treating emotional disorders. Patients may develop a problem with tolerance after taking these drugs for an extended period of time (they need larger and larger doses). In general, antidepressants are preferred to tranquilizers for treating mood disorders.
- Lithium, from the salt lithium carbonate, is a special category of drug. It is used successfully to calm patients who suffer from bipolar disorder (depression alternating with manic excitement). The patient on lithium needs to be carefully monitored since too much of this drug is toxic and too little is noneffective.

Electroconvulsive Therapy

Electroconvulsive therapy (ECT) is a procedure occasionally used for cases of prolonged major depression. This is a controversial treatment in which an electrode is placed on one or both sides of the patient's head, and brief current is turned on causing a convulsive seizure. A low level of voltage is used in modern ECT and the patient is administered a muscle relaxant and an anesthesia. Advocates of this treatment state that it is a more effective way to treat severe depression than the use of drugs. It is not effective with disorders other than depression, such as schizophrenia and alcoholism.

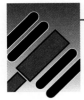

LEGAL AND ETHICAL ISSUES

The medical assistant must be cautioned against offering false hopes to a terminally ill patient. Promises, such as "I'm sure the doctor will make you better. He's done this before with patients who have your condition," can not only cause emotional anxiety for the patient, but may also result in litigation if the patient believes that this is a promise the physician has made. Never guarantee a cure.

The medical assistant has a responsibility to alert the physician to any threat of suicide the patient makes.

PATIENT EDUCATION

Patients will receive instructions on self care after such procedures as a colostomy shortly after the procedure while they are still in the hospital. Many patients are still recovering from an anesthetic and weakness when they receive instruction in the hospital. The medical assistant may see the patient in the office or handle a question over the telephone. At this time the medical assistant should reinforce the necessity for good hygiene habits and repeat the procedure for self-care. When possible preprinted material should be available to send home with patients or family members regarding necessary self-care. The medical assistant can reinforce healthy habits for coping with stress.

Summary

There are physical conditions and disabilities which cause the patient discomfort, but are not the presenting problem when they arrive in the physician's office. The medical assistant must remain flexible and be able to handle all unusual situations. It is vital that all health care workers keep up with literature that relates to their field. The medical assistant will want to read his or her association journal, *Professional Medical Assistant,* to remain current in the field.

Competency Review

1. Define and spell the glossary terms for this chapter.
2. What are Kubler-Ross's five stages of dying and why are they important to know?
3. What instructions might you give to a blind person when requesting a urine sample?
4. What are the key points in teaching about ostomy care?
5. Describe how to communicate to a profoundly deaf patient that he or she must remove all clothing and put on a patient gown.
6. Describe how you use the 8 health habits to cope with stress.

PREPARING FOR THE CERTIFICATION EXAM

Test Taking Tip — Completely fill in the bubble space on a computer-generated answer sheet. A small dot cannot always be picked up by the grading equipment.

Examination Review Questions

1. The five stages of dying do not include
   (A) denial
   (B) bargaining
   (C) brainstorming
   (D) depression
   (E) anger

2. A mental disorder which is characterized by delusions and hallucinations is
   (A) cognitive disorder
   (B) dissociative disorder
   (C) anxiety disorder
   (D) personality disorder
   (E) schizophrenia

3. An emotional disorder that impairs a person's judgement and concept of reality is
   (A) psychosis
   (B) neuroses
   (C) delusion
   (D) manic-depression
   (E) depression

4. A cerebrovascular accident (CVA) caused by a clot forming in the body and traveling to the brain is called
   (A) compression
   (B) cerebral hemorrhage
   (C) cerebral thrombosis
   (D) cerebral embolism
   (E) contusion

5. A surgical opening created into the small intestine for the purpose of allowing waste material to drain is called
   (A) colostomy
   (B) stoma
   (C) ileostomy
   (D) iliostomy
   (E) colorectal opening

6. A feeding tube is
   (A) placed into a vein
   (B) placed into one of several areas of the digestive system
   (C) intended to have fluids run through as quickly as possible to avoid clotting
   (D) used only for cancer patients
   (E) is administered through a port in the wrist

7. What symptom(s) should the patient with a feeding tube report to the physician?
   (A) nausea
   (B) vomiting
   (C) diarrhea
   (D) cramps
   (E) all of the above

8. Which of the following is a dangerous condition for a patient with a cast?
   (A) cast becomes dirty
   (B) cast becomes wet
   (C) limb becomes swollen
   (D) limb itches
   (E) none of the above

9. What is the best way to help a blind patient?
   (A) take the patient by the arm and lead him or her into an examination room
   (B) speak loudly to the patient so he or she can hear you since the patient can't read your lips
   (C) offer your arm for the patient to take
   (D) allow the patient to remain independent by doing as little as possible to help
   (E) tell the patient not to go outside without assistance

10. When assisting patients who have a terminal disease, the best method is to
    (A) allow them to talk about it
    (B) don't allow them to dwell on the depressing subject of death
    (C) encourage them by telling them they look wonderful and they will get better
    (D) advoid them
    (E) none of the above

ON THE JOB

Amy Freeman is a new medical assistant who has recently graduated and passed the CMA examination. She studied Dr. Kubler-Ross's five stages of dying and believes they make sense. Renee Baker, a young mother of two small children, has an appointment to see Dr. Williams for follow-up care after having been diagnosed with terminal ovarian cancer. Renee bitterly tells Amy that she is angry at the doctors for not diagnosing her condition sooner; angry at God for allowing this to happen; angry at her husband for not being more supportive; and angry at herself for not demanding better health care.

Since Renee has opened up to Amy about her feelings, Amy wants to try to help her. What should Amy do?

What is your response?

1. Keeping in mind Dr. Kubler-Ross's five stages of dying, what exactly should Amy say to Renee?
2. Does Amy have a responsibility to inform the physician?

References

Anderson, K., and Anderson, L. *Mosby's Pocket Dictionary of Medicine, Nursing & Allied Health.* Chicago: Mosby, 1994.

Badash, S. and Chesebro, D. *Introduction to Health Occupations.* Upper Saddle River, NJ: Brady/Prentice Hall, 1997.

Eysenck, H. "Prediction of Cancer and Coronary Heart Disease Mortality by Means of a Personality Inventory: Results of a 15-year Follow-up Study." *Psychological Reports.* 1993, 72, 499-516.

Eysenck, H. "The Prediction of Death From Cancer by Means of Personality/Stress Questionnaire: Too Good to Be True?" *Perceptual and Motor Skills.* 1990, 71, 216-218.

Fremgen, B. *Medical Terminology.* Upper Saddle River, NJ: Brady/Prentice Hall, 1997.

Greenwald, H. *Who Survives Cancer?* Berkeley: University of California Press, 1992.

Heller, M. and Krebs, C. *Delmar's Clinical Handbook for Health Care Professionals.* New York: Delmar, 1997.

Maddux, J. "The Mythology of Psychopathology: A Social Cognitive View of Deviance, Difference, and Disorder." *The General Psychologist.* Summer, 1993, 29, 34-45.

Nurse's Pocket Companion. Springhouse, PA: Springhouse Corporation, 1993.

Pediana, R. "Wound Care: Preparing to Heal." *Nursing Times.* 88:27, 1992.

Stoll, A., Tohen, M., and Baldessarini, R. "Increasing Frequency of the Diagnosis of Obsessive-compulsive Disorder: A Reply." *American Journal of Psychiatry.* 1993, 150, 682-683.

Taber's Cyclopedic Medical Dictionary, 18th ed. Philadelphia: PA. 1997.

Wade, C. and Tavris, C. *Psychology.* New York: HarperCollins College Publishers, 1996.

Zucker, E. *Being a Homemaker/Home Health Aide.* Upper Saddle River, NJ: Brady/Prentice Hall, 1996.

Workplace Wisdom

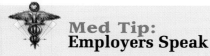

Med Tip:
Employers Speak

Demonstrate strong interpersonal skills and a mature level of courtesy, tact, and professionalism required to deal with patients, providers, and co-workers.

Exhibit strong communication skills and good judgment necessary to elicit information from patients in order to triage telephone calls and distinguish emergent, urgent, and routine problems.

Rita Geller, Compensation Specialist
Beth Israel Deaconess Medical Center
Boston, Massachusetts

Exhibit the ability to assess the patient's condition and triage him into the proper place in line and with the proper professional. Be prepared to assess and prioritize tasks.

Rachael Wallace, RN
Nurse Administrator
Howard Brown Health Center
Chicago, Illinois

When appropriate, demonstrate independence by being able to function on your own; be self-directed—don't wait for someone to tell you what to do.

Barbara Rodriguez, BSN
Staff Development Coordinator
Assistant Director of Nursing
University of Miami Hospitals
and Clinics/
Sylvester Comprehensive Cancer Center
Miami, Florida

Show a willingness to assist colleagues. Be alert to see what colleagues need. Do not say, "But, that's not my job." Show a sense of teamwork.

Linda Warren, RN, BS
Coordinator of Nursing Services
University of Michigan Health System
Chelsea Family Practice
Chelsea, Michigan

Keep patients as comfortable as possible.

Laurie Brenner
Director, Human Resources
Seton Medical Group
St. Agnes Health Care
Baltimore, Maryland

MEDICAL ASSISTANT ROLE DELINEATION CHART

Highlight indicates material covered in this chapter

ADMINISTRATIVE

ADMINISTRATIVE PROCEDURES

- Perform basic clerical functions
- Schedule, coordinate, and monitor appointments
- Schedule inpatient/outpatient admissions and procedures
- Understand and apply third party guidelines
- Obtain reimbursement through accurate claims submission
- Monitor third-party reimbursement
- Perform medical transcription
- Understand and adhere to managed care policies and procedures
- *Negotiate managed care contracts (adv)*

PRACTICE FINANCES

- Perform procedural and diagnostic coding
- Apply bookkeeping principles
- Document and maintain accounting and banking records
- Manage accounts receivable
- Manage accounts payable
- Process payroll
- *Develop and maintain fee schedules (adv)*
- *Manage renewals of business and professional insurance policies (adv)*
- *Manage personal benefits and maintain records (adv)*

CLINICAL

FUNDAMENTAL PRINCIPLES

- Apply principles of aseptic technique and infection control
- Comply with quality assurance practices
- Screen and follow up patient test results

DIAGNOSTIC ORDERS

- Collect and process specimens
- Perform diagnostic tests

PATIENT CARE

- Adhere to established triage procedures
- Obtain patient history and vital signs
- Prepare and maintain examination and treatment areas

- Prepare patient for examinations, procedures, and treatments
- Assist with examinations, procedures, and treatments
- Prepare and administer medications and immunizations
- Maintain medication and immunization records
- Recognize and respond to emergencies
- Coordinate patient care information with other health care providers

GENERAL (TRANSDISCIPLINARY)

PROFESSIONALISM

- Project a professional manner and image
- Adhere to ethical principles
- Demonstrate initiative and responsibility
- Work as a team member
- Manage time efficiently
- Prioritize and perform multiple tasks
- Adapt to change
- Promote the CMA credential
- Enhance skills through continuing education

COMMUNICATION SKILLS

- Treat all patients with compassion and empathy
- Recognize and respect cultural diversity
- Adapt communications to individual's ability to understand
- Use professional telephone technique
- Use effective and correct verbal and written communications
- Recognize and respond to verbal and non-verbal communications
- Use medical terminology appropriately
- Receive, organize, prioritize, and transmit information
- Serve as liaison
- Promote the practice through positive public relations

LEGAL CONCEPTS

- Maintain confidentiality
- Practice within the scope of education, training, and personal capabilities
- Prepare and maintain medical records
- Document accurately
- Use appropriate guidelines when releasing information
- Follow employer's established policies dealing with the health care contract
- Follow federal, state, and local legal guidelines
- Maintain awareness of federal and state health care legislation and regulations
- Maintain and dispose of regulated substances in compliance with government guidelines
- Comply with established risk management and safety procedures
- Recognize professional credentialing criteria
- Participate in the development and maintenance of personnel, policy, and procedure manuals
- *Develop and maintain personnel, policy, and procedure manuals (adv)*

INSTRUCTION

- Instruct individuals according to their needs
- Explain office policies and procedures
- Teach methods of health promotion and disease prevention
- Locate community resources and disseminate information
- *Orient and train personnel (adv)*
- *Develop educational materials (adv)*
- *Conduct continuing education activities (adv)*

OPERATIONAL FUNCTIONS

- Maintain supply inventory
- Evaluate and recommend equipment and supplies
- Apply computer techniques to support office operations
- *Supervise personnel (adv)*
- *Interview and recommend job applicants (adv)*
- *Negotiate leases and prices for equipment and supply contracts (adv)*

SOURCE: Reprinted by permission of the American Association of Medical Assistants from the *AAMA Role Delineation Study: Occupational Analysis of the Medical Assisting Profession.*

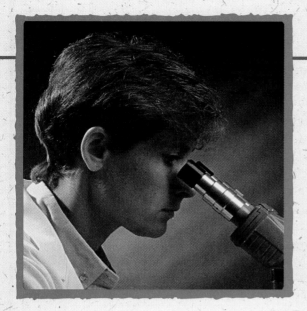

25

Microbiology

CHAPTER OUTLINE

LEARNING OBJECTIVES

After completing this chapter, you should:
1. Define and spell the glossary terms for this chapter.
2. List and describe 10 laboratory safety rules.
3. Explain the basic requirements of OSHA relating to laboratory safety.
4. Explain the parts of a microscope and how to use this equipment.
5. Describe the process for obtaining a specimen from the respiratory tract.
6. Discuss the importance of CLIA for the POLs.
7. Describe the process for culturing an organism.
8. Explain the characteristics of a good QA program.
9. Describe several examples of test kits.

CLINICAL PERFORMANCE COMPETENCIES

After completing this chapter, you should perform the following tasks:
1. Set-up and adjust a microscope for use.
2. Demonstrate the correct method for carrying a microscope.
3. Perform a Gram stain.
4. Perform a culture using an agar plate.
5. Explain the procedure for collecting a stool specimen.
6. Collect a throat culture.
7. Collect a sputum specimen.

Glossary

aerobes Microorganisms that are able to live only in the presence of oxygen.

agglutination Clumping.

anaerobes Microorganisms able to survive without oxygen.

cultures The propagation of microorganisms or of living tissue cells in special media that are conducive to their growth, and/or the process by which organisms are grown on media and identified.

Culturette Self-contained culturing packet system that readily adapts to most office specimen collections from the throat, nose, eye, ear, rectum, wound, and urogenital sites; it has a sterile, disposable plastic tube containing a cotton-tipped applicator swab and a sealed ampule of Stuart's holding medium.

cytology The science that deals with the formation, structure, and function of cells.

feces Evacuation of the bowels. Also referred to as stool.

gelatin culture The culture of bacteria on a gelatin medium, such as agar.

histology The study of the microscopic structure of tissue.

incubation In bacteriology, this is the period of culture development or the time it takes from placing an inoculated agar plate in an incubator or "oven" to when the microorganisms start to grow.

inoculate To inject or transfer a microorganism, serum, or toxic material into the body, culture, medium, or slide.

media A substance on which microorganisms may grow; those most commonly used are broth, gelatin, and agar.

microbiology The scientific study of microorganisms.

microbes Small organisms including bacteria, protozoa, algae, fungus, and defined viruses.

microorganisms Minute living organisms such as bacteria, virus, protozoa, and fungus that are not visible to the human eye without a microscope.

microscopic Visible only by using a microscope.

negative Culture that fails to reveal the suspected organism.

pathogens Disease producing microorganisms.

positive Culture that reveals the suspected organism.

pure culture Culture of a single form of microorganism uncontaminated by other organisms.

serologic Pertaining to the study of the serum component of the blood.

smears Bacteria spread on a surface, as a microscopic slide or a culture medium.

smear fixation Holding or fastening a bacterial specimen to a slide; adhering a smear to a glass slide by a fixative or heat.

specimen(s) A part of something intended to show the kind and quality of the whole, as a specimen of urine.

sputum The substance expelled by coughing or clearing the bronchi. Can be used as a specimen for culturing to discover possible causative agents of respiratory disease.

stool Evacuation of the bowels; waste matter used as a specimen for culturing to discover possible diseases. Also referred to as feces.

streak culture Spreading of the bacteria by drawing a wire containing the inoculum across the surface of the medium.

swab Cotton or gauze on the end of a slender stick used for cleansing, applying remedies, or obtaining tissue or secretions for bacteriologic examination.

viable Capable of living.

WARNING!

For all patient contact, adhere to Standard Precautions (see pages 342–373). Wear protective equipment as indicated.

The field of **microbiology** is the fascinating study of living organisms (microorganisms) which are too small to be seen with the naked eye. The invention of the microscope by Leeuwenhoek in 1680 allowed mankind to observe for the first time a variety of **microbes**, the small organisms found in stagnant water and from scrapings of Leeuwenhoek's teeth. **Cytology**, the study of cells, and **histology**, the study of tissue, both require the use of the microscope.

Louis Pasteur, the father of microbiology, developed methods for actually culturing and identifying microbes in the laboratory.

The medical assistant is responsible for collecting **specimens**—samples of blood, urine, or sputum—and instructing the patients about the collection process. Specimens are a part of something intended to show the kind and quality of the whole, for example a specimen of urine. In some offices, the medical assistant will also test the specimens if there is a clinical laboratory on site. In other situations, the specimens will be sent to outside laboratories for testing. No matter what process is used for testing, careful handling of equipment and specimens is required for the medical assistant's safety.

Laboratory Safety

An important part of laboratory safety is infection control. Medical assistants must be aware of the presence of harmful **microorganisms** or **pathogens** capable of causing disease in the medical environment. Necessary precautions must be taken to prevent their spread to co-workers and patients. It is important for medical assistants to know what causes infection, how it spreads, and what can be done to prevent transmission.

Our environment is full of **microscopic** organisms referred to as microbes or microorganisms, which include bacteria, protozoa, parasites, fungi, and algae that are only seen through a microscope. (For a more thorough discussion of these microorganisms see Chapter 19.) The majority of microbes are non-pathogenic and many can be found residing in the human body, such as in the mouth and throat. These are called the normal flora.

The human body is the perfect environment for growth of microorganisms: moist, dark inside, temperature at 98.6° F, nutrient-rich, with a *p*H that is not too acidic or too alkaline.

Microorganisms can be classified as heterotrophs, which feed on other organic matter, and autotrophs, which feed on inorganic matter. We can further classify microorganisms into **aerobes,** which need oxygen to grow, and **anaerobes,** that grow best in the absence of oxygen.

Microbes capable of causing disease are called pathogens or pathogenic organisms. If a pathogen enters the body, and the conditions are favorable for it to multiply and cause disease, the resulting condition is called an infection. Infection can be local, restricted to a small area, or systemic in which case the entire body is affected. The transmission or chain of infection requires three things: (1) a source of infection, for example contaminated equipment, (2) a means or mode of transmission, such as contaminated drinking water, an insect bite, or direct contact with an infected person, and (3) a susceptible host, such as an infant or elderly person with a weakened immune system.

Breaking the Chain of Infection

Preventing disease caused by microorganisms means providing a defense against the source and transmission of infection. Decontamination by general practices of asepsis (sanitization, disinfection, and sterilization) will stop infection at its source. Proper handwashing, wearing PPE (personal protective equipment) when indicated, and isolation procedures are excellent means of eliminating any transmission of pathogens. Maintenance of good hygiene, proper nutrition, and health will reduce or eliminate the susceptibility of potential hosts against common pathogens.

Safety Regulations

Providing quality care in an environment that is safe for employees as well as patients is an important responsibility of the health care team. While the Occupational Safety and Health Act (OSHA) has mandated that safe working conditions be assured to all employees, more specific regulations have been placed on laboratories.

Physicians' Office Laboratories (POLs)

Physicians' office laboratories (POLs), though not as equipped as full laboratories, make testing specimens convenient for both the patient and the doctor, but are no less immune to regulations. POLs may contain flammable and toxic chemicals, infectious waste material, and electrical equipment. Lab accidents can occur such as hazardous spills, glassware breaks, biological or chemical hazards, and electrical equipment failure.

OSHA law requires employers to make an inventory of all hazardous equipment and toxic substances used in the workplace. OSHA requires each medical facility to have a written Hazard Communication Program which outlines infection control for protection against HepB and HIV. As part of the program employers must post Material Safety Data Sheets (MSDA) for all hazardous substances and equipment, and properly label the container of all hazardous chemicals.

Clinical Laboratory Improvement Act (CLIA)

POLs are also subject to the Clinical Laboratory Improvement Act (CLIA). CLIA intends to regulate all human testing and this applies to anyone performing testing on human specimens for the diagnosis, prevention, or treatment of disease or health problems. CLIA regulations include specific guidelines for quality control, quality assurance, recordkeeping, and personnel qualifications.

The Health Care Financing Administration (HCFA) and Centers for Disease Control (CDC) regulate CLIA standards at the federal level, but states can seek to implement their own standards provided that the state standards are equivalent to federal standards.

The degree of applicable federal and state regulations of the POL depends on the complexity of the tests performed. Three categories of testing have been established. They are

- Waiver tests (simple, stable tests that require a minimum degree of judgment and interpretation, for example visual color comparison pregnancy tests).
- Moderate complexity tests (which make up approximately 75% of lab tests).
- High complexity tests (most of which are performed by pathologists and/or doctors in a specific field of medical science).

Moderate and highly complex POLs must meet specific standards for personnel training and experience. Table 25-1 describes safety rules that assist with safe laboratory practice.

Quality Assurance

Laboratory testing is an important part of patient diagnosis and medical care. Doctors rely on test results and they expect the process of testing to be carefully monitored from the beginning to end with the quality remaining consistent. For this reason it is necessary to set policies and procedures to ensure that patient preparation, specimen procurement, handling and labeling, and preserving specimens are accurate. These established policies and procedures (required by CLIA) fall under an overall process called Quality Assurance or QA (see Chapter 6 for further discussion of quality assurance). Quality Assurance is an ongoing program designed to monitor and evaluate the quality of patient care. Characteristics of a laboratory QA program would include

1. Written policies on the standards of patient care and professional behavior.
2. A Quality Control (QC) program.
3. A training and continuing education program.
4. An instrument maintenance program.
5. Documentation requirements.
6. Evaluation methods and frequency requirements.
7. Corrective action taken.

Quality Control

Quality Control (QC) is a component of a QA program and is a form of procedure control. This means that if standards are followed during a given procedure, results will be consistent. Laboratory QC methods include

1. Running control samples for each test performed.
2. Reagent management.
3. Instrument calibration.
4. Documentation.
5. Preventive maintenance of the equipment.
6. Patient preparation and specimen collections procedures.

Laboratory Equipment

Microscopes are frequently used in the medical office to examine urine sediment, vaginal and bacteriological smears, which are performed by spreading bacteria on a surface such as a slide, and differentials. This optical instrument magnifies structures unseen by the naked eye for the purpose of counting, naming, or differentiating. See Figure 25-1 for an example of a microscope.

TABLE 25-1 Laboratory Safety Rules

1. Wear appropriate PPE (personal protective equipment) in the lab only. Do not wear lab coats, masks, and gloves outside of the lab.

2. Avoid hand-to-mouth contact or hands touching the eyes, nose, or ears while in the lab.

   a. No pens, pencils placed in mouth or behind the ears.

   b. No food or drink in lab or lab refrigerator.

   c. Never apply cosmetics such as lipstick or lip balm or handle contact lens while in the lab.

3. Dress appropriately.

   a. Never wear long chains, dangling earrings, or bracelets.

   b. Always tie back hair.

   c. Keep fingernails short, well manicured, with no polish or artificial nails.

   d. Wear comfortable, sturdy shoes with nonslip soles - no sandals, open-toed shoes or heels.

4. Do not mouth pipette to draw material up through a pipette using suction from the mouth.

5. Do not store caustic material above the eye level.

6. Locate fire extinguishers in the lab and know how to use them.

7. Be sure hands are dry when transferring reagent bottles.

8. Keep First-Aid manual and supplies available.

9. Avoid inhaling any chemical substance that might cause injury to nasal membranes or lungs.

10. Never use chipped, broken, or cracked glassware.

11. Follow written clean up policies and procedures for spills.

12. Discard contaminated material in appropriate container.

The Microscope

The components of a microscope are

1. Eye piece(s) (monocular or binocular) with magnification printed on them.
2. Adjuster for eye width.
3. Body tube (directional light source).
4. Arm (used in carrying the microscope).
5. Revolving nosepiece (holds objectives and rotates for selection).
6. Objectives (magnification printed on each objective: 10× - low power; 40× - high dry; and 100× or oil immersion).
7. Mechanical stage (movable device that holds slide).
8. Stage (platform that slide sets on).
9. Mechanical stage adjustment (two knobs that control vertical/horizontal movement of slide).
10. Coarse/fine adjustment knobs (small knob atop larger knob that adjusts stage up and down for focusing).
11. Substage condenser (lens system used to increase light for sharper focus).
12. Diaphragm (adjustable aperture like a camera shutter that controls the amount of light).
13. Light source (illuminator set in base).
14. Rheostat (regulates intensity of the light).
15. Base (holds illuminator, rheostat, and microscope upright and used while carrying microscope).

Using the Microscope

The magnification of an object is calculated by multiplying the objective magnification with the eye piece magnification. On low power, magnification would be 10× (the objective) times 10× (the eye piece) equaling 100× magnification. The procedure for using the microscope follows.

It is important to use the correct lens for the type of microscopic work to be done. For example, the low power objective is used to view epithelial cells, such as skin scrapings; the high dry setting is used for urine RBCs (red blood cells), WBCs (white blood cells) or blood RBCs; oil immersion for differentials (stained with Wright's stain) or bacteria slides (stained with Gram stain). Microscopic work on the high dry setting is done with a cover glass on the specimen slide.

Care and Maintenance of the Microscope

Microscopes are delicate instruments that will last for many years if maintained properly. The following rules need to be adhered to:

1. Follow cleaning requirements during mandatory daily maintenance.
2. Always use two hands to carry a microscope: one hand to hold the arm of the microscope while using the other hand to support the base.
3. Clean oculars, objectives, and stage using only lens paper and lens cleaner.
4. Keep extra light bulbs on hand.

5. Document inspections and repairs in log book.
6. Store with electrical cord wrapped loosely around base.
7. Cover the microscope with a dust cover when it is not in use.

Specimen Collection

One of the first priorities of quality control (QC) is proper specimen collection. Any incorrect steps could result in a contaminated or altered specimen. The first step is proper patient preparation. There are many tests that require special preparation to obtain accurate results for diagnosis. It is up to the medical assistant to make sure the patient understands and complies with these instructions by doing two things: (a) carefully read and explain the instructions, answering any questions the patient might have and (b) give written instructions for the patient to follow or refer to at home. Figure 25-2 illustrates a medical assistant explaining a laboratory procedure to a patient.

The second important step is to follow the six basic rules or guidelines for specimen collection.

Stool Specimen Collection

The presence of microbial organisms, such as ova and parasites (O & P), may be determined by testing feces or stool, the waste product from the bowel. The specimen is usually obtained in the early morning or by using a rectal swab. The patient should be instructed to defecate into a stool

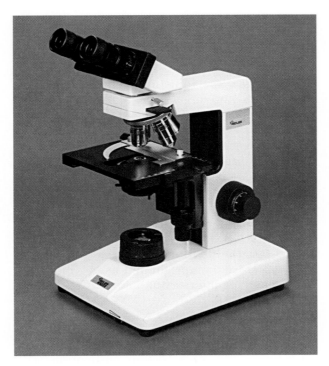

Figure 25-1   Clinical binocular microscope.

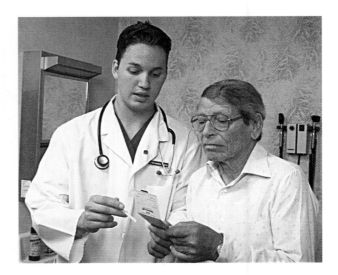

Figure 25-2   Medical assistant explains to patient how to use a collection specimen kit.

PROCEDURE: Using the Microscope

**Terminal Performance
Competency:** Student will observe a slide under the microscope using 10×, 40×, and 100× oil immersion using the correct procedure.

Equipment and Supplies

Microscope

Slide (prepared with specimen to be examined)

Lens paper/lens cleaner

Dust cover for microscope

Note: Follow Standard Precautions and safety guidelines when working with body fluid samples. Use care to avoid splashing or spilling body fluids. Wipe up all spills using guidelines established by OSHA.

Procedural Steps

1. Make sure the stage is in the down position before starting.
2. Place prepared slide on stage.
3. Turn light on.
4. Rotate nosepiece to 10× objective directly over slide.
5. Use coarse adjustment knob to raise stage until objective is close to slide on stage.
6. Look through eyepiece and adjust coarse focus knob until microscope field is seen (this will look like a round circle of bright light).
7. Use fine adjustment knob for clearer image.
8. Open diaphragm, adjust rheostat to focus if necessary.
9. Raise or lower condenser to alter light refraction (usually lower the condenser when using low power objective).
10. Observe.
11. Lower stage to change objective to 40× and re-adjust. Use oil on 100× oil immersion.
12. When finished, always lower stage before removing slide.
13. Turn off light.
14. Clean eye pieces and objectives with lens paper and oil immersion lens with lens cleaner. Xylene can be used sparingly to clean metal parts.
15. Unplug electrical cord and wrap around base.
16. Cover microscope with dust-cover.

Guidelines: Specimen Collection

The basic rules for specimen collection are

1. Confirm the identity of the patient by asking the patient to state his or her name and spell, if necessary.
2. Screen the patient to determine if pretest preparation was followed.
3. Use appropriate collection technique by observing proper cleaning and aseptic procedures to control contamination.
4. Select the proper containers for collection that comply with the reference lab (outside laboratory).
5. Label the specimen accurately at the time of collection.
   - Patient's full name
   - Date
   - Time of collection
   - Type of specimen
   - Your initials
6. Fill out the requisition form for the reference lab and double-check that the information matches the label.

specimen container or by using a bedpan, if available, placed over the toilet. The stool specimen samples should be taken from several different parts of the stool since microorganisms (such as ova and parasites) or occult blood may be in one portion of the stool and not another. The procedure for collecting a stool specimen follows.

PROCEDURE: Collecting a Stool Specimen

**Terminal Performance
Competency:** Instruct a patient how to collect a stool sample using the following correct infection control and procedure.

Equipment and Supplies

Labeled sterile specimen container with lid

Bedpan or container for collection of stool

Tongue depressor

Mailing container

Labels

Laboratory request form

Gloves

Hazardous waste container

Note: Follow Standard Precautions and safety guidelines when working with body fluid samples. Use care to avoid splashing or spilling body fluids. Wipe up all spills using guidelines established by OSHA.

Procedure Steps

1. Wash hands.
2. Assemble equipment.
3. Identify patient and explain the procedure, giving written instructions as well.
4. Instruct patient to defecate in container or bedpan, if available.
5. Apply gloves.
6. Using tongue depressor, take small amount of stool from different parts of the specimen and place in sterile container making sure no other contaminants are included (toilet paper, urine, etc.) and replace lid.
7. Refrigerate the specimen if not able to immediately process test or mail to outside lab facility.
8. Fill out lab request form and wrap around container securing with a rubber band.
9. Place in proper mailing container.

Charting Example

2/14/XX   9 AM   Stool specimen obtained for O & P. Specimen labeled and sent to lab.
M. King, CMA

If Hemmoccult Sensa Test is to be used by the patient at home, instruct the patient to write name, date, and doctor on label of booklet, collect a small amount of stool and place in one of the circles on back of booklet, obtain another sample from a different area of the stool and place this sample on the other circle. Patient should close booklet and take to the doctor's office immediately.

See Figure 25-3 for test for occult blood.

Respiratory Tract Specimen

Specimens obtained from the respiratory tract may include a throat swab using a cotton tipped or sputum culture. To obtain a throat culture it is necessary to utilize the Culturette, a self-contained collection system. The Culturette system is a disposable, clear plastic tube that contains a sterile cotton-tipped applicator swab and a sealed plastic vial of medium (broth containing nourishment for bac-

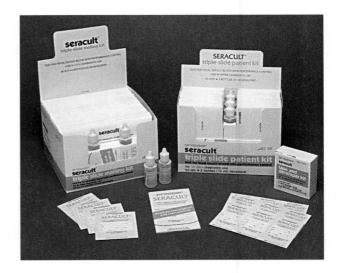

Figure 25-3   Test for occult blood.

teria and a preservative). This system is used to obtain many types of specimens, from sites such as the throat, nose, or eyes, to wounds, genital, or urethral areas. It is important that these types of specimens, collected in Culturettes, be transported immediately so that microorganisms remain viable, or capable of living, when they reach the laboratory.

The purpose of obtaining a throat and/or nasopharyngeal culture is that it can isolate and identify a disease such as strep throat or Candida (thrush). Have the patient face the light and open their mouth as wide as possible. Using a tongue depressor, hold the patient's tongue down and firmly roll the swab across the infected area(s) of the patient's throat being careful not to touch teeth, tongue, or inner cheek. A physician's order

is necessary for this test. The procedure for collecting a throat or nasopharyngeal culture follows. Sterile swabs are pictured in Figure 25-4.

To obtain a sputum specimen, which is the mucous substance expelled by coughing or clearing the bronchi, the patient must be carefully instructed to cough deeply when getting up in the morning and "spitting" the coughed up material into a sterile container. Explain to the patient that this should not be saliva from the mouth. The purpose for obtaining a sputum specimen is to isolate and diagnose diseases such as streptococcal pneumonia, haemophilus, and tuberculosis. Refer to the procedure for obtaining a sputum specimen in this chapter. See Chapter 26 for information regarding urine specimen collection.

PROCEDURE: Collecting a Throat or Nasopharyngeal Culture Using Culturette System

Terminal Performance
Competency: Collect a throat or nasopharyngeal culture without contaminating the specimen.

Equipment and Supplies
Culturette system
Tongue depressor
Gloves
Hazardous waste container
Note: Follow Standard Precautions and safety guidelines when working with body fluid samples. Use care to avoid splashing or spilling body fluids. Wipe up all spills using guidelines established by OSHA.

Procedural Steps
1. Wash hands.
2. Assemble equipment and Culturette system.
3. Identify patient and explain procedure.
4. Apply gloves.
5. Position patient facing a light source and have the patient open his or her mouth as wide as possible. The gag reflex may be diminished if the patient says, "Ah."

6. Remove sterile swab from Culturette.
7. Depress tongue, insert swab, and roll it firmly across back of patient's throat or nasopharyngeal area where infected using care not to contaminate swab on the teeth, lips, tongue, or inside of cheeks.
8. Insert swab into plastic vial containing Stuart's medium making sure swab is soaked.
9. Place in labeled mailing/transporting envelope and staple shut if necessary.
10. Complete laboratory request form and secure to envelope with rubber band.
11. Wash hands.
12. Transport immediately.

Charting Example
2/14/XX   9 AM   Throat culture obtained. Specimen labeled and sent to lab.
M. King, CMA

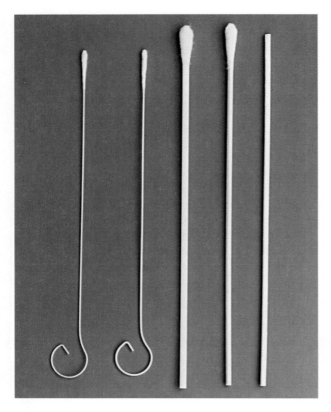

Figure 25-4   Sterile swab collection.

Specimen collection containers are pictured in Figure 25-5.

Culture Preparation

Pathogens can be observed in specimens of blood, feces, cerebrospinal fluid, mucus, urine, sputum, or other substances from the body. There are several techniques used to microscopically identify characteristics in specimens. These examination techniques include wet mount, smear, and Gram stain. The procedure for performing a wet mount culture follows.

The use of stained smears in microbiology is extensive. The color and shape (morphology) of microorganisms in smears can be observed, for example in vaginal and nasopharyngeal specimens. The medical assistant should know how to prepare a smear and have a general knowledge of the Gram stain and why it is used. The Gram stain, because several colors are used, will differentiate or separate, bacteria into two groups: Gram-positive and Gram-negative. Different bacteria stain differently, depending on the compounds in their walls. Gram-positive bacteria retain the crystal violet-blue color and Gram-negative bacteria retain only the safarnine color of pink. Thus, Gram-positive

(violet) bacteria can be distinguished from Gram-negative bacteria. Precautions must be taken in Gram staining in that temperature, age of specimen, or incubation, which is the amount of time for the microorganism to grow, could cause a change in Gram-positive bacteria. Gram stains must always be followed by culture for microorganism identification.

The staining properties, shape, and size can sometimes be used to identify pathogens in specimen samples. Also seen under the microscope, other than color, are the morphologic classification of bacteria, or shape and size. Bacilli are rod-shaped cells found singly, or in groups. Cocci are round bacteria found singly, in pairs (diplococci), in strings (streptococci), or in clusters (staphylococci). Spirillum, curved or spiral rods, can be arranged singly or in strands. Some bacteria can produce resistant forms called spores under adverse environmental conditions. Spores can lie dormant for thousands of years and when conditions are right, revert back to active form. This trait makes it difficult to destroy these pathogenic bacteria.

Refer to the procedures for preparing a smear and for preparing a Gram stain presented in this chapter.

See Figure 25-6A-F for an example of one method of performing a Gram stain and Table 25-2 for examples of pathogenic bacteria.

Culture Growth

Pathogens are further identified by growing cultures, which are the propagation of microorganisms, taken from the same specimen as used for the smear. Colonies of bacteria can be grown only on certain media, a liquid or gel-like (gelatin culture) substance, such as agar, containing nutrients. Media will either inhibit or encourage the growth of certain pathogens and are classified as differential, enrichment, or supportive. Pathogens are often identified by how they grow on a particular medium. An example of this would be streptococci bacteria causing "strep throat." Mucus swabbed from a sore throat and placed in a medium that contains blood will produce pinpoint-sized colonies that have a transparent ring around each, which is the result of hemolysis or bursting of red blood cells by the streptococci in the surrounding medium.

Table 25-3 lists common culture media and microorganisms that can be isolated on each and Figure 25-7 illustrates blood agar plate and equipment.

The key in growing cultures on media is to isolate pathogenic colonies of organisms from normal flora. To isolate colonies the agar must be streaked

PROCEDURE: Obtaining a Sputum Specimen

**Terminal Performance
Competency:** Obtain a sputum specimen using correct procedure.

Equipment and Supplies
Sterile labeled sputum container with lid
Lab requisition form
Gloves
Hazardous waste container
Note: Follow Standard Precautions and
safety guidelines when working with
body fluid samples. Use care to avoid
splashing or spilling body fluids. Wipe up
all spills using guidelines established by
OSHA.

Procedural Steps
1. Wash hands and apply gloves (if
   collecting sputum specimen from
   patient).
2. Identify patient.
3. Explain the procedure and give
   written instructions that the patient
   can take home, if necessary.

  a. Cough deeply (first thing in the
   morning) and expel fluid into
   center of container.
  b. Make sure no other fluids find
   their way into the cup, such as
   tears, nasal mucus, or saliva.
  c. Fit lid securely and write the time
   and date the specimen was
   obtained.
  d. Bring specimen into doctor's office
   as soon as possible or place in a
   refrigerator for no longer than two
   hours.
4. Label envelope with information,
   staple shut, and transport
   immediately.
5. Wash hands.

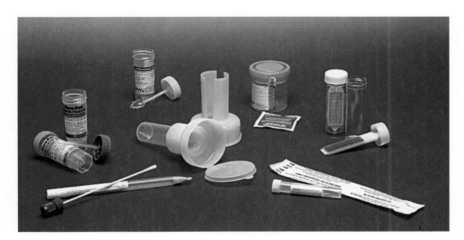

Figure 25-5 Specimen
collection containers.

properly. The specimen is transferred by rubbing
the swab across one small area of the agar near the
edge. Next, a wire inoculating loop is sterilized
under a Bunsen burner flame, cooled, and used to
streak through the area already inoculated and
onto a clear area of the agar in a zigzag motion. The
wire loop is then sterilized again, cooled, and is
used to streak through the zigzag area onto the remainder of un-inoculated agar with the same technique as before. This is called streaking for isolation (**streak culture**).

After inoculation, the "lid" of the Petri dish is
replaced and the agar plate inverted and placed
into an incubator. Figure 25-8 depicts an example
of an incubator. The inversion of the agar plate allows moisture to collect on the "lid" of the Petri

PROCEDURE: Wet Mount Culture

**Terminal Performance
Competency:** Successfully perform a wet mount culture.

Equipment and Supplies
- Clean, dry slide
- Cover slip
- Saline
- Specimen from a Culturette applicator or swab
- Paper/pen
- Microscope
- Gloves

Note: Follow Standard Precautions and safety guidelines when working with body fluid samples. Use care to avoid splashing or spilling body fluids. Wipe up all spills using guidelines established by OSHA.

Procedural Steps
1. Wash hands and apply gloves.
2. Label dry slide with patient's name and date.
3. Inoculate the dry slide by rolling swab containing specimen across surface.
4. If specimen is too thick, place a drop of saline solution on top of specimen.
5. Place coverslip on top of smeared slide.
6. Observe immediately under the microscope.
7. Special stains may be used to enhance characteristics.
8. Note on paper what is observed, remove slide, dispose of properly.
9. Remove gloves and wash hands.
10. Chart findings on patient's record.

PROCEDURE: Preparing a Smear

**Terminal Performance
Competency:** Be able to prepare a smear for microscopic examination without error.

Equipment and Supplies
- Slides
- Specimen from Culturette applicator or inoculating loop
- Bunsen burner
- Inoculating loop (or swab)
- Microscope
- Oil immersion
- Gloves
- Hazardous waste container

Note: Follow Standard Precautions and safety guidelines when working with body fluid samples. Use care to avoid splashing or spilling body fluids. Wipe up all spills using guidelines established by OSHA.

Procedural Steps
1. Wash hands and apply gloves.
2. Assemble equipment.
3. Label clean slide with patient's name and date.
4. Inoculate slide by transferring specimen to slide with an inoculating loop or swab.
5. Allow slide to air dry for 20 to 30 minutes.
6. Hold the slide with thumb forceps and pass slide over Bunsen burner flame. This heat "fixes" the specimen to the slide, known as smear fixation. Let the slide cool.
7. Slide is then ready to be stained.

**Terminal Performance
Competency:** Correctly prepare a slide for a Gram stain to differentiate a Gram-positive organism from a Gram-negative organism.

Equipment and Supplies

Gram-stain kit with decolorizer

Culture specimen

Slides

Bunsen burner

Staining rack

Water wash bottle

Water

Immersion oil

Stopwatch

Gloves

Slide stand

Paper towels

Hazardous waste container

Note: Follow Standard Precautions and safety guidelines when working with body fluid samples. Use care to avoid splashing or spilling body fluids. Wipe up all spills using guidelines established by OSHA.

Procedural Steps

1. Wash hands and apply gloves.
2. Assemble equipment.
3. Make a smear, air dry the smear, and heat fix.
4. Place slide on staining rack, smear side up.
5. Pour crystal violet solution all over the slide, let stand 1 minute.
6. Tilt slide to drain excess and rinse with water.
7. Pour Gram's iodine stain all over the slide, let stand 1 to 2 minutes.
8. Tilt slide to drain excess and rinse with water.
9. Gently pour decolorizer with alcohol-acetone all over slide for 15 seconds or until color blue stops running.
10. Rinse with water.
11. Pour safranine stain all over slide, let stand 30 seconds.
12. Tilt slide to drain excess and rinse with water.
13. Stand slide on end on paper towel or in slide drying rack, air dry.
14. Examine under microscope, using oil immersion lens and oil.

---

dish and not on the culture itself. The culture is allowed to grow in the incubator at 37° Celsius for a 24-, 48-, or 72-hour period. A secondary culture can be obtained by selecting an isolated colony from the initial agar plate and placing it onto another media plate. This provides a pure culture in that it only contains a single type of organism. Identification of the organism is made by using the pure culture to prepare special stains and by performing various biochemical tests.

Instruments such as Vitek and Autobac use automated technology to facilitate organism identification. The BAC-T Screen Bacteruria-Pyuria Detection Device is an automated system that immediately determines if significant numbers of bacteria are present in a urine specimen, avoiding the 24 to 48 hour wait for complete growth and identification.

Sensitivity Testing

Once the pathogenic organism is identified on the culture, it is necessary to determine which antibiotics will be effective in killing this bacteria. This method of detection is called sensitivity testing. A Petri dish with Mueller-Hinton agar and antibiotic disks are used. The Mueller-Hinton agar is inoculated with the pure culture specimen in overlapping strokes and the antibiotic disks are placed in a circle on top of the inoculated agar. The lid of the Petri dish is replaced, inverted, and placed in the incubator for 24 hours. After 24 hours, the bacterium will have grown all over except around those disks that inhibit its growth. These zones around the disks are measured to determine the susceptibility of the organism to each particular antibiotic disk. After the most effective antibiotic

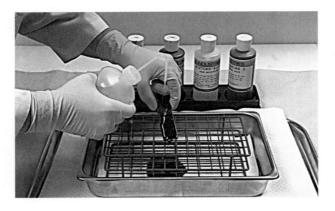

Figure 25-6 A   Rinse: start.

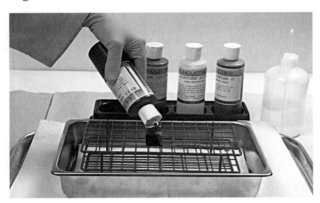

Figure 25-6 B   Gram stain.

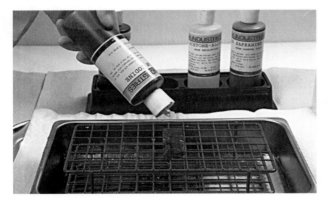

Figure 25-6 C   Iodine.

Figure 25-6 A-F   Gram-stain procedure.

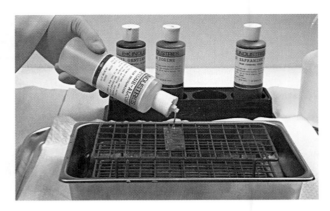

Figure 25-6 D   Acetone.

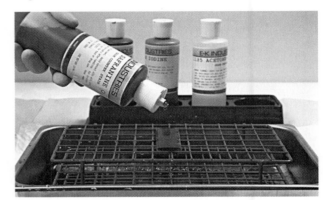

Figure 25-6 E   Safranine.

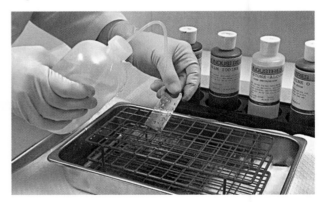

Figure 25-6 F   Rinse: finish.

TABLE 25-2   **Pathogenic Bacteria**

Structural Classification	Gram-Stain Classification	Bacterium	Diseases Caused
Bacilli	Gram-positive	Bacillus	Anthrax
	Gram-positive	Clostridium	Botulism, tetanus
	Gram-negative	*Enterobacteriaceae*	

TABLE 25-3 Culture Media and Isolates

Common Culture Media	Isolates
Blood agar	Most bacteria
Chocolate agar	*Neisseria, Haemophilus*
EMB	Gram-negative bacteria
MacConkey agar	Gram-negative bacteria
Thioglycollate broth	Anaerobic microorganisms
GN broth	Fecal microorganisms

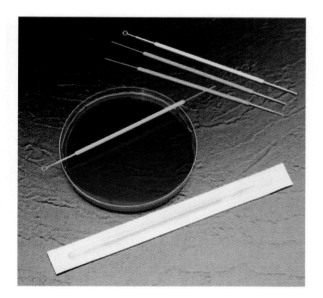

Figure 25-7 Blood agar plate and equipment for culture.

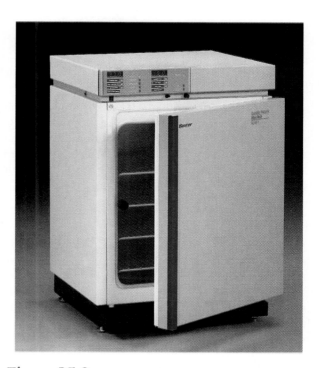

Figure 25-8 An example of an incubator.

is identified, the patient is started on drug therapy. See Figure 25-9 for an illustration of culture technique.

Serological Testing

Serology is the study of antigen and antibody reactions of the body's immune system. The body's ability to recognize a foreign substance (antigen) and produce an antibody against it is called the immune response. Antibodies are specific for stopping a particular antigen.

This antigen-antibody reaction is a frequently used testing tool and is used for tests, such as pregnancy, rheumatoid arthritis, mononucleosis, and strep. This testing is serologic since it studies or tests the serum component of the blood. These testing kits contain all equipment and supplies necessary and assist the medical assistant in en-

suring that reagents are fresh and quality control is maintained. The kits standardize testing, thus ensuring accuracy, precision, and quality control. It is absolutely essential to follow the exact manufacturer's directions. Serological testing refers to the testing, or study, of the serum component.

Strep Tests

The Group A Strep Screen is a test being done frequently in POLs. It is especially efficient in the pediatric office because it is self-contained and can be done while the patient waits. This screen is an antigen detection test for beta hemolytic streptococci (Group A) and follows the general procedure for antigen-antibody agglutination tests which

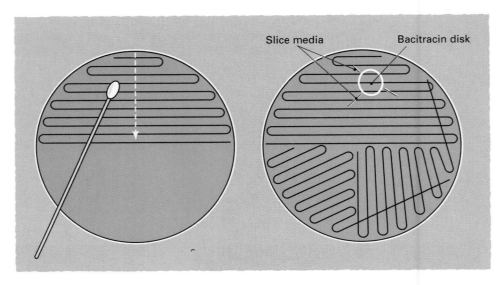

Figure 25-9 Culture technique.

produce a clumping of cells. One such test, called Q-test STREP, is a commercially prepared diagnostic testing kit that includes detailed instructions and contains reagents as well as controls and quality control suggestions. See Figure 25-10 for an example of a strep test kit.

Pregnancy Tests

Pregnancy tests are based on the presence or absence of a hormone called human chorionic gonadotropin or HCG. Immunologic tests of the reaction between serum or urine HCG and commercially prepared human chorionic gonadotropin antibody are the most commonly used. The two methods are: the direct agglutination test and the agglutination inhibition test.

A slide test kit using the direct agglutination method is as follows: Reagent latex particles provided in the container are coated with serum anti-HCG (antibody to HCG) and are incubated with the patient's urine. If an antigen-antibody reaction occurs, the latex particles will agglutinate (clump together) and the test is positive. If agglutination does not occur, the test is negative.

For the agglutination inhibition test, anti-HCG reagent (a commercially prepared serum) is incubated at the same time with the patient's urine or serum. If HCG is present, an antibody-antigen reaction occurs that neutralizes the anti-HCG serum. HCG coated latex particles are added, and if the anti-HCG has been neutralized, no agglutination will occur and the test is positive. If neutralization has not occurred, the anti-HCG is free to react with the latex particles and agglutination occurs, meaning the test is negative.

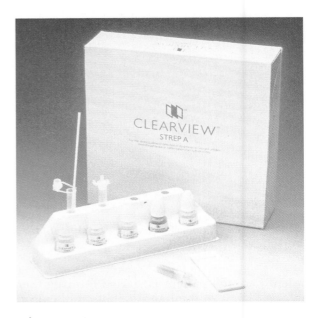

Figure 25-10 Example of a strep test kit.

It is important to always run positive and negative controls with each test to ensure accurate

Med Tip: Pregnancy tests are about 90% accurate and can detect low levels of HCG in early pregnancy; however, positive pregnancy tests may result from conditions other than pregnancy. Tumors of the ovaries can increase the concentration level of HCG and cause a positive reading.

readings. Sources of error include failure to follow directions, improper storage, or contaminants in the specimen. Newer kits are offering indicator signs, such as plus and minus signs, to reduce error in interpreting agglutination tests.

There are a variety of other serological test kits available. Examples are the test kit for Virogen Herpes Slide Test shown in Figure 25-11 and Figure 25-12 the Chemcard™ Cholesterol Test.

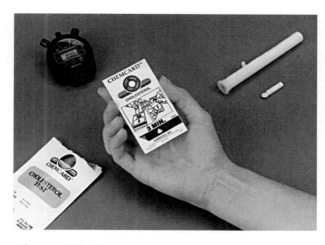

Figure 25-12   Chemcard™ Cholesterol Test.

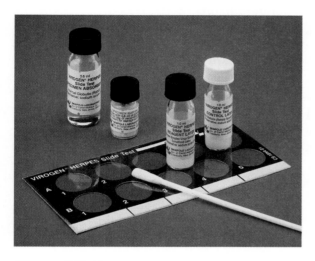

Figure 25-11   Virogen Herpes Slide Test.

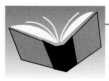

LEGAL AND ETHICAL ISSUES

Confidentiality regarding any patient testing is paramount. Careful labeling of specimens will assist in protecting the patient and physician from an incorrect diagnosis.

Since many of the microorganisms present in specimens taken in the office set-

ting are pathogenic, the medical assistant has an ethical responsibility to avoid carrying the microbes outside of the laboratory. This requires strict adherence to policies regarding wearing PPE and hand washing.

PATIENT EDUCATION

The role of the medical assistant in the education of the patient regarding the careful handling of all specimens and testing materials cannot be overemphasized. There is a danger of contamination with microorganisms to everyone coming into contact with the specimen if the patient has not carefully practiced hand washing and other infection control measures when obtaining the specimen.

Some patients are reluctant to collect specimens and the medical assistant can do much to allay their fears by explaining the value of specimen collection. The calm, professional attitude the medical assistant displays while explaining the collection of sputum and stool (feces) may mean the difference between a useful specimen and a contaminated one.

Summary

Microbiology, as practiced by the medical assistant in the physician's office laboratory (POL), is one of the most important aids in diagnosis for the physician. By correct processing and testing of patient specimens, an early diagnosis and treatment of disease can take place. The medical assistant plays an important role in the process.

Competency Review

1. Define and spell the glossary terms for this chapter.
2. How would you explain to a patient the method for collecting a stool specimen in their home?
3. Write a policy for your office regarding safe laboratory habits.
4. Create a sign that can be used in your clinical laboratory to remind personnel about the six basic lab rules.

PREPARING FOR THE CERTIFICATION EXAM

Test Taking Tip — Break test preparation into small bites. Never try to learn an entire chapter at one time.

Examination Review Questions

1. Which of the following statements is TRUE about laboratory safety?
   (A) caustic material is best stored at eye level
   (B) always have a pencil ready to use by placing it behind your ear
   (C) if you can't see blood, it's not present
   (D) remove PPE when leaving lab area
   (E) wear PPE outside of lab to protect street clothes

2. All of the following information should be included on a lab slip EXCEPT:
   (A) date specimen is obtained
   (B) time specimen is obtained
   (C) time specimen is sent to lab
   (D) physician's name
   (E) patient's name

3. Material taken for a throat culture can include the following areas
   (A) throat
   (B) back of tongue
   (C) mucous on inside of cheeks
   (D) teeth
   (E) all of the above contain microorganisms and can be used for a throat culture

4. Material for a sputum specimen is collected from what area?

   (A) mouth
   (B) throat
   (C) lungs and bronchial tubes
   (D) nose
   (E) pharynx

5. What type of culture requires the use of a concave depression on the slide?
   (A) gelatin culture
   (B) stab culture
   (C) streak culture
   (D) hanging drop culture
   (E) smear culture

6. What should you look for when identifying bacteria?
   (A) cocci will be round
   (B) streptococci are seen as strings of cocci
   (C) staphylococci are seen as clusters of cocci
   (D) there may be spores present
   (E) all of the above are correct

7. Microscopic slides are placed on what portion of the microscope?
   (A) diaphragm
   (B) stage
   (C) substage

(Continued)

(D) revolving nosepiece

(E) rheostat

8. What federal regulation provides guidelines for quality assurance and control, recordkeeping, and personnel qualification in the clinical laboratory?

(A) OSHA

(B) CDC

(C) CSC

(D) CLIA

(E) CIA

9. General rules of laboratory include all of the following EXCEPT

(A) store caustic materials at below eye level

(B) do not wear your PPE outside of the lab

(C) dry hands before handling reagent bottles

(D) use mouth suction, when possible, to pipette

(E) check glassware for chips

10. When working with the microscope, which of the following is correct?

(A) carry the microscope with one hand using only the arm of the microscope

(B) 10× setting is used for oil immersion

(C) 40× is used for a high power, dry specimen

(D) lower stage after removing slide

(E) all of the above are correct

ON THE JOB

You have been invited as a guest lecturer to speak to a group of medical assisting students who are about to enter into the area of study concerning microbiology. You have been specifically asked to discuss how to care for and operate the microscope.

What is your response?

1. Draft an outline you would use when discussing the use of the microscope.

2. What are some of the precautions you would mention?

3. Describe 10 general safety precautions to be followed when using a microscope that you would instruct the students about.

References

American Medical Association. *Current Procedural Terminology.* Chicago: American Medical Association, 1996.

Belsey, R., Mulrow, C., Sox, H. "How to Handle Baffling Test Results." *Patient Care.* May 30, 1993.

"CDC Summarizes Final Regulations for Implementing CLIA." *American Family Physician.* 45:6, 1992.

Chernecky, C., Krech, R., and Berger, B. *Laboratory Tests and Diagnostic Procedures.* Philadelphia: W. B. Saunders, 1993.

Fishbach, F. *A Manual of Laboratory & Diagnostic Tests.* Philadelphia: Lippincott, 1996.

Marshall, J. *Medical Laboratory Assistant.* Upper Saddle River, NJ: Brady/Prentice Hall, 1990.

Stucke, V. *Microbiology for Nurses.* Philadelphia: W. B. Saunders, 1992.

Tietz, N. *Clinical Guide to Laboratory Tests,* 2nd ed. Philadelphia: W. B. Saunders, 1990.

Tietz, N., Conn, R., and Pruden, E. *Applied Laboratory Medicine.* Philadelphia: W. B. Saunders, 1992.

Walters, N., Estridge, B., and Reynolds, A. *Basic Medical Laboratory Techniques.* New York: Delmar Publishers, Inc., 1990.

MEDICAL ASSISTANT ROLE DELINEATION CHART

Highlight indicates material covered in this chapter

ADMINISTRATIVE

ADMINISTRATIVE PROCEDURES

- Perform basic clerical functions
- Schedule, coordinate, and monitor appointments
- Schedule inpatient/outpatient admissions and procedures
- Understand and apply third party guidelines
- Obtain reimbursement through accurate claims submission
- Monitor third-party reimbursement
- Perform medical transcription
- Understand and adhere to managed care policies and procedures
- *Negotiate managed care contracts (adv)*

PRACTICE FINANCES

- Perform procedural and diagnostic coding
- Apply bookkeeping principles
- Document and maintain accounting and banking records
- Manage accounts receivable
- Manage accounts payable
- Process payroll
- *Develop and maintain fee schedules (adv)*
- *Manage renewals of business and professional insurance policies (adv)*
- *Manage personal benefits and maintain records (adv)*

CLINICAL

FUNDAMENTAL PRINCIPLES

- Apply principles of aseptic technique and infection control
- Comply with quality assurance practices
- Screen and follow up patient test results

DIAGNOSTIC ORDERS

- Collect and process specimens
- Perform diagnostic tests

PATIENT CARE

- Adhere to established triage procedures
- Obtain patient history and vital signs
- Prepare and maintain examination and treatment areas

- Prepare patient for examinations, procedures, and treatments
- Assist with examinations, procedures, and treatments
- Prepare and administer medications and immunizations
- Maintain medication and immunization records
- Recognize and respond to emergencies
- Coordinate patient care information with other health care providers

GENERAL (TRANSDISCIPLINARY)

PROFESSIONALISM

- Project a professional manner and image
- Adhere to ethical principles
- Demonstrate initiative and responsibility
- Work as a team member
- Manage time efficiently
- Prioritize and perform multiple tasks
- Adapt to change
- Promote the CMA credential
- Enhance skills through continuing education

COMMUNICATION SKILLS

- Treat all patients with compassion and empathy
- Recognize and respect cultural diversity
- Adapt communications to individual's ability to understand
- Use professional telephone technique
- Use effective and correct verbal and written communications
- Recognize and respond to verbal and nonverbal communications
- Use medical terminology appropriately
- Receive, organize, prioritize, and transmit information
- Serve as liaison
- Promote the practice through positive public relations

LEGAL CONCEPTS

- Maintain confidentiality
- Practice within the scope of education, training, and personal capabilities
- Prepare and maintain medical records
- Document accurately
- Use appropriate guidelines when releasing information
- Follow employer's established policies dealing with the health care contract
- Follow federal, state, and local legal guidelines
- Maintain awareness of federal and state health care legislation and regulations
- Maintain and dispose of regulated substances in compliance with government guidelines
- Comply with established risk management and safety procedures
- Recognize professional credentialing criteria
- Participate in the development and maintenance of personnel, policy, and procedure manuals
- *Develop and maintain personnel, policy, and procedure manuals (adv)*

INSTRUCTION

- Instruct individuals according to their needs
- Explain office policies and procedures
- Teach methods of health promotion and disease prevention
- Locate community resources and disseminate information
- *Orient and train personnel (adv)*
- *Develop educational materials (adv)*
- *Conduct continuing education activities (adv)*

OPERATIONAL FUNCTIONS

- Maintain supply inventory
- Evaluate and recommend equipment and supplies
- Apply computer techniques to support office operations
- *Supervise personnel (adv)*
- *Interview and recommend job applicants (adv)*
- *Negotiate leases and prices for equipment and supply contracts (adv)*

SOURCE: Reprinted by permission of the American Association of Medical Assistants from the *AAMA Role Delineation Study: Occupational Analysis of the Medical Assisting Profession.*

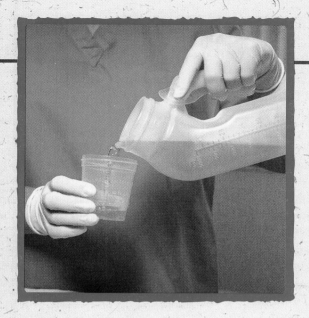

26

Urinalysis

LEARNING OBJECTIVES

After completing this chapter, you should:
1. Define and spell the glossary terms for this chapter.
2. List six types of urine specimens that can be collected.
3. Describe the steps for collecting a clean-catch urine specimen.
4. List 5 items included in a physical analysis of a urine specimen.
5. List 6 items included in a chemical analysis of a urine specimen.
6. Describe the procedure for measuring specific gravity using a urinometer.
7. Be able to state normal values for specific gravity and pH.
8. List what is included in organized and unorganized sediment.
9. Discuss quality control.

CLINICAL PERFORMANCE COMPETENCIES

After completing this chapter, you should perform the following tasks:
1. Instruct a patient on a routine urine sample, morning specimen, timed specimen, two-hour postprandial test, and clean-catch midstream specimen.
2. Measure specific gravity using a urinometer and refractometer.
3. Perform a chemical examination of urine using a Multistix, Clinitest, and Tes-Tape.
4. Be able to discuss pH results.
5. Be able to prepare a microscope slide for examination of sediment.
6. Do physical, chemical, and microscopic analyses.

Glossary

aromatic   Pleasant, natural odor.

catheterization   Inserting a sterile tube into the bladder to withdraw urine or into a vein for a procedure.

circumcised   Foreskin surrounding the glans penis has been removed surgically.

***Escherichia coli* (E. coli)**   A bacillus present in the colon or intestinal tract. Can cause infections when it is present in the urinary tract.

fetid   Foul odor.

first morning specimen   The first voided urine of the day upon arising.

glomerulonephritis   Kidney disease which involves inflammation and lesions of the glomeruli.

glucosuria/glycosuria   The presence of sugar (glucose) in the urine.

hematuria   The presence of blood in the urine.

high-powered field (hpf)   High power magnification of the microscope.

incontinent   Unable to control the passing of urine or feces.

labia   Two folds of tissue on either side of the female vaginal opening.

low power field (lpf)   Low power magnification of the microscope.

normal value(s)   The amount of a substance that is normally present. There can also be a range for normal value.

nosocomial infection   Infection acquired in a hospital.

occult blood   Blood in such small quantity that it can only be seen under a microscope or detected by a specific test (for example, Multistix test).

oliguria   Reduction of urine, scant amount.

parasites   An organism that lives within another organism.

pathology   Disease process.

perineal care   Cleansing the area between the vulva and the anus and within the vulva in a female and between the scrotum and the anus in a male.

random sample   The selection of one sample from a large group. In urinalysis it means any sample taken throughout the day.

refractometer   Used to measure the specific gravity of urine.

sediment   The substance settling to the bottom of a fluid.

specific gravity (S.G.)   Weight of a substance compared with an equal volume of water.

squamous epithelial cells   Flattened scale-like cells attached at the edges which line the bladder. Commonly seen in microscopic examinations.

turbidity   Having a cloudy appearance.

two hour postprandial   Two hours after eating a meal.

urinary meatus   Opening from the urethra to the outside of the body.

urinary retention   Inability to urinate.

urinalysis (U/A)   Refers to the testing of urine for the presence of infection or disease. The testing may be physical, chemical, or microscopic.

urinometer   Used to measure specific gravity of urine.

void   To pass urine.

WARNING!

For all patient contact, adhere to Standard Precautions
(see pages 342–373). Wear protective equipment as indicated.

One of the most common laboratory procedures is the routine urinalysis. This specimen is collected by the patient but the medical assistant must carefully explain how to collect the urine sample. This simple test can give the doctor valuable information about many functions of the body, including kidney function.

Asepsis

Asepsis plays a major role in urinalysis. When handling urine or containers of urine you must follow universal blood and body-fluid precautions. This means you will wear nonsterile gloves, lab coats, and goggles and carefully avoid contaminating the testing equipment with urine. Refer to Chapter 19 for a thorough discussion of asepsis or infection control.

Collecting the Specimen

The patient will need to provide more than just a few drops of urine. See Figure 26-1 for an example of a urine specimen collected in a container. Generally at least 10 mL of urine are necessary for proper testing.

Types of Specimens

1. Routine (random) sample
2. Morning specimen—first voided
3. Timed specimen
4. Two-hour postprandial
5. Clean-catch midstream
6. Catheterized specimen

Routine (*Random*) Sample

A routine (random) sample of urine is collected in a nonsterile container. The patient should be in-

Med Tip: Remember that many patients do not know or understand medical terminology. Terms such as void, micturition, and urination, which all mean basically the same thing, may not be understood by many of your patients. For example, "passing water" is a phrase that many elderly patients use when they discuss their own urination.

structed against using empty containers from home that have contained food products since this may contaminate the specimen. A random sample of urine can be collected any time during the day when the patient is in your office. This sample would be

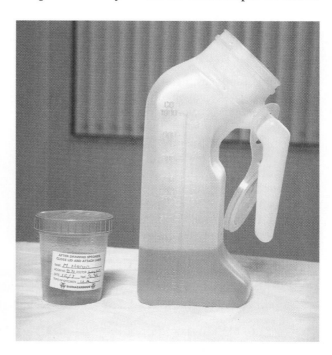

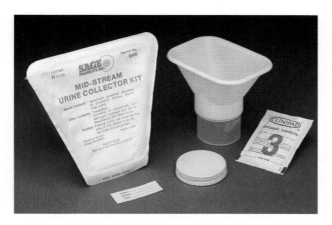

Figure 26-1   Urine specimen containers.

Collecting a Routine Urine Specimen

1. Provide the patient with a nonsterile container which is labeled with the patient's name and date.

2. Ask the patient to use the bathroom and void into the container. Tell the patient to only fill the container two-thirds of the way to avoid spillage.

3. Explain where you want the patient to leave the container with urine. Generally, the container is placed on paper toweling to avoid contamination of a work area.

4. Wearing nonsterile gloves, take the specimen and test the urine immediately.

5. If you are not able to test the specimen within 30 minutes, place it in the refrigerator. Urine should be at room temperature before testing.

used only for a routine screening since urine will change its composition during the day. See the instructions for collecting a routine urine specimen.

Morning Specimens—First Voided

Patients may be asked to collect a sample of urine the first time they urinate in the morning since it is the most concentrated urine. This is called a first morning specimen. It is used for pregnancy testing, urine culturing, and microscopic examinations. The patient is instructed to collect this specimen at home and bring it into the office. These specimens should be examined within thirty minutes to one hour after collection since the urine can undergo changes. If the sample cannot be examined right away, it should be refrigerated. The doctor may want you to add a preservative to the urine container.

Timed Specimens

Timed specimens are used when the doctor wants urine samples taken at specific intervals during the day. For instance, twenty-four hour urine specimens would be collected during a specific twenty-four hour period of the day. Every drop of urine the patient produces must be placed in a container and saved for this test. This test is used to determine the glomerular filtration rate of the kidneys (creatinine clearance) and for a chemical analysis to test hormone levels. The instructions for collecting a twenty-four hour urine specimen follow.

Obtaining a urine specimen for an infant or young child requires special equipment. See Figure 26-2 for an example of a baby's urine collector.

Two-Hour Postprandial

A two-hour postprandial urine specimen is collected two hours after a meal is eaten. This is used for diabetic testing.

Clean-Catch Midstream Specimen

A clean-catch midstream specimen may be necessary if the urine is going to be examined for microorganisms or cultured for bacterial growth. You will have to provide the patient with clear instructions so they do not contaminate the specimen. See instructions for obtaining a clean-catch midstream specimen.

Catheterization

Catheterization is sometimes necessary to collect a sterile specimen of urine. This procedure is not generally performed by a medical assistant, however, a discussion of the process follows since the medical assistant may be called on to assist. In this procedure, a catheter or sterile thin tube is inserted into the bladder via the urethra to withdraw urine (Figures 26-4 and 26-5). Some reasons for doing this procedure are:

Collecting a Twenty-four Hour Urine Specimen

1. Explain why the patient is being asked to save all urine for twenty-four hours.

2. Give the patient a container large enough to hold all their urine. Generally, a one gallon container is used. Label the container with the patient's name, date and time the collection begins and ends on the laboratory slip.

3. The test usually begins at 7 A.M. Tell the patient to discard (throw away) the first voided urine so that the bladder is empty when the test begins. The test will be over at 7 A.M. the next morning. It is very important that the patient collects the last 7 A.M. specimen. If the test begins at any other time, have the patient write the exact time on the container.

4. Instruct the patient not to urinate directly into the container but, rather, into a container with a spout, such as a large measuring cup. The urine is then poured into the large 24-hour container. Caution the patient against spilling any urine outside of the collection container.

5. The urine must be kept cool to preserve it. The 24-hour container should be placed in a container of ice or portable cooler during collection. Tell the patient to keep the urine cool during transport for testing, also.

6. The patient is instructed where to take the specimen at the end of a 24-hour period. It must be taken in for testing immediately.

- To obtain a sterile urine specimen.
- To determine the amount of urine remaining in the bladder (residual urine) after the patient has attempted to empty the bladder by voiding. The patient is asked to void normally. Since this amount is often measured, you will have to provide the patient with a container that is calibrated. The patient is then catheterized by trained personnel and the remaining amount of urine is the residual. With this procedure there is risk of a nosocomial (hospital acquired) infection for the patient, so great care must be taken to maintain sterile conditions.
- To obtain a urine specimen when it cannot be obtained naturally through voiding. For instance, if a patient is incontinent—unable

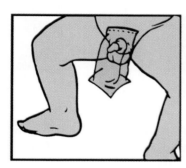 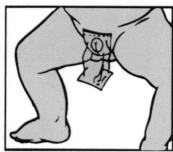

Figure 26-2 Baby's urine collector.

Collecting a Clean-Catch Midstream Specimen

Equipment: sterile urine container, 4 cotton balls or cleansing towelettes, soap and water, or midstream urine kit. (*Note:* Towelettes are preferred for cleansing since cotton balls may leave minute fibers.)

1. Instruct the patient to wash hands and remove underwear if necessary.

2. Cleansing the area:
   For female patients: Use one hand to spread apart the labia and perform perineal care by washing inside the labia at the urinary meatus (opening) with a soap moistened cotton ball or cleansing towelette. Instruct the patient to wash herself from the front to the back of her labia area. Use a fresh cotton ball or cleansing towelette for each side of the meatus. Then use a fresh cotton ball or towelette to wipe across the meatus once. Tell the patient to continue to hold the labia apart during the entire process. *Note:* Instruct the patient using lay terms since not all patients understand the terms *labia* and *urinary meatus.*
   For male patient: Instruct the patient to pull the foreskin back, if he is not circumcised, and hold it back while he is cleaning the penis and during urination. (The foreskin surrounding the glans penis is surgically removed when a male is circumcised.) Tell the patient to use a moistened cotton ball or cleansing towelette in a circular motion to clean the head of the penis and around the urinary meatus. Then use a fresh cotton ball or towelette to wipe directly across the urinary meatus.

3. Rinse the area to remove the soap. Dry the area with a fresh cotton ball using the front to back wiping method. This is not necessary when using towelettes (which most clean-catch urine kits include).

4. Instruct the patient to start to void urine into the toilet while holding labia apart. Then tell the patient to stop voiding and place the urine container in a position to catch the remaining urine "midstream." The inside of the container should not be touched by the patient since it is sterile.

5. When the cup is 2/3 filled, the patient should take the cup away and void the last urine into the toilet. The "mid-stream" urine has now been collected since the first and last of the patient's urine was voided into the toilet. See Figure 26-3 for an example of a container for clean-catch urine specimen.

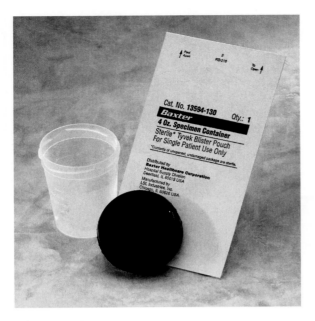

Figure 26-3 Container for clean-catch urine specimen.

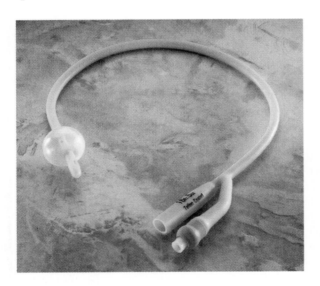

Figure 26-4 Foley catheter.

to control the passing of urine—it may be necessary to catheterize the patient for a urine specimen or drug test. Also used to relieve urinary retention.

- To empty the bladder completely before surgery or diagnostic tests.

Routine Analysis

Urinalysis refers to the testing of urine for the presence of infection or disease. A routine urinalysis is divided into three categories: physical characteristics, chemical examination, and microscopic analysis. Table 26-1 contains a list of items included in each category.

In general, a routine urinalysis will include a description of color and appearance, pH reaction (acidity/alkalinity), specific gravity, chemical analysis for glucose and protein and microscopic examination of the sediment. Sediment is the substance that settles to the bottom of a fluid.

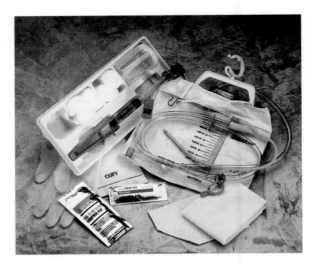

Figure 26-5 Foley catheter tray.

Physical Characteristics

The physical characteristics observed in a urine analysis include: appearance (clarity/turbidity), color, odor, quantity or volume, and specific gravity. A discussion of each of these characteristics as well as a description of the procedures and equipment used to test these characteristics follows.

Appearance

The appearance of the specimen may range from clear to cloudy. Terms that are used to describe appearance include: clear, slightly cloudy, cloudy with sediment, cloudy with shreds. Turbidity, or cloudiness, may be caused by bacterial infection, cells, yeast or vaginal contaminants. Your description should explain exactly what you see. It's important to remember that a clear specimen may become cloudy when crystals form during the cooling process.

Color

The normal color of urine is straw but due to the concentration of a specimen the color will vary from almost colorless to amber. Brown or black generally indicates a serious disease process. For

TABLE 26-1   Routine Analysis Categories

Physical	Chemical	Microscopic
Appearance (clarity/turbidity)	Reaction *pH*	Cells
Color	Protein	Blood = RBC, WBC
Odor	Glucose	Squamous epithelial cells
Quantity (24 hr. only)	Blood	Spermatozoa
Specific Gravity	Ketone	Transitional epithelial cells
	Bilirubin	Casts
	Urobilinogen	Hyaline
	Nitrite	Cellular
	Leukocytes	Granular
		Waxy
		Crystals
		Acid
		Alkaline
		Contaminants
		"Artifacts"
		Other:
		Bacteria
		Parasites
		Yeasts

example, greenish-brown urine may indicate a liver disorder such as hepatitis.

Many factors influence the color of urine including: food, medications, and disease. Foods such as beets will give urine a distinctive color. Abnormal color does not always indicate pathology or disease.

Odor

While normal odor may not be recorded, an abnormal odor can be an important finding. Urine normally has what is called an aromatic odor. Odors may be caused by disease, diet (foods) or bacteria. For instance, patients with uncontrolled diabetes may have a "fruity" odor to their urine due to ketones (products of fat metabolism). A fetid or foul odor may indicate infection or old urine. An ammonia smell may be due to infection.

As urine sits (such as in a diaper) you may smell an ammonia odor due to the bacteria breaking down the urea to form ammonia. Large amounts of asparagus in your patient's diet could result in urine with a strong odor.

Med Tip: If you notice a urine specimen has an unusual color, ask what medications the patient is taking or what foods he or she has eaten recently. Some medications and foods affect urine color, for example, beets may impart a red color. Also, a urine specimen from a menstruating woman may have physical evidence of blood from vaginal contamination.

Quantity (Volume)

The amount or volume of urine is not measured on a routine sample. It is measured in certain tests and procedures such as a timed specimen (24 hr.) and as part of the catheterization process. The normal quantity of urine for an adult during a 24 hour period will vary between 700 and 2000 mL with the average being around 1500 mL or 3 pints. However, this will vary according to fluids taken by the patient. Excessive urine production can be an indication of disease such as diabetes and some kidney disorders.

Oliguria (decreased amount of urine production) can be caused by excessive perspiration, diarrhea, bleeding, decreased fluid intake and kidney disease. Anuria or the complete absence of urine production can result from urinary tract obstruction or renal failure. The patient's intake and output (I & O) of fluid may have to be monitored. This is done by keeping a record of the amount of fluids taken in and the measurement of all urine excreted.

Specific Gravity

Specific gravity (SG) is the weight of a substance in relation to the weight of that same amount of distilled water. Water is used as the standard and has a specific gravity of one (1.000). The normal specific gravity of urine will vary between 1.010 and 1.030 depending on how concentrated the specimen is. If the reading falls below or above this normal range, it may indicate that the kidney's ability to dilute or concentrate the urine is not functioning properly. An abnormal result could be an indication of kidney disease. Dilute urine (for example S.G. 1.005), which is found in diseases such as diabetes mellitus and in patients on a salt restricting diet, has lower specific gravity. Further tests would be indicated.

Med Tip: The concentration of urine changes during the day depending on how much fluid is taken. Specific gravity is considered a rough measure of the amount of substances dissolved in the urine.

Urinometer Method Laboratories use the urinometer, dipstick, or refractometer methods to measure specific gravity (Figure 26-6).

The urinometer has a float with a bulb of mercury at the bottom which is attached to a stem that has a calibrated scale from 1.000 to 1.040. The uri-

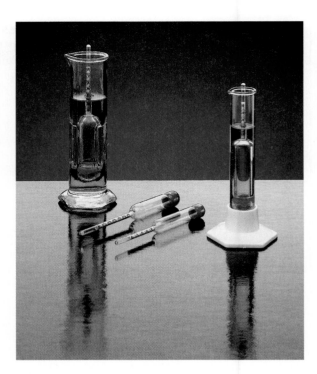

Figure 26-6   A urinometer is used to measure specific gravity.

nometer is a fragile device and shaking it can cause an incorrect reading. The calibration of the urinometer should be checked daily to make sure it has not changed. Using distilled water, the urinometer should calibrate at 1.000. If the calibration is off, replace the urinometer.

Note: On a short term basis you can use a miscalibrated urinometer by adjusting for the error. For example, if the urinometer reads 1.003 in distilled water, then subtract .003 from the urine reading.

If an unusually high reading is taken, wash the urinometer in cold water to remove all urine residue. Then test it in cold water and retest the urine sample. Someone may not have thoroughly cleaned the urinometer which would result in an incorrect test for your specimen. The procedure for using a urinometer to measure specific gravity follows.

Refractometer Method Another method used for determining specific gravity (S.G.) is the refractometer method. This method uses light, a prism, and a calibrated scale on the refractometer to measure the concentration level of the specimen (Figure 26-8 A and B).

It is necessary to know the normal values for a substance, for example, the amount of glucose or ketones normally present in urine or its natural

**Terminal Performance
Competency:** Student must perform procedure without error and not more than .01 difference from instructor's reading.

Equipment and Supplies

Biohazardous waste container

Blood and body fluid protection—lab coat, goggles, nonsterile gloves

Distilled water

Paper, pen/pencil

Patient record

Tube/cylinder

Urine specimen

Urinometer

Note: Follow Standard Precautions and safety guidelines when working with urine samples. Use care to avoid splashing or spilling urine. Wipe up all spills using guidelines established by OSHA.

Procedural Steps

1. Wash hands.
2. Put on gloves and protective clothing.
3. Assemble equipment and materials.
4. Make sure the urine is mixed well by swirling it in the urine container.
5. Pour room-temperature urine into the cylinder to the two-thirds to three-quarter full mark.
6. Place the cylinder on a level surface. Do not hold the cylinder in your hand. Ideally the meniscus should be at eye level (Figure 26-7). Gently float the urinometer in the urine with a spinning motion using the thumb and index finger.
7. When the spinning stops, read the S.G. at the point where the lower part of the meniscus crosses the urinometer line. Reading at the top of the meniscus or bottom of it is determined by whether the urine is clear or cloudy. If clear read at bottom; if cloudy read at top.
8. Duplicate the reading at least once to check accuracy.
9. Record the reading on a piece of paper.
10. Discard the urine according to OSHA guidelines.
11. Remove gloves and protective clothing, and dispose of them properly.
12. Wash hands.
13. Document findings in patient record. Bill using correct CPT code for procedure.
14. Clean work area and equipment according to OSHA guidelines.

Charting example:

4/23/XX   1:00 pm   S.G. 1.012
                                        M. King, CMA

color, "straw color," in order to evaluate the test findings of a specific specimen. Table 26-2 contains the normal values for a urine sample.

Chemical Analysis

Testing for chemicals in the urine can tell us more about the condition of the patient (Figures 26-9 through 26-12). This is used in addition to the physical examination. The most commonly used techniques are reagent strips or dipsticks. They are plastic strips which have chemicals implanted on small pads along the strip. The strips are then "dipped" into the urine and the results, or color changes of the chemicals, are compared to charts with normal and abnormal values. These color charts are generally on the dipstick container. Dipstick tests are available for *p*H, protein, glucose, ketones, blood, bilirubin, urobilinogen, nitrite, leukocytes, specific gravity, and others. These tests provide information about the functioning of the kidneys, liver, and other organs.

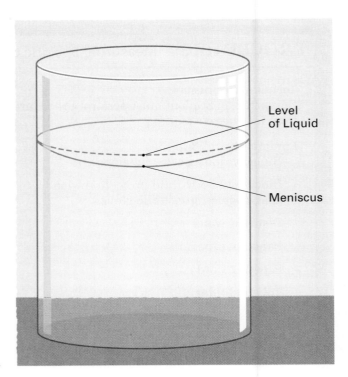

Figure 26-7   Meniscus.

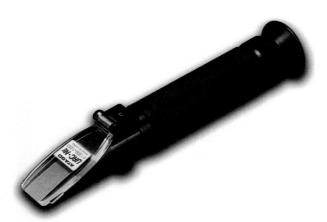

Figure 26-8   (A) Portable Digital Refractometer from Vee-Gee Scientific.

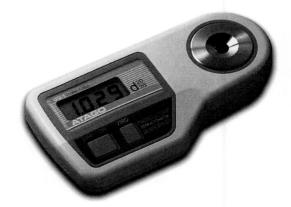

(B) Standard Refractometer Uri-con NE Refractometer from Vee-Gee Scientific.

Med Tip: Remember that the strip must not touch the side of the dipstick container when you are comparing it to the color chart. Touching the container with the urine covered dipstick will contaminate the container.

The reagent strips are used once and then discarded into a hazardous waste container. The reaction times after the chemical stick is moistened with urine are short. You will have to time the reading of each test. For instance, the reading for glucose can be read after waiting 30 seconds. The container of the test you are using will state the reaction times for each test. There are also tests available using test tablets and paper tapes.

The Clinitest uses a chemical tablet and color reaction chart to assist in determining the presence of certain sugars (lactose and galactose) in the urine. This test is generally not used any longer for insulin monitoring since it is not specific for glucose.

PROCEDURE: Measuring Specific Gravity (S.G.) With a Refractometer

**Terminal Performance
Competency:** Student must perform procedure without error and not more than .01 difference from instructor's reading.

Equipment and Supplies

Antiseptic cleaner

Biohazardous waste container

Blood and body fluid protection—lab coat, goggles, nonsterile gloves

Distilled water

Medicine dropper/pipette

Paper, pen/pencil

Paper towels

Prism

Refractometer (and cover plate if not attached to refractometer)

Urine specimen

Note: Follow Standard Precautions and safety guidelines when working with urine samples. Use care to avoid splashing or spilling urine. Wipe up all spills using guidelines established by OSHA.

Procedural Steps

1. Wash hands.
2. Put on gloves and protective clothing.
3. Assemble equipment and materials.
4. Before using the refractometer, perform a quality control check by using a sample of distilled water first. The value with distilled water should be 1.000.
   a. Clean the prism and refractometer cover with distilled water. Wipe dry.
   b. Close the cover. Using the medicine dropper or pipette, place a drop of distilled water on the notched area of the cover. If the refractometer does not have an attached cover, place the water directly onto the prism, and then place a cover plate on top of the prism.
   c. Tilt the refractometer to allow light to enter. Read the specific gravity by noting the division line between the light and dark area. This reading should be 1.000. If it is not, retest with fresh distilled water.
5. To test the urine sample, swirl the urine specimen gently to avoid splashing. Using the medicine dropper remove a small sample and place 1-2 drops onto the notched area of the cover.
6. Follow instructions in step "4c" to read the specific gravity.
7. Record the reading on a piece of paper.
8. Discard the urine according to OSHA guidelines.
9. Remove gloves and protective clothing, and dispose of them properly.
10. Wash hands.
11. Document findings in patient record. Bill using correct CPT code for procedure.
12. Clean work area and equipment according to OSHA guidelines.

Charting example:

4/23/XX   1:00 pm   S.G. 1.012
                         M. King, CMA

Reaction *p*H

The *p*H of a solution indicates acidity or alkalinity. This reaction is measured on a scale ranging from 0 to 14 with a 7 being the neutral point (Table 26-3). On this scale *0* represents the highest level of acidity and 14 represents the highest level of alkalinity.

Urine voided by patients on a normal diet is slightly acidic at around a *p*H of 6.0. Normal kidneys can produce urine ranging from 4.5 to 8. A *p*H

TABLE 26-2 Normal Values for Urinalysis Testing

Element	Normal Findings
Color	Pale yellow to deep gold
	Straw colored
Odor	Aromatic
Appearance	Clear
Specific Gravity	1.010-1.030
pH	5.0-8.0
Protein	Negative to trace
Glucose	None
Ketones	None
Occult Blood	Negative
Leukocytes	Negative
Nitrite	Negative
Bilirubin	Negative

lower than 7.0 is common in urinary tract infections, metabolic or respiratory acidosis, diets that are high in fruits or vegetables and the administration of some drugs such as sodium bicarbonate. A pH higher than 7.0 is common in fever, phenylketonuria, high protein diets, and when taking large amounts of ascorbic acid (Vitamin C). If a specimen is allowed to stand for a long time, bacteria will grow and the urine will test alkaline.

Protein

Urine may normally contain some protein after a person has been exposed to the cold, strenuous muscular activity, or eating large amounts of protein. However, the presence of protein may indicate preeclampsia (toxemia) in a pregnant woman, congestive heart failure, or glomerulonephritis for example. Glomerulonephritis is a kidney disease which involves inflammation and lesions of the glomeruli.

Glucose

Small amounts of glucose may be present in the urine after eating a high carbohydrate diet. This will return to normal if there are no disease factors present. Other reasons for the presence of glucose include poorly controlled diabetes, pregnancy, stress, the use of some medications (such as corti-

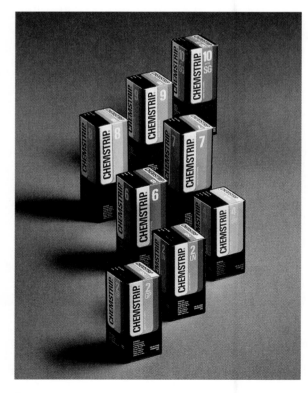

Figure 26-9   Ames Multistix chemical reagent strips.

PROCEDURE: Testing for Sugar in the Urine Using Tablets

Terminal Performance
Competency: Student will perform procedure without error.

Equipment and Supplies

Antiseptic cleaner

Biohazardous waste container

Body and body fluid protection—lab coat, goggles, nonsterile gloves

Clean glass test tube

Clinitest tablets

Distilled water

Medicine dropper/pipette

Urine specimen

Note: Follow Standard Precautions and safety guidelines when working with urine samples. Use care to avoid splashing or spilling urine. Wipe up all spills using guidelines established by OSHA.

Procedural Steps

1. Wash hands.
2. Apply gloves and protective clothing.
3. Assemble equipment and materials.
4. Using the medicine dropper or a pipette, remove a small amount of urine from the urine specimen container. Place five drops into a clean test tube.
5. Add 10 drops of water. Mix together using the pipette, being careful not to splash the urine.
6. Drop one Clinitest tablet into the urine/water solution. Observe the solution as it "boils" in the test tube without shaking the tube. Do not touch the bottom of the tube during this chemical process since it becomes very hot.

7. Fifteen seconds after the reaction (boiling) stops, gently shake the tube to mix the contents.
8. Immediately compare the color of the liquid against the color chart on the side of the Clinitest container by matching the color in the tube with one on the chart. *Note:* Do not touch the test tube of urine to the Clinitest bottle since this will contaminate the outside of the bottle. Ignore any additional color changes after the fifteen second period.
9. Discard the urine according to OSHA guidelines.
10. Remove gloves and protective clothing, and dispose of them properly.
11. Wash hands.
12. Document findings in patient record. Clinitest can be reported either as a percentage or as trace-4+.
13. Clean work area and equipment according to OSHA guidelines.

    For example:

    1/4% or trace

    1/2% or 1+

    3/4% or 2+

    1% or 3+

    2% or 4+

Charting example:

| 10/19/XX | 4:00 pm | Clinitest 2+ |
| | | M. King, CMA |

---

costeroids or aspirin), infection, and Cushing's syndrome. Glucose will begin to "spill" into the urine when the blood glucose level exceeds 160 to 180 mg/100 mL. This is the basis for the urine glucose tests (Figure 26-13). Glucosuria or glycosuria refers to an abnormal amount of sugar in the urine. This is mainly seen in diabetes mellitus. If the pa-

tient has taken large amounts of Vitamin C a false positive test for glucose may result.

Blood

While a few red blood cells seen in the urine under the microscope are normal, the presence of occult (hidden) blood in the urine may indicate some

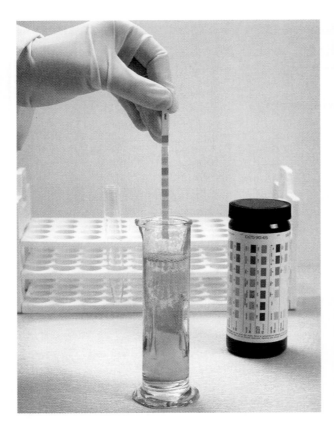

Figure 26-10 (A) Dip reagent strip into urine and withdraw.

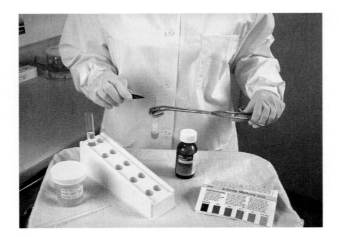

Figure 26-11 Testing urine with Clinitest tablets.

anemias, medications such as blood thinners, arsenic poisoning, reactions to transfusions, trauma, burns and convulsions. Hematuria is the presence of blood in the urine.

Ketone

Usually ketone bodies are not present in the urine. Ketone in the urine represents improper met-

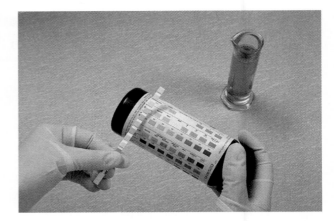

(B) Compare color change on reagent strip to chart on side of container.

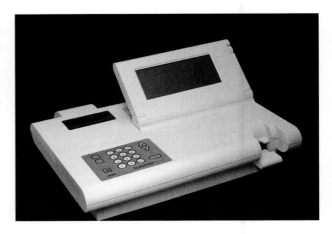

Figure 26-12 Clinitec 100.

abolism of fats. Conditions associated with ketone in the urine are poorly controlled diabetes, dehydration, starvation, ingestion of large amounts of aspirin and sometimes after a general anesthesia.

Bilirubin

When hemoglobin breaks down bilirubin is one of the products. Hemoglobin is converted to bilirubin in the liver and then to urobilinogen in the intestines. It is generally not found in the urine. Its presence may be one of the first signs of liver disease and such diseases as mononucleosis. A large amount of bilirubin in the urine will cause a change in color ranging from a yellow-brown to a green-orange. Light will cause bilirubin to decompose and specimens must be kept away from light until they are tested.

Urobilinogen

This can be found in urine in small amounts under normal conditions. However, it may be increased as a result of red blood destruction and in liver dis-

TABLE 26-3　Reaction pH Measured on a Scale of 0-14

Acidity 0-7	Neutral 7	Alkalinity 7-14
Acid Range 0-1-2-3-4-5-6-**7**	**7**	**Alkaline Range** **7**-8-9-10-11-12-13-14

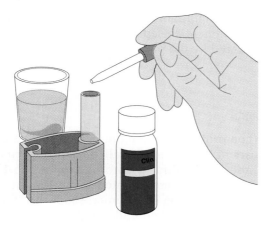

Clinitest

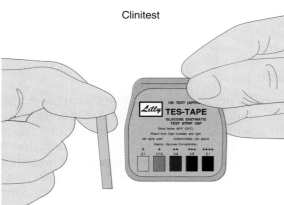

Tes-Tape

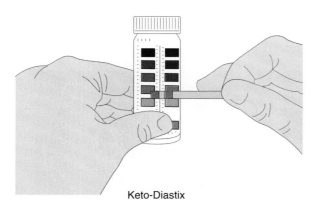

Keto-Diastix

Figure 26-13　Types of diabetic urine tests.

ease. The reagent strip for testing will show a positive test when the color changes from orange through green to dark blue. The lack of any urobilinogen may mean an obstruction of the bile duct.

Nitrite

Nitrites in the urine indicate a urinary tract infection. Nitrites occur in the urine when bacteria break down nitrite. However, a negative nitrite test may still mean there is a bacterial infection but it is not strong enough to break down the nitrite. The organism responsible for most urinary tract infections, especially in women, is *Escherichia coli* (**E. coli**) which can occur from the presence of bowel material finding its way into the urinary meatus and up into the tract to the bladder. E. Coli is nitrite positive. A false positive can occur by allowing a specimen to sit too long at room temperature so that the bacteria are allowed to grow. Refrigerating the specimen, if you cannot test it right away, will help to eliminate this problem. False negatives can also occur.

Leukocytes

Normally there should be no leukocytes—white blood cells (WBCs)—present in the urine. These occur when there is a urinary tract infection.

Microscopic Examination

The third type of examination included in the routine urinalysis is the microscopic examination. This identifies the type and approximate number of organisms present in the urine specimen. Microscopic examination helps the physician to determine a disease process. In some states or areas, medical assistants do not perform microscopic exams on urine. Some physicians may send urine specimens to outside labs for testing.

　　The sediment in urine consists of organized sediment containing red blood cells, white blood cells, epithelial cells, casts, bacteria, parasites, yeast, fungi, and spermatozoa. The unorganized sediment is generally all chemical material. It includes crystals and amorphous materials—materials having no definite shape. The type of specimen used for this analysis is a freshly voided specimen. If possible, the specimen should be clean-catch to avoid any contamination.

Generally, you will find one or two white blood cells and red blood cells and a few epithelial cells per high-power field (hpf). This is not considered to be abnormal. High-power field (hpf) refers to the high power magnification setting on a microscope that greatly enlarges images for viewing.

Cells

More than one or two red blood cells (RBC) per hpf is abnormal. Their presence must always be reported since this could indicate serious conditions such as trauma to the urinary system, hemorrhagic diseases, or tumor. Red blood cells are pale, round, have no nucleus, or core, and are nongranular. White blood cells, greater than 5 per hpf is abnormal and may be due to a contamination of the specimen. White blood cells contain a nucleus and are larger than red blood cells with a granular appearance. See Figure 26-14 for an illustration of blood cells.

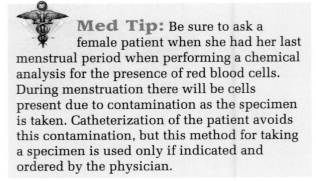

Med Tip: Be sure to ask a female patient when she had her last menstrual period when performing a chemical analysis for the presence of red blood cells. During menstruation there will be cells present due to contamination as the specimen is taken. Catheterization of the patient avoids this contamination, but this method for taking a specimen is used only if indicated and ordered by the physician.

Casts

When protein forms in the kidney tubules and appears in the urine it is called casts (Figure 26-15). These are classified according to what substance is in them. Casts are counted using the low-power field (lpf) setting of the microscope, but the types of cast are identified under high-power magnification. Hyaline casts must be observed under low light and their presence can indicate kidney disease. Red blood casts indicate disease and occur in glomerulonephritis.

Bacteria

Normally urine does not contain bacteria. A specimen could become contaminated during collection or with vaginal secretions from the female patient. A urinary tract infection is indicated by bacteria in the urine. If the specimen also contains white blood cells, this may indicate an infection as opposed to contamination of the specimen. Urine cultures are commonly used to aid in the diagnosis of a urinary tract infection (UTI) and/or to determine the effectiveness of an antibiotic prescribed for a patient with a UTI.

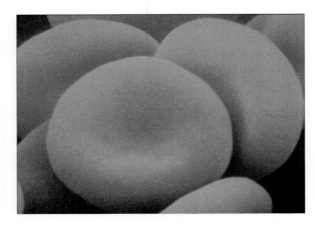

Figure 26-14   Blood cells.

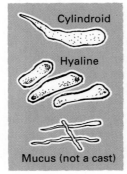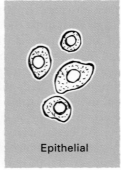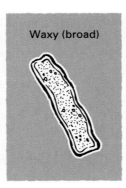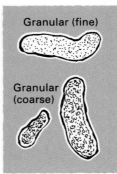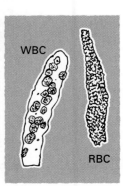

Figure 26-15   Urine casts come from protein that forms in the kidney.

Yeast

Yeast may be present in the urine of females who have a vaginal yeast infection (moniliasis). It also can be an indication of disease such as diabetes mellitus.

Parasites

Parasites are organisms that live within other organisms. They may be present in urine due to contamination from vaginal or bowel excretions.

Spermatozoa

Spermatozoa, the male sex cell, can appear as a contaminant in urine of the female after sexual intercourse. Sperm may occasionally be seen in the male's urine.

Crystals

The type and number of crystals depends on the pH of the urine. This is generally not a cause for concern since crystals will naturally form as urine cools.

Contaminants

Various materials can contaminate urine specimens such as clothing fibers, mucous threads, and hair. Before the urine can be examined under the microscope, it must be centrifuged. This means it has to be placed in a centrifuge machine and subjected to a spinning motion which separates liquids of different densities (Figure 26-16). This action produces a solid sediment that can then be examined under the microscope. Use the procedure presented here for preparing and per-

---

PROCEDURE: Performing a Microscopic Urine Specimen Examination

Terminal Performance Competency: Perform microscopic examination of urine sediment for casts and cells within a 1% error deviation from instructor.

Equipment and Supplies

Biohazardous waste container

Body and body fluid protection—lab coat, goggles, nonsterile gloves

Capillary pipette

Centrifuge

Centrifuge tube

Microscope

Microscope slide

Paper, pen/pencil

Sedi-stain (optional)

Urine specimen

Note: Follow Standard Precautions and safety guidelines when working with urine samples. Use care to avoid splashing or spilling urine. Wipe up all spills using guidelines established by OSHA.

Procedural Steps

1. Wash hands.
2. Put on gloves and protective clothing.
3. Assemble equipment and materials.

4. Mix the specimen gently to stir up the sediment that has settled to the bottom.
5. Place 10 mL of urine into the centrifuge tube. Place cap on tube. Place the tube in the centrifuge and balance this with another tube of 10 mL of water on the opposite side of the machine.
6. Set centrifuge timer for 5 minutes.
7. After the centrifuge has stopped, remove the tube and pour the supernatant fluid (the clear liquid left on the top of the specimen after centrifuging) off leaving only the sediment.

   Alternate method: Some medical assistants prefer using stain (such as Sedi-stain) to help identify sediment more easily. Place 1 drop of the commercially prepared stain in the test tube.
8. Mix the sediment by holding the top of the tube and tapping with a finger. Be sure that all material left in the tube, after pouring off the supernatant fluid, is mixed thoroughly for the correct reading.

9. Use a capillary pipette to transfer one drop of sediment to a clean slide.

10. Cover the drop of sediment with a coverslip.

11. Place the slide on the microscope stage.

12. Focus under low power and reduced light for casts and epithelial cells.

13. Carefully examine the coverslip for anything abnormal paying close attention to the edges which are where casts migrate.

14. Examine five fields using low power. Select one field from each corner of the coverslip and a fifth field from the center. Count the number of casts or abnormalties seen in each field. If there is nothing in one field, then record zero. Average the count from the five fields for the final result.

15. In the same five fields, use the high-power magnification and adjust for more light. Count RBCs, WBCs, round, transitional, and squamous epithelial cells. Squamous epithelial cells are flattened scale-like cells attached at the edges. They are used as lining throughout the body. Average the count from the five fields for the final result.

16. Also observe crystals, bacteria, sperm, yeast, and parasites. Report them as few, moderate, or many.

17. Discard the urine according to OSHA guidelines.

18. Remove gloves and protective clothing, and dispose of them properly.

19. Wash hands.

20. Document findings in patient record. Bill using correct CPT code for procedure.

21. Clean work area and equipment according to OSHA guidelines.

Charting example:
Note: Medical assistants are not expected to perform a microscopic examination. They may be requested by the physician to prepare the field to step number 11. The physician will chart all findings.

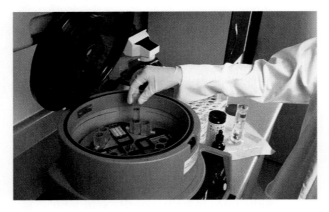

Figure 26-16 The centrifuge is used in microscopic analysis.

forming a microscopic examination of a urine specimen .

Quality Control

Quality control means that you continually check to make sure that tests, reagents, procedures and personnel are producing accurate re-

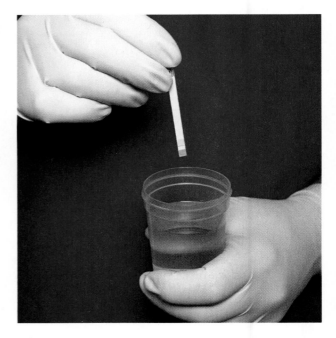

Figure 26-17 Dipstick for testing urine.

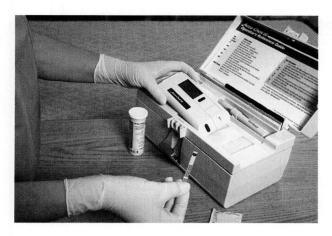

Figure 26-18 Equipment for testing urine (ACCU-Check III).

sults (Figures 26-17 and 26-18). Refer to Chapter 6 for a discussion of quality assurance (control) and follow the quality control guidelines for your particular laboratory/office.

The tests you use for urinary *p*H, protein, blood, glucose, ketones, bilirubin, nitrite, urobilinogen and specific gravity should be checked periodically by using solutions which contain a known amount of each of these substances. Ames Company produces quality control tests such as TEK-Chek. It is important to follow the directions that are supplied by the manufacturer for using this testing material (Figure 26-19). Document control results in the quality control log.

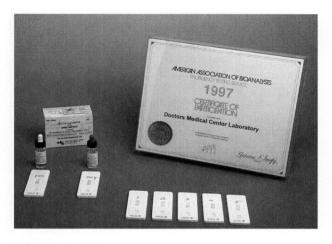

Figure 26-19 Quality control testing is a continual process.

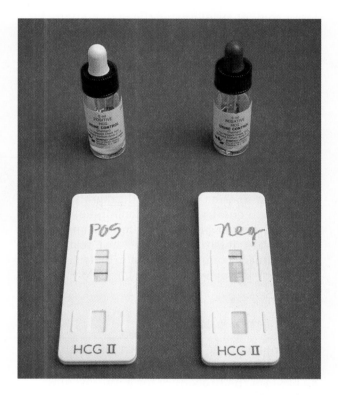

LEGAL AND ETHICAL ISSUES

The importance of accuracy in labeling all specimens cannot be stressed enough. It can be a serious and costly mistake to confuse patients' specimens. If you have any doubt about the ownership of the specimen then re-collect it. *Never guess.* Aseptic technique is paramount when handling any specimen of body fluids. All mailing containers must be handled using aseptic technique to prevent contamination for others handling the specimens. Patient confidentiality must be protected when leaving a message for the patient regarding a test result.

PATIENT EDUCATION

The medical assistant may be the only individual to instruct the patient about how to collect a urine specimen. It is important to make sure that patients understand all the terms that are used during the explanation. Also, provide written instructions for anything the patient must do at home. Post other instructions in the lab's toilet collection area.

The patient needs to understand how to properly cleanse the labia in the female and the foreskin in the male for clean-catch specimens. Patients need a clear description of what "mid-stream" means. You will need to emphasize the need for refrigeration of any specimens that are not immediately brought into the office.

Many patients are sensitive about body elimination. Keep in mind the patient's desire for modesty as you explain all procedures. Patient education for obtaining urine specimens should be conducted out of the hearing distance of other patients.

Summary

Urinalysis (UA) is one of the most common laboratory procedures performed by a medical assistant. Because urine is a bodily fluid, universal precautions, including aseptic technique, must be followed. Proper patient instructions are the first step toward insuring accurate test results. The three primary components of a urinalysis include the physical (appearance, color, odor, volume, specific gravity), chemical (*p*H, protein, glucose, blood, ketones, bilirubin, urobilinogen, nitrite, leukocytes), and microscopic (cells, casts, bacteria, yeast, parasites, spermatozoa, crystals, contaminants) examinations. Quality control—the final step in an accurate urinalysis—consists of checking the tests, reagents, and the procedures performed.

Competency Review

1. Define and spell the glossary terms for this chapter.
2. Explain the procedure for a microscopic examination of urine.
3. Discuss two types of commercial products for doing chemical analysis of urine specimens.
4. Why do we measure specific gravity?
5. Under what conditions can a urinometer give a false result?
6. What is a "fruity" odor in urine? In what disease condition is it found?
7. What is the purpose of catheterization?
8. Why is the twenty-four hour urine specimen kept cool? Describe several ways to keep it cool.
9. How can parasites move from the bowel to the urinary tract?

PREPARING FOR THE CERTIFICATION EXAM

Test Taking Tip — Set a timer when you review for an exam. Know that when 20 minutes are up you must have completed reviewing a certain section. This will force you to concentrate on what you are reading and reviewing.

Examination Review Questions

1. When handling a patient's urine, a medical assistant must follow universal handling of fluid precautions meaning
   (A) aseptic procedures must be followed
   (B) gloves and a lab coat must be worn
   (C) gloves, lab coat, and goggles must be worn
   (D) A and B
   (E) A, B, and C

2. Which of the following statements regarding the collection of a routine (random) urine sample is FALSE?
   (A) it is collected in a nonsterile container
   (B) it can be collected any time during the day
   (C) it should remain at room temperature at all times prior to testing
   (D) At least 10 mL of urine should be collected
   (E) the container should be labeled with the date and the patient's name

3. A 24-hour urine specimen would be an example of a _____ specimen
   (A) morning
   (B) timed
   (C) postprandial
   (D) clean-catch
   (E) clean-catch midstream

4. Fetid, in regards to urine, would refer to the
   (A) odor
   (B) color
   (C) quantity
   (D) turbidity
   (E) specific gravity

5. The normal specific gravity of urine, which measures the ability of the kidneys to concentrate urine, ranges from
   (A) 1.000 to 1.005
   (B) 1.005 to 1.010
   (C) 1.010 to 1.020
   (D) 1.010 to 1.030
   (E) 1.010 to 1.040

6. Glycosuria, an abnormal condition, is the presence of _____ in the urine
   (A) white blood cells
   (B) red blood cells
   (C) sugar
   (D) bacteria
   (E) parasites

7. Which of the following statements is TRUE?
   (A) urine voided by healthy patients on a normal diet is slightly acidic
   (B) urine voided by healthy patients on a normal diet is slightly alkaline
   (C) a pH greater than 7.0 is common in the presence of a UTI
   (D) a pH lower than 7.0 is common if a patient is consuming large amounts of Vitamin C
   (E) all of the above

8. The presence of which of the following may signal the onset of liver disease?
   (A) leukocytes
   (B) erythrocytes
   (C) ketones
   (D) bilirubin
   (E) nitrites

9. Sediment in urine, both organized and unorganized, includes
   (A) casts, cells, and crystals
   (B) casts, cells, bacteria, parasites, yeast, and fungi
   (C) casts, cells, bacteria, parasites, yeast, fungi, and spermatozoa
   (D) casts, cells, bacteria, parasites, yeast, fungi, spermatozoa, and crystals
   (E) casts, cells, bacteria, parasites, yeast, fungi, spermatozoa, crystals, and amorphous material

(Continued on next page)

10. Which of the following statements is TRUE?
   (A) casts are visualized microscopically under high power
   (B) cells are visualized microscopically under low power
   (C) crystals are visualized microscopically under low power
   (D) the findings are charted after averaging what has been seen in 5 fields
   (E) the findings are charted after averaging what has been seen in 10 fields

ON THE JOB

Jose is an elderly patient of Dr. Juarez, a board certified urologist. He has a history of recurrent UTIs dating back more than 10 years. When Jose becomes symptomatic, he has been instructed to call Dr. Juarez's office and schedule a urinalysis.

Dr. Juarez's receptionist has just received a call from Jose. He says he knows he is supposed to come in for a urine test, but that he just wants a prescription phoned in to his pharmacy instead. The receptionist asks Emilia, Dr. Juarez's medical assistant, to take the call from Jose.

Emilia listens as Jose recounts that he is experiencing dysuria–painful, burning urination. She asks him to come in to the office for a urinalysis, explaining that, as per the standing order, a clean-catch midstream specimen needs to be collected.

Jose repeated to Emilia that he does not want to come in to the office. "Why can't you call in a prescription for Bactrim . . . That's what I took last time and it helped."

What is your response?

1. Should the responsibility for this call have fallen on Emilia or should the receptionist have either handled the call herself or passed it on to Dr. Juarez?
2. What, if anything, could or should Emilia say to Jose to persuade him to come in for the urinalysis?
3. Might the cost of the procedure be a factor in the reason why Jose does not want to have a urinalysis and, if so, what, if anything, can Emilia do or say about the cost?
4. Is it appropriate in this case, given the patient's extensive history, to indeed call in a prescription for Bactrim?
5. If not, how should Emilia handle Jose's request for the prescription?
6. If so, what procedure should Emilia follow in order to arrange for a prescription for Jose?
7. How should this telephone call be charted?
8. What, if anything, should Dr. Juarez be told about the conversation with Jose?

References

Chernecky, C., Krech, R., and Berger, B. *Laboratory Tests and Diagnostic Procedures.* Philadelphia: W. B. Saunders, 1993.

Fishbach, F. *A Manual of Laboratory & Diagnostic Tests.* Philadelphia: Lippincott, 1996.

Fremgen, B. *Medical Terminology.* Upper Saddle River, NJ: Brady/Prentice Hall, 1997.

Greenberg, A., editor. *Primer on Kidney Diseases.* New York: Academic Press, 1994.

Marshall, J. *Medical Laboratory Assistant.* Upper Saddle River, NJ: Brady/Prentice Hall, 1990.

Nurse's Pocket Companion. Springhouse, PA: Springhouse Corporation, 1993.

Straasinger, S. *Urinalysis & Body Fluids.* Philadelphia: F. A. Davis, 1994.

Taber's Cyclopedic Medical Dictionary, 18th ed. Philadelphia: F. A. Davis, 1997.

Tietz, N., Conn, R., and Pruden, E. *Applied Laboratory Medicine.* Philadelphia: W. B. Saunders, 1992.

Tietz, N. *Clinical Guide to Laboratory Tests,* 2nd ed. Philadelphia: W. B. Saunders, 1990.

The Regents/Prentice Hall Medical Assistant Kit: Laboratory Processes. Upper Saddle River, NJ: Brady/Prentice Hall, 1993.

Walters, N., Estridge, B., and Reynolds, A. *Basic Medical Laboratory Techniques.* Albany, NY: Delmar, 1990.

MEDICAL ASSISTANT ROLE DELINEATION CHART

Highlight indicates material covered in this chapter

ADMINISTRATIVE

ADMINISTRATIVE PROCEDURES

- Perform basic clerical functions
- Schedule, coordinate, and monitor appointments
- Schedule inpatient/outpatient admissions and procedures
- Understand and apply third party guidelines
- Obtain reimbursement through accurate claims submission
- Monitor third-party reimbursement
- Perform medical transcription
- Understand and adhere to managed care policies and procedures
- *Negotiate managed care contracts (adv)*

PRACTICE FINANCES

- Perform procedural and diagnostic coding
- Apply bookkeeping principles
- Document and maintain accounting and banking records
- Manage accounts receivable
- Manage accounts payable
- Process payroll
- *Develop and maintain fee schedules (adv)*
- *Manage renewals of business and professional insurance policies (adv)*
- *Manage personal benefits and maintain records (adv)*

CLINICAL

FUNDAMENTAL PRINCIPLES

- Apply principles of aseptic technique and infection control
- Comply with quality assurance practices
- Screen and follow up patient test results

DIAGNOSTIC ORDERS

- Collect and process specimens
- Perform diagnostic tests

PATIENT CARE

- Adhere to established triage procedures
- Obtain patient history and vital signs
- Prepare and maintain examination and treatment areas

- Prepare patient for examinations, procedures, and treatments
- Assist with examinations, procedures, and treatments
- Prepare and administer medications and immunizations
- Maintain medication and immunization records
- Recognize and respond to emergencies
- Coordinate patient care information with other health care providers

GENERAL (TRANSDISCIPLINARY)

PROFESSIONALISM

- Project a professional manner and image
- Adhere to ethical principles
- Demonstrate initiative and responsibility
- Work as a team member
- Manage time efficiently
- Prioritize and perform multiple tasks
- Adapt to change
- Promote the CMA credential
- Enhance skills through continuing education

COMMUNICATION SKILLS

- Treat all patients with compassion and empathy
- Recognize and respect cultural diversity
- Adapt communications to individual's ability to understand
- Use professional telephone technique
- Use effective and correct verbal and written communications
- Recognize and respond to verbal and nonverbal communications
- Use medical terminology appropriately
- Receive, organize, prioritize, and transmit information
- Serve as liaison
- Promote the practice through positive public relations

LEGAL CONCEPTS

- Maintain confidentiality
- Practice within the scope of education, training, and personal capabilities
- Prepare and maintain medical records
- Document accurately
- Use appropriate guidelines when releasing information
- Follow employer's established policies dealing with the health care contract
- Follow federal, state, and local legal guidelines
- Maintain awareness of federal and state health care legislation and regulations
- Maintain and dispose of regulated substances in compliance with government guidelines
- Comply with established risk management and safety procedures
- Recognize professional credentialing criteria
- Participate in the development and maintenance of personnel, policy, and procedure manuals
- *Develop and maintain personnel, policy, and procedure manuals (adv)*

INSTRUCTION

- Instruct individuals according to their needs
- Explain office policies and procedures
- Teach methods of health promotion and disease prevention
- Locate community resources and disseminate information
- *Orient and train personnel (adv)*
- *Develop educational materials (adv)*
- *Conduct continuing education activities (adv)*

OPERATIONAL FUNCTIONS

- Maintain supply inventory
- Evaluate and recommend equipment and supplies
- Apply computer techniques to support office operations
- *Supervise personnel (adv)*
- *Interview and recommend job applicants (adv)*
- *Negotiate leases and prices for equipment and supply contracts (adv)*

SOURCE: Reprinted by permission of the American Association of Medical Assistants from the *AAMA Role Delineation Study: Occupational Analysis of the Medical Assisting Profession.*

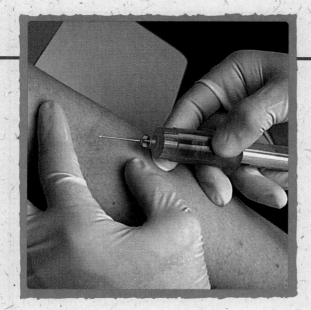

27

Hematology

Chapter Outline

Learning Objectives

After completing this chapter, you should:
1. Define and spell the glossary terms for this chapter.
2. List the components of blood, including the liquid and cellular portions and the functions of each.
3. Describe how to prepare a patient for collection of a blood specimen via venipuncture and capillary puncture methods.
4. Describe how to collect a blood specimen via venipuncture and capillary puncture methods.
5. Discuss how to process a blood specimen for routine testing in a physician's office.
6. Explain how to perform an automated white blood cell count, red blood cell count, and a hemoglobin determination.
7. State the normal values for each of the blood tests discussed.

Clinical Performance Competencies

After completing this chapter, you should perform the following tasks:
1. Demonstrate the proper procedure for obtaining a venous blood sample using the vacuum tube method.
2. Demonstrate the proper procedure for obtaining a capillary blood sample using a manual or spring-loaded lancet device.
3. Perform a microhematocrit test on a whole blood sample.
4. Demonstrate the proper procedure to make, stain, and read a differential blood slide.
5. Perform an erythrocyte sedimentation rate on a whole blood sample.
6. Accurately document the results of routine blood tests.

Glossary

agranulocyte(s) Type of white blood cell with a clear cytoplasm.

anemia Decrease in the number of circulating red blood cells.

antibodies Proteins that defend the body against infection.

anticoagulant Substance which prevents blood from clotting (EDTA and heparin).

antigen Foreign substance which stimulates the production of antibodies.

buffy coat The white colored layer which forms between the packed red blood cells and the plasma after centrifuging a whole blood sample; composed of white blood cells and platelets.

capillaries Tiny blood vessels which connect arterioles and venules.

centrifuge An instrument used to separate blood into its liquid and solid components.

dehydration Loss of body water which can become life-threatening if not corrected.

electrolytes Ionized salts in the blood, such as Na, K, and Cl.

erythrocytes A red blood cell (RBC).

granulocytes Type of white blood cell in which the cytoplasm contains granules.

hemacytometer Instrument used to count red and white blood cells.

hematology Study of blood and blood-forming tissues.

hematoma Collection of blood underneath the skin, for example a bruise.

hematopoiesis Formation of blood cells.

hemoglobin Carries oxygen and an iron containing pigment which gives an RBC its color.

hemolyzed Refers to the destruction (hemolysis) of blood cells.

leukemia Cancerous condition with elevated numbers of white blood cells.

leukocytes A white blood cell (WBC).

oxyhemoglobin Combination of oxygen and hemoglobin; carries oxygen to the tissues.

phagocytosis Process in which white blood cells (WBCs) ingest and digest foreign material.

phlebotomy Blood collection using the venipuncture method.

plasma The liquid portion of blood, contains fibrinogen.

platelets A cell which aids in the blood clotting process, for example thrombocyte.

polycythemia A condition where there are too many red blood cells (RBCs) in blood.

reticulocyte An immature red blood cell containing a nucleus. Red blood cells containing granules or filaments in an immature stage of development.

serum The liquid portion of blood which contains no fibrinogen.

thrombocytes *See platelet.*

venipuncture The process of withdrawing blood from a vein.

WARNING!

For all patient contact, adhere to Standard Precautions (see pages 342–373). Wear protective equipment as indicated.

Hematology is the study of blood and blood forming tissues. The goal of this study or blood testing is to examine the components of blood to detect pathological conditions and to determine a course of treatment.

Blood analysis is a vital tool used routinely in the physician's office. Doctors rely heavily on accurate lab results. Therefore, medical assistants must know how to collect, handle, and analyze a blood specimen properly. This requires a basic, but thorough, understanding of the blood's components and the various, routine tests performed.

Blood Formation

Hematopoiesis, the formation of blood cells, begins at the stem cell level during fetal development. All blood cells originate from the hematopoietic stem cell but mature into seven individual cells:

1. Red blood cells (erythrocytes)
2. White blood cells (5 types)
   - Neutrophilic segmented cell
   - Lymphocyte
   - Monocyte
   - Eosinophil
   - Basophil
3. Platelets (thrombocyte)

Hematopoiesis occurs primarily in the bone marrow of the adult. In addition, the lymph nodes form lymphocytes, one type of white blood cell.

Blood Components

Blood is a specialized tissue consisting of a cellular component (red blood cells, white blood cells, and platelets) and a liquid component (plasma). The average adult has 5.5 to 6 liters of blood.

Liquid Component

Plasma transports substances in the blood to different parts of the body. It is the clear straw-colored liquid portion of the blood which comprises approximately 55% of the total blood volume and contains fibrinogen. Fibrinogen converts to fibrin during the clotting process. A clot is then formed. Serum is the liquid portion of blood containing no fibrin. The serum portion of blood is extracted from the liquid portion that does not contain the clot.

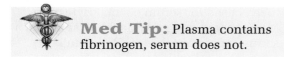

Med Tip: Plasma contains fibrinogen, serum does not.

Ninety percent of plasma is water while 10% is solid substances or solutes. Examples of solid substances include plasma proteins: albumin, globulin, fibrinogen, and prothrombin; electrolytes: sodium (Na), potassium (K), and chloride (Cl); nutrients: glucose, amino acids, lipids, and carbohydrates; metabolism waste products: urea, lactic acid, uric acid, creatinine; respiratory gases: oxygen and carbon dioxide; and miscellaneous substances: hormones, antibodies, enzymes, vitamins, and mineral salts.

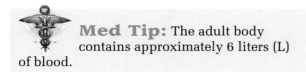

Med Tip: The adult body contains approximately 6 liters (L) of blood.

Cellular Components

The largest cellular portion of blood consists of red blood cells (RBCs) or erythrocytes. RBCs are non-nucleated, biconcave discs which live for 120 days before they are hemolyzed, or destroyed, by the liver. The biconcave shape provides a greater surface area which allows an increased oxygen carrying capacity.

Most of the RBC is composed of hemoglobin (Hb or Hgb), which gives the RBC its red color. The function of hemoglobin is two-fold. First it carries oxygen from the lungs to the tissues. Then it carries carbon dioxide, a waste product, from the tissues to the lungs to be expelled from the body via exhalation. When oxygen combines with hemoglobin in the lungs, oxyhemoglobin is formed. Arterial blood has a higher concentration of oxygen, hence the bright red color. In contrast, venous blood has low levels of oxygen hence the deep red color.

The second largest cellular portion consists of white blood cells (WBCs) or leukocytes. The range of leukocytes in the adult is 4.5-11 thousand/mm^3. WBCs are slightly larger than RBCs and live between a few hours and several days. There are five types of WBCs, all containing a distinct nucleus. Also, WBCs can be categorized into granulocytes (neutrophilic segmented cell, eosinophil, and basophil), which contain granules in the cytoplasm and agranulocytes (monocyte and lymphocyte), which have no granules in cytoplasm.

The white blood cell's primary function is to defend the body against disease. To function, the WBC must leave the circulating blood and enter into the tissues. Each WBC has a specific function. The monocyte and the neutrophilic segmented cell (the "seg") engulf foreign material, such as bacteria and dead tissue cells, through a process called phagocytosis. Both the eosinophil and basophil play an important role in allergic reactions.

Lastly, the lymphocytes produce antibodies in response to an antigen. Antibodies help protect the body against infection.

Platelets, or thrombocytes, are cellular fragments which aid in clotting. They comprise the third major cellular portion of blood. Normally, there are between 150,000-400,000 platelets/mm^3.

Blood Specimen Collection

In all cases, laboratory testing of blood, as well as the collecting of specimens, is strictly controlled by OSHA regulations, and the CDC's Standard Precautions must be followed at all times. CLIA '88 regulations set the standard for laboratory testing, including the professional training of technicians. (See Chapters 6 and 26 for more information regarding CLIA.)

The type and amount of specimen needed for blood analysis will dictate the method of collection. If a small amount is needed, then the sample could be obtained via capillary puncture. Conversely, if a larger volume is needed, a **venipuncture** would be performed. For example, a physician requests a complete blood count (CBC). The medical assistant should perform a venipuncture to obtain at least 5 cc of blood. The entire 5 cc will not be processed/tested, but must be collected to have an adequate representation of the tissue.

Venipuncture

A medical assistant can perform a venipuncture, or **phlebotomy,** using one of 2 methods: the vacuum tube method or the less common needle and syringe method.

Method

Most medical assistants prefer the vacuum tube method because multiple samples can be easily collected in a short period of time (Figures 27-1 and 27-2). The needle and syringe method is best when drawing blood from small, fragile veins. Small veins may collapse if a large sample is being collected. Care should be taken to expel all the air from the syringe prior to puncture.

Equipment

Figure 27-3 shows the equipment needed for a venipuncture. All equipment should be assembled and the vacuum tubes should be checked for their expiration date. Expired tubes may not have a vacuum. Also, Figure 27-3 shows the various colored-stopper tubes available. Each colored stopper, except red, contains a different **anticoagulant,** or additive, which keeps blood from clotting.

> **Med Tip:** If the proportion of blood to anticoagulant is not correct, RBC shrinkage may occur. Any vacutainer tube containing an additive must be filled completely.

1. Red: Tube contains no anticoagulant and has a sterile interior, blood will clot and

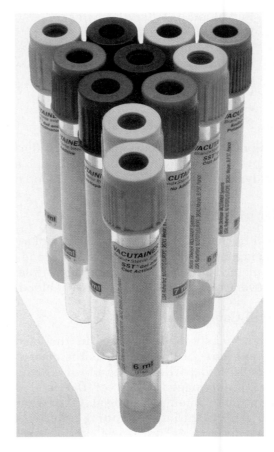

Figure 27-1 Vacutainer evacuated specimen tubes with Hemogard® Closure blood collection tubes.

yield serum after centrifugation. A red top tube is used for serum chemistry testing.

2. Marbled (red and gray/black): Also called a serum separator tube (SST), this tube contains a gel which will permanently separate the serum from the clot after centrifugation. It also contains a clot activator.

3. Lavender/Purple: Tube contains ethylenediamine tetra-acetic acid (EDTA), used if whole blood or plasma is needed, commonly used for a CBC or a glycosolated hemoglobin.

4. Green: Tube contains heparin, used if whole blood or plasma is needed, not used often for routine testing in a physician's office.

5. Light blue: Tube contains sodium citrate, used if whole blood or plasma is needed, commonly used for a PT (prothrombin time) or PTT (partial thromboplastin time).

6. Gray (not shown): Tube contains potassium oxylate, used if whole blood or

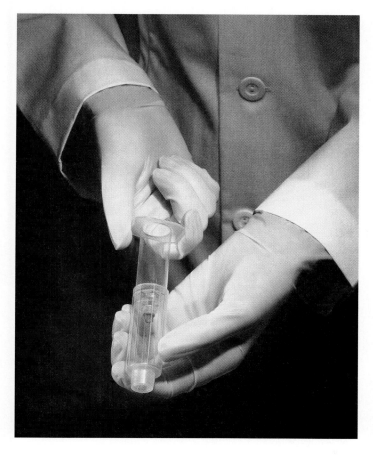

Figure 27-2 Vacutainer® Brand safety lock needle holder.

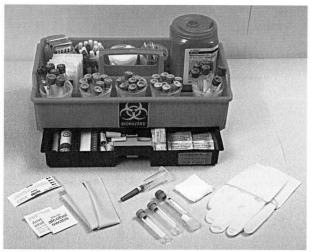

Figure 27-3 Venipuncture equipment.

plasma is needed, commonly used for a GTT (glucose tolerance test).

Vacutainer tube sizes include 5 mL, 7 mL, 10 mL, and 15 mL. The amount of blood needed for each test will vary, therefore the tube size will also vary.

Sites

The antecubital space, at the junction where the upper and lower arm meets, is the site of choice in the adult for a few reasons: the veins are easy to access, relatively large, and usually easy to locate.

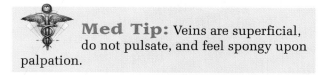

Med Tip: Veins are superficial, do not pulsate, and feel spongy upon palpation.

Figure 27-4 shows the anatomy of an arm for venipuncture. The vessel of choice is most often the median cephalic vein located in the antecubital space.

Patient Preparation

Routine blood tests performed in a physician's office require very little patient preparation. Patients are required to fast for 12-14 hours for a glucose tolerance test, a cholesterol and a triglyceride level. No fasting is required for a complete blood count. See Figure 27-5 A-D for an illustration of venipuncture equipment.

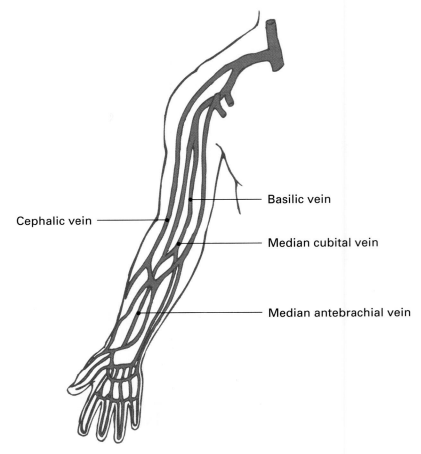

Cephalic vein

Basilic vein

Median cubital vein

Median antebrachial vein

Figure 27-4 Anatomy of an arm for venipuncture.

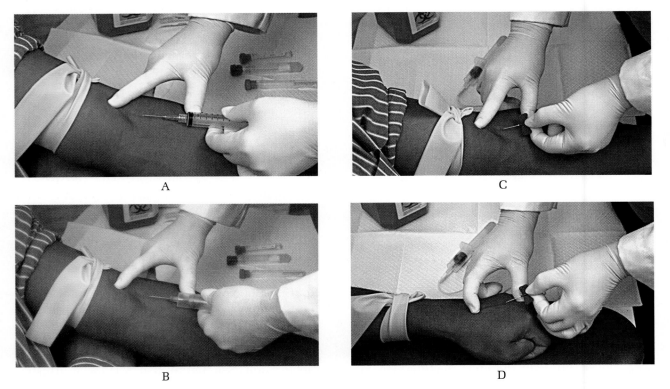

A

C

B

D

Figure 27-5 A-D Venipuncture equipment.

PROCEDURE: Venipuncture (Vacutainer Method)

**Terminal Performance
Competency:** Be able to perform venipuncture by correctly assembling, locating, and entering vein and withdrawing blood sample.

Equipment and Supplies

Biohazard sharps container

Vacutainer tubes

Multi-sample needle

2×2 gauze squares

Alcohol pads

Latex gloves

Vacutainer sleeve

Tourniquet

Band-Aid

Cotton balls

Adhesive

Ink pen

Lab coat

Patient record

Ammonia ampules

Note: Follow Standard Precautions and safety guidelines when working with blood samples. Use care to avoid splashing or spilling blood. Wipe up all spills using guidelines established by OSHA.

Procedural Steps

1. Wash hands.

2. Assemble equipment (refer to Figure 27-6 A).

3. Identify the patient and explain the procedure. Ensure the patient is either sitting or lying down. ***Rationale:*** Explaining the procedure helps decrease anxiety. A sitting or lying down position is safer if the patient becomes faint (prevent falls).

4. Screw the vacutainer needle into the plastic sleeve (Figure 27-6 B). Insert the tube into the other end of the sleeve. The top of the colored stopper should reach the thin guide line on the sleeve. Do not press tube. If the tube exceeds the line, discard the tube; it may not have a vacuum.

5. Apply the rubber tourniquet about two inches above the antecubital space. Place the middle of the tourniquet on the posterior (elbow) side of the arm. Crisscross the ends. While holding one end stable, tuck the other end in. This creates a tie which can be quickly released with one hand. In addition, the tourniquet should apply enough tension to engorge the vein with blood.

6. Apply latex examination gloves.

7. The arm should be in an extended position with the palm facing up and comfortably resting on a soft surface or towel (Figure 27-6 D). Palpate the vein with your fingertips (Figure 27-6 E). If a vein cannot be felt in one arm, try the other.

8. Wipe the site with alcohol pad in a circular pattern beginning at the insertion site. Let alcohol evaporate (Figure 27-6 F). Cleanse your gloved finger with alcohol in case you need to re-palpate after site is cleansed.

9. Stabilize the vein by placing thumb of nondominant hand two inches below insertion site and pull skin toward hand. ***Rationale:*** Veins are superficial and may roll when needle is inserted.

10. While holding onto the sleeve with your dominant hand, insert needle smoothly and rapidly at a 15 degree angle with the bevel up. The needle only needs to be inserted just past the bevel. If inserted too far, it will puncture both vein walls. Also keep needle in line with the vein.

11. While stabilizing the sleeve push the tube into the sleeve. Use your thumb to push the tube and hold sleeve with index and middle finger on the flange. ***Rationale:*** The sleeve must be perfectly stable or needle

(Continued on next page)

will damage the fragile vein and will result in a **hematoma** (bruise).

12. Allow the tube to fill. The vacuum will automatically fill tube 3/4 full.

13. Remove the tube very carefully without moving the needle and apply a second tube if needed. Gently roll the tube 5-6 times after removing it from the sleeve to allow the blood to mix with the additive. If both a red and purple tube are needed, collect the red tube that contains no additive first (Figure 27-6 I).

14. After removing the last tube, release the tourniquet.

15. Remove the needle while covering the site with a gauze square. Immediately have patient apply firm, continuous pressure using a cotton ball or gauze square (Figure 27-6 J). **Rationale:** Firm, continuous pressure will decrease chance of **hematoma**, or bruise, formation.

16. Discard needle in sharps container (Figure 27-6 K). Never recap needle if sharps container is available. **Rationale:** Recapping a needle is the most common cause of a needle stick. The main dangers from blood due to a needle stick are from Hepatitis B and AIDS.

17. Gently invert all tubes collected 8-10 times in a figure eight pattern. **Rationale:** RBCs are fragile and may hemolyze if handled improperly.

18. Assess the patient. Check the venipuncture site for bleeding, then apply some cotton and a strip of adhesive or Band-Aid (Figure 27-6 L). Ask if the patient is dizzy or lightheaded. **Rationale:** If patient is dizzy or lightheaded, he or she may faint when attempting to stand.

19. Label tubes with patient's name, date, time, ID number, specimen type, tests to be done, and phlebotomist's initials. Fill out laboratory requisition sheet (Figure 27-6 M).

20. Remove gloves. Wash hands.

21. Record procedure on patient's medical record.

Charting Example

2/28/XX 1 PM Withdrew 10 mL of blood from L arm, no complications. Sent blood to in-office lab for CBC.   M. Smith, RMA

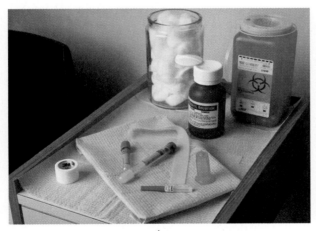

A

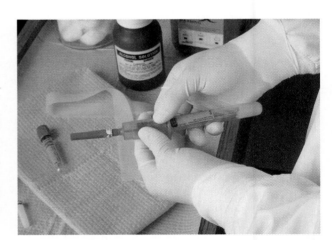

B

Figure 27-6 A-M   Venipuncture procedure. *(Continued)*

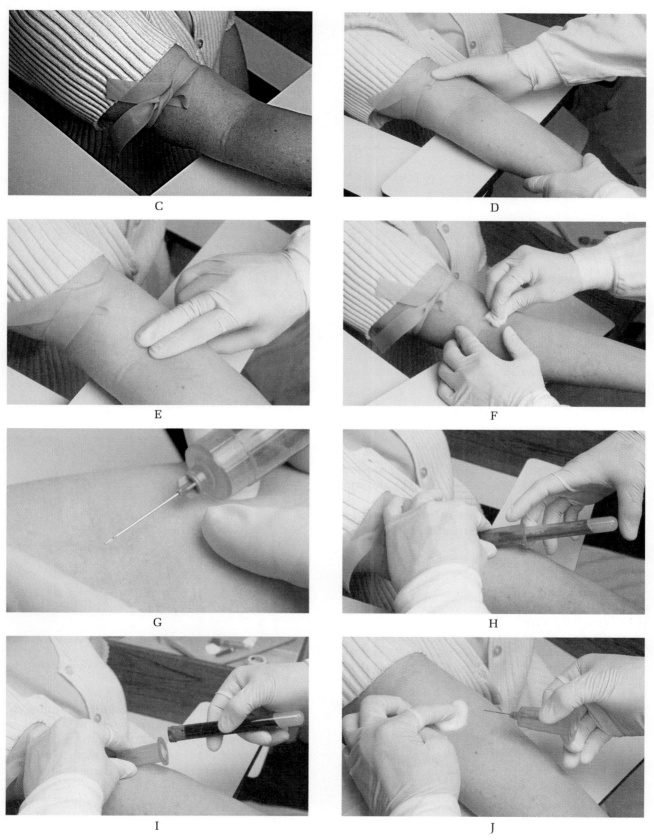

Figure 27-6 A-M Venipuncture procedure. *(Continued on next page)*

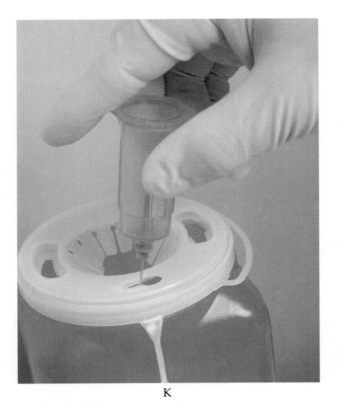

K

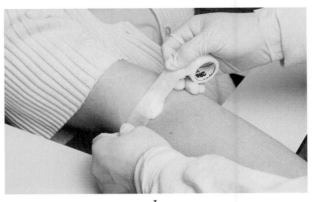

L

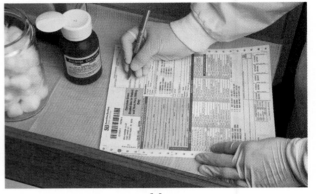

M

Figure 27-6 A-M   (continued)

Capillary Puncture (manual)

Capillaries are small blood vessels which are the bridges between arterioles and venules. Oxygen and carbon dioxide are exchanged at the capillary level. Small amounts of blood can easily be obtained in a capillary puncture, or a "finger stick" (Figure 27-7).

Puncture Sites

Capillary puncture sites are shown in Figure 27-8 for both the infant and adult. Avoid the index finger because the skin is thicker than on the ring or great finger. An infant's fingers are not large enough to provide an adequate sample. Therefore the plantar surface, medial, and lateral edges of the heel are used.

> **Med Tip:** Always use the patient's nondominant hand for a finger puncture.

Equipment and Supplies

Figure 27-9 shows the equipment needed for a finger stick. Either a manual or automatic lancet can be used. The primary advantage of the automatic

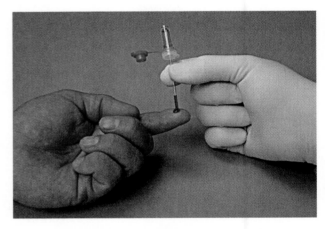

Figure 27-7   A "finger stick" is useful for obtaining small amounts of blood.

lancet is the depth of the puncture is controlled by the spring-loaded mechanism, thereby causing less pain to the patient (Figure 27-10). Both lancets have sharp, pointed blades which are used once, then immediately discarded into the sharps container.

> **Med Tip:** If blood spills on the table, it should be cleaned with a 10% bleach solution made fresh daily.

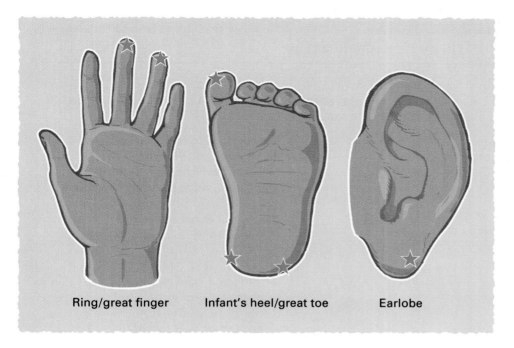

Figure 27-8 Capillary puncture sites.

Ring/great finger   Infant's heel/great toe   Earlobe

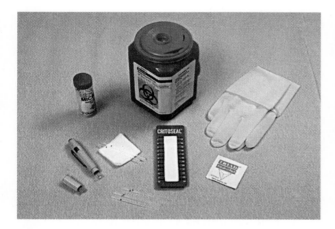

Figure 27-9 Capillary stick equipment.

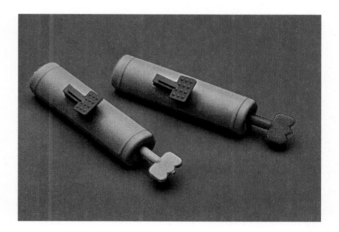

Figure 27-10 Spring-activated lancet from Lukens® Medical Corporation.

Routine Blood Tests

Blood analysis is a routine and vital tool. The medical assistant performs basic tests in a physician's office. A medical lab technician (MLT) or medical technologist (MT) is trained to perform more sophisticated lab tests. (Refer to CLIA regulations in Chapters 6 and 26 for more information regarding control of laboratory testing standards and professional training requirements for technicians.) Figures 27-12 and 27-13 display different types of hemotology analyzing systems.

Physicians often request a complete blood test (CBC). A CBC may vary between offices but usu-

ally consists of the following tests: a microhematocrit, a hemoglobin determination, a white blood cell count, a red blood cell count, a platelet count, and a differential white blood cell count (diff).

Diabetics must monitor their blood regularly. One type of machine used to measure blood glucose, the One Touch Profile Diabetes tracking system, is shown in Figure 27-14).

Microhematocrit Procedure

The microhematocrit (Hct or "crit") provides the physician with reliable information about the patient's red blood cell volume. For example, a low

PROCEDURE: Capillary Puncture (manual)

**Terminal Performance
Competency:** Perform a capillary stick using a lancet or spring-loaded lancet following correct aseptic technique and obtaining an adequate sample without error.

Equipment and Supplies

Biohazard sharps container

Latex gloves

Alcohol pad

2×2 gauze square

Lancet or spring-loaded lancet

Capillary tubes

Sealing clay

Ammonia ampules

Band-aid

Lab coat

Note: Follow Standard Precautions and safety guidelines when working with blood samples. Use care to avoid splashing or spilling blood. Wipe up all spills using guidelines established by OSHA.

Procedural Steps

1. Wash hands. *Rationale:* Handwashing helps prevent the spread of infection.
2. Assemble equipment.
3. Identify the patient and explain the procedure. Have the patient either sitting or lying.
4. Apply latex gloves.
5. Select either the ring or great finger on the non-dominant hand. Wipe the site with an alcohol pad. Let alcohol evaporate.
6. Remove plastic protective tip to expose the lancet.
7. Grasp patient's hand and gently squeeze the finger one inch below the puncture site.
8. Puncture the site using a quick, jabbing motion across the fingerprints to obtain a full round drop of blood (Figure 27-11A). Do not puncture the direct center of the finger pad since the skin is generally tougher there. Immediately discard lancet in sharps container. (A spring-loaded lancet may also be used.)
9. Wipe away the first drop of blood with a gauze square. *Rationale:* The first drop contains alcohol and tissue fluid and will not provide accurate test results (Figure 27-11B).
10. Obtain the sample using a microhematocrit capillary tube (Figure 27-11C). The finger may be gently massaged to increase blood flow. Seal one end of capillary tube in clay sealer (Figure 27-11D).
11. Apply a clean gauze over the site and ask patient to apply firm, continuous pressure until the bleeding stops. *Rationale:* Firm, continuous pressure will decrease hematoma formation.
12. Assess patient and the site. Apply a Band-Aid, if needed. Ask patient if he/she is dizzy or lightheaded.
13. Remove gloves and wash hands.
14. Record procedure on patient's medical record.

Charting Example

2/28/XX 1:30 PM   Performed capillary puncture on L ring finger, no complications.

M. Smith, RMA

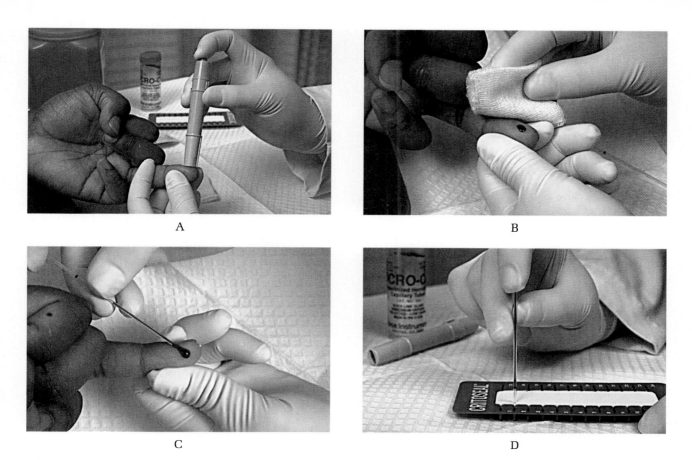

A

B

C

D

Figure 27-11 A-D Capillary stick.

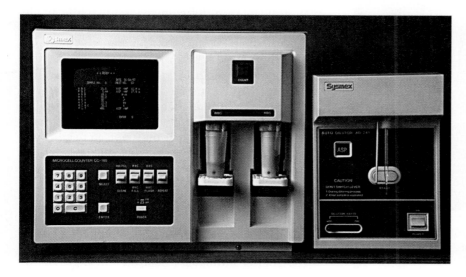

Figure 27-12 Whole Blood
Analyzer from B. Warling.

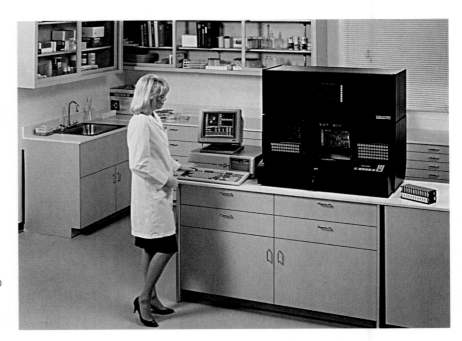

Figure 27-13 The COULTER©
STKS Hematology Analyzer
System, courtesy of Coulter
Corporation, Miami, Florida.

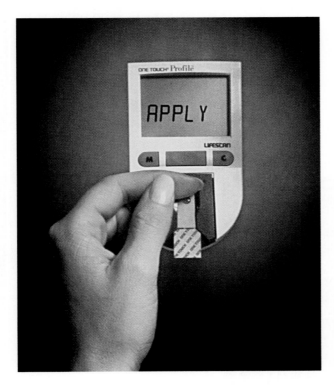

Figure 27-14 ONE TOUCH Profile Diabetes
Tracking System. Courtesy LifeSpan, Inc.

Med Tip: Some centrifuges
contain a built in Hct Reader which
can be used instead of the card.

Hct may indicate anemia—a decrease in the number of circulating RBCs—or hemorrhage, while an elevated Hct may indicate dehydration or polycythemia. A centrifuge is used to separate blood into its liquid and solid components.

Hemoglobin Determination

Hemoglobin (Hgb) determination provides the physician with valuable information. A low Hgb may indicate iron-deficiency anemia while an elevated reading is present with severe burns. Normal values for the adult female are 12-16 g/dl and in the male 14-18 g/dl.

Hemoglobin can be measured manually in a physician's office using a hemoglobinometer or by using an automated blood analyzer (Figures 27-16, 17, and 18). Since the manual method has a wide margin of error, it may not be used. Refer to the manufacturer's instruction booklet for directions.

White Blood Cell Counts

Normal white blood cell (WBC) or leukocyte range in the adult is 4.5-11 thousand/mm^3. An elevated level usually indicates infection and if grossly elevated can indicate leukemia, while a low value may indicate an immunodeficiency problem or a viral infection.

A WBC count can be performed by the medical assistant either manually or using an automated blood analyzer. Just like the hemoglobin de-

PROCEDURE: Microhematocrit

**Terminal Performance
Competency:** Student will perform a microhematocrit or a capillary blood sample using proper aseptic technique without error.

Equipment and Supplies
Biohazard sharps container

Latex gloves

Capillary tubes

Sealing clay

Microhematocrit centrifuge

Whole blood

Hematocrit card or other reader

Note: Follow Standard Precautions and safety guidelines when working with blood samples. Use care to avoid splashing or spilling blood. Wipe up all spills using guidelines established by OSHA.

Procedural Steps
1. Wash hands and apply latex gloves.
2. Assemble equipment as shown in Figure 27-15A.
3. Fill two capillary tubes 3/4 full. The blood specimen can be obtained from a vacuum tube of anticoagulated blood using a plain capillary tube or directly from a finger stick site using a heparinized capillary tube. Seal one end in the sealing clay.
4. Place capillary tubes in centrifuge with the sealed ends against the rubber gasket (Figure 27-15B). If more than one patients' blood is being tested, mark down the number of the slot the patient's tube is in. Spin for 3-5 minutes at 10,000 rpm's. (Always check manufacturer's recommendations for proper time and speed.) After centrifuging the sample will be separated into 3 layers:

  - Top layer is the plasma
  - Middle layer, or the buffy coat, which is made of WBCs and platelets
  - Bottom layer of packed RBCs

5. Remove tubes immediately after centrifuge stops. **Rationale:** If tubes aren't removed immediately, blood may begin to mix together.
6. Determine results. Use the Hct card by placing the sealing clay just below the zero line. Then match the top of the plasma with the 100 line. Read results directly below buffy coat.
7. Discard tubes into sharps container.
8. Remove gloves and wash hands.
9. Record the value as a % on the patient's medical record.

Charting Example
2/28/XX	1:45 PM	Hct 47%.
		M. Smith, CMA

termination is commonly done on an automated machine, so is the WBC count. Each automated machine has its own directions. (Always follow directions exactly as recommended and only use after receiving proper training.) Figure 27-19 displays one type of blood analyzer.

Red Blood Cell Count

Normal red blood cell (RBC) count in the adult female is 4.5-5.0 million/mm^3 and in the adult male is 5.0-6.0 million/mm^3. An increase in the number of circulating RBCs may indicate polycythemia, while a decrease may indicate anemia.

A manual RBC count is very similar to the manual WBC count. Both require small samples of blood to be diluted in special solutions. Then it is placed on a hemacytometer which is placed on a microscope used to count red and white blood cells.

Automated testing for RBCs is more common than manual testing. Directions will be found in the machine's procedure manual.

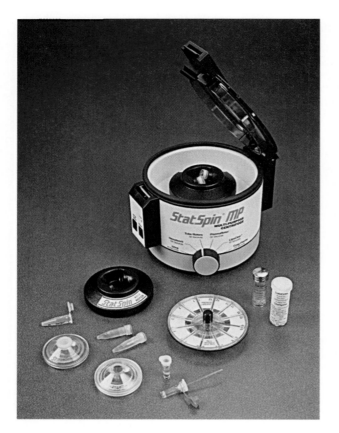

Figure 27-15 A   Centrifuge and supplies.

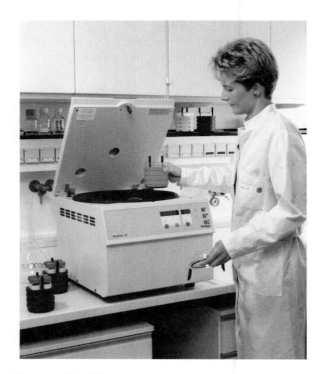

Figure 27-15 B   Loading centrifuge.

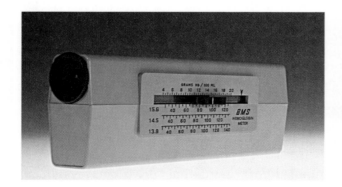

Figure 27-16   Hemoglobinometer.

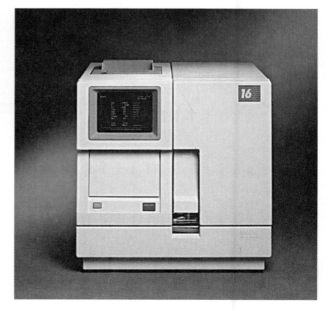

Figure 27-17   Nova 16 Analyzer.

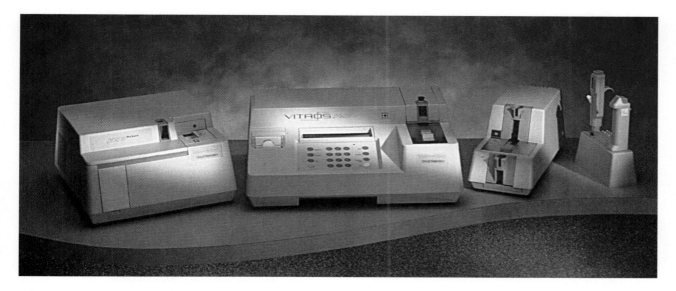

Figure 27-18   VITROS® DT60 II system from Johnson & Johnson Clinical Diagnostics.

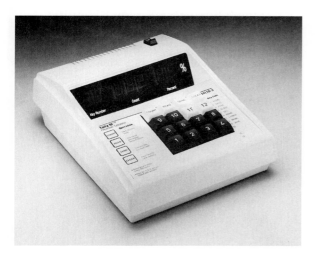

Figure 27-19   Electronic Tabulator, Scientific Products, Tally III.

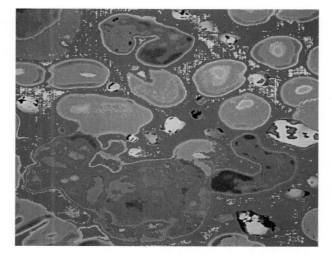

Figure 27-20   Computer visualization of RBCs and WBCs 400 ×s real life size.

Differential White Blood Cell Count

A differential white blood cell count, or "a diff," determines the percentages of each type of WBC, RBC morphology, and platelet estimation. A manual differential WBC count is a skill which takes practice in order for the medical assistant to become proficient. Using a bright light, focus the blood cells using 100× (oil immersion) under the microscope. Be certain to focus near the feathered edge where the cells are one-cell layer thick. Cells will appear distorted if viewing in an area where the cells overlap each other.

Figure 27-20 shows a super computer visulization—400×Life—of RBCs and WBCs in an excessive (diabetic) volume of complex sugars unbroken down (yellow).

Red Blood Cells

The most numerous salmon-colored structures are the red blood cells. They should appear slightly oval with a slightly pale center, and no nuclei or inclusions. If a RBC has a nucleus, it is an immature RBC or a **reticulocyte.** If RBCs appear normal, this is recorded as "normal RBC morphology."

PROCEDURE: Slide Preparation

Terminal Performance Competency: Student will prepare a slide for a differential white blood cell count using correct aseptic procedure without error.

Equipment and Supplies
Clean, glass slides
Whole blood (EDTA)
Latex gloves
Biohazard container
Eye dropper
Wright's stain
Lab coat
Ink pen
Patient record

Note: Follow Standard Precautions and safety guidelines when working with blood samples. Use care to avoid splashing or spilling blood. Wipe up all spills using guidelines established by OSHA.

Procedural Steps

1. Wash hands and apply latex gloves.
2. Assemble equipment.
3. Obtain a whole blood sample using EDTA as the anticoagulant of choice. Blood must be mixed thoroughly before use.
4. Using a dropper place one drop of room temperature blood on the end of a clean, glass slide (Figure 27-21 A).
5. Using the short side of another clean, glass slide, back the slide to the drop of blood. Allow the blood to spread across the short side of the slide (Figure 27-21 B). Holding the spreader slide at a 30 degree angle, spread the blood across the length of the slide (Figure 27-21 C). Use gentle,

continuous pressure, and a smooth gliding motion to create a smear as pictured in Figure 27-21 D. Notice the smear has a thick side which gradually changes to a thin side. The thin side has a feathered edge, and the blood covers 1/2-3/4 the length of the slide.

6. Allow the slide to air dry on a rack (Figure 27-22 A). *Rationale:* Air drying will not distort cells.
7. Label on the frosted edge of the slide with patient's name and the date.
8. Stain slide using Wright's staining method. Flood slide with stain for exactly 45 seconds or amount of time indicated by manufacturer (Figure 27-22 B).
9. Rinse with distilled water as in Figure 27-22 C. Rinse until water is clear (Figure 27-22 D).
10. Allow slide to air dry before examining under the microscope.
11. Abnormal findings may need to be referred to a laboratory technician for analysis. Record results on the patient's medical record.

Charting Example
2/28/XX   2:15 PM Differential cell count: neutrophils 62%, lymphocyte 28%, monocytes 5%, Eosinophils 5%, Basophils 0%, RBC morphology-normal, adequate platelet estimation.   M. Smith, RMA.

Platelets

Platelets are the smallest of all the formed blood elements. They are one-half the size of an erythrocyte. The least numerous purple-staining structures are platelets. They should appear as if they have a rough, outer edge and contain many small granules. At times, they appear singly and other times, they clump together. There are between 200,000-300,000 per cubic millimeter in the body. Normally, there are between five and twenty platelets in one field of view. If this number is counted, then record as "adequate platelet estimation."

White Blood Cells

Each of the five white blood cells have distinct characteristics which enables the medical assistant

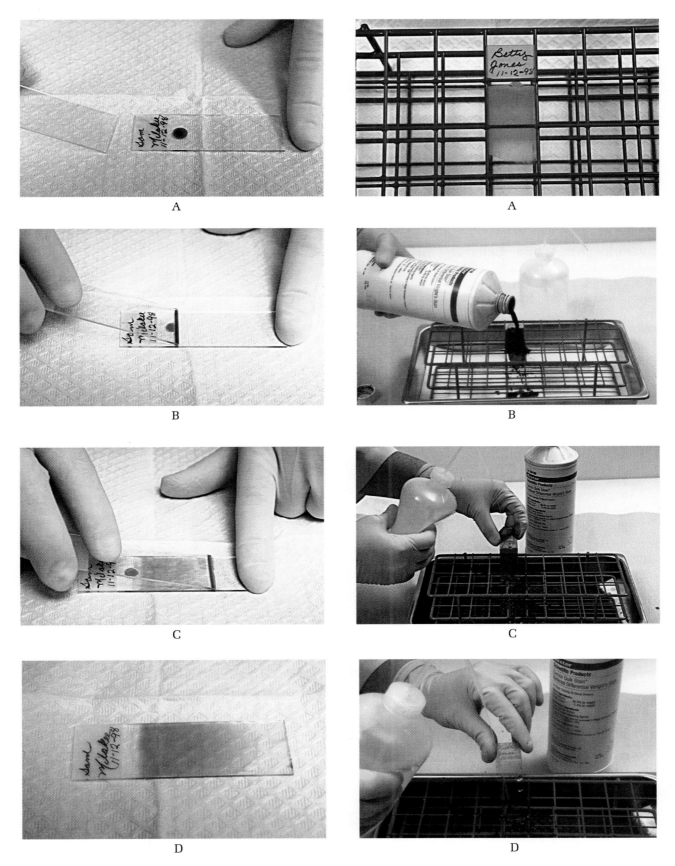

Figure 27-21 A-D Blood smear.

Figure 27-22 A-D Wright staining process.

to identify them. The Wright's stain method is responsible for these characteristics. One hundred WBCs should be counted. All cell types are then expressed as percentages of the total 100 cell count. Normal values for an adult are

- Neutrophils   50-70%
- Eosinophils   1-4%
- Basophils   0-1%
- Lymphocytes   20-35%
- Monocytes   3-8%

Values may differ between manual and automated methods.

Granulocytic White Cells The neutrophilic segmented cell, or the "seg" is the most numerous WBC. Characteristics include small cytoplasmic granules that stain pink or lilac and a multi-lobed nucleus with small strands connecting each of the purple staining lobes.

- A band neutrophil or a stab cell is an immature seg. The band appears similar to the seg except the nucleus is a non-segmented, curved, "band-like" structure. Cytoplasmic granules stain pale blue to pink.
- An eosinophil has a segmented nucleus and large, round, bright reddish staining granules found in the cytoplasm.
- A basophil is seldom seen in a diff count. This WBC has an S-shaped nucleus and large, irregularly shaped purplish-blue granules which almost cover the nucleus.

Agranulocytic White Cells

- Lymphocytes have a single round or lightly indented nucleus which almost completely fills the cell. The cytoplasm is clear and stains a pale blue. Lymphocytes are the smallest WBC.
- Monocytes are the largest WBC and have a distinct kidney-bean shaped nucleus. The cytoplasm is abundant, clear and stains a grayish-blue.

 Med Tip: To readily identify a WBC, note:

1. Size of the cell.
2. Size and shape of the nucleus.
3. Color and characteristics of the cytoplasm.

Erythrocyte Sedimentation Rate

The erythrocyte sedimentation rate measures the rate at which RBCs settle at the bottom of a tube. The tube, usually the Winthrobe tube, is calibrated in mm/hr (Figure 27-23). The rate at high RBCs fall to the bottom is the ESR.

Normal ESR in the adult is 0-20 mm/hr. An increased value may indicate inflammation. An ESR is not a diagnostic, definitive test, and it is done in conjunction with other tests. For example, when used with tests called the rheumatoid factor and an antinuclear antibody test (ANA), disorders, such as rheumatoid arthritis or fibromyalgia, may be diagnosed.

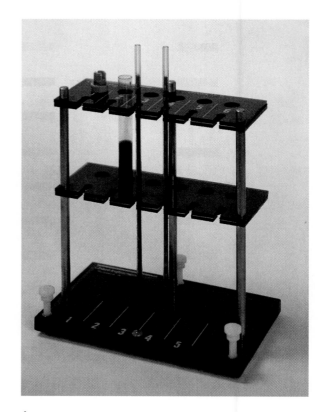

Figure 27-23   Winthrobe Tube and Westergren Test are used to measure the ESR.

PROCEDURE: ESR (Winthrobe Method)

Terminal Performance
Competency: Student will perform an erythrocyte sedimentation rate (ESR) using the Winthrobe tube method and aseptic technique without error.

Equipment and Supplies
Latex gloves
Whole blood (EDTA)
Winthrobe tube
Winthrobe rack
Ink pen
Patient's record
Lab coat
Biohazard sharps container
Note: Follow Standard Precautions and safety guidelines when working with blood samples. Use care to avoid splashing or spilling blood. Wipe up all spills using guidelines established by OSHA.

Procedural Steps
1. Wash hands and apply latex gloves.
2. Assemble equipment.
3. Obtain a whole blood sample using a purple top tube. Mix well. ***Rationale:*** EDTA is the anticoagulant of choice.
4. Slowly fill Winthrobe tube with blood. Avoid air bubbles. ***Rationale:*** Air bubbles will distort the results.
5. Adjust meniscus of specimen to the zero line at the top of the tube.
6. Maintain the tube in an upright vertical position for one hour.
7. After one hour record the number of RBCs that settle. Read ESR on same side of tube of zero line at the top.
8. Remove gloves and wash hands.
9. Record procedure on the patient's medical record.

Charting Example
2/28/XX   2:00 PM   ESR (Winthrobe Method) 10 fall of cells/hr.

M. Smith, RMA

LEGAL AND ETHICAL ISSUES

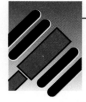

It is legal in most states for a medical assistant to perform a venipuncture. Check with the local American Association of Medical Assistants (AAMA) chapter for specifics in your state. When performing basic in-office lab tests, the medical assistant must keep all results confidential. Confidentiality is a moral and ethical obligation for all health care team members.

Many patients become apprehensive and anxious regarding venipuncture. The medical assistant should keep a confident, professional attitude and explain the procedure, if needed, to decrease patient fears. Since venipuncture is an invasive procedure, the steps must be followed exactly. Every effort should be made to maintain sterile technique.

In addition, the medical assistant should strictly adhere to OSHA regulations and the Centers for Disease Control (CDC) Standard Precautions. This helps to ensure patient and medical assistant safety. CLIA '88 regulations set the standard for laboratory testing and the need for proper training before performing any tests (Chapters 6 and 26).

PATIENT EDUCATION

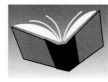

Routine blood tests performed in a physician's office require very little patient preparation.

However, patients must be told in advance of fasting requirements. For example, patients are required to fast for 12-14 hours for a glucose tolerance test while no fasting is required for a complete blood count.

Patients are much less anxious when having a procedure involving invasive equipment, such as needles, if the procedure is explained in a calm, caring manner.

Summary

The proper collection, handling, and processing of blood specimens are vital to reliable test results. In addition, it is critical that a medical assistant have a thorough understanding of patient preparation and the theory of blood formation, including the cellular and liquid components of blood. Last, knowledge of and competency in, the performance of routine blood tests—CBCs, differentials, hemoglobins, microhematocrits, ESRs—are essential to proper patient care.

Competency Review

1. Define and spell the glossary terms for this chapter.
2. List, in order, the steps for performing a venipuncture.
3. Prepare a list of the different types of venipuncture collection tubes. Explain what makes them unique; for which tests they are commonly used; and in which order they should be used.
4. Make a list of the types of white blood cells and the values of each of these expected to be found in a normal differential.
5. Create a list of the normal values, by male and female if applicable, for WBC, RBC, microhematocrit, hemoglobin, and ESR.

PREPARING FOR THE CERTIFICATION EXAM

Test Taking Tip — Keep a list of key words or important concepts and review them again one hour before the exam.

Examination Review Questions

1. A collection of blood below the surface of the skin is called a
   (A) hematoma
   (B) hemolysis
   (C) hematemesis
   (D) hematuria
   (E) hematology

2. Which type of blood collection tube contains a clot activator and a gel which permanently separates the serum from the clot after centrifugation?
   (A) red top
   (B) purple top
   (C) green top
   (D) marbled top
   (E) gray top

3. The best vein to use in order to obtain a venous sample of blood is the
   (A) median cephalic
   (B) median cubital
   (C) basilic vein
   (D) accessory cephalic
   (E) small vein in the hand

4. The most commonly used anticoagulant for blood tests is
   (A) heparin
   (B) potassium oxylate
   (C) sodium citrate
   (D) potassium citrate
   (E) EDTA

5. When drawing blood for a PT and/or a PTT, which type of blood collection tube should be used?
   (A) red top
   (B) purple top
   (C) green top
   (D) light blue top
   (E) gray top

6. If an angle of more than 15 degrees is used when inserting a needle into a patient's arm
   (A) the needle may not puncture the vein
   (B) the needle may break
   (C) the needle may go through both vein walls
   (D) the blood sample will hemolyze
   (E) a significant degree of pain will be caused

7. If the blood collection tube is pushed past the thin guideline on the plastic sleeve the
   (A) blood will hemolyze
   (B) needle will dull
   (C) vacuum may be compromised
   (D) blood will enter the tube too quickly
   (E) blood sample will be contaminated

8. Another name for a capillary puncture is a
   (A) finger stick

(B) arterial blood draw

(C) phlebotomy

(D) arterioles draw

(E) venipuncture

9. The purpose behind applying pressure and a gauze or bandage after a capillary puncture is to

(A) prevent an infection by keeping the site sterile

(B) decrease the likelihood of a hematoma

(C) cause a sterile clot to form

(D) prevent the spread of infection

(E) reassure the patient that the procedure has ended

10. When performing an ESR, the sample should sit for

(A) 20 minutes

(B) 40 minutes

(C) 60 minutes

(D) 80 minutes

(E) 90 minutes

ON THE JOB

It is Wednesday. Drs. Joseph and Burg are not seeing patients, but the office is open for blood draws. Angie, a medical assistant, is in the office alone.

Matt, a 17 year old upcoming college Freshman, has just arrived to have his labs done so that Dr. Joseph can complete Matt's college physical. He is extremely nervous, although he is trying very hard to put up a cool front. Angie tries to reassure Matt, but the more she tries, the more nervous he gets. At Matt's urging to "just get it over with," Angie decides to go ahead and draw his blood. Unfortunately, as soon as the first collection tube begins to fill with blood, Matt notices it and slumps forward. He has fainted.

What is your response?

1. What is the very first thing that Angie should do?

2. Was Angie at all negligent in drawing Matt's blood given that he was extremely nervous?

3. Does the fact that Matt is a minor influence how Angie should handle this situation? If so, how?

4. Does Matt have some level of complicity in this incident? If so, describe.

5. Is this considered a medical emergency? Why or why not?

6. Would the situation have been different or handled differently, if Angie wasn't alone?

7. Does an incident report of some sort need to be filed? If so, what should be included and who should receive a copy?

References

American Red Cross. *Basic Criteria for Blood Donors.* Columbus, Ohio: American Red Cross, 1993.

Belsey, R., Mulrow, C., Sox, H. "How To Handle Baffling Test Results." *Patient Care.* May 30, 1993.

Brown, S. "Behind the Numbers on the CBC." *RN.* February, 1990.

"CDC Summarizes Final Regulations for Implementing CLIA." *American Family Physician.* 45:6, 1992.

Chernecky, C., Krech, R., and Berger, B. *Laboratory Tests and Diagnostic Procedures.* Philadelphia: W. B. Saunders, 1993.

Fishbach, F. A *Manual of Laboratory & Diagnostic Tests.* Philadelphia: Lippincott, 1996.

Garza, D., and Becan-McBride, K. *Phlebotomy Handbook.* Stamford, CT: Appleton & Lange, 1996.

Kresten, F. "Using Blood Glucose Meters: What You and Your Patient Need to Know, Part III." *Nursing.* May, 1993.

Marshall, J. *Medical Laboratory Assistant.* Upper Saddle River, NJ: Brady/Prentice Hall, 1990.

Pagana, K. and Pagana, T. *Mosby's Diagnostic and Laboratory Test Reference.* St. Louis: Mosby Year Book, 1992.

Palko, T. and Palko, H. *Laboratory Procedures for the Medical Office.* New York: Glencoe Co., 1996.

Tietz, N. *Clinical Guide to Laboratory Tests,* 2nd ed. Philadelphia: W. B. Saunders, 1990.

Tietz, N., Conn, R., and Pruden, E. *Applied Laboratory Medicine.* Philadelphia: W. B. Saunders, 1992.

Turgeion, M. *Clinical Hematology:* Theory and Procedures Boston: Little, Brown, 1993.

MEDICAL ASSISTANT ROLE DELINEATION CHART

Highlight indicates material covered in this chapter

ADMINISTRATIVE

ADMINISTRATIVE PROCEDURES

- Perform basic clerical functions
- Schedule, coordinate, and monitor appointments
- Schedule inpatient/outpatient admissions and procedures
- Understand and apply third party guidelines
- Obtain reimbursement through accurate claims submission
- Monitor third-party reimbursement
- Perform medical transcription
- Understand and adhere to managed care policies and procedures
- *Negotiate managed care contracts (adv)*

PRACTICE FINANCES

- Perform procedural and diagnostic coding
- Apply bookkeeping principles
- Document and maintain accounting and banking records
- Manage accounts receivable
- Manage accounts payable
- Process payroll
- *Develop and maintain fee schedules (adv)*
- *Manage renewals of business and professional insurance policies (adv)*
- *Manage personal benefits and maintain records (adv)*

CLINICAL

FUNDAMENTAL PRINCIPLES

- Apply principles of aseptic technique and infection control
- Comply with quality assurance practices
- Screen and follow up patient test results

DIAGNOSTIC ORDERS

- Collect and process specimens
- Perform diagnostic tests

PATIENT CARE

- Adhere to established triage procedures
- Obtain patient history and vital signs
- Prepare and maintain examination and treatment areas

- Prepare patient for examinations, procedures, and treatments
- Assist with examinations, procedures, and treatments
- Prepare and administer medications and immunizations
- Maintain medication and immunization records
- Recognize and respond to emergencies
- Coordinate patient care information with other health care providers

GENERAL (TRANSDISCIPLINARY)

PROFESSIONALISM

- Project a professional manner and image
- Adhere to ethical principles
- Demonstrate initiative and responsibility
- Work as a team member
- Manage time efficiently
- Prioritize and perform multiple tasks
- Adapt to change
- Promote the CMA credential
- Enhance skills through continuing education

COMMUNICATION SKILLS

- Treat all patients with compassion and empathy
- Recognize and respect cultural diversity
- Adapt communications to individual's ability to understand
- Use professional telephone technique
- Use effective and correct verbal and written communications
- Recognize and respond to verbal and non-verbal communications
- Use medical terminology appropriately
- Receive, organize, prioritize, and transmit information
- Serve as liaison
- Promote the practice through positive public relations

LEGAL CONCEPTS

- Maintain confidentiality
- Practice within the scope of education, training, and personal capabilities
- Prepare and maintain medical records
- Document accurately
- Use appropriate guidelines when releasing information
- Follow employer's established policies dealing with the health care contract
- Follow federal, state, and local legal guidelines
- Maintain awareness of federal and state health care legislation and regulations
- Maintain and dispose of regulated substances in compliance with government guidelines
- Comply with established risk management and safety procedures
- Recognize professional credentialing criteria
- Participate in the development and maintenance of personnel, policy, and procedure manuals
- *Develop and maintain personnel, policy, and procedure manuals (adv)*

INSTRUCTION

- Instruct individuals according to their needs
- Explain office policies and procedures
- Teach methods of health promotion and disease prevention
- Locate community resources and disseminate information
- *Orient and train personnel (adv)*
- *Develop educational materials (adv)*
- *Conduct continuing education activities (adv)*

OPERATIONAL FUNCTIONS

- Maintain supply inventory
- Evaluate and recommend equipment and supplies
- Apply computer techniques to support office operations
- *Supervise personnel (adv)*
- *Interview and recommend job applicants (adv)*
- *Negotiate leases and prices for equipment and supply contracts (adv)*

SOURCE: Reprinted by permission of the American Association of Medical Assistants from the *AAMA Role Delineation Study: Occupational Analysis of the Medical Assisting Profession.*

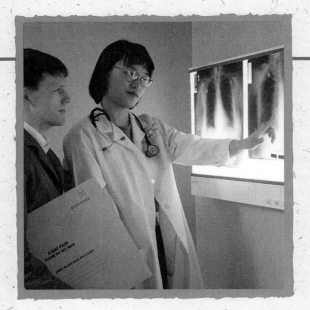

28

Radiology

LEARNING OBJECTIVES

After completing this chapter, you should:
1. Define and spell the glossary terms for this chapter.
2. List and explain the 4 basic positions during x-ray procedures.
3. Discuss positron emission tomography (PET), computerized tomography (CT), magnetic resonance imaging (MRI) and ultrasound.
4. Define and discuss the use for radiology, radiation therapy, and nuclear medicine.
5. Describe the safety precautions to take for health care workers and patients relating to x-ray procedures.
6. Describe the process and medical use of fluoroscopy.
7. List 4 side effects of radiation therapy.
8. List 6 x-ray procedures that require preparations ahead of time. Describe the preparations.
9. Discuss the proper methods for storage of x-ray film and x-rays.

CLINICAL PERFORMANCE COMPETENCIES

After completing this chapter, you should perform the following tasks:
1. Prepare the patient who is receiving a radiologic procedure.
2. Provide instructions relating to x-ray procedures.
3. Identify safety hazards relating to radiology.
4. Demonstrate precautionary measures to take relating to radiology and nuclear medicine.
5. Position the patient correctly for an AP, PA, and lateral film (if permitted to do so in your state).

Glossary

angiography X-ray visualization of the heart and blood vessels after the injection of a radiopaque material into the blood vessels.

claustrophobia Fear of closed-in or narrow spaces.

cumulative Each exposure to a substance is added to the effect of all previous exposures.

fluoroscope Device used to project an x-ray image on a special screen to allow for visual examination.

fluoroscopy Visual examination of internal body structures using a fluoroscope. Many fluoroscopy procedures require the use of a contrast medium.

nuclear medicine Medical discipline that uses radioactive isotopes in the diagnosis and treatment of disease.

radioactive Ability to give off radiation as the result of the disintegration of the nucleus of an atom.

radiation Use of radioactive substances for the diagnosis and treatment of disease.

radiologist Physician who specializes in the practice of radiology.

radiology Branch of medicine which uses radioactive substances and visualization techniques for the diagnosis and treatment of disease.

radiopaque Substance which does not allow the passage of x-rays or other radiant materials. Bones are considered radiopaque and show up as white on exposed x-ray film.

x-rays Electromagnetic radiation of shorter wavelength than visible light rays; able to pass through opaque bodies.

WARNING!

For all patient contact, adhere to Standard Precautions (see pages 342–373). Wear protective equipment as indicated.

The study of radiology includes an understanding of the use of x-rays, diagnostic radiology, radiation therapy, and nuclear medicine. The medical assistant will require additional training in order to assist with radiologic procedures.

Med Tip: In some states only licensed personnel are permitted to assist with radiologic procedures. However, the medical assistant should understand the purpose of the various procedures and the preparation necessary for them in order to provide patient instruction.

Radiology

Radiology is the branch of medicine that uses radioactive substances and various techniques for visualizing the internal structures of the body for the diagnosis and treatment of disease. Radiology uses x-rays, radioactive substances, and other forms of radiant energy such as ultraviolet rays.

Radiology can be divided into three specialties: diagnostic radiology, radiation therapy, and nuclear medicine. A discussion of various x-ray, fluoroscopic, and radiologic procedures follows.

Principles of X-rays

X-rays were discovered by Wilhelm Röentgen, a German physicist, in 1895. X-rays were formerly called roentgen rays after their discoverer. They are produced when electrons, traveling at a high speed strike against certain materials, such as heavy metals. The x-ray, which is not visible to the human eye, is produced by electromagnetic radiation that has a shorter wave length than visible light. X-rays can penetrate most materials and therefore are useful for making photographic images for diagnostic purposes. They are used in the procedures of radiography and fluoroscopy.

X-ray film is produced by projecting x-rays through organs or structures of the body onto photographic film. Some structures and tissue, such as bone, are more **radiopaque**, which allows fewer x-rays to pass through, than other tissues such as skin. Thus the bone leaves a shadow on the film which can be examined for defects.

X-rays which are able to penetrate the body are able to change the basic structure of body cells. Thus they have been useful in the diagnosis and treatment of tumors.

Fluoroscopy

Fluoroscopy is a technique in radiology for visually examining a portion of the body or the function of an organ using a **fluoroscope**. This technique allows the **radiologist** to have immediate images which can be used to assess heart function, such as in the procedure of cardiac catheterization. The moving image that is seen on the fluoroscope can then be filmed using a radiograph (x-ray).

Contrast media are often used during fluoroscopic procedures to better visualize organ function and abnormalities.

The Use of a Contrast Medium

A contrast medium is a radiopaque substance, which does not allow the passage of x-rays, but facilitates radiographic imaging of internal structures that are difficult to visualize on a regular x-ray or fluoroscopic screen. The body structure or organ with the contrast medium, such as the gallbladder, is seen in contrast to adjacent structures.

Med Tip: The patient must always be asked about any known allergies, such as to iodine, before a contrast medium is used or an invasive procedure with the insertion of dye is begun.

Contrast media include liquids such as barium, powders, air and gas. They are administered orally, by injection (parenterally), or through an enema into the rectum. The contrast medium acts to convert an organ or structure into an opaque area. In this way, the actual function of that particular organ or structure can be visualized under fluoroscopy or by film.

Barium sulfate and iodine are positive contrast media which means they have more density and thus can absorb more radiation. These will appear white on x-ray images. This is in contrast to air which is a negative contrast medium allowing more x-rays to pass through.

Barium Sulfate Barium sulfate consists of a chalky compound which is mixed with water and flavoring until it is the right consistency for a patient to drink or for a technician to administer as an enema. Barium sulfate is used for fluoroscopic examination of the gastrointestinal tract.

Iodine Contrast Compounds Iodine compounds used to form radiopaque compound are used for thyroid studies, pyelograms, angiograms, and cholecystograms. This compound should not be used if the patient is allergic to iodine. In addition, iodine radiopaque compounds interfere with nuclear medicine thyroid studies. Therefore these two types of studies should not be performed during the same time period.

Negative contrast media include air, carbon dioxide and other gases. These will appear black on x-rays. This media is used to visualize the spinal cord, as in a myelogram, and joints. The introduction of gas and air into the body can result in severe headaches following such procedures as myelograms. Negative contrast studies have largely been replaced with the use of the magnetic resonance imaging (MRI).

Fluoroscopic Procedures

Fluoroscopic procedures include the gastrointestinal series (upper GI and lower GI), intravenous pyelogram (IVP), cholecystogram, and mammography.

Gastrointestinal (GI) Series A GI series is a fluoroscopic study of the digestive tract using a contrast media to detect abnormalities such as tumors, ulcers, polyps, and diverticulosis. An upper gastrointestinal (upper GI) series is an examination of the esophagus, stomach, duodenum, and small intestine. A procedure called a barium swallow outlines the esophagus, stomach, and small intestine as it moves through the system after the patient drinks a barium mixture. A lower gastrointestinal (lower GI) series is the administration of a barium enema which outlines the colon and rectum on a radiographic picture.

The patient should receive written instructions for these procedures. In addition, the medical assistant should explain the instructions and the procedure. Careful preparation is necessary for good results on these procedures. If the patient's digestive tract is not properly prepared and cleaned, the procedure may have to be repeated. This results in added expense, time, and patient discomfort. Guidelines are provided for patients who will undergo upper and lower GI series.

1. The patient should not eat or drink after midnight since the stomach must be empty for this procedure. No water should even be swallowed while brushing teeth. The physician may order that no morning medications should be taken.
2. The patient should be instructed not to smoke since this can stimulate gastric secretions.
3. The patient will have to undress and put on a patient gown.
4. A barium sulfate drink is prepared for the patient to drink. This may be flavored but will still retain a slightly chalky taste.
5. The patient will stand in front of the fluoroscopic screen while drinking the mixture. The radiologist will observe the progress of the barium as the patient drinks.
6. The patient is then placed on an x-ray table which will tip into various positions for additional views. Permanent x-rays are taken during which the patient will be told to hold his or her breath.
7. The procedure may last for several hours during which time the barium will move out of the stomach and into the small intestine.
8. The patient may resume normal eating after the examination but should be reminded to drink water to assist in flushing out the remaining barium, as this may cause constipation. The stool may remain chalky for a couple of days.

Intravenous Pyelogram (IVP) or Intravenous Urogram

The intravenous pyelogram, also called a pyelogram, is an radiologic examination of the kidneys, ureters, and bladder. The patient will be instructed to eat a low-residue diet and drink plenty of water the day before the procedure. The patient will be allowed nothing by mouth (NPO) after midnight. A cathartic, such as castor oil or citrate of magnesia, may be ordered along with an enema to be taken the night before the examination.

The patient will need to undress and wear a patient gown for this procedure. A contrast medium containing iodine is injected into the vein (IV). This substance may cause the patient to have a warm, flushed feeling and a metallic taste in the mouth. The patient should be instructed to notify the radi-

The colon and rectum need to be free of stool for a clear view of the area on x-ray.

Day Before the Examination

1. The patient may be instructed to eat only a low-residue diet for several days before the procedure and then only clear liquids (such as water and clear soup) on the day of the lower GI.
2. A cathartic such as castor oil or citrate of magnesia may be ordered to be taken at 4 PM the day before the procedure. Enemas need to be taken until the return fluid is clear.

Day of the Examination

1. The patient must undress and wear a patient gown for the procedure. Another cleansing enema may be given before the procedure.
2. The patient lies on his or her side on the x-ray table while the technician gives an enema of barium sulfate. The patient is asked to retain or hold the enema within the rectal and colon area.
3. The patient is then moved or tipped into different positions on the table while the radiologist observes the flow of barium on the fluoroscope. Periodically radiographs (x-rays) are taken during the procedure.
4. The patient is asked to expel the barium into the toilet. Then a final x-ray is taken of the empty bowel.
5. The patient may return to a regular diet after this procedure. Whitish stools may be present for one or two days after the procedure. The patient should be encouraged to drink water to flush out the remaining barium with stool.

ologist if there are any unusual symptoms, such as shortness of breath or itching, which could indicate an allergic reaction to the dye.

The patient is then tipped into various positions on the x-ray table in order for the radiologist to view the dye as it flows through the urinary system. The patient may be asked to urinate, and then have one final x-ray taken. After the examination, the patient can return to a normal diet. He or she should be encouraged to drink water to flush out the contrast medium through the kidneys.

Cholecystogram

A cholecystogram is a radiologic examination of the gallbladder using a contrast medium, usually iodine. This procedure is done to detect abnormalities such as the presence of gallstones. The patient is instructed to have a fat-free meal the evening before the procedure and nothing by mouth (NPO) after midnight.

The contrast medium, in the form of pills, is taken after dinner. The patient is instructed to take one pill at a time every few minutes with water. In some facilities, the contrast medium is administered by intravenous (IV) injection.

The patient undresses and wears a patient gown for this procedure. An initial x-ray is taken to see if the gallbladder is visible. A study is then conducted using the fluoroscope. Radiographs (x-rays) are taken also. After this portion of the procedure the patient is asked to eat a fatty meal. This meal stimulates the gallbladder to empty. Another x-ray is taken 1 hour after this meal. The patient can resume a normal diet after the procedure is complete. The contrast medium is eliminated through the intestines. This procedure has been replaced by ultrasound in many facilities.

Radiology Procedures Not Requiring Contrast Media

There are several other diagnostic radiologic examinations that do not require the use of a contrast material, such as barium. These examinations or films require that the patient is positioned properly, however, no prior preparation, such as enemas, is required. One of these procedures is the mammogram.

Mammography Mammography is the radiology examination of the soft tissue of the breast to provide identification of benign and malignant neoplasms (tumors). Contrast medium is not used for this procedure. The patient should be instructed not to use underarm deodorant, talcum powder, body lotion or perfume since these could affect the image clarity.

The patient stands in front of the x-ray equipment and the technician positions the patient carefully in order to have all breast tissue examined under x-ray. The patient should be instructed to follow the technician's direction regarding placement of hands, arms, and body position. Patient's of childbearing age are given a lead apron to wear during the procedure.

Each breast is compressed by the mammography equipment in order to spread the tissue for better viewing. The x-rays are directed at angles into the breast tissue. The procedure takes a few seconds for each view with the entire procedure lasting about a half hour. Some patients may feel discomfort during the procedure due to pressure during the breast compression. The discomfort is over as soon as the compression is completed (less than a minute).

Women over the age of 40 are advised by the American Cancer Society to have a yearly mammogram for early detection of breast cancer. Figure 28-1 shows a woman receiving a mammogram and Figure 28-2 shows a doctor viewing mammographies.

Other procedures not requiring contrast media include films of the abdomen; bone; chest; kidneys, ureters, and bladder (KUB); and paranasal sinuses. They are described in Table 28-1.

Tomography

Tomography, or the sectioning of the body using roetgenography, allows the technician to penetrate

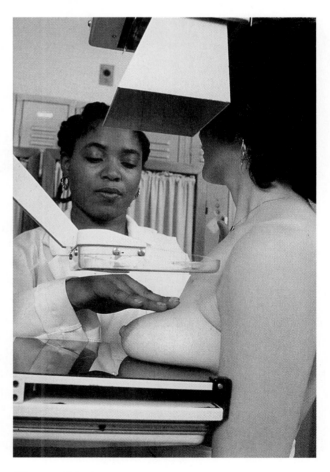

Figure 28-1 Women receive regular mammograms to detect cancer early.

dense areas of the body that could not otherwise be visualized. It is a valuable diagnostic tool for identifying and discovering space-occupying lesions such as those found in the brain, liver, gallbladder, and spleen. Tomography has the ability to remove, or blur out, areas that are not within the plane being examined. It is especially valuable in evaluating malignant conditions in the lungs and bones.

Computerized tomography (CT) and magnetic resonance imaging (MRI) have largely replaced the use of tomography except in areas where these two techniques requiring expensive equipment are not available.

Positron Emission Tomography (PET)

Positron Emission Tomography (PET) is a computerized radiographic method that uses radioactive substances to examine the metabolic activity within the body.

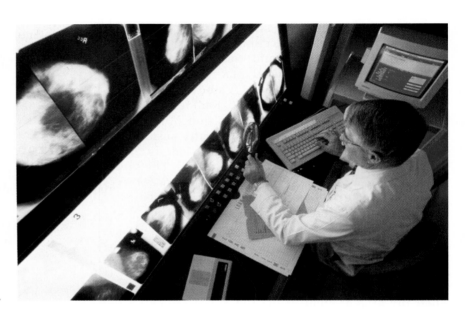

Figure 28-2   Mammographies.

TABLE 28-1   Radiology Procedures Not Requiring Contrast Material

Type	Description and Use
Abdomen	Flat plate or survey of abdomen used for suspected tumors, hematomas, enlarged organs, or abscesses.
Bone	X-ray studies of bones for suspected abnormalities from disease or trauma such as fractures, and tumors. Commonly performed spinal x-rays are: Cervical x-ray in neck area. Thoracic x-ray in middle back. Lumbosacral x-ray in lower back.
Chest	Routine chest x-rays are taken to rule out any abnormality and to pick up hidden disease in the lungs and some cardiac abnormalities (for example, cardiomegaly). The patient assumes the posteroanterior erect position and a lateral position.
Kidneys, ureters, bladder	This abdominal x-ray studies the kidneys, ureters, and bladder (KUB); abdominal wall; pelvic bones; and unusual masses.
Paranasal sinuses	X-ray of the sinuses found within the maxillary, frontal, ethmoid, and sphenoid bones for signs of infection, inflammation, and abnormalities.

In PET the patient is either injected with or inhales a chemical, such as glucose, which carries a radioactive substance. This substance then emits positively charged particles, called positrons, that combine with negatively charged electrons found within the body. The rays that are produced are converted into color-coded images that indicate the degree of metabolic activity. PET is used to assist in the treatment of epilepsy, brain tumors, stroke, Alzheimer's disease, blood flow and metabolism of the heart and blood vessels. The radioactive elements used in PET are short-lived which results in minimal radiation exposure for patients.

Computerized Tomography (CT)

In computerized tomography (CT), formerly called computerized axial tomography (CAT scan), a thin x-ray beam penetrates the body tissues at angles to produce a film representing a detailed cross section of tissue structures. This procedure is painless, noninvasive, and requires no special preparation. In this procedure a narrow beam of x-ray rotates in a continuous 360-degree motion around the patient to slice the body in cross-sectional angles. The computer then calculates various factors including tissue absorption and displays a printout that determines the density of tissue. In this way tissue masses, such as tumors, bone displacement, and fluid accumulation are detected.

CTs are useful when there is conflicting information about the cause of a patient's condition. They are also useful for defining exactly where radiation therapy must be directed for tumor masses. Other uses for CT include: detecting cerebral abnormalities, such as tumors, hematomas, childhood cancers, and abdominal masses, and surveying difficult to visualize glands, such as the pituitary gland and tissue. The CT scanner is able to scan the entire body in 15 to 20 minutes which allows for up to 20 patients to be scanned in one day. For some CT procedures, a contrast medium is used so the patient may be instructed to have nothing by mouth (NPO) for 4 hours before the procedure.

Magnetic Resonance Imaging (MRI)

One of the newest imaging technologies, magnetic resonance imaging (MRI), has changed the field of radiology. There is no ionizing radiation used and the MRI has no known risks. The MRI uses a powerful magnetic field to visualize internal tissues, organs, and structures. The images produced with this technique are excellent. All areas of the body can be scanned using the MRI. See Figure 28-3 for a color-enhanced image from MRI.

The signal or nuclear magnetic resonance that is produced by the MRI varies with different body tissues. These signals are processed within the computer and form a visual image. An MRI scan can be of the body in total or they can be seen as slices which give the viewer a three-dimensional view of tissues or organs. This can be useful for tumor detection.

Patient preparation consists of explaining the procedure to the patient including a description of the chamber in which the patient is placed. The

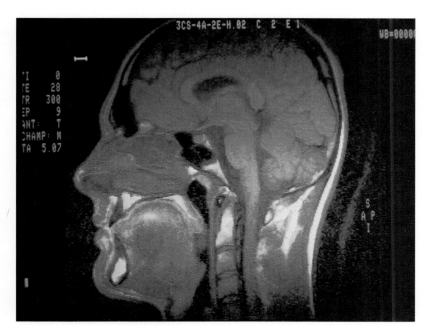

Figure 28-3   Color-enhanced image from MRI.

chamber consists of a large cylindrical electromagnet into which the patient is rolled on a pallet and then sealed within. This allows the entire patient's body to come into contact with the electromagnetic field. The procedure, while painless, can be upsetting to patients who have claustrophobia, or are afraid of closed in spaces (Figure 28-4). In this case, the patients may need to be given a medication to promote relaxation.

There are some limitations to the use of the MRI. It is not possible to view the hard portion of bone for visualizing fractures and other abnormalities. For this the CT and general x-rays are still used. In addition, the strong magnetic field is not appropriate for patients who have pacemakers or metallic clips on blood vessels. The patient should be instructed to:

1. Remove all jewelry, eye shadow, and metallic objects, such as watches, belts, hearing aids, and hairpins.
2. Identify which devices, if any, have been inserted within his or her body, such as pacemakers, dental implants, surgical staples, intrauterine devices, joint or bone pins or prosthesis, metallic clips on blood vessels, or metal fragments, for example, from gunshots. These will all be present on the scan and can interfere with magnetic conduction. In addition, metallic clips on blood vessels can become loosened.

3. Leave credit cards or devices which contain metallic or magnetic code strips outside the MRI chamber.
4. Use a patient gown if the patient's clothing has zippers or metal snaps.

The technician is not in the chamber with the patient during the procedure. The patient should be told that the technician will be in constant contact with the patient via a microphone and camera. The patient should be instructed to remain still during the procedure. An MRI scan takes from 20 to 60 minutes depending on the amount of the body to be scanned.

Digital Radiology

Digital radiology is the use of standard fluoroscopy which is digitized and stored into computer bits, processed, and then converted into an image on a television or video monitor screen. The image is stored on a videotape or digital disc. Digital angiography is used for cardiac and pulmonary arteries and structures, and head and neck angiograms. A discussion of angiography follows.

Angiography

Angiography is the x-ray visualization of the internal anatomy of blood vessels after a radiopaque material has been injected into the blood vessels. This procedure is used to assist in the diagnosis of

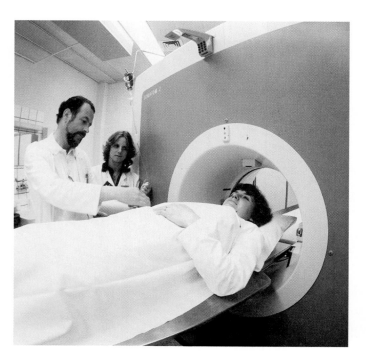

Figure 28-4 MRI equipment.

many conditions including myocardial infarction (MI or heart attack), cerebrovascular accident (CVA or stroke), renal artery stenosis as a cause of hypertension and clots and stenosis in arteries in the lower extremities and abdomen, aneurysm of the aorta, and pulmonary emboli or clots.

Contrast medium is injected into an artery or vein by way of a catheter and threaded through the vessel until it reaches the correct site. Since iodine is used as the contrast medium, the patient should be tested for allergy to iodine before the procedure begins. The patient is monitored for a few hours after the procedure for any signs of bleeding from the puncture site.

Diagnostic Digital Ultrasound

Ultrasound is the use of high frequency sound waves causing 20,000 cycles per second to image internal structures. Ultrasound imaging consists of projecting a beam of sound waves into the body which results in the wave bouncing back as it comes into contact with a structure, such as a fetus. This produces an outline of the internal structure. Ultrasound has valuable medical applications, such as in fetal monitoring and detecting abnormalities, such as gallstones, tumors, and heart defects. It is used to scan organs such as the liver, heart, kidneys, thyroid, gonads, and blood vessels. Ultrasound is not used to image the lungs, brain, or skeleton since they are made of or surrounded by bone which sound waves cannot penetrate.

Ultrasound differs from diagnostic radiology in that no ionizing radiation is used. In addition, ultrasound is a painless noninvasive procedure and has been widely accepted as a safe examination of delicate tissues and the fetus. Fetal ultrasound is commonly performed to detect the presence of multiple pregnancies, fetal and placental positioning, and internal organ development. The use of ultrasound is not recommended simply to determine gender of the fetus.

To perform an ultrasound procedure, a conduction material such as water, special jelly, or oil is used to conduct the sound waves into the body. An instrument called a transducer with a conduction head is then placed on or near the skin. As the sound waves pass through the skin, they bounce off the body tissues or fetus and remit an echo reflection of the image back to the instrument. These echoes of the body tissue or fetus are then recorded as a series of dots on an oscilloscope, which is an instrument that displays a visual picture. The record that is produced is called an echogram or a sonogram. The patient is often able to view the sonogram on the screen as it occurs. A print-out of this visual picture can then be printed for the patient's record. In some cases, a copy of this print-out is also given to the mother. In most cases, it will require some interpretation. The medical assistant should not attempt to explain the results of a sonogram to the patient.

Med Tip: An ultrasound procedure will frequently be referred to as a sonogram or an echogram. It is wise to use a complete description when discussing an ultrasound procedure, such as fetal ultrasound, or echocardiogram, which detects heart abnormalities, or echoencephalogram for observing the brain.

Patient preparation for the ultrasound examination is minimal. The patient should wear loose fitting clothing or clothing that is easy to remove since the procedure is performed over bare skin. During a fetal ultrasound, the patient is instructed not to urinate right before the test since a full bladder displaces the intestines and allows for a better view of the uterus. In fact, the patient may be asked to drink water just prior to the examination if the bladder is empty. For an ultrasound of the gallbladder or liver, the patient may be asked not to eat for several hours before the procedure.

Ultrasound is also used in physical therapy and discussed in Chapter 30. See Figure 28-5 and Figure 28-6 for illustrations of an ultrasound unit from Chattanooga Group, Inc. and of a patient receiving an ultrasound treatment.

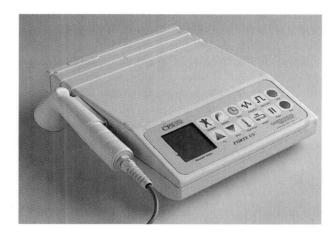

Figure 28-5 Forte CPS Series™ Ultrasound Unit.

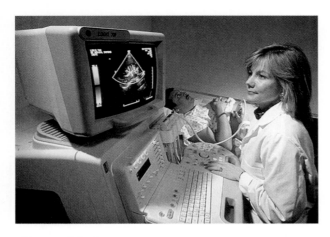

Figure 28-6 Ultrasound being performed on a patient.

Radiation Therapy

Radiation is the use of a radioactive substance in the diagnosis and treatment of disease.

> **Med Tip:** The medical assistant should be familiar with the radiation process in order to answer the patient's questions. Any questions from a patient relating to the chance for success or cure, as a result of receiving radiation therapy, should be referred to the physician.

When radiation is used to treat cancers or other conditions, it is called radiation therapy. Radiation therapy is the process of administering a particular dosage of radiation to a specific area on the patient's body for the purpose of killing diseased cells. Radiation actually alters the cells so they cannot reproduce and thus eventually die leaving no new cells to develop. Both diseased and normal cells are altered with radiation. Diseased cells are eventually destroyed. However, normal or healthy cells are able to repair themselves and regrow new cells.

The tumors are located through the use of CT and ultrasound. The boundary of the tumor can be localized by these radiologic procedures. Radiation therapy is administered after the tumor is well defined.

Patients receive radiation therapy for a variety of types of cancers including: cancer of the ovaries, testes, skin, larynx, and oral cavity. Hodgkin's disease, Wilms' tumor (a type of kidney tumor found in children), and retinoblastoma are also treated with radiation therapy. For some types of malignancies, such as cervical cancer, a combination of radiation and chemotherapy is used.

Radiation therapy may cause side effects in some patients including hair loss, skin changes, nausea and diarrhea, and irritation of the mucous membranes in the mouth, throat, bladder, vagina, and chromosome changes.

Nuclear Medicine

Nuclear medicine is that branch of medicine that uses radioactive isotopes in the diagnosis and treatment of disease. Radioactive refers to the ability to give off radiation as the result of the disintegration of the nucleus of an atom. Isotopes are chemical elements which may have several forms but identical properties.

Radioactive isotopes of iodine, cobalt and other elements are used in nuclear medicine for the treatment of tumors and for nuclear imaging of certain parts of the body. Radionuclides, isotopes whose nuclei (central core) are undergoing decay, are administered to patients intravenously or orally. The radionuclides then travel to a point within the body that attracts them, such as the thyroid, and create an image or "outline" of that organ or tumor (abnormality). Radionuclides have a short life which results in very few side effects for the patient.

A concentration of radionuclides is referred to as either "hot" or "cold." If the radionuclide is in an area with an abnormality, it is referred to as "hot." If the radionuclide does not concentrate into a tumor, but, instead, is situated in the surrounding area, it is referred to as "cold." Both hot and cold areas can indicate the presence of abnormalities.

The process of studying an area with a concentration of a radioactive substance is called scanning. The thyroid, liver, and brain are frequently evaluated using a scanning process. Scanning requires the administration of the radionuclide in an intravenous (IV) injection. The scan will then take place at intervals of time for up to 72 hours.

If a radioisotope is used in a high dose for treatment, then the patients may have symptoms that are similar to those found with radiation. These include: hair loss, nausea, diarrhea, mucous membrane irritation (mouth, throat and bladder), and chromosome changes.

Preparing and Positioning the Patient

The medical assistant may be the person who will prepare the patients for x-ray examinations. Patients should be requested to remove all metallic materials such as jewelry, belt buckles, watches, eyeglasses, hairpins, earrings, and hearing aids. In some x-rays of the head, mouth, and neck, the patient may have to remove dentures.

Explain the type of x-rays that will be taken and the approximate amount of time the patient will spend in the radiology area or department.

> **Med Tip:** Patients are much less likely to complain about the long waiting periods required for some radiology procedures, such as barium examinations, if they have information ahead of time regarding why there will be a waiting period. For example, "There will be a time delay, perhaps up to an hour, while the barium moves throughout your system."

For many radiology exams the patient will be asked to undress and wear a patient gown. Since the patient is not able to have jewelry on their person, a safe container or locker should be provided for personal belongings.

The patient may need assistance in getting onto the x-ray table. A footstool should be available if the table is high. X-ray tables do not have side rails. If there is a concern that the patient may become confused, then someone must remain in the room with the patient until the procedure begins. The x-ray technician should be told about the patient's confused state.

Positioning

The position of the patient is critical for an accurate x-ray. The position of the patient and the po-
sition of the x-ray beam need to be known ahead of time by the technician. See Table 28-2 for an explanation of positions used in radiology.

> **Med Tip:** The patient may ask you about the results of the x-ray after the procedure is complete. State that the physician will discuss the results with the patient as soon as the film has been developed and interpreted.

For some x-ray procedures special patient preparation must be performed before the patient can be examined. These are described in Table 28-3.

Scheduling Guidelines

The medical assistant often has the responsibility for scheduling the patient and providing instruction for radiologic procedures. If the procedure is performed in a facility other than the medical office, you may have to call to make the appointment. The patient's name, type of insurance with precertification or approval number, the referring physician's name, and type of radiologic procedure to be performed need to be stated.

When multiple procedures need to be scheduled, it is important to remember the sequence of scheduling. Attention to sequencing is important since some procedures, such as those that require the use of contrast medium, may interfere with others. In addition, the patient may not be able to tolerate multiple procedures on one day. In general, examinations which do not require the use of

TABLE 28-2 Radiology Positions

Position	Description
Anteroposterior (AP)	The x-ray beam is directed from front to back. Patient may be standing or supine. The front of the patient will face the x-ray equipment and the patient's back will be near the film plate.
Posteroanterior (PA)	The x-ray beam is directed from back to front. Patient will be standing upright. Patient's back will face the x-ray equipment and their front will be near the film plate.
Lateral	The x-ray beam is directed toward one side of the body. In a RL (right lateral) position, the patient's right side is near the film plate and the left side is near the x-ray equipment. In a LL (left lateral) position, the patient's left side is near the film plate.
Oblique	The patient is turned at an angle to the film plate so the x-ray beam can be directed at areas that would be hidden on an AP, PA, or lateral x-ray.

TABLE 28-3 X-ray Procedures Requiring Special Preparations*

Procedure	Preparation
Angiogram	No breakfast if morning examination. No lunch if afternoon examination.
Barium enema (Lower GI)	Enemas until the bowel return is clear the evening before the examination. May order rectal suppository in the morning or a cathartic, such as 2 oz. of castor oil or citrate of magnesia, at 4:00 PM the day before the x-ray. Clear liquids and jello for dinner. Nothing by mouth (NPO) after midnight.
Barium meal (Upper GI)	NPO after midnight.
Bronchogram	NPO.
Cholecystogram (GB series)	Light supper of nonfatty food, such as fruits and vegetables without butter or fat, the evening before x-ray. Gallbladder tablets (prescribed by physician) are taken with water after supper. NPO except for water until x-ray on following day.
Computerized tomography (CT)	NPO for 4 hours before x-ray if a contrast media is used.
Intravenous cholangiogram	NPO.
Intravenous pyelogram (IVP)	Three Dulcolax tablets or 2 oz. castor oil 4 PM day before x-ray. Eat light supper. NPO after midnight.
Myelogram	NPO.
Retrograde pyelogram	Enemas or laxatives evening before x-ray. NPO for 8 hours before procedure.
Ultrasound	May require a full bladder or laxatives depending on the type of ultrasound.

*Preparations may vary at different facilities.

contrast medium are performed before those examinations which do use contrast mediums. For example, an abdominal x-ray would be taken before a barium enema.

Many examinations require long waiting periods between filmings, because it takes time for the contrast medium to move through portions of the body. This should be carefully explained to patients in order for them to schedule their time appropriately. The patient may have to allow a full morning for a series of x-ray procedures.

Safety Precautions

Excessive exposure to radiation causes tissue damage and side effects. Overexposure to radiation may result in a lowered red blood cell and white blood cell count since the blood forming organs and bone marrow are altered. Other dangers of radiation include burns, damage to ovaries and testes, fetal damage (especially during the first three months of pregnancy), and cancer.

Since x-rays have a potential for danger to both the patient and the health care personnel, special precautions must be taken. Lead has been proven to be an effective barrier to an x-ray beam. Lead aprons and gloves are provided for personnel coming into close contact with x-ray equipment.

Radiation is discussed in terms of primary and secondary radiation. Primary radiation is that which strikes the patient for either therapeutic reasons or for an x-ray examination. Once that primary beam strikes the patient, it can then become secondary radiation as it bounces off the patient. Secondary radiation is the strongest closest to the patient. Therefore, x-ray technicians do not remain next to the patient during the x-ray process. They stand behind a lead shielded divider. The x-ray rooms are lined with metal (1-inch thick) as a precaution against x-ray beams escaping from the room. Some facilities have a red light that flashes

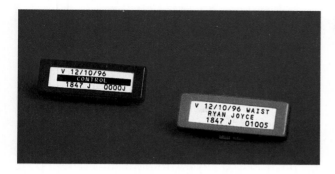

Figure 28-7 Radiation badge.

when x-ray equipment is being used to warn others not to enter.

A film badge, called a dosimeter, is worn on the outer clothing of all personnel working with or near radiologic equipment (see Figure 28-7). The badge records the level and intensity of radiation exposure. It is periodically examined to assure the health care worker is not exposed to excessive radiation since radiation exposure is cumulative. (Each exposure is added to the effect of all previous exposures.)

Guidelines are provided here for safeguarding the safety of health care workers and patients.

Processing X-ray Film

All film development takes place in the darkroom of the facility since exposure to light can ruin the film. Both manual and automated processing methods are used. The automated processing method is able to meet quality control standards since the equipment can be tested frequently for accuracy. Automated processing may take anywhere from 90 seconds to 10 minutes depending on the equipment used. The film is fed into the processor which transports the film through processing chemicals, dries the film, and moves it out of the equipment for the radiologist to view and read.

Storage and Records

X-ray materials to be used in radiologic procedures must be kept in special storage containers which will protect the film from damage due to light, heat, chemical fumes, and moisture. In order for film to remain fresh, it needs to be kept in a dry, cool place within its sealed package. X-ray film should be stored on end to prevent pressure damage from stacking film. The expiration dates, which are printed on the top end of the package, can be seen clearly when stored on end. X-ray developer is also kept in a cool location which is

Guidelines: Maintaining Personnel Safety

1. Wear a film badge on outer clothing at all times when you are exposed to any form of x-rays. Do not wear a patient gown or lead shield over the badge. These badges are submitted for routine—usually weekly—evaluation of the levels of radiation exposure.
2. Health care personnel should stay behind a lead shield in a lead-lined room when the x-ray is in use.
3. A sign or lighted display should be visible when x-ray equipment is in use.
4. All equipment should be inspected on a frequent, routine basis to check for radiation leakage.
5. The patient should not be held or supported during radiologic procedures. There are devices which can be used to hold and position the patient.
6. If it is necessary to remain in the room with the patient, the attendant should wear a protective lead apron and rubber gloves containing a lead lining. The attendant should face the patient with the lead apron between the patient and the attendant.
7. Periodic blood tests may be required by facilities to determine the presence of blood abnormalities from radiation exposure.

Guidelines: Maintaining Patient Safety

1. Ask if the patient has recently been exposed to x-rays from other examinations or through work-related activities.
2. If the patient is female, inquire about the possibility of a pregnancy. If the patient is pregnant, report this to the physician before scheduling or assisting with any x-ray procedure. It is important to obtain a release, or even a pregnancy test, prior to some x-ray procedures due to liability concerns.
3. Place a lead shield over the patient's abdominal and reproductive organs in patients who are of childbearing age, children, and patients who are pregnant.
4. Patients must be carefully positioned. Positioning of the patient is critical for the proper film accuracy. Only perform this procedure if you have been fully instructed and trained (and are authorized to do so in your state).

moisture-free since damage to this fluid can affect the quality of the film. The film packages are only opened in the "dark room" of the medical facility since light will destroy the film imaging ability.

All film records are maintained in a record/log book that is kept in the x-ray room. Entered in this record book are the identification number, name of the patient, date, type, and x-rays which were taken. Each film taken will have an identification number which is created by placing lead letters or numbers in the film holder, or cassette, at the time the x-ray is taken (time of exposure). These numbers will identify the name of the physician, date, and name of the patient. This data will then be permanently on the film after it is processed.

Films that have been processed should be stored in special envelopes and filed in specially designed film cabinets. They are usually filed alphabetically. If a chronological numbering system is used based on the identification number of each film, a master log must be maintained. If a film has to be removed from the file cabinet, an insert explaining where the film was sent is filed in place of the film within the file cabinet.

Ownership of the Film

The medical assistant is frequently called upon to explain the ownership of film to the patient. Although the patient has paid for the film, it is the property of the medical facility or hospital that performed the x-ray. Written reports prepared by the radiologist are sent to other physicians at the request of the patient but the film generally remains in the original office or hospital. The reason for this is simple: if the film remains in one location, it can always be accessed for future examination and comparison. Once it leaves the originating facility, it can be misplaced and lost.

Physicians are able to loan their films to referring physicians for further examination. The patient has to sign a release of records form for this to take place, but the film must then be returned to the original facility. Since films are a permanent record of the patient at a particular moment, they need to be preserved carefully. It is possible, in some locations, for the patient to obtain a duplicate copy of a film. The patient would have to pay for the copy to be made.

LEGAL AND ETHICAL ISSUES

To protect the patient and the physician always have a written order for every procedure. For invasive procedures, a written consent from the patient is necessary before the procedure can be performed.

The procedures discussed in this chapter would not ordinarily be a part of the medical assistant's routine work assignment. Assisting with radiologic procedures requires extra training and practice. The medical assistant must refrain from assisting with or performing advanced procedures without adequate training.

In some states, the medical assistant is not allowed to assist with radiologic procedures. If in doubt about the practice and laws within your state, always check with your local medical assistant organization or call the AAMA located in Chicago, Illinois.

PATIENT EDUCATION

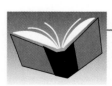

Thorough instructions for radiologic procedures include explanations, such as the need for the patient to administer cleansing enemas and to avoid the use of deodorants and powders for some procedures. The correct time and place for the procedure must be stressed. The informed patient is better able to cooperate during the preparation stage for radiologic procedures.

Clear instructions ultimately save time and money for all involved since clear patient instructions help to prevent the need for having to repeat procedures.

The role of the medical assistant is to reinforce instructions that have already been given to the patient by the physician or the radiology therapist. You should not provide advice for the patient without permission of the physician.

Summary

The use of radiology in medical practice makes it possible to view internal body structures and functions and therefore assist in diagnosis and treatment. These procedures include radiology, radiation therapy, and nuclear medicine. There are inherent risks to the patients, technicians, and the medical assistants in performing these procedures. The use of proper safety precautions can greatly reduce or eliminate these risks altogether.

Competency Review

Note: These competencies may only be practiced by a medical assistant if permitted by state law.

1. Define and spell the glossary terms for this chapter.
2. Prepare the patient for a radiology procedure by correctly positioning the patient for the AP, PA, RL and LL.
3. Explain radiologic procedures and preparations to patients.
4. Demonstrate safety precautions relevant to radiology procedures.
5. Describe a film badge and its use.
6. Demonstrate how to store x-ray film in the office.

PREPARING FOR THE CERTIFICATION EXAM

Test Taking Tip — Set a timer when you review for an examination. Know that when 20 minutes are up, you must have completed the review of a certain section. This will force you to concentrate on what you are reading and reviewing.

Examination Review Questions

1. An example of a contrast medium is
   (A) lidocaine
   (B) epinephrine
   (C) sodium chloride
   (D) barium oxylate
   (E) barium sulfate

2. Which of the following procedures, relating to x-rays, are NOT performed by medical assistants?
   (A) instruct the patient
   (B) handle x-ray film
   (C) position the patient
   (D) interpret x-ray film
   (E) prepare the patient

3. Secondary radiation is
   (A) emitted by the direct x-ray beam
   (B) scattered from the patient being x-rayed
   (C) emitted through the radiology room walls
   (D) the second beam of x-ray coming from equipment

   (E) none of the above

4. A patient is scheduled for an IV pyelogram. This is an examination of the
   (A) gallbladder
   (B) small intestine
   (C) kidneys, ureters, and bladder
   (D) colon
   (E) pyloric sphincter of the stomach

5. A patient is scheduled for a cholecystogram. This is an examination of the
   (A) gallbladder
   (B) small intestine
   (C) kidneys, ureters, and bladder
   (D) colon
   (E) pyloric sphincter of the stomach

6. If a patient notices a white stool after having a lower GI, what advice can be given?
   (A) drink plenty of fluid(s)
   (B) eat a large meal

(Continued on next page)

(C) take an antacid product

(D) take a laxative

(E) only the physician can give medical advice

7. A radiologic procedure that does not require a contrast medium is

(A) IVP

(B) mammogram

(C) LGI

(D) UGI

(E) cholecystogram

8. Symptoms the patient should NOT expect after having radiation treatments are

(A) hair loss

(B) nausea

(C) diarrhea

(D) hemorrhage

(E) irritated throat

9. NPO means

(A) nothing by mouth except water

(B) nothing by mouth after the procedure

(C) only clear fluids

(D) nothing by mouth

(E) nothing except medications

10. A patient who is having a cholecystogram will take the dye

(A) as oral tablets

(B) in enema form

(C) in liquid form

(D) as a barium sulfate drink

(E) no dye is used in this procedure

ON THE JOB

Marge Riley, an overweight 50 year old woman with a history of abdominal pain, has been scheduled for a barium enema and a cholecystogram on Monday morning. She states she has board meetings every Monday morning at which breakfast is served and that she will come in for her x-rays after the meeting is over. Marge indicates that she doesn't understand why she needs these procedures.

What is your response?

1. What, if anything, would you tell the patient regarding her need for these procedures?

2. How would you describe these procedures to the patient?

3. What combination of teaching methods would you use to explain the procedures?

4. You are still concerned, after explaining everything to Marge, that she won't follow the instructions. What do you do?

References

Anderson, K., ed. *Mosby's Medical, Nursing, and Allied Health Dictionary,* 4th ed. Chicago: Mosby, 1994.

Fremgen, B. *Medical Terminology.* Upper Saddle River, NJ: Brady/Prentice Hall, 1997.

Grimaldi, P. "Screening Mammography Is Back." *Nursing Management.* 22:4, 1991.

Monroe, D. "Patient Teaching for X-ray and Other Diagnostics." *RN.* September, 1990.

Schroeder, S., Krupp, M., Tuerney, L. *Current Medical Diagnosis and Treatment.* Norwalk, CT: Appleton & Lange, 1990.

Snopeck, A. *Fundamentals of Special Radiographic Procedures,* 3rd ed. Philadelphia: W.B. Saunders, 1992.

Taber's Cyclopedic Medical Dictionary, 18th ed. Philadelphia, PA: F.A. Davis, 1997.

Tempkin, B. *Ultrasound Scanning: Principles and Protocols.* Philadelphia: W.B. Saunders, 1993.

Workplace Wisdom

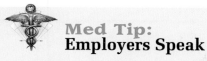

Med Tip:
Employers Speak

Be willing and able to perform many functions especially in back office situations.

Nicole Shepherd, Recruiter
Parkland Health and Hospital System
Dallas, Texas

Maintain skill level—through classes and ongoing training.

Daniel A. Staifer
Human Resources Generalist
Henry Ford Health System/
Henry Ford Wyandotte Hospital
Wyandotte, Michigan

Attend In-service and Training Sessions whenever possible, even though they may not be required. Keep skills up to date.

Barbara Rodriguez, BSN
Staff Development Coordinator
Assistant Director of Nursing
University of Miami Hospitals and Clinics/
Sylvester Comprehensive Cancer Center
Miami, Florida

Give evidence of the desire to grow beyond the position. It shows initiative and a serious commitment to the choice of the health care profession.

Laurie Brenner
Director, Human Resources
Seton Medical Group
St. Agnes Health Care
Baltimore, Maryland

MEDICAL ASSISTANT ROLE DELINEATION CHART

Highlight indicates material covered in this chapter

ADMINISTRATIVE

ADMINISTRATIVE PROCEDURES

- Perform basic clerical functions
- Schedule, coordinate, and monitor appointments
- Schedule inpatient/outpatient admissions and procedures
- Understand and apply third party guidelines
- Obtain reimbursement through accurate claims submission
- Monitor third-party reimbursement
- Perform medical transcription
- Understand and adhere to managed care policies and procedures
- *Negotiate managed care contracts (adv)*

PRACTICE FINANCES

- Perform procedural and diagnostic coding
- Apply bookkeeping principles
- Document and maintain accounting and banking records
- Manage accounts receivable
- Manage accounts payable
- Process payroll
- *Develop and maintain fee schedules (adv)*
- *Manage renewals of business and professional insurance policies (adv)*
- *Manage personal benefits and maintain records (adv)*

CLINICAL

FUNDAMENTAL PRINCIPLES

- Apply principles of aseptic technique and infection control
- Comply with quality assurance practices
- Screen and follow up patient test results

DIAGNOSTIC ORDERS

- Collect and process specimens
- Perform diagnostic tests

PATIENT CARE

- Adhere to established triage procedures
- Obtain patient history and vital signs
- Prepare and maintain examination and treatment areas

- Prepare patient for examinations, procedures, and treatments
- Assist with examinations, procedures, and treatments
- Prepare and administer medications and immunizations
- Maintain medication and immunization records
- Recognize and respond to emergencies
- Coordinate patient care information with other health care providers

GENERAL (TRANSDISCIPLINARY)

PROFESSIONALISM

- Project a professional manner and image
- Adhere to ethical principles
- Demonstrate initiative and responsibility
- Work as a team member
- Manage time efficiently
- Prioritize and perform multiple tasks
- Adapt to change
- Promote the CMA credential
- Enhance skills through continuing education

COMMUNICATION SKILLS

- Treat all patients with compassion and empathy
- Recognize and respect cultural diversity
- Adapt communications to individual's ability to understand
- Use professional telephone technique
- Use effective and correct verbal and written communications
- Recognize and respond to verbal and non-verbal communications
- Use medical terminology appropriately
- Receive, organize, prioritize, and transmit information
- Serve as liaison
- Promote the practice through positive public relations

LEGAL CONCEPTS

- Maintain confidentiality
- Practice within the scope of education, training, and personal capabilities
- Prepare and maintain medical records
- Document accurately
- Use appropriate guidelines when releasing information
- Follow employer's established policies dealing with the health care contract
- Follow federal, state, and local legal guidelines
- Maintain awareness of federal and state health care legislation and regulations
- Maintain and dispose of regulated substances in compliance with government guidelines
- Comply with established risk management and safety procedures
- Recognize professional credentialing criteria
- Participate in the development and maintenance of personnel, policy, and procedure manuals
- *Develop and maintain personnel, policy, and procedure manuals (adv)*

INSTRUCTION

- Instruct individuals according to their needs
- Explain office policies and procedures
- Teach methods of health promotion and disease prevention
- Locate community resources and disseminate information
- *Orient and train personnel (adv)*
- *Develop educational materials (adv)*
- *Conduct continuing education activities (adv)*

OPERATIONAL FUNCTIONS

- Maintain supply inventory
- Evaluate and recommend equipment and supplies
- Apply computer techniques to support office operations
- *Supervise personnel (adv)*
- *Interview and recommend job applicants (adv)*
- *Negotiate leases and prices for equipment and supply contracts (adv)*

SOURCE: Reprinted by permission of the American Association of Medical Assistants from the *AAMA Role Delineation Study: Occupational Analysis of the Medical Assisting Profession.*

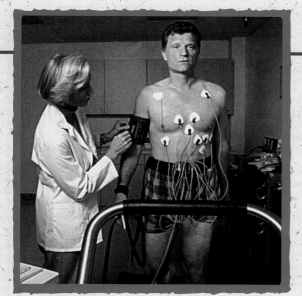

29

Electrocardiography and Pulmonary Function

LEARNING OBJECTIVES

After completing this chapter, you should:
1. Define and spell the glossary terms for this chapter.
2. Practice within the scope of education, training and personal capabilities.
3. Conduct oneself in a courteous and diplomatic manner.
4. Treat all patients with empathy and impartiality.
5. Prepare and maintain examination and treatment area.
6. Prepare patients for procedures.
7. Assist physician with examinations and treatments.
8. Perform selected tests that assist with diagnosis and treatment.
9. Document accurately.
10. Maintain and operate electrocardiogram and pulmonary function equipment.
11. Identify by name and function the controls on an electrocardiograph machine.
12. Name the standard 12 leads and the locations of their sensors.
13. State the cause and correction of artifacts.
14. Name six abnormalities that can be detected in an electrocardiogram.
15. Explain Forced Vital Capacity (FVC), Forced Expiratory Volume in 1 second (FEV1) and Maximal Midexpiratory Flow (MMEF).
16. Differentiate between obstructive and restrictive pulmonary disease.

CLINICAL PERFORMANCE COMPETENCIES

After completing this chapter, you should perform the following tasks:
1. Prepare the patient and obtain a clear and accurate electrocardiograph tracing.
2. Obtain a clear and accurate recording of a patient's pulmonary function.
3. Correctly attach patient to holter monitor.

Glossary

amplitude   Degree of variation from zero or the baseline, up or down, in recording electrical output of the heart. Also called voltage.

artifact(s)   In reference to EKGs, these are deflections caused by electrical activity other than from the heart; irregular and erratic markings.

baseline   No electrical charge or activity; return to zero; flat on electrocardiogram recording. Also known as isoelectric line.

cardiac cycle   One heartbeat, designated arbitrarily as P, Q, R, S, and T, consisting of contraction and relaxation of both atria and ventricles; one pulse.

cardiac rate   Pulse rate, number of beats or contractions per minute.

channel(s)   On a machine capable of receiving more than one signal at once, a channel is the pathway for one signal.

deflection   Deviation, up or down, from zero or the isoelectric line.

depolarized (depolarization)   Discharge of electrical activity that precedes contraction.

depolarization, atrial   Discharge of electrical activity in the upper heart chambers.

depolarization, ventricular   Discharge of electrical activity in the lower chambers.

electrocardiogram   Record of electrical activity of the heart; voltage with respect to time.

electrocardiograph   Machine used to record electrical activity of the heart.

electrode(s)   Device that detects electrical charges. Also know as sensor.

electrolyte   Material applied to the skin to enhance contact between skin and the sensor.

endocardium   Lining of the heart.

interval   Time between beginning of one phase and beginning of the next phase.

isoelectric line   *See baseline.*

lead(s)   An electrical connection to the body to receive data from a specific combination of sensors.

myocardium   Heart wall composed of muscle and fibrous tissue.

obstructive lung disease   Those diseases that obstruct the flow of air out of the lungs characterized by generally slow expiratory rate and increased residual volume.

pacemaker   The portion of cardiac electrical tissue that establishes the beat; the sinoatrial node; also the artificial equipment used when the natural pacemaker fails.

pericardium   A double-walled sac that encloses the heart.

polarized   State of electrical charge in living cells.

pulmonary volume tests   Under constant conditions, the patient breathes with extreme inhalations and exhalations, and the amount of gas inhaled or exhaled is recorded.

QRS complex   Multiple waves or deflections occurring in a group.

repolarization   Return to polarization from the depolarized state; return to rest.

repolarization, atrial   Return to polarization of the upper heart chambers.

repolarization, ventricular   Return to polarization of the lower chambers.

restrictive lung disease   Those diseases that prevent the expansion of the lungs, diminish the total lung capacity, vital capacity, and inspiratory capacity.

segment   Time from the end of one phase to the beginning of another phase.

sensitivity   Ability of the equipment to detect a change in amplitude; normally a state of one.

sensors   *See electrode.*

standardization   Test performed to document a machine's compliance with the international agreement.

tracing   Recording.

voltage   *See amplitude.*

wave   *See deflection.*

Within the thorax or chest are the major organs of both respiration and circulation. These two systems work very closely together; both are vital for survival, and a problem with one is likely to cause a problem with the other. Because many patients suffer with disorders of these two systems, both primary care physicians and specialists monitor and treat these pa-

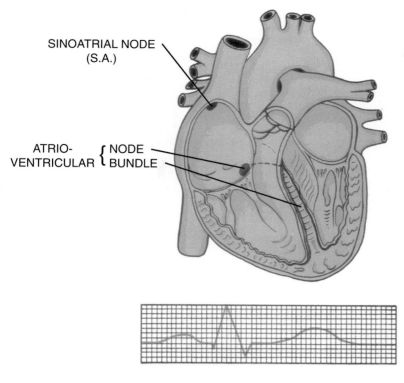

SINOATRIAL NODE
(S.A.)

ATRIO-
VENTRICULAR { NODE
{ BUNDLE

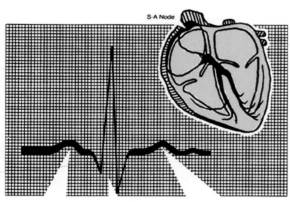

S-A Node

P wave	QRS complex	T wave
corresponds to contraction of the atria	correlates to ventricles contracting	represents preparation for next series of complexes

Figure 29-1   The heart and an electrocardiogram tracing.

tients, and the tests performed to evaluate their status are performed frequently by a medical assistant. Figure 29-1 shows the heart and an electrocardiogram.

Assessment of the heart and lungs begins when any patient visits the physician, whether they are sick or well. A stethoscope is used to evaluate the sounds made as the heart works. These sounds represent the closing of the valves and usually occur close together followed by a pause, as in "lubb-dubb . . . lubb-dubb. . . ." S1 designates the first sound and represents the closing of the tricuspid and bicuspid (mitral) valves. S2 results from the closing of the aortic and pulmonary valves (Figure 29-2). The physician notes on the patient record any abnormalities in heart sounds and rhythm.

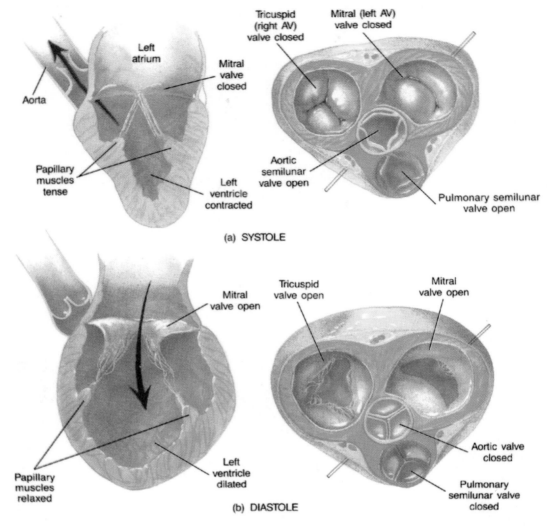

Figure 29-2   Heart valves.

When more specific cardiac documentation is needed, an **electrocardiogram** (ECG or EKG) is made. The electrocardiogram is a *tracing*, or recording, of electrical activity as it moves through the heart. Thus, it is a recording with respect to time. The physician orders this painless, non-invasive test when the heart sounds are unusual, the rhythm is irregular, the patient has any heart related complaints or has a condition that might affect the heart or be due to the heart. A recording will also be made to serve as a reference with which to compare future recordings in evaluating any changes. This may be called a baseline electrocardiogram, not to be confused with the baseline in the recording itself.

Heart Structure and Function

Located between the lungs behind the sternum, the heart is a hollow triangular organ enclosed within a double-walled sac called the **pericardium**. The middle layer or **myocardium** makes up most of the heart wall and is composed of interconnected muscle and fibrous tissue. The **endocardium** lines the upper chambers, or atria, and lower chamber, or ventricles, of the heart.

Blood circulates throughout the body and returns from the general circulation by way of the superior and inferior vena cava, to the right atrium, moving in one direction through the heart. When the right atrium is full, the atrium contracts and blood is pumped into the right ventricle through the tricuspid valve. Upon filling, blood is pumped by contraction of the right ventricle through the semilunar valves into the pulmonary artery going to the lungs. There, blood is oxygenated and returned to the left atrium through the four pulmonary veins. When that chamber is full, it contracts and blood is squeezed into the left ventricle through the mitral (bicuspid) valve. In the left ventricle, blood will enter the aortic semilunar valve and move into all parts of the body except the lungs.

Heart valves act as gates to prevent the backward flow of blood. They open and shut in response to the changing pressure brought about by cardiac contraction and relaxation. The contraction and relaxation of the chambers occurs in sequence because electrical impulses move smoothly along the electrical conduction system of the heart.

This conduction system involves the movement of charged particles or ions during different phases. Minerals (sodium, potassium, and calcium) are responsible for smooth contractions and consistent rhythm. At rest, the cells of the heart are **polarized**; that is, they are charged with energy (negative inside the cell and positive outside). As the cells are stimulated to contract, the mineral particles move like a wave and the charge within the cells changes to positive inside and negative outside. The cells are **depolarized** and contraction occurs. The cells then return to a resting state, called **repolarization**, as their electrical charge returns to the original negative inside and positive outside.

The four major components of this conduction system are the sinoatrial (SA) node, atrioventricular (AV) node, the bundle of His with the right and left bundle branches, and the Purkinje fibers. The heartbeat is controlled by rhythmic impulses that arise in the SA node and move through the conduction system. The SA node, located in the right atrium, is made of modified myocardial cells and acts like a battery. It is known as the **pacemaker** of the heart because it establishes the pace. It may accelerate or slow the rate under the influence of the autonomic nervous system.

The conduction system carries the impulse from the SA node and spreads it through the atria, causing them to contract. Contraction of the atria is called **atrial depolarization**. The impulses reach the atrioventricular or AV node (also made of modified myocardial cells) where they are momentarily delayed. During this delay, the atria rest and recover. This is known as atrial recovery, atrial rest, or **atrial repolarization**. The impulse passes from the AV node down the bundle of His as it divides into 2 bundle branches, carrying the impulse along both sides of the interventricular septum. The bundle branches spread to form a network, the Purkinje system, that distributes the impulse to all parts of the ventricular muscle, resulting in ventricular contraction or **ventricular depolarization**. Ventricular depolarization follows atrial repolarization, and is followed by a period of ventricular recovery known as **ventricular repolarization** or rest. There is a brief pause, and the cycle begins again. Atrial and ventricular depolarization plus atrial and ventricular repolarization comprise the **cardiac cycle**, one pulse and one heart beat.

A unique property of cardiac muscle is that all conductive tissue has the potential to serve in the role of pacemaker; that is, any area can set the **cardiac rate** if the SA node fails. Under abnormal circumstances, such as when damage has occurred, other areas may assume the role of pacemaker. Slower rhythms will be generated by the AV node (40 to 60 beats per minute), by the bundle of His (less than 40 beats per minute), and by the Purkinje system. But normally the SA node generates the controlling impulses at a resting rate of 60 to 80 beats per minute.

The Electrocardiogram

As the electrical changes are passed through the cardiac conduction system, they also spread throughout the body and can be detected by **sensors**, or **electrodes**, placed on the skin. These sensors will be placed on arms, legs, and specific places across the chest. Wires from sensors on the skin transmit these minute changes via a patient cable to the **electrocardiograph** machine; the machine amplifies them and converts electrical energy to mechanical action, causing movement of a writing instrument, the stylus. When there is no energy being recorded, there is no movement of the stylus, and a **baseline** or **isoelectric line** or straight flat line appears. Movement away from the baseline is called a **deflection** or **wave**. The waves or deflections may go up (positive) or down (negative) from the baseline and represent **amplitude** or **voltage**. An increase in voltage will cause a larger deflection. Smaller deflections mean only a small amount of voltage is being detected and recorded. The deflections are arbitrarily labeled P, Q, R, S, and T. (Sometimes a small U wave follows the T wave. This is considered normal and is most probably due to a potassium deficiency.) A normal cardiac cycle is one series of PQRST waves. The P represents atrial depolarization, the QRS complex represents ventricular depolarization, and the T is repolarization.

On an ECG, the horizontal axis (line) represents time; a slower heart rate will have more space between the PQRST complexes. On a patient with a faster heart rate, the cardiac cycles will be closer together. When a heart skips a beat, there is a long flat line between PQRSTs. Additionally, the amount of space between the P wave and the QRS complex indicates the time required for the conduction system to carry the impulse from the SA node to the Purkinje fibers.

Recordings are made from a variety of perspectives or angles known as **leads**. Each lead will record from a specific combination of sensors. When completed, the 12 lead electrocardiograph produces a three dimensional record of cardiac impulses. The pattern of deflections will appear quite different on each lead. The pattern of deflections recorded, voltage or amplitude and time, assists the physician in evaluating the status of the patient's heart.

In some instances, it may be necessary to enlarge or shrink the recording. Under ordinary circumstances, a recording is made in **sensitivity** 1 (This represents a 10 mm deflection per 1 millivolt of electricity). The size is doubled in sensitivity 2 or halved in sensitivity 1/2.

Time and the Cardiac Cycle

The P wave represents the impulse that originated in the sinoatrial node and spread throughout the atria. It is atrial depolarization. If the P wave is present in normal size and shape, it can be assumed that the stimulus originated in the SA node.

Normally, the P-R **interval** (time from the beginning of P to the beginning of QRS) is between 0.12 and 0.20 seconds (3 to 5 small boxes on the EKG graph paper). A deviation from these times could represent pathology. This interval represents the time it takes for the impulse to cross the atria and the atrioventricular node and reach the ventricles. A P-R interval that is too short means the impulse has reached the ventricles through a shorter than normal pathway. If the interval is too long, a conduction delay in the AV node might be assumed.

The **QRS complex** represents the time necessary for the impulse to travel through the bundle of His, the bundle branches, and the Purkinje fibers to complete ventricular activation or contraction, known as ventricular depolarization. This usually takes less than 0.12 seconds (3 small boxes).

Repolarization of the ventricles is represented by the ST segment and the T wave. The ST **segment** is normally flat (on the isoelectric line or baseline) or is only slightly elevated.

The T wave represents a part of recovery of the ventricles after contraction. Usually the QRS complex and the T wave point in the same direction. T waves that are opposite in direction from the QRS may indicate pathology. While the medical assistant should not try to interpret the electrocardiogram, a knowledge of what is normal in the cardiac cycle is helpful.

ECG Machines

There are a great variety of machines in use, but all should be calibrated to align with the international standard. This means that the paper moves at the same speed of 25 mm per second and, given the same amount of electrical energy, the recording stylus will move the same distance (1 mv of electricity input will cause the stylus to deflect 10 mm), thus giving uniform recordings worldwide. **Standardization** is a means of verifying that each machine deflects 10 mm in response to 1 mv of electricity in sensitivity 1.

Older models are manual; you must tell the machine what to do. You may record from arms and legs in fairly rapid succession, but you must move the chest sensor and record from each lead, then move the sensor again. Computerized models have automatic features so you may only need to push a button. You place all sensors on the patient at the beginning of the procedure and the computer switches from lead to lead in rapid succession. These automated machines can be overridden by the operator if there is a need for manual controls. Many computerized models can record from more than one lead at once, to save time. Each is recorded in a separate channel or pathway for the signal, and typically these machines record 3 channels at once. Some other machines have a built-in interpretive feature as in Figure 29-3 and will print out a statement as to the status of the heart. Others can connect directly via fax with a regional office that will carry out the interpretation function and fax results to your office. Many automated machines require that you type in pertinent patient data such as height, weight, age, blood pressure, and prescription drugs being taken.

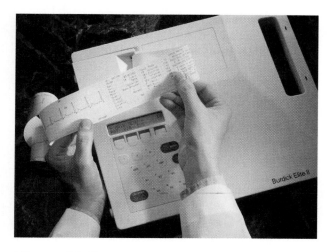

Figure 29-3 Single channel electrocardiograph.

It is your responsibility to produce a clear and accurate tracing from each patient, so you must be familiar with the machines in your office. Read the manufacturer's instructions for the machine before using. Knowledge of the control panel will help you produce a tracing that is clear, accurate, and easily read.

- *Main power switch (off/on).* Allow for a warm-up of 2 minutes (or whatever is specified by the manufacturer) before using.
- *Record switch.* This switch moves the paper at the standard "run 25" speed (25 mm/sec). EKGs are usually recorded at this speed. Another option is "run 50" (50 mm/sec or twice as fast). This is used when the heart rate is so rapid that interpretation requires that it be stretched out.
- *Lead selector.* This determines from which sensors the machine will record. Standard (limb) leads: Record from 2 sensors placed on all extremities. Augmented leads: Record from the midpoint between 2 limb sensors to a third limb sensor. Chest leads (also called precordial leads): Record from various positions on the thorax.
- *Standard adjustment screw.* Increases or decreases the size of the deflection in response to 1 mv electricity.
- *Sensitivity control.* Allows the operator to increase or decrease the recording size in order to enlarge or shrink the deflections to fit on the paper. When changing from the international standard of sensitivity 1 to sensitivity of 1/2 or 2, the operator needs to include a standard for the interpreter's information.

- *Standard button.* Allows verification of calibration to the international standard.
- *Stylus control.* Centers the recording in the middle of the page or the center of each channel by moving the stylus.
- *Stylus heat control.* Increases or decreases heat and adjusts for the sharpest tracing.
- *Marker.* Indicates, by a code, which lead is being recorded.

Electrocardiogram Paper

There are "time" markers printed on all electrocardiogram paper, referred to as 3 second markers. Look for them at the top of single channel paper and between **channels** in multichannel paper.

A heated stylus melts the light colored coating and reveals the black base of this special electrocardiogram paper. The stylus temperature is adjustable with a screwdriver; if it becomes too hot, a hole will be burned in the paper. If it is not hot enough, insufficient coating is removed and the line revealed is very faint. The paper is also pressure sensitive and must be handled carefully. Note that it is marked in small squares with a light line and in larger squares with a darker line. The small squares are 1 mm square and represent 0.1 mv of voltage in the height, and .04 seconds time in the width. The larger squares are 5 mm square and represent 0.5 mv of voltage in the height, and 0.20 seconds time in the width. Thus the paper records both time (horizontally) and voltage (vertically).

Heart Rate

It is possible to estimate the heart rate from an electrocardiogram. Some offices have a protocol that states you should record some additional cycles if the heart rate is above or below certain numbers. Many cardiologists also expect you to perform an exact calculation of the heart rate before you place the recording in the patient record or on the doctor's desk. Here are two methods for estimation of the heart rate and one for exact calculation.

Note the "3 second markers" that are printed by the manufacturer on the paper. To estimate the cardiac rate (beats per minute) from the tracing use the "6 second method." Begin at one 3 second marker and go to the right for two additional markers, a total of 6 seconds. Count the number of QRS complexes between the first and third markers and add a zero. This is your estimated ventricular rate per minute. A similar atrial estimate can be made by counting the P waves between these markers. This estimate is accurate even if the rhythm is irregular (arrhythmia).

The heart rate can also be estimated by locating a QRS complex close to a 5 mm line, the darker line on the paper. Move to the next deflection at the right or the left, counting how many 5 mm lines intersect the tracing before the next QRS complex. Count off at each 5 mm line, beginning at the deflection near the 5 mm line and saying "zero, 300, 150, 100, 75, 60, 50." Stop counting when you reach the next QRS complex. This "count-off method" is an estimate of the ventricular rate. This estimate is accurate only for the complexes where it was done.

To get the exact calculation of the heart rate, recall that the paper moves at a standard speed of 25 mm/second, so it will move at 1500 mm/minute (25 mm × 60 seconds = 1500). An exact calculation of ventricular heart rate is achieved by counting the mm boxes between two QRS complexes and dividing that number into 1500. For instance, if there are 20 mm between two QRS complexes, 1500 divided by 20 equals 75 beats per minute. An exact calculation of atrial heart rate is achieved by counting the mm boxes between two P waves and by dividing that number into 1500. These calculations are accurate only for the complexes where they were done.

Rate is the same as beats per minute. Rhythm is the regularity of the occurrence of those beats. Ventricular rhythm is determined by measuring the distance between QRS complexes. There should be a fairly consistent space between complexes. Atrial rhythm is determined by measuring the distance between P waves. There should be a fairly consistent space between waves. Again, train yourself to look at the rhythm while you are recording. Some offices have protocols about what extra tracings to record in the event the rhythm appears irregular to you.

Sensor Placement

The EKG machine records the cardiac cycle through sensors placed on the patient's bare skin. Sensors are placed over the fleshy part of the inner aspect of both lower legs and both upper arms or forearms, avoiding the bony prominences. These locations are abbreviated LA for left arm, RA for right arm, LL for left leg and RL for right leg. The RL sensor serves as an electrical reference point and is not actually used in the recording. If you have a patient on whom you cannot place the sensor as planned, you must place the sensors on both extremities symmetrically. For

example, a patient in a cast up to the knee requires that both sensors be placed above the knee. If a hand and forearm are amputated, both arm sensors are placed on the upper arm. The chest sensor, abbreviated with V, is used in six locations, with a number following the V, as in V1, V2, and so forth. Placement of chest sensors must be anatomically correct. Figure 29-4 A-H shows the 12-lead ECG.

By recording from different combinations of sensors, the electrical activity of the heart is seen from different angles. A lead selector switch or lead indicator selects the combination of sensors for that lead. One sensor is used for chest (unipolar) leads. A combination may be two sensors, as with standard limb (bipolar) leads, or 3 sensors, as with augmented limb leads.

With many sensors and many views possible, you will need to indicate on the tracing from which lead you are recording. An international marking system has been devised using dashes and dots. Some machines automatically mark the code just above the cardiac tracing. Others require manual marking with the international code. Table 29-1 lists *limb, augmented,* and *chest* leads indicating proper placement and marking codes.

It is beneficial to memorize the sensors used in the limb and augmented leads. Then, if you have difficulty getting a clear recording from one lead, you do not have to look at all the sensors, only those involved. Some find it easier to remember all the leads and the sensors being recorded using Table 29-1 or by picturing Einthoven's triangle, as in Figure 29-5.

Patient Preparation

A well informed patient is more cooperative and less anxious. Explain the equipment and procedure as well as what you will expect the patient to do. The surroundings should be pleasant and the table wide enough for adequate support. Patients will need to be bare to the waist so privacy should be provided for disrobing. Offer female patients a gown, to be worn with the opening at the front. In addition, you will need access to bare skin on the lower legs. Patients have to remove socks or stockings. Roll long pant legs out of the way. Position the patient comfortably supine with a pillow under the head, and another under the knees, if needed, to eliminate back strain. Jewelry usually does not interfere with sensor placement. Prepare the skin where the sensors will be applied. Any area that has been treated with talcum powder or skin lotion must be rubbed with alcohol to remove

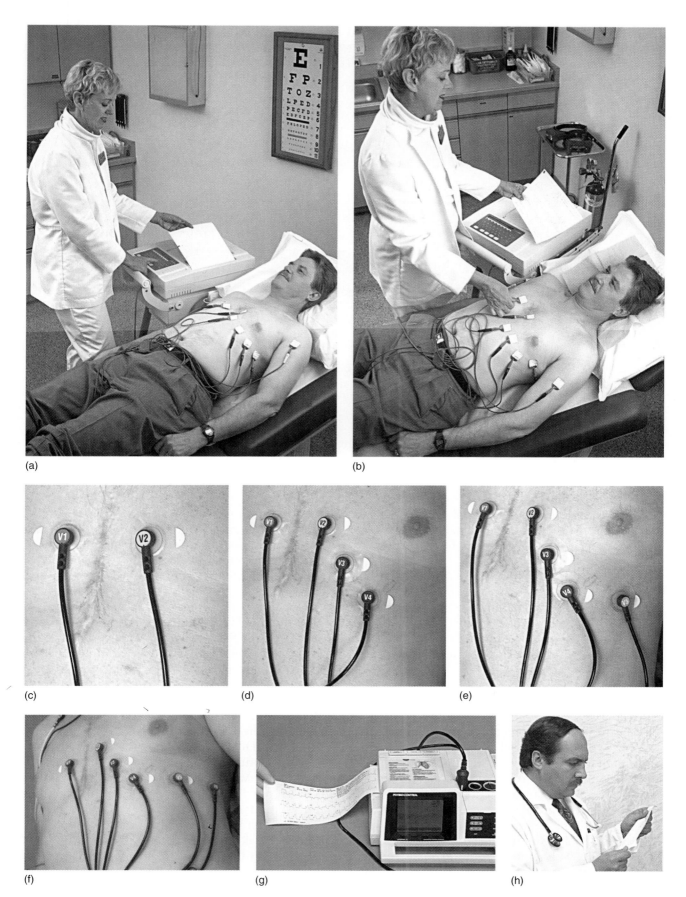

Figure 29-4 A-H Sensors of a 12-lead ECG.

TABLE 29-1   Sensor (Lead) Placement and Marking Codes

Limb Leads	Placement	Abbreviation	Marking Code
Lead I	Right arm to left arm	RA - LA	•
Lead II	Right arm to left leg	RA - LL	••
Lead III	Left arm to left leg	LA - LL	•••
Augmented Leads			
aVR	RA-midpoint (LA-LL)	(LA-LL) RA	-
aVL	LA-midpoint (RA-LL)	(RA-LL) LA	- -
aVF	LL-midpoint (RA-LA)	(RA-LA) LL	- - -
Chest Leads	**Placement**		**Marking Code**
V1	4th intercostal space, right sternal border		- •
V2	4th intercostal space, left sternal border		- • •
V3	Midway between V2 and V4		- • • •
V4	5th intercostal space, mid-clavicular left		- • • • •
V5	Left anterior axillary fold horizontal to V4		- • • • • •
V6	Left mid-axillary horizontal to V4 and V5		- • • • • • •

Note: The right leg is never used for the tracings, but is an electrical ground.

the residue. Some shower gels leave sufficient moisturizer as a residue that interfere with sensor contact and this must be removed with alcohol. Then the electrolyte sensors may be applied.

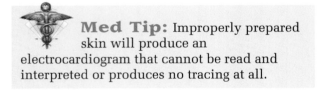 **Med Tip:** Improperly prepared skin will produce an electrocardiogram that cannot be read and interpreted or produces no tracing at all.

The Procedure

If you are to obtain a clear recording of the patient's cardiac cycle, you will need a machine, calibrated and in good working order with a supply of special paper. You may also need a screwdriver for adjustment of stylus temperature and the standard control screw. A patient gown should be available for female patients. You will also need the sensors to place on the skin and a supply of electrolyte or conduction cream, gel, or pads to improve the contact between the skin and

electrodes. The sensors may be metal plates that attach with rubber straps or they may be small suction cups called Welch electrodes. These will need to be cleaned between patients to prevent the accumulation of electrolyte. Adhesive disposable sensors that contain electrolyte are also available.

To begin, assemble the necessary supplies, plug the machine into a properly grounded outlet, allow for it to warm-up, and verify that the machine is operational and in compliance with the international standard. Using manual controls, run the machine at "run 25" and push the standard button briefly to release 1 millivolt of electricity. Stop the machine and count the small boxes covered by the deflection of the stylus. The 1 mv of electricity should have caused a positive deflection of 10 mm. If not, adjust the standard screw with a screwdriver until the deflection is precisely 10 mm, or call your service representative.

Identify, interview, and instruct the patient. Following skin preparation, the electrolyte and sensors may be applied. There are many forms of electrolyte, including gel, lotion and paste. Each

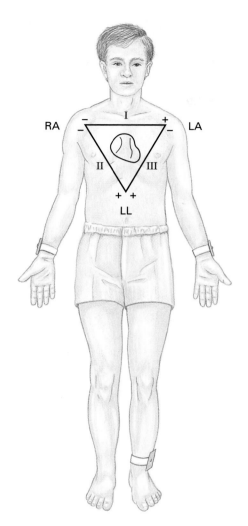

Figure 29-5   Einthoven's triangle.

rapid succession because the computerized machines can switch from one lead to another quickly.

office selects one that is compatible with the type of sensors they are using and their machines. The most recent development is a disposable gummy sensor containing electrolyte. It requires that small alligator clamps be added to the sensor wires. These clip onto the edge of the sensor.

The procedure to attach the sensors will vary slightly, depending on the machine you are using. Some sensors are secured with a rubber strap. One electrolyte saturated pad is placed on the skin and the sensor plate strapped over it. The limb sensors are attached and the first six leads are recorded, one at a time. Then the one chest sensor is moved from position to position as each lead is recorded. Newer machines use a small amount of electrolyte lotion and suction cup sensors, referred to as Welch electrodes. Electrolyte and all sensors are placed on the skin at once. All 12 leads are run in

The placement of chest sensors must be precise. It is possible to complete this task without unnecessary exposure for female patients. The landmarks you will need to palpate or view are the sternum, the fourth intercostal space, both clavicles, and the left axilla. Stand on the left side of the patient and expose the sternum. Locate the right clavicle and the space immediately inferior to it. This is a supracostal space; that is, it is above the first rib and does not count as an intercostal space. Proceed toward the feet at the right edge of the sternum and, using the tips of your fingers, palpate the first rib and first intercostal space, second rib and intercostal space, and so forth until you feel the fourth intercostal space. This space at the right sternal margin is the location of V 1. V 2 is at the same level on the left side of the sternum. Next, you will need to locate V 4 to find V 3. From the middle of the left clavicle, draw an imaginary line towards the feet, stopping one intercostal space below the level of V 2. This is V 4 (5th intercostal space, mid-clavicular left). Lift a female patient's gown up from the hemline in respect of patient privacy. V4 must be at the base of the breast and, in some patients, under the breast. In males, it should be about nipple level. Now you can locate V 3 midway between V 2 and V 4. It is on a rib. V 5 is at a point where 2 imaginary lines intersect. Continue to work under the patient's gown. Draw a line from the front of the left axillary fold toward the feet, parallel to the table on which the patient is lying. Draw another line toward the table from V 4. Where these lines intersect is V 5. V 6 is at the mid-axilla, in line with V4 and V5. You will need to practice locating the landmarks and sensor sites on different body sizes and shapes. Remember to keep your female patients covered.

Arrange the patient cable to follow body contours, avoiding coils. Connect the patient cable and begin to record by performing a standard. For manual machines, select the STD lead, "run 25", and push the standard button. Stop the machine and count the boxes included in the deflection. You should have 10 mm. If more or less, adjust the standard control as needed with a screwdriver. Then use the lead selector knob and select the leads in sequence, running a six inch strip, marking the lead code, if necessary. The length of the tracing you will need depends on how your office mounts single channel cardiograms. Have information about your mounting format before you begin to record. Adjust the stylus to the center of the paper. For automatic machines, depress "auto run" and adjust the stylus to the center of each channel. Record the tracing, using problem-solving skills. When the cardiogram is completed, remove the sensors and wipe the electrolyte from the patient's skin. Dismiss the patient. Clean the machine. Mount the electrocardiogram, if necessary, and transfer the patient information. Sign or initial your work.

Med Tip: The medical assistant is responsible for adhering to the international agreement for sensor placement, recording and coding for leads.

Making Adjustments

A satisfactory tracing is one that is accurate, readable, clear, travels down the center of the page, and has a baseline that is consistently horizontal. If the baseline begins to drift upward or downward, use the position control knob to return it to the center of the page. Observe whether the tracing remains within the graph portion of the paper. If the deflections are so large that they exceed the upper and lower limits of the graph, you will have to reduce the sensitivity from 1 to 1/2. This will make the tracing half as large, and you will need to include a standard to let the interpreter know what you have done. 1 mv of electricity will cause a deflection of 5 mm in sensitivity 1/2. However, if your tracing in sensitivity 1 is so tiny that it is not readable, increase the size by changing the sensitivity from 1 to 2. Again, place a standard on the page to let the physician know that you have made a change. 1 mv of electricity will cause a deflection of 20 mm in sensitivity two.

Since the paper moves through the machine at the rate of 25 mm per second, an option available in recording is to move the paper twice as fast, or at 50 mm per second. This would only be necessary if the cardiac cycles were compacted by a very rapid heart rate. In this case, a better quality cardiogram would be produced if the cycles were stretched out. Mark the tracing to indicate you have changed the speed. In machines that mark the lead with an international code, the code marks are stretched out; the dots appear as dashes, and the dashes are long ones.

The multi-channel machines produce an EKG very quickly, on a single sheet of paper about 8 inches by 11 inches. You will have to center three baselines. A sensitivity or speed change affects all three channels.

Knowledge of the leads and their sensor locations will help the medical assistant to trace back to the source any irregular or erratic markings, known as **artifacts**. You can also perform other troubleshooting techniques during the recording process. Failure to make the necessary corrections will result in an unsatisfactory or no tracing. The physician will not be able to read and interpret such a recording.

Artifacts

Occasionally, the sensors will detect electrical activity from a source other than the heart. These deflections or artifacts impair accurate interpretation of the tracing. The medical assistant needs to find the cause of the artifact and correct it. The different causes of artifacts and how to correct them include:

1. *Somatic tremor.* A tense muscle or a muscle contraction, even one that you cannot see, is called somatic tremor. It may result from patient discomfort, tension, chills, and talking or moving. Calm and reassure the patient. Suggest that the patient relax, breathe normally, and not talk. If necessary, place the patient's hands palm-side down under the hips. This is especially helpful if the patient is not relaxed on the narrow table. This position is also best for patients with a tremor disorder. They will display the least artifacts in this position.

2. *Wandering baseline, baseline shift.* This artifact is caused by poor sensor contact with the skin, such as when sensors are dirty or applied too tightly or too loosely, when lotion or talcum prevents good contact with the skin, or when the patient cable slips toward the floor, pulling on

PROCEDURE: Recording A 12 Lead Electrocardiogram

**Terminal Performance
Competency:** Will be able to perform an ECG, obtaining a satisfactory tracing with 100% accuracy, without assistance.

Equipment and Supplies
ECG machine with sensors, patient cable, power cord
ECG Paper
Electrolyte
Alcohol
Screwdriver for adjustments, if needed
Patient gown, if needed

Procedural Steps
1. Wash hands.
2. Assemble necessary supplies.
3. Attach and plug in the power cord.
4. Verify that the machine is operational and positioned properly.
5. Identify, interview, and instruct the patient. Offer female patients a gown, to be worn with the opening down the front.
6. Position the patient flat on a table with a pillow under the head and one under the knees if needed.
7. Prepare the electrode sites and attach the electrodes:

- Limb electrodes should be applied over the fleshy part of the inner aspect of lower legs and forearms.
- Chest leads should be applied as illustrated in Figure 29-6 A and B.

8. Connect the patient cable.
9. Instruct the patient to relax, breathe normally, and refrain from speaking.
10. Standardize the machine.
11. Adjust the stylus to the center of the paper or the center of each channel.
12. Record—For automatic machines, depress AUTO-RUN; for manual machines, select the leads in sequence and use RUN 25. Use your problem-solving skills if you encounter any artifacts.
13. Mark the leads, if necessary.
14. Remove the sensors; wipe electrolyte from the patient's skin.
15. Dismiss the patient.
16. Wash hands.
17. Clean the machine, straps, and sensors.
18. Mount the electrocardiogram and transfer the patient information.
19. Chart the procedure in the patient's record. Sign or initial your work.

Charting Example
3/11/XX 2:10 PM 12-lead ECG performed.
M. King, CMA

---

the lead wires. You need to readjust, reapply, or clean the sensors, and place the patient cable securely on the table.
3. *AC (alternating current) interference.* The current in wires and equipment may leak into the room and be picked up by the patient's body and the recording machine. This appears in the recording as small regular spikes or static, and is due to improper grounding, nearby electrical equipment in use, or twisted and coiled

lead wires. Ground the machine properly. Unplug other electrical equipment in the area. Move the machine to the patient's feet and away from walls containing cables. You may have to wait until a procedure in an adjacent room, such as an x-ray, is completed.
4. *Erratic stylus.* Loose or broken lead wires cause the stylus to thrash erratically, and go off the page. Repair the wires, replace them or call for service on the equipment.

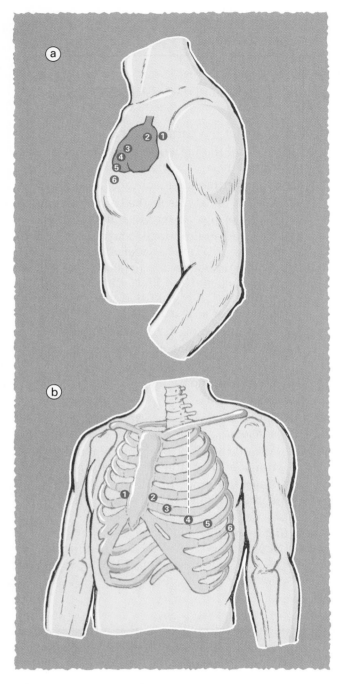

Figure 29-6 A and B   Placement of chest leads.

Mounting an Electrocardiogram

Machines that record one lead at a time produce a tracing that is 6 or 12 feet long. To have a document that will fit into the patient record, use a mounting device. Manufacturers make heavy paper folders with pockets or self-stick areas la-

beled for each of the leads. There are many different forms available. Knowing the form you will use for mounting will help avoid the waste in obtaining a longer tracing than you need. Select the best part of the recording for that lead. It must have a straight baseline and no artifacts. Cut and trim it, and place it in the appropriate area of the folder. Double check your work to make certain you have read the international code for leads correctly. Repeat the process until all 12 leads have been properly mounted. Employer preference will determine where to place the standardization. Machines that record from 3 leads at once do not require mounting. The final product fits nicely into a patient record.

What is Normal?

A normal sinus rhythm means that each heartbeat has 3 distinct waves, a P wave, a T wave, and between the two, a QRS complex where the Q is a downward deflection, the R is an upward deflection, and the S is a downward deflection following an R. The beats come at regular intervals, indicating the impulse originates in the SA node. Within the lead being recorded, each cardiac cycle appears the same as previous cycles.

Abnormalities

Occasionally a tracing will reveal an abnormality caused by cardiac pathology in the patient. An observant medical assistant will recognize the more common abnormalities and draw them to the attention of the physician or follow office protocol, which often calls for an additional recording in a particular lead. A few examples are listed in Table 29-2. Figures 29-7 A-D illustrate varying paper runs of EKGs.

Cardiology Specials

There are a few EKG-related diagnostic procedures performed regularly in the primary care office or in cardiology. The first two are additional lengths of tracings, and may be part of written office protocol for cardiograms.

A rhythm strip will be run in Lead II for 20 seconds on the physician's request or, in some instances, if the medical assistant sees anything that appears abnormal on the tracing. This is not cut and mounted, but carefully folded and given to the physician for interpretation.

TABLE 29-2 Abnormalities Caused by Cardiac Pathology

Abnormality	Description
Sinus tachycardia	There are over 100 beats per minute; cycles are normal.
Sinus bradycardia	There are less than 60 beats per minute; cycles are normal.
Sinus arrhythmia	Normally seen in children and young adults, all aspects of the EKG are normal except the irregularity. The space between QRS complexes is not equal. The heart rate increases on inspiration and decreases on expiration.
Premature atrial contractions or PACs	There is an early P wave occurring before expected, usually from a source outside the sinus node. Therefore P waves are distorted.
Paroxysmal atrial tachycardia or PAT	This is a common arrhythmia, usually seen in young adults with normal hearts. There are no visible P waves because they are hidden by the T wave of the previous cycle. The atrial rate is between 140-250/minute. In many ways it looks on the ECG like repeated PACs.
Atrial flutter	This rapid fluttering of the upper chambers appears on the electrocardiogram like the pattern of teeth on a saw. The atrial rate is 250-350/minute. Not all the impulses are conducted through the AV node because they are coming too fast. There is some "blockage" at the AV node. This is one type of heart block.
Atrial fibrillation	There are as many as 350 irregular P waves and 130-150 irregular QRS complexes per minute.
AV heart block	The node is diseased and does not conduct the impulse well. There are three types. First degree where the PR interval is prolonged, second degree where some waves do not pass through to the ventricles, and third degree or complete AV block where the atria and ventricles beat independently.
Premature ventricular contractions or PVCs	The wide QRS complexes occur without preceding P waves. They may be caused by electrolyte imbalance, stress, smoking, alcohol or toxic reactions to drugs and in a majority of patients who have had a heart attack.
Ventricular tachycardia	Three or more consecutive PVCs. Usually originating below the SA node, the complexes are wide and bizarre in appearance.
Ventricular fibrillation	The waves are irregular and rounded, the contractions uncoordinated. Death may occur in as little as 4 minutes.
MI or myocardial infarction	There are broad and deep Q waves. Old injury: The ST segment is usually depressed below the baseline. New Injury: The ST segment is usually elevated above the baseline. Angina pectoris is the name for the syndrome of pain and oppression in the anterior chest due to heart tissue being deprived of oxygen. If this pain lasts 20-30 minutes, suspect a myocardial infarction in which the heart tissue is actually dying.

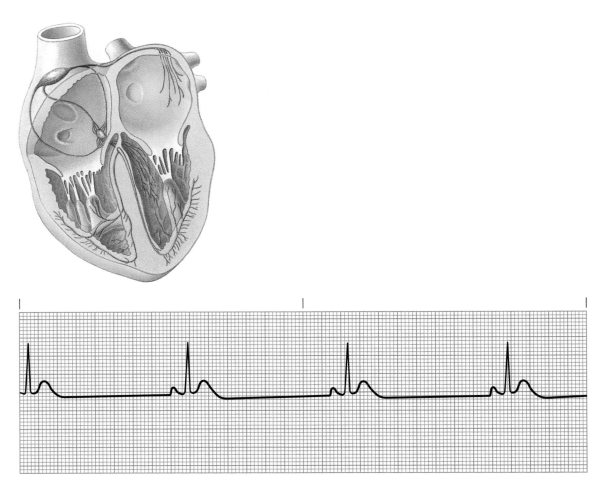

Figures 29-7 A   Sinus bradycardia.

An inspiration strip is run on Lead II for 10 seconds with the patient holding his or her breath. This is of greatest value when, as the patient breathes, your tracing shows wandering baseline. This will eliminate any respiratory impact on the tracing.

Exercise Tolerance Testing

A stress test or treadmill is an evaluation of the heart's response during moderate exercise following a 12 lead electrocardiogram. This may be used to evaluate patients with a high risk for developing heart disease, or known to have early heart disease, and for patients about to begin a strenuous exercise program. This test is also done on patients who have cardiac complaints when exercising and as an evaluation of their rehabilitation following cardiac surgery. Figure 29-8 shows a technician discussing the EKG read-out with the patient.

The patient should be prepared before the scheduled day with instructions to wear comfortable exercise or walking shoes and loose fitting clothes. The patient should know that ECGs will be recorded as he or she walks at a carefully prescribed pace in the presence of the physician. Increases in rate or incline will be made but the patient should not feel discomfort or shortness of breath. The medical assistant prepares the patient, connects the patient to the recording devices (ECG, heart rate, BP) and frequently checks blood pressure during the test. The physician evaluates the effect of exercise on the heart rate, blood pressure, and the electrocardiogram.

Because there is always the risk of cardiac arrest, the medical assistant becomes responsible for maintaining emergency equipment that might be needed and having it in the room at the time of the test. Oxygen equipment, a defibrillator, an airway, intravenous solutions, and medications should be periodically checked and replaced, if outdated or not functioning. Figure 29-9 shows the patient being closely observed during a stress test.

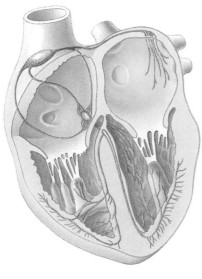

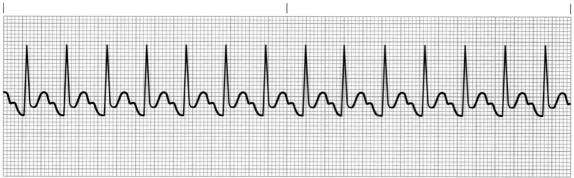

Figures 29-7 B   Sinus tachycardia.

Holter Monitor

The Holter monitor is performed when the ECG is not conclusive or the cardiac irregularity was not captured on the tracing. The Holter monitor records cardiac activity while the patient is ambulatory for at least a 24 hour period. A small tape recorder and a patient diary are used to detect heart irregularities that are infrequent and not detected on the standard 12-lead cardiogram. It may be set to record continuously and/or to record when the patient presses an "event" button at the onset of symptoms. A medical assistant may instruct the patient and apply the chest sensors.

Patient preparation should stress the importance of the diary. Patients carry out all routine daily activities except showering or bathing. They must also avoid areas of high voltage as the tape will be affected. Patients use the diary to record their activities during the day. They also indicate in the diary or by depressing an "event

button" when they experience any cardiac symptoms, such as chest pain, shortness of breath, or palpitations. See Figure 29-10 A and B for an example of the Holter monitor with and without the patient.

The five special disposable chest sensors are attached more securely than in the 12 lead electrocardiogram because they must remain in place during all activity. In addition to the usual skin preparation to remove oils, areas for attachment may have to be shaved and an abrasive skin cleaner used. Peel off the cover on the adhesive backing and attach one sensor to each of the following locations:

- 3rd intercostal space 2 or 3 inches to the right of the sternum
- 3rd intercostal space 2 or 3 inches to the left of the sternum
- 5th intercostal space at the left sternum margin

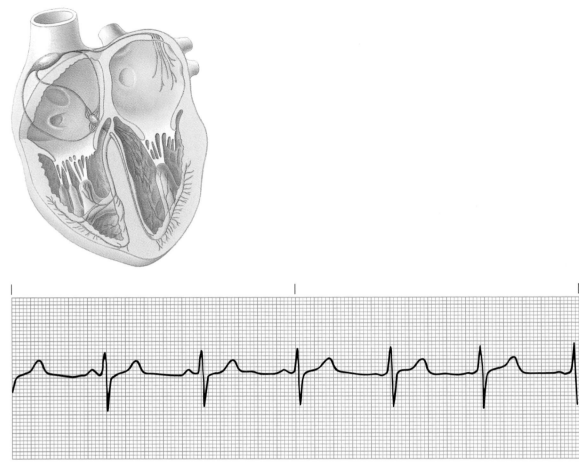

Figures 29-7 C   Wandering pacemaker.

- 6th intercostal space at the right anterior axillary line
- 6th intercostal space at the left anterior axillary line

Pulmonary Function

Pulmonary function tests are performed to evaluate lung volume and capacity, to assist in the differential diagnosis of patients with suspected pulmonary dysfunction (obstructive or restrictive disease processes), and to assess the effectiveness of drug therapies. These tests may be done by physicians devoted to primary care or allergy, or by a specialist in lung diseases (pulmonologist).

Sometimes patients complain of difficulty breathing after minimal exertion, or shortness of breath. Other patients have no symptoms or may have been diagnosed with asthma, chronic bronchitis, emphysema, cystic fibrosis or a combination of these. An awareness of the long-term effects of smoking and exposure to occupational or environmental toxins has increased the frequency with which this assessment is performed. Because lung disease tends to worsen with age, it is important to make a diagnosis early and, thereby, slow the rapid loss of function that occurs without treatment. Allergic patients may undergo a status change quite suddenly. Pulmonary patients can expect to have pulmonary function tests performed quite frequently.

Pulmonary Volume Tests

The first part of the procedure is to discover the amount of air the lungs move normally, and how much lung space is available after a normal inhale and a normal exhale. These are called pulmonary volume tests and there are four of them:

- Tidal Volume is abbreviated VT. It is the amount of air inhaled or exhaled during normal breathing (about 500 ml).

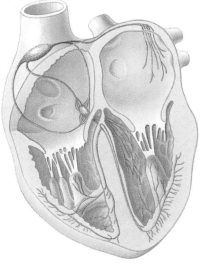

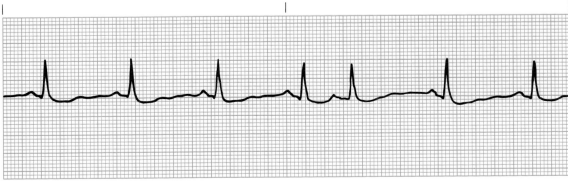

Figures 29-7 D   Premature artrial contractions.

- Expiratory Reserve Volume is abbreviated ERV. This is the amount of air that can be forcibly exhaled after a normal exhale.
- Inspiratory Reserve Volume is abbreviated IRV. It is the amount of air that can be forcibly inspired after a normal inhale.
- Residual Volume is abbreviated RV. It is the volume of air left in the lungs at the end of an exhale (around 1200 ml).

From these volume tests, pulmonary capacity can be calculated, based on two or more volumes. Capacities include:

- Total Lung Capacity, or TLC, is the volume of the lungs at peak inspiration, and is equal to the sum of the four volumes above.
- Vital Capacity, or VC, is the amount of air that can be exhaled following forced inspiration and includes maximum expiration.
- Inspiratory Capacity, or IC, is the amount of air that can be inhaled after normal expiration.

- Functional Residual Capacity, or FRC, is the amount of air remaining in the lungs after a normal expiration.

Total Lung Capacity and Functional Residual Capacity will increase in obstructive lung disease (those diseases that obstruct the flow of air out of the lungs and generally slow expiratory rate and increase residual volume). Patients with asthma have a decreased ability of the lungs to deflate during expiration. In restrictive lung disease the volumes are decreased because expansion of the lungs is prevented, thereby diminishing total lung capacity, vital capacity, and inspiratory capacity.

These tests are performed by a Respiratory Care Specialist, usually in a hospital setting, as ordered by the Pulmonologist. The capacities are included here because, in working with the specialist and pulmonary patient, you encounter the terms and volumes. It is helpful to know what they describe. To continue monitoring the effects of respiratory disease, an evaluation can be carried out by the medical assistant in an office or clinic.

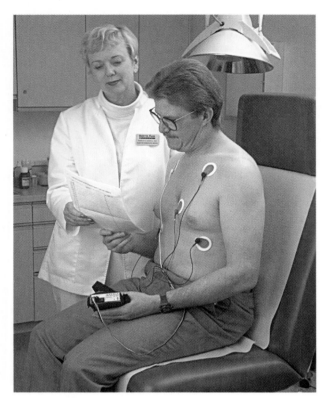

Figure 29-8 Technician with EKG read-out.

Volume Capacity Spirometry

A diagnostic spirometer is employed to evaluate the patient's ability to ventilate during a maximum forced exhale. This device measures and records the volume exhaled and the time required to do so. This air movement is recorded on special paper with vertical second marks and horizontal liter marks in one of three ways:

- Forced Vital Capacity (FVC)—Amount of air exhaled after maximum inspiration or one of the two timed FVCs
- Forced Expiratory Volume in 1 second (FEV1)—Amount of air exhaled on 1st second of FVC maneuver
- Maximal Midexpiratory Flow (MMEF)— Average flow rate during middle half of FVC

Figure 29-11 shows one type of spirometer.

Patient Preparation

The patient must have accurate instructions and reassurance with questions answered. Generally, preparation begins when the patient schedules the appointment. Patients should eat lightly and not

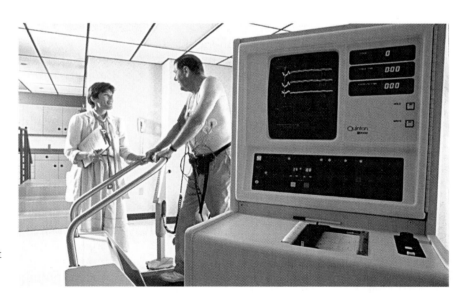

Figure 29-9 The patient must be observed very closely during a stress test.

PROCEDURE: Treadmill Stress Test

Terminal Performance
Competency: Will be able to apply monitors, instruct the patient, monitor and record ECG, BP, and heart rate periodically and make adjustments to the treadmill as requested with 100% accuracy, without assistance.

Equipment and Supplies
Treadmill
Sensors
Blood pressure monitor

Procedural Steps
1. Assemble necessary supplies.
2. Plug in the power cord and turn on the machine.
3. Verify that the treadmill is operational.
4. Identify, interview, and instruct the patient. Offer female patients a gown, to be worn to open down the front.
5. Perform a baseline ECG.
6. Disconnect the patient cable from the ECG machine.
7. Attach a sphygmomanometer to the patient's arm.
8. Permit the patient to walk about the room or on the slow moving treadmill to see what it feels like.
9. Connect the patient to all recording devices.
10. The physician will determine the pace and incline of the treadmill.
11. Record BP, ECG, and heart and respiratory rate periodically as you observe the patient's face for redness, difficulty breathing, chest pain, and so on.
12. When the test is completed, clean the patient's skin and assist with dressing as needed.
13. Organize the documentation into the patient record.

Charting Example
3/11/XX   2:10 PM   Stress test performed
and tolerated well.   M. King, CMA

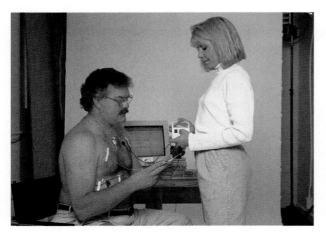

Figure 29-10 A   Holter monitor with patient.

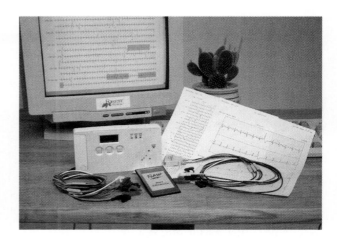

Figure 29-10 B   Holter monitor equipment.

PROCEDURE: Applying a Holter Monitor

**Terminal Performance
Competency:** Will be able to apply a Holter monitor, instruct the patient and obtain a satisfactory recording with 100% accuracy, without assistance.

Equipment and Supplies
Holter monitor with sensors, patient cable
Patient activity diary
Fresh batteries
Blank recording tape
Adhesive tape
Razor
Alcohol

Procedural Steps
1. Assemble necessary supplies.
2. Install new batteries and a blank tape.
3. Verify that the machine is operational.
4. Identify, interview, and instruct the patient.
5. Have the patient remove clothing to the waist (female patients may wear a gown opened down the front) and sit on an examination table.
6. Prepare the electrode sites and attach the electrodes.
7. Attach the wires so that they point toward the feet and connect the patient cable.
8. Secure each sensor with adhesive tape.
9. Connect the patient cable to the ECG machine and record a baseline cardiogram.
10. Assist the patient with replacing his or her shirt. Extend the cable between the buttons or under the hem.
11. Place the recorder in the carrying case and either attach to the patient's belt or to the shoulder strap. Check that there is no tension on the wires.
12. Plug the cable into the recorder.
13. Record the starting time in the diary.
14. Confirm an understanding of what the patient is to do.
15. Confirm the time for return to the clinic for removal of the Holter monitor.
16. Dismiss the patient.
17. Chart the procedure in the patient's record. Sign or initial your work.

Charting Example
3/11/XX   2:10 PM Holter monitor applied and instruction given. Will return in 24 hours.   M. King, CMA

---

smoke prior to the test, and should avoid using analgesics or bronchodilators for 24 hours prior to the test, if the physician so orders.

Spirometry Procedure

When the patient arrives for the procedure, obtain his or her height, weight, and vital signs. Reassure patients that they will be given time to rest if dyspnea or fatigue occur during the test. The test will be stopped if the patient experiences any chest pain, palpitations, nausea, or wheezing. After a basic test, some patients are asked to breathe an aerosolized bronchodilator, and the physician evaluates the value of the drug in causing an increase in capacity. The graphic test results become part of the patient's permanent record.

Spirometric measurements depend upon patient effort, which, in turn, depends on the coaching of the medical assistant. Generally, 3 good measurements are performed and the best is considered for evaluation. Patients usually need some practice with wrapping their lips around the disposable mouthpiece and forcibly exhaling. Next, the patient may wish to experiment with a

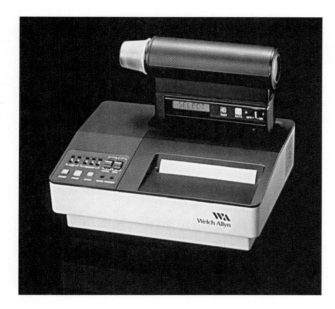

Figure 29-11 One type of spirometer.

standing versus sitting position. Since it makes no difference with the results, the choice depends on patient comfort.

Med Tip: Remind the patient that it is important to blow hard and fast from the very beginning, as if all the candles on the birthday cake were not extinguished. The patient should avoid doubling over at the waist. Demonstrate the maneuver and have the patient practice. Then begin, reminding the patient to take as deep a breath as possible, blast the air out hard and fast, and keep blowing, blowing, blowing until told to stop.

There are a variety of spirometers available in the marketplace, but they must meet minimum standards for acceptable performance. When using automated computerized machines, the spirometry procedure is complicated by the necessity of dealing with the computer program. You must enter patient data into the computer, such as age, height, weight, vital signs, medication, and so forth, depending on the machine and the computer program used. The machine usually makes predictions about what the graphic representation should look like.

The basic spirometry procedure is as follows: Plug in and turn on the machine, allowing it to warm up. Verify that the equipment is operational. Explain the procedure to the patient. The patient will breathe in and out through a mouthpiece. The quantity of this air is measured and the nose is kept shut with a nose clip. Apply the nose clip to the patient's nose and allow the patient to adjust it for comfort. Set the machine according to the manufacturer's guidelines. Have the patient take a big breath in. Have the patient place the mouthpiece in his or her mouth and seal the lips around the mouthpiece. Push the start button at the same time as you instruct the patient to "blow". Have the patient exhale as hard, fast, and long as possible, while you coach to "blow, blow, blow. . . ." Most machines will have you stop at this point—you have recorded the forced vital capacity, forced expiratory volume at 1 second, and the mean expiration flow rate. With a few other machines, the patient must record an inhale. Keeping the tube in his or her mouth, have the patient take a big breath in. Have the patient exhale normally. Remove the noseclip and mouthpiece, permitting the patient to rest. Repeat this procedure as often as needed, up to eight attempts. Submit the best of three acceptable trials to the physician.

There are changes anticipated with lung disease. Note that in obstructive disease, more time is required for a complete exhale, and in a restrictive pattern, maximum exhale is reached quickly but the volume is small.

With the test results, the patient's pulmonary measurement is compared to the predicted values for the patient's height, weight, age, race and sex by the physician who takes into account the patient's clinical status at the same time. Clinical status refers to the patient's physical condition at the time of the test. A fever, asthma attack, poor night's sleep, scoliosis, or any of a number of other variables could affect the pulmonary function results. A prediction indicator result of 85% to 100% would indicate no impairment; 75-85% would be slight impairment, and so on.

Peak Flowmeter

A patient may use a flowmeter at home to monitor breathing and assist the physician with determining the medication regimen that is most effective. On a "good" day, the patient blows as hard as possible into the device to establish a goal or baseline against which to compare other expiratory attempts.

PROCEDURE: Performing Spirometry

Terminal Performance
Competency: Will be able to obtain spirometric results (instruct the patient and obtain a satisfactory recording) with 100% accuracy, without assistance.

Equipment and Supplies
Functioning spirometry machine
Nose clip
Mouthpiece

Procedural Steps
1. Plug in and turn on the machine; verify that the equipment is operational.
2. Explain the procedure to the patient.
3. Apply the noseclip to the patient's nose.
4. Set the machine according to the manufacturer's guidelines. All spirometers will be different even though they operate on the same principle. Some require movement of parts.
5. Have the patient take a big breath in.
6. Have the patient place the mouthpiece in his or her mouth and seal his or her lips around the mouthpiece.
7. Push the start button at the same time as you give instructions to the patient.
8. Have the patient blast breath out as hard, fast, and long as possible.
9. Repeat the procedure to get three good trials, up to eight attempts.
10. Submit to the physician the best of three trials. Some computerized machines will select the best attempt and print it.

Note: All equipment, including tubing and disposable mouthpieces should be properly cleaned or disposed of after use, using Standard Precautions.

Charting Example
3/11/XX   2:10 PM   Spirometry performed
with 3 good results.   M. King, CMA

Oximeter

For patients suffering from cardiac and pulmonary disorders it may be necessary to determine the oxygen content of the blood. An electronic device called an oximeter, which can be clipped on the bridge of the nose, the forehead, earlobe, or to the tip of a finger, determines the oxygen concentration in arterial blood. A pulse oximeter is illustrated in Figure 29-12.

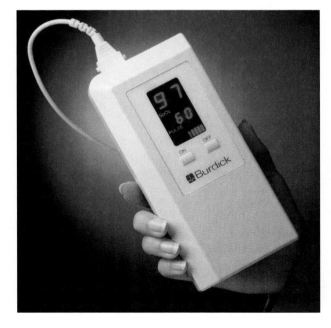

Figure 29-12   Burdick 100 Pulse Oximeter.

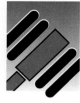

LEGAL AND ETHICAL ISSUES

Provide an appropriate explanation to reinforce the physician's explanation of the necessary procedure. Accurate understanding assists the patient in giving expressed or written consent and in being cooperative.

Perform your cardiac and pulmonary diagnostic tasks quickly and accurately. Improper technique or error could affect the patient's diagnosis and treatment. However, if an error is made, admit it and seek to put things right, even if it is embarrassing to you.

The patient's right to privacy and dignity must be considered at all times. Many procedures performed by the internist and specialist are uncomfortable for the patient. The medical assistant must respect the patient's need for privacy during these tests.

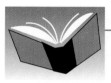

PATIENT EDUCATION

Patients with pulmonary disease may need some educational materials on breathing exercises, a moderate exercise program, the avoidance of inhaled irritants, and the use of an inhaler. As you work in these areas you will pick up some interesting tips from other patients that you can pass along.

Many patients need dietary guidance, especially regarding the reduction of salt and cholesterol, and some will need information about weight loss and moderate exercise programs. Never give out materials or educational information without the specific direction of the physician.

Summary

The use of electrocardiography and spirometry for the early diagnosis and treatment of heart and lung disease has contributed to the lengthened life expectancy of many patients and has improved their quality of life. Accuracy in carrying out your duties during these tests will provide the physician with the best possible data to make that diagnosis and institute the correct treatment.

Competency Review

1. Define and spell the glossary terms for this chapter.
2. Describe how to maintain and operate electrocardiograph equipment; pulmonary function equipment.
3. Identify by name and the location of their sensors the standard 12 leads on an electrocardiograph machine.
4. Name and describe six abnormalities that can be detected in an electrocardiogram.
5. Explain Forced Vital Capacity (FVC), Forced Expiratory Volume in 1 second (FEV1), and Maximal Mixexpiratory Flow (MMEF).
6. Explain the difference(s) between *obstructive* and *restrictive* pulmonary disease.

Test Taking Tip — When studying a textbook in preparation for an examination, write in the margin of the book the important word or concept covered in each paragraph. Then do a final quick study for the examination by just reviewing the notes in the margin.

Examination Review Questions

1. An artifact in leads 1, 2, and AVR would cause you to recheck the sensors attached to which body part?
   (A) chest
   (B) left arm
   (C) left leg
   (D) right arm
   (E) right leg

2. When performing an EKG on a patient with a right lower leg cast, the leg sensors are placed
   (A) on the left leg
   (B) on both upper legs
   (C) on both upper arms
   (D) on the bottom of the feet
   (E) they are eliminated

3. An electrocardiogram is a
   (A) recording of the voltage with respect to time
   (B) recording of the mechanical action of the heart
   (C) technique for making recordings of heart activity
   (D) machine used to make cardiac tracings
   (E) recording of the size of the heart

4. Normally, a complete EKG consists of ___sensors and ___leads
   (A) 10, 10
   (B) 8, 10
   (C) 6, 12
   (D) 12, 10
   (E) 10, 12

5. The SA node is located in or on the
   (A) right atrium
   (B) right ventricle
   (C) apex
   (D) valve between the right atrium and right ventricle
   (E) septum between the atria

6. The portion of the EKG that relates to ventricular depolarization is the
   (A) P wave
   (B) QRS complex
   (C) T wave
   (D) U wave
   (E) P-R interval

7. A standard limb lead monitors voltage from
   (A) any limb sensor
   (B) any two limb sensors
   (C) the chest sensor
   (D) two of the following: RA, LL, RL
   (E) two of the following: RA, LA, LL

8. The little "spark" that begins or starts the heart beat originates in the
   (A) Purkinje fibers
   (B) Vagus nerve
   (C) SA node
   (D) AV node
   (E) artificial pacemaker

9. The correct order of stimulation in the electrical conduction system of the heart is
   (A) AV node, SA node, bundle of His, bundle branches, Purkinje network
   (B) SA node, AV node, bundle of His, bundle branches, Purkinje network
   (C) Bundle of His, AV node, SA node, bundle branches, Purkinje network
   (D) Purkinje network, Purkinje fibers, SA node, AV node
   (E) bundle of His, SA node, AV node, bundle branches, Purkinje network

10. Leads 1, 2, and 3 (I, II, III) are called
    (A) standard limb or bipolar leads
    (B) Welch sensors
    (C) augmented leads
    (D) chest leads
    (E) precordial leads

ON THE JOB

Mrs. Nagle has just arrived at the office stating, that prior to getting dressed this morning, she forgot to read the directions she was given and applied talcum powder. After assuring Mrs. Nagle that she can still take the test, you provide her with a patient gown and direct her to remove her clothing including her stockings. You also direct her to remove the talcum powder.

During the procedure, Mrs. Nagle asked why you used the "cold paste" and why she had to remove her stockings and the talcum powder. How did you answer these questions? And more important, how *did you explain to her that the doctor wants her to wear an ambulatory monitor and that she will be wearing it when she leaves the office today?*

What is your response?

1. State the patient explanation and preparation you would give for a patient having his or her first cardiogram.
2. Explain to Mrs. Nagle what an ambulatory monitor does and what she will be expected to do.
3. Why does she need to have a 12 lead cardiogram first?

References

Bledsoe, B., Cherry, R., and Porter, R. *Intermediate Emergency Care*. Upper Saddle River, NJ: Brady/Prentice Hall, 1995.

Clinical Skillbuilders. *ECG Interpretation*. Springhouse, PA: Springhouse Corporation, 1990.

Cohn, E. and Gilroy-Doohan, M. *Flip and See ECG*. Philadelphia: W.B. Saunders Co., 1996.

Ehrat, Karen, S. *The Art of EKG Interpretation*. Dubuque, IA: Kendall/Hunt Publishing Co., 1993.

Grant, H., Murray, R., Bergeron, J., O'Keefe, M., and Limmer, D. *Emergency Care*. Upper Saddle River, NJ: Brady/Prentice Hall, 1995.

Hafen, B., Karren, K., and Mistovich, J. *Prehospital Emergency Care*. Upper Saddle River, NJ: Brady/Prentice Hall, 1996.

Potter, P. and Perry, A. *Fundamentals of Nursing—Concepts, Process and Practice*, 3rd ed. St. Louis: Mosby Year Book, 1993.

Ruppel, Gregg, *Manual of Pulmonary Function Testing*, 5th ed. St. Louis: C.V. Mosby Co., 1993.

Taber's Cycolpedic Medical Dictionary, 18th ed. Philadelphia: F.A. Davis Company, 1997.

Thaler, M. *The Only EKG Book You'll Ever Need*. Philadelphia: J. B. Lippincott Company, 1995.

MEDICAL ASSISTANT ROLE DELINEATION CHART

Highlight indicates material covered in this chapter

ADMINISTRATIVE

ADMINISTRATIVE PROCEDURES

- Perform basic clerical functions
- Schedule, coordinate, and monitor appointments
- Schedule inpatient/outpatient admissions and procedures
- Understand and apply third party guidelines
- Obtain reimbursement through accurate claims submission
- Monitor third-party reimbursement
- Perform medical transcription
- Understand and adhere to managed care policies and procedures
- *Negotiate managed care contracts (adv)*

PRACTICE FINANCES

- Perform procedural and diagnostic coding
- Apply bookkeeping principles
- Document and maintain accounting and banking records
- Manage accounts receivable
- Manage accounts payable
- Process payroll
- *Develop and maintain fee schedules (adv)*
- *Manage renewals of business and professional insurance policies (adv)*
- *Manage personal benefits and maintain records (adv)*

CLINICAL

FUNDAMENTAL PRINCIPLES

- Apply principles of aseptic technique and infection control
- Comply with quality assurance practices
- Screen and follow up patient test results

DIAGNOSTIC ORDERS

- Collect and process specimens
- Perform diagnostic tests

PATIENT CARE

- Adhere to established triage procedures
- Obtain patient history and vital signs
- Prepare and maintain examination and treatment areas

- Prepare patient for examinations, procedures, and treatments
- Assist with examinations, procedures, and treatments
- Prepare and administer medications and immunizations
- Maintain medication and immunization records
- Recognize and respond to emergencies
- Coordinate patient care information with other health care providers

GENERAL (TRANSDISCIPLINARY)

PROFESSIONALISM

- Project a professional manner and image
- Adhere to ethical principles
- Demonstrate initiative and responsibility
- Work as a team member
- Manage time efficiently
- Prioritize and perform multiple tasks
- Adapt to change
- Promote the CMA credential
- Enhance skills through continuing education

COMMUNICATION SKILLS

- Treat all patients with compassion and empathy
- Recognize and respect cultural diversity
- Adapt communications to individual's ability to understand
- Use professional telephone technique
- Use effective and correct verbal and written communications
- Recognize and respond to verbal and non-verbal communications
- Use medical terminology appropriately
- Receive, organize, prioritize, and transmit information
- Serve as liaison
- Promote the practice through positive public relations

LEGAL CONCEPTS

- Maintain confidentiality
- Practice within the scope of education, training, and personal capabilities
- Prepare and maintain medical records
- Document accurately
- Use appropriate guidelines when releasing information
- Follow employer's established policies dealing with the health care contract
- Follow federal, state, and local legal guidelines
- Maintain awareness of federal and state health care legislation and regulations
- Maintain and dispose of regulated substances in compliance with government guidelines
- Comply with established risk management and safety procedures
- Recognize professional credentialing criteria
- Participate in the development and maintenance of personnel, policy, and procedure manuals
- *Develop and maintain personnel, policy, and procedure manuals (adv)*

INSTRUCTION

- Instruct individuals according to their needs
- Explain office policies and procedures
- Teach methods of health promotion and disease prevention
- Locate community resources and disseminate information
- *Orient and train personnel (adv)*
- *Develop educational materials (adv)*
- *Conduct continuing education activities (adv)*

OPERATIONAL FUNCTIONS

- Maintain supply inventory
- Evaluate and recommend equipment and supplies
- Apply computer techniques to support office operations
- *Supervise personnel (adv)*
- *Interview and recommend job applicants (adv)*
- *Negotiate leases and prices for equipment and supply contracts (adv)*

SOURCE: Reprinted by permission of the American Association of Medical Assistants from the *AAMA Role Delineation Study: Occupational Analysis of the Medical Assisting Profession.*

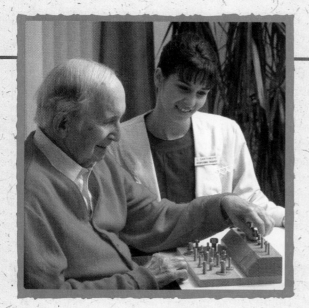

30

Physical Therapy and Rehabilitation

LEARNING OBJECTIVES

After completing this chapter, you should:
1. Define and spell the glossary terms for this chapter.
2. Differentiate between a psychiatrist and a physical therapist.
3. Describe ten modalities used in physical therapy.
4. Discuss ten range of motion exercises
5. Describe the difference between ultraviolet radiation, diathermy, and ultrasound.
6. List and discuss three applications of heat and cold therapy and their uses.
7. State the physiologic reactions to the applications of heat and cold. State any contraindications.
8. Differentiate between electromyography, evoked potential studies and somatosensory evoked potentials.
9. Describe the two-point, three-point, and four-point gait in crutch walking.
10. Describe proper body mechanics.

11. List and discuss five pieces of adaptive equipment used in rehabilitation.
12. Describe AROM and PROM.

CLINICAL PERFORMANCE COMPETENCIES

After completing this chapter, you should perform the following tasks:
1. Apply the hot and cold applications discussed in this chapter using correct safety precautions.
2. Describe the desired and undesired effects of hot and cold applications.
3. Teach the three crutch walking gaits to a patient/partner.
4. Determine the correct measurement for crutches on a patient.
5. Design patient education materials for patients requiring the following physical therapy applications at home.
   a. Hot compress
   b. Hot soak
   c. Heating pad
   d. Cold compress
   e. Ice bag
   f. Cold chemical pack
   g. Crutches
   h. Range of motion exercises
6. Demonstrate proper lifting techniques using good body mechanics.
7. Assist a patient/partner in learning to use a walker and cane.
8. Transfer a patient from the wheelchair to the examination table.
9. Demonstrate PROM and AROM.

Glossary

diagnostic   A type of test, series of tests, or an evaluation to determine the extent of an illness or disease.

diathermy   Use of heat-inducing wavelengths to provide muscle relaxation and therapy.

erythemia   Redness of the skin.

exudate   Accumulation of fluid, pus, or serum in a cavity or tissue which may become hard and crusty.

massage   To apply pressure with hands.

physiatrist   A physician specializing in physical medicine and rehabilitation.

physiatry   Medical specialty of physical medicine and rehabilitation.

prosthesis   An artificial body part.

rehabilitation   Process of assisting patient to regain a state of health and the highest level of function possible.

suppuration   Process of pus formation due to infection.

WARNING!

For all patient contact, adhere to Standard Precautions
(see pages 342–373). Wear protective equipment as indicated.

Physical medicine, the branch of medicine which is called **physiatry**, is the therapeutic use of physical agents for the diagnosis, treatment, management and prevention of diseases and debilitating illnesses.

The treatments prescribed by a **physiatrist**, sports medicine specialist, or a physician are usually carried out by a physical therapist. Physical therapists are licensed professionals who carry out the physician's orders and teach patients the correct use of equipment and body mechanics to prevent further injury or disability. Physical therapy is the medical specialty that involves treating disorders with the use of physical means and methods. These methods consist of rehabilitation, restoration, and the prevention of disabilities. See Figure 30-1 physical therapist assisting patient on parallel bars.

Conditions Requiring Physical Therapy

Table 30-1 lists conditions which may require physical therapy and the services of a physical medicine specialist.

The goal of physical therapy is to restore as much function as possible after an illness, surgery, or injury. Figure 30-2 illustrates a therapist assisting a patient to regain mobility and strength after amputation.

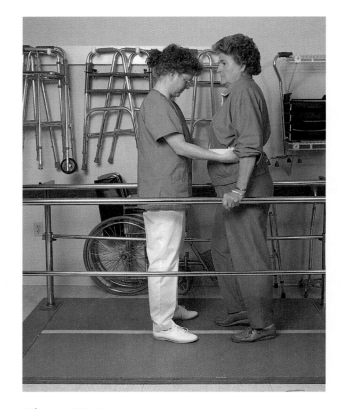

Figure 30-1   Physical therapist assisting patient on parallel bars.

TABLE 30-1 **Conditions Treated by Physical Therapy**

Disorder/Pathology	Description
amputation	Removal of an extremity due to injury or disease.
arthritis	Inflammation of a joint which usually occurs with pain and swelling.
back pain	Pain along, and radiating from, the spinal column area resulting from back strain, muscular weakness, and/or disease or pathology of the spinal cord such as a slipped intervertebral disc.
burn	Damage to the skin as a result of first-, second-, and third-degree burns resulting in strictures, decreased mobility, and/or stiffness.
	first-degree: Damage to superficial layer of skin or outer layer of epidermis with no scarring but resulting in erythemia.
	second-degree: Damage extending through the epidermis and into the dermis, causing vesicles and scarring.
	third-degree: Damage to full thickness (epidermis and dermis) and into underlying layers of the skin with scarring.
bursitis	Inflammation of the bursa between bony prominences and muscles or tendons.
cardiovascular disease	Disease(s) of the circulatory and cardiac systems.
cerebral palsy	Nonprogressive paralysis due to defects in the brain or birth trauma.
cerebrovascular accident (CVA)	Hemorrhage or clotting in the brain which can result in unconsciousness or paralysis. This is also called a stroke.
fracture	Broken bone.
multiple sclerosis	Inflammatory disease of the central nervous system. It generally strikes adults between the ages of 20 and 40. There is progressive weakness and numbness.
muscular dystrophy	Wasting disease of the muscles.
neck trauma	Damage to neck muscles and nerves as the result of trauma or injury (for example, whiplash from auto accident) resulting.
osteoporosis	Disease that results in a reduction of bone mass which frequently occurs in postmenopausal women. Can result in back pain and fractures.
paraplegia	Paralysis of the lower portion of the body.
Parkinson's disease	Chronic nerve disease with fine tremors, slow gait, muscular weakness, and rigidity.
poliomyelitis	Acute viral disease that causes an inflammation of the gray matter of the spinal cord, resulting in paralysis in some cases. Has been brought under partial control through vaccinations.
quadriplegia	Paralysis of all four extremities of the body.
	(Continued on next page)

TABLE 30-1 Conditions Treated by Physical Therapy *(Continued)*

Disorder/Pathology	Description
rheumatoid arthritis	Form of arthritis with inflammation of the joints, swelling, stiffness, and pain.
sprain	Pain and disability caused by trauma to a joint. A ligament may be torn in severe sprain.
strain	Trauma to a muscle from excessive stretching or pulling.
tendinitis	Inflammation of a tendon resulting in pain, tenderness, and lack of mobility.

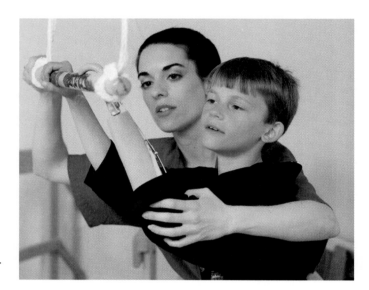

Figure 30-2 Therapist assisting an amputee patient to regain mobility and strength after an amputation.

Physical Therapy Methods

Methods used in physical therapy include massage, exercise, heat and cold, electricity, ultraviolet radiation, ultrasonic diathermy, hydrotherapy, hot paraffin, and manipulation. These treatment methods are used to improve circulation, strengthen muscles, improve circulation, and assist the patient in learning to perform all the activities of daily living.

Massage

Massage is kneading or applying pressure by hands to a part of the patient's body to promote muscle relaxation and reduce tension. Massage can consist of the simple act of rubbing an injection site to stimulate absorption and reduce pain. It can also refer to techniques such as kneading, rolling, stroking, and tapping the skin which are performed by persons skilled in the art of massage.

Massage is considered a form of passive exercise since it is usually performed by someone other than the patient. Terminology related to massage follows:

- Effeurage—Light stroking movement which may be performed in a circular pattern.
- Friction—Rubbing or deep stroking that produces an increase in circulation and mild heat within the tissues.
- Petrissage—Kneading or a rolling method of massage which requires pressing the muscles.
- Tapotement—Light tapping or percussion that is performed with the sides of the hands in a cupping position to relieve congestion.

Massage is useful in the healing process by increasing circulation to the injured body part. In addition, massage can help restore mobility, decrease swelling, relax muscle spasms, and reduce pain.

Exercise Therapy

Exercise programs are conducted to maintain or regain fitness through a planned activity of muscles and joints. Effective exercise programs can help increase or establish lost muscle tone, improve circulation, relieve stress, correct poor posture and body alignment, and increase endurance.

Regular exercise programs, at least three times a week for 20 to 30 minute periods, are recommended for normal adults. Patients with known medical problems should have a medical consultation with their physician who can evaluate their medical condition and recommend appropriate exercise.

Med Tip: When a physician orders an exercise program for a patient, the patient must be taught how to do exercises by demonstration, rather than just being told to get some exercise.

Various Types of Exercise

- Aerobics - Exercise designed to strengthen the cardiopulmonary system.
- Isotonic - Exercise that maintains uniform (unchanging) tension or tones the muscles upon stimulation.
- Isometric - Exercise involving muscle contractions with the muscles fixed in place so that the tension occurs without noticeable movement.
- Stretching - Exercise that results in muscle elongation.

Med Tip: Avoid recommending exercise programs to patients. The exercise component of a patient's treatment must be ordered and supervised by the physician.

Range of Motion

Patients who have suffered from a temporary or permanent loss of mobility will need instruction on range of motion (ROM) exercises. These exercises can help to maintain muscle tone and flexibility. The medical assistant may need to demonstrate range of motion exercises for the patient's family members if the patient is unable to perform the exercises alone. Based on the ability of the patient, the physician may order one of the following types of range of motion exercises:

- Active range of motion (AROM): The patient is able to move all limbs through the entire range of motion unassisted.
- Passive range of motion (PROM): The patient must have someone else move their limbs through the range of motion exercises because they are unable to do it.
- Active assist range of motion (AAROM): The patient participates to a limited extent in range of motion exercises. They will require assistance.

Figures 30-3 A-G illustrates range of motion exercises. Before beginning range of motion exercises, guidelines similar to the ones provided here should be explained to the patient. The patient and the patient's family should be given printed range of motion instructions and precautions to take home with them.

Guidelines: Range of Motion

1. Each exercise should be performed three times, unless otherwise ordered by the physician.
2. A logical sequence of exercises should be followed so that every muscle and joint receives some movement. In general, ROM exercises begin with the head and move down the body.
3. The patient should attempt to do as much as he or she are able to without assistance.
4. Never force any body part beyond its normal range. Do not exercise to the point of pain.
5. Exercise should not be performed if a joint is reddened, swollen, or painful.
6. Limbs should be supported at all the joints when exercising.

Range of Motion Exercises

Range of motion (ROM) exercises are used to develop and strengthen muscles and joints. The classifications of range of motion exercises are listed in Table 30-2. Some range of motion exercises are illustrated in Figure 30-4.

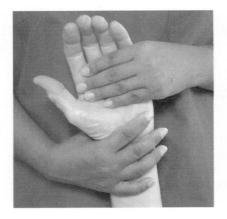

A   Radial deviation.

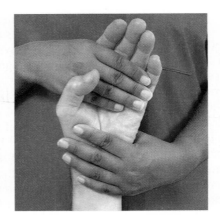

B   Ulnar deviation.

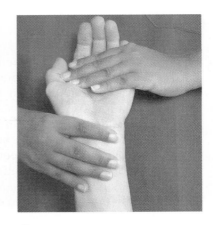

C   Extension.

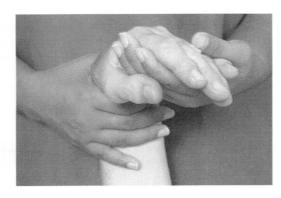

D   Flexion.

Figure 30-3 A-D   Exercise each wrist.

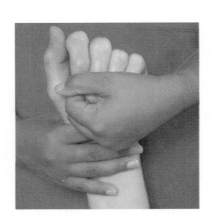

E

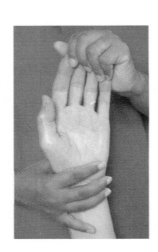

F

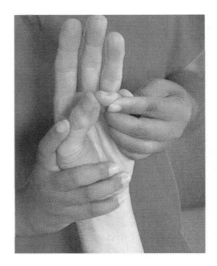

G

Figure 30-3 E-G   Exercise each finger.

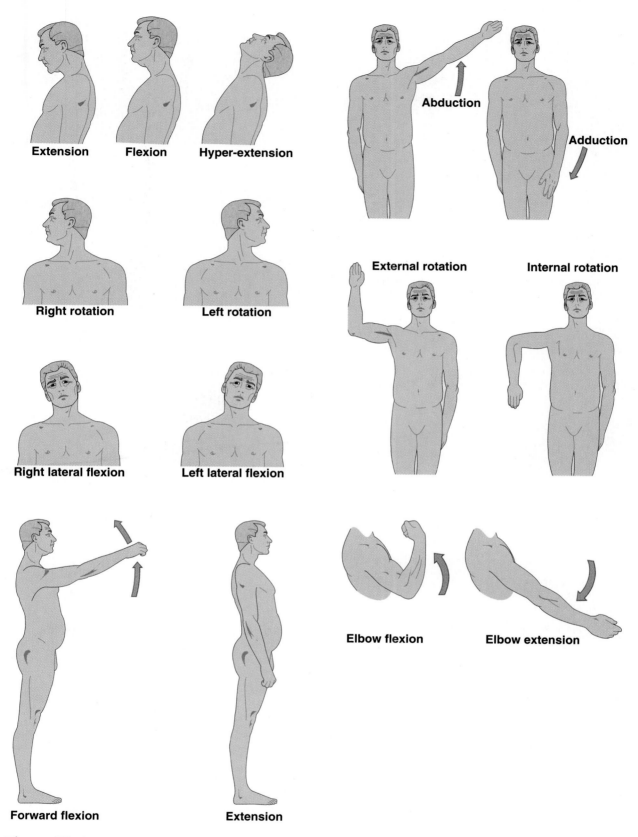

Extension   Flexion   Hyper-extension

Right rotation   Left rotation

Right lateral flexion   Left lateral flexion

Forward flexion   Extension

Abduction

Adduction

External rotation   Internal rotation

Elbow flexion   Elbow extension

Figure 30-4   Range of motion exercises.

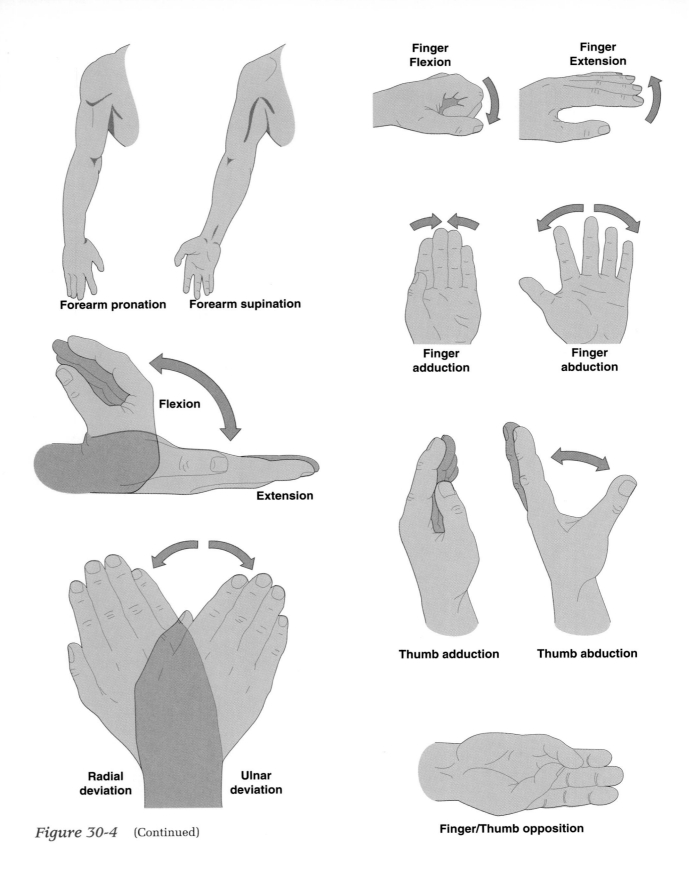

Forearm pronation   Forearm supination

Finger Flexion   Finger Extension

Flexion

Extension

Finger adduction   Finger abduction

Radial deviation   Ulnar deviation

Thumb adduction   Thumb abduction

Finger/Thumb opposition

Figure 30-4   (Continued)

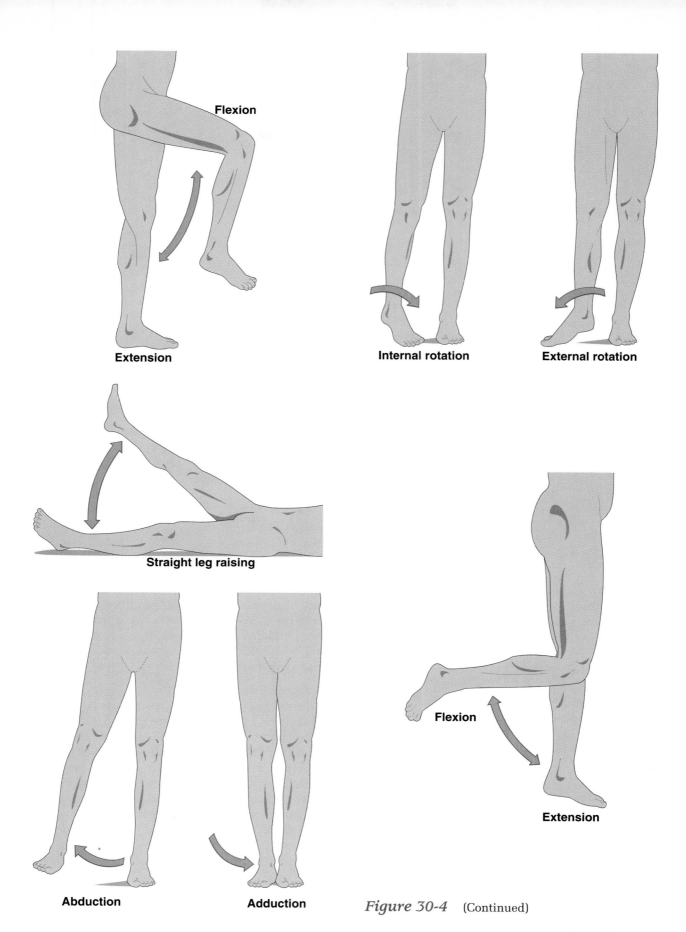

Figure 30-4 (Continued)

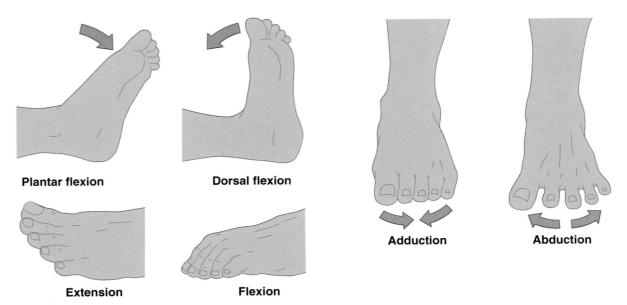

Plantar flexion   **Dorsal flexion**   **Adduction**   **Abduction**

Extension   **Flexion**

Figure 30-4 (Continued)

TABLE 30-2 **Classification of Range of Motion Exercises**

Classification	Description
active range of motion (AROM)	Patient performs exercises without the assistance of someone else.
active resistance	Patient applies movement while another person applies resistance. Used for muscle building and testing patient's strength.
aided exercise	Patient receives some assistance from another person.
passive range of motion (PROM)	Therapist puts patient's joints through a full range of motion without assistance from the patient.

Terminology which is used when discussing movement produced by muscles in range of motion exercises is listed in Table 30-3.

Med Tip: Most terminology relating to muscle movement is in pairs with opposite meanings. For example, abduction and adduction; pronation and supination; and eversion and inversion.

Application of Heat and Cold

The medical assistant may have responsibility for providing patient teaching in the use of heat and cold for therapeutic purposes. In some cases the medical assistant will apply these devices in the office setting.

Heat and cold are used to treat conditions resulting from trauma and infection. Heat and cold, when used therapeutically, are applied for short periods of time (usually 15-30 minutes). Circulation can be impaired if either hot or cold applications remain on a body part for an extended period of time.

Heat Applications

Heat is often used to hasten the healing process. The application of heat to a body part causes dilation of blood vessels and allows more blood to circulate to injured tissues. A condition of **erythema**, or redness of the skin, is caused when the capillaries become congested with blood. This increased circulation assists in providing the body with oxygen and nutrients necessary for repair and healing. Tissue metabolism increases and then healing can occur.

Heat can also assist in relieving pain and muscle spasms. In addition, heat can also be used to soften hard crusts of **exudate** produced by damaged body tissues. The application of heat, in particular moist heat, can hasten the **suppuration** process to relieve the internal buildup of pus formation.

TABLE 30-3　Terminology for Movement Produced By Muscles

Term	Description
abduction	Movement away from the midline of the body.
adduction	Movement toward the midline of the body.
circumduction	Movement in a circular direction from a central point.
dorsiflexion	Backward bending (as of hand or foot).
eversion	Turning outward.
inversion	Turning inward.
extension	Movement that brings limb into or toward a straight condition.
hyperextension	Extreme or abnormal extension or stretching.
flexion	The act of bending.
opposition	Ability to move the thumb into contact with the other fingers.
plantar flexion	Bend sole of foot; point toes downward.
pronation	Turn downward or backward as with the hand or foot; to lie in a prone position is to be face downward.
rotation	The process of turning.
supination	To turn the palm or hand anteriorly; To turn the foot inward and upward. To lie in the supine position is to be face upward.
gait	Manner of walking.

Med Tip: Heat is not recommended as the first treatment for an acute inflammation or injury. In many cases of acute injury, cold application for a brief period of time is the recommended treatment as ordered by physicians.

Heat application can take the form of either moist or dry applications to produce a dilatation of blood vessels in the skin. This causes muscle relaxation in the deeper regions of the body and increases circulation, which aids healing. *Note:* Hot soaks, often containing a medicated solution, are applied to hasten healing or cleanse open wounds.

Moist application is one in which the water actually touches the skin such as in a tub or with a warm compress (pad) of water. Examples of moist heat applications include warm Sitz baths, tub baths, and warm soaks. A dry application of heat is the application of heat without water such as with a heating pad. See Figure 30-5 for illustration of applying heat and ice. *Note:* Any soft, absorbent cloth, such as a washcloth, small towel, disposable woven towels, or gauze squares, can be used as a hot compress. Applying a hot compress to an open wound requires the use of sterile procedures.

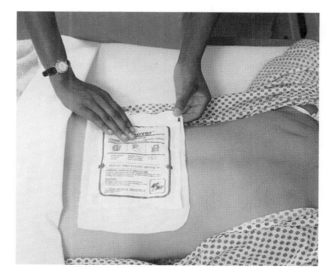

Figure 30-5　Applying heat and ice.

PROCEDURE: Applying a Hot Compress

**Terminal Performance
Competency:** Student will perform and document procedure without error.

Equipment and Supplies

Soaking solution (or water) as ordered by physician

Basin

Bath thermometer

Absorbent cloths such as washcloths or gauze squares

Waterproof cover such as plastic wrap

Procedural Steps

1. Wash hands.
2. Assemble equipment. If an open wound is present, use sterile equipment and Standard Precautions.
3. Identify and explain procedure to patient.
4. Fill the basin half full of water or medicated solution prepared according to directions of physician.
5. Request patient to remove any necessary clothing since compresses are performed on bare skin. Assist patient if necessary.
6. Check temperature of the solution with bath thermometer. Temperature range for an adult is between 105°F and 110°F (41° and 44°C).
7. Position the patient into a comfortable well-supported position.
8. Place the cloths in basin of hot water or solution. Wring out one cloth until it is wet but not dripping.
9. Gradually place the compress on the patient's body part. Ask the patient to tell you how the temperature feels.
10. Frequently test the temperature of the solution. Replace the water as it cools with more warm water.
11. Time the procedure according to the physician's order (15-30 minutes). Check the patient periodically for any signs of a change in redness, swelling, or pain.
12. Gently dry the affected body part.
13. Instruct patient on any further care such as warm compresses at home.
14. Place towels in laundry. If an open wound is present, then handle the linens according to Standard Precautions.
15. Clean all equipment.
16. Wash hands and return equipment.
17. Document procedure in patient's record.

Charting Example

6/14/XX   3:00 PM Hot compress at 105°F applied to left thigh 20 minutes. Skin slightly pink after application. Pt. states there is pain relief. Instructed on application of hot compresses at home.

M. King, CMA

PROCEDURE: Application of Hot Soak

Terminal Performance
Competency: Student will perform and document procedure without error.

Equipment and Supplies
Soaking solution or water as ordered by physician
Basin or tub
Pitcher
Bath thermometer
Towels

Procedural Steps
1. Wash hands.
2. Assemble equipment. If an open wound is present, use sterile equipment and Standard Precautions.
3. Identify and explain procedure to patient.
4. Fill the basin or tub half full of water or medicated solution prepared according to directions of physician.
5. Request patient to remove any obstructing clothing since soaks are applied to bare skin. Assist patient if necessary.
6. Check temperature of the solution with bath thermometer. Temperature range for an adult is between 105°F and 110°F (41° and 44°C).
7. Position the patient into a comfortable well-supported position.
8. Pad the side of the basin or tub with a towel to support the patient's body from rubbing on the edge.
9. Gradually place the patient's body part (for example, an extremity) into the solution. Ask the patient to tell you how the temperature feels.
10. Frequently test the temperature of the solution. Using the pitcher, remove part of the liquid every 5 minutes and replace with hot water. Pour the hot water at the edge of the basin or tub and protect the patient by placing your hand between the patient's body part and the hot water as it is poured. Swirl the water while pouring to mix the hot and cool fluid together.
11. Time the procedure according to the physician's order (15-30 minutes). Check the patient periodically for any signs of a change in redness, swelling, or pain.
12. Gently dry the affected body part.
13. Instruct patient on any after care such as further warm soaks at home.
14. Place towels in laundry. If an open wound is present, then handle the linens according to Standard Precautions.
15. Clean all equipment.
16. Wash hands and return equipment.
17. Document procedure in patient's record.

Charting Example
1/15/XX   1:00 PM Hot water soak at 105°F applied to left foot for 30 minutes. Skin slightly pink after application. Pt. states there is pain relief. Instructed on application of hot water soaks at home.

M. King, CMA

Heat hydrotherapy is the use of warm water as a therapeutic, or healing, treatment. This can be done in baths, swimming pools, and whirlpools. The whirlpool is a bath in which there is continuous jets of hot water reaching the body surfaces. This promotes circulation and flexibility of muscles and joints.

Dry heat, which does not produce moisture, includes infrared radiation (heat lamps), electric light bulbs, electric heating pads, hot water bottles, chemical hot packs, and aquamatic (K-matic) pad.

Hot Paraffin Hot paraffin, a form of heat treatment, involves placing the extremities into hot wax to relax the muscles and promote healing. The temperature of the paraffin, or wax, has to be controlled carefully to prevent burning. Paraffin treatments are usually performed by licensed physical

---

PROCEDURE: Application of a Heating Pad

Terminal Performance
Competency: Student will perform and document procedure without error.

Equipment and Supplies
Heating pad with protective covering (or pillowcase)

Note: Perform preliminary check of the heating pad to determine that the wires are in good condition without bending.

Procedural Steps

1. Wash hands.
2. Assemble and test the equipment.
3. Identify and instruct patient concerning the procedure. Patient should be cautioned against using pins, bending the heating elements within the pad, or lying on the pad. *Rationale:* Pins should never be used in a heating pad either to secure a pad to its cover or to attach the pad to the patient's clothing. Pins can puncture the heating pad elements and cause an electrical shock. Lying on the pad may cause heat to accumulate in that area and burn the patient.
4. Place heating pad in protective covering or pillowcase.
5. Connect the heating pad to an electric plug. Set the temperature selector at the setting as ordered by the physician (low or medium).
6. Place the heating pad over the patient's affected area. Ask the patient to tell you how it feels. *Rationale:* The pad should be warm but not uncomfortable or "hot."
7. Instruct the patient regarding the proper temperature setting. Tell them not to change the setting. *Rationale:* Some patients, such as the elderly, have poor circulation and may not feel the heat of the pad.
8. Leave the heating pad in place for the amount of time ordered by the physician (15-20 minutes). Check the patient periodically for any signs of a change in redness, swelling, or pain.
9. Remove the pad when procedure is complete. Instruct patient on any after care such as further heat treatments at home.
10. Place protective covering in laundry.
11. Wash hands and return equipment.
12. Document procedure in patient's record.

Charting Example
1/12/XX 9:00 AM Heating pad on medium setting applied to left elbow for 20 minutes. Erythema noted over application site. Pt. states there is pain relief and increased mobility in elbow joint. Instructed on application of heating pad at home.

M. King, CMA

therapists using standard paraffin bath equipment.

This therapy is useful for patients with rheumatoid arthritis to relieve the pain and stiffness in joints. The hand or limb is inserted into hot melted paraffin which has been heated to 126°F. The hand is dipped in the hot paraffin until there is a thick coating. It is left in place for 15 to 30 minutes. The relief after this treatment is longer lasting than in some other forms of moist heat treatment. *Note:* there is a danger of burns if the temperature of the paraffin is not carefully monitored.

Cold Applications

Cold applications result in constriction of blood vessels, which is the opposite affect of warm applications. Constriction of blood vessels is very useful to prevent or reduce swelling, such as in the case of a sprain. The blood flow is actually slowed and this reduces the amount of body fluids carried into an injured part, such as a leg. An additional benefit of cold applications may be the reduction of pain. In addition, cold applications are used to control bleeding due to the slowing of blood circulation. Examples of both moist and dry applications are illustrated in Table 30-4.

Cold, or cryotherapy, is using cold for therapeutic purposes. Cold applications can be applied to a body part, such as with an ice bag after a tooth extraction or tonsillectomy. In addition, cold applications can be placed on the entire body to reduce an elevated body temperature. Cold applications consist of cold compresses, soaks, ice packs, and hypothermia blankets. Ice in a bag or container (ice packs) is used to treat localized conditions.

Chemical cold packs are self-contained packets containing a small amount of water in an inner bag, which when released into a chemical contained in the outer bag, results in a chemical reaction causing the bag to be cold. This pack can be used as an alternative to an ice pack.

PROCEDURE: Application of Cold Compress

Terminal Performance
Competency: Student will perform and document procedure without error.

Equipment and Supplies
Water
Absorbent cloths or gauze squares
Waterproof cover or plastic wrap
Basin
Ice

Procedural Steps
1. Wash hands.
2. Assemble the equipment. If an open wound is present, use sterile equipment and Standard Precautions.
3. Identify and instruct patient concerning the procedure.
4. Fill the basin 1/2 full of cold water. Add ice cubes and compresses.
5. Wring out compress until it is wet but not dripping. Gently place the compress on the patient's affected body part. Wrap the compress in plastic or waterproof covering to prevent dripping.
6. Check the compress every 3-5 minutes and replace with another cold compress. Add more ice as the water becomes warm.
7. Leave the compress in place for the time specified by the physician (usually 15-20 minutes).
8. Gently dry the affected body part.
9. Place linens in proper container. Clean equipment.
10. Wash hands and return equipment.
11. Document procedure in patient's record.

Charting example:
10/23/XX   10:00 AM Cold compresses applied to right ankle for 20 minutes.
Swelling decreased after treatment.
Erythema noted over application site.
Instructed on application of cold compress at home.   M. King, CMA

PROCEDURE: Application of Ice Bag

Terminal Performance
Competency: Student will perform and document procedure without error.

Equipment and Supplies
Ice bag with a protective cover (or small hand towel)
Ice chips or crushed ice

Procedural Steps
1. Wash hands.
2. Assemble and test the equipment.
3. Identify and instruct patient concerning the procedure.
4. Fill the ice bag 1/2 to 2/3 full of ice. Expel air by squeezing the empty 1/2 of ice bag. Replace cap.
5. Dry the bag and place into protective covering or small hand towel.
6. Place the ice bag over the patient's affected body part. Ask the patient how the ice bag feels.
7. Refill the bag with ice as needed.
8. Leave the ice bag in place for the time specified by the physician (usually 15-20 minutes).
9. Clean equipment. Allow bag to air dry.
10. Wash hands and return equipment.
11. Document procedure in patient's record.

Charting Example
2/14/XX   2:00 PM Ice bag applied to contusion on right forehead. Swelling reduced after 20 minutes. Erythema noted in treatment area. Instructed on application of ice bag at home.   M. King, CMA

PROCEDURE: Application of Cold Chemical Pack

Terminal Performance
Competency: Student will perform and document procedure without error.

Equipment and Supplies
Cold chemical pack
Soft cloth

Procedural Steps
1. Wash hands.
2. Assemble the equipment.
3. Identify and instruct patient concerning the procedure.
4. Shake the bag to allow crystals to fall to the bottom. Squeeze until the inner bag ruptures. Shake bag to mix contents. The bag should become cold immediately and remain cold for about 30 minutes.
5. Place bag inside a soft cloth.
6. Place cloth protected bag over patient's affected body part.
7. Check patient every 3-5 minutes.
8. Leave the cold pack in place for the time specified by the physician (usually 15-20 minutes).
9. Discard ice pack in proper waste container after use.
10. Wash hands.
11. Document procedure in patient's record.

Charting Example
7/31/XX   2:00 PM Cold pack applied to left cheek over molar area for 20 minutes. Swelling decreased after treatment. Instructed on application of chemical pack at home.   M. King, CMA

TABLE 30-4 Moist and Dry Applications

Moist Heat	Dry Heat
Compress (warm or cold)	Heat lamp
Sitz bath	Aquamatic K-pad
Tub Bath	Warm-water bottle
Soaks: (warm or cold)	Commercial warm pack
Cool wet packs	Commercial cold pack
	Ice cap or bag
	Hypothermia blanket

Patient safety and comfort are a concern when using either warm or cold applications. The patient must be cautioned to test all warm applications before applying to avoid burning the skin. The skin of elderly patients is especially conducive to burning since their nerve endings lose some sensitivity during the aging process. Parents must be reminded to carefully test all warm applications on themselves before placing it on an infant or child. Ice bags and heating pads (including the Aquamatic K-pad) should be wrapped in a small towel or cotton cloth before applying to the skin to prevent damaging the skin. Electrical equipment, such as heating pads, should not come into contact with water.

Ultraviolet Radiation

Ultraviolet radiation is the use of rays from natural sources, such as the sun, and artificial sources, such as sun lamps, for healing purposes. Ultraviolet rays stimulate the growth of new epithelial cells and are capable of killing bacteria.

These rays are used therapeutically for the treatment of disorders such as psoriasis. Disorders caused by bacteria such as acne and pressure sores are treated effectively with this therapy. The goal of the treatment is to produce a small redness on the skin to stimulate circulation and kill bacteria.

Ultraviolet ray lamp treatment must be carefully controlled since they can cause severe sunburn and even second and third degree burns.

Both the timing of the exposure and the distance of the lamp from the patient must be carefully controlled. A patient can receive a second degree burn after 1 to 2 minutes of exposure to a lamp set at 30 inches from the patient. Patients do not feel this type of burn occurring so they cannot warn the operator to stop treatment.

Treatment is ordered by the second such as a 20-second treatment with the lamp placed at least 30 inches from the patient and directed only on the area to be treated. Eye protection in the form of dark goggles should be worn by both patient and medical assistant to protect the eyes from ultraviolet ray exposure.

The patient should never be left unattended during this procedure. If you have to leave the room during the treatment then turn off the lamp until you return. There is a great danger of severe burns if the timing is not exact.

Diathermy

Diathermy is the therapeutic use of high-frequency currency which induces an electrical field within a portion of the body. This generates heat in various parts of the body and increases blood flow to aid in healing. Diathermy is useful in treating muscular disorders and for the treatment of tendinitis, arthritis, and bursitis.

The diathermy machine placement must be carefully controlled according to the manufacturer's instructions. Some machines are placed one inch from the patient's skin and may have a built-in spacer to assist with exact placement. Others have applicators with pads which require a towel to be placed between the applicator pad and the patient.

Patients will be able to feel the heat as it is generated from this treatment. The operator must continually monitor the patient's sensations from the diathermy. Any area of skin breakdown or inflammation must be avoided during diathermy treatment since these areas are sensitive to burning.

Since diathermy creates an electrical field which is attracted to metal, patients with metal implants, such as hip replacements, cannot receive this treatment due to danger of burns. Patients must be told to remove all metal jewelry, hairpins, and buckles before treatment. They must sit on a wooden, not metal, chair or treatment table.

> **Med Tip:** Remember that all metal becomes hot during diathermy treatment. Severe burns can result if precautions are not observed.

Diathermy treatments have to be carefully timed according to physician's instructions. Treatments are usually from 15 to 30 minutes in length. The patient should be instructed that they will feel warmth which should not be uncomfortable. They must be instructed to tell the operator immediately if they feel uncomfortable. Due to the danger inherent in diathermy treatment, it has been replaced in many facilities with ultrasound, which is safer.

Ultrasound

Ultrasound is sound energy which results from high-frequency sound waves penetrating deep tissue layers. Ultrasound waves have the ability to vibrate at the rate of one million times per second which produces a mechanical effect and a heating effect. The mechanical effect, or vibration, produces an effect on connective tissues such as ligaments and tendons. The heat produces an effect on all body tissues except bone, which reflects the heat back. Ultrasound treatments are usually ten minutes or less in length as ordered by the physician. The patient may require several ultrasound treatments to receive benefit.

Ultrasound is used effectively to treat pain, relax muscle spasm, stimulate circulation in patients with vascular disorders, relax tendons and ligaments, and break up calcium deposits and scars. Ultrasound treatments are used in conjunction with other treatments such as medications to relieve back spasms.

Ultrasound is administered via a machine attached to an applicator head which is placed directly on the skin. A conducting medium, such as a special gel or mineral oil, must be placed on the skin to conduct the ultrasound into the body. The ultrasound operator applies the ultrasound head to the patient's skin using a steady up and down motion. The operator must keep the ultrasound head in continuous motion over the body part since tissue damage can occur if it is held in one place for a prolonged pe-

riod of time. Patients should be asked if they have any implants, such as a hip or joint replacement, since the ultrasound could loosen the implant.

Manipulation

A variety of devices, including splints and slings, are used by the physical therapist. These devices are prescribed by the physician, however, the physical therapist provides the initial instruction on using the devices to the patient. In a general practice setting, the medical assistant will assist the physician with these devices. The medical assistant will provide continuing education and support the patient when he or she is seen in the physician's office. Various splints and slings are used by the physical therapist to immobilize damaged bones and tissues.

Physical Therapy Assistive Devices

Equipment used to assist recovery from physical disorders or disabilities includes adaptive equipment, wheelchairs, walkers, canes, crutches, and special furniture such as shower chairs and geriatric chairs.

Crutches

Crutches are metal or wooden supports to assist a person with walking. Crutches should have a rubber tip at the end to prevent slipping on a smooth floor surface. The two most common types of crutches are:

1. Axillary crutch—Tall crutch with shoulder rests and handgrips that reaches from the ground to under the axilla. These crutches are commonly used for persons who have suffered a fractured leg.
2. Lofstrand or Canadian crutch (forearm crutch)—Shorter version of the axillary crutch that is a single aluminum tube that fits snugly around the patient's forearm and has a hand grip to use for weight bearing. This crutch allows the patient to release the hand grip to use the hand and still have the crutch held in place with the cuff on the arm. This is the crutch of choice for persons with cerebral palsy and paraplegia.

Measuring for Axillary Crutches

Axillary crutch measurement has to be taken carefully to prevent pressure damage to the axillae. If the crutch is too long it may cause pressure on the brachial plexus (nerve running under the axilla and down the arm). The patient may develop a condition known as crutch palsy resulting in muscle weakness in the arm, wrist, and hand. Crutches that are too short can result in the patient having to bend forward while walking. Back pain, nerve damage, and injury to the axilla and palms of the hands can occur if the crutches are improperly fitted. The steps for measuring axillary crutches follow:

1. Have the patient wear walking shoes and stand straight.
2. Place the crutch tips 6 inches to the side and 2 inches in front of each foot.
3. Adjust the crutch, using the bolts and nuts at the sides of the crutch, so that the axillary bars are 3 finger-widths below the axilla. Measure this by inserting your own fingers between the patient's axilla and the crutch bar.
4. Next adjust the handgrips so the patient can flex his or her elbows at a 30 degree angle when the crutch is in place and the patient's hands are on the hand bars.

Teaching the patient how to use crutches and proper crutch-walking gaits is one of the responsibilities of the medical assistant. Instructions should be provided in writing to a patient who is using crutches, in addition to actual instruction and demonstration. The following guidelines will be helpful in preparing patient instructions for using crutches.

Med Tip: Remind patients to remove all throw rugs and obstacles from their homes and work spaces while they are using crutches.

Guidelines: Using Crutches

1. Instruct the patient to keep his or her head up, abdomen in, feet straight, with a slight (5 degree) bend at the knee joint. Remind the patient to look ahead and not down while walking with crutches. This will prevent the patient from bending forward or leaning over while walking.
2. The basic crutch stance is the tripod to provide a firm base of support. The tripod stance occurs when the feet are slightly apart, and the tips of the crutches are 6 inches in front of and 6 inches to the side of the toes. An imaginary line drawn from the two crutch points to an area behind the center of the feet will form a triangle (tripod).
3. The patient should practice standing so that balance is maintained, and weight is placed on the palms of the hands at the hand bars, and not on the axilla.
4. The distance between the top of the crutch and the axilla should be three finger lengths. If not, adjust the crutch using the nuts and wing bolts on the side of the crutches.
5. Do not rest body weight on the axillary bars for more than one or two minutes to prevent injury on the brachial plexus.
6. Take small steps and swing through when first learning to use crutches. The crutches should only move about 12 inches forward with each step. When taking larger steps, the crutches may slip causing a patient to fall.
7. Check the rubber tips frequently for cracks. They can easily be replaced.
8. The shoulder and hand bars can be padded for extra comfort with either sponge rubber or a soft cloth. The patient should then remeasure and adjust the crutches for the correct length.
9. Crutches should always be moved forward and to the side so the feet or foot can swing through.
10. Look forward and straight ahead while using crutches.
11. Periodically check the wing nuts and bolts to maintain tightness.
12. Report any tingling or numbness in the arms to the physician at once.

Crutch Walking Gaits

The type of crutch gait, or walk, that a patient will use depends on the amount of weight bearing the patient's leg or legs will support, his or her muscular coordination, and physical condition. In a crutch walking gait, each foot and crutch is called a point. For example, with a two-point gait, two points of the total four points (two legs and two crutches) are in contact with the ground during each step. The patient should be encouraged to use a slow gait. Common gaits include the four-point, three-point, two-point, swing-to and swing-through gaits. Figure 30-6 illustrates crutch walking.

Four-point Gait The four-point gait is a slow and steady gait. This is considered the safest of all gaits since the patient always has three points of support in contact with the ground at all times. This gait is used for patients who may have muscular weakness and some lack of coordination.

To use this gait the right crutch is moved forward, then the left foot, then the left crutch, and then the right foot. This is repeated over and over. The patient must be able to move each leg separately to use this gait.

Three-point Gait The three-point gait is used when one leg is stronger than the other or when there is no weight bearing on one leg. To use this gait the patient must be able to support his or her full weight on one leg. The crutches are moved forward and the weaker leg is brought through the crutches. This gait requires good coordination and muscle strength. This gait is used by patients who are amputees without a prosthesis, with musculoskeletal disorders (for example fractures) or who have had recent leg surgery.

Two-point Gait The two-point gait is faster moving than the four point gait. There are two types of this gait.

1. Put both crutches ahead and move the body forward by hopping with one foot.
2. The second type of two-point gait occurs when a crutch and the opposite foot are moved forward at the same time, for example the left crutch and the right leg. This is partial weight-bearing and can be used by patients who can bear some weight on each foot.

Swing-to Gait To use this gait the patient moves the crutches forward and then swings the legs up

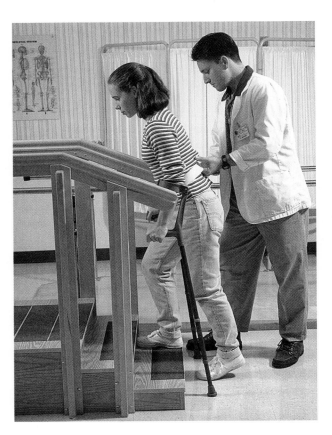

Figure 30-6   Crutch walking.

to the same point. Good muscular control is needed for this gait since there is a tendency to lose one's balance and fall forward with this gait.

Swing-through Gait To use this gait the patient moves the crutches forward, as in the swing-to gait, and then swings the legs past the crutches. This provides a good base of support. It is a gait that allows for fast movement.

Both the swing-to and swing-through gaits are used by paraplegic patients who are using the forearm type of crutches or by patients with a generalized leg weakness.

Sitting

The patient using crutches should be instructed on how to manipulate the crutches and support their legs as they sit down.

1. The patient should face forward and back into a straight-back chair with arm rests until their legs touch the chair seat.
2. The crutches should be placed in the hand on the strong side of the body opposite the weak leg.

3. The patient should grasp the chair arm with the other hand and lower himself or herself gently into the chair.

Standing

The patient should be instructed to follow four points when moving from a sitting to a standing position with the use of crutches.

1. Place the crutches in the hand on the strong side of the body to use as support.
2. Move their body forward in the chair.
3. Grasp the arm of the chair with the hand on the affected side.
4. Push up to a standing position.

Diagnostic Testing

To determine the presence or full extent of disabling disease, the physician may order evaluative, or **diagnostic** testing. This may include an examination of the following:

- Muscle strength
- Muscle coordination
- Mobility of joints
- Neuromuscular function
- Circulation and sensory function

Neuromuscular evaluation may include tests such as electromyography (EMG), nerve conduction studies (NCS), and evoked studies such as brainstem auditory evoked response (BAER) and somatosensory evoked potentials (SEP) to pick up abnormalities such as diseases of the peripheral nerves, muscles, and spinal cord.

Electromyography (EMG)

Electromyography (EMG) consists of using an electromyograph to test the electrical activity of muscles. The electromyograph consists of electrodes, an oscilloscope to visually produce the waves of muscle activity, an amplifier and loudspeaker, an electrical stimulator, and a camera. The patient may receive sedation before this test is conducted since there can be a painful stimulation from the electric current. The EMG consists of inserting a fine-gauge needle electrode through the skin and into a muscle and then sending a small amount of electric current into the muscle.

The electrical activity of the muscle is recorded on a paper graph or on film. This permanent record is then evaluated to determine the ad-

equacy of muscle activity. Abnormal EMG test results can indicate a congenital or an acquired disease condition of the muscles, for example one caused by a virus.

Evoked Potential Studies

Responses within the brain to external stimuli such as light, sound, and touch is called an evoked potential study. These tests are considered noninvasive since no equipment or needle is inserted into the body. Two types of evoked potential studies are described below.

- Brainstem auditory evoked response (BAER) is used to assess the auditory nerve pathways. This is useful in diagnosing auditory tumors and lesions.
- Somatosensory evoked peripheral nerves (SEP) is used for diagnosing nerve function defects in peripheral nerves, for example in the legs.

Rehabilitation

Rehabilitation is the process of assisting a patient to regain a state of health and the highest level of function possible. Injury, illness, and conditions such as multiple sclerosis cause patients to lose mobility and self-esteem.

The rehabilitation process is a holistic approach to a concern for every aspect of the patient's well being, not just the present disease or injury. The goal of rehabilitation is to restore as much function as possible for the patient. In addition, the patient is assisted to resume activities of daily living, such as feeding, toileting, and providing as much care for oneself as possible.

Rehabilitation after a long illness or a debilitating disease causing muscle loss and atrophy, requires patience from everyone involved: the patient, family members, and care givers. Rehabilitation programs are useful for the following conditions/diseases:

- Surgery (for example hip and knee replacements)
- Trauma, such as broken bones, which result in long periods of inactivity and/or muscle weakness
- Catastrophic illness such as stroke
- Disease conditions resulting in muscle atrophy or disuse such as multiple sclerosis and muscular dystrophy

A formal rehabilitation program begins as soon as the acute phase of an illness or disease has passed. Short-term and long-term goal setting takes place based on the physician's orders and the patient's willingness to cooperate.

A short-term goal would include such items as learning crutch walking, and learning range of motion exercises. Long-term goals aim at independence, and the patient acquiring a feeling of confidence.

Adaptive Equipment

Equipment used to facilitate rehabilitation from physical disorders or disabilities, such as a stroke, includes adaptive equipment: wheelchairs, walkers, canes, and special furniture such as shower chairs and geriatric chairs. Adaptive equipment also includes a variety of utensils, such as eating utensils molded to fit the patient's hand and dishes with a wide edge to prevent spilling (see Chapter 24, Figure 24-2 A). There are long handled devices for reaching items on the floor (see Chapter 24, Figure 24-2 B).

Canes

Several types of wooden and aluminum canes are available. The aluminum canes are adjustable for height using the nut and wing bolts. The wooden canes have to be purchased to size or cut to the correct length. All canes should have a rubber tip on the end to prevent slipping.

Canes are used by patients who have a one-sided muscle or bone weakness, or need assistance with balance. Three common types of canes are the standard cane, four-point (quad) cane, and the tripod cane.

A standard cane has a curved neck for ease of gripping. It provides support for patients who need only slight assistance. The tripod (3-point) and quad (four-point) canes have a wide base with three or four points to provide a steady support. The neck is bent with a T-shaped handle.

The hand grip of the cane should be at the level of the hip joint with the elbow flexed at an angle of 25-30 degrees.

Walkers

Walkers are assistive devices made of aluminum which provide a base of support for patients who need help with balance and walking. They are used by geriatric patients to aid with mobility. The

Guidelines: Using a Single Cane (or Crutch)

1. Hold the cane (or single crutch) on the opposite side of the injury or affected limb. As the affected leg moves forward the cane (or crutch) on the opposite side will move forward to provide support.
2. The cane (or single crutch) should be placed 6 inches in front of and slightly to one side of the unaffected side.
3. The elbow should be slightly flexed during weight bearing.
4. The affected limb and cane should be moved forward together 6-10 inches. The weight should be placed on the strong foot and leg.
5. As the unaffected foot moves forward, the weight is shifted to the weak/affected foot and cane. Thus the cane will provide support for weight bearing on the weaker leg.
6. This procedure is repeated using small steps.

walker should be adjusted to the patient's height with the height of the walker just below the patient's waistline.

A stationary walker must be picked up by the patient, moved forward, and then used as a base of support while the patient walks into it. This requires strong arm muscle development. A walker with wheels can be used by patients who have good coordination and balance. This walker can be dangerous since there is a tendency for it to move too quickly causing the patient to lose his or her balance and fall.

There are walkers with wheels that have a bar the patient presses to unlock the wheels; if the patient lets go of the bar the wheels lock, thus preventing the walker from moving away from the patient.

Wheelchairs

Wheelchairs are hand manipulated and power-driven and many patients operate their own wheelchairs. However, not all patients are able to (nor should they) operate their own wheelchairs (Figure 30-7). For example, an individual who is paralyzed on one side may not be able to operate his or her own wheelchair, and obviously the blind or frail patient will need assistance (Figure 30-8).

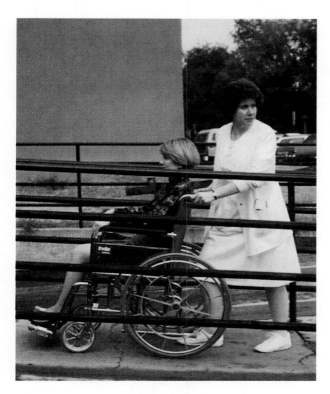

Figure 30-7 Wheelchairs are moved down ramps backwards.

Wheelchair Transfer

Always think of moving patients as the process of transferring them from one place to another. In many cases, the patient is familiar with the techniques necessary for the transfer and will be able to assist the medical assistant.

A person who is paralyzed on one side of the body (hemiplegia) or who has a general weakness can be moved from a wheelchair by a process of pivoting the patient so that he or she can use the stronger leg to assist you. Explain that this transfer technique is used to prevent injury to the patient and to the individual assisting with the transfer, for example back injury (Figure 30-9). Figure 30-10 is an example of moving a patient from a wheelchair to a sitting position, such as on a bed.

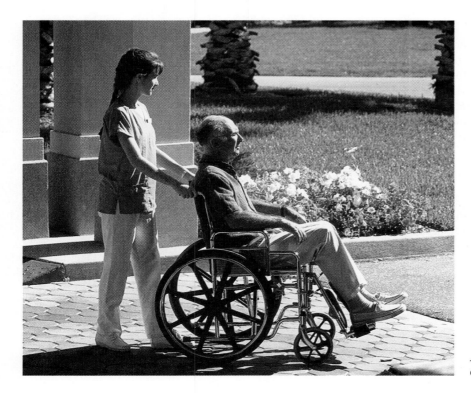

Figure 30-8 Assisting a disabled patient.

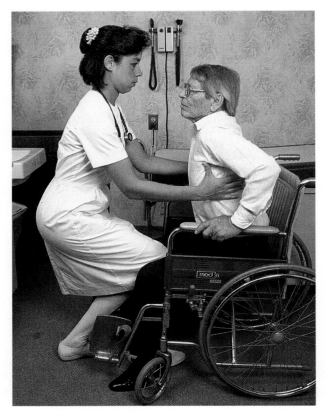

Figure 30-9 Medical assistant assists patient out of wheelchair.

Special Furniture

Special furniture for patients needing assistance includes shower chairs, made of aluminum or plastic, which allow the patient to sit while taking a shower. The geriatric chair, a wheeled chair that reclines with an attached tray for meals, is useful for patients who can feed themselves but may not be able to sit securely in a regular chair.

Role of the Physical Therapist

A physical therapist receives special training in assisting patients with the use of exercises and equipment related to regaining body motion. The therapist is skilled at using special equipment for strengthening muscles, measuring and fitting a prosthesis (artificial body part), and the use of assistive devices such as crutches, walkers, and canes.

Role of the Occupational Therapist

An occupational therapist is a vital member of the rehabilitative team with a focus on increasing the

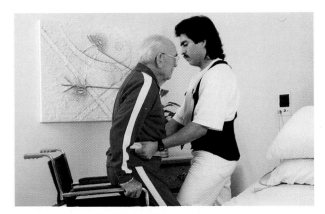

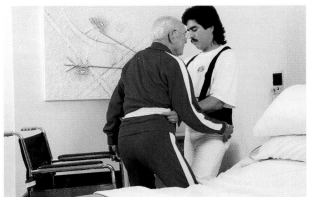

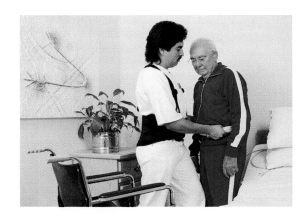

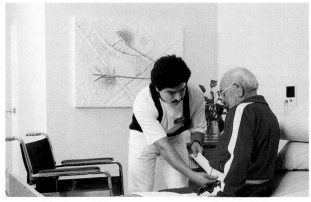

Figure 30-10 Moving a patient from a wheelchair to a sitting position.

PROCEDURE: Wheelchair Transfer to Chair or Examination Table

Terminal Performance
Competency: Student will move the patient from a wheelchair to a chair or examination table without error.

Equipment and Supplies
Chair or examination table
Gait belt, if needed
Step stool, if needed

Procedural Steps

1. Wash hands.

2. Identify the patient and introduce yourself.

3. Explain what you are going to do before you start. Discuss what the patient will do to assist you.

4. Place the wheelchair at a 45 degree angle to the chair or examination table. This provides a shorter distance to pivot the patient from the wheelchair.

5. Put the wheelchair brakes into the lock position on both sides. Move the foot pedals up and out of the way so the patient has a clear path to move forward. The patient's legs should be moved off the pedals by supporting the ankle and lower leg. Gently place the patient's feet on the floor and have the patient shift forward in chair, if possible.

6. Make sure the examination table or chair is stable before attempting the transfer.

7. Position yourself near the patient's nonparalyzed side so you can provide support and the patient can use his or her stronger limb. You will move the patient toward the stronger side. Do not refer to the patient's "good" or "bad" side.

8. Place one of your feet forward to establish a firm base of support for your body. Move down toward the patient while keeping your back straight.

9. Have the patient place his or her hands on the arm supports on the wheelchair. Then, ask the patient to lean forward and push up as you assist the patient to a standing position, on the count of three.

10. Position yourself so that the patient's paralyzed leg is between your knees. Support the paralyzed leg with your knees, if necessary, so the leg will not slip as the patient stands.

11. Place your hands under the patient's armpits and help the patient to stand. Use the muscles in your legs to push your body upward. Do not bend over and use back muscles. *Note:* a "gait belt" can be placed around the heavy patient's waist for lifting.

12. Allow the patient to stand for a few moments before attempting to move into a chair or onto an examination table.

13. Assist the patient to pivot (turn) toward the nonparalyzed side by pivoting your own body as you hold the patient under their armpits. Do not twist your body. Turn it as a unit.

14. Gently lower the patient into a chair by bending your knees and keeping your back straight.

15. If the patient must move up onto an examination table and can assist you, then support the weak side as the patient places his or her stronger leg onto the step stool. Pivot the patient around so he or she can then sit on the edge of the table. Encourage the patient to move back on the table to eliminate the danger of falling.

16. If the patient is unable to assist you, then ask for another assistant to hold one side of the patient as you support the other side. Count aloud "one," "two," "three," and then lift the patient together. Do not attempt to lift—by yourself—a patient who is unable to help you.

17. When assisting the patient into a supine position, support the paralyzed leg gently onto the table.

18. Never leave a physically challenged (disabled) patient unattended.

patient's ability to function within his or her own environment. This therapist assists the patient to relearn and to acquire activities of daily living. The occupational therapist functions in the following areas: mobilization, teaching activities of daily living skills, and coordination and strength tolerance.

- Mobilization activities include assisting patients to maintain balance, reach, grasp, move, and turn while sitting.
- Teaching activities of daily living include bathing, dressing, feeding, grooming, homemaking, and leisure activities.
- Coordination, strength and activity tolerance includes teaching the patient techniques to use all physical resources without tiring quickly as well as techniques to conserve strength.

Speech Therapy

A speech therapist works with children and adults to help patients regain lost speech as a result of illness or disease. In addition this therapist works with the hearing impaired to evaluate and train in using speech, sign language, finger-spelling, and residual hearing to communicate. See (Figure 30-11) for an example of speech therapy.

One of the most useful devices to aid communication for hearing impaired children and adults is the use of sign language. Signing, the nonverbal method of communicating with the hands and fingers, exists in many forms. Examples of sign language follows:

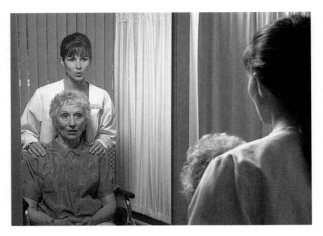

Figure 30-11   Speech therapy.

- American Sign Language (ASL) is a method of communicating in which the hands and fingers are used to indicate words and concepts. This is used by both the deaf and speech-impaired persons.
- Finger-spelling is the use of various hand and finger shapes and positions that represent the written alphabet. These positions can be strung together to form words.
- Signing Exact English (SEE-2) is translating English into signs. American Sign Language (ASL) is used in combination with other sign languages and finger-spelling to correspond exactly to the spoken word.
- Speech-reading is the ability to watch a person's mouth and word formation during speaking to interpret what they are saying. This is also referred to as lip-reading.

LEGAL AND ETHICAL ISSUES

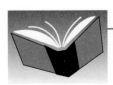

Many of the procedures described in this chapter are beyond the scope of practice of the medical assistant beginning his or her first job. Additional training and practice is required before teaching a patient to use crutches, for instance. In some states, only a licensed physical therapist is able to perform many of the procedures discussed. The medical assistant must remember that with many procedures he or she is "assisting" another licensed person such as the physician, nurse or physical therapist. Always check with your local or state medical association regarding the laws in your state if there is any doubt. The patient's safety must always be placed first.

PATIENT EDUCATION

The medical assistant plays an important role in educating the patient with physical therapy needs. In many cases the medical assistant is the only person providing instructions regarding commonly ordered procedures relating to the application of heat and cold.

A team approach, including all members of the health care team, patient and family, is the ideal structure for patient education when handling physical disabilities.

Summary

Physical therapy involves the use of physical measures, equipment, and body movement to promote mobility, circulation, restore normal function, and relieve pain. The medical assistant, working under the supervision of a physician, is able to teach the patient about proper body mechanics, exercise, and the application of various therapeutic devices such as heat and cold applications. In some cases the medical assistant will apply these devices.

Competency Review

1. Define and spell the glossary terms for this chapter.
2. Instruct a partner on the two-point, three-point, and four-point crutch walking gait.
3. Create patient education materials for the application of hot and cold applications.
4. Using a partner demonstrate PROM. Demonstrate AROM yourself.
5. Demonstrate the proper method for wheelchair transfer.
6. Talk to a local physical therapist about a typical day in his or her practice.
7. Describe the following testing methods: electromyography (EMG), nerve conduction studies (NCS), evoked potential studies (EPS), and brainstem auditory evoked response (BAER).
8. Describe four methods of sign language.

PREPARING FOR THE CERTIFICATION EXAM

Test Taking Tip — Do not look for tricks in examination questions. Examinations are meant to be a determination of your knowledge of the subject.

Examination Review Questions

1. A licensed professional who teaches a patient the correct use of equipment and body mechanics to prevent further injury or disability is referred to as a/an
   (A) speech therapist
   (B) occupational therapist
   (C) physical therapist
   (D) psychotherapist
   (E) respiratory therapist

2. Which of the following does moist heat application include?
   (A) hypothermia blanket
   (B) aquamatic K-pad
   (C) warm-water bottle
   (D) heat lamp
   (E) Sitz bath

3. The electrical activity of a muscle is recorded by using which test?
   (A) somatosensory evoked potentials (SEP)
   (B) electromyography (EMG)
   (C) evoked potential studies (EPS)
   (D) brainstem auditory evoked response (BAER)
   (E) none of the above

4. Rehabilitative programs are useful for treating all of the following EXCEPT
   (A) catastrophic illness, for example stroke
   (B) trauma
   (C) acute illness
   (D) diseases resulting in muscle atrophy
   (E) chronic illness

5. The process which provides a medicinal or healthful effect is called
   (A) suppuration
   (B) erythemia
   (C) therapeutic
   (D) contraindicated
   (E) supination

6. When applying hot compresses, the correct temperature is
   (A) 90° F
   (B) 105° F

(Continued on next page)

(C) 115° F

(D) 120° F

(E) 125° F

7. Movement that bends a body part backward is

   (A) inversion

   (B) supination

   (C) pronation

   (D) dorsiflexion

   (E) rotation

8. When the patient faces downward, this is called

   (A) inversion

   (B) supination

   (C) pronation

   (D) dorsiflexion

(E) rotation

9. Range of motion exercise performed without assistance from another person is

   (A) AROM

   (B) PROM

   (C) active resistive

   (D) A and B

   (E) none of the above

10. The crutch-walking gait used when a patient is able to bear weight on both legs is

   (A) two-point

   (B) three-point

   (C) four-point

   (D) swing-to

   (E) swing-through

ON THE JOB

Jenny Watmore, a recently graduated medical assistant, employed by Dr. Cory in his orthopedic practice, has been asked to assist Mr. Ivy from the wheelchair onto the examination table. Mr. Ivy, a recovering stroke patient, is being seen by Dr. Cory to be evaluated for an assistive walking device. Mr. Ivy, who is 80 years old, is weakened on the left side of his body from the cerebrovascular accident (CVA). He weighs 200 pounds and is reluctant to provide much help to Jenny when she has to transfer him from the wheelchair to the examination table.

What is your response?

1. What should Jenny do?
2. Describe the body mechanics that Jenny should use.
3. What patient education does Mr. Ivy need?
4. What documentation should Jenny provide on Mr. Ivy's record?

References

Corwin, D. and Miller, C. "Get Your Patient Off on the Right Foot." *RN.* November, 1990.

Lane, P., LeBlanc, R. "Crutch Walking." *Orthopedic Nursing.* 9:5, 1990.

Lewis, C. and McNerney, T. *Exercise Handouts for Rehabilitation.* Gaithersburg, MD: Aspen, 1993.

Reed, K. *Quick Reference to Occupational Therapy.* Gaithersburg, MD: Aspen, 1991.

Workplace Wisdom

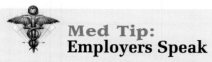

Med Tip:
Employers Speak

Maintain a professional look and attitude from the first interview throughout your employment.

Linda Warren, RN, BS
Coordinator of Nursing Services
University of Michigan Health System
Chelsea Family Practice
Chelsea, Michigan

Take every opportunity for new training regardless of how unnecessary it may seem. It may be the key to keeping your job or making yourself more marketable.

Daniel A. Staifer
Human Resources Generalist
Henry Ford Health System/
Henry Ford Wyandotte Hospital
Wyandotte, Michigan

When you are in the process of completing a job application, take enough time to be neat and thorough. Complete every line of the application form and attach a resume if possible.

Linda Davis-Rogers
Recruiter
Sharp Health Care
San Diego, California

Your success will be influenced by your true dedication to the cause of helping and working with the patient population.

Charlotte Stein
Employment Specialist
Saint Luke's Medical Center
Cleveland, Ohio

Following a job interview, show assertiveness and ambitious persistence by calling back to check on the job status. But, understand that there is a fine line between persistence and pushiness. Send a simple thank you note.

Linda Davis-Rogers
Recruiter
Sharp Health Care
San Diego, California

Understand and practice situational interviewing in which you are given a situation and asked how you would handle the situation.

Example: A patient who has just been seen on the third floor walks up to you on the first floor and asks, "What do I do with this specimen?"

Wrong answer: "Go back to the third floor and they will tell you."

Correct answer: "Let me find out. I will call them for you."

Denise Williams
Staffing Specialist (Radnor Office)
University of Pennsylvania
Health System
Philadelphia, Pennsylvania

MEDICAL ASSISTANT ROLE DELINEATION CHART

Highlight indicates material covered in this chapter

ADMINISTRATIVE

ADMINISTRATIVE PROCEDURES

- Perform basic clerical functions
- Schedule, coordinate, and monitor appointments
- Schedule inpatient/outpatient admissions and procedures
- Understand and apply third party guidelines
- Obtain reimbursement through accurate claims submission
- Monitor third-party reimbursement
- Perform medical transcription
- Understand and adhere to managed care policies and procedures
- *Negotiate managed care contracts (adv)*

PRACTICE FINANCES

- Perform procedural and diagnostic coding
- Apply bookkeeping principles
- Document and maintain accounting and banking records
- Manage accounts receivable
- Manage accounts payable
- Process payroll
- *Develop and maintain fee schedules (adv)*
- *Manage renewals of business and professional insurance policies (adv)*
- *Manage personal benefits and maintain records (adv)*

CLINICAL

FUNDAMENTAL PRINCIPLES

- Apply principles of aseptic technique and infection control
- Comply with quality assurance practices
- Screen and follow up patient test results

DIAGNOSTIC ORDERS

- Collect and process specimens
- Perform diagnostic tests

PATIENT CARE

- Adhere to established triage procedures
- Obtain patient history and vital signs
- Prepare and maintain examination and treatment areas

- Prepare patient for examinations, procedures, and treatments
- Assist with examinations, procedures, and treatments
- Prepare and administer medications and immunizations
- Maintain medication and immunization records
- Recognize and respond to emergencies
- Coordinate patient care information with other health care providers

GENERAL (TRANSDISCIPLINARY)

PROFESSIONALISM

- Project a professional manner and image
- Adhere to ethical principles
- Demonstrate initiative and responsibility
- Work as a team member
- Manage time efficiently
- Prioritize and perform multiple tasks
- Adapt to change
- Promote the CMA credential
- Enhance skills through continuing education

COMMUNICATION SKILLS

- Treat all patients with compassion and empathy
- Recognize and respect cultural diversity
- Adapt communications to individual's ability to understand
- Use professional telephone technique
- Use effective and correct verbal and written communications
- Recognize and respond to verbal and non-verbal communications
- Use medical terminology appropriately
- Receive, organize, prioritize, and transmit information
- Serve as liaison
- Promote the practice through positive public relations

LEGAL CONCEPTS

- Maintain confidentiality
- Practice within the scope of education, training, and personal capabilities
- Prepare and maintain medical records
- Document accurately
- Use appropriate guidelines when releasing information
- Follow employer's established policies dealing with the health care contract
- Follow federal, state, and local legal guidelines
- Maintain awareness of federal and state health care legislation and regulations
- Maintain and dispose of regulated substances in compliance with government guidelines
- Comply with established risk management and safety procedures
- Recognize professional credentialing criteria
- Participate in the development and maintenance of personnel, policy, and procedure manuals
- *Develop and maintain personnel, policy, and procedure manuals (adv)*

INSTRUCTION

- Instruct individuals according to their needs
- Explain office policies and procedures
- Teach methods of health promotion and disease prevention
- Locate community resources and disseminate information
- *Orient and train personnel (adv)*
- *Develop educational materials (adv)*
- *Conduct continuing education activities (adv)*

OPERATIONAL FUNCTIONS

- Maintain supply inventory
- Evaluate and recommend equipment and supplies
- Apply computer techniques to support office operations
- *Supervise personnel (adv)*
- *Interview and recommend job applicants (adv)*
- *Negotiate leases and prices for equipment and supply contracts (adv)*

SOURCE: Reprinted by permission of the American Association of Medical Assistants from the *AAMA Role Delineation Study: Occupational Analysis of the Medical Assisting Profession.*

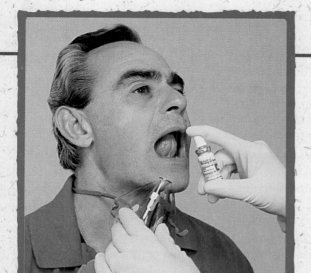

31

Pharmacology

LEARNING OBJECTIVES

After completing this chapter, you should:

1. Define and spell the glossary terms for this chapter.
2. Differentiate between the legal (generic), commercial (trade) and chemical name for a drug.
3. Know the precautions to be observed when administering drugs.
4. Describe the drug reference books which should be in all physician's offices.
5. List the "six rights" to medication administration.
6. List the five schedules of the Controlled Substances Act.
7. Know the conditions under which a medical assistant may administer medications.
8. Cite the information that must be charted when administering a medication.

Glossary

addiction An acquired physical and psychological dependence on a drug.

anaphylactic shock A life-threatening reaction to certain foods, drugs, and insect bites in some people. This can cause respiratory distress, edema, rash, convulsions, and eventually unconsciousness and death if emergency treatment is not given.

broad-spectrum The ability of a drug to be effective against a wide range of microorganisms.

Bureau of Narcotics and Dangerous Drugs (BNDD) An agency of the federal government, used to enforce drug control.

chemotherapy Use of chemicals, including drugs, to treat or control infections and diseases; commonly used to treat cancer by killing the cancer cells.

contraindicated A condition in which the use of a drug should not be used.

dilute To weaken the strength of a substance by the addition of something else.

drug tolerance A decrease in susceptibility to a drug after the continued use of the drug.

Food and Drug Administration (FDA) The official federal agency with responsibility for the regulation of food, drugs, cosmetics, and medical devices. It is a part of the US Department of Health and Human Services.

generic name Common name by which a drug or product is known (for example, aspirin).

habituation The development of an emotional dependence on a drug due to repeated use.

hemostatic Any drug, medicine, or blood component that stops bleeding, such as vasopressin, vitamin K, or whole blood.

idiosyncrasy An unusual or abnormal response to a drug or food by an individual.

parenteral Medication route other than the alimentary canal (oral and rectal). Parenteral routes include subcutaneous, intravenous, and intramuscular.

pharmacist A druggist or one who is licensed to prepare and dispense drugs.

pharmacology The study of drugs, their origins, nature, properties and effects on the living organism.

Physician's Desk Reference (PDR) A book used as a quick reference on drugs.

placebo An inactive, harmless substance used to satisfy a patient's desire for medication. This is also used in research when given to a control group of patients in a study in which another group receives the actual drug. The effect of the placebo versus the drug is then observed.

prophylaxis The prevention of disease. A medication, such as an antibiotic, can be used to prevent the occurrence of an infection prior to surgery (as opposed to antibiotics given to treat an infection).

side effect(s) A response to a drug other than the effect desired.

toxicity The extent or degree to which a substance is poisonous.

untoward effect An undesirable side effect.

United States Pharmacopeia-National Formulary (USP-NF) A drug book listing all the official drugs that are authorized for use in the United States. This is used in medical facilities and physicians' offices as a reference.

WARNING!

For all patient contact, adhere to Standard Precautions (see pages 342–373). Wear protective equipment as indicated.

Pharmacology is the study of drugs, their origin, characteristics, and effects. The drugs used in the study of pharmacology are products of many different sources including: plants, animals, minerals, and synthetics.

Some drugs, such as vitamins, are naturally found in the foods we eat. Others, such as hormones, are obtained from animals. Penicillin and some of the other antibiotics are developed from molds which are a form of plant life. Many drugs, such as those used in chemotherapy, are synthetically formed by artificial means in the laboratory. Chemotherapy refers to the use of chemicals, including drugs, to treat or control infections and diseases. Chemotherapy is commonly used to treat cancer by killing the cancer cells.

Drugs prescribed to treat an infection are known as antibiotics; drugs prescribed or measures taken to prevent disease from occurring, for example drugs given to a patient prior to surgery, are prophylactics. Prophylaxis is prevention of disease through the prescribing of drugs and/or treatment.

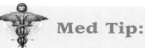

Med Tip:

| generic name | = | lower case | Example: acetaminophen |
| brand/trade name | = | Capitalized | Example: Tylenol |

Med Tip: The term drug and medication have the same meaning. However, the general public considers the term "drug" or "drugs" to mean a narcotic-type of medication. The term can also mean the use of illegal chemical substances. For purposes of medical terminology, the use of the word "drug" means a medication.

Drug Names

A drug may be known by as many as three different names: the generic name, the brand or trade name, and the chemical name. The generic term for a drug is the single name for identifying a drug. This is recognized by pharmaceutical companies and is considered the legal term for the drug. An example of a generic name for a drug would be tetracycline. The drug under the generic name can be manufactured by many companies which then place their own brand name on the drug.

The brand or trade name is also referred to as the proprietary name. This is the commercial name that is patented by the pharmaceutical company that manufactures the drug. If the brand name is patented by the company, no other company can use that name for 17 years. Other drug companies can manufacture and patent the drug, but it must be under their own brand name. For example, Achromycin V, which is used to treat infection, is a brand name Lederle Laboratories uses for the generic drug, tetracycline. Tylenol is the brand name for acetaminophen. One drug can be manufactured by several companies under many brand names. Brand names are used by the pharmaceutical companies for advertising the drugs.

Generic drugs are usually priced lower than the brand name drug. However, not every drug is available generically and drug levels may not be as closely regulated in generic drugs as they are in brand name drugs. The physician can indicate on the prescription if the druggist may substitute a generic drug for a brand name. In some cases, the physician will prefer that a particular brand named drug be used if he or she believes it to be more effective than the generic drug.

The chemical name is the chemical formula for that particular drug. It is difficult for the lay person to comprehend and is used by the manufacturer and pharmacists. Pharmacists are licensed to prepare and dispense drugs. In the example above, the chemical name for Achromycin V is tetracycline hydrochloride (HCL). HCL after the term stands for the abbreviation for hydrochloride.

Med Tip: A physician can order a drug by either its generic or brand name. In general the generic drug is less expensive than the brand name drug. Many physicians will order the generic drug to save money for the patient. Never guess at the name of a drug if you are asked to interpret a physician's prescription. Always ask!

Regulations and Standards

The Food and Drug Administration (FDA), a department within the Federal Department of Health and Human Services, ultimately enforces drug sales and distribution. The actual control of drugs is stipulated by the Federal Food, Drug, and Cosmetic Act of 1938. This act was initiated to ensure the safety of food, drugs, and cosmetics that are sold within the United States borders. The Controlled Substance Act of 1970 regulates the manufacture and distribution of the drugs which are capable of causing dependence and the Bureau of Narcotics and Dangerous Drugs (BNDD) is the agency of the federal government which is authorized to enforce drug control.

References

There are two major resources for drug information and facts—the *Hospital Formulary* and the *Physician's Desk Reference* (PDR). The *Hospital Formulary* contains up-to-date information about drugs and their usage. It is published by the American Hospital Formulary Service and used extensively by pharmacists. The *Physician's Desk Reference* or *PDR* is an easy to use resource and should be in every physician's office or medical facility. The *PDR* is published by a private company and is sent free of charge to medical offices and hospitals. In addition to the well know book version, the *PDR* is also available on computer disk and CD-ROM. It lists drug products with addresses of manufacturers, generic and chemical name listings, and other valuable information.

Med Tip: It is critical that patients receive the correct drug. Since it is not possible to list or remember all the drug names, you must acquire the habit of looking up any drug name you do not recognize in the *Physician's Desk Reference* (PDR). Every medical office or medical facility should have a copy of this book and update it each year.

Other books which are helpful include the *United States Pharmacopeia-National Formulary (USP-NF)*. This is a drug book listing all the official drugs that are authorized for use in the United States.

Legal Classification of Drugs

Drugs are classified as prescription and nonprescription drugs and controlled substances. A description of each of these categories follows. It is important for the medical assistant to be knowledgeable about these specific categories and to keep current with state and federal regulations that are published regarding a change of status of drugs, for example from "prescription" to "nonprescription."

Prescription Drugs

A prescription drug can only be ordered by a person who is licensed to dispense medications, such as physicians. These drugs must include on the label the words, "Caution: Federal Law prohibits dispensing without prescription." Antibiotics such as penicillin and heart medications such as digoxin are only available by prescription. A prescription is the written explanation to the pharmacist regarding the name of the medication, the dosage and the times of administration. A prescription can also be given verbally to the pharmacist by a licensed physician.

Nonprescription Drugs

A nonprescription drug is also referred to as an "over-the-counter" (OTC) drug. They are easily accessible in drug stores without a prescription. There are many medications or drugs that can be purchased without a prescription. Examples would include aspirin and antidiarrheal medications.

Some of these OTC drugs, for example cortisone ointments, required a prescription until recently. If taken incorrectly, some OTC drugs can be unsafe since they may react negatively with a prescription drug the patient is taking. For instance, aspirin taken along with an anticoagulant, such as Coumadin, can cause internal bleeding in some people. Antacids which are available as OTC drugs should not be taken with tetracycline since they interfere with the absorption of tetracycline into the body. Milk can have the same effect on tetracycline. It is best to allow the physician and the pharmacist to advise on the proper OTC drugs.

Controlled Substances

Certain drugs are controlled if they have a potential for **addiction** or abuse. The control of these drugs is enforced by the Drug Enforcement Agency (DEA). Controlled substances must be kept under lock and key. An accurate count of all narcotics is kept in a record called the "narcotic's log." The date and person to whom the drug was administered along with the signature of the person administering the drug are recorded. Most states do not allow medical assistants to administer narcotics.

The expiration dates of all medication in stock should be examined monthly. Do not place medications in waste containers. They are generally destroyed by pouring down a drain or flushing down a toilet. Two people should be present when controlled substances are destroyed. Both signatures are then placed on the narcotics log. Some more commonly controlled substances are:

TABLE 31-1 **Schedule for Controlled Substances**

Level	Description	Comment
Schedule I	Highest potential for addiction and abuse. Not accepted for medical use. Example: Marijuana, heroin, and LSD	Not prescribed drugs.
Schedule II	High potential for addiction and abuse. Accepted for medical use in the US. Example: Codeine, cocaine, morphine, opium, and secobarbital	A DEA licensed physician must complete the required triplicate prescription forms entirely written in his or her own handwriting. The prescription must be filled within seven days and it may not be refilled. In an emergency, the physician may order a limited amount of the drug by telephone. These drugs must be stored under lock and key if they are kept on the office premises. The law requires that a dispensing record of these drugs be kept on file for two years.
Schedule III	Moderate to low potential for addiction and abuse. Example: Butabarbital, anabolic steroids, and APC with codeine	A DEA number is not required to write a prescription for these drugs but the physician must hand write the order. Five refills are allowed during a six month period and must be indicated on the prescription form. Only the physician can give telephone orders to the pharmacist for these drugs.
Schedule IV	Lower potential for addiction and abuse than Schedule III drugs. Example: Chloral hydrate, Phenobarbital, and diazepam	A medical assistant may write the prescription order for the physician, but it must be signed by the physician. Five refills are allowed over a six month period of time.
Schedule V	Low potential for addiction and abuse. Example: Low-strength codeine combined with other drugs to form cough suppressant	Inventory records must be maintained on these drugs also.

- anabolic steroids
- APC with codeine
- butabarbital
- chloral hydrate
- cocaine
- codeine
- diazepam
- heroin
- LSD
- marijuana
- morphine
- opium
- phenobarbital
- secobarbital

The controlled drugs are classified into five schedules which indicate levels of abuse. The schedules are listed Schedule I through Schedule V. They are listed in Table 31-1.

General Classes of Drugs

The classification of drugs relates to their action on the body. Table 31-2 presents a comprehensive list of names of drug classifications with descriptions of the use, or function, for each classification. Table 31-3 contains a similar list of drug classifications and provides specific examples of each drug type.

TABLE 31-2   Drug Classification Names and Descriptions of Use

Name	Use
adrenergic	Increases the rate and strength of the heart muscle. Acts as a vasoconstrictor, dilates bronchi, dilates pupils and relaxes muscular walls. Used to treat asthma, bronchitis and allergies.
adrenergic blocking agent	Increases peripheral circulation, decreases blood pressure and vasodilation. Used to treat hypertension.
analgesic	Relieves pain without the loss of consciousness. These may be either narcotic or non-narcotic. Narcotic drugs are derived from the opium poppy and act upon the brain to cause pain relief and drowsiness. For example, morphine.
anesthetic	Produces a lack of feeling which may be of local or general effect depending on the type of administration.
antacid	Neutralizes acid in the stomach.
antianxiety	Relieves or reduces anxiety and muscle tension. These are used to treat panic disorders, anxiety, and insomnia.
antiarrhythmic	Controls cardiac arrhythmias by altering nerve impulses within the heart.
antibiotic	Destroys or prohibits the growth of microorganisms. These are used to treat bacterial infections. They have not been found to be effective in treating viral infections. Antibiotics must be taken regularly for a specified time period to be effective.
anticoagulant	Prevents or delays blood clotting. Also referred to as blood thinners. These may be administered by intravenous injection, such as with the drug heparin. Oral drugs, such as warfarin, cannot be taken along with aspirin since the interaction between the two medications could cause internal bleeding.
anticonvulsant	Prevents or relieves convulsions. Drugs such as phenobarbital reduce excessive stimulation in the brain to control seizures and other symptoms of epilepsy.
antidepressant	Prevents or relieves the symptoms of depression. These drugs are also used in the prevention of migraine headaches.
antidiabetic	Drugs that control diabetes by regulating the level of glucose in the blood and the metabolism of carbohydrates and fat.
antidiarrheal	Prevents or relieves diarrhea.
antidote	Counteracts the effects of poisons.
antiemetic	Controls nausea and vomiting. These generally act upon the vomiting center in the brain.
antifungal	Kills fungus.
antihelminthic	Kills parasitic worms.
antihistamine	Counteracts histamine and controls allergic reactions.

(Continued)

Name	Use
antihypertensive	Prevents or controls high blood pressure. Some of these drugs act to block nerve impulses that cause arteries to constrict and thus increase the blood pressure. Other drugs slow the heart rate and decrease its force of contraction. Still others may reduce the amount of the hormone aldosterone in the blood that is causing the blood pressure to rise.
anti-inflammatory	Counteracts inflammation.
antineoplastic	Kills normal and abnormal cancerous cells by interfering with cell reproduction.
antipruritics	Relieves itching.
antipyretic	Reduces fever.
antiseptic	Prevents the growth of microorganisms.
antitussive	Controls or relieves coughing. Codeine is an ingredient in many prescription cough medicines. It acts upon the brain to control coughing.
astringent	A substance that has a constricting or binding effect by coagulating proteins on a cell's surface. This may be used to stop hemorrhage.
bronchodilator	Dilates or opens the bronchi (airways in the lungs) to improve breathing.
cardiogenic	Strengthens the heart muscle.
cathartic	Causes bowel movements to occur. These drugs may have a strong purging action and can become habit forming.
contraceptive	Used to prevent conception.
decongestant	Reduces nasal congestion and swelling.
diuretic	Increases the excretion of urine which promotes the loss of water and salt from the body. This can assist in lowering blood pressure, therefore, these drugs are used to treat hypertension. Potassium in the body may be depleted with continued use of diuretics. Potassium-rich foods, such as bananas, kiwi, and orange juice along with medications for potassium deficiency, can help correct this deficiency.
emetic	Induces vomiting.
estrogen	A hormone used to replace estrogen lost during menopause. Estrogen is responsible for the development of secondary sexual characteristics and is produced by the ovaries.
expectorant	Assists in the removal of secretions from the bronchopulmonary membranes.
hemostatic	Controls bleeding.
hypnotic	Produces sleep or hypnosis.
hypoglycemic	Lowers blood glucose level.
immunosuppressive	Suppresses the body's natural immune response to an antigen. This is used to control autoimmune diseases such as multiple sclerosis and rheumatoid arthritis.

(Continued on next page)

TABLE 31-2 *(Continued)*

Name	Use
laxative	Used to promote normal bowel function.
miotic	Constricts the pupils of the eye.
muscle relaxant	Produces the relaxation of skeletal muscle.
mydriatic	Dilates the pupils of the eye.
narcotic	Produces sleep or stupor. In moderate doses this drug will depress the central nervous system and relieve pain. In excessive doses it will cause stupor, coma and even death. Can become habit-forming (addictive).
purgative	Stimulates bowel movements.
psychedelic	Drugs such as lysergic acid diethylamide (LSD) that can produce visual hallucinations.
sedative	Produces relaxation without causing sleep.
stimulant	Speeds up the heart and respiratory system. Used to increase alertness.
tranquilizer	Used to reduce mental anxiety and tensions.
vaccine	Given to promote resistance (immunity) to infectious diseases.
vasodilator	Produces a relaxation of blood vessels to lower blood pressure.
vasopressor	Produces the contraction of muscles in the capillaries and arteries which elevates the blood pressure.
vitamin	Organic substances found naturally in foods that are essential for normal metabolism. Most have been produced synthetically to be taken in pill form.

Routes and Methods of Drug Administration

The method by which a drug is introduced into the body is referred to as the route of administration (Figure 31-1). In general the routes of administration are

1. *Oral:* This method includes all drugs that are given by mouth. The advantages are ease of administration and a slow rate of absorption via stomach and intestinal wall. The disadvantages include slowness of absorption and destroying of some chemical compounds by gastric juices. In addition, some medications, such as aspirin, can have a corrosive action on the stomach lining.
2. *Sublingual:* These are drugs that are held under the tongue and not swallowed. The medication is absorbed as the saliva dissolves it. Nitroglycerin to treat angina or chest pain is administered by this route.
3. *Parenteral:* This is an invasive method of administering drugs since it requires the skin to be punctured by a needle. The needle with syringe attached is introduced either under the skin, into a muscle, vein, or body cavity. Table 31-4 lists the methods for parenteral administration and provides a description of each method.

Additional methods (other than parenteral) for administering medication are given in Table 31-5.

Drugs must be administered by a particular route in order to be effective. Sometimes there is a variety of routes by which a drug can be administered. For instance, the female hormone estrogen can be administered orally in the form of a pill or topically in the form of a skin patch. Table 31-6 lists numerous forms in which medications are prepared and routes through which they are administered.

TABLE 31-3 Classification of Drugs by Type or Usage With Examples

Type/Usage	Example
adrenergic	Isuprel (isoproterenol)
	Sudafed (pseudoephedrine hydrochloride HCL)
adrenergic blocking agent	Aldomet (methyldopa)
	Inderal (propranolol HCL)
analgesic	Advil (ibuprofen)
	Acetophen (aspirin)
	Darvon (propoxyphene HCL)
	Dilaudid (hydromorphine HCL)
	Demerol (meperidine HCL)
	Talwin (pentazocine HCL)
	Tylenol (acetaminophen)
anesthetic	Carbocaine (mepivacaine HCL)
	Novocaine (procaine HCL)
	Nupercaine (dibucaine HCL)
	Xylocaine (lidocaine HCL)
antacid	Milk of Magnesia (magnesia magma)
	Mylanta (aluminum hydroxide)
	Maalox (aluminum hydroxide)
antianxiety	Valium (diazepam)
antiarrhythmic	Digoxin (digoxin)
	Norpace (disopyramide)
	Pronestyl (procainamide HCL)
antibiotic	
Aminogylcosides	Garamycin (gentamicin sulfate)
	Kantrex (kanamycin)
	Mycifradin Sulfate (neomycin sulfate)
	Nebcin (tobramycin sulfate)
	Neobiotic (neomycin sulfate)
Cephalosporins	Ancef (cefazolin sodium)
	Anspor (cephradine)

(Continued on next page)

TABLE 31-3 *(Continued)*

Type/Usage	Example
Cephalosporins	Ceclor (cefaclor)
	Duricef (cefadroxil)
	Keflix (cephalexin)
	Keflin (cephalothin sodium)
Penicillins	Amoxil (amoxicillin)
	Bicillin (penicillin G potassium)
	Duracillin (penicillin G procaine)
	Polycillin (ampicillin)
Tetracyclines	Acromycin (tetracycline HCL)
	Declomycin (democlocycline)
	Terramycin (oxytetracycline)
	Vibramycin (doxycycline Hyclate)
anticholinergic	Atropine (atropine sulfate)
	Banthine (methantheline bromide)
	Donnatol (belladonna)
anticoagulant	Coumadin (warfarin sodium)
anticonvulsant	Dilantin (phenytoin sodium)
	Phenobarbital (phenobarbitol)
antidepressant	Elavil (amitriptyline HCL)
antidiabetic	Insulin and oral medications: Precose and Metformin
antidiarrheal	Kaopectate (kaolin and pectin mixture)
	Lomotil (diphenoxylate)
antiemetics	Atarax (hydroxyzine HCL)
	Compazine (prochlorperazine)
	Dramamine (dimenhydrinate)
	Phenergan (promethazine HCL)
antifungal	Mycostatin (nystatin)
antihelminthics	Vermox (mebendazole)
antihistamine	Adrenalin (epinephrine)
	Benadryl (diphenhydramine)

(Continued)

Type/Usage	Example
antihistamine	Chlor-Trimeton (chlorapheneramine maleate)
	Dimetane (brompheniramine maleate)
antihypertensives	Aldomet (methyldopa)
	Catapres (clonidine HCL)
	Lopressor (metoprolol tartrate)
	Minipress (prazosin HCL)
anti-inflammatory	Aspirin (acetylsalisylic acid)
	Indocin (indomethacin)
	Motrin (naprosyn)
	Nalfon (fenoprofen calcium)
	Naproxen (naprosyn)
antineoplastic	Cytoxan (cyclophosphamide)
	Fluorouracil (5FU)
	Adriamycin (doxorubicin HCL)
antipruritic	Calamine lotion (calamine)
	Hydrocortone (hydrocortisone sodium phosphate)
antipyretic	Advil (ibuprofen)
	Aspirin (acetylsalicylic acid)
	Tylenol (acetaminophen)
antiseptic	Cidex (glutarldehyde)
	pHisoHex (hexachlorophene)
antitussive	Codeine (codeine phosphate)
bronchodilator	Alupent (metaproterenol sulfate)
	Brethine (terbutaline sulfate)
	Isuprel (isoproterenol HCL)
	Theolair (theophylline)
contraceptive	Ortho-Novum 10/11-21 (estrogen with progestogen)
	Enovid-E 21 (estrogen with progestogen)
decongestant	Neo-Synephrine (phenylephrine HCL)
	Sudafed (pseudoephedrine HCL)
diuretic	Diuril (chlorothiazide)

(Continued on next page)

TABLE 31-3   *(Continued)*

Type/Usage	Example
diuretic	Hygroton (chlorthalidone)
	Lasix (furosemide)
emetic	Ipecac syrup
estrogen	Estrace (estrogen)
expectorant	Robitussin (guaifenesin)
hormone	Testosterone
	Premarin, estrogen
hypnotic	Seconal (secobarbital)
hypoglycemic	Precose (oral)
	Metformin (oral)
laxative	Dulcolax (bisacodyl)
muscle relaxant	Valium (diazepam)
	Robaxin (methocarbamol)
narcotic	Demerol (meperidine HCL)
	Percodan
purgative	Ex-Lax (phenolphthalein)
psychedelic	LSD (lysergic acid diethylamide)
sedative and hypnotic	Amytal (amobarbital)
	Butisol (butabarbital sodium)
	Nembutal Sodium (phenobarbital)
	Seconal Sodium (secobarbital sodium)
	Valium (diazepam)
stimulant	Dexedrine (dextroamphetamine sulfate)
tranquilizer	Haldol (haloperidol)
vasodilator	Isordil (isorbide dinitrate)
	Nitro-bid (nitroglycerin)
	Nitrostat (nitroglycerin)
vasopressor	Levophed (norepinephrine)
vitamin	Vitamin A
	Vitamin C
	Vitamin D
	Vitamin K

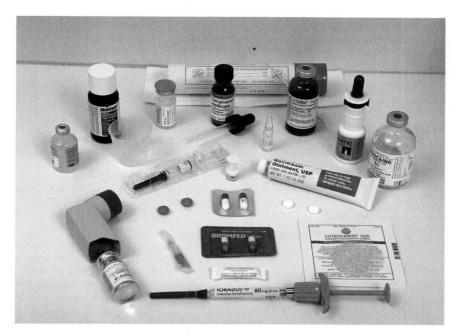

Figure 31-1 Different types of medication require different routes of administration.

TABLE 31-4   Methods for Parenteral Administration of Drugs

Method	Description
Intradermal	A very shallow injection just within the top layer of skin. This is a method commonly used in skin testing for allergies and tuberculosis.
Subcutaneous (SC)	An injection under the skin and fat layers. The middle of the upper, outer arm is usually used.
Intramuscular (IM)	An injection directly into the muscle of the buttocks or upper arm (deltoid). This method is used when there is a large amount of medication or it is irritating.
Intravenous (IV)	An injection into the veins. This route can be set up so that there is a continuous administration of medication, usually post-op a major surgery or during a major procedure.
Intrathecal	Injection into the meninges space surrounding the brain and spinal cord.
Intracavity	Injection into a body cavity such as the peritoneal and chest cavity.

Frequently Administered Drugs

New drugs are constantly being developed, researched, tested, and distributed by the pharmaceutical (drug) companies. As a result, broad spectrum antibiotics, that have the ability to be effective against a wide range of microorganisms, are frequently prescribed instead of a less-complex drug that targets more specific microorganisms.

Fifty of the most frequently dispensed drugs as listed in the *American Druggist* are noted in Table 31-7 along with the classification or group to which each belongs. The drugs are listed by brand name.

Side Effects of Medications

In addition to the desirable effects for which drugs are prescribed, there are undesirable side effects for all medications. In some cases these side effects can be lethal for the patient, so it is important to take these untoward (undesirable) effects seriously.

Some side effects are as simple as an individual patient's idiosyncrasy or reaction to the

TABLE 31-5   Non-parenteral Methods for Administering Drugs

Method	Description
Rectal	The drug is introduced directly into the rectal cavity in the form of suppositories or solution. Drugs may have to be administered by this route if the patient is unable to take them by mouth due to nausea, vomiting, and surgery of the mouth.
Inhalation	This category of drugs includes those that are inhaled directly into the nose and mouth. Aerosol sprays are administered by this route.
Topical	These drugs are applied directly to the skin or mucous membranes. They are distributed in ointment, cream or lotion form. These drugs are used to treat skin infections and eruptions. Transdermal patches, for example nicotrol, estraderm, and nitoderm.
Vaginal	Vaginal tablets and suppositories are used to treat vaginal yeast infections and other irritations.
Eye drops	Drugs placed into the eye to control eye pressure in glaucoma. Used during eye examinations to dilate the pupil of the eye for better examination of the interior of the eye. Also used to treat infections.
Ear drops	Drugs placed directly into the ear canal for the purpose of relieving pain or treating infection.
Buccal	Drugs, such as nitroglycerin for anginal pain, which are placed under the lip or between the cheek and gum.

TABLE 31-6   Routes of Drug Administration

Form	Route	Form	Route
aerosol	Inhalation	pills	Oral
caplets	Oral	powders	Topical
capsules	Oral	skin patch	Topical
elixir	Oral	spansules	Oral
liniment	Topical	spray	Oral, topical
lotion	Topical	suppository	Rectal, vaginal
lozenges	Oral	syrup	Oral
ointment	Topical	tablet	Oral

medication. See Table 31-8 for some medications that have a negative interaction with food products. In some cases, the effects are quite obvious, for example a rash, indicating an allergy to a medication. In other cases, the side effects are hidden and may require laboratory testing to detect. Some specific side effects to drugs include:

1. Anaphylactic shock is a life-threatening reaction in some people to a drug, food, or insect bite. This can cause severe respiratory distress, edema, convulsions, unconsciousness, and even death if untreated.

2. Drug tolerance that results in a decrease of a drug's effectiveness, may result after a continued use of the drug, such as in the case of an antibiotic. Another drug to which the patient has not yet developed a tolerance, will have to be prescribed. This is a problem when antibiotics are over prescribed for ailments, such as colds,

TABLE 31-7 Frequently Administered Drugs

Brand Name	Type	Brand Name	Type
1. Amoxil	antibiotic	26. Lopressor	beta-blocker
2. Lanoxin	cardiotonic	27. Lasix	diuretic
3. Zantac	antiulcer	28. Voltaren	nonsteroidal anti-inflammatory
4. Xanax	tranquilizer		
5. Premarin	hormone (estrogen)	29. Darvocet-N	analgesic (narcotic)
		30. Dilantin	anticonvulsant
6. Cardizem	cardiotonic	31. Monistat	antibiotic (antifungal)
7. Ceclor	antibiotic	32. Augmentin	antibiotic (pencillin)
8. Synthroid	hormone (thyroid)	33. Micronase	oral hypoglycemic agent
9. Seldane	antihistamine		
10. Tenormin	beta-blocker	34. Feldene	nonsteroidal anti-inflammatory
11. Vasotec	antihypertensive	35. Micro-K	potassium supplement
12. Tagamet	antiulcer	36. Provera	hormone (progestin)
13. Naprosyn	nonsteroidal anti-inflammatory	37. Motrin	nonsteroidal anti-inflammatory
14. Capoten	antihypertensive	38. Mevacor	cholesterol-lowering
15. Ortho-Novum 7/7/7	synthetic hormone	39. Triphasil	synthetic hormone
		40. Prozac	antidepressant
16. Dyazid	diuretic	41. Lo/Ovral	synthetic hormone
17. Ortho-Novum	synthetic hormone	42. Valium	tranquilizer
18. Proventil	bronchodilator	43. Retin-A	antiacne
19. Tylenol with codeine	analgesic (narcotic)	44. Cipro	antibiotic
		45. E-Mycin	antibiotic
20. Procardia	calcium channel blocker	46. Maxzide	diuretic
21. Calan	calcium channel blocker	47. Coumadin	anticoagulant
		48. Carafate	antiulcer
22. Ventolin	bronchodilator	49. Timoptic	beta-blocker
23. Inderal	beta-blocker	50. Slow-K	potassium supplement
24. Halcion	sedative		
25. Theo-Dur	bronchodilator		

TABLE 31-8   Drug-Food Interactions

Drug	Negative Reaction to Food
Accutane	Dairy products and food increase absorption.
Achromycin V	Dairy products and food interfere with absorption of tetracycline.
Apresoline	Food increases the plasma levels of the drug.
Antihypertensive drugs	Licorice decreases effect.
Hismanal	Food reduces absorption by 60%.
Bacampicillin HCL	Food decreases drug absorption.
Caffeine	Caffeine-containing beverages and food may cause irritability, nervousness, sleeplessness and rapid heartbeat.
Calcium gluconate	Cereals, bran, rhubarb, and spinach interfere with calcium absorption.
Capoten	Food reduces drug absorption by 30% to 40%.
Ceftin	Food increases drug absorption.
Coumadin	Diet high in vitamin K decreases prothrombin time.
Declomycin	Dairy products and food interfere with absorption.
Dicumarol	Diet high in vitamin K decreases prothrombin time.
Digoxin	Food high in bran fiber reduces availability of drug.
Erythromycin	Food interferes with absorption.
Feosol	Dairy products and eggs inhibit iron absorption.
Ibuprofen	Food reduces rate of absorption.
Inderal	Food increases availability of drug.
Monopril	Food slows rate of absorption.
Pepcid	Food increases availability of drug.
Plendil	Grapefruit juice doubles the concentration.
Procardia XL	Food alters rate of absorption.
Sinemet	High protein diet impairs absorption.
Synthroid	Soybean formula (in infants) causes excessive stools.
Xylocaine	Food enhances danger of aspiration due to topical anesthesia which may impair swallowing.

which will clear up naturally. An increase in the dosage of a drug beyond the recommended amount may result in a condition known as **toxicity** from that drug.

3. **Habituation**, or dependence on a drug, may develop to habit-forming drugs, such as laxatives and narcotics.

In general, unexpected side effects range from a rash and/or itching to drowsiness, runny nose, constipation, dizziness, headache, temporary ringing in the ears (tinnitus), blurred vision, loss of appetite, nausea, and vomiting.

The patient should be instructed to call the physician if these side effects are persistent or troublesome (Figure 31-2). The physician may ad-

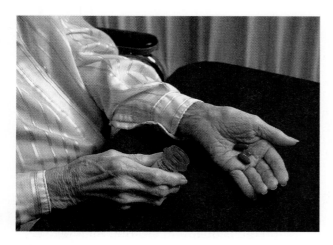

Figure 31-2   Older adults may need special assistance with medications.

just the medication dosage or change to a similar medication with fewer side effects. In all cases, patients should be instructed not to adjust the dosage themselves or stop taking the medication without consulting the physician. A placebo, which is an inactive harmless substance, such as a sugar pill, may occasionally be used by a physician to satisfy a patient's desire for unnecessary medication.

Drug Use During Pregnancy

Since the thalidomide tragedy during the 1950's when thousands of malformed babies were born after their mothers took this sedative during pregnancy, there has been better research and testing of drugs. Today most drugs carry special warnings concerning medication use during pregnancy either on the label or in the enclosed literature insert.

There are very few drugs that are approved for use during pregnancy. Even aspirin carries its dangers. Therefore it is especially important for women of child-bearing age to be warned about the risks. Fetal development during the first trimester is particularly at risk.

A woman should be asked for the date of her last menstrual period and whether she could be pregnant before she is administered any medication. Women should be cautioned to advise their physicians when there is a possibility of pregnancy.

Drug Use and the Breast Feeding Mother

Medications that a nursing mother takes do appear in breast milk. She should be instructed to breast feed before taking any medication since the blood levels are highest immediately after ingestion.

With a physician's permission, there are some medications, such as medication to control epilepsy, that the nursing mother can continue to take. However, there are medications which are contraindicated. This means the medications are so dangerous for the infant that the mother must stop breast feeding and place her baby on bottle feedings while she is taking any of these medications. These contraindicated medications include:

- Tetracyclines
- Chloramphenicol
- Sulfonamides (during the first 2 weeks postpartum)
- Oral anticoagulants
- Iodine-containing drugs
- Antineoplastics

A nursing mother should avoid taking any medication without talking to her physician first.

How to Read a Prescription

A prescription is not difficult to read once you understand the symbols that are used. Symbols and abbreviations based on Latin and Greek words are used in order to save time for the physician. For example, the abbreviation "po" meaning "to be taken by mouth" comes from the Latin words *per os* which mean by mouth. There are seven main parts to a prescription:

1. Patient's name, address, age (if a child), and date appear on the top line.
2. The superscription, consisting of the symbol Rx from the Latin term *recipe,* means "take thou." This symbol is usually preprinted on the prescription form.
3. The inscription specifies the name of the drug, actual ingredients, and the amount per dose.
4. The subscription tells the pharmacist how to mix the drug and the number of doses to supply to the patient.
5. The signa (Sig.) from the Latin term *signa,* means "mark." The instructions that should be given to the patient are stated here.
6. The physician's name, address, telephone number and DEA number. In some cases, all except the signature are printed at the top of each prescription blank. A prescription becomes a legal document when signed by the physician.
7. And finally, the number of times that the prescription can be refilled.

1. Medications/drugs can only be administered to a patient under the supervision of a licensed physician. To do otherwise is considered "practicing medicine without a license." The medication order must be written and signed on the patient's medical record by the physician.
2. The medical assistant acts as the liaison or intermediary between the physician and the patient. Some of the duties include ordering, storing, rotating, and checking expiration dates on medications.
3. Medications must be checked three times before administration.

The "Three Befores" are:

- Before medication is removed from the medication cabinet
- Before medication is poured or drawn up into a syringe
- Before medication is returned to the cabinet

4. Medications cannot be returned to the container once they have been removed. If they are not administered, they must be discarded.
5. Remember the "six rights" for administering medications (Figure 31-3).

The "Six Rights" are:

- Right patient
- Right medication
- Right dosage
- Right route
- Right time
- Right documentation

6. Keep a record of all allergies on the patient's medical record. Often these allergies are noted on the front of the medical record as well as within the medical record.
7. The documentation on the patient's medical record must include the following:
   a. Name of the medication
   b. Dosage
   c. Route of administration
   d. Date of administration
   e. Site of administration
   f. Signature of the person administering the medication along with initials designating the person's status, for example CMA or RMA
8. All narcotics must be recorded into a record maintained for that purpose. This is referred to as "logging a narcotic." Every narcotic must be accounted for.
9. Be careful that you administer the medication by the correct route. Methods of administration include:
   a. Oral (by mouth)
   b. Sublingual (under the tongue)
   c. Buccal (in the cheek)
   d. Rectal (inserted into the anal cavity)
   e. Vaginal (inserted into vaginal canal)
   f. Parenteral (by injection)
   g. Topical (applied to the skin)
   h. Inhalation (by breathing the medication)
   Medical assistants do not administer medications by the following routes:
   a. Intrathecal (into the meninges space)
   b. Intracavity (into a body cavity)
   c. Intravenous (IV) (into a vein)
10. Medication labels should be clean and readable. If they become soiled, unreadable, or fall off the container they must be discarded.
11. If you are not familiar with a particular medication, you must look it up in the *PDR*. Never violate this rule.
12. Know the side effects for the medication you are administering.
13. Always advise the patient to take the complete number of dosages ordered in the prescription. This is especially important when using antibiotics.
14. Advise the patient to only use medication for the member of the family or person it was prescribed for.

Figure 31-4 is an example of a prescription. In this example, the physician has ordered the medication Estrace which is a form of the hormone estrogen. The prescription tells the pharmacist to give 100 (dtd C) tablets, and orders a 1 mg dosage which is to be taken once a day (1 q am). The instruction to the pharmacist is to refill the prescription 3 times and not to substitute with another (generic) medication.

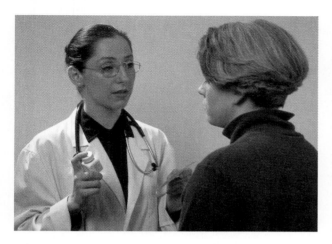

Figure 31-3 Remember the "Six Rights" when administering medications.

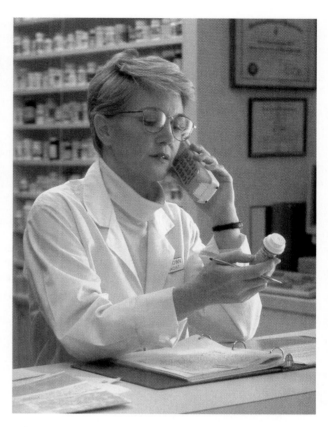

Figure 31-5 Speak with the pharmacist about any questions you have about prescription medications.

Beth Williams, MD
Windy City Clinic
123 Michigan Avenue
Chicago, IL 60000
Telephone (200) 555-9876

Name _Jane Doe_   Age _56_

Address _____

Date _2/14/xx_

Rx   _Estrace   1 mg_

Sig.   _i   q̄ ^AM_
Disp. # 100

Substitution Permissible _____ M.D.

"Prescriber must hand-write "Brand Necessary" or "Brand Medically Necessary" in the space below in order for a brand name product to be dispensed." _Brand Necessary_

B Williams MD M.D.

Refill   0   1   2   (3)   4   5   6

Figure 31-4 Sample prescription.

On some prescriptions, the physician will give a "prn" refill order meaning that the prescription can be refilled as needed. The physician will fill in the name, address, age of the patient and date. The physician must also sign his or her name at the bottom of the prescription. A blank prescription cannot be handed to a patient. Be sure that prescription blanks are not left out but in a secure place.

The physician's instructions to the patient will be placed on the label. The pharmacist will also include instructions about the medication and alert the patient to side effects of the medication that the patient may experience. These side effects may need to be reported to the physician. In addition, any special instructions regarding the medication (for example "take with meals" or "do not take along with dairy products") will also be supplied by the pharmacist. The label on the medication container must always be checked to match the prescription. If in doubt always question the pharmacist (Figure 31-5).

Some prescriptions can be filled by telephone. At such times, the patient's record should be pulled for the physician and the refill order or new medications prescribed should be documented.

Abbreviations Used in Pharmacology

Medical abbreviations are used extensively in pharmacology. The general public cannot usually decipher prescriptions due to the use of medical abbreviations. You will have to assist your patients with their questions.

> **Med Tip:** Many abbreviations have multiple meanings such as "od" which can mean either once a day (od) or right eye (OD) depending on whether the letters are small or capitalized. Care must be taken when reading abbreviations since some may be written too quickly making them difficult to decipher. Never create your own abbreviations. Some of the most common abbreviations used in pharmacology are listed in Table 31-9.

TABLE 31-9 Common Abbreviations Used in Pharmacology

Abbreviation	Meaning	Abbreviation	Meaning
@	At	dil	Dilute
ā	Before	dtd#	Give this number
aa	Of each	Dx	Diagnosis
ac	Before meals	dr	Dram
AD	Right ear	elix	Elixir
ad lib	As desired	emul	Emulsion
alt dieb	Alternate days	et	And
alt hor	Alternate hours	ext	Extract/external
alt noc	Alternate nights	Fe	Iron
am, AM	Morning	fl	Fluid
amt	Amount	G	Gauge
ante	Before	gal	Gallon
aq	Aqueous (water)	g	Gram
AS	Left ear	gr	Grain
AU	Both ears	gt	One drop
Ba	Barium	gtt	Two or more drops
bid	Twice a day	H	Hour/hypodermic
C	100	hs	Hour of sleep
c̄	With	IM	Intramuscular
cap(s)	Capsule(s)	inj	Injection
cc	Cubic centimeter	IV	Intravenous
d	Day	k	Potassium
DC, disc	Discontinue	kg	Kilogram
d/c, DISC	Discontinue	L	Liter
disp	Dispense		*(Continued)*

Abbreviation	Meaning	Abbreviation	Meaning
L	Left	qh	Every hour
liq	Liquid	qhs	Every night
M ft	Make	qid	Four times a day
mug	Microgram	qm	Every morning
mg	Milligram	qod	Every other day
mL	Milliliter	®	Right
mitt#	Give this number	Rx	Take
mm	Millimeter	s or s̄	Without
noct	Night	SC	Subcutaneous
non rep	Do not repeat	SOB	Shortness of breath
NPO	Nothing by mouth	Subc, SubQ	Subcutaneous
NS	Normal saline	Sig.	Label as follows/directions
noc	Night		
O	Pint	sl	Under the tongue
od	Once a day/daily	sol	Solution
OD	Right eye	ss or s̄s̄	One-half
o m	Every morning	stat	At once/immediately
OS	Left eye	subling	Sublingual
OU	Both eyes	suppos	Suppository
OTC	Over the counter	susp	Suspension
oz or ℥	Ounce	syr	Syrup
pc	After meals	T, tbsp	Tablespoon
per	With	tab	Tablet
PM	Evening	tid	Three times a day
po	By mouth	tinc/tr	Tincture
prn	As needed	top	Apply topically
pt	Pint	tsp	Teaspoon
pulv	Powder	u	Unit
q	Every	ung	Ointment
q2h	Every two hours	UT	Under the tongue
qam	Every morning	ut dict, UD	As directed
qd	Once a day/every day	wt	Weight

LEGAL AND ETHICAL ISSUES

You must always remember that even though you work under the supervision of a physician as a medical assistant, nevertheless, you are still legally and ethically responsible for your own actions. The physician must report any known patient drug abuse. As the medical assistant, you may be the first person to become aware of a patient's problem. It is therefore your ethical responsibility to inform the physician.

You have a responsibility for maintaining accurate records for all narcotic use. State laws regarding what a medical assistant may and may not do vary from state to state. You must become familiar with the laws in your own state. In addition, careful triple-checking of all medications before administering them, remaining current on all medications which are prescribed in your office, and remembering the "six rights" of drug administration will help to protect you legally and ethically. Never administer a medication with which you are unfamiliar.

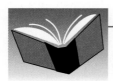

PATIENT EDUCATION

Patient education is especially important when working with medications. Instructions regarding the type of medication prescribed, dosage, side effects, and reaction with foods must be clearly explained. You may have to develop teaching materials and aids, such as a written schedule indicating when medications should be taken, to assist patients who have difficulty remembering.

It is the medical assistant's responsibility to keep the physician informed of all medications patients have indicated they are taking, as well as any allergies the patients may have to specific medications. Patients have to be instructed to throw out all out-dated medications. Patients must be warned to keep medications out of the reach of children, and, of course, never to share their medicines with others.

Summary

The medical assistant works directly under the supervision of the physician. This relationship needs to be well understood with regard to medication administration. The medical assistant must know the legalities concerning the limitations of his or her credentials. A medical assistant may administer medications only when they have been prescribed and documented on the patient's medical record by a licensed physician. At no time can the medical assistant prescribe even the simplest of drugs, for example an aspirin. A medical assistant can lose his or her certification for "practicing medicine without a license."

In addition to knowing how drugs are classified—prescription, nonprescription, and controlled substances—the medical assistant must have a thorough knowledge of dosage, abbreviations, and side effects relating to medications. In whatever situation you work, be sure to follow the federal, state, and local regulations regarding the administration, storage, inventory, and dispensing of drugs.

Competency Review

1. Define and spell the glossary terms for this chapter.
2. Name the governmental agency which enforces drug sales and distribution.
3. Describe the differences between the legal, commercial, and chemical names for a drug.
4. List 10 of the 14 precautions to observe when administering medications.
5. Name a reference book that is one of the most frequently used sources of information when administering medications in the physician's office.
6. Name the federal act that controls the use of drugs causing dependency.
7. List the "six rights" to medication administration.
8. Discuss the "three befores" that must take place before dispensing medication.
9. Describe what you would do when a patient indicates a drug allergy.
10. State under what conditions a medical assistant may administer a medication.
11. Define "logging a narcotic."
12. List the information that must be charted when administering a medication.
13. Explain the functions of the following types of medication: diuretic, bronchodilator, antiemetic, hypnotic, sedative, anti-inflammatory agent, vasodilator, anti-convulsive, anesthetic, analgesic, antacid, antibiotic, anticoagulant, antihistamine.
14. Write out the following prescription instructions:
    a. Pravachol, 20 mg., Sig. i qd @ noc, dtd 30, refill 3x, no sub.
    b. Lanoxin 0.125 mg., Sig. iii stat, then ii a AM, dtd C, refills prn.
    c. Synthroid 0.075 mg., Sig. i qd, C, refill x4.
    d. Norvasc 5 mg., i q am, dtd 60, refillable.

PREPARING FOR THE CERTIFICATION EXAM

Test Taking Tip — Wear a watch when you study for an exam or take a test. Pace yourself so that you can work quickly not spending too much time on any one question.

Examination Review Questions

1. The chemical name for the OTC medication Aleve is
   (A) acetaminophen
   (B) naproxen sodium
   (C) Naprosyn
   (D) Tylenol
   (E) Aldomet

2. According to the Drug Enforcement Agency, controlled substances
   (A) can be addictive
   (B) may have the potential for abuse by a patient
   (C) must be kept under a lock and key
   (D) (the dispensation of) must be recorded in a narcotic's log
   (E) all of the above

3. An example of a Schedule IV drug is
   (A) Xanax
   (B) morphine
   (C) Vicodin
   (D) MS Contin
   (E) Tylenol with codeine

4. Capoten, which is an ACE inhibitor, is classified as an
   (A) antibiotic
   (B) anti-inflammatory
   (C) antipruritic
   (D) antihypertensive
   (E) antipyretic

5. Which of the following is a method for the administration of a drug by means of an injection under the skin and fat layers?
   (A) intradermal
   (B) intramuscular
   (C) subcutaneous
   (D) intravenous
   (E) intrathecal

(Continued on next page)

6. A non-parenteral method for administering drugs would be
   (A) inhalation
   (B) topical
   (C) vaginal
   (D) buccal
   (E) all of the above

7. The "Six Rights" a medical assistant must observe when administering medications include the right medication, documentation, and
   (A) time
   (B) route
   (C) dosage
   (D) patient
   (E) all of the above

8. Which, if any, of the following routes of administration may not be used by a medical assistant?
   (A) ID
   (B) IV
   (C) IM
   (D) Z-track IM
   (E) SC

9. Which part of a prescription precedes the instructions that should be given to the patient?
   (A) Sig.
   (B) Rx
   (C) superscription
   (D) inscription
   (E) subscription

10. A common abbreviation, used in pharmacology, that means "as needed" is
   (A) aa
   (B) ac
   (C) prn
   (D) ante
   (E) NS

ON THE JOB

Dr. Waring is in solo practice. When she is on vacation, she arranges for Dr. Dumphey to cover her patients. Dr. Dumphey's medical assistant, Theresa, has just received a call from a patient of Dr. Waring's.

The patient is an elderly woman, with multiple medical problems, who is experiencing what may be a reaction to a medication that Dr. Waring prescribed 2 days ago for bronchitis. Her symptoms include nausea, upset stomach, dizziness, headache, rash on her chest, and extreme exhaustion. Theresa senses that the patient may be exhibiting some disorientation to time and place as it is difficult to elicit consistent responses from her regarding her medications.

The patient is reporting to Theresa that the newest medication she has been taking is Bioxin. The other medications she says she takes include Prinivil, Cardizem CD, Premarin, Prilosec, Robaxin, Zocor, Prozac, Ambien, Fosamax, Seldane and aspirin. The patient does not know the dosage of any of these medications, but is willing to "open up her bag of medicine" and read each prescription label to Theresa. What should Theresa do?

What is your response?

1. Does Theresa have an obligation, as Dr. Dumphey's medical assistant, to handle this situation with this patient or should Dr. Waring simply be notified?

2. Is this an emergency situation, or potential emergency situation and, if so, what should Theresa do immediately?

3. Since the patient seems disoriented, should Theresa even trust in what the patient is reporting? Would it be appropriate for Theresa to speak to a member of Theresa's family, perhaps, in this regard?

4. Should Theresa have the patient read the label of each of her medications?

5. Consider the newly prescribed medication, Bioxin, that the patient is taking. Could this medication cause the adverse reaction that the patient is reporting?

6. Given the other medications that the patient is reporting taking, could Bioxin be interacting with any of them and, therefore, causing an adverse reaction?

References

Anderson, K., and Anderson, L. *Mosby's Pocket Dictionary of Medicine, Nursing, & Allied Health.* Chicago: Mosby, 1994.

Bledsoe, B., Clayden, D. and Papa, F. *Prehospital Emergency Pharmacology,* 4th ed. Upper Saddle River, NJ: Brady/Prentice Hall, 1996.

Hemby, M. *Medical Assisting Review.* Upper Saddle River, NJ: Brady/Prentice Hall, 1995.

Hitner, H. and Nagle, B. *Basic Pharmacology for Health Occupations,* 3rd ed. New York: Glencoe, 1994.

Levine, G. *Pocket Guide to Commonly Prescribed Drugs.* Stamford, CT: Appelton & Lange, 1996.

Lewis, M. and Tamparo, C. *Medical Law, Ethics, and Bioethics in the Medical Office.* Philadelphia: F.A. Davis Company, 1993.

Moore, H. and Best, G. *Drug Calculations.* Upper Saddle River, NJ: Prentice Hall, 1995.

Nurse's Pocket Companion. Springhouse, PA: Springhouse Corporation, 1993.

Physicians' Desk Reference, 44th ed. Oradell, NJ: Medical Economics, 1990.

Prescription Drugs. Lincolnwood, IL: Publications International, Ltd., 1995.

Professional Guide to Drugs. Horsham, PA: Intermed Communications, Inc., 1991.

Schwinghammer, T. *Pharmacology: A Patient Focused Approach.* Stamford, CT: Appelton & Lange, 1997.

Spratto, G. and Woods, A. *Nurse's Drug Reference.* Boston: Delmar, 1997.

Stringer, J. *Basic Concepts in Pharmacology.* St. Louis: McGraw-Hill, 1996.

Taber's Cyclopedic Medical Dictionary, 18th ed. Philadelphia, F.A. Davis Company, 1997.

Watts, E. *Pharmacology for Medical Assistants.* Upper Saddle River, NJ: Prentice Hall, 1987.

MEDICAL ASSISTANT ROLE DELINEATION CHART

Highlight indicates material covered in this chapter

ADMINISTRATIVE

ADMINISTRATIVE PROCEDURES

- Perform basic clerical functions
- Schedule, coordinate, and monitor appointments
- Schedule inpatient/outpatient admissions and procedures
- Understand and apply third party guidelines
- Obtain reimbursement through accurate claims submission
- Monitor third-party reimbursement
- Perform medical transcription
- Understand and adhere to managed care policies and procedures
- *Negotiate managed care contracts (adv)*

PRACTICE FINANCES

- Perform procedural and diagnostic coding
- Apply bookkeeping principles
- Document and maintain accounting and banking records
- Manage accounts receivable
- Manage accounts payable
- Process payroll
- *Develop and maintain fee schedules (adv)*
- *Manage renewals of business and professional insurance policies (adv)*
- *Manage personal benefits and maintain records (adv)*

CLINICAL

FUNDAMENTAL PRINCIPLES

- Apply principles of aseptic technique and infection control
- Comply with quality assurance practices
- Screen and follow up patient test results

DIAGNOSTIC ORDERS

- Collect and process specimens
- Perform diagnostic tests

PATIENT CARE

- Adhere to established triage procedures
- Obtain patient history and vital signs
- Prepare and maintain examination and treatment areas

- Prepare patient for examinations, procedures, and treatments
- Assist with examinations, procedures, and treatments
- Prepare and administer medications and immunizations
- Maintain medication and immunization records
- Recognize and respond to emergencies
- Coordinate patient care information with other health care providers

GENERAL (TRANSDISCIPLINARY)

PROFESSIONALISM

- Project a professional manner and image
- Adhere to ethical principles
- Demonstrate initiative and responsibility
- Work as a team member
- Manage time efficiently
- Prioritize and perform multiple tasks
- Adapt to change
- Promote the CMA credential
- Enhance skills through continuing education

COMMUNICATION SKILLS

- Treat all patients with compassion and empathy
- Recognize and respect cultural diversity
- Adapt communications to individual's ability to understand
- Use professional telephone technique
- Use effective and correct verbal and written communications
- Recognize and respond to verbal and nonverbal communications
- Use medical terminology appropriately
- Receive, organize, prioritize, and transmit information
- Serve as liaison
- Promote the practice through positive public relations

LEGAL CONCEPTS

- Maintain confidentiality
- Practice within the scope of education, training, and personal capabilities
- Prepare and maintain medical records
- Document accurately
- Use appropriate guidelines when releasing information
- Follow employer's established policies dealing with the health care contract
- Follow federal, state, and local legal guidelines
- Maintain awareness of federal and state health care legislation and regulations
- Maintain and dispose of regulated substances in compliance with government guidelines
- Comply with established risk management and safety procedures
- Recognize professional credentialing criteria
- Participate in the development and maintenance of personnel, policy, and procedure manuals
- *Develop and maintain personnel, policy, and procedure manuals (adv)*

INSTRUCTION

- Instruct individuals according to their needs
- Explain office policies and procedures
- Teach methods of health promotion and disease prevention
- Locate community resources and disseminate information
- *Orient and train personnel (adv)*
- *Develop educational materials (adv)*
- *Conduct continuing education activities (adv)*

OPERATIONAL FUNCTIONS

- Maintain supply inventory
- Evaluate and recommend equipment and supplies
- Apply computer techniques to support office operations
- *Supervise personnel (adv)*
- *Interview and recommend job applicants (adv)*
- *Negotiate leases and prices for equipment and supply contracts (adv)*

SOURCE: Reprinted by permission of the American Association of Medical Assistants from the *AAMA Role Delineation Study: Occupational Analysis of the Medical Assisting Profession.*

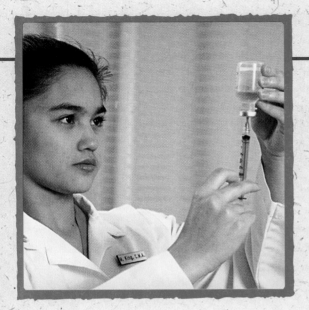

32

Administering Medications

LEARNING OBJECTIVES

After completing this chapter, you should:
1. Define and spell the glossary terms for this chapter.
2. State the difference between the apothecary and the metric systems.
3. Correctly calculate medication dosage using mathematical equivalents.
4. State four rules for calculating pediatric dosage.
5. Describe the OSHA standards relating to needle sticks.
6. Correctly describe the procedure for the administration of oral medications.
7. Correctly describe the procedure for the administration of parenteral medications.
8. List the standard needle lengths and gauges.
9. List and define the four sites for intramuscular injections (IM).
10. State the rationale for using the Z-track injection method.
11. State the names of ten drugs commonly found in the medical office.
12. List the precautions used when administering an injection to an infant or small child.

CLINICAL PERFORMANCE OBJECTIVES

After completing this chapter, you should perform the following tasks:
1. Correctly calculate drug dosage.
2. Prepare a medication for injection using the correct sterile technique.
3. Correctly inject medication into the deltoid, gluteus medius, and vastus lateralis muscles using the proper needle and syringe.
4. Correctly inject medication using the subcutaneous route of administration.
5. Correctly administer an intradermal injection using the proper needle and syringe.
6. Correctly administer a medication using the Z-track method.
7. Instruct a patient on the use of vaginal medications.
8. Instruct the patient on the use of rectal medications.

Glossary

apothecary system A system of weights and measures, used by physicians and pharmacists, that is based on these basic units of measurements: grain (gr.), gram (g), and dram (℥), for example. This system has been replaced by the metric system whenever possible.

handbreadth Use the size and surface of one's hand to measure distance on a patient for injection purposes.

metric system A system of weights and measures based upon the meter as the unit of measurement. This system uses the decimal system.

untoward effect An unexpected or adverse reaction of a patient to a medication.

WARNING!

For all patient contact, adhere to Standard Precautions (see pages 342–373). Wear protective equipment as indicated.

One of the most important functions for the medical assistant is administering medications. Pharmacology and drug therapy involve the skills and expertise of many health care professionals including the physician, pharmacist, nurse, and medical assistant. The role of the medical assistant in administering the correct medication at the correct time and in the proper amount is a critical part of the process. Before proceeding with this chapter, review the "three befores" and the "six rights" of drug administration discussed in Chapter 31.

Weights and Measures

Two systems of weights and measurements are used to calculate dosages: apothecary and metric. The medical assistant must be familiar with both systems since drugs may be ordered in one system but contain a label in another system. You will have to be able to easily convert from one system to another. In addition, there are common household measurements, such as teaspoon (t) and tablespoon (T), which are used even though they are not considered medical measurement units. These household measures are useful when instructing patients.

The Apothecary System

The **apothecary system** is considered to be the oldest system of measurement. Dry weight equivalent is 1 grain = 1 gram of wheat. The basic units of weight are grain (gr), gram (g), dram (℥), ounce (℥), and pound (lb). Fluid measurements using the apothecary system are called minims (mn), fluid dram (fl ℥), fluid ounce (fl ℥), pint (pt), quart (qt), and gallon (c). Some of common household measures, for example pint, quart, and gallon, are based on the apothecary system.

Roman numerals are used when numbering in this system. For example, 3 grains would be gr iii and 4 ounces would be ℥ iv. The apothecary system also uses fractions such as 1/4, 1/2, 2/3. Therefore three-fourths of a grain would be gr 3/4. The unit of measurement (gr) is placed before the dosage in the apothecary system.

The Metric System

The **metric system** is used more widely for prescriptions. This system of measurement is based on the decimal system. This means that all the numbers are derived by either multiplying or dividing by the power of 10. In the metric system, the liter (l) means volume, gram (g) stands for weight, and meter (m) represents length. See Table 32-1 for common abbreviations for weights and measures.

When using the metric system, the dosage is written as a decimal with the unit of measurement (such as mL) following.

See Table 32-2 for commonly used equivalents.

Table 32-3 lists some common household measures.

For a comparison of the three systems for liquid measurements see Table 32-4.

Drug Calculation

Some offices and clinics keep a supply of medications which are referred to as stock medications. The physician may order a medication dosage for

TABLE 32-1 Common Abbreviations for Weights and Measures

Apothecary System			Metric System	
Symbol/Abbreviation		**Meaning**	**Symbol/Abbreviation Weights**	**Meaning**
gtt	drop	drop	mg	milligram
m	Min	minim	gm	gram
ʒ	dr	dram	**Symbol/Abbreviation Volume**	**Meaning**
	f dr	fluid dram		
℥	oz	ounce	L	liter
	fl oz	fluid ounce	mL	milliliter
O	pt	pint	cc	cubic centimeter
C	gal	gallon		
	gr	grain		

Guidelines: Conversion Within the Metric System

1. There is no change necessary to change milliliters into cubic centimeters. They are equal to each other.
2. To change grams to milligrams, multiply grams by 1000 or move the decimal point 3 places to the RIGHT.
3. To change milligrams to grams, divide milligrams by 1000 or move the decimal point 3 places to the LEFT.
4. To convert liters to milliliters, multiply liters by 1000 or move the decimal point 3 places to the RIGHT.
5. To convert milliliters to liters, divide milliliters by 1000 or move the decimal point 3 places to the LEFT.

 Med Tip: By placing the greater than (>)or less than (<) signs between the units, you can see which way to move the decimal point.

a patient that is different from the dosage of the medication you keep in stock.

You may have a conversion chart to use when calculating the correct dosage from a stock dosage. However, it is necessary for you to know how to arrive at the correct calculation of a dose so that you can double-check for accuracy.

Calculating the correct amount of drug to give a patient depends on many factors including pa-

tient's age, weight, and current state of health. In addition, you will need to know what other medications the patient is taking since some drugs will be either weakened or strengthened in combination with other drugs.

After receiving the medication order from the physician, the medical assistant should check to see if the order and the medication label are written in the same system of measurement. In other words, is everything in the metric system or in the apothecary system? If a combination of the two systems has been used (for example, physician's order is written in the metric system and the medication label is in the apothecary system), you will have to use a conversion chart as in Tables 32-2 and 32-4.

Dosages can be calculated using either the formula method or by ratios. Both methods will be explained in this chapter. You should use the method that is easiest for you.

Review of Math Principles

In order to understand the methods used for drug calculations, you must refresh your memory concerning mathematics. Remember that there is a relationship between fractions, ratios, percentages, and decimals. Refer to Table 32-5 for examples of some mathematical equivalents.

For example, the fraction 1/2 is the same as the ratio 1:2 (one-to-two). A ratio is another way of expressing a fraction. This is also the same as the percentage 50% and the decimal .50.

Using ratios is one method for calculating the correct drug dosage from a stock dosage. We

TABLE 32-2   **Commonly Used Equivalents for the Apothecary and Metric Systems**

Measure Apothecary	Equivalent Metric
1 gr	65 mg or 0.065 g
5 gr	325 mg or 0.33 g
10 gr	650 mg or 0.67 g
15 or 16 gr	1 g
15 or 16 m	1.00 mL or cc
1 dram	4 mL
1 oz	30 cc, 30 mL, 8 tsp, 8 drams, 3 tbsp
1 lb	450 g
1 lb	0.4536 kg
1 minim (m)	0.06 mL
4 m	0.25 mL
Liquid Measure	
1 fl dr	4 mL
2 fl dr	8 mL
2.5 fl dr	10 mL
4 fl dr	15 mL
1 fl oz	30 mL
3.5 fl oz	100 mL
7 fl oz	200 mL
1 pt	500 mL
1 qt	1000 mL
60 gtts	4 mL

would compare the amount of drug the physician ordered to the amount we have on hand (stock medications).

To determine a percentage from a fraction, divide the numerator (top number) by the denominator (bottom number). The decimal number that results can then be converted into a percentage by moving the decimal point two spaces to the right.

For example:
1/2 = 1 ÷ 2 = .50
.50 = 50.0% or 50%

When you have two ratios to compare, you then have a proportion. A proportion resulting from the fraction 1/2 or ratio 1:2 could be 10/20 = 1/2 or 10:20 :: 1:2. The proportion is read as 10 divided by 20 equals 1 divided by 2, or ten is to twenty as one is to two. Even though the numbers may be larger, the actual proportions or relationship to each other is the same. If you know three numbers in the above equation (10/20 = 1/2 or 10:20 :: 1:2), you can solve for the fourth, or unknown quantity by using mathematic principles. We use the symbol x for the unknown quantity. For example: 10/20 = 1/x

TABLE 32-3   Common Household Measures

Measure	Equivalent
60 gtts. (drops)	1 teaspoon (tsp.)
3 tsp	1 Tablespoon (T.)
2 T	1 oz
4 oz	1 small juice glass
8 oz	1 cup (C) or glass
16 T. or 8 oz	1 C
2 Cups	1 pint (pt)
2 pints	1 quart (qt)
4 quarts	1 gallon

TABLE 32-4   Comparison of Household/Apothecary/Metric Liquid Measurements

Household	Apothecary	Metric
1 drop	1 minim (m)	0.06 mL
1 tsp.	1 fl dr (fl ℥)	4-5 mL
1 T	4 fl dr (fl ℥)	15-16 mL
2 T	1 fl oz (fl ℥)	30-32 mL
1 cup or glass	8 fl oz (fl ℥)	250 mL
2 cups or glasses	16 fl oz/ 1 pt	500 mL
4 cups or glasses	1 qt	1000 mL = approximately 1 liter

TABLE 32-5   Example of Mathematical Equivalents

Fraction	Ratio	Percent	Decimal
1/4	1:4	25%	.25
1/2	1:2	50%	.50
2/3	2:3	66%	.66
3/4	3:4	75%	.75
7/8	7:8	88%	.88
1/100	1:100	1%	.01
1/200	1:200	.5%	.005
1/1000	1:1000	.1%	.001

Cross-multiply to find the unknown quantity. To cross-multiply means to multiply the top number against the opposite bottom number. Therefore $10 \times x = 1 \times 20$. Restate this to $10x = 20$. Since we want to find the value of x, we need to have it stand alone. If we divide both sides of the equation by the same number, we can have x stand alone. Therefore, $10x \div 10 = 1x$ or x. Next divide the other side of the equation by 10. $20 \div 10 = 2$. This means that $x = 2$.

$$\frac{10}{20} \diagdown\!\!\!\!\diagup \frac{1}{x} = 10 \times x = 20 \times 1$$
$$10x = 20$$
$$\frac{10x}{10} = \frac{20}{10}$$
$$1x = 2$$
$$x = 2$$

Another method is to convert $\dfrac{10}{20} = \dfrac{1}{x}$ into the ratio $10:20 :: 1:x$.

Then, multiply the extremes (two outer numbers 10 and x) by each other and the means (the two inner numbers 20 and 1) to solve for x (the unknown).

$$10 : 20 :: 1 : x$$
$$10 \times x = 20 \times 1$$
$$10x = 20$$
$$20 \div 10 = 2$$
$$2 = x$$
$$2 \text{ cc} = x$$

To prove this answer is correct multiply the extremes and multiply the means. If the answer is correct, they will be equal.

$$10 : 20 :: 1 : 2$$
$$10 \times 2 = 20 \times 1$$
$$20 = 20 \quad \text{Proven}$$

Problem: Physician's order is to give 80 mg of Lasix. The supply on hand states that there is 40 mg/cc.

$$80 \text{ mg} : x \text{ cc} :: 40 \text{ mg} : 1 \text{ cc}$$
$$80 \times 1 = 40 \times x$$
$$80 = 40x$$
$$x = 2 \text{ cc}$$

2 cc of Lasix needs to be administered to give an 80 mg dose using the Lasix in stock (40 mg/cc).

Calculating Dosages

Using the concepts about ratios you have just reviewed, it is possible to calculate dosages using a formula. To find an amount of a drug that is needed to administer set up the following formula (proportion).

Calculation Formula:
$$\frac{\text{available strength}}{\text{ordered strength}} = \frac{\text{available amount}}{\text{amount to give}}$$

- Available strength = The potency (strength) of the drug you have in stock.
- Available amount = (What actually contains the drug.)

For instance, a vial marked 1000 mg/cc. means that in every 1 cc. of liquid there is contained 1000 mg of medication. An oral pill that contains 10 gr. means that 10 grains of medication are in every pill.

- Ordered strength = The potency or strength the physician has ordered in this prescription.
- Amount to give = This is the unknown amount (x) or the amount that you will be solving the problem to find.
  Using this formula we can solve the following problem.

Physician's order: Give 500 mg of a drug.
Available: A vial which contains 1000 mg/cc.

Calculation Formula:
$$\frac{\text{available strength}}{\text{ordered strength}} = \frac{\text{available amount}}{\text{amount to give}}$$

Strength of the drug in the vial = 1000 mg/cc.
Available amount = 1 cc
Ordered Strength = 500 mg
Amount to give = x

$$\frac{1000 \text{ mg}}{500 \text{ mg}} = \frac{1 \text{ cc}}{x}$$
$$1000 \times x = 500 \times 1$$
$$1000x = 500$$
$$\frac{1000x}{1000} = \frac{500}{1000}$$
$$1x = 5/10 = 1/2 \text{ cc} = 0.5 \text{ cc}$$

You would fill the syringe with 0.5 cc of liquid to give you the physician's order of 500 mg of medication. To solve a problem using other forms of medication, such as tablets, use the same formula.

Physician's order: Give 10 grains of medication.
Available: Tablets containing 2.5 grains each.

Calculation Formula:

$$\frac{\text{available strength}}{\text{ordered strength}} = \frac{\text{available amount}}{\text{amount to give}} =$$
$$\text{HAVE/WANT}$$

2.5 gr = 1 tablet
10 gr x (no. of tablets)
$2.5 \times x = 10 \times 1$
$2.5x = 10$
$$\frac{2.5x}{2.5} = \frac{10}{2.5}$$
$1x = 4$ tablets

Another formula that is frequently used is D/H × Quantity.

D = Desired or ordered dose
H = Supply on hand or available supply
Q = Quantity available

Problem: The physician ordered Penicillin 250 mg. The bottle from the supply you have in stock is labeled "Penicillin 500 mg per cc."

Solution: Set up the formula
$$\frac{\text{Desired}}{\text{Hand}} \times \text{Quantity}$$

The physician's order is placed in the Desired (D) space and the supply you have on hand is placed in the Hand (H) space. The quantity per cc is placed in the Quantity (Q) space.

$$\frac{D}{H} \times Q = \frac{250}{500} \times 1$$
Divide 250 by 500 $\times \frac{1}{1} = 0.5$ cc.

The answer is 0.5 cc or 1/2 a cc.

Rules for Conversion

Remember that in converting from one system to another the equivalencies are only going to be approximate. It may be necessary to round off the amounts. A simplified list of conversions that you may wish to memorize is found in Table 32-6. It is based on Table 32-2.

Guidelines: Conversion

1. To change grains to grams, divide by 15.
2. To change ounces to cubic centimeters (cc's), multiply by 30.
3. To change grains to milligrams (mg), multiply by 60. (Only use this rule when you have less than one grain.)
4. To change kilograms to pounds, multiply by 2.2.
5. To change cubic centimeters (cc's) to ounces, divide by 30.
6. To change drams to milliliters (mL), multiply by 4.
7. To change cubic centimeters (cc) or milliliters (mL) to minims, multiply by 15 or 16.
8. To change minims to cubic centimeter's (cc's), divide by 15 or 16.
9. To convert drams to grams, multiply by 4.

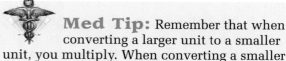

Med Tip: Remember that when converting a larger unit to a smaller unit, you multiply. When converting a smaller unit to a larger unit, you divide.

TABLE 32-6   **Conversion List**

Apothecary	Metric
15 or 16 minims (m)	1 mL or 1 cc
1 fluid dr	4 mL or cc
1 fluid oz	30 mL or cc
1 quart	1000 mL or cc
1/60 grain	1 milligram (mg)
1 grain	0.065 gram
15 grains	1 gram
2.2 pounds	1 kilogram

Calculating Pediatric Doses

Adult medications are generally not suitable for children even if the dosage is changed. However, there are situations when only an adult dose is available. In that event, a child's—pediatric—dosage can be calculated using the adult dosage as the base.

Determining the correct dosage for a child is the responsibility of the physician. You may be asked to assist by performing the calculations. However, this can only be done under the supervision of the physician.

There are several rules or "laws" for calculating pediatric dosage which bear the names of the person who developed the rule. These include Clark's Rule, Fried's Law, Young's Law, and West's Nomogram.

Clark's Rule

Clark's Rule is based on the weight of the child. Many physicians favor using this rule since children's weight at a particular age can vary greatly from one child to another. The formula for Clark's Rule is:

$$\text{Pediatric dose} = \frac{\text{child's weight in pounds}}{150 \text{ pounds}} \times \text{adult dose}$$

To use Clark's Rule divide the weight of the child by 150 pounds. Multiply this number by the adult dose to arrive at the pediatric dosage. For example: Penicillin is ordered for a child weighing 35 pounds. The average dose for an adult is 360 mg. How many mg. will the child receive?

$$\frac{35}{150} \times 360 \text{ mg} = 83.9 \text{ mg}$$

To convert the mg into cc's use the $\frac{D}{H} \times Q$ formula.

Fried's Law

Fried's law applies to children under the age of one year. The principle is based on the age of the child in months as compared to a child who is 12 1/2 years old. Fried's assumption is that a 12 1/2 year old child could take an adult dose. The formula for using Fried's Law is:

$$\text{Pediatric dose} = \frac{\text{child's age in months}}{150 \text{ months}} \times \text{adult dose}$$

First, convert 12 1/2 years into months (150 months) since the calculation will be done using months of age as the base. Then, take the patient's age in months and divide it by 150. Multiply this number by the adult dose of the medication to determine what the appropriate pediatric dose would be.

Physician's order:
Child's age: 6 months
Pediatric Dose:

Young's Rule

Young's Rule is used for children who are over 1 year of age. The formula for Young's Rule is:

$$\text{Pediatric dose} = \frac{\text{child's age in years}}{\text{child's age in years} + 12} \times \text{adult dose}$$

To use this formula divide the child's age in years by the same number plus 12. Multiply this number by the adult dose to determine the correct pediatric dosage.

Problem: An adult dose of Phenobarbitol is 30 mg. What would it be for a four year old child?

Solution: $\frac{4}{4 + 12} \times 30 \text{ mg} = 7.5 \text{ mg}$

West's Nomogram

The West's Nomogram is considered the most accurate of all the methods. This method is preferred for sick and underweight children. The nomogram can be used for both infants and children. The nomogram chart is found in pediatrician's offices, medical textbooks and dictionaries.

West's Nomogram is the preferred method of most physicians for calculating pediatric dosage since it is based on a calculation of the child's body surface area (height and weight). The body surface area (BSA) is expressed in square meters (m^2). The nomogram chart has three columns (see Figure 32-1). To calculate the child's BSA a straight line is drawn from the patient's height in inches or centimeters across the columns to the patient's weight in kilograms or pounds. This straight line will intersect on the BSA column. The reading at this point of intersection will give the BSA average. Once the BSA average is found, then a calculation using the formula below is done to calculate the child's dose. The formula for using West's Nomogram is:

$$\text{Pediatric dose} = \frac{\text{basic surface area of child}}{1.73 \text{ square meters}} \times \text{adult dose}$$

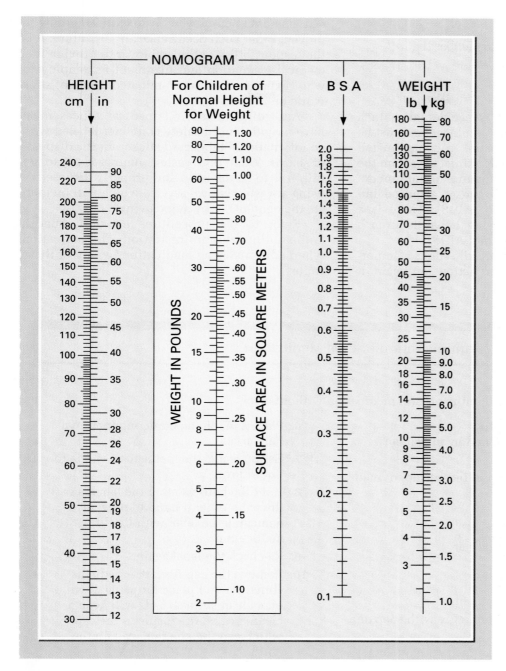

Figure 32-1 Nomogram Chart.

To use this formula you must use West's Nomogram chart. The basic surface area (BSA) for the child has been calculated on the chart. Find the child's weight and height on the chart. Lay a ruler or a paper's sharp edge across the chart and find the point of intersection where the child's weight and height intercept the BSA. Take this calculation and divide it by 1.73 square meters. Then, multiply this number by the adult dose to find the pediatric dosage.

Administration Procedures: OSHA Standards

The Occupational Safety and Health Administration (OSHA) has established guidelines for disposal of contaminated needles and syringes. In addition, OSHA's bloodborne pathogens standard has provisions for medical follow-up procedures that health care workers must take if they have experienced a puncture with a contaminated needle.

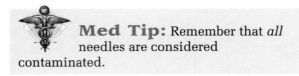

Med Tip: Remember that *all* needles are considered contaminated.

If a medical assistant is accidentally stuck with a contaminated needle, a physician must be notified immediately. Exposure to contaminated needles carries with it a risk of infection from the hepatitis B virus (HBV) or the human immunodeficiency virus (HIV) which causes acquired immune deficiency syndrome (AIDS). There is a greater incidence of acquiring hepatitis from a contaminated needle stick than AIDS.

Immediate reporting of needle sticks is important so that early testing and action can begin. It can also assist employers in determining how to prevent other such occurrences in the future. It is the responsibility of the employer to provide free medical evaluation and treatment for employees who experience a contaminated needle stick while on the job.

According to law all medical offices must have a rigid, locked safety container labeled with an international biohazard sticker for the disposal of sharps. When this waste container is 2/3 to 3/4 full, it is to be removed and properly disposed of using a waste removal service which will incinerate the contents or by autoclaving.

Refer to the procedures for oral, buccal, and sublingual administration of medication when administering medication by any of these routes.

PROCEDURE: Administration of Oral Medication

Terminal Performance
Competency: Able to administer oral medication without error.

Equipment and Supplies
Medication order signed by physician
Oral medication
Calibrated paper cup or receptacle for medication
Water in glass
Patient instruction sheet
Biohazard waste container
Pen

Procedural Steps
1. Assemble equipment.
2. Wash hands thoroughly with soap and running water.
3. Select the correct medication using the "three befores." If you are not familiar with the medication, look it up in a reference book, read the package insert, and/or consult the physician.
4. Always double-check the label to make sure the strength is correct since medications are manufactured with different strengths.
5. Correctly calculate the dosage in writing. Double-check your calculations with someone else.
6. Place a medicine cup/container on a flat surface.
7. Gently shake the medication if it is in liquid form.
8. Hold the bottle so that the label is in the palm of your hand to prevent damaging the label with liquid medication.
9. Re-check the label again.
10. Remove the cap from the medicine container and place it upside down on a clean surface. This will keep a clean area on the inside of the cap which can then be replaced on the bottle.
11A. *Liquid medication:* Hold the calibrated medicine cup at eye level and pour the medication into the cup stopping at the correct dosage line. Pour the medication away from the label side of the bottle. If too much medication is poured into the calibrated cup, do not return it to the bottle. Discard it into a sink.
11B. *Tablet or capsule medication:* Shake out the correct number of tablets or pills into the bottle cap. Then place

them in the medicine cup. If you accidentally pour out an extra tablet, do not return it to the medication bottle. Discard it.

12. Check the medication again to make sure the dosage is the same as the medication order.

13. Replace the cap on the medication bottle and return the bottle to the storage shelf.

14. Take the prepared medication and a glass of water to the patient.

15. Identify the patient both by stating his or her name and examining any printed identification such as a wrist name band or medical record. Ask the patient if he or she has any allergies (Figure 32-2).

16. Remain with the patient until the medication has been swallowed.

17. Provide the patient with written follow-up instructions if further medication is to be taken.

18. Chart the medication administration on the correct patient's record noting the time, medication name, dosage, route (oral procedure), and your name. After giving the medication to the patient, it is best to have the patient wait in the office for 30 minutes.

Charting Example

2/14/XX	1 PM	ASA, 500 mg, po.
		N. Young, RMA

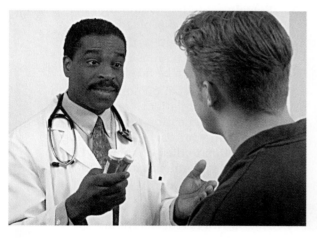

Figure 32-2 Provide patient instruction as needed.

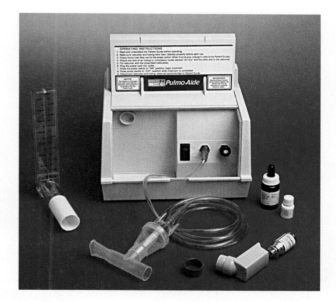

Figure 32-3 A nebulizer with a medication inhaler.

Another method for administering oral medications is via an inhaler or nebulizer which discharges the medication into the respiratory track. See Figure 32-3 for an example of a nebulizer with a medication inhaler.

The procedure for insertion of a rectal or vaginal suppository provides instruction for administering (inserting) medication into the rectum or vagina.

Parenteral Medication Administration

The term parenteral means to administer medication by injection. The advantages to using the parenteral route for medication administration include

PROCEDURE: Administration of Sublingual or Buccal Medication

Terminal Performance
Competency: Be able to administer without error a medication to a patient under the tongue or between the cheek and gum as ordered by the physician.

Equipment and Supplies
Medication order signed by physician on the patient's medical record
Oral medication
Paper cup or receptacle for medication
Patient instruction sheet
Biohazard waste container
Pen

Procedural Steps
1. Assemble equipment.
2. Wash hands thoroughly with soap and running water.
3. Select the correct medication using the "three befores."

If you are not familiar with the medication look it up in a reference book, read the package insert and/or consult the physician.

4. Always *double-check* the label to make sure the strength is correct since medications are manufactured with different strengths.
5. Correctly calculate the dosage in writing. Double-check your calculations.
6. Place a medicine cup/container on a flat surface.
7. Shake the tablet ordered into the bottle cap and then into a medication container.
8. *Check the dosage again* against the medication order.
9. Replace the cap on the medication bottle and return the bottle to the storage shelf after reading the label again.
10. Identify the patient both by stating his or her name and examining any printed identification, such as a wrist name band or medical record. Ask the patient if he or she has any allergies.
11A. *Sublingual medication:* Have the patient place the tablet under the tongue. Instruct the patient not to swallow until the tablet has dissolved.
11B. *Buccal medication:* Have the patient place the tablet between the cheek and gum area. Instruct the patient not to swallow until the tablet is dissoled.
12. Tell the patient not to take fluids until the tablet is dissolved.
13. Remain with the patient until the medication has dissolved.
14. Provide the patient with written follow-up instructions if further medication is to be taken.
15. Chart the medication administration on the correct patient's record noting the time, medication name, dosage, route, and your name. After giving the medication to the patient, it is best to have the patient wait in the office for 30 minutes.

Charting Example
2/14/XX   9 AM Nitroglycerin tab 1,
(gr. 1/100) subling., P = 60
N. Young, RMA

(1) fast absorption of the medication into the system, (2) introduction of medications into the system which cannot otherwise be absorbed through the digestive system, and (3) ability to administer medication to the patient whose condition will not tolerate oral medications.

The disadvantages include (1) inability to remove the medication once it has been injected, (2) potential for infection via the needle, and (3) trauma to tissue from the needle and harsh medications.

The routes for injection include intradermal (ID), subcutaneous (subq), and intramuscular (IM). The Z-track method is also used for intramuscular injections. A fourth route for the administration of parenteral medications is by intravenous (IV) fluids.

PROCEDURE: Administration (Insertion) of a Rectal or Vaginal Suppository

Terminal Performance
Competency: Be able to insert a suppository without error as ordered by the physician.

Equipment and Supplies
Medication order signed by physician
Lubricant
Water
Biohazard waste container
Patient instructions
Vaginal suppository and supplies:
    Vaginal suppository or cream
    Sterile gloves
    Sanitary napkin
Rectal suppository and supplies:
    Rectal suppository
    Nonsterile gloves
    4 × 4 gauze square
Pen

Procedural Steps

1. Assemble equipment.
2. Wash hands thoroughly with soap and running water.
3. Select the correct medication using the "three befores."

If you are not familiar with the medication, look it up in a reference book, read the package insert and/or consult the physician.

4. Always double-check the label to make sure the strength is correct since medications are manufactured with different strengths.
5. Correctly calculate the dosage in writing. Double-check your calculations with someone else.
6. Check the dosage again against the medication order.
7. Replace the cap on the medication bottle and return the bottle to the storage shelf or refrigerator after reading the label again.
8. Identify the patient both by stating his or her name and examining any printed identification, such as a wrist name band or medical record.

Ask the patient if he or she has any allergies.

9. Give patient a gown or sheet. Have the patient remove all clothing from the waist down.

10A. *Rectal suppository:* Have the patient lie on left side, if possible, with top leg bent. Drape a sheet over the patient. Put on nonsterile gloves. Open the suppository wrapper and place suppository on a gauze square. Moisten the suppository with a small amount of lubricant or water. With one hand separate the buttocks. Pick up the suppository with the other hand. Ask the patient to breathe slowly as you insert the suppository from 1 to 1 1/2 inches through the rectal sphincter. Hold the buttocks together and instruct the patient not to bear down or push out the suppository. Wipe the anal area with the gauze and discard gauze into a biohazard waste container. Have the patient remain in the side position for around 20 minutes until the suppository melts.

10B. *Vaginal suppository:* Have the patient assume the dorsal recumbent position with legs apart. Drape the patient. Open the sterile glove pack on a flat surface leaving the gloves in place. Use the inside of the glove wrapper as a sterile field. Peel open the suppository container and drop the suppository onto the inside of the glove wrapper. If an applicator is provided drop it onto the sterile surface also. Glove using sterile technique. With one gloved hand separate the labia minora and hold it in place. Using the other hand insert the suppository one finger length into the vagina. If an applicator is used, place the suppository into the

(continued on next page)

applicator and insert it in a downward direction. Instruct the patient to remain in this position for at least 10 minutes for the suppository to dissolve. Place applicator into the glove wrapper. Remove one glove by pulling inside out from the cuff. With the remaining gloved hand, roll the contaminated wrapper and contents. Hold these waste items as you remove the remaining glove over them. Dispose of all materials into a biohazard waste container. Give the patient a sanitary napkin.

11. Remain with the patient until the medication has dissolved.

12. Provide the patient with written follow-up instructions if further medication is to be taken.

13. Chart the medication administration on the patient's record noting the time, medication name, dosage, injection site, route and your name.

Charting Example

2/26/XX   9 AM   Ducolax 15 mg. Rectal
                     supp.   M. King, CMA

Medical assistants do not administer medications by this route. Figure 32-4 illustrates the angle of needle insertion for these four types of injections.

Equipment Used for Medication Administration

Equipment for dispensing parenteral medications will vary slightly from office to office. Generally you will need to make sure that you have the correct needle gauge, needle length, syringe size and type.

Needle Gauge

Gauge of the needle refers to the actual width of the needle. The gauge ranges from size 14 (largest) to 28 (smallest). The most common gauges for subcutaneous (subq) injections are 25 and 26. Large gauge needles (20-23) are used for intramuscular (IM) injections when a thick or viscous medication, such as penicillin, is administered. You will not generally use a needle larger than a 20 gauge when administering medications. These larger gauge needles are used for venipuncture and blood transfusions. Smaller gauge needles (27-28) are used when a small needle opening is needed. This smaller size is used for giving intradermal (ID) injections when a small amount of medication is placed within the top layer of the skin.

Needle Length

In addition to the size of the needle opening (gauge), the length of the needle is important. Needle sizes

Med Tip: Remember the smaller the number the larger the needle opening. Carefully select the correct gauge needle for the type of injection to be administered. A large gauge needle can cause tissue damage and pain for the patient if used for anything other than an intramuscular injection.

vary from 3/8 inch to 4 inches in length. The length of needle selected depends upon the route used and the area of the body to be injected. See Figure 32-5 for an example of a hypodermic needle.

Med Tip: The correct needle length is extremely important since you will be placing the entire needle, up to 1/8 inch of the hub, into the patient. If the needle is too long there is a danger of touching the patient's bone.

The 3/8 inch needle is used for intradermal injections when a very short needle is needed to insert within the skin. Subcutaneous needles are 1/2 or 5/8 inches in length. A longer needle is not necessary or advised since a longer needle could be inserted beyond the subcutaneous layer. A longer (1-inch, 1 1/2 inch, 2 inch, or 3 inch) needle is used for injection into a muscle. The actual length

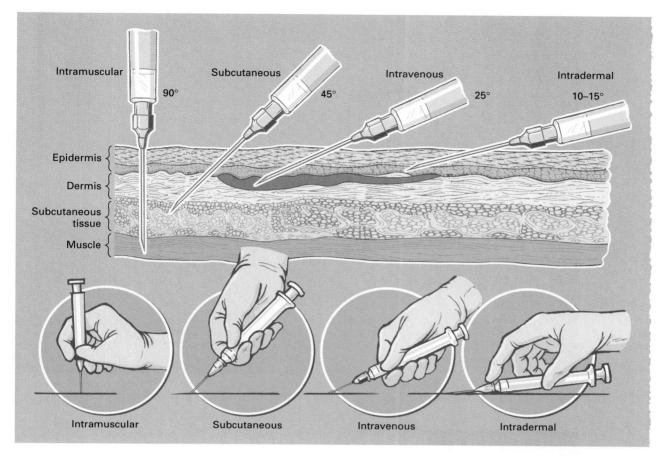

Figure 32-4   Angle of needle insertion for four types of injection.

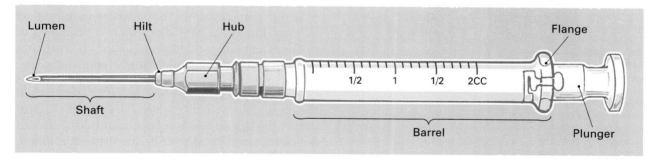

Figure 32-5   A hypodermic needle.

used would depend on the size and weight of the patient and the muscle that is used.

Syringes

Syringes come in a variety of sizes. They are selected based on the type and the amount of medication to be dispensed. The U 100 syringe is the most commonly used insulin syringe. Figures 32-6 A-D show different types of syringes.

The smallest syringe is the tuberculin syringe. It is a long narrow syringe holding only 1 cc (mL) of medication. The tuberculin syringe is calibrated in one hundredths (1/100) of a milliliter and minims. It is used for tuberculosis testing and when small amounts of medication are needed, such as in skin testing for allergies.

The insulin syringe is a small syringe that is calibrated into "Units (U)" especially for the administration of insulin. Since insulin is

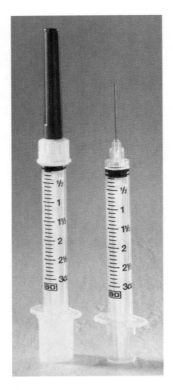

Figure 32-6 A   Med-Saver syringe.

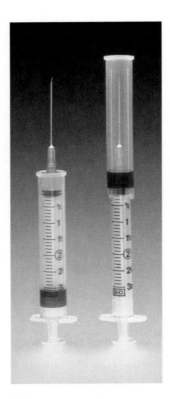

Figure 32-6 B   Safety-Lok syringe.

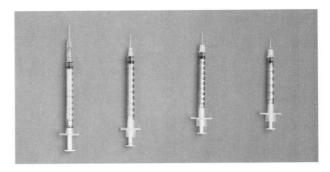

Figure 32-6 C   Insulin syringes.

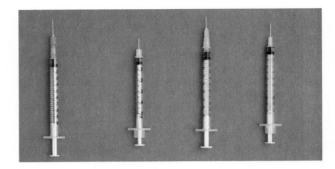

Figure 32-6 D   Tuberculin syringes.

administered by its concentration of insulin rather than by cubic centimeters the calibrations are in units.

Larger syringes are available that hold 2 cc (mL), 3 cc (mL), 5 cc (mL), 10 cc (mL), and up to 60 cc (mL) of medication. The most commonly used syringe is the 3 cc (mL) size which is calibrated in tenths of a mL (cc) and minims. Table 32-7 provides a summary of needle and syringe sizes.

Disposable syringes with needles attached come in peel-apart paper wrappers. There is a rigid sheath which protects the needle. Once the sheath protecting the needle has been removed it should not be replaced using your hands since an accidental needle stick can occur. See Figure 32-7 for an example of a biohazard sharps container.

Med Tip: Never put the syringe and needle down on any surface after completing the injection. A portable biohazard sharps container should be within reach so that the needle can immediately be discarded. The most critical time for a needle stick incident is immediately *after* the injection.

TABLE 32-7   **Summary of Needle and Syringe Sizes**

Route	Gauge	Length	Syringe to Use
Intradermal (ID)	27-28	3/8 inch	tuberculin
Subcutaneous (subq)	25-26	1/2, 5/8 inch	tuberculin; 2 cc; or insulin
Intramuscular (IM)	20-23	1-3 inch	2-5 cc
Deltoid (IM)	25	1/2 inch	2 cc
Vastus lateralis	25	5/8 inch	2 cc

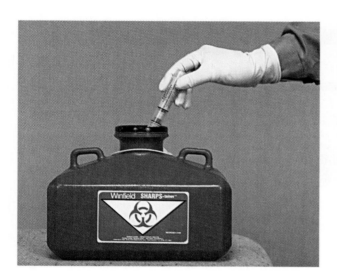

Figure 32-7   Biohazard sharps container.

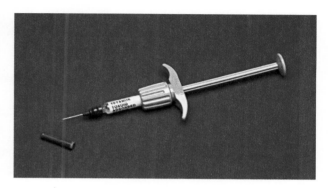

Figure 32-8   Tubex cartridge system.

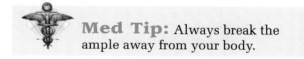

Med Tip: Always break the ample away from your body.

Using a Prefilled Cartridge Injection System

Some drug manufacturers package medications in single-dose glass cartridges which can be placed into a special cartridge holder. You can use the cartridge holder over and over again. The advantage to this system is that the dose is already correctly drawn into the cartridge which eliminates the need to withdraw medication from a vial or bottle. The cartridge holder is sturdy and long-lasting. This system can save money for the office. See Figure 32-8 for an illustration of the Tubex cartridge system. The Medi-jector needle-free insulin delivery system is illustrated in Figure 32-9 .

Ampule

An ampule is a small sealed glass tube which contains medication. An ampule generally contains a single dose of liquid medication and is packed in a storage container to prevent breakage. There is generally an indentation in the neck of the ampule which is the weak point.

Single-dose and Multi-dose Vials

Single-dose and multi-dose vials (bottles) containing fluid medication are small bottles with rubber stoppers on the top. The rubber stopper on the top of the vial allows you to enter the vial with a needle and syringe to withdraw more than one dose.

The single-dose vial is meant to be discarded after withdrawing one dose. Both types of vials will contain instructions concerning the total amount of fluid in the vial. In addition, the instruction will state what the dosage is in each cc of fluid. It is good practice to review the procedure for withdrawing medication from a single-dose and a multi-dose vial before performing the procedure.

Sites for Intramuscular Injections

An intramuscular (IM) injection can be administered in one of four major sites. These sites or muscles are the deltoid, vastus lateralis, dorsogluteal,

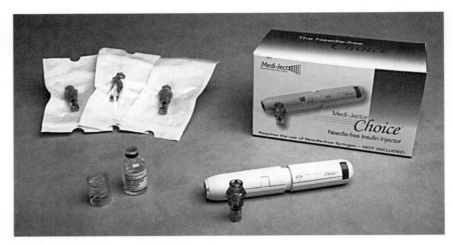

Figure 32-9 Medi-jector needle-free insulin delivery system.

PROCEDURE: Using an Ampule

Terminal Performance Competency: Be able to correctly open and withdraw medication from an ampule.

Equipment and Supplies
Ampule containing medication
Soap
Alcohol sponge
Needle
Syringe
Hazard waste container
Pen

Procedural Steps
1. Do not open the ampule until you are ready to withdraw the fluid. *Note:* Always follow the "three befores" when checking medications against the medication order.
2. Thoroughly wash hands with soap and running water.
3. Snap your thumb and middle finger gently against the tip of the ampule to move all the medication away from the neck and into the bottom of the ampule. (Figure 32-10 illustrates breaking a glass ampule.)
4. Clean the neck of the ampule using an alcohol swab.
5. Use gauze between ampule and thumbs when breaking ampule. Using one hand to hold the bottom of the vial, snap the top off with the other hand using a gauze square to prevent a cut when the glass neck breaks.
6. If the top of the ampule does not snap off easily, you may have to use a file to create a cut or "score" the ampule at the neck. The glass ampule should then break easily at this point.
7. Insert a needle (attached to a syringe) into the ampule and withdraw the fluid without touching the sides of the ampule.
8. Withdraw all the medication from the ampule. It may be necessary to tip the ampule slightly to withdraw all the fluid.
9. Discard the broken ampule into a hazard waste container.

---

and ventrogluteal. A description of each muscle follows, including the location of the muscle and the medication circumstance to which the muscle is best suited.

Deltoid Muscle

The deltoid muscle is located at the top of the arm on the upper, outer surface. This is a small muscle mass which is not a good site for a large

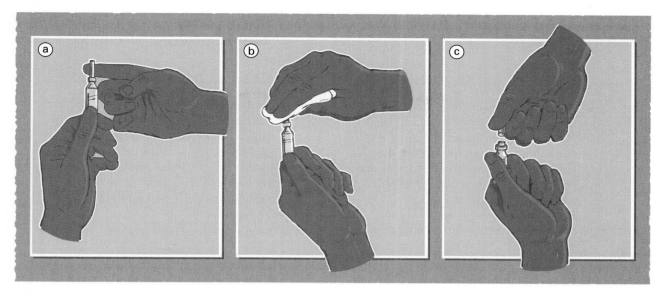

Figure 32-10 Breaking a glass ampule containing medication.

PROCEDURE: Withdrawing Medication From a Single-dose and Multi-dose Vial

**Terminal Performance
Competency:** Be able to correctly withdraw medication from a single-dose and a multi-dose vial.

Equipment and Supplies
Disposable gloves
Biohazard waste container
Biohazard sharps container
Soap
Needle
Syringe
Alcohol sponge
Medication vial
Pen

Procedural Steps
1. Check the medication using the "three befores" technique before beginning. Compare the medication vial (bottle) against the physician's order.
2. Select the correct syringe and needle depending on the type of medication and location for the injection site.
3. Thoroughly wash hands with soap and running water.
4. Roll the medication vial between your hands to mix any medication that has settled on the bottom.
5. Wipe the rubber stopper with an alcohol sponge firmly in a circular motion. Then set the vial on a clean surface while you prepare the syringe.
6. Remove the protective cap from the needle on the syringe. Maintain the sterility of the inner surface of the protective cap since it will be needed to cover the needle again after you have filled the syringe. Figure 32-11 A-E shows the steps involved in filling a syringe.
7. Withdraw the syringe plunger and allow air to enter the syringe in an amount equal to the amount of medication to be withdrawn. Since the vials are vacuum sealed, this will allow for easier withdrawal of fluid.

(Continued on next page)

8. Turning the vial upside down at eye level, using care not to touch the rubber stopper, insert the needle into the rubber stopper and inject the air into the vial. Be extremely cautious concerning contamination as you enter the multiple-dose bottle. *Rationale:* There is an increased danger of contamination since the multiple-dose vial may be entered more than once by several people.

9. Keeping the upside down vial at eye level, slowly withdraw the correct amount of fluid medication. *Rationale:* Rapid withdrawal of fluid may cause air bubbles to form in the syringe.

10. While the needle is still in the vial, check to make sure that the dosage is accurate. Any air bubbles in the syringe will give you an inaccurate dose since they take up the space needed for medication. To remove air bubbles, flick your fingers against the side of the syringe until the air bubbles go back into the tip of the syringe. Expel these bubbles back into the vial and withdraw more medication until the dosage is accurate.

11. Remove needle from vial.

12. If you have accidentally withdrawn too much fluid then discard the excess fluid by shooting it into a sink or waste receptacle. Never return medications to the vial or bottle from which they came.

13. Check the medication vial after you have withdrawn the dosage to make sure you are correct. This is the last step of the "three befores" for checking medications. Also, check to see if the multi-dose vial needs to be refrigerated after opening.

Med Tip: Remember: once you have withdrawn medication into a syringe, there is no way to tell by simply looking if it is the correct medication. You must double check the medication vial after you withdraw the needle from it and before you put the vial away.

amount of medication. This muscle is commonly used for injections such as tetanus boosters in adults. The deltoid muscle can be used for older children, but it should not be used for infants and small children since the muscle is not well-developed.

The deltoid muscle is found by measuring two fingerbreadths below the acromion process of the shoulder. The back surface of the arm should be avoided since the major blood vessels and nerves in the upper arm are located in the posterior portion of the arm. A 23-gauge, 1-inch needle is most commonly used for injection into this site. Use a 25 gauge, 5/8 inch needle for a small arm.

Vastus Lateralis Muscle

The vastus lateralis, or thigh muscle, is located on the upper outer thigh and is part of the quadriceps muscle group. This site is considered to be the safest site for an intramuscular (IM) injection since there are fewer major blood vessels located there. The vastus lateralis muscle lies below the greater trochanter of the femur and within the upper lateral quadrant of the thigh (Figure 32-12).

This muscle is well developed in the infant and is recommended by the American Academy of Pediatrics as the preferred site for all infants and children. Children's immunization are commonly administered into the vastus lateralis muscle in the thigh. Table 32-8 gives a recommended schedule of children's immunizations.

In the adult, the vastus lateralis extends from the middle of the anterior (front) thigh to the middle of the lateral thigh. The measurement at the top is one handbreadth below the greater trochanter and one handbreadth above the knee. A handbreadth is measured using the size and surface of the hand. The patient may be either in a sitting or supine position.

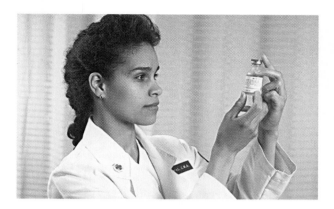

Figure 32-11 A Read the label on the medication bottle.

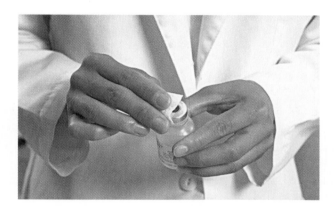

Figure 32-11 B Clean the top of the bottle.

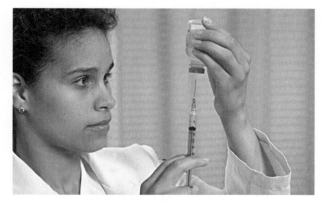

Figure 32-11 C Invert bottle and inject the same amount of air into the bottle as amount of medication to be withdrawn.

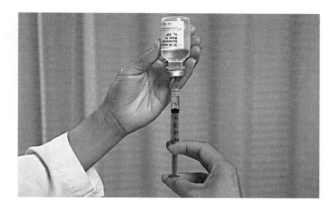

Figure 32-11 D Keeping the bottle inverted, draw the correct amount of medication into the syringe.

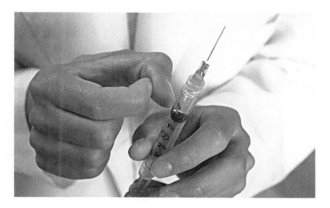

Figure 32-11 E Remove the needle from the bottle and expel the air or tap out the air bubbles.

Dorsogluteal (Gluteus Medius) Muscle

The dorsogluteal muscle is the muscle most commonly used when a deep intramuscular (IM) injection is needed for injecting irritating or viscous (thick) medications such as antibiotics. Since there is a danger of damage to the sciatic nerve in this area, many physicians prefer the vastus lateralis muscle be used for adults' and children's intramuscular injections. The vastus lateralis site is used for infants since their gluteus medius muscle is not well-developed.

This injection needs to be done carefully using landmarks to avoid injecting near the sciatic nerve (Figure 32-13). The patient should be asked to lie in the prone position. Ask the patient to point his or her toes inward which will cause the muscles to relax. To avoid the sciatic nerve draw an imaginary line from the greater trochanter of the femur to the posterior superior iliac spine. You can feel these bone prominences on the patient. Give the injection above and lateral to the imaginary line. See Figure 32-14 for an illustration of the needle position for an IM injection. You can also divide the buttocks

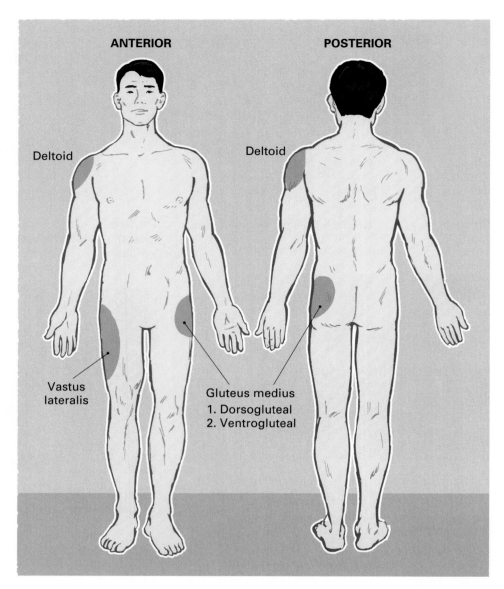

Figure 32-12 Sites for intramuscular injections.

into four imaginary quadrants and inject into the upper outer quadrant (Figure 32-15).

Ventrogluteal (Gluteus Medius) Muscle

The ventrogluteal site is considered safer than the dorsogluteal site since the gluteus medius muscle does not contain major nerves and blood vessels. This site is considered to be safe for infants, children, and adults.

When injecting into the left side of the patient, the site is located by placing the palm of the right hand on the greater trochanter and the index finger on the anterior superior iliac crest. Next, stretch the index finger as far as possible along the iliac crest. Then, spread the middle finger away from your index finger. The injection is made in the V that is formed by middle and index fingers (Figure 32-16). Always use the hand opposite the patient's side, for example your left hand and patient's right gluteus medius, when using this method to determine the injection location.

Sites for Subcutaneous Injection

The subcutaneous injection is given just under (sub) the skin (cutaneous). The injection is given into adipose tissue rather than into muscle. This method is ideal when a small dose of a non-

TABLE 32-8 Schedule of Child Immunizations

Age	Immunizations
Birth	HBV (hepatitis B) #1
2 months	DPT (Diptheria, pertussis, tetanus) #1
	Oral Polio #1
	HBV #2
	Hib (*Haemophilus influenzae*) #1
4-5 months	DPT #2
	Oral Polio #2
	Hib #2
6 months	DPT #3
	Oral Polio #3
	HBV #3
1 year	MMR (Measles, Mumps, Rubella)
	TB test
1 1/2 year	DPT Booster
	Oral Polio Booster
	Rubeola (measles) one dose only
4-6 years	DPT Booster
	Oral Polio Booster

irritating medications, such as in immunizations, insulin, and analgesics, are given. Table 32-9 lists insulin types and duration of action. The deltoid area and upper back are commonly used. However, when the injection is self-administered by the patient, other sites are commonly used, such as the thighs and abdomen. See Figure 32-17 for an illustration of the sites for subcutaneous injection.

The subcutaneous injection is usually administered at a 45-degree angle with the exception of insulin and heparin which are given at a 90-degree angle (Figure 32-18). When a medication is frequently administered, for example insulin, the sites must be rotated. A record of the rotation sites is kept in the patient's medical record. The patients must also be instructed on how to maintain their own rotation at home. See Figure 32-19 for an example of rotation sites.

When allergy medication is administered, the patient should be asked to remain in the of-

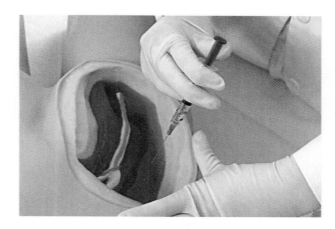

Figure 32-13 Care must always be taken to avoid injecting too close to the sciatic nerve.

fice for an additional 30 minutes following the injection, in case the patient has a reaction to the medication.

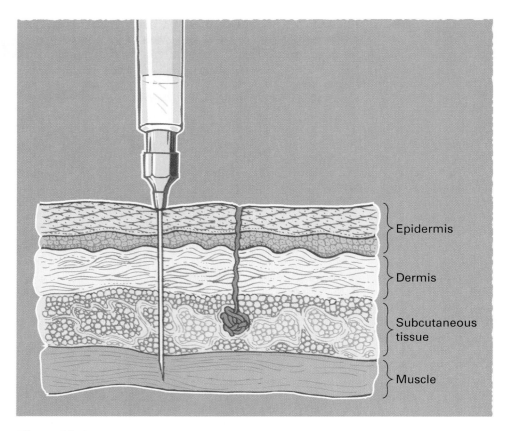

Figure 32-14   Needle position for an intramuscular injection.

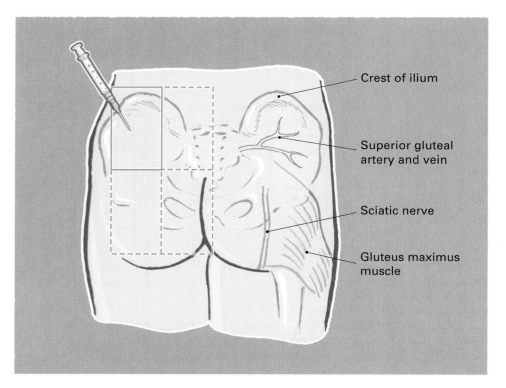

Crest of ilium

Superior gluteal artery and vein

Sciatic nerve

Gluteus maximus muscle

Figure 32-15   Injecting the upper outer quadrant of the buttocks.

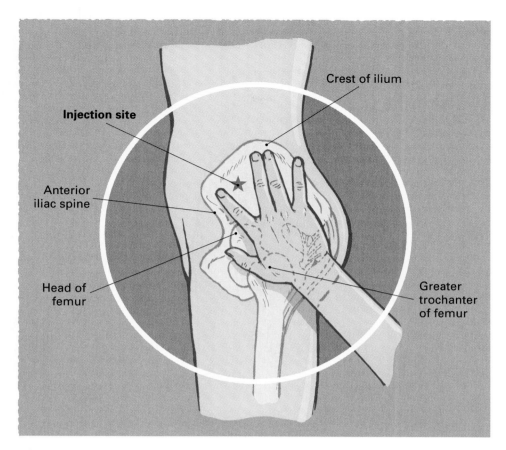

Figure 32-16   Injecting the ventrogluteal muscle.

Labels in figure:
Crest of ilium
Injection site
Anterior iliac spine
Head of femur
Greater trochanter of femur

Parenteral Injections: Intramuscular (IM) and Subcutaneous (SC)

The basic procedure for parenteral injections is similar for both intramuscular and subcutaneous injections. The administration sites and needle gauge and lengths differ. Follow this procedure when administering subcutaneous and intramuscular injections.

Intramuscular Injections: Z-track

The Z-track method for injecting medications into the muscle is used for irritating medications, for example ferrous sulfate (iron). This method involves pulling aside the skin, injecting the medication, and then allowing the skin to move back over the injection site. This will help to prevent irritating medications from causing tissue damage by seeping from the muscle into the subcutaneous tissue. See Figure 32-22 for illustration of Z-track injection.

The Z-tract method is only used for injections into the gluteus medius muscle of the buttocks.

Do not massage the area over the injection site after withdrawing the needle. Advise the patient to walk around which will encourage absorption of the medication. Chart whether the injection was administered into the right or left buttock so that you know to rotate to the other side when you give the next injection. Tell the patient not to rub the area.

Intradermal Injection

The intradermal injection is commonly used for allergy skin testing in which a minute amount of material is injected within the top layer of skin to determine a patient's sensitivity. Since just the top level of skin is entered, a small "wheal" or bubble which contains the injection fluid appears on the skin. Don't rub the area after giving the injection.

The intradermal injection is also the method of administration for the tuberculosis (TB) test. The TB test is "read" 48 hours after it has been administered. Reading consists of a medical professional examining the injection site for any signs of reaction, such as elevated wheal or redness, to the tuberculin material.

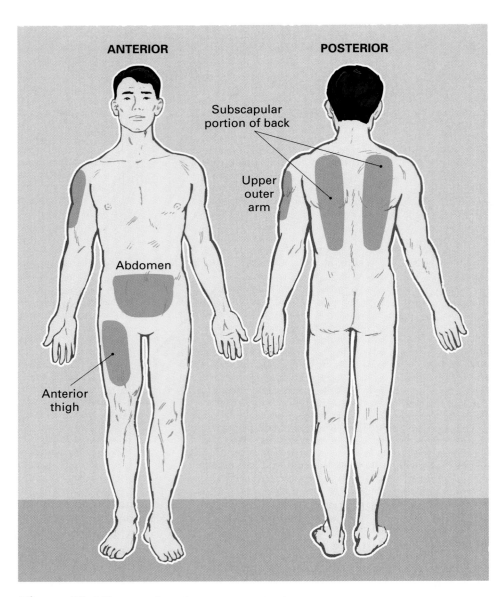

Figure 32-17   Sites for subcutaneous injection.

Injectable Drugs Used in the Medical Office

Many physician's offices and clinics keep a stock of injectables locked in the medication cabinet. Table 32-10 lists some of the most commonly stocked injectable drugs. The emergency medications which are found at the end of the list may be kept in an emergency cart or special locked cabinet. See Figure 32-25 for examples of injectable drugs.

Giving Injections to Infants and Children

Be sure to obtain the parent's permission before giving any child an injection. If the physician has examined the child and then ordered the injection while the parent is present and not objecting, this constitutes permission.

A child should be told that he or she is going to receive some medicine that will help them. Tell the child honestly that there will be a slight sting but it will be over soon. A child who can count may find that by counting slowly to ten, the procedure will go more quickly. Some children like to have a small bandage applied after they have received an injection.

When giving an infant or child an injection be sure to have another adult (assistant or parent) restrain the child. If the child were to suddenly move while the needle is in their body severe damage could occur. It is extremely difficult

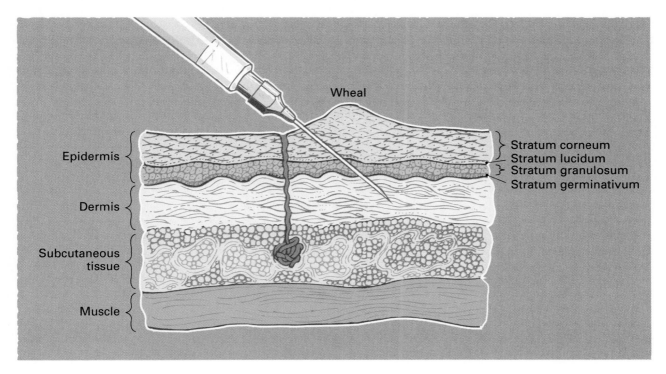

Figure 32-18   Needle position during subcutaneous injections.

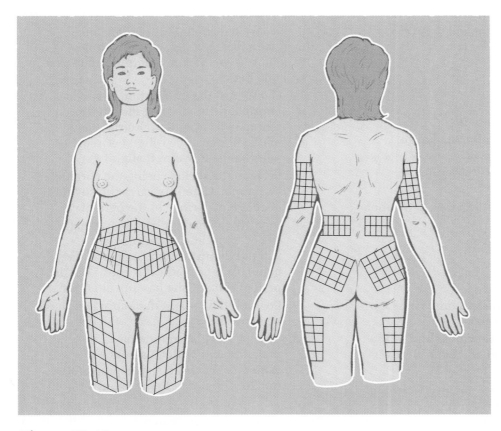

Figure 32-19   Rotation sites for administering insulin.

TABLE 32-9 Insulin Types and Duration of Action

Insulin Name	Type	Common Name	Action Onset	Action Peak	Action Duration
Crystalline	Rapid action	Regular	1 hour	2-4 hr	6-8 hr
Semilente	Rapid	Regular	1 hour	4-10 hr	12-16 hr
Humilin-R	Rapid	—	15 min	1 hr	6-8 hr
Isophane	Intermediate	NPH	2-4 hr	6-15 hr	24-48 hr
Insulin Zinc Suspension	Intermediate	Lente	2-4 hr	6-15 hr	24-48 hr
Humilin-N	Intermediate	—	1 hr	4 hr	24 hr
Protamine Zinc	Slow action	PZI	3-6 hr	12-20 hr	24-36 hr
Ultralente	Slow	PZI	8 hr	12-24 hr	36 hr +

PROCEDURE: Administration of Parenteral (Subcutaneous (SC) or Intramuscular (IM) Injection)

Terminal Performance
Competency: Be able to administer SC and IM injections without error.

Equipment and Supplies
  Medication order signed by physician
  Vial of medication
  Nonsterile gloves
  Alcohol sponges
  Biohazard sharps container
  Biohazard waste container
  Subcutaneous injection: 25-gauge, 5/8-inch needle for small arm; 23-gauge, 1-inch needle for average arm
  Disposable 3-mL syringe
  Intramuscular injection: 22g, 1 1/2-inch needle
  Disposable 3-mL syringe
  Pen

Procedural Steps
  1. Thoroughly wash hands with soap and running water.
  2. Apply nonsterile gloves and follow universal blood and body-fluid precautions.
  3. Select the correct medication using the "three befores."

Note: Always double-check the label to make sure the strength is correct since medications are manufactured with different strengths, for example 250 mg/cc and 500 mg/cc.

  4. Gently roll the medication between your hands to mix any medication that may have settled. Refrigerated medication can be rolled between your hands to warm it slightly.
  5. Prepare the syringe using the correct technique. Carefully carry the covered needle and syringe to the patient.
  6. Identify the patient both by stating his or her name and examining any printed identification, such as a wrist name band or medical record. Ask the patient if he or she has any allergies.
  7. Position the patient depending on the site you are using.
  8. Using a circular motion clean the patient's skin with an alcohol sponge. Wipe the skin with a sweeping motion from the center of the area outward.

(Continued)

This prevents recontamination of the injection site by the alcohol sponge. Figure 32-20 illustrates the sites for administering an injection.

9. Once again check the medication dosage against the patient's order to determine if this is the correct time to administer the dose (one of the "six rights").

10. Remove the protective covering from the needle using care not to touch the needle. If you accidentally touch the needle, excuse yourself to the patient, then return to the preparation area and change the needle on the syringe. If you are using a self-contained syringe and needle unit that does not come apart, discard the entire syringe with the medication and start the process over again. ***Rationale:*** A contaminated needle can cause a severe infection in an already ill patient. Remember: the patient's safety is your first priority.

11. When you are prepared to administer the injection, place a new alcohol sponge or a cotton ball between two fingers of your nondominant hand so that you can easily grasp it when you are through with the injection.

12. Firmly grasp the syringe in your predominant hand similar to the way a pencil is held.

13A. *To administer a subcutaneous injection:* With your nondominant hand, pick up the skin at the injection site and form a small mass of tissue. This will aid in the needle entering only the subcutaneous tissue.

13B. *To administer an intramuscular injection:* With your nondominant hand stretch the skin tightly where you will insert the needle. Pulling the skin taut allows the needle to enter the skin more easily. (If the patient is thin or a child you would pinch the muscle into a bundle and squeeze as

the needle is inserted. In this way you would avoid going deeper than the muscle and touching a bone.)

14. Grasping the syringe in a dart-like fashion insert the entire needle with one swift movement.

15A. *For subcutaneous injection:* Insert into the subcutaneous tissue at a 45-degree angle.

15B. *For intramuscular injection:* Insert needle directly into the muscle at a 90-degree angle. ***Rationale:*** The selection of the correct size needle is important since you will be inserting the entire needle into the patient.

16. Do not move the needle once you have inserted it. If the needle is pushed in further, contaminants are carried into the skin from the exposed needle.

17. Aspirate to determine if you have entered a blood vessel. To do this pull back slightly on the plunger with the hand holding the syringe while holding the needle steady in the muscle. If blood appears in the hub area of the syringe it means that you are in a blood vessel. You will then have to withdraw the needle using correct technique and discard the syringe containing the blood and medication. Begin the procedure again with step 1 and fresh supplies. ***Rationale:*** You may not administer a subcutaneous or intramuscular injection intravenously into a blood vessel.

18. If you do not see a return of blood in the syringe when you aspirate, slowly inject the medication without moving the needle. Do not move the needle until you have completed injecting all the medication. See Figure 32-21 for illustrations of intramuscular injection. *Note:* Insert and withdraw the needle quickly to minimize pain *but* administer the medication slowly.

(Continued on next page)

PROCEDURE: Administration of Parenteral (Subcutaneous (SC) or Intramuscular (IM)) Injection *(Continued)*

19. Taking the alcohol sponge (or cotton ball) from between the last two fingers of your nondominant hand place it over the area containing the needle. Withdraw the needle at the same angle you used for insertion using care not to stick yourself with the needle.

20. With one hand place the sponge firmly over the injection site. With the other hand discard the needle in a biohazard sharps container.

21. You may gently massage the injection site to assist absorption and ease pain for the patient.

22. Make sure the patient is safe before leaving him or her unattended.

Observe the patient for any untoward effect of the medication for at least 15 minutes.

23. Correctly dispose of all materials.

24. Remove gloves into biohazard bag and wash your hands.

25. Chart the medication administration on the patient's record noting the time, medication name, dosage, injection site, route, lot # on immunizations, and your name.

Charting Example

2/14/XX   1:30 PM   Penicillin G. procaine, 600,000 unit   IM Right gluteus.

M. King, CMA

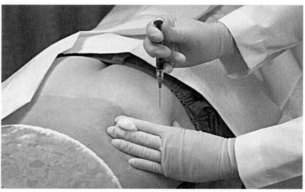

A

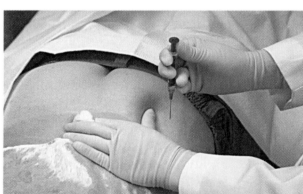

B

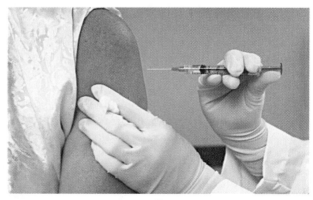

C

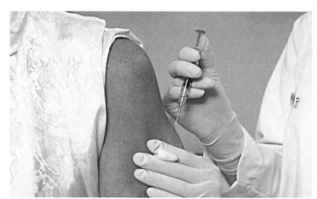

D

Figure 32-20 A-F   Sites for administering medication.

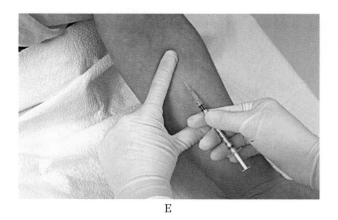

E

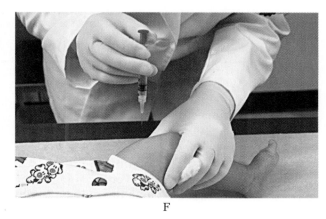

F

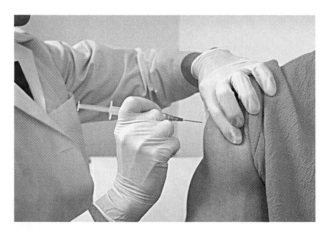

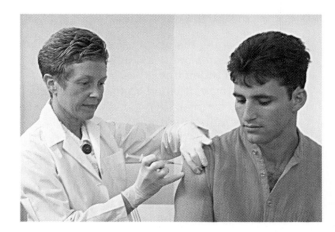

Figure 32-21   Intramuscular injections.

PROCEDURE: Administration of a Z-track Injection

Terminal Performance
Competency: Be able to administer Z-track injection using proper technique without error.

Equipment and Supplies
   Alcohol sponges
   Biohazard sharps container
   Biohazard waste container
   Disposable gloves
   Medication order signed by the
   physician
   Pen
   Sterile needle and syringe
   Vial of medication

Procedural Steps
   Follow steps **1** through **15** of the procedure
   for administration of an intramuscular
   injection.

16. After withdrawing the medication from the vial, change to a fresh needle. This will eliminate any irritating medication that may be within the needle from coming into contact with the patient's tissue until the needle is placed into the muscle layer.

17. When ready to administer the medication, pull the skin of the buttock to one side and hold it in place with your nondominant hand. You may wish to use a dry gauze sponge if the skin is slippery.

(Continued on next page)

18. With your dominant hand and using a dart-like grip on the syringe, insert the needle up to the hub quickly into the gluteus medius muscle. Do not move the needle once it is in place.

19. While still maintaining a firm hold on the taut skin with your nondominant hand, pull back on the plunger of the syringe to check for a blood return with the fingers of the hand holding the syringe. To do this simply move your fingers up the syringe, while keeping the needle steady within the patient's buttocks, until your thumb and index finger reach the top of the plunger. If blood appears in the hub of the syringe, then using correct technique, withdraw the syringe, discard, and begin with step 1 again.

20. If there is no return of blood, then very slowly inject the medication into the muscle.

21. Wait several seconds after injecting the medication before you withdraw the needle. Cover the area with the alcohol sponge and withdraw the needle at the same angle of insertion. Wait at least 10 seconds before releasing the skin being held by the nondominant hand.

22. Do not massage the area. Observe the patient for at least 15 minutes for any untoward reaction. You may advise the patient to walk around to assist in the absorption process of the medication.

23. Correctly dispose of all materials.

24. Remove gloves and wash your hands.

25. Chart the medication administration on the patient's record noting the time, medication name, dosage, injection site, route and your name.

Charting Example
2/14/XX   3:30 PM   Iron dextran, 50 mg-
Z-track into left gluteus. No C/O pain.
N. Young, RMA

---

for one person to restrain an uncooperative child while giving an injection. Always get help before you begin. If the parent seems to be disturbed by the procedure, then ask the parent to wait outside.

The preferred site for an infant's or child's injection is in the vastus lateralis muscle of the thigh (top of the thigh). In the case of an infant, you may find it is possible to secure the baby by placing your nondominant arm across the baby or use a papoose type of wrapping while you inject into his or her thigh.

The areas to avoid are: buttocks and deltoid muscle. The buttocks is avoided in infants since the sciatic nerve is quite large and could be entered accidentally. The gluteus medius is underdeveloped in children until they begin to walk. Similarly, the deltoid muscle is not well-developed in babies.

Charting Medications

Parenteral medications are charted using the same documentation as for oral medications: name of medication, dosage, route, date, site, and signature of person administering the medication. It is also necessary to document that you have provided instructions to the patient regarding follow-up care. Examples of charting follow.

9/10/XX 9:00 AM, nitroglycerin, I tab. sublingually. Written instructions given to pt. Precautions explained. Told to call progress in to office at 1:00 PM today.   M. Richards, CMA.
1/19/XX 11:00 AM, Monistat-3, 200 mg. Vaginal. Pt. given written instructions for follow-up care.
M. Richards, CMA.
10/10/XX 1:00 PM Mantoux test, 0.01 mL. Tuberculin Purified Protein Derivative, L forearm, subq., Small wheal noted. Pt. instructed not to rub or cover the area and to return for reading in 48 hours.
M. Richards, CMA.

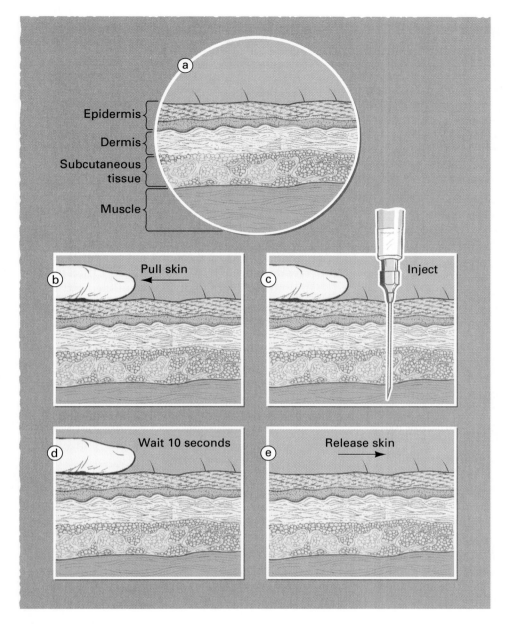

Epidermis

Dermis

Subcutaneous
tissue

Muscle

Pull skin

Inject

Wait 10 seconds

Release skin

Figure 32-22   An example of the Z-track method
of injection.

PROCEDURE: Administration of an Intradermal Injection

**Terminal Performance
Competency:** Be able to correctly administer an intradermal injection without error as ordered by the physician.

Equipment and Supplies
Disposable gloves
Biohazard sharps container
Alcohol sponges
Sterile needle
Sterile syringe
Vial of medication
Medication order signed by physician
Pen

Procedural Steps

I. Preparation:

1. Thoroughly wash hands with soap and running water.

2. Apply nonsterile gloves and follow universal blood and body-fluid precautions.

3. Select the correct medication using the "three befores."
   Always double-check the label to make sure the strength is correct since medications are manufactured with different strengths, for example 1:10, 1:100, or 1:1000 dilutions.

4. Gently roll the medication between your hands to mix any medication that may have settled. Refrigerated medication can be rolled between your hands to warm it slightly.

5. Prepare the syringe using the correct technique. Carefully carry the covered needle and syringe to the patient.

6. Identify the patient both by stating his or her name and examining any printed identification such as a wrist name band or medical record.

7. Select the proper site (center of forearm, upper chest or upper back). See Figure 32-23 for intradermal skin injection sites.

8. Using a circular motion clean the patient's skin with an alcohol sponge. Wipe the skin with a sweeping motion from the center of the area outward. This prevents recontamination of the injection site by the alcohol sponge.

9. Allow time for the antiseptic on the sponge to dry to reduce the possibility of it reacting with the medication.

10. Once again check the medication dosage against the patient's order to determine if this is the correct time to administer the dose (one of the "six rights").

11. Remove the protective covering from the needle using care not to touch the needle. If you accidentally touch the needle then excuse yourself to the patient. Return to your preparation area and change the needle on the syringe. If you are using a self-contained syringe and needle unit that does not come apart, you will have to discard the entire syringe with the medication and start the process over again. (Remember: The patient's safety is your first priority. A contaminated needle can cause a severe infection in an already ill patient.)

II. Injection:

12. Hold the syringe between the first two fingers and thumb of your dominant hand with the palm down and the bevel of the needle up. Figure 32-24 A-F illustrates the steps used to administer an intradermal skin test.

13. Hold the skin taut with the fingers of your nondominant hand. If you are using the center of the forearm, then place the nondominant hand under the patient's arm and pull the skin taut. This will allow the needle to slip into the skin more easily.

14. Using a 15-degree angle insert the needle through the skin to about

(Continued)

1/8 inch. The bevel of the needle will be facing upward and covered with skin. The needle will still show through the skin. Do not aspirate.

15. Slowly inject the medication beneath the surface of the skin. A small elevation of skin (wheal) will occur where you have injected the medication.

16. Quickly withdraw the needle. With the other hand discard the needle into the biohazard sharps container.

III. Patient follow-up:

17. Do not massage the area.

18. Make sure the patient is safe before leaving him or her unattended. Observe the patient for any untoward effect, such as an allergic reaction to

the medication, for at least 20 to 30 minutes. Tell the patient not to rub the area.

19. Correctly dispose of all materials.

20. Remove gloves and wash your hands.

21. Chart the medication administration on the patient's record noting the time, medication name, dosage, injection site, route, appearance of the intradermal site after injection and your name.

Charting Example

2/14/XX   10 AM   Mantoux (PPP) tuberculin test, 0.10 mL ID Right anterior forearm. Instructed to return on 2/16 to have test read.

M. King, CMA

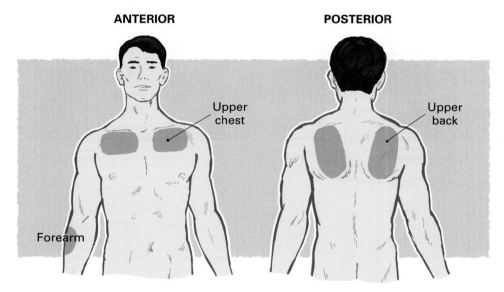

ANTERIOR

POSTERIOR

Upper chest

Upper back

Forearm

Figure 32-23   Intradermal skin injection sites.

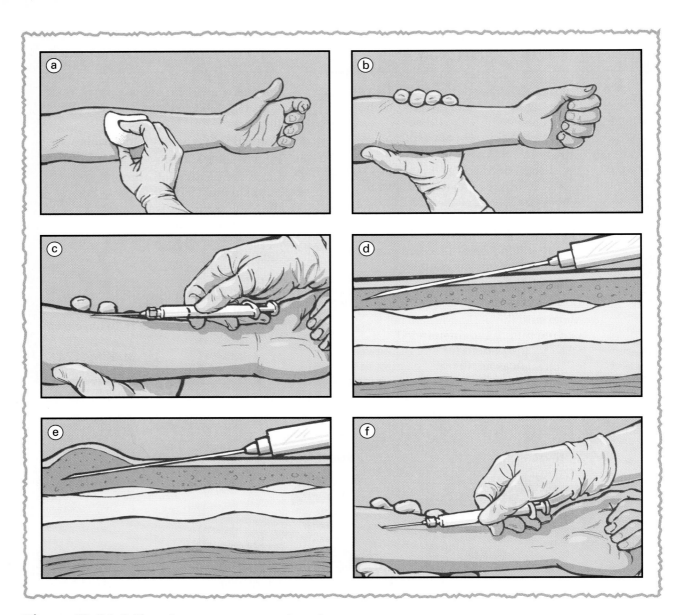

Figure 32-24 A-F   Administering an intradermal
skin test.

TABLE 32-10 Injectable Drugs Commonly in Stock in the Medical Office

Name Generic	Trade Name	Route	Usage
Amitriptyline HCL	Elavil	IM	Depression
Bropheniramine maleate	Dimetane	IM/SC	Allergy
Chlorpromazine HCL	Thorazine	IM	Psychosis
Diazepam	Valium	IM	Anxiety
Dimenhydrinate	Dramamine	IM	Nausea/Vomiting
Diphenhydramine	Benadryl	IM	Allergic reaction
Diphtheria, tetanus toxoid	Same name	IM	Immunization active vaccine
Furosemide	Lasix	IM	Edema
Gentamicin sulfate	Garamycin	IM	Infection
Heparin sodium	Same name	SC	Prevent clotting
Hydromorphine HCL	Dilaudid	SC/IM	Severe pain
Lidocaine HCL 1%, 2%	Xylocaine	SC	Anesthetic for minor surgery
Prochlorperazine	Compazine	IM	Psychosis
Promethazine HCL	Phenergan	IM	Nausea/Vomiting
Sodium Chloride with benzyl alcohol 0.9%	Sodium Chloride Bacteriostatic		Diluent for injection
Tetanus & diphtheria toxoids	Same name	IM	Immunization active vaccine
Tetanus antitoxin	Same name	IM	Prevention passive vaccine
Tetanus immune globulin	Hyper-Tet	IM	Prevention passive vaccine
Tetanus toxoid	Same name	IM	Immunization active vaccine
Tuberculin protein derivative	Tine test	ID	Tuberculin testing
Water for injection	Same name		Diluent for injection
Emergency Drugs Bretylium Tostlate	Bretylol	IV	Arrhythmia
Epinephrine		IV SC	Cardiac arrest Allergic reaction
Norepinephrine	Levophed	IV	Hypotension
Sodium Bicarbonate		IV	Acidosis
Electrolytes/Ringer's 1000 cc		IV	Dehydration

ID = intradermal; IM = intramuscular; SC = subcutaneous; IV = intravenous (*Note:* Only physician and nurse may administer intravenous medications.)

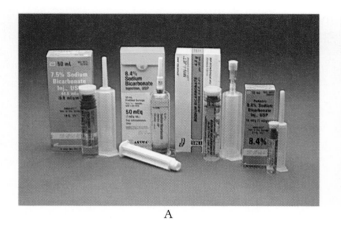

A

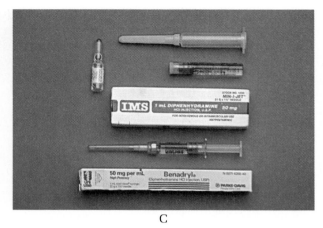

C

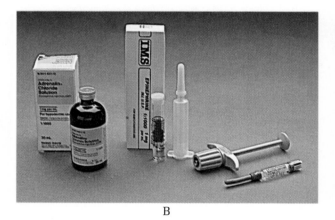

B

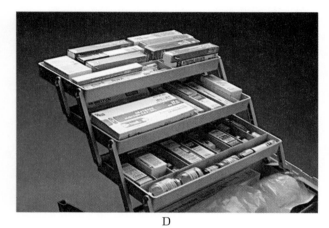

D

Figure 32-25   Injectable drugs.

LEGAL AND ETHICAL ISSUES

The medical assistant must use careful aseptic technique when administering injections to patients. There is a danger of pain and infection for the patient with improperly administered drugs. There is also the danger of liability for both the physician and medical assistant. The ethical issue of always placing the patients needs first is of paramount importance when administering medications.

Verbal orders, in which the medication order is told to the MA, must be recorded and then signed by the physician and the medical assistant. No medication can be administered to a patient without the written order of a physician. The medical assistant must be willing to say, "I'm sorry, but I'm not allowed to perform that procedure without the doctor's order."

The medical assistant must constantly seek clarification on orders and dosage calculations. A thorough knowledge of drug interactions and side effects is necessary before dispensing any medication. The medical assistant has a responsibility to look up any unfamiliar medication. Failure to do so puts the physician and the medical assistant in jeopardy. Do not perform the administration of a medication with which you are unfamiliar. Never give a parenteral injection if you have not been trained in the procedure.

Pediatric medication administration is especially susceptible to liability since even a small error can result in major problems for the child. All calculations should be reviewed and double-checked with the physician or a nurse.

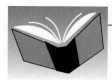

PATIENT EDUCATION

The physician will be the first to discuss medications with the patient. It is the medical assistant's responsibility to reinforce what the physician has explained. Some clarification of what the physician has said may be needed. It is especially important that the patients know why they are taking medications. Do not assume anything when teaching about medication administration. There is a risk that the patient will not take the medication or will take it incorrectly if the patient did not understand the explanation.

Medication names, dosages, expected results, and side effects have to be carefully explained in language the patient will understand. The inserts that are placed into sample drug packets can be helpful to patients. However, they may need to be interpreted for the patient. You may have to provide simple line drawings for patients who are hearing impaired or cannot understand your verbal explanation. This instruction should be documented.

Patients may not understand the metric or the apothecary systems for calculating dosage. It is important for the medical assistant to easily move between the metric, apothecary, and household systems of measure, in order to be able to explain medication dosage in terms of household measures, if necessary.

Special emphasis must be placed on the need to take all the medication that is prescribed. For example, antibiotics must be taken for the entire length of time or they will be ineffective and the infection may reoccur. In many cases, dietary instructions will be needed along with an explanation of drug administration. For example, a patient who is taking a diuretic should know that it depletes sodium which may require the need for extra potassium. This can be replenished with foods, such as bananas and kiwis.

Summary

The medical assistant must be able to calculate dosages correctly since any error has the potential to be fatal to the patient. Also, observing the "three befores" before dispensing medication and the "six rights" before administering medication, can help to reduce errors. Any errors must be immediately reported in order for the physician to handle the situation. Failure to report an error compounds the seriousness of the error.

Thorough preparation of the patient who is to receive an injection can help to eliminate unnecessary pain. Injections are always given under the supervision of a physician. This means that in addition to writing the order for the medication, the physician must be physically present in the facility when you are administering the drug. This can be critical when giving allergy tests or medications since a minute amount of medication can cause a life-threatening allergic response in a sensitive patient.

Competency Review

1. Define and spell the glossary terms for this chapter.
2. What are the "six rights" for drug administration?
3. State what you would do if Mrs. Lopez, age 88, refuses to cooperate while receiving an injection.
4. State what you would do if Billy Mendez, age three, refuses to cooperate while receiving a tetanus shot.
5. State what you would do if you have drawn up a narcotic that is not needed.
6. State what you would do if you see a small amount of blood appear in the syringe as you withdraw the plunger.

PREPARING FOR THE CERTIFICATION EXAM

Test Taking Tip — Move quickly through the exam so that you have time to review your answers. One of the most common examination errors is to misread a question. You will need time to double-check that you haven't missed a key word, such as "always," "never," or "except."

Examination Review Questions

1. The two systems of weights and measurements that are used to calculate medication dosages are
   (A) metric and apothecary
   (B) metric and pounds
   (C) metric and ounces
   (D) apothecary and pounds
   (E) apothecary and ounces

2. Cubic centimeters are equal to
   (A) ounces
   (B) grams
   (C) drams
   (D) milliliters
   (E) millimeters

3. In liquid measures, one fluid ounce is equal to
   (A) 1 mL
   (B) 10 mL
   (C) 30 mL
   (D) 100 cc
   (E) 30 cc

4. In regard to medication, available strength refers to
   (A) what actually contains the medication
   (B) the potency of the medication in stock
   (C) the potency the physician has ordered
   (D) the amount of medication that should be administered
   (E) the calculated strength

5. According to the rules for converting from one system of measurement to another, to change
   (A) grains to milligrams, multiply by 60
   (B) grains to grams, multiply by 15
   (C) cc's to ounces, divide by 50
   (D) cc's to mL, divide by 15
   (E) drams to grams, multiply by 2

6. What is the preferred method of most physicians for calculating pediatric dosages?

   (A) Young's Rule
   (B) Fried's Law
   (C) West's Nomogram
   (D) Clark's Rule
   (E) none of the above

7. When administering oral or sublingual medication
   (A) assemble all of the equipment and use aseptic technique
   (B) select the correct medication using the "three befores"
   (C) double-check the label on the medication
   (D) A and B
   (E) A, B, and C

8. In regard to the administration of parenteral medication, a smaller gauge needle is used for which type of injection?
   (A) intramuscular
   (B) Z-track
   (C) subcutaneous
   (D) intradermal
   (E) intravenous

9. Since the entire needle, up to the hub, must go into the patient, what length needle should be used for an intradermal injection?
   (A) 3/8 inch
   (B) 4/8 inch
   (C) 5/8 inch
   (D) 6/8 inch
   (E) 1 inch

10. Which site, because there are fewer major blood vessels, is considered the safest for an intramuscular injection?
   (A) vastus lateralis
   (B) deltoid
   (C) dorsogluteal
   (D) ventrogluteal
   (E) gluteus medius

ON THE JOB

Latoya is a medical assistant in Dr. Reed's office. Dr. Reed is a board certified pediatrician licensed to practice medicine in the state of Illinois.

A patient, a 4 year old boy, has been brought in by his baby-sitter for an emergency appointment because of severe nausea and vomiting. He weighs about 30 pounds. Dr. Reed is concerned that the child might be dehydrated.

Dr. Reed, upon examination of the child, orders 2.5 mg. of Compazine, rectally, stat. He asks Latoya to administer the medication. The child is upset and crying and appears very fearful of Latoya. Latoya is concerned about being able to administer the medication to the child given his behavior.

What is your response?

1. How should Latoya proceed in order to follow Dr. Reed's instructions?
2. Does the fact that this is the state of Illinois effect Latoya's ability to fulfill this order?
3. Since the boy's baby-sitter has brought him to the office and is in charge of his care, must Latoya still obtain parental permission before administering the Compazine?
4. Because the child is extremely anxious and upset, should Latoya ask another medical assistant to help administer the medication or might this further alarm the child?
5. Does the prescribed dosage of Compazine seem like the proper one given the child's age and weight?
6. How would Latoya confirm that the dosage is correct?
7. Generally, suppositories are kept refrigerated in Dr. Reed's office. If the Compazine is, indeed, refrigerated, what must Latoya do first?
8. As she prepares to administer the Compazine, what procedure, step by step, must Latoya follow in order to correctly administer this medication rectally?
9. Is the administration, including patient instructions, any different given that the patient is a child?

References

Anderson, K., and Anderson, L. *Mosby's Pocket Dictionary of Medicine, Nursing, & Allied Health.* Chicago: Mosby, 1994.

Bledsoe, B., Clayden, D., and Papa, F. *Prehospital Emergency Pharmacology,* 4th ed., Upper Saddle River, NJ: Brady/Prentice Hall, 1996.

Dickerson, P. "10 Tips for Easing the Pain of Intramuscular Injections." *Nursing.* 28:8, 1992.

Hitner, H. and Nagle, B. *Basic Pharmacology for Health Occupations,* 3rd ed. New York: Glencoe, 1994.

Keen, M. "Get on the Right Track with Z-track Injections." *Nursing.* 20:8, 1990.

Levine, G. *Pocket Guide to Commonly Prescribed Drugs.* Stamford, CT: Appelton & Lange, 1996.

Monaghan, J., ed. "IM and SC Injections." *Patient Care.* 24:16, 1990.

Moore, H. and Best, G. *Drug Calculations.* Upper Saddle River, NJ: Brady/Prentice Hall, 1995.

Newton, M. "Reviewing the Big Three Injection Routes." *Nursing.* 22:2, 1992.

Physician's Desk Reference, 44th ed. Oradell, NJ: Medical Economics, 1990.

Schwinghammer, T. *Pharmacotherapy: A Patient Focused Approach.* Stamford, CT: Appelton & Lange, 1997.

Taber's Cyclopedic Medical Dictionary, 18th ed. Philadelphia: F.A. Davis, 1997.

Taylor, H. "Patient's Deserve Painless Injections— Z-track Techniques." *RN.* March, 1992.

US Department of Health and Human Service. *Parent's Guide to Childhood Immunizations.* Atlanta: Centers for Disease Control, January, 1992.

MEDICAL ASSISTANT ROLE DELINEATION CHART

Highlight indicates material covered in this chapter

ADMINISTRATIVE

ADMINISTRATIVE PROCEDURES

- Perform basic clerical functions
- Schedule, coordinate, and monitor appointments
- Schedule inpatient/outpatient admissions and procedures
- Understand and apply third party guidelines
- Obtain reimbursement through accurate claims submission
- Monitor third-party reimbursement
- Perform medical transcription
- Understand and adhere to managed care policies and procedures
- *Negotiate managed care contracts (adv)*

PRACTICE FINANCES

- Perform procedural and diagnostic coding
- Apply bookkeeping principles
- Document and maintain accounting and banking records
- Manage accounts receivable
- Manage accounts payable
- Process payroll
- *Develop and maintain fee schedules (adv)*
- *Manage renewals of business and professional insurance policies (adv)*
- *Manage personal benefits and maintain records (adv)*

CLINICAL

FUNDAMENTAL PRINCIPLES

- Apply principles of aseptic technique and infection control
- Comply with quality assurance practices
- Screen and follow up patient test results

DIAGNOSTIC ORDERS

- Collect and process specimens
- Perform diagnostic tests

PATIENT CARE

- Adhere to established triage procedures
- Obtain patient history and vital signs
- Prepare and maintain examination and treatment areas

- Prepare patient for examinations, procedures, and treatments
- Assist with examinations, procedures, and treatments
- Prepare and administer medications and immunizations
- Maintain medication and immunization records
- Recognize and respond to emergencies
- Coordinate patient care information with other health care providers

GENERAL (TRANSDISCIPLINARY)

PROFESSIONALISM

- Project a professional manner and image
- Adhere to ethical principles
- Demonstrate initiative and responsibility
- Work as a team member
- Manage time efficiently
- Prioritize and perform multiple tasks
- Adapt to change
- Promote the CMA credential
- Enhance skills through continuing education

COMMUNICATION SKILLS

- Treat all patients with compassion and empathy
- Recognize and respect cultural diversity
- Adapt communications to individual's ability to understand
- Use professional telephone technique
- Use effective and correct verbal and written communications
- Recognize and respond to verbal and non-verbal communications
- Use medical terminology appropriately
- Receive, organize, prioritize, and transmit information
- Serve as liaison
- Promote the practice through positive public relations

LEGAL CONCEPTS

- Maintain confidentiality
- Practice within the scope of education, training, and personal capabilities
- Prepare and maintain medical records
- Document accurately
- Use appropriate guidelines when releasing information
- Follow employer's established policies dealing with the health care contract
- Follow federal, state, and local legal guidelines
- Maintain awareness of federal and state health care legislation and regulations
- Maintain and dispose of regulated substances in compliance with government guidelines
- Comply with established risk management and safety procedures
- Recognize professional credentialing criteria
- Participate in the development and maintenance of personnel, policy, and procedure manuals
- *Develop and maintain personnel, policy, and procedure manuals (adv)*

INSTRUCTION

- Instruct individuals according to their needs
- Explain office policies and procedures
- Teach methods of health promotion and disease prevention
- Locate community resources and disseminate information
- *Orient and train personnel (adv)*
- *Develop educational materials (adv)*
- *Conduct continuing education activities (adv)*

OPERATIONAL FUNCTIONS

- Maintain supply inventory
- Evaluate and recommend equipment and supplies
- Apply computer techniques to support office operations
- *Supervise personnel (adv)*
- *Interview and recommend job applicants (adv)*
- *Negotiate leases and prices for equipment and supply contracts (adv)*

SOURCE: Reprinted by permission of the American Association of Medical Assistants from the *AAMA Role Delineation Study: Occupational Analysis of the Medical Assisting Profession.*

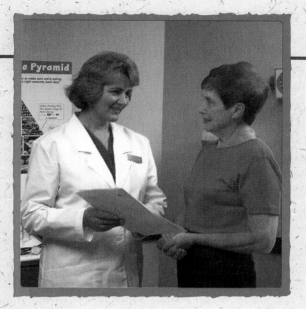

33

Patient Education and Nutrition

CHAPTER OUTLINE

LEARNING OBJECTIVES

After completing this chapter, you should:

1. Define and spell the glossary terms for this chapter.
2. List and describe 5 mechanisms on how adults learn.
3. State 10 teaching methods and strategies to use for patient education.
4. Discuss 6 tips for clear writing.
5. Describe the 4 changes that take place as people age.
6. Describe the process used when developing a teaching plan.
7. Discuss some of the reasons for noncompliance with patient education.
8. Define metabolism.
9. Describe the 6 classifications of foods.
10. Discuss the difference between saturated and unsaturated fats.
11. Discuss the difference between LDL and HDL in cholesterol.
12. Describe the food guide pyramid and state its importance for patient education.
13. Discuss calories as the term relates to proteins, carbohydrates and fats.
14. State the formula for determining the % of calories in a food that are supplied by fat.
15. List and discuss 10 important dietary guidelines.
16. State 10 diet modifications and why they are ordered by the physician.

CLINICAL PERFORMANCE COMPETENCIES

After completing this chapter, you should perform the following tasks:

1. Develop a patient teaching plan.
2. Develop a patient follow-up plan.
3. Design patient teaching materials
4. Use the food pyramid to design a healthy eating plan.

digestion The process by which food is broken down mechanically and chemically in the alimentary canal.

hydrogenation A process of changing an unsaturated fat to a solid saturated fat by the addition of hydrogen.

ingested Food or drink taken orally.

monosaccharides A simple sugar that cannot be decomposed further, such as fructose, or glucose.

nutrient(s) Food or any substance that supplies the body with elements necessary for metabolism.

obesity An abnormal amount of fat on the body of an individual who is 20% over the average weight for his or her age, sex, or height.

predisposes The tendency or susceptibility to develop a certain disease or condition.

regimen A systematic plan of activities.

O ne of the rights patients have is to receive instructions on how they can manage their own health needs. The medical assistant is often the person of choice to provide patient education. Patients become familiar with the medical assistant who escorts them into the exam room, is often present during the examination process, and who they will see when the exam is complete. This familiarity and comfort level of the patient assists in the learning process.

The medical assistant will also be called upon to provide nutrition education for patients. A good knowledge of nutrition is necessary to understand the correct balance of nutrients that is necessary in a daily diet. The second half of this chapter provides a thorough presentation of nutrition.

Patient Education

Most of the patients you will be teaching will be adults. If children do need instruction, their parents should be present so they can reinforce the teaching. Most patient education concepts apply to both the child and adult learner. There are specific learning concepts that relate to the adult based on language skills, previous experience, and motivation.

How Adults Learn

Adult learning is an active process and adults prefer to participate actively. Therefore, activities and techniques that call for participation, such as role playing, will achieve more learning faster than those that do not, for example lecture.

Learning must be self-directed for adults. Therefore the clearer and more relevant the statement of desired outcomes, the more learning that will take place. Any learning that is applied immediately by the patient is retained longer. Practical application of learning is desired by most adult learners.

The adult often prefers a group learning atmosphere because of the group mutual support it offers. In order for learning to be effective it must be reinforced. This can be done either through the group or by the teacher. Weight loss centers have used this technique effectively.

Learning new material is facilitated when it is reinforced by material that is already known. For instance, when instructing a new colostomy patient on the necessity for meticulous handwashing before and after handling the colostomy material, it is important to build upon the patient's previous knowledge of handwashing.

Motivational incentives for adult learners are health, improved appearance, pride of accomplishment, self-confidence, and praise from others. In addition to frequent praise, the adult learner learns more rapidly when he or she is made aware of progress. The time an adult spends on learning is related to many factors, including:

- Number of years spent in school
- Reading level
- Use of vocabulary
- Satisfaction with previous attempts to learn
- Health status of family members

Teaching Methods and Strategy

Table 33-1 describes several teaching methods that can be used effectively for adults and children. In some cases a combination of methods may prove more useful.

It is recommended that a combination of teaching techniques be used for patient education. For example, when instructing a newly-diagnosed diabetic patient, a combination of

TABLE 33-1   Patient Teaching Methods

Method	Description	Advantage	Disadvantage	Usefulness
Lecture	Formal report or instructions delivered to the patient with little interaction between teacher and learner	Efficient No limit to number of learners	No interaction to handle individual learner confusion May be boring for learner	Patients who need general knowledge (new mothers) Large groups (stop-smoking, weight reduction)
Role Play	Short play in which the learner participates in "playing out" the story	Learner sees how others might do something Learner involvement	Time consuming Learner must be willing to "play" the role	Patients with chronic diseases (hypertension, diabetes) Patient learning new interactions (how to direct home health aid) Handling unusual situations which cannot be demonstrated, such as calling "911" in an emergency
Case Problems	Applies information to real situations	Believable Concrete rather than abstract	Significant facts may be missing Effectiveness depends on teacher	Patients who must apply new knowledge (patient with angina, new mothers, diabetes) Convincing the patient that he or she can successfully do something since others have
Demonstration/Return Demonstration	Showing patients how to do something and then immediately having them do the same procedure	Presents standards for performance both visual and oral Allows learner to know it can be done	May be difficult to see Limited to small group Patient may be nervous	Patients who need to understand cause and effect Patients who must learn new skills (colostomy care, diabetic injections, baby care, CPR)

(Continued on next page)

TABLE 33-1 (*Continued*)

Method	Description	Advantage	Disadvantage	Usefulness
Contracting	Setting up goals with clear behaviors and responsibilities for the patient	Requires learner involvement Promotes learner's strengths Identifies acceptable goals	Requires learner decision-making May be threatening Time-consuming	Patients with chronic disease Well patients who wish to change health habits
Use of Significant Other	Teaching a close relative/friend the same information the patient receives	Provides learner support and reinforcement Learning continues at home	Other person must be willing to help Other person may be a negative influence Other person may foster dependence	Elderly and disabled patients Patients whose compliance is in question
Past Experiences	Building learning on what has been learned in the past rather than creating a new set of knowledge	Identifies potential problems Makes the patient more comfortable	Depends on ability to recall Requires insight	Patients who are anxious or overwhelmed Patients who must change behavior (take medication, use proper diet, exercise)
Group Teaching	Bringing together patients who have common learning needs	Efficient and economical Participants support each other Participants are actively involved	Group may digress Some cultures discourage open discussion Transportation may be a problem Difficult for all to agree on a time	Patients and families with common learning needs (weight reduction, smoking cessation) Patients with chronic disease Preoperative patients School-aged children

(Continued)

Method	Description	Advantage	Disadvantage	Usefulness
Programmed Instruction	Printed instructions that force the learner to understand one concept before going on to the next Every correct response builds toward the next question; can be computer-assisted	Active learner participation Individual pacing Provides immediate feedback	May be impersonal and boring Patient must be literate Lack of personal involvement between patient and teacher Patient must be self-motivated	Self motivated learners Encouraging independence Reading level
Simulations (Games)	To create a pretend scenario for learning purposes	Involves the patient in the learning process Non-threatening Allows patients to see knowledge previously learned	Some patients dislike competition Some patients do not like games Some patients have difficulty following directions or with abstract ideas	Adults and children with acute problems (broken bones), chronic problems (asthma, heart disease), or health promotion issues (dental care, weight control)
Tests of Knowledge	Short questions that relate to the patient's knowledge of the subject	Evaluates patient's knowledge at that moment Gives patient a feeling of accomplishment Raises patient's consciousness of what they were unaware of	May make patients anxious Time-consuming Embarrassed by lack of knowledge	Adults and children who must apply knowledge (diabetic patient, surgical patient with dressing)

(Continued on next page)

Method	Description	Advantage	Disadvantage	Usefulness
Printed Handouts	Brochures or instruction sheets printed for the main purpose of imparting knowledge to the patient	Promotes consistency Gives visual reinforcement	Must be accompanied by verbal teaching Difficult to create since they require clarity and simplicity	Well patients (health maintenance literature) Patients who must remember difficult information (presurgical instructions, medication information)
Diagrams	Picture models of concepts	Offers visual reinforcement Attracts attention of the patient Shows proportions and relationships	Must be accurate May require artistic skill to produce	Preschoolers People with limited reading or vocabulary levels
Models	A miniature (usually) representation of an object produced in a substance, such as clay or plaster	Encourages patient participation Offers direct application of skill	May be expensive	School-age children Adults practicing a skill (CPR, breast self-exam, bathing a child)
Film	A video, slide presentation or moving picture	Recreates real-life situations Effective for patients with limited reading skills	Too fast for the elderly adult May be expensive Takes time to set up and run	Groups of patients Health maintenance material (nutrition, preventive dentistry) Video in waiting room

brief lecture, models of anatomical sites for injections, demonstration/return demonstration of injection procedure, use of significant others, printed handouts, diagrams of injection site rotation, and videos might all be used at different points in the educational process. Table 33-2 provides an extensive list of tips on how to prepare printed material that is easier for patients to read.

The guidelines for effective health instruction provide additional means for improving instruction.

Using language and communication skills that are not suited to the learner creates roadblocks to effective patient learning. Some roadblocks to effective patient learning are

- Ordering, commanding, and directing the patient to learn
- Warning or threatening
- Moralizing or preaching ("ought to do," "should do")
- Judging
- Criticizing
- Name-calling, stereotyping, labeling
- Sarcasm

Teaching the Older Adult

Older adult patients' abilities, motivations, and social circumstances differ from younger patients. Their intellectual capacity does not diminish; in fact, it only changes. Some changes that take place as a person ages include increased amount of time required or slower processing of new material, decreased short-term memory, decreased dexterity, and increased anxiety over new situations

One type of intellectual ability is based on the intelligence absorbed during life, for example vocabulary, arithmetic, and the ability to reflect on and evaluate past experience. This type of intelligence can increase with age. Therefore, the older person is able to learn quickly if the learning requires information acquired in the past. When teaching the older adult, it is wise to explore past experiences using concrete examples, such as "Tell me how you calculate the amount of food you eat on your diabetic diet."

Slowed Processing Time

Older patients need more time to think through and absorb new information, therefore the medical assistant should break down information into small units. When teaching from a list of things, take time to explain each item on the list. For example, when the instructions state, "Call your doctor for the following reasons: temperature over 99 degrees, drainage from the incision, inability to take the medication, or pain," each of these reasons should be explained separately. These explanations should be accompanied by a description of the relationship of each item to the patient's problem.

TABLE 33-2   Tips for Clear Writing

1. Begin the material with a short introduction to state the purpose and to orient the reader.

2. Use titles and headings to clearly define the topics.

3. Use boldface, italics, or underlining to emphasize important words and ideas.

4. Use a summary paragraph to end a section or recap a point.

5. Use one important idea per paragraph.

6. Start each paragraph with a strong topic sentence.

7. Vary the length of sentences.

8. Use frequent examples to clarify ideas with which the reader may not have had experience.

9. Use active rather than passive voice.

10. Avoid polysyllabic words whenever possible. Use shorter words.

11. Avoid using a specialized vocabulary such as medical terminology.

12. Avoid abbreviations except when commonly understood.

1. Always address the patient by name. Do not use the patient's first name unless you have asked permission.

2. Be well organized. Have all materials, models, and brochures together so that you will not have to leave the patient during the education process.

3. Have either a verbal or written order from the physician for teaching medical procedures, such as self-injection.

4. Assume the patient can learn. Do not equate intelligence level with educational level. Avoid talking down to patients.

5. Write or print instructions large enough to be clearly read by the patient.

6. Do not overwhelm the patient with technicalities. The patient does not have to know everything you know.

7. Do not use medical abbreviations when discussing medical procedures or conditions with patients.

8. Define necessary medical terms for patients using simple explanations. Never use "street language" to discuss bodily functions. However, you may have to adapt some medical terms, such as urination, to more common terms or expressions, for example "passing water," if the patient does not understand.

9. Correct patient errors in the learning process without harsh judgment. Reemphasize the correct information.

10. Avoid teaching by performing the procedure over and over for the patient. Give a demonstration of a procedure, such as drawing up insulin for the diabetic patient. Then, allow the patient to immediately practice. If the technique is not perfect, reinforce learning by having the patient perform the procedure again.

11. Establish a quiet, unhurried, non-threatening atmosphere for patient education. It should not be conducted in a waiting room or hallway.

12. Remember that if a patient is facing you as you demonstrate a procedure, such as bathing a baby or giving CPR, the patient's hands will be reversed when performing the procedure. Whenever possible, have the learner stand next to you during a one-on-one demonstration.

13. Avoid criticism. Always stress the positive with comments, such as "You're doing fine. Let's try it one more time."

Decreased Short-term Memory

The older adult patient can remember easily things that happened in the past but may have difficulty remembering new information that was acquired yesterday. Learning then becomes very frustrating for them. The medical assistant should work with the patient to devise methods to reinforce instruction or prod the memory. The new information should be linked to a well-known past experience when possible. Always attempt to reinforce old ways of doing things rather than introducing new behavior. For example, when teaching the signs and symptoms of an infection to an older diabetic patient, ask the patient to recall the symptoms experienced in the past with an infected wound or cut.

Decreased Dexterity

Due to arthritis and other physical changes some elderly patients are not able to do the same things they could when they were younger. Advising an overweight elderly patient who uses a cane and is on a reduction diet to get more exercise by walking for one hour a day may not be appropriate for them.

Some procedures requiring small muscle dexterity such as flossing teeth and opening medication bottles are almost impossible for the elderly person with arthritis. Adaptive equipment may have to be advised for these patients (see Chapter 24).

Increased Anxiety Over New Situations

The elderly patient must be given a feeling of confidence by the medical assistant. This can alleviate some of the anxiety over a new learning situation. When the patient sees that they are able to manage the situation they will relax and learning will take place.

Teaching methods to use for the older adult range from handouts with large print, to video and audiovisual displays. Slow moving slides are preferable to a fast video or movie since the slide can be stopped to reinforce learning. Role playing can be useful as long as the patient's energy level can be maintained.

Family members should be included in the teaching process whenever possible. The elderly person is accustomed to being in control and may not wish to learn anything new if he or she does not see the advantage.

> **Med Tip:** Elderly patients may not like to be addressed by their first name. Use the more formal style of address, for example Miss., Mrs., or Mr. followed by the patient's surname unless the patient instructs you otherwise.

Developing a Teaching Plan

An effective teaching plan for both the adult and child learner must include desired outcomes. A teaching plan that the medical assistant develops for a condition, such as hypertension (high blood pressure), can be used with some adaptations for all patients with hypertension. Table 33-3 illustrates a sample teaching plan.

Handling Noncompliance

Noncompliance in following a physician's orders can seriously jeopardize a patient's health and recovery. For instance, a patient with hypertension who fails to take prescribed medication, can develop uncontrolled hypertension, stroke and/or heart attack. In addition, health care costs escalate with noncompliance.

Several groups of patients, including those who have had heart by-pass or hemodialysis, have been followed-up to determine their compliance level. In both situations the compliance levels were around 50%. Lack of compliance may be indicated by failure to (1) take medication as ordered, (2) return for follow-up appointments, (3) practice dietary changes, and (4) follow an exercise programs. On the other hand, patients with cystic fibrosis, a serious disease causing respiratory problems and failure, were found to be more than 80% compliant with their medication regimen. This compliance was attributed to the possibility that these patients and their families perceived the consequences for failure to take cystic fibrosis medications were very serious.

Noncompliance with instructions is a problem for all age groups but children have the least problem as long as their parents are compliant and assist them. Patients who have formed a positive relationship with their health care provider,

physician, and other staff, such as the medical assistant, have been found to be more compliant.

One of the best methods to encourage patient compliance is through the effect of knowledge or education. For instance the cystic fibrosis patients mentioned above were more compliant after realizing the seriousness of their disease.

In addition to having greater knowledge, the patient must also want to comply. The medical assistant can reinforce learning, and reduce noncompliance, by working out a follow-up plan with regular evaluation of progress. This plan will include an objective stating what the patient should be able to do along with a date indicating when the objective should be accomplished. Table 33-4 is an example of a patient-education-follow-up plan.

Nutrition

Nutrition includes all the processes involved in using foods for growth, repair, and maintenance of the body. The nutrition process includes ingestion, digestion, absorption, and metabolism. Some nutrients are capable of being stored in the body and can be used when the food intake is insufficient. Other nutrients such as vitamin C are not stored and need to be continually replenished.

Interest in nutrition has been around for a long time. Debilitating diseases such as scurvy, rickets, and beriberi were found to be caused by deficiencies in the diet. Scurvy was discovered to be a disease of sailors and others who did not receive fresh fruits and vegetables for long periods of time. When sailors began to take lemons and limes along on their sea voyages, the symptoms of scurvy (hemorrhages, anemia, weakness, sallow complexion) disappeared. A lack of vitamin C was the culprit. Rickets, caused by a deficiency of vitamin D, produced bowed legs in young babies and children until this vitamin was added to milk to fortify it. Beriberi, more commonly found in rice-growing regions, caused neurologic and cardiovascular abnormalities until thiamin was added to the diet of patients.

The cures for these diseases resulted from research into what people were eating. The study of nutrition is performed by nutritionists and dietitians. Nutritionists provide information on foods and nutrition. Dietitians promote good health through proper diet and the use of diet in the treatment of disease.

It has been said that the typical American diet contains too much fat, too many calories, too

TABLE 33-3   Sample Teaching Plan for Hypertension

Purpose: To give the patient and family information about the causes of hypertension, recognition of symptoms, and steps to control hypertension.

Content:

I.   Basic anatomy and physiology of the heart and blood vessels.

II.   What is hypertension?

III.   Symptoms of hypertension.

IV.   Risk factors related to hypertension.

V.   Situations that might precipitate hypertension.

VI.   Home treatment for hypertension.

VII.   Handling medications.

VIII.   Reasons to contact the physician.

IX.   Follow-up.

X.   Community Resources/Support Groups.

Learner Objectives:

I.   The patient describes the anatomy and physiology of the heart muscle and blood vessels in simple terms.

    A. The heart muscle is a strong hollow organ that acts as a pump. It pumps blood throughout the body and lungs.

    B. Blood vessels throughout the body carry oxygen to the tissues and cells.

    C. When the blood vessels become narrowed or do not function properly it can cause the heart to work harder. Eventually, pressure within the vessels will rise.

II.   The patient states in simple terms the definition and causes of hypertension.

    A. Hypertension is an elevation in blood pressure in which the systolic pressure is 140 mm Hg or above and the diastolic pressure is 90 mm Hg or above.

    B. An elevated blood pressure reading is a signal that there is a problem which could affect the heart action or even cause a stroke.

    C. Hypertension (high blood pressure) may be caused by a buildup of fatty substances (cholesterol) on the lining of the blood vessels that feed the heart.

III.   The patient states the most common symptoms of hypertension.

    A. This is generally a "silent" disease which means there are few or no symptoms.

    B. The patient may feel very well.

    C. The best indicator is an elevated blood pressure reading on several occasions.

    D. May have headaches or dizziness.

    E. Patient's symptoms are _____.

(Continued)

IV.   The patient defines risk factors and describes controllable and uncontrollable risk factors.

A. Risk factors are habits or characteristics that increase the probability of developing a narrowing of the blood vessels.

B. Controllable factors are

1. Obesity (20% over the average weight for the age, sex, and height)

2. Cigarette smoking

3. Increased amount of fatty substances in the blood

4. Stress

5. Lack of exercise

6. Diet

C. Uncontrollable factors are

1. Family history

2. Diabetes

3. Patients over the age of 50

D. Patient's risk factors are

Controllable _____

_____

Uncontrollable _____

_____

V.   Patient states situations that may precipitate hypertension.

A. Diet heavy in fats and salt

B. Stress

C. Smoking

D. Family history

E. Age

F. Lack of exercise

G. Patient's hypertension may be precipitated by the following:

_____

_____

VI.   The patient states the home treatment of hypertension.

A. Monitor blood pressure with home equipment. Record blood pressure readings.

B. Take medications on a regular basis at the same time every day.

C. Adjust diet by eliminating salt and fat and reducing calorie intake.

(Continued on next page)

TABLE 33-3 Continued

    D. Monitor weight

    E. Use stress reduction techniques

    F. Moderate exercise

VII. The patient states how to handle medications.

    A. Patient must call physician for a prescription renewal every 3 months.

    B. Patient must have a supply of medication on hand when traveling.

    C. Patient must come in to have blood pressure checked by physician every 2 weeks.

VIII. The patient states reasons to contact the physician or go to the emergency room.

    A. Dizziness or fainting.

    B. Blood pressure reading of 160/98 or higher.

IX. The patient provides the following:

Physician #: _____

Emergency Room #: _____

If the patient and/or significant others are unable to complete some or all of this teaching plan, document evaluation in progress notes on chart.

TABLE 33-4 Patient-Education-Follow-up Plan

Objective	Performance	Date Needed
Objective 1. Self-administer insulin injections	1. Understand types of insulin	2/14/19XX
	2. Practice drawing up insulin (X3)	2/14/19XX
	3. Practice on anatomical model (X3)	2/16/19XX
	4. Demonstration on patient by instructor using saline	2/18/19XX
	5. Return demonstration using saline	2/18/19XX
	6. Injection of insulin	2/18/19XX
	7. Follow-up to check technique	3/1/19XX

much cholesterol, too much salt, not enough fiber, and insufficient complex carbohydrates. Nutritionists believe that many Americans receive more than 40% of their daily calories from fats. The best diet is a well balanced eating plan with the correct proportion of the major nutrients (Figure 33-1). A well-nourished person is better able to ward off infection, remain more alert, and may even be able to live longer.

Digestion

Digestion is the actual process the body undergoes when it converts food into chemical substances that can be absorbed into the blood and used by the body tissues and organs. The actual digestive process is accomplished by physically breaking down, diluting, and dissolving food substances. In the process they are also chemically

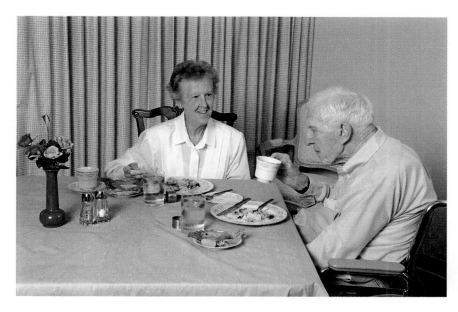

Figure 33-1   Sharing a meal with someone may improve the appetite.

split into simpler compounds. For example, proteins are broken down into amino acids; carbohydrates are broken down into monosaccharides (simple sugars); and fats are absorbed as fatty acids and glycerol (glycerin).

Actual digestion takes place in the alimentary canal also referred to as the digestive system (Figure 33-2). Accessory organs including the salivary glands, liver, gallbladder, and pancreas provide essential enzymes for digestion through their secretions. Water, minerals, some vitamins, and some of the carbohydrates in fruit are absorbable as soon as they are ingested.

The average adult stomach holds about 1 1/2 quarts of food and liquid. The stomach will reach a peak in the digestive process 2 hours after a meal and may take 3-5 hours to empty into the small intestine. It may take 20 minutes for the brain to register that food has entered the system. The digestion process is influenced by emotions as well as the enzyme and chemical actions of the digestive system. A quiet, calm atmosphere at meal time can enhance the digestive process.

Metabolism

Metabolism is the sum of all physical and chemical changes that take place within the human body. Metabolism is the process of changing food, air, water and other materials into substances absorbed into the body through the blood and respiratory system. Specific enzymes that are required to maintain metabolism are amino acids, carbohydrates, vitamins and essential trace minerals.

Approximately 23% of all the energy released by nutrients is used by the body to carry on its normal functions, such as respiration, digestion, reproduction, muscular movement, circulation, and cellular regrowth. The remaining 75% of the energy becomes heat. Eating and drinking the wrong foods can negatively affect metabolism.

Med Tip: We might like to blame a sluggish metabolism for a tendency to put on weight. However, it is rare for a person to have a metabolism that predisposes him or her to gain weight. A person is considered to be predisposed to a certain condition or disease when he or she has a tendency or susceptibility to develop the condition or disease due to the family's medical history regarding such conditions.

Classification of Nutrients

Nutrients are the organic and inorganic chemical substances found in foods that supply the body with necessary elements for metabolism. Certain nutrients (carbohydrates, fats, and proteins) provide energy; other nutrients (water, electrolytes, minerals and vitamins) are essential to the metabolic process.

There are six main classifications of nutrients and a total of over 50 nutrients that are

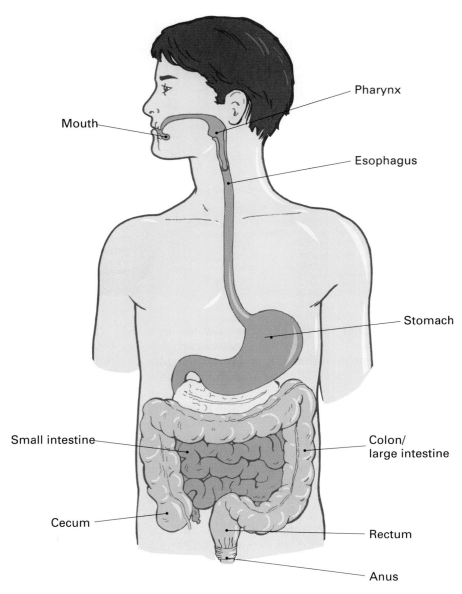

Mouth

Pharynx

Esophagus

Stomach

Small intestine

Colon/
large intestine

Cecum

Rectum

Anus

Figure 33-2 The digestive system.

required for the human body to function properly. These nutrients must be consumed in a diet on a daily basis. The six classifications of nutrients are

1. Carbohydrates
2. Protein
3. Fat
4. Water
5. Vitamins
6. Minerals

Carbohydrates

The main source of energy from foods is from carbohydrates. Carbohydrates are the sugars (simple carbohydrates), starches (complex carbohydrates), and fiber (cellulose) that are found mainly in plants. They are stored in the body as glycogen in virtually all tissues but mainly in the liver and muscles. They form an important source of reserved energy in the body.

Sugars include simple sugars (monosaccharides of glucose, galactose, and fructose) and complex sugars (disaccharide of sucrose, lactose or milk sugar, and maltose). Starches are polysaccharides which are reduced to glucose during the digestive process and transported into the blood.

Carbohydrates provide 4 calories of energy for every gram of carbohydrate. Complex carbohydrates are considered ideal foods for a healthy diet since they are generally low in fat, high in fiber, and are a good source for vitamins and minerals. An excess of carbohydrates are stored in the body as fat.

Sources of simple carbohydrates (simple sugars) are

- Refined table sugar, honey, jelly, syrup, candy
- Natural sugar in fruits and vegetables

Sources of complex carbohydrates (starches) are

- Vegetables (yams, potatoes, broccoli, carrots, peas, beans)
- Citrus fruits (oranges, grapefruit, lemons, limes)
- Whole grains, cereals, and pastas

Nutritionists recommend that only 10% of the body's calorie requirements should come from refined sugar. Complex carbohydrates should provide 50% to 60% of the daily calorie requirements.

Protein

Proteins are called the "building blocks" of the body since they form the base of every living cell. A protein is linked together, much like a chain, with 20 amino acids. Eleven of the amino acids can be produced by the body. However nine amino acids, referred to as essential amino acids, must be obtained from the diet.

The nine essential amino acids are only found in complete proteins which includes proteins from animal sources, such as meat, cheese, eggs, fish, and milk. Incomplete proteins, which cannot supply the body with all the essential amino acids include vegetable proteins, such as peas, beans, and wheat. Fortunately, various combinations of the incomplete proteins can supply the essential amino acids, for example legumes and rice. It is recommended that 12% to 15% of the daily calories consumed come from proteins.

Proteins are necessary for

- Producing energy (four calories of energy for every gram of protein consumed).
- Promoting growth and repair of tissues.
- Providing the framework for bones, muscles, and blood.

Fats

Fats, also called lipids, are fatty acids which can be chemically classified as saturated or unsatu-rated. Fats do not dissolve in water. Some fat is necessary in the diet since the fat-soluble vitamins A, D, E, and K are all carried into the blood system by way of fats. There are also two critical fatty acids, linoleic and linolenic, which are "essential" to the diet.

Saturated fat is produced by animal sources, such as meat, eggs, lard, and dairy products and certain oil producing plants such as coconuts and palms. Many commercially prepared cakes, cookies, and non-dairy creamers contain hidden saturated fat. Saturated fat has many negative effects on the body including raising the level of blood cholesterol. It is recommended that no more than 10% of the daily calorie intake should come from saturated fat. Fat reduction can also reduce the risk of disease, for example certain types of cancer, heart disease, and stroke.

Unsaturated fats are of two types: polyunsaturated fat and monounsaturated fat. Polyunsaturated fat is found in vegetable oils and fish oils (Omega-3 fatty acids). Unsaturated fat is normally liquid at room temperature but can be converted into a solid fat through the process of hydrogenation. Hydrogenation turns liquid unsaturated fat into margarine by adding hydrogen.

Monounsaturated fat is considered to be a more desirable type of unsaturated fat since it has the ability to lower cholesterol levels and LDLs. Monounsaturated fats include canola oil, olive oil, and peanut oil. Fats, in moderation, are beneficial for the body. These fats

- Are a concentrated source of energy (9 calories of energy for every gram of fat consumed)
- Aid in the transportation of soluble fat-vitamins A, D, E, and K
- Serve as a source of energy
- Provide some taste to foods
- Satisfy appetite
- Provide lubrication for skin and internal tissues
- Are stored for future energy use

Unfortunately, many Americans are eating more fat in their diet than they need. Many foods contain hidden fat. Fat content is indicated on many foods. However, food labeling can be confusing and misleading. A high fiber muffin may actually contain polyunsaturated fat, eggs, sugar, and very little fiber. See Table 33-5 for an example of food labeling components mandated by the Department of Health and Human Services and the US Department of Agriculture.

TABLE 33-5 Food Label for Snack Crackers

Food Labeling Components	
Nutrition Facts	
Serving Size 16 Crackers (29g)	
Servings Per Container About 4	
Amount Per Serving	
Calories	140
Calories from Fat	50
	% Daily Value*
Total Fat 6g	9%
Saturated Fat 1g	6%
Polyunsaturated Fat 0.5g	
Monounsaturated Fat 2.5g	
Cholesterol 0mg	0%
Sodium 170mg	7%
Total Carbohydrate 19g	6%
Dietary Fiber 2g	
Protein 2g	
Vitamin A	0%
Vitamin C	0%
Calcium	2%
Iron	4%
* Percent Daily Values are based on a 2,000 calorie diet. Your daily values may be higher or lower depending on your calorie needs.	

	Calories	2,000	2,500
Total Fat	Less than	65g	80g
Sat Fat	Less than	20g	25g
Cholesterol	Less than	300mg	300mg
Sodium	Less than	2,400mg	2,400mg
Total Carb.		300mg	375g
Dietary Fiber		25g	30g

Water

Water is considered a vital nutrient that is necessary for survival. The human body can survive for several weeks without food, but cannot live more than a few days without water. Water is an inorganic nutrient with no caloric value. Approximately two-thirds of the body is water.

The average human body is composed of between 50 to 60 percent water. The male body has more water than the female due to the greater muscle mass of the male, which can hold more water. The female body, on the other hand, contains a greater percentage of fat than the male body. Fat does not hold as much water as muscle tissue does.

There are a variety of sources for water in the body. Water is found in most fruits and vegetables, ingested as a liquid beverage, or occurs naturally as a result of metabolism. The function of water in the body is described in Table 33-6.

The recommended daily amount of water to be ingested is six to eight glasses. Since water occurs in many foods, such as fruits, vegetables, meats, crackers, and even desserts, most people ingest enough water on a daily basis. Water intake is kept in balance with fluid output through the skin, lungs, urine, and feces. Individuals vary in their requirements for water depending on

- Age
- Body size
- Exercise
- Climate
- Pregnancy
- Illness
- Metabolic rate
- Diet

Vitamins

Vitamins are organic substances that are essential for metabolism, growth, and development of the body. They are not sources of energy but they are required for health. There are a variety of conditions that increase the need for vitamins above the usual recommended dose. These include pregnancy, lactation, excessive use of alcohol, and some illnesses.

In general, most of the vitamins cannot be formed in the body with the exception of vitamin A which is formed from carotene. Vitamin D is formed by the action of ultraviolet light on the skin (sunlight) and vitamin K by bacteria of the intestines.

Vitamins are generally identified by their alphabetic letter. The two main classifications of vitamins are: fat-soluble (A, D, E, and K) and water-soluble (B and C). This is important in patients who have diseases that interfere with the digestion of fat, such as in celiac disease, since they will eventually develop a deficiency in the fat-soluble vitamins. The human body cannot manufacture vitamin C therefore it must be taken in foods—citrus fruits—or as a supplement.

Sources for water-soluble vitamins are

- Vitamin B1—liver, eggs, pork, wheat germ, yeast-enriched cereals, nuts
- Vitamin B2—milk, liver, egg white, yeast, wheat germ, almonds
- Vitamin B6—wheat bran, molasses, liver, soybeans, bananas, raisins
- Vitamin B12—beef, liver, milk, shellfish, cheese
- Niacin—liver, poultry, enriched cereals, tuna, peanuts
- Biotin—egg yolks, legumes, meat

TABLE 33-6   **Function of Water in the Body**

Water is used by the body to
• Carry oxygen and nutrients to cells
• Regulate body temperature
• Prevent dehydration
• Replace water lost through perspiration, respiration, urination, and defecation
• Remove waste products from cells
• Protect organs and tissues

- Folacin—legumes, green leafy vegetables
- Pantothenic Acid—legumes, grains
- Vitamin C—citrus fruits, raw vegetables, strawberries

Sources of fat-soluble *vitamins are*

- Vitamin A—green and yellow vegetables, animal foods, egg yolks, cheese
- Vitamin D—milk, butter, margarine, sardines, fish liver oils, sunlight
- Vitamin E—wheat germ, corn oil, soybeans
- Vitamin K—green leafy vegetables, liver, cabbage, cauliflower

Vitamins can be destroyed in foods through improper storage and prolonged cooking. They do provide essential organic substances. See Table 33-7 for a further description of individual vitamins.

Minerals

Minerals are inorganic elements which are neither of animal nor of plant origin. They are found throughout the body but mainly in bones and teeth and compose 5% of the body. The two classifications of minerals are: macrominerals (major minerals) and microminerals (trace minerals). The macrominerals include calcium, magnesium, phosphorus, sodium, potassium, chlorine, and sulfur. Macrominerals are required in greater amounts than the trace minerals iron, iodine, copper, manganese, cobalt, fluorine, zinc, selenium, chromium, nickel, tin and vanadium. Minerals are found in the following sources:

- Vegetables and fruits for calcium, iron, phosphorus, copper, and iodine.
- Milk and leafy vegetables for calcium
- Balanced diet

Minerals do not supply calories or energy. See Table 33-7 for more information on minerals.

Cholesterol

There is currently much controversy surrounding cholesterol. Cholesterol is a fat-like material that is normally found in the body. It is essential for the function of body systems, such as the nervous system, formation of cell membranes, and many hormones.

Cholesterol is found in only two sources: the human body and in animal sources. There is no cholesterol from plants. Animal sources of choles-

Med Tip: There are many popular books on the market discussing methods for reducing cholesterol which your patients may have read. They will ask your opinion about various diets and medications. Always remind them to discuss these questions with the physician.

terol provide saturated fat which may contribute to elevated blood cholesterol in humans.

Cholesterol moves into and out of the body cells within compounds called lipoproteins. These lipoproteins are classified into either high-density lipoproteins (HDLs) or low-density lipoproteins (LDLs). HDLs are the "good cholesterol" and LDLs are the "bad cholesterol." LDLs are bad since they carry most (60%-70%) of the cholesterol into the blood stream. This cholesterol is deposited into blood vessels and can lead to a narrowing of the blood vessels which leads to heart disease and stroke. HDLs are good because they only contain 20% to 30% of the blood cholesterol and carry cholesterol away from the arteries. It is believed that the higher the HDL level in the blood, the lower is the risk for a cardiovascular disease.

An increase in cholesterol level has been tied to an increased risk for heart disease: heart attack and stroke. There is evidence indicating that unsaturated fats (olive oil and canola oil) may help to lower the amount of cholesterol in the blood. It is important to examine food labels for the amounts of both cholesterol and saturated fat. Many foods contain no cholesterol but have a large amount of saturated fat which can lead to cholesterol buildup in the body.

Balanced Diet

The key to a balanced diet is eating a variety of foods in the correct amount. Eating food as recommended in the food guide pyramid published by the US Department of Health and Human Services, will be adequate for good health. The size of portions and numbers of servings will depend on the age, size, and exercise level of the individual. See Figure 33-3 for an illustration of the basic food groups.

Food Guide Pyramid

A revised food guide pyramid was introduced in 1992 by the United States Department of Agriculture to replace the old "basic four" food

TABLE 33-7 Vitamins and Minerals

Vitamins/Nutrient	Source	Function Deficiency	Toxicity	Recommended Dietary Allowance (RDA)
Vitamin A (carotene): Necessary for formation and maintenance of skin, mucous membranes, teeth and hair, and normal vision	Egg yolk, fish liver oils, liver, green leafy or yellow vegetables, yellow and orange fruits, dairy products	Night blindness, fatigue, scaly skin	Headache, skin peeling, bone thickening, liver and spleen enlargement	5000 IU* per day
Vitamin B1 (thiamine): Carbohydrate metabolism, nerve cell function, heart muscle function	Dried yeast, whole grains, meat (liver and pork), nuts, enriched cereals, potatoes, legumes	Beriberi, fatigue, mental confusion		1.5 mg** per day
Vitamin B2 (riboflavin): Releases energy during protein metabolism	Milk, cheese, eggs, liver, enriched cereals, almonds	Anemia, dermatosis, skin cracks		1.2 mg per day
Vitamin B6 (group): Nitrogen and protein metabolism, assists in building body tissue	Dried yeast, liver, whole-grain cereals, fish, legumes, bananas, avocados	Anemia, seborrheic dermatitis, nervous system disorders convulsions, skin cracks	Nerve damage	2 mg per day
Vitamin B12 (cyanocobalamin): nervous system function, metabolism of fat and protein, cell development	Milk products, seafood, meat, liver, cheese	Pernicious anemia, fatigue, nervousness		6 mcg*** per day
Niacin (nicotinic acid): Carbohydrate, fat, and protein metabolism	Dried yeast, fish, liver, meat, legumes, enriched cereals, eggs, peanuts, poultry	Pellagra, dermatosis, glossitis, CNS dysfunction, fatigue		20 mg per day
Vitamin C (ascorbic acid): Needed to build bones, muscles, blood vessels, and connective tissue. Aids in iron absorption	Citrus fruits, tomatoes, broccoli, potatoes, cabbage, green peppers, berries, strawberries	Scurvy, loose teeth, hemorrhages, gingivitis, fatigue	Nausea and diarrhea	60 mg per day

(Continued on next page)

TABLE 33-7 (Continued)

Vitamins/Nutrient	Source	Function Deficiency	Toxicity	Recommended Dietary Allowance (RDA)
Vitamin D: Necessary for calcium and phosphorus absorption, bone and tooth development and maintenance, helps maintain nervous system and heart muscle action	Fortified milk, butter, margarine, eggs, fish liver oils, liver, sunlight	Rickets, tetany, loss of bone calcium	Diarrhea, weight loss, renal failure	400 IU per day
Vitamin E: Protects blood cell membranes, body tissues and fatty acids from destruction	Vegetable oil, wheat germ, margarine, egg yolk, leafy vegetables, legumes, cereals	Anemia, nerve damage, RBC hemolysis, muscle damage		30 IU per day
Vitamin K: Normal blood coagulation, prothrombin formation	Leafy vegetable, liver, pork, vegetable oils, fruit, dairy	Hemorrhage in newborn and in person taking blood thinner		No RDA for vitamin K
Biotin: metabolism of protein, carbohydrates, and fats	Yeast, liver, kidney, egg yolk, nuts, legumes, cauliflower	Dermatitis, glossitis		0.5 mg per day
Folic Acid: RBC production	Dried legumes, green leafy vegetables, organ meats	Anemia, GI disorders, mouth cracks		0.4 mg per day
Pantothenic Acid: Aids in energy release from carbohydrates and fats	Whole grains, meats, vegetables, fruits, legumes	Muscle cramps, fatigue, vomiting		10 mg per day

Minerals	Source	Function Deficiency	Toxicity	Recommended Dietary Allowance (RDA)
Calcium: Bone and tooth formation, muscle contractility, blood coagulation, myocardial conduction, neuromuscular function	Milk and milk products, meat, fish, eggs, beans, cereals, fruits, vegetables, tofu, fortified orange juice	Hypocalcemia, tetany, neuromuscular excitability, osteoporosis	Hypercalcemia, kidney stones, renal failure	800 mg per day
Chromium: Part of glucose tolerance factor (GTF)	Brewer's yeast and widely distributed in other foods	Impaired glucose tolerance in malnourished children and diabetics		No RDA
Cobalt: Part of vitamin B12 molecule	Green leafy vegetables	Anemia in children		20 mg per day

(Continued)

Minerals	Source	Function Deficiency	Toxicity	Recommended Dietary Allowance (RDA)
Copper: enzyme component	Oysters, organ meats, nuts, dried legumes, whole-grain cereals	Anemia in malnourished children		0.3 mg/kg per day
Fluorine: Bone and tooth formation	Coffee, tea, fluoridated water	Dental caries	Mottling and pitting of permanent teeth	No RDA
Iodine: Thyroxine (T4) and tri-iodothyronine (T3) formation, necessary for energy formation	Seafood, iodized salt, dairy products	Goiter, cretinism	Myxedema	150 mcg per day
Iron: Hemoglobin, enzymes	Soybean flour, kidney, beef, liver, beans, peaches	Anemia		30 mg per day
Magnesium: Bone and tooth formation, nerve conduction, muscle contractility, enzyme activity	Green leafy vegetables, cereals, nuts, wheat bran, grains, seafood, chocolate	Neuromuscular irritability, weakness	Hypotension, respiratory failure, cardiac disturbances	280 mg per day
Phosphorus: Bone and tooth formation, acid-base balance	Milk, cheese, meat, fish, poultry, cereals, nuts, legumes	Irritability, weakness, blood cell disorders		300 mg per day
Potassium: Muscle activity, nerve transmission, intracellular acid-base balance, water retention	Milk, bananas, kiwi, raisins, vegetables	Hypokalemia, paralysis, cardiac arrhythmia (irregular heartbeat)	Hyperkalemia, paralysis, cardiac arrhythmia	2000 mg per day
Sodium: Maintain acid-base balance, muscle contractility, nerve transmission	Meat (beef, pork), cheese, sardines, olives, potato chips, table salt	Hyponatremia, muscle cramping	Hypernatremia, coma, confusion, high blood pressure	500 mg per day
Zinc: Growth, wound healing, component of insulin and enzyme	Vegetables	Growth retardation		30 mg per day

* IU = international units
** mg = milligram
*** mcg = microgram

NUTRIENT CLASS	BODILY FUNCTION	FOOD SOURCES
CARBOHYDRATES 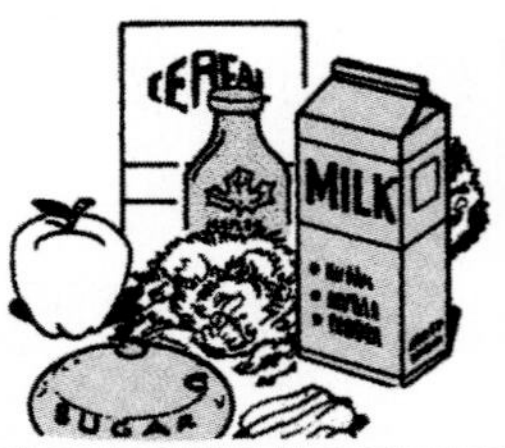	Provides work energy for body activities, and heat energy for maintenance of body temperature.	Cereal grains and their products (bread, breakfast cereals, macaroni products), potatoes, sugar, syrups, fruits, milk, vegetables, nuts.
PROTEINS 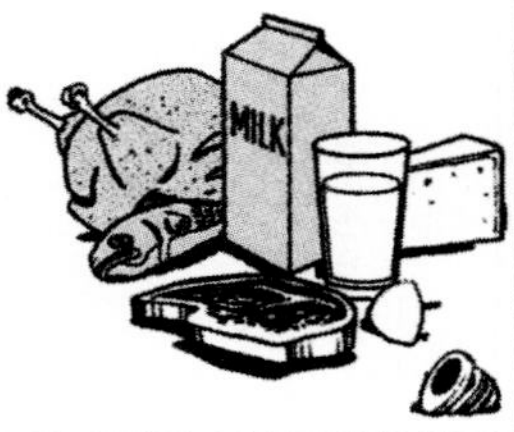	Build and renew body tissues; regulate body functions and supply energy. Complete proteins: maintain life and provide growth. Incomplete proteins: maintain life but do not provide for growth.	Complete proteins: Derived from animal foods — meat, milk, eggs, fish, cheese, poultry. Incomplete proteins: Derived from vegetable foods — soybeans, dry beans, peas, some nuts and whole–grain products.
FATS 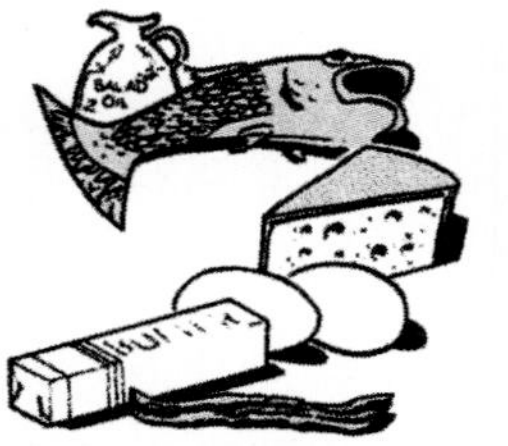	Give work energy for body activities and heat energy for maintenance of body temperature. Carrier of vitamins A and D, provide fatty acids necessary for growth and maintenance of body tissues.	Some foods are chiefly fat, such as lard, vegetable fats and oils, and butter. Many other foods contain smaller proportions of fats — nuts, meats, fish, poultry, cream, whole milk.
MINERALS Calcium 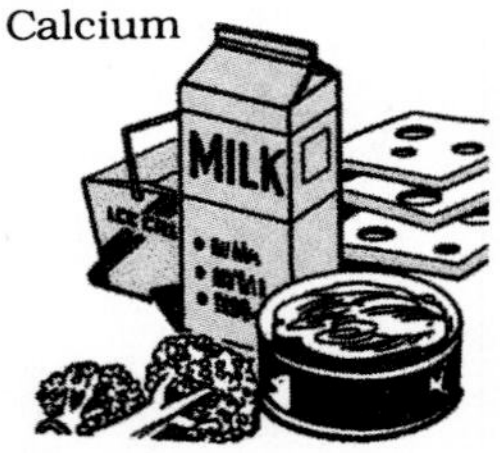	Builds and renews bones, teeth, and other tissues; regulates the activity of the muscles, heart, nerves; and controls the clotting of blood.	Milk and milk products except butter; most dark green vegetables; canned salmon.
PHOSPHORUS 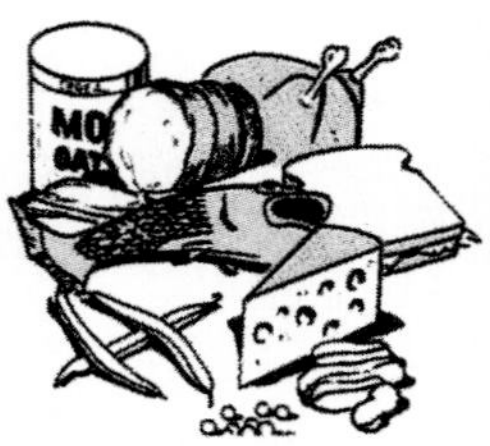	Associated with calcium in some functions needed to build and renew bones and teeth. Influences the oxidation of foods in the body cells; important in nerve tissue.	Widely distributed in foods; especially cheese, oat cereals, whole–wheat products, dry beans and peas, meat, fish, poultry, nuts.

Figure 33-3 (A)   A balanced diet begins with eating foods from the basic food groups.

groups from 1946. The food pyramid is divided into six categories:

1. Breads, cereals, rice, grains and pasta
2. Vegetables
3. Fruits
4. Milk, yogurt, cheese
5. Meat, poultry, fish, dry beans
6. Fats and oils, and sweets

Figure 33-4 illustrates the six categories of the food pyramid. The foods placed in the largest por-

NUTRIENT GLASS	BODILY FUNCTIONS	FOOD SOURCES
MINERALS (continued) Iron 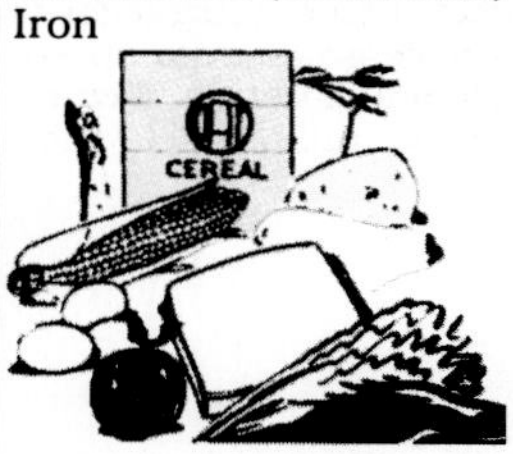	Builds and renews hemoglobin, the red pigment in blood which carries oxygen from the lungs to the cells.	Eggs, meat, especially liver and kidney; deep–yellow and dark green vegetables; potatoes, dried fruits, whole–grain products; enriched flour, bread, breakfast cereals.
Iodine 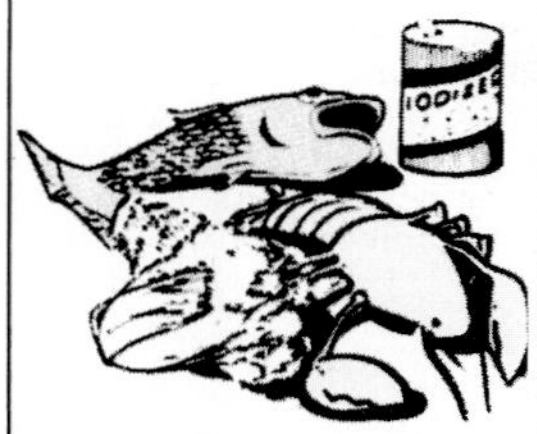	Enables the thyroid gland to perform its function of controlling the rate at which foods are oxidized in the cells.	Fish (obtained from the sea), some plant–foods grown in soils containing iodine; table salt fortified with iodine (iodized).
VITAMINS A 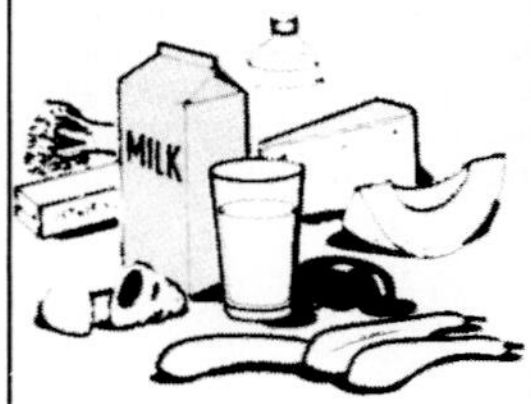	Necessary for normal functioning of the eyes, prevents night blindness. Ensures a healthy condition of the skin, hair, and mucous membranes. Maintains a state of resistance to infections of the eyes, mouth, and respiratory tract.	One form of vitamin A is yellow and one from is colorless. Apricots, cantaloupe, milk, cheese, eggs, meat organs, (especially liver and kidney), fortified margarine, butter fish-liver oils, dark green and deep yellow vegetables.
B Complex B_1 (Thiamine) 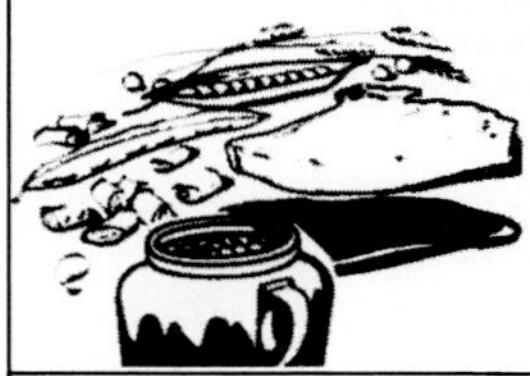	Maintains a healthy condition of the nerves. Fosters a good appetite. Helps the body cells use carbohydrates.	Whole–grain and enriched grain products; meats (especially pork, liver and kidney). Dry beans and peas.
B_2 (Riboflavin) 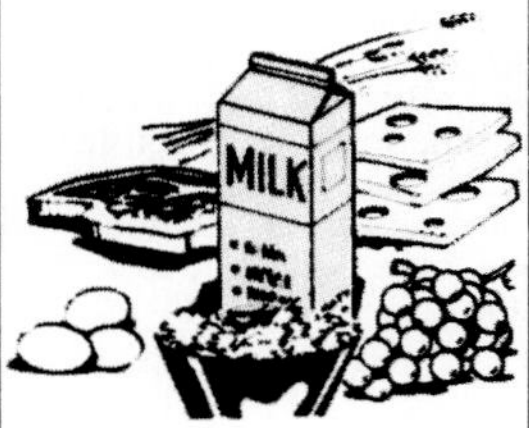	Keeps the skin, mouth, and eyes in a healthy condition. Acts with other nutrients to form enzymes and control oxidation in cells.	Milk, cheese, eggs, meat (especially liver and kidney), whole grain and enriched grain products, dark green vegetables.

Figure 33-3 (B)

tion of the pyramid (breads, cereals, fruits, and vegetables) should be consumed in the largest quantities. Fats, oil, and sweets at the top of the food pyramid should be eaten in very small amounts or not at all. A healthy diet should include a wide variety of foods. Patients can better understand the entire nutritional process if they see the food pyramid. Many offices have a large poster on the wall.

Recommended Dietary Allowances (RDAs)

The Food and Nutrition Board of the National Academy of Sciences of the US government has created standards of recommendations for the amount of protein, vitamins, minerals, and weights that Americans should try to maintain for good nutrition. These standards periodically

NUTRIENT CLASS	BODILY FUNCTIONS	FOOD SOURCES
VITAMINS (Continued) Niacin 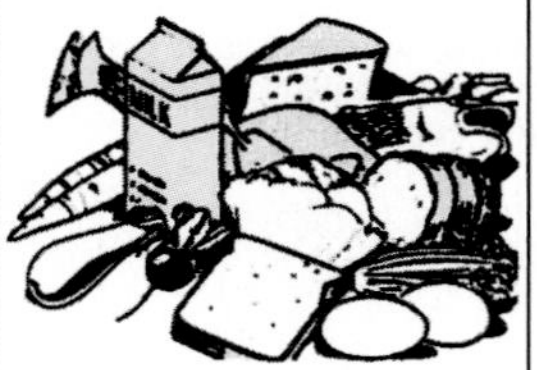	Influences the oxidation of carbohydrates and proteins in the body cells.	Liver, meat, fish poultry, eggs, peanuts; dark green vegetables, whole–grain and enriched cereal products.
B$_{12}$ 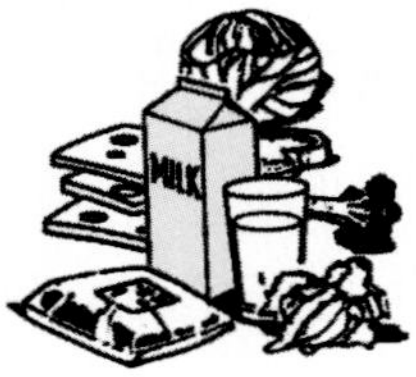	Regulates specific processes in digestion. Helps maintain normal functions of muscles, nerves, heart, blood — general body metabolism.	Liver, other organ meats, cheese, eggs, milk, leafy green vegetables.
C (Ascorbic Acid) 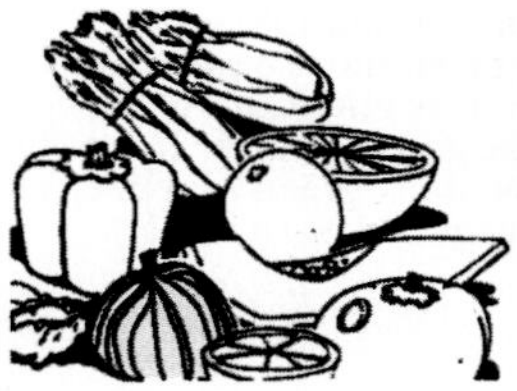	Acts as a cement between body cells, and helps them work together to carry out their special functions. Maintains a sound condition of bones, teeth, and gums. Not stored in the body.	Fresh, raw citrus fruits and vegetables — oranges, grapefruit, cantaloupe, strawberries, tomatoes, raw onions, cabbage, green and sweet red peppers, dark green vegetables.
D 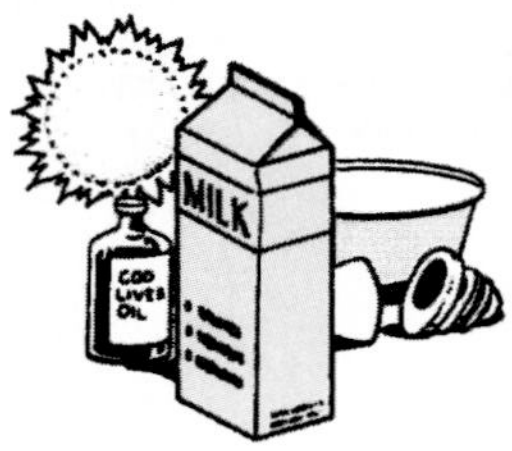	Enables the growing body to use calcium and phosphorus in a normal way to build bones and teeth.	Provided by vitamin D fortification of certain foods, such as milk and margarine. Also fish–liver oils and eggs. Sunshine is also a source of vitamin D.
WATER 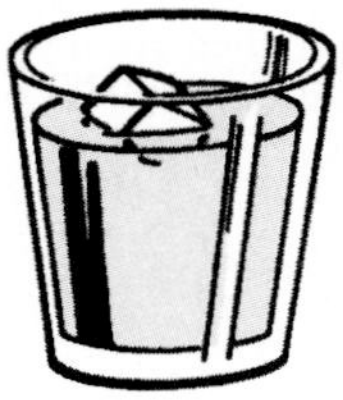	Regulates body processes. Aids in regulating body temperature. Carries nutrients to body cells and carries waste products away from them. Helps to lubricate joints. Water has no food value, although most water contains mineral elements. More immediately necessary to life than food — second only to oxygen.	Drinking water, and other beverages; all foods except those made up of a single nutrient, as sugar and some fats. Milk, milk drinks, soups, vegetables, fruit juices. Ice cream, watermelon, strawberries, lettuce, tomatoes, cereals, other dry products.

Figure 33-3 (C)

change as the weight ranges and protein needs are reviewed. The charts can be ordered through the National Academy Press, Washington, DC.

Calories

The intake of food is measured in terms of the energy that it produces. A calorie is a measurement of a unit of heat that provides energy. The definition of a calorie is the amount of heat (energy) required to raise the temperature of 1 kg of water 1 degree Celsius.

All food (except water) generates energy in the body. Daily calorie requirements of individuals will vary based on a variety of factors including: gender, age, weight, and activity level. Men generally need more calories than women; the young need more calories than older adults; heavier people require more calories to maintain their weight; and active people require more

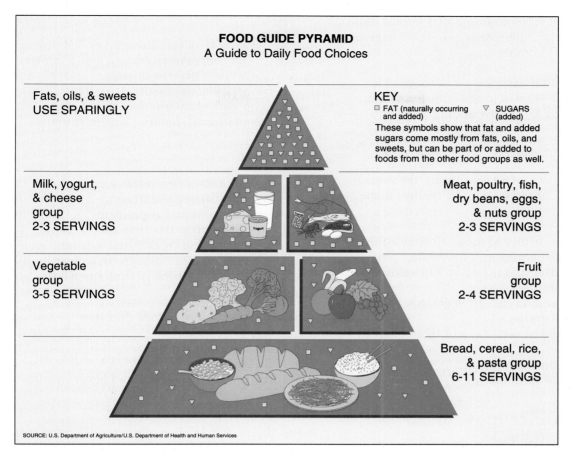

FOOD GUIDE PYRAMID
A Guide to Daily Food Choices

Fats, oils, & sweets
USE SPARINGLY

KEY
□ FAT (naturally occurring and added)   ▽ SUGARS (added)
These symbols show that fat and added sugars come mostly from fats, oils, and sweets, but can be part of or added to foods from the other food groups as well.

Milk, yogurt, & cheese group
2-3 SERVINGS

Meat, poultry, fish, dry beans, eggs, & nuts group
2-3 SERVINGS

Vegetable group
3-5 SERVINGS

Fruit group
2-4 SERVINGS

Bread, cereal, rice, & pasta group
6-11 SERVINGS

SOURCE: U.S. Department of Agriculture/U.S. Department of Health and Human Services

Figure 33-4   The food pyramid.

calories because they tend to burn calories faster than individuals that are inactive. Women require more calories during periods of pregnancy and lactation.

When more calories are taken in than are consumed, they are stored as fat. Overall body weight will increase when this happens on a consistent basis. When fewer calories are taken in than are needed, stored calories are used and the body weight will decrease.

Calories come from the protein, carbohydrate and fats in food. To determine the amount of energy generated by the food eaten use the following figures*:

- Proteins = 4 calories of energy per gram
- Carbohydrate = 4 calories of energy per gram
- Fat = 9 calories of energy per gram

Note: These figures are just for the protein, carbohydrate, and fat content of foods and not the total weight, including fluid, of the food.

Determining the Number of Calories in Food

Using a cookie that contains 1 g of protein, 4 g of carbohydrates and 4 g of fat, calculate the total number of calories.

1. 1 g protein $\times$ 4 calories = 4 calories
2. 4 g of carbohydrates $\times$ 4 calories = 16 calories
3. 4 g of fat $\times$ 9 calories = 36 calories

Total Calories = 4 + 16 + 36 = 58 calories per cookie.

Determining the % of Calories Supplied by Fat

Use this formula when you want to determine the % of calories in a food supplied by fat:

1. Fat calories = Grams of fat $\times$ 9
2. $\dfrac{\text{Fat calories}}{\text{Total calories}} \times 100$ = percentage of calories from fat

Using the previous example of a cookie containing 58 calories, determine the percentage of calories supplied from fat.

1. $4 \times 9 = 36$ fat calories
2. $\frac{36}{58} \times 100 = 62.1\%$ of the calories that are supplied by fat in this cookie

Dietary Guidelines

Under normal disease-free conditions, the average person should observe the following dietary guidelines:

1. Eat a wide variety of foods to acquire the necessary vitamins and minerals.
2. Choose a diet that is low in fat, saturated fat, cholesterol.
3. Eat a diet that is rich in vegetables, fruits, and whole grains.
4. Limit intake of salt. Try not to add salt to food.
5. Use sugar in moderation.
6. Use alcohol in moderation.

Dietary Modifications

The normal (regular) diet can be modified to adjust to specific patient conditions, such as pregnancy, recovery from surgery, gastrointestinal upset, allergies, dental work and disease conditions such as diabetes mellitus. A modified diet for health reasons is called a therapeutic diet. Diets can be modified based on calorie content, level of spice and salt content, bulk, nutrients, consistency, and intervals between meals.

Therapeutic diets need to be carefully explained to patients. In some cases, the physician will refer the patient to a registered dietitian (RD) who can discuss all the aspects of a therapeutic diet with the patient.

The medical assistant will often provide dietary education for patients in the medical office. Since life style changes must be made to comply with some of the diets the patient must be motivated to change. All the principles of adult education need to be considered when teaching patients about dietary changes. Figure 33-5 is an example of a prenatal education and counseling form that addresses dietary changes and modifications and other plans of care during pregnancy.

Clear Liquid Diet

A clear liquid diet contains no solid food or milk products. A clear liquid diet is frequently required

 Med Tip: Remember that only a physician or registered dietitian can prescribe a diet. Other health care professionals, such as medical assistants, assist with patient instruction. Avoid any recommendation of dietary plans to patients.

before certain laboratory tests, examinations or surgery. It may also be prescribed for a patient suffering from gastrointestinal problems. A clear liquid diet is frequently the first diet a patient is placed on after having surgery and a general anesthetic. Patients must not remain on a clear liquid diet for an extended period of time since it has little nutritional value.

Foods included on the clear diet are

- Clear soup and broth
- Plain gelatin
- Black Coffee, tea, carbonated beverages

Full Liquid Diet

A full liquid diet is often prescribed for patients who are unable to chew and/or digest solid food. This may be due to gastrointestinal problems, infections, or oral surgery. This diet is also prescribed as the next diet step for patients who have been on a clear liquid diet.

Foods recommended on a full liquid diet are

- All liquids allowed on a clear diet
- Fruit and vegetable juices
- Strained fruit
- Soup (creamed or strained)
- Milk and milkshakes
- Ice cream

As with the clear liquid diet, a full liquid diet is not to be used for extended periods of time.

Mechanical Soft Diet

The mechanical soft diet is recommended for patients who have dental problems, such as a lack of teeth, or who have difficulty swallowing. This diet is often recommended when patients are recovering from surgery.

Foods included on this diet are

- All soups
- All liquids

- Cooked vegetables
- Canned fruit
- Ground meat and vegetables
- Tender fish and poultry

Bland Diet

A bland diet contains no seasonings or fibers that are irritating. This diet is prescribed for patients who have gastrointestinal problems and allergies. Foods that are gas-forming (such as cabbage), contain caffeine or spices, or are high in fiber are eliminated.

Foods included in a bland diet are

- Mildly flavored foods
- Low fiber foods
- Milk products
- Cooked fruit
- Non-citrus juices

BRAT Diet

Children suffering from uncontrolled gastrointestinal upsets can become dehydrated more easily than adults due to the depletion of body fluids. Physicians often recommend that mothers use foods on the BRAT diet since they are easily digested and do not cause further upsets.

BRAT stands for

B = bananas
R = rice
A = applesauce
T = toast

This combination of foods is prescribed for small children who suffer from vomiting, nausea, and diarrhea. Children should be seen by the physician if symptoms continue.

High Protein Diet

A high protein diet is recommended for patients recovering from bone injuries. This diet can aid in healing. Protein foods such as meat, dairy products, and legumes need to be eaten along with a variety of fruits and vegetables for a balanced diet. Often a high protein drink is included for the patient.

Diabetic Diet

A therapeutic diet designed for diabetic patients must consider several factors including:

1. Type of insulin therapy the patient receives
2. Severity of the diabetes
3. Activity and exercise level
4. Ability for activity
5. Calories necessary to maintain the patient's weight

A food exchange system is often used for diabetic patients. This allows for variety in their diet since the patient is able to select foods they prefer. Foods are grouped into the same 6 categories discussed in the food pyramid: Breads, fruits, vegetables, meat, milk, and fat.

Each food plan must be prescribed for the individual patient. All diabetic diets should be placed in writing for the patient. The medical assistant will be asked to reinforce the eating plan with the patient.

High Residue/Fiber Diet

The high fiber diet is used to treat patients with existing problems as well as to provide prevention for heart disease. New research is demonstrating that a diet high in fiber is effective in preventing colon cancer.

Dietary fiber is thought to provide protection against diabetes, breast and colon cancer, gallbladder disease, constipation, irritable bowel syndrome, hemorrhoids, and diverticulosis. Fiber may also reduce the level of cholesterol within the blood thereby protecting against heart disease. The recommended daily intake of fiber is between 20 to 30 grams. Dietary fiber is not found in animal products or dairy products.

Fiber sources are

- Raw fruits and vegetables
- Whole-grain breads and cereals
- Legumes

Low Residue Diet

A low residue diet is also called a low fiber diet. This diet is useful for a variety of patients including those with colitis, diarrhea, indigestion, or a colostomy.

Some low residue foods are

- Cooked vegetables and stewed fruit
- Bananas are the only raw fruit allowed
- Lean beef, lamb, chicken and turkey
- Cooked cereal
- Eggs
- Soups, all except creamed soups

Foods not allowed on a low residue diet are

- Fried food
- Milk or milk products
- Seasonings

Low-Fat/Low-Cholesterol Diet

The average American diet contains between 30-50g of fat per day. A low-fat diet is aimed at keeping the fat content between 20–30g of fat. This diet is recommended for patients who have an intolerance to fat, for example patients with gallbladder, pancreatic, and/or liver disease. A low-fat diet has been found to reduce the risk of colon, breast, and prostate cancer, heart disease, and obesity.

Foods recommended on a low-fat/low-cholesterol diet are

- Fruits and vegetables
- Skim milk
- Whole grain breads and cereals
- Only desserts such as angel food cake, graham crackers, and no-fat wafers

Foods not allowed on a low-fat/low-cholesterol diet are

- All fried foods
- Visible fat
- Butter and margarine

Low-Sodium/Low-Salt Diet

Therapeutic diets vary in the amount of salt restrictions. Restrictions vary from mild to moderate and severe. Diets are restricted in salt for patients with hypertension, heart and kidney disease. Salt restriction is also recommended for patients on weight reduction diets since an excess of salt/sodium in the diet promotes water retention.

Mild sodium-restricted diets allow between 3000 to 5000 mg of sodium per day. Many foods, especially processed foods, contain salt. A mild sodium-restricted diet (2000-3000 mg) would result in an allowance of 1/2 teaspoon of table salt per day and a very limited amount of foods containing salt.

A moderate salt-restricted diet allows 1500-2000 mg of sodium per day. This diet allows 1/2 teaspoon of table salt, but all processed and canned foods containing salt are prohibited. No salt is allowed in food preparation. This is the most frequently prescribed level of salt restriction.

A severe salt-restricted diet of 500 mg per day would limit all table salt use, cooking salt, and include only salt-free products in the diet. This diet is difficult to maintain using purchased foods. Patients are recommended to increase the use of fresh fruits and vegetables and to read labels carefully when on severe salt-restricted diets.

Calorie Content Diet

Weight reduction diets are often prescribed for patients whose health is affected by excess weight. Gaining excess body fat can lead to serious health problems, such as high blood pressure, heart disease, and diabetes.

A 1200-calorie diet using a balance of the 5 food groups and low-fat foods will result in weight loss. For a healthy diet patients are recommended to have at least 4 choices from the starch/bread group; 5 meat or meat substitute choices; 2 vegetable choices; 2 fruit choices; 2 skim milk choices; and not more than 3 fat choices. These choices add up to 1200 calories. Examples of these foods are listed in Table 33-8.

Patients are encouraged to keep a food diary of all they eat in a day. Table 33-9 contains a sample food diary format.

Healthy Food Choices

Healthy food choices include eating less fat, more high-fiber foods, using less salt, and eating less sugar.

Eat Less Fat

- Eat smaller servings of meat. Eat poultry and fish more often. Choose lean cuts of red meat.
- Prepare all meats by roasting, broiling, or baking. Trim off all visible fat. Be careful of added sauces or gravy.
- Remove skin from all poultry.
- Avoid all fried foods. Avoid adding fat during cooking.
- Eat fewer high-fat foods such as cold cuts, bacon, sausage, hot dogs, butter, margarine, salad dressing, nuts, lard, and solid shortening.
- Drink skim or low-fat milk.
- Eat less ice cream, cheese, sour cream, whole milk, cream, and other high-fat dairy products.

Eat More High-Fiber Foods

- Choose dried beans, peas, and lentils more often.
- Eat whole grain breads, cereals, crackers.
- Eat more vegetables, raw and cooked.
- Eat whole fruit in place of fruit juice.

TABLE 33-8 Basic Food Group Choices for a 1200-Calorie Eating Plan

Starch/Bread

Each of these equals one starch/bread choice (80 calories) and contains one gram of fat. For weight reduction limit to 4-6 choices a day.

½ cup pasta or barley

⅓ cup rice or cooked dried peas or beans

1 small potato

1 slice bread or 1 roll

½ cup starchy vegetables (corn, peas, or winter squash)

4-6 crackers

½ English muffin, bagel, hamburger/hot dog bun

½ cup cooked cereal

¾ cup dry, unsweetened cereal

3 cups popcorn, unbuttered, not cooked in oil

Vegetables

Each of these equals one vegetable choice (25 calories). Two or more servings are recommended per day.

½ cup cooked vegetables

1 cup raw vegetables

½ cup tomato/vegetable juice

Meat and Substitutes

Each of these equals one meat choice (75 calories). Five to six servings are recommended per day.

1 oz. cooked poultry, fish, or meat

¼ cup salmon or tuna, water packed

¼ cup cottage cheese

1 tablespoon peanut butter

1 egg (limit to 3 per week)

1 oz. low-fat cheese, such as mozzarella or ricotta

Each of these equals 2 meat choices (150 calories). Fat content varies for meat but should be limited to a total of 18 fat grams for meat per day.

1 small chicken leg or thigh

½ cup cottage cheese or tuna

Each of these equals 3 meat choices (225 calories)

1 small hamburger

1 small pork chop

½ chicken breast

1 medium fish filet

Cooked meat about the size of a deck of cards

Fruit

Each of these equals one fruit choice (60 calories). Two servings a day are recommended.

1 fresh medium fruit

1 cup berries or melon

½ cup fruit juice

½ cup canned fruit in juice without sugar

¼ cup dried fruit

Fat

Each of these equals one fat choice (45 calories and 5 grams of fat each). Fat should be limited to 3 servings per day.

1 teaspoon margarine, oil, mayonnaise

2 teaspoons diet margarine or diet mayonnaise

1 tablespoon salad dressing

2 tablespoons reduced-calorie salad dressing

TABLE 33-9 Sample Food Diary

Your Food Choices

Calories Each Day: _____

Meal Time:	Meal Time:	Meal Time
_____	_____	_____
_____	_____	_____
_____	_____	_____
_____	_____	_____
_____	_____	_____
_____	_____	_____
_____	_____	_____

Snack Time:	Snack Time:	Snack Time:
_____	_____	_____
_____	_____	_____

- Try high fiber foods such as oat bran, barley, brown rice, bulgar, and wild rice.

Use Less Salt

- Reduce the amount of salt you use in cooking.
- Try not to put salt on food at the table.
- Eat fewer high-salt foods such as canned soups, ham, hot dogs, pickles, sauerkraut, and foods that taste salty.
- Eat fewer convenience and fast foods.

Eat Less Sugar

- Avoid adding table sugar, syrup, honey, jam, jelly, candy, sweet rolls, fruit canned in syrup, regular gelatin desserts, pie, cake with icing, and other sweets.
- Avoid regular soft drinks. One 12-ounce can has nine teaspoons of sugar!
- Choose fresh fruit or fruit canned in natural juice or water.
- If desired, use sweeteners that do not have calories, such as saccharin or aspartame, instead of sugar.

Food Supplements

Physicians prescribe protein-vitamin-mineral food supplements when patients are debilitated due to disease processes, such as AIDS, or they are unable to tolerate a normal diet. In some cases, the liquid supplement may have to be given through a tube feeding until the patient is strong enough to drink the supplement. Supplements to the diet should only be used under the direction of a physician.

Exercise

Exercise and physical activity should be included as part of the patient's health plan. Activity helps to metabolize the fat in the diet so that it does not become stored in the body.

Alcohol

Alcohol is not considered a food product but it does contain calories and lowers the rate at which calories are burned. Consumption of alcohol is not recommended since there are associated problems, such as alcoholism, auto accidents, family and work disruptions.

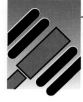

LEGAL AND ETHICAL ISSUES

Use caution in providing dietary information to patients. Only provide the instructions you are trained to give to the patient. Referring the patient to a registered dietitian (RD) or the physician for specific information may be necessary. It is an unsafe practice to recommend diets to patients. Only the physician or registered dietitian is licensed to prescribe a diet.

Follow-up is essential when providing patient instructions. For example, if a patient was still under the influence of anesthetic, when care instructions were given following the day-surgery, the patient may not understand the need to report bleeding. A follow-up telephone call, several hours after the patient has returned home, can protect the patient, the physician, and yourself.

Providing patient information which is not ordered by the physician can result in legal problems also. Providing a patient with information for an alternative form of treatment resulted in a nurse being suspended for 6 months and charged with unprofessional conduct in Idaho in 1976. This case was later reversed in 1979 ("News: Tuma Case Reversed." *Am J Nurs,* 79:1144, 1979). However, much anguish could have been prevented if the nurse had sought the counsel of her physician/employer before providing patient instruction which was not ordered.

The medical assistant has an ethical obligation to teach the patient even if there is a strong suspicion the patient will not comply with instructions. The best legal protection you can give to the patient, your physician/employer, and yourself is to do nothing for which you are not trained.

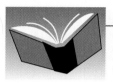

PATIENT EDUCATION

The medical assistant plays a key role in the patient's nutritional education. The medical assistant must be prepared to provide an explanation of the actual diet, purposes of the diet, nutritional needs of the patient, and steps to assist in compliance.

Dietary education will have to be explained in terms the patient can understand. It is always bet-

ter to place key points in writing for the patient. All dietary instruction needs to be individualized for the patient. Include the family, when possible, in all dietary instructions. Spouses are often responsible for cooking the foods that are included in the patient's diet. Every attempt should be made to include foods the patient likes in order for better dietary compliance.

Summary

One of the vital tasks of a medical assistant is to provide patient education, as needed, and as directed by a physician. An example would be nutritional planning for a diabetic patient. Being cognizant of adult learning, various teaching methodology and strategies, and the procedures for developing an effective

teaching plan facilitates this process. In addition, the medical assistant often plays a critical role in handling noncompliant patients. For example, a diabetic patient who will not adhere to the prescribed diet. Again, patient education is one of the most effective means of resolving such a difficult situation.

Competency Review

1. Define and spell the glossary terms for this chapter.
2. Design a patient teaching chart based on the "food pyramid" to illustrate the 6 classifications of nutrients.
3. Develop a sample menu for three days based on the food pyramid.
4. Determine the number of calories in a piece of pie that has 1 g of protein, 8 g of carbohydrates, and 9 fat grams.
5. Take a food label from a package of cereal and list the number of calories, total fat, cholesterol, sodium, total carbohydrates, dietary fiber, sugars, protein and vitamins.
6. Write a one-day food plan for the following therapeutic diets: full liquid, mechanical soft, high fiber, moderate salt restrictive, and 1200 calorie.
7. Maintain a weekly diary of your weekly intake of food. Analyze each food group usage.

PREPARING FOR THE CERTIFICATION EXAM

Test Taking Tip — Multiple choice questions should take a little less than 1 minute to answer. Practice answering multiple choice questions by timing yourself using a watch with a sweep second hand.

Examination Review Questions

1. _____ is an example of a water-soluble vitamin.
   - (A) vitamin A
   - (B) vitamin B
   - (C) vitamin D
   - (D) vitamin E
   - (E) vitamin K

2. The recommended percentage of foods from proteins in the daily diet is
   - (A) 5%
   - (B) 8%
   - (C) 12%
   - (D) 30%
   - (E) 50%

3. A BRAT diet has been ordered for Emily Miller, who is 2 years old. What foods will be included on that diet?
   - (A) baby cereal
   - (B) milk
   - (C) strained meats
   - (D) bananas and rice
   - (E) vegetables

4. When restricting food on a 1200-calorie diet that is being adapted for a diabetic patient using food exchange lists, what needs to be remembered?
   - (A) the food pyramid
   - (B) the amount of exercise the patient does
   - (C) 1200 calories may be too restrictive for a diabetic patient
   - (D) Vitamins A, B, C, D, E, K
   - (E) all of the above

5. An example of a complex carbohydrate is
   - (A) jelly
   - (B) table sugar
   - (C) orange
   - (D) syrup
   - (E) honey

6. Which of the following statements about cholesterol is TRUE?
   - (A) all cholesterol is bad
   - (B) good cholesterol is low-density lipoproteins (LDL)
   - (C) there is no evidence that high cholesterol intake is linked to disease
   - (D) cholesterol is an essential element normally found in the body
   - (E) the information, "cholesterol 0mg," on a food label, means that there is no fat present

7. The most effective combination of teaching methods for the older adults is
   - (A) lecture, printed materials, models
   - (B) lecture, return demonstration, programmed instruction
   - (C) role play, group teaching, return demonstration
   - (D) video, test of knowledge, group teaching
   - (E) all of the above

8. When writing instructional booklets to teach diabetics nutritional planning, which statement is TRUE?
   - (A) use of medical terminology is fine as long as a detailed definitions are given
   - (B) sprinkle material with medical abbreviations so the patient will know this is medical education
   - (C) combine several ideas into one grouping in order to save space
   - (D) avoid using too many examples
   - (E) none of the above is true

9. Which statement about carbohydrates is NOT TRUE?
   - (A) they are the body's main source of energy
   - (B) they provide 4 calories of energy for every gram of carbohydrate

(Continued on next page)

(C) they include the nine essential amino acids

(D) they include sugar, syrup, and jam

(E) they include wheat germ, pasta, and sweet potatoes

10. Which situation is a potential legal dilemma for the CMA?

(A) the patient asks for information regarding an alternative treatment for breast cancer

(B) the patient asks for a list of the foods that her baby, who has diarrhea, can eat

(C) the patient is discharged after day-surgery for a hernia repair with only an instructional pamphlet

(D) the patient states that he or she won't follow instructions, so none are given

(E) all of the above

ON THE JOB

Jacob Freeman, is a CMA in the office of Dr. Luo, an internist. Dr. Luo has asked Jacob to develop a teaching plan for Mr. Young, who is 70. Mr. Young was operated on for colon cancer one year ago and has been handling his own colostomy care since that time. He has also been the caregiver for his 75 year old wife, Adele, who is recovering from the effects of a stroke and diabetes. Adele is also a patient of Dr. Luo. She has had frequent infections of a leg ulcer caused by the bacteria E. coli. Dr. Luo is concerned that Mr. Young has been contaminating his wife's leg with E. coli from his colostomy when he changes her dressing.

What Is Your Response?

1. Is there anything about Mr. Young that might preclude him from properly caring for himself or his wife?

2. If so, can it be addressed in the teaching plan?

3. Consider that two issues need to be addressed: (1) Mr. Young's self-care and (2) the care he provides for his wife, particularly her leg ulcer. Should two teaching plans be designed? Why or why not?

4. Given this scenario, what is the very first issue that Jacob should address with Mr. Young?

5. Should Mr. Young's wife be involved in the implementation of the teaching plan?

6. Describe in detail the teaching plan, follow-up plan, and any instructional materials for Mr. and Mrs. Young.

References

Brown, I. "Cholesterol and the Consumer." *Nursing Times.* 86:31, 1990.

Eating Healthy Foods. Alexandria, VA: American Diabetes Association, 1988.

Exchange Lists. Chicago: American Dietetics Association, 1995.

Taber's Cyclopedic Medical Dictionary, 18th ed. Philadelphia, F. A. Davis Company, 1997.

Woldrum, K., Ryan-Morrell, V., Towson, M., Bower, K., Zander, K. *Patient Education.* Rockville, MD: Aspen Systems Corporation, 1985.

MEDICAL ASSISTANT ROLE DELINEATION CHART

Highlight indicates material covered in this chapter

ADMINISTRATIVE

ADMINISTRATIVE PROCEDURES
- Perform basic clerical functions
- Schedule, coordinate, and monitor appointments
- Schedule inpatient/outpatient admissions and procedures
- Understand and apply third party guidelines
- Obtain reimbursement through accurate claims submission
- Monitor third-party reimbursement
- Perform medical transcription
- Understand and adhere to managed care policies and procedures
- *Negotiate managed care contracts (adv)*

PRACTICE FINANCES
- Perform procedural and diagnostic coding
- Apply bookkeeping principles
- Document and maintain accounting and banking records
- Manage accounts receivable
- Manage accounts payable
- Process payroll
- *Develop and maintain fee schedules (adv)*
- *Manage renewals of business and professional insurance policies (adv)*
- *Manage personal benefits and maintain records (adv)*

CLINICAL

FUNDAMENTAL PRINCIPLES
- Apply principles of aseptic technique and infection control
- Comply with quality assurance practices
- Screen and follow up patient test results

DIAGNOSTIC ORDERS
- Collect and process specimens
- Perform diagnostic tests

PATIENT CARE
- Adhere to established triage procedures
- Obtain patient history and vital signs
- Prepare and maintain examination and treatment areas

- Prepare patient for examinations, procedures, and treatments
- Assist with examinations, procedures, and treatments
- Prepare and administer medications and immunizations
- Maintain medication and immunization records
- Recognize and respond to emergencies
- Coordinate patient care information with other health care providers

GENERAL (TRANSDISCIPLINARY)

PROFESSIONALISM
- Project a professional manner and image
- Adhere to ethical principles
- Demonstrate initiative and responsibility
- Work as a team member
- Manage time efficiently
- Prioritize and perform multiple tasks
- Adapt to change
- Promote the CMA credential
- Enhance skills through continuing education

COMMUNICATION SKILLS
- Treat all patients with compassion and empathy
- Recognize and respect cultural diversity
- Adapt communications to individual's ability to understand
- Use professional telephone technique
- Use effective and correct verbal and written communications
- Recognize and respond to verbal and non-verbal communications
- Use medical terminology appropriately
- Receive, organize, prioritize, and transmit information
- Serve as liaison
- Promote the practice through positive public relations

LEGAL CONCEPTS
- Maintain confidentiality
- Practice within the scope of education, training, and personal capabilities
- Prepare and maintain medical records
- Document accurately
- Use appropriate guidelines when releasing information
- Follow employer's established policies dealing with the health care contract
- Follow federal, state, and local legal guidelines
- Maintain awareness of federal and state health care legislation and regulations
- Maintain and dispose of regulated substances in compliance with government guidelines
- Comply with established risk management and safety procedures
- Recognize professional credentialing criteria
- Participate in the development and maintenance of personnel, policy, and procedure manuals
- *Develop and maintain personnel, policy, and procedure manuals (adv)*

INSTRUCTION
- Instruct individuals according to their needs
- Explain office policies and procedures
- Teach methods of health promotion and disease prevention
- Locate community resources and disseminate information
- *Orient and train personnel (adv)*
- *Develop educational materials (adv)*
- *Conduct continuing education activities (adv)*

OPERATIONAL FUNCTIONS
- Maintain supply inventory
- Evaluate and recommend equipment and supplies
- Apply computer techniques to support office operations
- *Supervise personnel (adv)*
- *Interview and recommend job applicants (adv)*
- *Negotiate leases and prices for equipment and supply contracts (adv)*

SOURCE: Reprinted by permission of the American Association of Medical Assistants from the *AAMA Role Delineation Study: Occupational Analysis of the Medical Assisting Profession.*

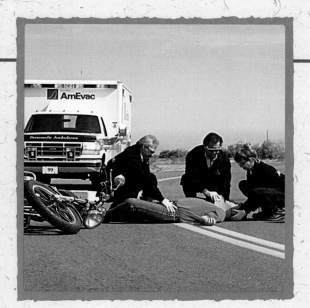

34

Emergency First Aid

CHAPTER OUTLINE

LEARNING OBJECTIVES

After completing this chapter, you should:
1. Define and spell all of the glossary terms for this chapter.
2. List the emergency priorities for a patient who is found to be apneic and pulseless.
3. Describe the differences between first, second and third-degree burns.
4. Discuss the difference between treating complete and incomplete airway obstruction in an adult.
5. State the difference between immediate history and overall medical history.
6. Give the legal name for the primary responsibility of any caregiver, whether on the job or not.
7. List three examples of histories that would worry you about the patient who presents with a persistent nosebleed.
8. Explain when you would attempt to remove an impaled object and when not.
9. Discuss the differences between the four kinds of musculoskeletal injuries.
10. Name and explain the sequential steps you would take during the first minute after finding a patient seated in an examination room who looks like he's in cardiac arrest.
11. List at least ten things that might cause a patient to seize.
12. Describe the differences in pathophysiology between heat stroke and heat exhaustion.
13. Explain why you would want to place an unconscious patient on his left side.
14. Give the hand or finger placements for adult, child and infant CPR.
15. Discuss the two major kinds of diabetic crises, and explain why you would want to administer sugar for either one.
16. Compare and contrast at least five kinds of shock.

CLINICAL PERFORMANCE COMPETENCIES

After completing this chapter, you should perform the following tasks:
1. Correctly address the priorities for a patient who walks into the office with a medical emergency.
2. Conduct an emergency physical examination.
3. Elicit a good patient history without wasting time.
4. Respond appropriately to a patient who walks into the office complaining of a severe headache and then immediately goes into full-body seizure in front of you.
5. Correctly perform CPR on an adult, a child, and an infant.
6. Demonstrate the treatment for a patient in shock.
7. Take a good emergency history.
8. Demonstrate a common-sense approach to an unresponsive patient.
9. Demonstrate the correct procedure for irrigating the eyes to remove a foreign body.
10. Correctly perform aid for an obstructive airway on infant and adult, unconscious and conscious, victims.

Glossary

affect A patient's mood or emotional state.

allergen Any substance that triggers an allergic reaction.

aneurysm A weakening or out-pouching in the wall of an artery.

asphyxia Suffocation, inability to breathe.

aspirated Drawn in or out, by means of a vacuum. For example, a substance or an object being aspirated, or sucked, into the lungs.

benign Non-threatening, non-cancerous.

bradycardic Pertaining to an abnormally slow heart rate (< 60 beats/minute).

cardiogenic Pertaining to the heart. For example, shock related to heart failure.

convulsions Involuntary muscle contractions that may alternate between contraction and relaxation of muscles. May be generalized or localized (focal) and may be followed by a period of unresponsiveness.

ferrous Containing iron.

gag reflex Closure of the glottis and constriction of its associated musculature in response to stimulation of the posterior pharynx by an object or substance in that area.

generalized Involving the entire body or system; widespread.

hives Peculiar raised patches of skin surrounded by reddened areas, triggered by the release of histamine. Also called urticaria.

infarction Death of tissue, as in myocardial infarction or heart attack.

inspiration Inhalation.

localized Limited to a definable area of the body; focal.

myocardial Heart muscle, especially referring to the ventricles.

necrotic Refers to death of tissue, such as occurs with venoms of pit vipers and the brown recluse spider.

non-pleuritic Not related to the pleura, or membranes that lubricate the outer surfaces of the lungs. A pleuritic chest pain worsens when the patient takes a deep breath, and is not characteristic of a cardiac disorder.

occult Hidden, as in hidden bleeding.

orifices Openings, especially naturally occurring body surface openings.

pathologic Pertaining to a condition of disease or injury.

perfusion The process of bathing cells in healthy blood which is rich in nutrients, especially oxygen and glucose.

periosteum A membrane that covers the shaft of a long bone; promotes growth and healing.

reimplantation Reattachment of a severed limb or portion of a severed limb.

seizures Same as convulsions.

sublingual Beneath the tongue.

syncope Sudden loss of consciousness, which may be transient. Also called fainting.

systemic Pertaining to the body as a whole; affects the entire body.

tidal volume The volume of air inspired and expired during one normal respiratory cycle.

triage To determine the priority for handling patients with severe conditions or injuries. For example, the most severely injured patient with a chance for survival will be treated first.

xiphoid process The piece of cartilage that forms the lowermost tip of the sternum, and which functions as a major point of attachment for the abdominal muscles.

WARNING!

For all patient contact, adhere to Standard Precautions (see pages 342-373). Wear protective equipment as indicated.

Have you ever witnessed the actions of emergency crews at an auto accident scene, or maybe even at a shopping center where someone has had a serious medical emergency? Maybe you noticed how calm those people were; no running, no shouting, everybody with a job to do . . . almost automatic.

What makes that kind of performance possible under even the worst circumstances is the same thing that would make it possible for you, too: a rock-solid foundation in the basics. An understanding of what causes most medical emergencies. A knowledge of some basic first steps to take, no matter what is happening around you. And the will to help.

Equipped with those three things, you are ready to make that first contact with someone who has had a medical emergency. Find out how sick they are and what they really need. And make sure they get it. Those are the elements of emergency first aid, presented in the context of a medical as-

sistant, and laid out for you as a medical professional and team member.

A variety of medical emergencies are presented in this chapter. The physician must be notified immediately regarding all medical office emergencies. In some cases the Emergency Medical Services (EMS) system will need to be notified by calling *911*. Medical assistants are cautioned not to perform procedures outside their scope of practice. Figure 34-1 depicts common first aid practices being followed to

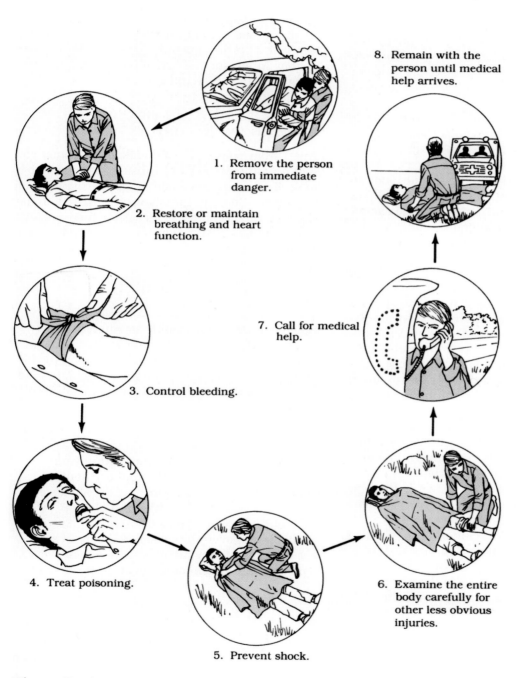

1. Remove the person from immediate danger.
2. Restore or maintain breathing and heart function.
3. Control bleeding.
4. Treat poisoning.
5. Prevent shock.
6. Examine the entire body carefully for other less obvious injuries.
7. Call for medical help.
8. Remain with the person until medical help arrives.

Figure 34-1 Medical emergency first aid.

ensure the safety of a person until medical help arrives.

The Emergency Medical Services System

You are an important part of your community's EMS system, and so is every other member of your community who knows how and when to use a telephone. When your good judgment tells you that you are looking at a patient whose problems are more than you can handle, inform the physician immediately, which may include calling *911*. In response, you will quickly obtain the help of people, equipment, and a communication system that are all designed for the kinds of emergencies that the office staff is not equipped to handle.

Typically such a system would employ you as a first-responder—someone who is trained to recognize medical conditions, initiate basic life support and access the system. Because you are a medical professional as well, they would look to you and your staff for detailed information about the patient's complaint, the immediate and overall history, medications and allergies, and the care you have administered. The EMS normally operate as follows.

Once you have accessed the system, you would inform the patient and any relatives that you have decided to have the patient transported to a hospital. You would continue your assessment and care until the arrival of an engine company from the fire department or an ambulance crew (depending on your system). The reason for the engine company is that there are many more fire engines than ambulances; and the engine company may include one or more paramedics. Even if not, all firefighters are trained and equipped as first-responders and/or emergency medical technicians (EMTs). Although they may not be capable to transport a patient, they have access to a communications network that includes police, ambulance paramedics, emergency departments, and advanced trauma, poison, pediatric and burn centers. They carry emergency equipment which you may not have, and they can provide the necessary staffing to handle a cardiac arrest. The ambulance crew may also be staffed by one or more paramedics depending on your system.

Paramedics can intubate, insert a tube into the trachea as an emergency airway, or start an IV in seconds, they have ample oxygen supplies and an assortment of emergency medications, and they

are licensed to perform some other invasive procedures. You may expect their professional courtesy, and you should return it. Figure 34-2 A-D illustrates EMTs establishing an airway.

EMS personnel are accustomed to working with health care professionals like yourself. You may expect one of them to seek you out, ask you and your staff for all the patient information you have, and make sure that your observations become part of the patient chart. In addition, this communicator will operate the radio system that connects your patient to the receiving hospital.

It may be a good idea for you to familiarize yourself with the capabilities of your area's EMS system in advance of an emergency by inviting them to your facility, introducing yourself, and exchanging tours.

Specialized Resources

Apart from your emergency response teams, you will occasionally need to consult with specialists in such areas as poison control, pediatrics, trauma and burns. Some of these consults will be under emergency conditions, so make sure there are telephone numbers displayed prominently near the phones in your office.

Guidelines for Providing Emergency Care

Emergency situations call for medicine that is unique to itself. During an emergency there may never be enough time, space, light, or equipment that you need. Certain guidelines are helpful and can minimize confusion and prevent fatalities in some emergencies.

Med Tip: Stay within your scope of practice, but use your imagination. For example, how do you keep from having to fiddle with a roll of tape? Fold the end of it when you stock it or put it away. Always put everything back in the exact spot it was taken from, and memorize where every piece of equipment or medical supply is kept.

Medical Emergencies

Medical assistants need to be able to handle emergencies in two ways. The most common way is on the telephone, when a patient's relative calls to ask

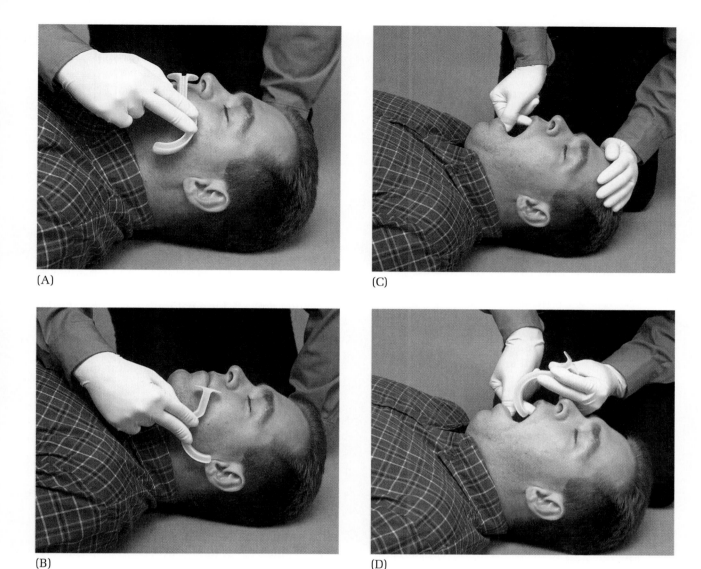

Figure 34-2 A-D EMTs establishing an airway.

for advice during an emergency outside the office. The other way is when an emergency occurs near the office and somebody brings the patient in.

In some states, triage, or assessing the emergency care needed by victims, is not within the scope of practice of the medical assistant. In these states the medical assistant should not work alone in the medical office.

Either way, in an emergency you need to be able to look at someone and quickly assess if they are ill and require emergency care. Or, harder still, you need to hear about them on the phone and make a decision on their behalf without being able to see them. You can ask your physician for advice anytime he or she is in the office. If you are alone in the office, you must make the decision to access the EMS by calling *911*.

The Primary Assessment

Every patient contact by every caregiver at every level begins with a few simple questions and a basic patient examination called the primary assessment. This assessment is critically important for the medical assistant, whose role it is to organize the process of caring for people.

The key to effective patient assessment is the combination of careful observation with automatic, medically sound routines that are applied in every patient situation. The following steps describe both.

Determine the Patient's Name, Approximate Age, and Sex

What is the patient's name? That may seem like an unimportant question, but you should always ask it first—for two reasons.

1. It tells you who you're dealing with, enables you to access patient records, and helps you to protect every patient against accidentally receiving the wrong care.

   All people have names, and all people are supposed to know their names even when not fully alert. A person who answers questions but does not know his or her name warrants immediate attention.
2. As you become a better observer over time, the way a patient answers to their name (or does not answer) can reveal a lot about how well their mind and body are functioning—and how sick they are.

When you ask somebody for their name, they must quickly go through an extensive neurologic process in order to give you a simple appropriate answer:

- They must hear you.
- They must localize the sound of your voice, using both ears and both eyes.
- They must be able to look at you with a symmetrical gaze and focus on you with both eyes.
- They must be able to reason that you are a caregiver, and then process the meaning of your words, hopefully in your own language (but maybe not).
- They must be able to remember their name, and formulate a meaningful response.
- They must be able to answer in coherent speech and with a symmetrical face.

In those two seconds, you may have learned a lot about this patient's mental function and maybe a lot more than that. How much more you learn depends on how well you observe other things such as facial signs, body language and overall affect.

When you ask for a patient's name, ask for the patient's medicine bottles at the same time. If they are available, the labels can provide the date of birth and the correct spelling of the name. The medicine labels can also provide some clues as to the medical history and the name(s) of one or more physicians.

Decide if the Patient Looks Sick

This is a question that needs to be answered and re-answered both early and throughout every patient contact.

Why early? Because if the patient is really sick, there is not time to ask a lot of questions. Why throughout contact? Because a patient's status can change in a matter of seconds. Either way, when you think somebody needs emergency help right away, interrupt everything else you're doing to intervene. Then, concentrate on getting help.

How do you tell if someone is really sick—maybe in danger of dying? The fastest way is to *look at the person.* When someone looks really sick to you, there is often something wrong with that individual. That does not mean everyone with intestinal flu symptoms is about to die (although some do). On the other hand, a patient who cannot be aroused or who cannot stay awake deserves serious concern. Does the patient seem too weak to stand up? Does the skin color seem very pale, or perhaps blue? Is the patient very sweaty for no apparent reason (such as, hot weather or recent exercise)? Is the patient bleeding uncontrollably, or struggling to breathe?

These are all signs of serious trouble. Stop everything else and alert your physician or nurse, right away. If they are not available, contact *911* and anticipate transport to an emergency department.

Med Tip: It is important to mention that bizarre forms of behavior may indicate serious medical emergencies and not just mental illness. Caregivers who observe what seem to be abnormal behaviors, especially in unfamiliar patients, should consider drugs or poisoning, high blood pressure, diabetes, head injuries, and/or shock. These are all potentially life-threatening processes.

Determine a Chief Complaint

Another way to find out if someone is really sick, if it's not obvious, is to determine his or her *chief complaint*. A patient's chief complaint is the main reason he or she is seeking medical help right now.

How do you obtain a chief complaint? *You watch for it.* Whether he mentions it or not, a patient who clutches his chest all the time may be having chest pain. A child who seems to carry, or "cradle," one elbow with the opposite hand may be having some pain in his or her clavicle or upper extremity. An infant who seems very quiet and who drools a lot may have a very sore throat.

How else do you obtain a chief complaint? In the case of difficulty breathing, *you listen for it.* A patient whose breathing seems noisy and labored and who does not waste words, may have a respiratory obstruction of some kind. Is the patient silent, to the point of not answering questions? Remember: when you cannot breathe, you do not talk. All of these are important findings which may change by the time help arrives. Your observations, which you should describe in your own words, are very important to an emergency caregiver.

How *else* do you obtain a chief complaint? In addition to the above techniques, and most importantly, *you ask for it.* Try hard to use *open-ended* questions that leave the patient free to choose his or her own words and gestures to describe how he or she feels.

Sometimes the complaint itself is all you need to know. There are some specific complaints that always warrant prompt attention, based on years of experience by thousands of emergency caregivers. They include the following:

- Trouble breathing (extremely labored or noisy, shallow, slow or absent)
- Severe or persistent bleeding
- Chest, neck, jaw or left arm pain that is unrelieved by rest, O_2 or nitrates

- Prolonged or recurrent seizures (especially in the unresponsive patient)
- Extreme weakness (especially if the patient gets dizzy on standing)
- Impending emergency childbirth
- Severe headache, unrelieved by aspirin or acetaminophen
- Severe abdominal pain
- Palpitations (patient is able to feel heart beating in chest)
- Major trauma (probably not seen in a physician's office)

In addition to this list, never ignore what you *think* you see, smell, or hear. For instance, findings such as skin colors and breath or body odors can indicate a variety of medical problems, including poisons, intestinal bleeding, cancer and diabetes (not to mention poor personal hygiene). All of these things can be crucial hints about a patient's chief complaint.

Med Tip: *Trust your instinct.* If you simply have a feeling that somebody is in danger of dying, you do not necessarily need to be able to explain it in medical terms. Contact your physician or nurse right away (or call *911*, if they are not available). Nobody will fault you if your suspicions turn out to be wrong.

There is one final note about the things that people complain about. Most of us do not know when we're going to die, but some patients get very accurate premonitions about it. When a patient looks into your eyes and tells you he thinks he's going to die—no matter what his complaint—believe him, and treat him as though his problem is a true emergency.

Very few people in medicine will ever criticize you for over-caring, unless you attempt something you're not licensed to do. Short of that, if a colleague does criticize your care, it will be nothing compared to the trouble you can get into for not caring.

Obtain the History

Whenever you question somebody, especially about something as important as their medical history, it is important for you to see, hear, and sense all of the key information they can give you in as brief a time as possible. That can challenge even the best interrogators, especially when it becomes necessary to get the information from someone other than the patient—an interpreter, for instance, or a parent (if the patient is a small child).

There are two kinds of history: the patient's *immediate* history (or history of the event), and the patient's *overall* medical history (or lifelong history). They're both extremely important, but try to keep them separate—both in your mind and in your questioning. Otherwise, you may confuse yourself and the people you work with.

The *immediate* history can reveal a lot about the nature of a problem. For instance, a patient who feels "dizzy" when she wakes up in the morning with a cold is a lot different than a patient who feels the same way after several episodes of dark-colored, foul-smelling diarrhea. Although both of these patients have the same complaint (dizziness), their histories differ. By itself, the first patient's history suggests an ear infection, while the second patient's history points to GI bleeding.

Some of the things you see and hear will only be seen and heard by you. For instance, a caller might tell you where their terrible headache is located, and then lose consciousness. That would make you a key witness. Your report would prompt the initial decisions and actions of an entire team of people who would then care for that patient.

The *overall*, or *past* medical history is just what its name implies: a medical story of a person's life, intended to consider everything remarkable that has ever happened to them medically. Sometimes it reveals clues that are essential to a diagnosis. For instance, a person who develops severe shortness of breath along with a simple chest cold might surprise you until you learn that the patient has only one lung.

The best way to gather the past medical history is to use a checklist, whether mental or written. The questions you ask may depend on your employer's standard procedures, but should probably be the same for every patient, no matter what their complaint. Specifically, they might include the following:

- Heart problems? (*Heart "attack"?*)
- Lung problems? (*Does the patient have both lungs?*)
- Kidney problems? (*Does the patient have both kidneys?*)
- Diabetes? (*Does the patient take insulin/has the patient had insulin today, and if so, when?*)
- High or low blood pressure (*which?*)
- Seizures?
- Fainting spells?

- Any possibility of pregnancy/ObGyn history/LMP? (*Normal?*)
- Previous similar events? (*When, treatment, outcome?*)

Except for allergies, this list of questions includes all of the conditions that most commonly kill people.

Not only during history-taking, but throughout all contact with patients and their relatives, involve all of your senses. In addition to hearing what people say, watch their eyes. Is somebody doing their best not to let you know that they are afraid to be in the doctor's office? Is somebody extremely concerned about their modesty, or does someone feel cold? Is someone expecting bad news about their spouse of 50 years? All of this is part of the history, and should be communicated to the physician or nurse who will be continuing your care.

The most frightening thing about any emergency is often the patient's perception of it. Try very hard to anticipate people's feelings, and to explain everything in plain language before it happens. Concentrate on people's comfort. And after you are finished with them, check up on them every few minutes, just to let them know how important they are. This is especially important if things are very busy.

Gather the Meds

Once you know the patient's complaint and something about his medical history, find out what medicines he or she takes. If you have not already, obtain the medicine containers and save them for whomever will continue your care. Later on, write them down. A smart caregiver can learn a lot about a patient from his medicine bottles. Not only that, but it can provide the names of the prescribing physicians.

The same is true of medicines that are used to treat people with diabetes, lung problems or high blood pressure. Knowing when a patient's medicines were prescribed (there should be a date on each label) is also helpful. It can reveal how recently the patient was treated by someone for each of his or her various problems, and it can indicate when a patient is taking too much medicine—or not enough.

Does the patient seem confused about their medicines? If so, your physician needs to know that. Sometimes all that needs to happen is for someone to explain things. If the patient takes a lot of different kinds of medicines, a daily organizer may be the solution. They come in various configurations, but most consist of rows and columns of small plastic boxes. And sometimes, as is the case with some elderly patients (who often have too many physicians and take too much medicine), the patient's whole list of medications needs to be re-evaluated and simplified.

Finally, a great many medical conditions are caused by medicines in the first place; either by interactions between them or by a patient's reaction to one or more of them.

Determine the Allergies

Most caregivers underestimate the importance of allergies. People die of their allergies. That happens all the time, and thousands of patients are violently allergic to some of the medicines that are dispensed every day. Many wear some kind of jewelry as a reminder, in the form of bracelets, wristbands or necklaces. Usually they are keenly aware of their allergies, but it happens sometimes during a medical crisis that a person will either forget about their allergies or become unable to communicate about them. It is good practice to check for warning tags and jewelry during the patient examination, even if a patient denies having any allergies.

Remember, too, that asthma is a kind of allergy, and that people with allergies tend to have more than just one of them. Be extra suspicious of allergies when a patient tells you their medical history includes asthma—or when, during your questions about medicines, you find a pocket inhaler.

Just as patients sometimes forget their allergies in times of crisis, physicians and nurses sometimes overlook them as well. A medical assistant's attention to details in times like those can save lives and prevent a lot of misery.

Primary Care Physician's Name

The name of a patient's primary care physician can be a great asset to any caregiver, and it's worth a fair amount of trouble—especially if the patient is in grave danger. Why?

Even though it may cost some time due to fruitless phone calls and digging through patient records, being able to contact a physician who knows a patient well can take all the mystery out of an emergency situation. However, never delay a patient's emergency care while trying to locate the primary care physician.

Do a Physical Examination

If a physician is not available, it makes sense to know how to do a good, quick, basic physical when someone looks sick to you.

When you do a quick physical assessment, start with the things that do not require the use of tools. One of the ways you communicate your concern for someone is by touch. *After asking permission* and *before you put your gloves on*, gently place the back of your hand or wrist first against the skin of the patient's forehead and then the cheek. Finally, grasp both of the patient's hands in your own, perhaps for less than a second. You will know immediately about the patient's skin moisture and temperature, and you'll be able to feel trembling or shivering that you may not be able to see. When people are nervous, their hands get clammy. But when a patient's face gets cold and moist, he or she is more than just nervous.

Look into the patient's eyes for a moment. Are the pupils about normal, and are they equal? Does the gaze seem symmetrical, or do you notice anything abnormal about the overall appearance of the eyes or face? Use a penlight, if available, to check the pupils of first one eye and then the other.

What is the patient's overall **affect** or apparent emotional state? Does the patient seem well nourished, articulate, dressed appropriately? angry or irritable? abnormally tired? Is the patient coughing or sneezing and can you hear his or her respirations? Does the patient seem to be holding onto a part of the body as though injured, or possibly cradling an aching head in his or her hands? When you walk the patient to the scale, do you notice anything unusual about his or her gait? What is your overall impression of how sick the patient is?

All of the physical observations you have made so far are potentially important, but chances are they have consumed as little as a minute.

Take the Vital Signs

Now, with the patient's permission, insert the thermometer. Count the respirations for about 30 seconds while the thermometer calculates the temperature. Then spend another 30 seconds checking the pulse, and follow that with the blood pressure. Record these readings on the chart. If the patient has a potentially serious complaint, or if you find anything in the vitals or the patient's appearance that concerns you, terminate the physical examination and notify the physician immediately. If the physician is unavailable, you should call *911*. Have the patient lie down on the examination table, and make him comfortable. Oxygen may need to be administered as ordered by the physician.

The Office Emergency Crash Cart

All of those tools should be instantly accessible, by anyone in your office. One practical way to make that happen is by means of a crash cart. A crash cart is usually based on a large roll-around tool box with drawers that can be used to store emergency medications, intubation equipment, needles and syringes and assorted small instruments as well as a resuscitator, a monitor/defibrillator, an oxygen supply, airways and suction. Especially in a small office, a crash cart can be brought to the side of any patient within moments of an emergency (also called a "code") (Figure 34-3).

Emergency supplies need to be checked routinely, for two reasons. First, emergency medicines do not tend to get used often, so they expire. The same is true of the batteries that power the monitor-defibrillator, laryngoscopes and suction device. When these items do get used, someone who is not currently dealing with the aftermath of an emergency needs to double-check them. And second, being able to use emergency equipment under the pressure of an emergency requires comfortable, hands-on familiarity with the equipment. When you do not handle many emergencies (as in the case of most physicians' offices), that kind of familiarity can only come from handling the equipment during daily checks.

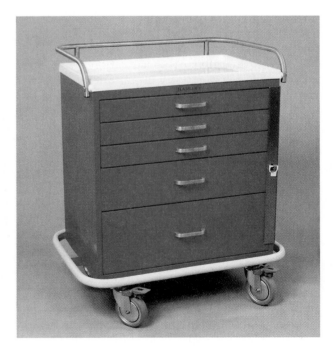

Figure 34-3   Crash Cart.

Finally, a crash cart needs to be outfitted with a physical checklist that names every drug container and every piece of equipment the cart contains. The checklist should provide space for a daily date and signature, and someone in the office should be accountable for maintaining the cart. But everyone who is likely to use the cart needs to check it personally as well, for the sake of their own performance.

> **Med Tip:** Everyone needs to know how to use the equipment and where it is stored. During a "code," is no time to be looking for equipment.

First Aid Kit

Although it has wheels, the crash cart normally stays inside the office. For patients who arrive in cars and can not come into the office—with broken legs, airway problems, or a bleeding problem, for example there also needs to be a first aid kit. Like the crash cart, it should be checked every day.

Ideally, the first aid kit should contain at least an assortment of airways, a bite block, a manual resuscitator, some splinting materials, bandages and dressings, and an assortment of tape. The first aid kit should be simple and compact. It should facilitate getting the patient into the controlled office environment. The contents of both the first aid kit and the crash cart should be determined by the physician and the office staff.

Emergencies

The following sections of this chapter outline the findings and treatment for the types of medical emergencies seen in the medical office. You should consider it an overview.

Airway Obstruction (*Foreign Body Airway Obstruction*)

The airway is so important to caregivers and patients alike. No priority in any branch of medicine is outranked by the airway; it's at the very top of every list. Normally, the airway does such a good job of protecting itself and keeping itself clean that its owner does not even feel it. But airway obstruction can be disastrous. How can you help the patient who comes in to the office choking on an obstruction? First of all, alert a fellow staff member to notify the physician immediately. The patient in Figure 34-4 exhibits the universal choking sign—both hands to the neck, possible facial reddening or cyanosis, and a look of panic (but no respiratory sounds).

Chances are that if the patient walks into the office with or without help, she does not have a complete airway obstruction. As soon as you see the patient, walk up to him or her calmly, look into her eyes and ask, "Are you choking?" If she can make any breathing sounds at all, do not do anything but reassure her. The last thing you want to do is to convert a partial obstruction into a complete one.

> **Med Tip:** Always remember to check the ABCs when giving emergency care: A = airway (Is the patient's airway open?), B = breathing (Can the patient breathe on his or her own?), and C = circulation (Has something interfered with normal blood flow?).

Heimlich Maneuver A patient with a complete airway obstruction will be vocally silent. Ask her if she's choking. If she nods yes, tell her you are about to help her. Walk around behind the patient, encircle her with your arms, locate her navel and the bottom end of her sternum (**xiphoid process**), and place the thumb-side of your closed fist against her abdomen directly between these two points. Grab your fist with your other (free) hand, and deliver a firm thrust into the patient's abdomen in an upward direction towards you (Figure 34-5). Keep doing that until the obstruction is removed (the patient will cough) or until she loses consciousness.

If the patient does become unconscious after you have administered one or more abdominal thrusts, ease her to the floor and place her on her back. Call for help and attempt ventilation. If ventilation does not work, grasp the mandible with your thumb and forefinger and pull it forward. Use the index finger of your other hand to sweep the mouth. Do not spend a lot of time at it, but see if you can retrieve an obstruction which may have been freed when the patient lost consciousness.

If you are not able to see and remove the obstruction, kneel astride the patient's thighs and place the heels of your hands (as though you were doing CPR) on the surface of her abdomen midway between her navel and xiphoid. Deliver five firm thrusts into her abdomen, aimed toward her chest (Figure 34-6). Try once again to

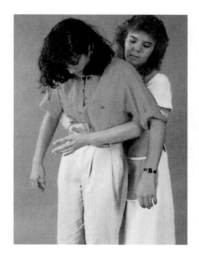

Figure 34-5 Heimlich maneuver.

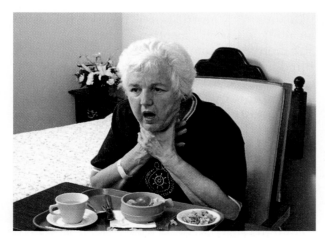

Figure 34-4 The universal choking sign.

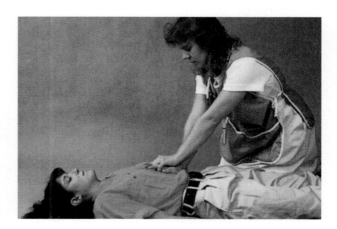

Figure 34-6 Chest thrusts are delivered with a firm thrust into the patient's abdomen in an upward motion.

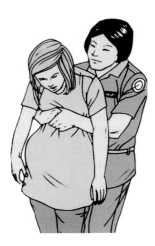

Figure 34-7 Chest thrusts are used on pregnant women and very large persons.

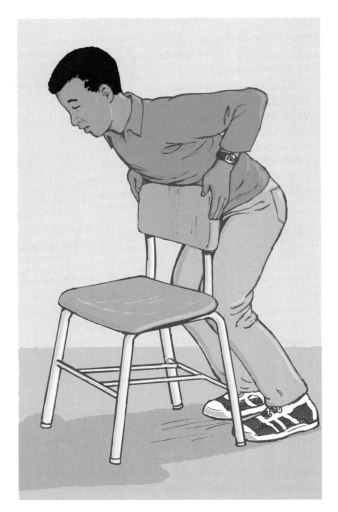

Figure 34-8 Self-administered Heimlich maneuver.

ventilate, and keep repeating these steps in sequence as quickly as you can until you can ventilate the patient.

Variations There are some patients in whom abdominal thrusts can cause injury. They are pregnant patients, infants, and very large persons. In those patients, you can achieve some success by performing chest thrusts or back blows instead of abdominal thrusts. If the pregnant patient (with a complete airway obstruction) is conscious, approach her from behind as before, encircle her chest with your arms, and place your fist against the middle of her sternum. Now grasp your fist with your free hand and deliver a single thrust against her sternum. Repeat the maneuver until the obstruction is cleared or she becomes unconscious. Figure 34-7 illustrates a chest thrust to be used on large persons and pregnant women.

If the patient becomes unconscious, attempt to ventilate. If ventilation does not work, do a jaw lift and finger-sweep. If that does not work, straddle her body as with the abdominal thrust on an unconscious patient, and deliver five chest thrusts to her mid-sternum. Start all over again, and continue the sequence as quickly as you can until the obstruction is cleared or until the physician or paramedic tells you to stop.

Figure 34-8 shows an individual performing a self-administered Heimlich maneuver. This is done by leaning over a chair rail and forcefully thrusting the rail into one's diaphragm until the obstruction is expelled.

The Small Child Airway obstructions in small children and infants are very common, because they put lots of things into their mouths. A child with an airway obstruction is treated the same as an adult, with one exception. Only remove an obstruction from a child's airway if you can see it. Blind finger-sweeps are not recommended.

The Infant The attempt to manage a complete airway obstruction in an infant is described in Table 34-1.

Med Tip: As with any procedure, practice is extremely important. Become re-certified in infant and adult CPR every year on a date that is easy to remember—such as your birthday.

TABLE 34-1   Airway Obstruction in Infants

Action	Description
1. Attempt to ventilate the infant.	Check for unresponsiveness by flicking the sole of the infant's foot with your finger. If that does not arouse the child, call for the physician or *911*. Open the airway. (Do not extend an infant's neck; a neutral position works fine.) Using mouth-to-mouth technique (if nothing else is available), attempt ventilation. If that fails, reposition the head and try again.
2. If you cannot ventilate. . . . Deliver back blows.	Place the infant face-down on your forearm with your fingers cradling the head, and rest your forearm on your thigh. Keep the child's head dependent. Using the heel of your free hand, deliver five back blows between the child's shoulder blades.
3. Initiate chest thrusts.	Using your forearms to sandwich the child's body, now place the child face-up on your opposite forearm and rest that forearm on your thigh on the same side. Place two fingers on the midline of the child's chest just below the nipple line and deliver five quick chest compressions, almost as though you were doing CPR.
4. Remove foreign body from infant's airway.	Repeat back blows and chest compressions in rapid sequence until the object is dislodged. Remove it immediately, but only if you can visualize it in the pharynx. If the child awakens, provide high-flow oxygen and encourage crying. If not, check for and support breathing as necessary. If you still cannot ventilate, quickly repeat the whole sequence until the obstruction is removed or until the physician or paramedic takes over.

All Patients Any patient who has lost consciousness as a result of an airway obstruction requires x-rays to verify that nothing was aspirated (sucked) into the lungs.

Abdominal Pain

The abdomen is a complex part of the body, packed with organs, vessels and spaces that are essential to life. Normally it conducts a thousand functions in complete silence, even tolerating our indiscretions without complaint. But when something does go wrong, the results can be catastrophic. While a thorough discussion of abdominal pain is beyond the scope of this text, some general concepts are essential to all caregivers.

First, all complaints of abdominal pain should trigger two thoughts: surgery and pregnancy (in females). Since so many abdominal complications can only be resolved by surgery, the patient who complains of abdominal pain should thereafter not ingest anything by mouth (NPO) pending a physician's diagnosis. And second, because of their potentially serious consequences, complications of pregnancy should always be considered a possibility in the female patient who complains of abdominal pain.

Findings With few exceptions, people's complaints of abdominal pain tend to be vaguely described and poorly localized. So, the process of solving abdominal mysteries is most often one of synthesizing many subtle findings, rather than finding the glaring ones. That can take some time, and since the physician will be going through the same assessment process anyway, there is no reason to put the patient through it twice.

Instead, take a look at the patient. Whatever the abdominal problem, is the patient in shock? Is the skin hot (infection?) or cold (bleeding?) Get a quick set of vitals, including the temperature. Does the patient need to lie down?

Without getting too involved, ask a few "payoff questions"—questions that can get you the most important information you need, quickly:

- Has there been vomiting?
- Irregularities of stool or urine?
- Any abnormal discharges? (from mouth, rectum, urinary tract)
- Changes in diet?

- Trouble breathing?
- Recent injury?
- Last menstrual period?
- Any possibility of pregnancy? (Be aware, patients don't always know or tell the truth about this.)

If you hear anything that makes you think this patient is bleeding, or if at any time you think you're dealing with someone who is in serious trouble for any reason, interrupt yourself and alert the physician. If the physician is not available, contact EMS.

Treatment Not all disorders related to the abdomen are emergencies. But most emergencies related to the abdomen are surgical and therefore, not performed in the physician's office. Apply oxygen at high flow, if ordered by the physician. Keep the patient flat with knees bent to relieve pain and calm. Contact EMS.

Allergic Reactions

The way our bodies respond to substances and pathogens in our environment is supposed to be automatic, unconscious and trouble-free. Except for an occasional bout of poison oak or mosquito attack, that's how life is for most of us. But for some, life is a constant struggle with allergies in the forms of discomfort, fear of environmental substances, and even the reality of sudden death.

Any one of us can discover a severe allergy at any time, but people with severe allergies tend to have many of them rather than just one or two. Fortunately, allergic emergencies are usually easy to recognize and not difficult to treat.

Findings Patients with an allergic reaction usually have red, warm skin. They may have some difficulty breathing, and parts of their body (like the face) may appear so puffy that family will say that they look like somebody else. The patient may have localized or widespread hives (irregular, white blotchy areas where the skin seems to be raised). If the breathing is a problem , you may hear respiratory wheezing even without a stethoscope. Usually, but not always, the patient will be able to describe an encounter with a substance to which he has a known allergy (an allergen). If not, and he says he has allergies to other substances, you can surmise that he is having an allergic reaction.

If the patient's systolic blood pressure is below 100 in addition to the above findings, you should probably get the patient to lie down, raise the lower extremities, and treat him or her for anaphylactic shock.

Treatment Treatment for an allergic reaction always begins with the same step: *break contact between the patient and the allergen.* If there is no clear information about what that is, remove the patient's clothing and suspect an allergy there. Do a thorough physical examination and make sure there is not a stinger somewhere, an ointment or cream, a new kind of hair spray, evidence of a recent injection, or some other substance or object that might be responsible. Find out about recent meals, especially if they included seafood. Consider the recent use of unfamiliar latex contraceptives (male or female). If the patient has a diaphragm in place, it should probably be removed by the patient or by a physician. Do whatever else is necessary to remove anything suspicious. Alert your physician and administer oxygen if ordered. Chances are that no matter how sick the patient appears, he or she will begin to respond within a minute or so to subcutaneous epinephrine (1:1000) (adrenaline). The medical assistant can prepare the epinephrine injection for the physician to administer. Some patients with a history of severe allergic reactions may be given a prescription for an epinephrine auto-injector like the one shown in Figure 34-9.

The patient who has been in shock, may require transport to a hospital; otherwise, that should not be necessary.

Amputation

Amputation of an extremity or body part is such a profound insult that these injuries do not tend to find their way into physicians offices until after they have been cared for in the Emergency Department (ED) of the nearest hospital. They are

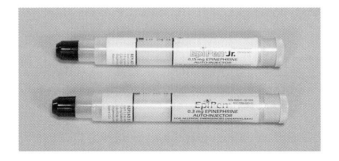

Figure 34-9 Epinephrine auto-injector.

fairly easy to care for, since the body normally reacts almost immediately to amputation by shutting down the blood flow to the severed extremity.

It is important to preserve the severed body part, because reimplantation is a standard procedure at most modern trauma centers. It can take place several hours after the incident, but the sooner the better. (Remember to take care of the patient first, and then the extremity.)

Findings The patient is likely to need a great deal of emotional support after the loss of a major extremity, as well as physical treatment for shock. The amputation may be the most obvious injury, and bleeding may be brisk at first. But consider the potential of other injuries as well, especially after a major amputation (for instance, of a lower extremity). Amputations may occur as isolated injuries, but they may also involve extraordinary amounts of force on the body as a whole.

Treatment Take care of the ABCs. Act quickly to protect the patient from further injury, and control any bleeding by means of direct pressure. Apply a pressure dressing to free your hands for other things, but watch for continued bleeding. Do not delay treatment for shock. Place the patient on high-flow oxygen as ordered by the physican. Be gentle. Keep him flat, elevate the injured extremity, and provide as much reassurance as you can.

After treatment for shock, what an amputee needs most is prompt transport to a trauma center along with the severed body part. Carefully remove any clothing from the part, place it in a sterile container (or a clean one, if necessary; a red infection control bag will do). Be sure to include any small pieces of tissue that you find along with the main portion. (Provide enough sterile normal saline solution, if available, to keep the parts submerged.) Label the container plainly with the contents and the time of packaging, and have it transported with the patient. You can reassure the patient and family significantly by informing them of the possibility of reimplantation—reattachment—without making any promises.

Asphyxia

It would be very unlikely for a patient suffering from traumatic asphyxia to survive a trip to a physician's office. Asphyxia, or suffocation, can occur as a result of almost any mechanical disruption of the organs or structures that enable us to breathe. Some examples include a ruptured lung or diaphragm, blockage of a major pulmonary vessel, crushed ribs, or a crushed trachea or larynx.

Findings This would be a patient who would instantly get your undivided attention. He would be blue from the clavicles upward. His neck veins would be very distended, and if he were conscious he might be struggling frantically to breathe but unable to do so. You would readily see that he has almost no tidal volume (the volume of air we exchange with each cycle of breathing).

Treatment Alert your physician immediately, and contact EMS even if the physician is available. Try to ventilate the patient with 100% oxygen as ordered by the physician. Allow the patient to remain in the position of choice. If the patient can be helped at all, it will be by means of an advanced procedure by a physician or a paramedic.

Birth (Emergency)

A pregnant patient may come into the medical office in active labor—the birth imminent. In this case, it is not wise for the patient to then leave the office and make the trip to the hospital for the delivery, particularly if the patient is unaccompanied or drove the vehicle herself. The EMS needs to be called in order to deliver the baby (if the mother has not delivered prior to the EMS's arrival) or provide care to the mother and baby immediately after birth, as well as provide transport to the hospital.

Childbirth is a normal process unless the mother is hemorrhaging or the baby is in fetal distress. This can be caused by a condition, such as a prolapsed umbilical cord or placenta previa, which is the blockage of the birth canal by the placenta.

Labor is the actual process of expelling the fetus from the uterus and through the vagina. The length of time for labor varies in women from a few hours to 24 hours or more. A mother who has had several previous births may deliver a baby very quickly. While she will have strong contractions just before the birth, there may have been few or no labor pains or contractions that she was aware of. When a mother who has delivered several babies (multipara) comes into the office in labor, be prepared to conduct an emergency childbirth.

The first stage of labor is referred to as the stage of dilation. During this stage the uterine muscles contract in an attempt to expel the fetus. During this process the fetus presses on the cervix and causes it to dilate or expand. When the cervix is completely dilated at 10 centimeters, the second stage of labor begins. The thinning of the cervix is

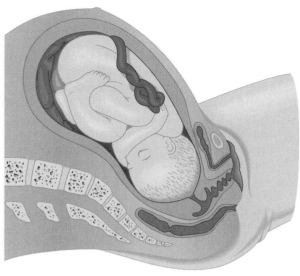

FIRST STAGE:
First uterine contraction to dilation of cervix

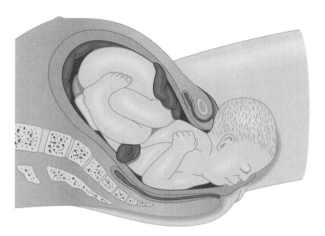

SECOND STAGE:
Birth of baby or expulsion

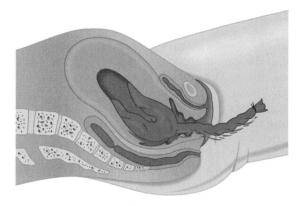

THIRD STAGE:
Delivery of placenta

Figure 34-10   Three stages of labor.

referred to as effacement. This stage ends with the birth of the baby. See Figures 34-10 and 34-11 for illustrations of the childbirth process. Generally the head of the baby appears first. This is referred to a crowning. In some cases, the baby's buttocks will appear first, and this is referred to as a breech birth. The last stage of labor is the placental stage, during which the placenta or afterbirth is delivered. Immediately after childbirth the uterus again begins to contract, causing the placenta to be expelled through the vagina.

Bites and Stings (Venomous and Non-venomous)

There are three common kinds of bites and a variety of stings that you may expect to see, depending on the area where you work. To some extent, the advanced resources for treating venomous bites and stings will be specialized to meet the needs of your area. For instance, antivenom serum which is specific to cottonmouth snakebites would probably not be common in

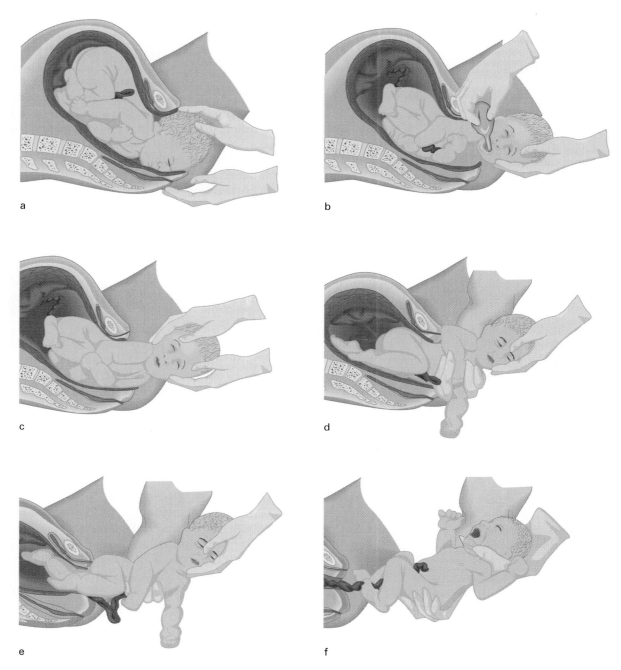

a

b

c

d

e

f

Figure 34-11 Delivery of fetus.

Denver, but it would be a necessity in Baton Rouge, Louisiana.

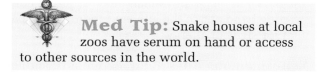

Med Tip: Snake houses at local zoos have serum on hand or access to other sources in the world.

Venomous Bites and Stings Fortunately, venomous creatures do not always inject venom when they bite. If they do, pain is usually immediate and intense, and swelling follows within minutes to hours. Other variables include:

* The type of creature that bit or stung the patient.
* The age and size of the patient.

- The location of the site of the sting or bite.
- The amount of activity following the bite. *(less is better)*
- The elapsed time since the bite. *(less is better)*

A complete discussion of all kinds of bites or stings is not within the scope of this text, but general descriptions follow.

There is not much you can do for the victims of most venomous bites or stings in the office setting. Most will require the resources of a trauma center and the kind of antivenin which is specific to their injuries. But it is important to recognize the appearance of injury sites that may not be associated with serious signs or symptoms until 12-24 hours or more after envenomation. It is also important to remember that even common insect stings may trigger severe allergic reactions, including anaphylactic shock in some patients.

Venomous Snakebite Most venom attacks are not fatal. Small children and elderly adults are most at risk, and so are victims of snakes with fangs in which the venom entered the blood stream very directly.

Findings: You can generally expect to see two kinds of poisonous snakebites, namely those from snakes with fangs and those from snakes without fangs. Snakes with fangs (for example rattlesnakes, copperheads, and cottonmouths) leave distinctive marks from well developed paired fangs, and the onset of pain and swelling is almost immediate. Be aware that the fang marks may look like abrasions or small cuts instead of puncture wounds. Snakes without fangs (for example coral snakes) inject their venom during a kind of chewing motion as they bite. Systemic signs—signs indicating that the entire body is effected—may not develop for many hours following these bites.

Treatment: Contact EMS. The treatment for snakebite is antivenin, administered at an ED or trauma center. If the remains of the snake are obtainable, arrange for them to be transported, sealed in a plastic bag, with the patient for accurate identification. Apply oxygen if ordered by the physician. Your physician may want to start an IV and monitor the patient for signs of allergy.

Venomous Spider Bite In most snake bite cases, the victims know what bit them and when. However, that is not always true of spider bites.

Findings (Brown recluse bite): Bites by the brown recluse spider are often painless for the first few hours. By the time you see one of these bites, it will have evolved into a small blister surrounded by a painful, reddened area of tissue that will eventually die without recognition and proper treatment by a physician.

Treatment: Early recognition and prompt treatment for brown recluse bites by a physician may prevent the development of a large necrotic ulcer (involving the death of tissue). There is no effective first aid, unless the patient is allergic to the venom. (See *allergies*.)

Findings (Black widow bite): Black widow venom is extremely potent, but fortunately this spider is not particularly aggressive. When it does bite, pain and swelling are immediate and intense, and systemic signs develop over several hours. Fatalities can occur in people who are already in poor health, especially those with high blood pressure. Systemic signs include nausea and vomiting, diaphoresis (sweating), hypertension and profound painful muscle spasms over large areas of the body adjacent to the bite, followed by decreased level of consciousness, paralysis and seizures.

Treatment: Contact EMS. This patient needs black widow antivenin, and because systemic complications are such a concern, the patient belongs in an ED. Apply oxygen if ordered by the physician. The physician may wish to administer an IV. He may also want to administer diazepam to control muscle spasms and seizures. Watch for signs of allergy. And finally, monitor the vital signs, especially the blood pressure.

Venomous Stings (Scorpions) Scorpions are found throughout the world. They are reclusive and mostly nocturnal and only a few species have produced human fatalities.

Findings: The venom of scorpions is neurotoxic and cardiotoxic. Pain at the injection site may progress to numbness, and the patient may exhibit a wide variety of neurologic signs. They include:

- Hyperactivity, especially in children.
- Muscular twitching.
- Slurred speech.
- Nausea & vomiting.
- Excessive salivation.
- Convulsions.

Treatment: Contact EMS. This patient may need antivenin, especially if you note a lot of neurologic signs. The physician may apply a constricting band above the site, and monitor the patient for signs of allergy.

Non-venomous Bites Bites are not all handled in the same way. Knowing which specific creature inflicted a bite can have everything to do with treatment.

Findings: Important findings include bleeding and whether there appears to be tissue missing. Missing tissue needs to be found quickly, if possible.

Treatment: The treatment for non-venomous bites does not vary much by type of bite. But it should be noted that there is probably no non-venomous bite more disfiguring or more prone to infection than a human one. Human bites are jagged and dirty, and are almost sure to produce scarring and infection. They are also very often associated with other kinds of trauma, both physical and emotional. Human bite victims are assault victims, and you should inform police when you encounter them.

Dog bites are also common, and should also result in a police contact, especially if the bite involves a child. In most places, any mammal bite results in mandatory containment of the animal and a rabies examination as soon as possible. Bites by other non-venomous creatures, such as birds or snakes, should be cared for like any other simple wound.

Severe Bleeding (Hemorrhage)

The patient who stumbles into your office with a bulky towel wrapped around an arm and leaving a trail of blood can be a real attention-getter. But for someone who does not see large volumes of blood every day, a small amount can look like a lot more than it really is.

Findings To the average person, external, visible arterial bleeding is a dramatic and frightening thing. But a smart caregiver knows how easy that is to fix, and how much more worrisome is the prospect of hidden bleeding, deep inside the abdomen, chest or head. The kinds of findings you need to be most alert for are the signs of hypovolemic shock. They are discussed under "Shock," later in this chapter .

In addition to shock, be alert for other signs of bleeding, system by system. Sometimes the first clues about hidden bleeding come from the nature of the pain associated with it. But headache is an important sign of bleeding inside the head; especially severe, debilitating headache of very sudden onset, with or without other neurologic findings. This kind of complaint should be considered a true emergency until ruled out by a neurologist using a CAT scan.

Another pain that should get your attention is a kind of sharp, stabbing pain that comes on suddenly, deep in the abdomen or between the shoulder blades, and is unrelieved by anything. This is the kind of pain that comes from a dissecting aneurysm of the aorta, which is the body's largest artery. The patient may have a history of high blood pressure. He is usually seen writhing in pain and will not be pacified. This kind of pain is associated with a spreading bubble between layers of the vessel. If it ruptures, the patient can bleed to death internally within a few minutes. Or, if the bubble is on the inside of the vessel, it can occlude the blood flow to a large area of the body.

Sometimes your biggest clues about the origin and seriousness of bleeding come from the patient's body orifices, or openings. If the bleeding is in the esophagus, you may find bright red undigested blood in the vomit, possibly mixed with brown, predigested blood. The patient who bleeds into his small intestines vomits brown, foul-smelling digested blood. Both of these patients will exhibit a characteristic breath odor of digested blood. The patient who bleeds into his lower GI tract may not vomit at all, but will report dark, tarry, foul-smelling diarrhea. And the patient who bleeds from the rectum discharges red blood rectally. People who are bleeding into their digestive systems tend to have firm, oversized abdomens. That results from the presence of gas produced as a byproduct of digested blood.

Patients who cough up pink or reddish-colored sputum, or who cough blood as opposed to vomiting it, tend to be bleeding somewhere in the airway. That includes the mouth, the nose, the pharynx, the trachea, and the mainstem bronchi and lungs.

Patients who appear to be in shock and whose abdomens are oversized and firm to the touch (with or without tenderness) may be bleeding into the abdomen. And finally, people whose urine seems bloody may be bleeding somewhere from their kidneys or elsewhere in their genitourinary system.

Treatment Fortunately, the body does a good job of controlling its own blood loss. When it fails, the most effective thing you can do is also the simplest. Direct pressure with a gloved hand over a bulky compress will stop almost any external bleeding, even arterial bleeding. Do not forget that persistent bleeding is just as important as rapid bleeding. Simple suspicion that a patient may be bleeding internally can be life-saving. That, and once again, treating for shock.

Pressure Points

Caregivers were once expected to memorize a list of points on the surface of the body where they could apply pressure (pressure points) in order to

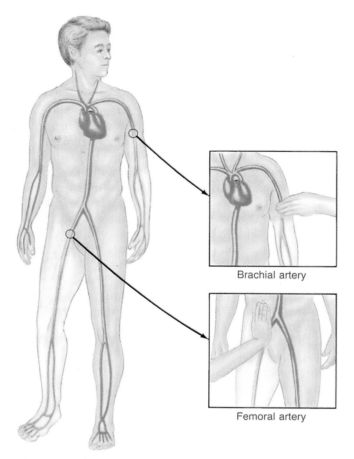

Figure 34-12 Pressure points in the body.

Brachial artery

Femoral artery

stop external bleeding (Figure 34-12). Applying pressure to pressure points is no longer recommended because direct local pressure is so much more effective. In theory, you can apply pressure almost anywhere you can feel a pulse and, if you apply enough pressure, stop the flow of blood in that artery. Unfortunately, this process is so uncomfortable for the patient and so seldom effective that most modern caregivers do not use it.

Never apply pressure directly on the carotid artery. Not only can this cause a stroke, but it also directly stimulates the vagus nerve, which slows the heart rate and can in some cases disrupt cardiac output altogether.

Breathing Emergencies

The respiratory system is a complex network of structures and organs that keeps us alive. In health it keeps itself clean, protects itself against infection and obstructions, and generally makes our breathing so easy that we are not even aware of it. But to many people breathing is a nonstop ordeal—both laborious and frightening.

You will see two kinds of breathing emergencies: those that occur suddenly in healthy people, and those that are based on complications of existing disorders. Some can be corrected in the physician's office, and some require emergency hospitalization. Determining which is which can be a challenge even for a well equipped physician. But it is not difficult to tell how sick somebody is by looking at them. And the most important steps in helping them are the same regardless of their disease process.

Foreign Body Airway Obstruction Obstruction of the airway by a foreign body is a common type of emergency, especially among small children and among people who attempt to eat while intoxicated. Airway obstruction is discussed separately earlier in this chapter.

Findings: People with respiratory disorders range in severity from the child with a cold to the busy wage-earner who comes in with a fever and a cough, to the 70-year-old ex-smoker who is panicky, struggling for her life, and is an ashen gray color. In each case, a caregiver looks at four basic things:

1. What is the patient's overall appearance?
2. What is the degree of effort?
3. What is the respiratory rate?
4. What are the respiratory sounds?

The urgency presented by a patient in this kind of distress can be so desperate that you may feel compelled to treat the patient immediately, thinking you have no time to assess anything. Actually, you can do the above assessment steps simultaneously as you initiate treatment. Since the physician's actions will depend on a set of accurate vital signs, the process of taking them—the vitals—can benefit the patient a great deal. By convincing the patient that the treatment he or she needs is about to be given, the patient may become less fearful and better able to cooperate in his or her own care.

Observe how the patient is communicating. Communication is our highest mental function, and it is a very reliable indicator of how well we are oxygenating our brains. Is the patient expressing spontaneous humor? If so, chances are the patient is not in grave distress. Is he or she ignoring you and concentrating only on breathing? That is not good, especially if the patient seems very tired (chances are, this patient will require intubation and artificial breathing by the EMS).

Between those two extremes are a series of communication levels you can look for. Simple observation takes no time. You can do it early in your contact with the patient (so you know how sick he is when he arrives) and several times dur-

TABLE 34-2 Communication (Mental Awareness) Levels

Range	Level	Description
Best	1	Spontaneous expression of humor.
	2	Spontaneous speech, even when not being questioned (note syllables per breath).
	3	Intelligible speech in response to questions only (responses are meaningful).
	4	Non-intelligible speech in response to questions (responses are not meaningful).
	5	Obeys commands appropriately, but does not answer questions.
	6	Reacts to commands, but does not obey them.
	7	Appears awake, but does not answer questions or obey commands.
	8	Falls asleep, but verbally arousable.
	9	Localizes/avoids noxious stimuli, but never wakes up.
	10	Localizes deep pain by trying to push it away.
	11	Withdraws from deep pain, but does not localize it.
	12	Postures in response to deep pain, but does not withdraw or localize it.
Worst	13	Totally unresponsive to any stimuli.

ing your contact with him (so you know if he's improving or getting worse). See Table 34-2 for a list of mental awareness levels indicating the ability to communicate and quality of communication ranging from best to worst.

In addition to these levels of mental awareness, pay attention to the number of syllables of speech a person uses with each breath. Somebody who spontaneously communicates using 10-15 syllables per breath is probably not having much respiratory trouble. But when the best your patient can muster is one or two syllables per breath, there's a problem. Again, this is a consideration that does not take any time away from other things you need to do. Of course, counting syllables does not mean you need to sit there and actually count with a watch. Instead, estimate an average, then re-estimate it from time to time.

Watch for trends. Was this person originally talking like a college professor, and now she's only grunting in response to your questions? That kind of change may be instantaneous, or it can occur very subtly over time. In the latter case, counting syllables is a good way to detect and monitor it.

Another important sign of shock is irritability. A patient who was nice to you on their arrival and gradually becomes more irritable with you as time goes by is getting worse (unless someone is ignoring them).

Med Tip: Try hard to tolerate behaviors of sick people that would normally make you angry. For instance, it's fairly common for people with cerebral irritability to curse or to abuse others verbally. Even people who have never said a bad word in their lives can become loud and can exhibit very foul language when their brain gets irritated. No matter what you do, avoid retaliating. None of this is intentional. Instead, try to protect the patient from injury, and have someone explain to family members what is happening while you continue to be a good caregiver.

Finally, remember that respiratory distress can either result from or cause cardiac disorders. These are patients who need to be monitored and who will probably require chest x-rays.

Treatment: When someone is scared to death, he or she needs to see caregivers as people who care and who can help. Explain everything you do before you do it. Apply oxygen as ordered by the physician. The EMS may apply high-flow oxygen via non-rebreather mask or, if the patient seems tired or mental ability seems impaired, assist the patient's ventilations (preferably with an oxygen-powered resuscitator). Continually offer

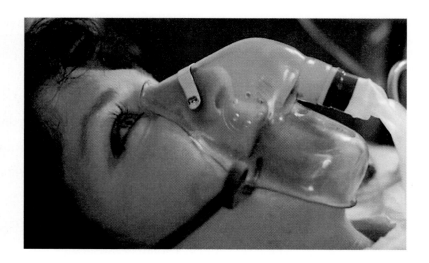

Figure 34-13   Application of oxygen mask.

reassurance so that the patient does not panic and remind the patient not to be afraid.

If the patient has a breathing disorder that can be treated in the office (for instance asthma or an allergic reaction), you can gradually cut back on your efforts to oxygenate them as their status improves and the physician orders the oxygen stopped. Other patients have bigger problems, such as emphysema, pneumonia or congestive heart failure. Your physician may be able to ease the distress of these patients somewhat, but after that these patients need transport to a hospital with treatment continuing en route. Still others are in such dire straits that they simply need to get to a hospital (for instance, the patient with a pulmonary embolus or a lung tumor).

All of these patients need the same kind of basic care. Any patient with difficulty breathing should be considered as a potential "code" patient. Get the cardiac monitor connected, and run a 12-lead ECG if you can. Have the crash cart ready. Figure 34-13 shows an oxygen mask being applied and Figure 34-14 illustrates mouth to mask ventilation.

Med Tip: If you have the luxury of help during an emergency, do not forget to warn them that you have a critical patient in Room Such-And-Such.

When paramedics arrive, inform them in detail about what changes you have seen, and in response to what treatment. See Figure 34-15 for an illustration of how to prepare the oxygen delivery system.

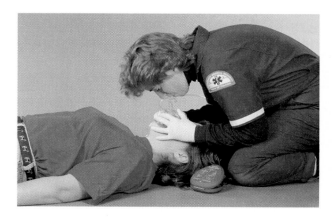

Figure 34-14   Mouth to mask ventilation.

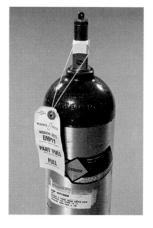

1. Select desired cylinder. Check label, "Oxygen U.S.P."

Figure 34-15   Preparing the oxygen delivery system. *(Continued)*

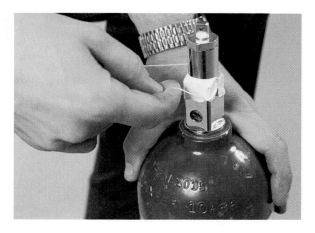

2. Remove the plastic wrapper or cap protecting the cylinder outlet.

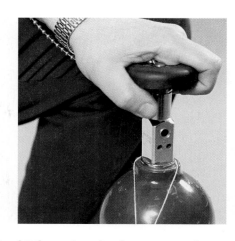

3. "Crack" the main valve for one second.

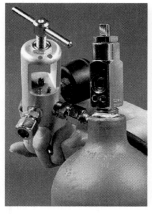 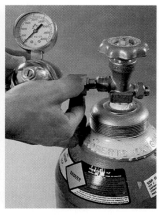

4. Select the correct pressure regulator and flowmeter. Pin yoke in shown on the threaded outlet on the right.

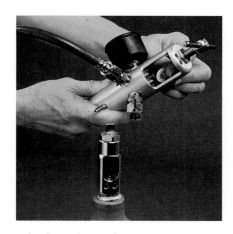

5. Place cylinder valve gasket on regulator oxygen port.

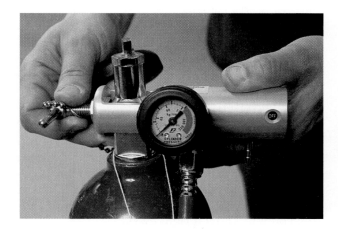

6. Make certain that the pressure regulator is closed.

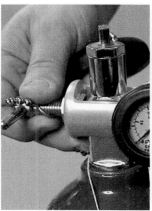 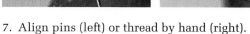

7. Align pins (left) or thread by hand (right).

Figure 34-15 Preparing the oxygen delivery system. *(Continued on next page)*

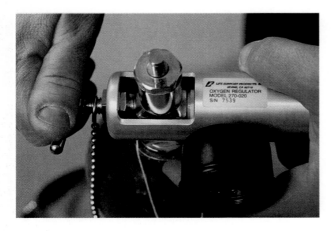

8. Tighten T-screw for pin yoke.

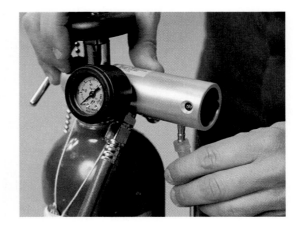

9. Attach tubing and delivery device.

Figure 34-15 (Continued)

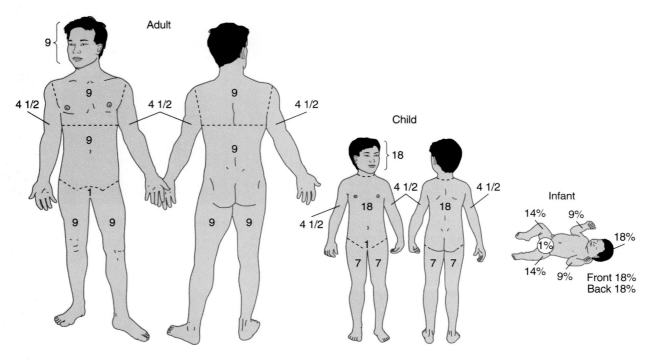

Figure 34-16 Rule of Nines for burns.

Burns

There simply is no form of trauma as painful, disfiguring, difficult to heal from, or as hard for caregivers to deal with as burns. Fortunately, the kinds of burns you will see in the office setting will probably not be the bad ones.

A burn injury occurs when an area of tissue is destroyed by the action of physical heat, chemical activity, high electrical current, or heavy exposure to radiation. The severity of a burn (and the likelihood of healing) depend on the amount and depth of tissue injury. Survival depends on those factors in addition to the amount of surface area that is destroyed. Chances are that when you are confronted with a burn that is too much for your office to handle, you will know it right away.

Destruction of skin surface is important because of all of the skin functions that are thereby lost: insulation, regulation of fluids, sensation, protection from infection, and overall appearance. All of these are crucial to life.

TABLE 34-3 **Classification of Burns**

Degree	Characteristics
First	Reddening, swelling of epidermis (like mild sunburn).
Second	Reddening, swelling of epidermis and outer dermis; blisters noted.
Third	Charring of all layers of skin and at least some deeper structures.

Findings As you might imagine after reading the second paragraph above, burns are classified in two basic ways: by surface area and by depth. The *Rule of Nines* is a useful tool for estimating surface area (Figure 34-16). In addition, Table 34-3 will give you a basic idea of burn severity by depth.

First and second-degree burns are extremely painful, even those involving very small areas. Third-degree burns tend not to be painful immediately because along with the entire dermis, this kind of burn destroys sensory nerve endings. But it also disrupts all of the normal functions of skin, including its self-regenerative properties and its ability to resist infection. Third-degree burns are profound injuries, even if they only involve a small amount of surface area.

Actually, there are some special considerations that also help determine the seriousness of a burn. They include

- The mortality of serious burns is higher for elderly patients and very young ones.
- The mortality is higher if the patient was burned in a closed area (partly due to the possibility of carbon monoxide poisoning and partly due to the possibility of airway burns).
- Burns of the genitalia are always considered serious, regardless of depth.
- Always consider the possibility of other injuries besides burns, especially in a patient who was burned in an auto or industrial accident.
- Patients with chemical burns should be bathed immediately with large amounts of water (Figure 34-17). If the burns resulted from an alkali substance, irrigation should be continued even in favor of transport to an ED for a minimum of 20 minutes. Contact EMS as soon as you encounter such a patient to be sure that if you are dealing with a hazardous substance that cannot be rendered harmless, you have access to the proper resources as early as possible.
- Electrical burns serious enough to leave marks on the body are considered serious burns, because of the probability of internal

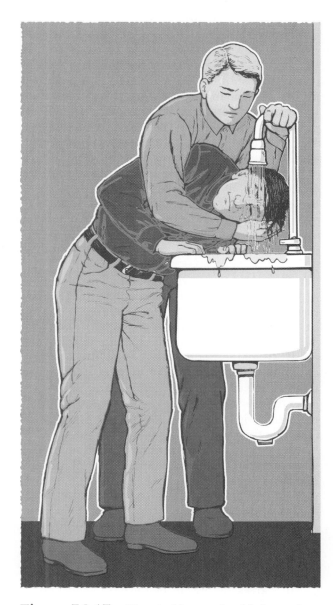

Figure 34-17 Chemical burns should always be flushed with large amounts of water.

injuries. (Electrocution by lightning is always considered serious until proven otherwise.)

These factors are all regarded as stand-alone admission criteria by trauma centers in most places.

Treatment Treatment for first-degree burns involving less than 10% of the body surface includes pain relief by means of cool water. That instantly relieves pain, but it is not appropriate for larger surface areas. Damaged skin may not be able to regulate body temperature, so the use of cooling measures over large surface areas can cause hypothermia. Analgesic creams and ointments are appropriate for use on first-degree burns only if ordered by the physician.

Cool water can also be used to soothe second-degree burns for small surface areas, as long as there are no broken blisters. Second-degree burns of any size should not be treated with creams or ointments, due to the risk of breaking blisters and the resulting potential of infection.

Burns of any kind that involve broken skin may need to be debrided (removal of dead or damaged tissue) by a physician. If third-degree burns are present in any amount, the patient warrants treatment at a trauma center. Burns should be dressed with dry sterile dressings, and pain should be managed with injectable analgesics as ordered. If the patient will be transported by paramedics, the paramedics will start the IV and administer analgesics via that route.

Upper airway burns constitute a dire emergency, and always warrant prompt intubation by EMS paramedics with the largest tube that can be inserted. The epiglottis can swell quickly and make intubation very difficult or impossible later on. If the patient sounds even slightly hoarse or complains of difficulty breathing, or if you notice stridor (noisy breathing) in any burn patient, consider the possibility of airway burns and notify the physician right away. Administer oxygen as ordered by the physician.

Large surface-area burns should be dressed with dry sterile sheets, wrapped entirely around the patient's body. These patients benefit most from prompt transport to a trauma center. All burn patients should be monitored for signs of shock, especially in the case of large surface area involvement.

Cardiac Arrest

Cardiac arrest is not an every day occurrence in the office. But because it is not, the experience can seem more intimidating than it needs to be. Try to think of a cardiac arrest patient as an unresponsive patient who requires extra steps of care.

Findings The patient in cardiac arrest is fairly easy to recognize, even from the other side of a room. Their skin color may be normal, but more often it is pale, gray or slightly blue. Most of all, they seem inappropriately quiet.

When you encounter someone who appears unresponsive, call the individual's name (if you know it or ask repeatedly, "Are you OK?") and shake the patient to establish responsiveness. This should wake the person up. If not, and the patient is not on an examining table, ease the patient to the floor and call loudly for the crash cart. Clear some furniture so you have room to work. It is difficult when you try to conduct an emergency code in a space where you do not have room for three people plus a supine patient. If possible, move the patient someplace where you will have room to work.

Treatment Place the patient on his back and hyperextend the neck, to quickly provide an airway. Is the patient breathing? Look, listen, and feel for air movement. Place your ear next to the patient's mouth and nose while you watch to see if the chest rises. If you do not see, hear or feel evidence of regular breathing, use a rescue mask or resuscitator to apply a seal around the patient's mouth and nose, and administer two full breaths.

Next, check for a carotid pulse with your three middle fingers, on your side of the patient's neck. If there is a pulse, but the patient is still not breathing, continue ventilating about 12 times a minute. If there is no pulse, place the heel of one hand over the midline of the lower third of the patient's sternum, place your other hand on top of the first hand, and administer 15 smooth chest compressions at a rate of 80-100 compressions per minute. (80-100 compressions is about what you get when you count aloud as follows: ONE thousand, TWO thousand, THREE thousand. . . .)

When you are with a patient who suddenly becomes unresponsive, shake the patient and shout. Establish an airway and begin CPR. Call for help loudly enough for someone in another room to hear you, and announce an emergency code in your location. Treat for unresponsiveness as above.

The patient who arrests in a physician's office has the best possible chance of surviving the arrest, especially if the physician is available and the staff can perform good CPR. But this is a patient who for a time can demand the total resources of an office. He may require an airway, intubation, and defibrillation by the EMS team as well as someone to handle the ventilations, someone to compress the chest, one or more IVs, a 12-lead ECG and constant monitoring of the rhythm, one or more defibrillations, suction, and a lot of oxygen. Paramedics will typically need to change portable tanks at least once. Figure 34-18 is an example of a defibrillator.

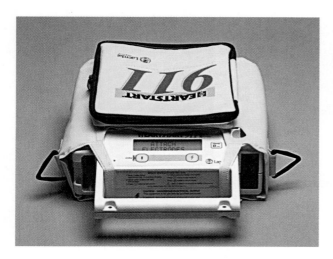

Figure 34-18 AED Defibrillator Headstart® *911* by Laerdol.

In addition, someone will need to take care of the patient's family and explain to the other patients what is happening. The arrest patient will definitely require transport to an ED, if he is not pronounced dead in the office.

Your EMS responders conduct codes, emergency procedures, every day. It is wise from a practical standpoint to alert them as early as possible and turn the arrest patient over to them so your other patients can receive the attention they need and deserve. Figure 34-19 A and B illustrates two-rescuer CPR.

CPR (Cardiopulmonary Resuscitation)

The patient whom you find unresponsive, apneic and pulseless will die unless you act quickly to control the airway, restart breathing and provide some form of circulation. These steps are not difficult, they make sense, they are likely to make a difference, and you can perform them easily.

Often, you can recognize the patient in cardiac arrest as soon as you enter a room. Something is wrong; the victim is just too quiet. But you do not want to perform CPR on a patient who does not need it. Make sure that does not happen, by adhering to the following sequence.

1. *Establish unresponsiveness.* Call the patient, if possible by name. Grasp him by the shoulder and shake him briskly. Ask in a firm voice, "Are you all right?" If the patient is merely asleep, this will usually get a response. If not, you know

you have a job to do. Alert your physician and staff that you need some help, and if the physician is not available, contact *911*. This patient will be going to a hospital.

2. *Establish a good airway.* Extend the patient's neck, to open the airway. This is a further check for responsiveness, but most importantly it creates a passage for air past the back of the patient's tongue to facilitate breathing and allow you to ventilate the patient during CPR.

3. *Check to see if the patient is breathing.* Look at the patient's chest. Does it rise and fall? Place your ear next to the patient's mouth and nose. Listen and feel for the sounds of breathing. Is the patient breathing? If so, he or she needs to be breathing regularly, not just occasionally, and you need to be able to hear and feel this patient breathing clearly and without question. If not, grab your plastic mouth guard, place it firmly over the patient's mouth and nose, and administer two full breaths through mouth to mouth resuscitation.

4. *Feel for a carotid pulse.* Find the patient's Adam's Apple with two fingers of one hand. Slide your fingers sideways, off of the Adam's Apple and into the groove in the patient's neck right next to the Adam's Apple. Feel for a pulse, for about five full seconds. Do you feel anything? If so, get some vitals. If not then begin cardiac compressions.

   Make sure you have room to work. If you will be doing CPR, remember that's not all you will be doing. Get the patient into a room where there will be plenty of space to do CPR if this can be done quickly. Do that immediately, before you initiate compressions. It is difficult to run a code in a small room, no matter what kind of resources you have. If EMS has not been contacted, ask someone to contact them even if you do have a physician available.

5. *Locate the site for chest compressions.* Make sure the patient is on his back on a flat, firm surface. Kneel or stand at a 90-degree angle to the patient's body. Palpate both ends of the patient's sternum. Place the heel of one of your hands parallel to and on top of the lower half of the patient's sternum.

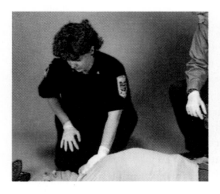

1. Determine unresponsiveness.

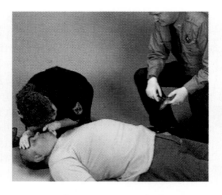

2. Open the airway. Look, listen, feel for 3-5 seconds.

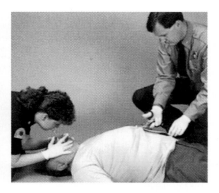

3. Ventilate twice (1.5 to 2.0 seconds per breath).

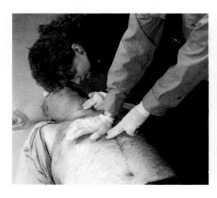

4. Determine pulselessness (no pulse). Locate CPR compression site.

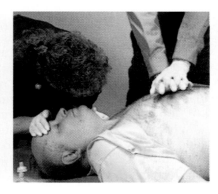

5. Say "No pulse." Begin compressions.

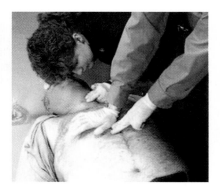

6. Check compression effectiveness. Deliver five compressions in 3-4 seconds (80-100 per minute).

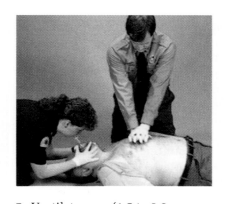

7. Ventilate once (1.5 to 2.0 seconds). Stop for mouth-to-mask ventilation.

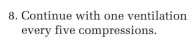

8. Continue with one ventilation every five compressions.

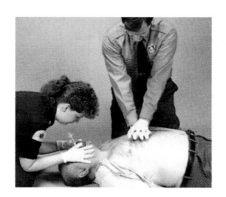

9. After ten cycles, reassess breathing and pulse. No pulse—say "Continue CPR." Pulse—say "Stop CPR."

Note: Assess for spontaneous breathing and pulse for 5 seconds at the end of the first minute, then every few minutes thereafter.

Figure 34-19 A Two-Rescuer CPR.

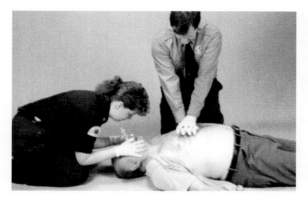

1. When fatigued the compressor calls for a switch. Give a clear signal to change.

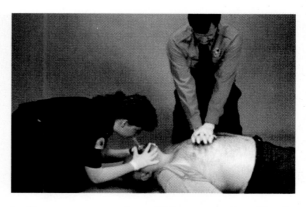

2. Compressor completes fifth compression. Ventilator provides one ventilation.

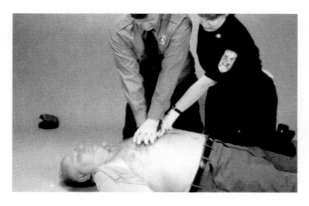

3. Ventilator moves to chest and locates compression site. Compressor moves to head and checks carotid pulse.

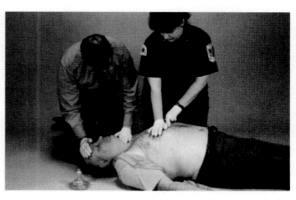

4. New compressor positions hands. New ventilator checks carotid pulse (5 seconds) and says "No pulse, continue CPR." (*Note:* Another breath is not given.)

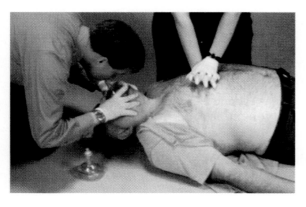

5. New compressor begins compressions and new ventilator breathes after every fifth compression (1.5 to 2.0 seconds for each breath).

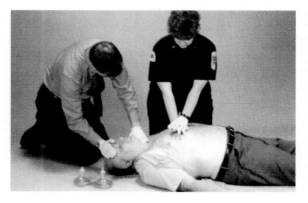

6. New ventilator and new compressor continue until compressor is fatigued and calls for a change.

Figure 34-19 B   Changing position.

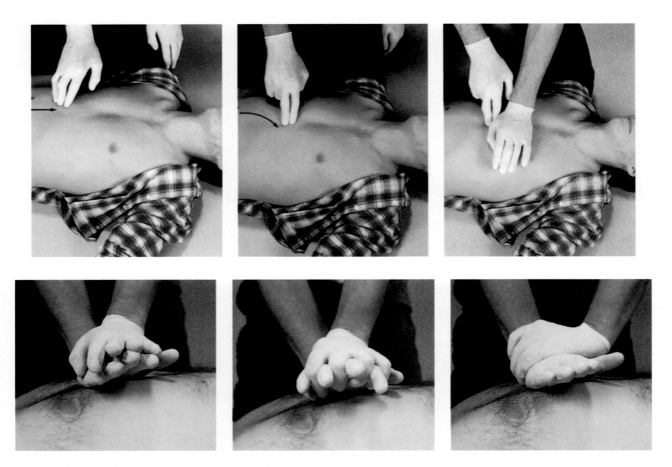

Figure 34-20   Location and position of hand during chest compressions.

6. *Compress.* Place the heel of your second hand on top of your first hand, straighten your arms and press downward on the patient's sternum. You should depress the sternum from 1.5-2 inches (Figure 34-20).

7. *Do that 15 times* in succession if you are alone, or five times if you have help. Either way, you should deliver compressions at a rate of 80-100 times per minute. Reassess pulses by taking the carotid pulse every few minutes. Except to reassess and unless you are relieved by others, do not interrupt CPR until the patient either resumes spontaneous life functions or is pronounced dead. Figure 34-21 A and B illustrates the step-by-step procedure of one-rescuer CPR.

Different Techniques for Children CPR works the same way for children and infants as it does for adults. But because of the obvious differences in a child's anatomy, you do not compress or ventilate a child as vigorously as you do an adult (Figure 34-22 A and B). In addition, since a child's smaller lungs and heart function at higher rates than those of an adult, those rates vary in pediatric CPR as well.

1. *Two fingers* are adequate to compress the sternum of an infant. Locate the compression point one finger-breadth below the nipple line, and depress only 1/2 to one inch .

2. *One hand* does it for a small child. Using the heel of one hand, depress the chest one to 1-1/2 inch. The location? Same as an adult.

Figure 34-23 provides a summary chart of adult-patient CPR. Table 34-4 outlines the basic differences in rates and ratios between adult, child, and infant CPR.

Cerebrovascular Accident (Stroke)

A stroke is an interruption in perfusion (the flow of oxygenated blood) to part of the brain. Apart from trauma, a stroke can result from a structural problem like blockage, spasm or rupture of a blood vessel, or from pressure produced by an expanding mass of some kind, such as a tumor, inside the skull.

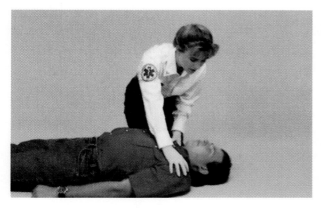

1. Establish unresponsiveness, and alert EMS. Position the patient and yourself.

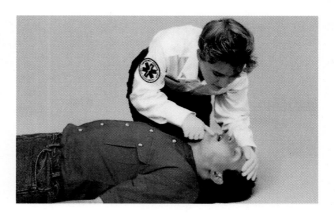

2. Establish an open airway.

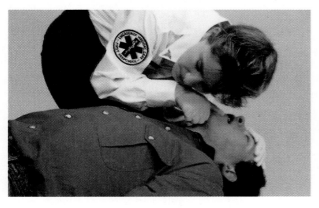

3. Look, listen, and feel for breathing (3-5 seconds).

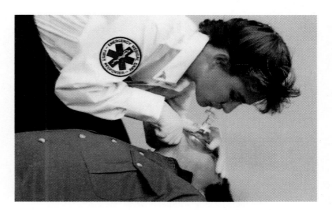

4. Ventilate twice (1.5 to 2.0 seconds per breath).

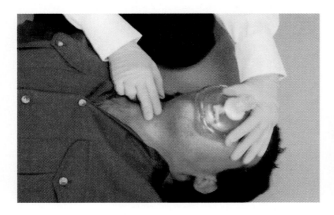

5. No pulse (5-10 seconds).

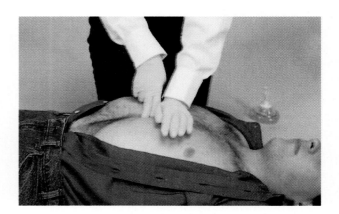

6. Locate compression site.

Figure 34-21 A and B One-Rescuer CPR.

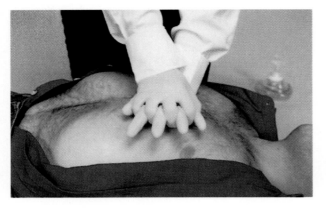

7. Position your hands.

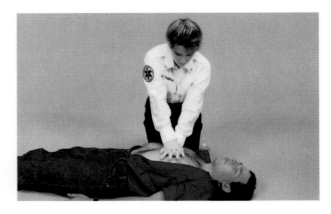

8. Begin compressions.

Compression rate is
80-100 per minute.

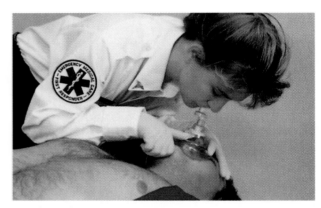

9. Ventilate twice.

Cycle = 2 ventilations
every 15 compressions.

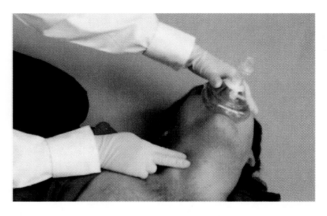

Note: If alone with an unresponsive infant or child, provide one minute of CPR before calling EMS dispatch.

10. Recheck pulse after 4 cycles, then every few minutes.

Figure 34-21 A and B   *(Continued)*

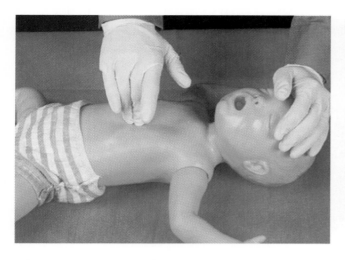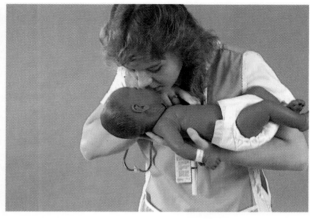

Figure 34-22 A and B   Infant compressions and ventilations.

Findings The brain cannot store oxygen or nutrients. As a result, almost immediately after the flow of blood is interrupted to a portion of the brain, there is a resulting disturbance in whatever function it controls. So, the signs of stroke can vary.

Stroke patients can experience anything from apnea to loss of speech and death. Perhaps the most common finding is some degree of one-sided numbness or paralysis. If the patient happens to be standing or sitting when a stroke occurs, they may fall and suffer injuries as a result. In addition, they may experience urinary or fecal incontinence, facial droop, unequal pupils, unconsciousness or seizures. Depending on the size, location and nature of the stroke, the patient's signs may be permanent or they may diminish or disappear completely.

Your observations are very important to a physician, because the diagnosis and treatment of brain disorders depends on the sequence of changes in the patient's appearance over time. In addition, there is a type of mild stroke called a transient ischemic attack (TIA) that may cause no lasting effects at all. TIAs can occur repeatedly, leading up to a major event that might be preventable with access to a good history. That kind of history could come from any careful observer who witnesses changes in a patient.

Treatment It would be rare for a stroke to occur while a patient is in a physician's office, but that does happen. The kinds of stroke patients who come into the office are more often the ones who have had a mild stroke at home, but who can then get into a car for the trip to the office. Either way, there is not much you can do for stroke patients, except take airway precautions, provide oxygen if ordered and keep them comfortable.

The patient who has suffered a stroke will need to be hospitalized. If your physician is not available, call for EMS promptly. While EMS is en route, take precautions in case the patient becomes worse. Be alert for unconsciousness, convulsions and apnea, but watch the patient for changes of any kind. The EMS paramedics would start an IV, monitor the ECG, and have suction available. Try to gather as much immediate and overall history as possible, and relay it accurately to the EMS team.

Chest Pain

A number of conditions can produce chest pain, and some of them are life-threatening. As a result, it would be best to take this complaint seriously anytime you encounter it.

Findings Although the history determines what is important about any chest pain, it is probably not wise for you to spend a lot of time asking history questions if your physician is readily available. Most physicians have their own techniques for analyzing chest pain anyway. But it is important to listen to what the patient says about the pain; what it feels like, when it came on, what makes it better or relieves it, and if it has ever occurred before. Generally, patients with chest pain who look sick are probably in trouble.

Do not panic, but do not waste time. Get a good set of vital signs, including a temperature. Promptly alert your physician, or contact EMS if the physician is not available. Connect the ECG, and get a 12-lead if you have time.

Treatment People with chest pain tend to be anxious, whether they show it or not. Give them

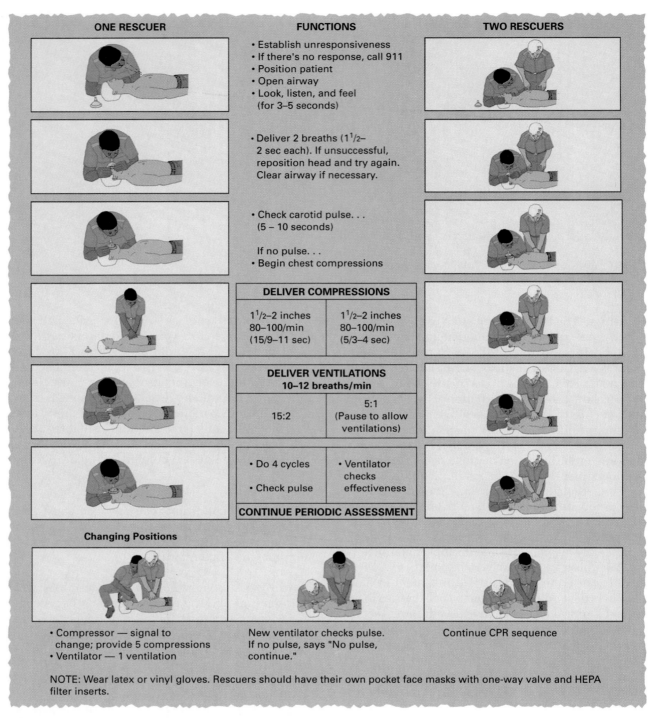

ONE RESCUER	FUNCTIONS	TWO RESCUERS

FUNCTIONS

- Establish unresponsiveness
- If there's no response, call 911
- Position patient
- Open airway
- Look, listen, and feel (for 3–5 seconds)

- Deliver 2 breaths (1½–2 sec each). If unsuccessful, reposition head and try again. Clear airway if necessary.

- Check carotid pulse. . . (5 – 10 seconds)

  If no pulse. . .
- Begin chest compressions

DELIVER COMPRESSIONS

1½–2 inches 80–100/min (15/9–11 sec)	1½–2 inches 80–100/min (5/3–4 sec)

DELIVER VENTILATIONS
10–12 breaths/min

15:2	5:1 (Pause to allow ventilations)

• Do 4 cycles • Check pulse	• Ventilator checks effectiveness

CONTINUE PERIODIC ASSESSMENT

Changing Positions

• Compressor — signal to change; provide 5 compressions • Ventilator — 1 ventilation	New ventilator checks pulse. If no pulse, says "No pulse, continue."	Continue CPR sequence

NOTE: Wear latex or vinyl gloves. Rescuers should have their own pocket face masks with one-way valve and HEPA filter inserts.

Figure 34-23 CPR adult-patient summary.

plenty of reassurance, and do what you can to keep them quiet and comfortable. Notify your physician immediately, and if the physician is not available, call for EMS. Administer oxygen if ordered by the physician.

If the patient's appearance or the vital signs indicate that the patient may be in shock, help them to lie down flat or on their left side. If the vitals seem about normal, place the patient on a bed or examination table that will support their head and chest in a raised position (about 45 degrees). If the blood pressure seems higher than normal and the patient is complaining of pain in the front of their chest that is not provoked by deep inspiration, the physician may order one sublingual (beneath the tongue) dose of nitroglycerin.

TABLE 34-4 Rates & Ratios: Adult Versus Pediatric CPR

Technique	Adult	Child	Infant
Compressions/Breaths	15:1 (1 technician) 5:1 (2 technicians)	5:1	5:1
Compressions/min.	80-100	100	100 or more
Compression depth (in.)	1.5-2	1-1.5	0.5-1
Breaths/min.	10-12	20	20
Breaths, duration (sec.)	1.5-2 (one breath every 5 sec.)	1-1.5 (one breath every 4 sec.)	1-1.5 (one breath every 3 sec.)
Hand(s) on sternum	2 hands/lower half	1 hand /lower half	2 fingers/lower third

TABLE 34-5 Problems Causing Seizures

Alcohol	Fever
Airway Obstruction/Apnea	Head Trauma
Brain Infection	Hypoglycemia
Brain Tumor	Hypovolemia
Cardiac Arrest	Hypoxia
Cardiac Rhythm Disturbance	Metabolic Disorder
Cerebral Edema	Overdose
Diabetes	Poisoning
Drugs	Poisoning
Drugs	Respiratory Arrest
Electrolyte Imbalance	Sepsis
Epilepsy	Stroke

Patients with chest pain can get very sick or go into cardiac arrest without warning. These are patients who need to be watched constantly as long as they are under your care.

Convulsions (Seizures)

Convulsions, or seizures, are produced by disorganized electrical activity in the brain and are characterized by involuntary muscle contractions that may alternate between contraction and relaxation of muscles. In some cases the convulsions are generalized, involving the entire body, or localized and limited to a specific area of the body. Convulsions can result from a number of problems or combinations of problems, listed in Table 34-5.

Findings By themselves, convulsions are not life-threatening. But the muscle spasms that come with full-body seizures can restrict breathing. Seizure patients may also bite their tongues causing bleeding and swelling, which can obstruct the airway. Finally, seizure patients are sometimes injured when their convulsions cause them to fall.

Once a seizure stops, especially a full-body seizure, it is normal for a patient to remain unconscious for as long as 15 minutes. During that time, most patients cannot control their secretions, for example urine, the way they would in normal sleep. In addition, whatever caused the first seizure may produce more.

Treatment A medical assistant can do two important things for a seizing patient. First, prevent injuries. Keep the patient from falling, and prevent the head from striking anything until the seizure stops. And second, pay close attention to what you see so you can describe it in your own words later on. Your observations will eventually be very important to the patient's neurologist.

Assess the patient's breathing and color, and estimate how long the seizure lasts. Once it stops, reassess breathing. If breathing seems inadequate or absent, the physician may order oxygen. Immediately alert the rest of your staff that you have an emergency in your location, and check for a pulse. If there is no pulse, initiate CPR and contact EMS.

If breathing seems adequate, note the patient's response, apply oxygen as ordered, and control the patient's secretions by placing them on their left side and allowing the secretions to drain. Listen for noise in the airway, and be prepared to assist the patient. Notify your physician. If the physician is not available, contact EMS and anticipate transport. Continue to assess the patient until they arrive, and communicate your findings to them.

Many caregivers feel compelled to wedge something between the patient's teeth, and that is a mistake. If the patient's teeth are clenched, do NOT try to force something between them or pry the mouth open. Broken teeth are expensive to repair, and they can become terrible airway obstructions. Observe the patient for breathing problems.

Once the patient begins to regain consciousness, explain to him what has happened (you may need to repeat yourself) and keep him as comfortable as possible, and if he does not have a history of seizures he will require transport to the ED. He may need extra reassurance, especially if he is incontinent or if this is his first seizure.

Diabetic Crisis

In health, insulin enables body tissues to produce energy from sugar. Several complex mechanisms maintain a constant balance between sugar and insulin in the blood. Diabetes is a disorder that disrupts this balance. It can occur in childhood or in later life. Some forms can be controlled by diet alone; others require treatment with oral or injectable medicines.

Most diabetics routinely monitor their blood sugar levels by means of small hand-held computers. Many inject themselves with insulin one or more times per day. But this produces a crude sugar-insulin balance at best, with levels that vary widely. Diabetics commonly miscalculate, forget, or simply get tired of the whole process and fail to comply with their treatment.

Diabetics can suffer two kinds of crises: insulin shock, which is a kind of *hypoglycemia* (too little sugar in the blood) and diabetic coma, a kind of *hyperglycemia* (too much sugar). Either condition can be fatal eventually, but insulin shock tends to evolve suddenly and can produce death within minutes. Insulin shock results when a diabetic takes his insulin but strays from his diet. It is probably the most common of all metabolic emergencies, and one of the most common true emergencies you will see in the office.

It is also possible for a diabetic to accidentally inject insulin into a small vein, rather than the fatty deposits beneath the skin where it is normally injected. The brain has no tolerance for an absence of sugar or oxygen, because it has no ready reserves to borrow from. When insulin is injected intravenously, its concentration in the blood can climb so quickly that any circulating sugar is absorbed by tissues all over the body almost immediately, and the brain is confronted by a sudden near-absence of sugar. Brain cells can begin to die in minutes.

Med Tip: Always remind diabetic patients to aspirate the syringe containing insulin before injecting to make sure they are not injecting insulin into a vein.

Unlike insulin shock, diabetic coma occurs when a diabetic either over-indulges in sugar, or ingests a normal amount of dietary sugar but fails to take his insulin (or other diabetic medication).

Findings Look for signs of shock in the absence of trauma, including pale skin, weakness, nausea/vomiting, and inappropriate sweating (which may be profound). The pulse may be normal or elevated, the blood pressure may be normal or low, and the respirations may be rapid and deep. The blood sugar, if you have access to it, may be either very low or very high. If there is no access to a good history, check for the presence of medical jewelry indicating the patient is a diabetic.

Treatment The immediate treatment for potential diabetic crisis of either type begins with checking the airway. Can the patient talk? The physician may check for a gag reflex by stimulating the back of the tongue with a tongue blade. If the patient can talk or has a positive gag reflex, the physician will order you to administer a small amount of sugar in any form by mouth. That can be in the form of fruit juice, candy, milk, or virtually anything sweet. If the patient does not have a gag reflex, nothing should be administered by mouth. If your physician is not available, contact EMS immediately.

If it happens that the patient is in diabetic coma, there will be no response to the sugar. If instead the problem is insulin shock, the patient will typically respond within 30 seconds or so. Either way, the patient will eventually need to be evaluated by a physician familiar with his case.

Epistaxis (Nosebleed)

Non-traumatic nosebleed may be messy and embarrassing, but it is usually a **benign** (non-life-threatening) occurrence caused by picking the nose or by blowing it forcefully. Nosebleed tends to occur most commonly in dry weather or in dusty conditions, and is usually easy to correct.

Bleeding from both nostrils tends to be more serious than bleeding from just one nostril. Nosebleed that occurs after a head injury and does not stop should be considered a serious emergency until proven otherwise. If there is no history of trauma, there are at least three other circumstances that should worry a caregiver about persistent nosebleeds. One is high blood pressure, especially in a patient who has recently changed or stopped taking medicines for high blood pressure. Another is a clotting disorder of some kind, and the third is a patient history of nosebleeds that have caused shock in the past.

Post-Trauma Findings If trauma is a possible factor, the physician in the medical office may not attempt to pack the nose or stop bleeding. In this case, contact *911* immediately and anticipate transport to the emergency department (ED). The paramedics will insert an oral airway if the patient is unresponsive (do not use a nasal airway in this kind of patient). Place the patient on high-flow oxygen by non-rebreather mask and stay with them. Monitor them carefully for changes in status.

Findings in the Absence of Trauma Nosebleeds severe enough to cause changes in a patient's vital signs are rare, but they do occur. If the patient's vital signs are normal in the absence of trauma, the patient should be seated upright. If the vital signs are compromised the patient should lie on the affected side and may need oxygen.

If the bleeding emerges from both nostrils, its origin is not in the nose but somewhere above it, and it requires the immediate attention of a physician or stat (immediate) transport to an emergency department. A nosebleed that em-

anates from one nostril is easily treated by a physician. To stop it, the physician will grasp a facial tissue by one corner and twist that corner firmly into a Christmas-tree shape about four inches long. Continuing to twist it, the pack is inserted deeply into the patient's affected nostril until the nostril is firmly packed. Then a wash cloth is placed over the patient's upper face and the patient is instructed to hold a chemical cold pack against the wash cloth so it fits the bridge of the nose like a saddle.

Bleeding should stop after only a few minutes, at which time the packing can be removed. If bleeding does not stop, electrocautery may be necessary. Your physician may be able to perform this treatment in the office, or the patient may require transport to an emergency department. Depending on the vital signs and degree of bleeding, that can usually be accomplished in a private vehicle if someone other than the patient is available to drive.

Fainting (Syncope)

Unresponsiveness deserves special respect from a caregiver, because there are so many serious disorders that cause it. Simple fainting (**syncope**) occurs often in some people and almost never in others. Fainting, or syncope, the sudden loss of consciousness, seems to be caused by a brief interruption in the body's ability to control the brain's circulation. When fainting does occur, it usually does so just after a patient has received an emotional shock of some kind. The patient usually collapses and becomes totally unresponsive, but within a minute, should awaken and return to normal function. Patients seldom become incontinent or seize as a result of simple fainting, but may be injured in the course of a fall. Table 34-6 lists some serious disorders that can produce fainting.

Findings The patient who has fainted can appear differently at different times after fainting. *Cyanosis is always a sign of shock, and should make you think of respiratory or cardiac arrest!* It would be very unlikely for a patient who has fainted for any reason to wake up suddenly and be completely alert. If that happens, you should probably consider two possibilities: that he was simply asleep, or that he was faking. If he really fainted, he should awaken gradually, seem confused, and have some difficulty remembering things. He may ask you the same questions over and over again.

Treatment There is always a reason for unresponsiveness and determining the reason is important.

TABLE 34-6 Disorders That Can Result in Fainting

Airway obstruction/apnea	Cerebral edema	Hyperglycemia	Seizure
Allergy	Diabetes	Hypovolemia	Sepsis
Assault	Drugs or alcohol ingestion	Hypoxia	Shock (any kind)
Brain infection	Electrolyte imbalance	Metabolic disorders	Stroke
Brain tumor	Epilepsy	Overdose	
Cardiac arrest	Head Trauma	Poisoning	
Cardiac rhythm disturbance	Hypoglycemia	Respiratory arrest	

However, early in your contact with any unconscious patient, your first concern should be to take care of the ABCs (airway, breathing, and circulation).

When you are with a patient who suddenly becomes unresponsive, consider an arrhythmia like V-fib or V-tach. Shake and shout. Establish an airway.

When you encounter a patient who already appears unresponsive, make sure he really is. Shake and shout. If there is no response, provide oxygen if the physician orders this. Check the ABCs, call for help. If the patient is breathing well but you cannot wake him, place him on his left side (so patient's secretions can drain; stomach contents probably will not), contact your physician. If your physician is not available, contact EMS. While you await their arrival, try to get a good set of vital signs and if possible obtain a blood sugar reading.

Never leave an unresponsive patient alone for more than a few seconds, and then never on an examination table that is not equipped with railings and/or restraining straps.

Foreign Bodies in Nose, Ear, or Eye

Foreign bodies in the nose and ear are common among children. They seldom present among adults, and they seldom represent serious medical emergencies. The kinds of objects children insert can be tough to extract when doing so depends on the patient's cooperation.

Foreign bodies in the eye are more common in adults, especially as a feature of industrial medicine and among motorcyclists. They can produce serious consequences in the absence of competent care.

Findings (nose or ear) While not common, incidents do occur involving impaled objects in the facial orifices of adults, largely as a result of domestic violence. Among children, it is much more common for small round objects such as BBs, jelly beans, coins, beans, and small objects to find their way into openings. Typically, the result is uncomfortable and the parents bring the child in because the child has become unusually cranky and has been fussing with the affected body part.

Treatment Impaled objects of any kind should never be removed by anyone but a physician. Objects impaled in the head should probably not be removed except at a trauma center.

Findings (eye) Metal or wood splinters are commonly found embedded in the eye and its surrounding membranes. Due to the extreme sensitivity of the area, they are never tolerated for long and you are likely to see them promptly. The sclera of the eye, will probably appear reddened and inflamed, and you may be able to see an object with the aid of an examination lamp.

Treatment The physician may be able to remove a small splinter by means of vigorous irrigation, as long as the object is not lodged in the cornea. Place the patient on his back or on the affected side, and place several absorbent towels beneath and around the area in which the physician will be working. Using one hand to hold the lids open, the physician will direct a small stream of sterile normal saline (0.9%) from the medial side (inner canthus) of the eye laterally. Even if the object is dislodged, the physician will examine the eye and may prescribe ophthalmic antibiotics in the form of drops to prevent infection.

All **ferrous** objects (those containing iron) that become lodged in the cornea warrant follow-up by an ophthalmologist as soon as possible (preferably on the same day). They tend to leave particles

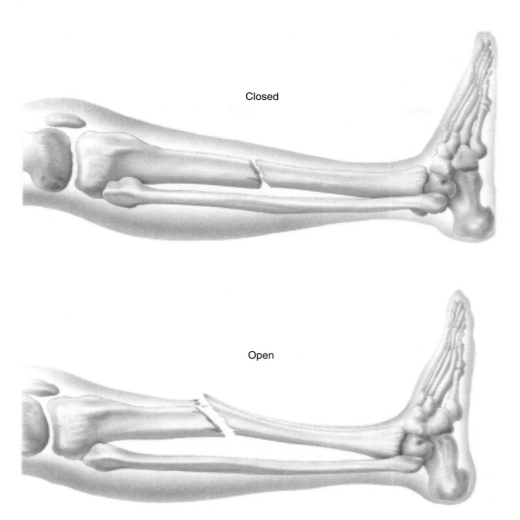

Closed

Open

Figure 34-24   Types of fractures.

and/or rusty residues embedded in the cornea which cannot be visualized in the office setting, and which must be removed at high magnification. If not removed, these residues can cause corneal ulcers that do not heal.

If your physician is unable to remove the object, patch both eyes. Inform the patient that he will need a ride to an ophthalmologist's office, and help him to arrange for that. If the object is large enough so the physician does not want to remove it, consider sending the patient to a trauma center. Keep the patient in an examination room with the lights off, to minimize eye movements, and contact EMS.

Fractures (Musculoskeletal Injuries)

You would probably not see the dramatic kinds of musculoskeletal injuries in a physician's office that can be diagnosed prior to x-rays. Those you do see will probably have been immobilized prior to the patient's arrival, either by the patient (cradling

a forearm, for instance) or by a family member. But all potential fractures are important, because broken bone ends are like broken glass. They can cause severe, permanent soft-tissue injuries during movement if mishandled (Figure 34-24).

Your physician's approach to splinting is something your staff needs to discuss in advance. It will vary somewhat depending on the physician's specialty. The following are some general principles.

Findings When does the physician suspect a fracture? Any patient who describes a forceful mechanism of injury that has produced pain, loss of use and/or swelling of a body part should be treated for a fracture until the x-rays say otherwise. That treatment may come from your physician, or your physician may decide to stabilize the injury temporarily and refer the patient to an orthopedist. So, you may have two roles in the treatment of fractures: to stabilize a patient who has not yet seen a physician, and to splint the patient

TABLE 34-7 Musculoskeletal Injuries

Type	Description
Fracture	Broken bone
Dislocation	Separated joint
Sprain	Torn or stretched ligament with swelling of area
Strain	Torn or stretched muscle or tendon

who has been seen by a physician and is being referred to a specialist.

When a patient comes into the office with a painful disability, pay attention to the history of the injury. How did it happen? How long ago? Does the patient have function and feeling in the injured area and, especially, distal to it? These findings may change later, and they are important to the physician. It is possible for swelling to cause permanent nerve damage.

Besides fractures, there are three other major kinds of musculoskeletal injuries. Prior to treatment by the physician, they should all be treated as fractures. They are dislocations, sprains and strains (in decreasing order of severity). Musculoskeletal injuries are described and compared in Table 34-7.

Treatment Do not waste time with a lot of elaborate splinting prior to the physician's examination. You do not want to obscure any injury from examination, either by the physician or the x-rays. Instead, pay attention tox how the patient immobilizes his own injury. Pillows and blankets are used to pad the injured area accordingly. Cold compresses minimize swelling. Do whatever you can to keep the patient comfortable and still.

Exercise special care to prevent a closed fracture from becoming an open one (in which there is protruding bone tissue). Open fractures usually require surgery; closed ones may not. If you do encounter an open fracture, sterility and moisture are both very important for healing to occur. Also be careful to preserve the membrane that covers the bone (periosteum). If there is protruding bone tissue, the physician may irrigate the area with sterile 0.9% normal saline solution. Follow that with a sterile dressing that has been moistened with the same solution (not water), and follow that with a sterile occlusive dressing. Keep any loose teeth or bone fragments in sterile saline, preferably in a sealed sterile container (you can cut the corner out of an IV bag, if one is available).

The kinds of injuries which need to be stabilized might involve joints or long bones. Do not try to straighten a joint injury. Instead, try to make the splint fit the injury. Then, to prevent movement, stabilize the bone above the injury and the bone below it. Be sure to pad for comfort, because the patient may be wearing the splint for several hours.

In the case of a long bone injury, the physician will try to stabilize the joint above the injury and the joint below it. You need to contact the EMS if the physician is unavailable.

The most versatile kind of splint is probably the vacuum type. A vacuum splint consists of a double-layered bag filled with round Styrofoam beads or pellets. It is wrapped around a patient's affected area and the air is pumped out of the bag. That squeezes the pellets closer to one another until they are unable to move—forming a rigid cast that fits the patient exactly but causes no inward pressure. Vacuum splints are available in a range of sizes, and are easy to sanitize. Their main disadvantage is that they tend to be expensive, so you need a system for retrieving them.

Ladder splints are cheaper, but they are less comfortable and they do not come in large sizes. A ladder splint is made of bendible steel wire and is roughly shaped like a ladder. You can bend one to fit almost anything, then use padding and elastic bandages to fasten it to a patient's ankle, elbow, wrist or forearm. You can also use more than one ladder splint at a time to stabilize the same injury.

Pillows make good splints for wrists, elbows, ankles and feet, and they are invaluable for use as temporary padding prior to the physician's examination.

1. The sling starts with a triangular piece of cloth that is 50 to 60 inches at its base and 36 to 40 inches on each side. Fold it to any width needed.
2. Check distal pulse, sensation, and motor function. Position sling over the chest. The point is toward the injured side and beyond the elbow with the upper end placed over the shoulder.
3. Bring the bottom end up and over the patient's injured arm. Keep the hand elevated above the elbow.
4. Tie the two ends together. Pad the knot with gauze or a small cloth to make sure it does not rest on the patient's neck. Reassess distal pulse and sensation.
5. Secure the point of the sling with a knot or pin to form a pocket for the elbow.
6. Fold another triangular piece of material to form a sling. Tie it around the patient. Be sure it is positioned to support the arm and to maintain elevation.

Cravat bandages have been used in an immense variety of applications, but since the development of conforming roller bandages like Kerlix and Kling not many people use them anymore. A cravat bandage is commonly fashioned into a sling, which is still the method of choice for supporting an injury of the shoulder girdle or upper extremity.

The value of cervical collars has been questioned vigorously in recent years. There is little in the medical literature that supports the use of anything but a few specialized versions of these devices during extrication from certain kinds of major trauma situations. In fact, they may have the effect of raising intracranial pressures.

Patients with suspected spinal injuries should be handled by EMS crews, who are specially equipped to handle those circumstances.

Fractures of the Neck and Back

You are not likely to see many spinal fractures in the office setting, and when you do they will probably not be striking in appearance. The reason is that spinal fractures almost always produce too much pain and loss of function to permit travel to a doctor's office. But all post-injury neck or back pain deserves respect. All people tolerate pain differently, and these are injuries that no caregiver wants to overlook or neglect when they do occur.

Findings There are two situations when you might see a patient in the office who has spinal fractures. One happens when the patient with a bone disorder suffers a pathologic, or disease-related fracture as a result of weakened bones. Pathologic fractures sometimes occur all by themselves, in the absence of external trauma. Cancer and osteoporosis patients are prone to pathologic fractures.

The other kind of spinal fracture you could encounter in the office is an occult fracture, which is so minor it seems stable. The patient with an occult fracture of the neck or back, for instance, might feel very sore or stiff, yet not be incapacitated. Occult fractures sometimes do not show up in x-rays. The spinous processes of the vertebrae are common sites of occult fractures; they are sometimes fractured by direct blows to the middle of the back or neck. Occult vertebral fractures are often associated with fractured heels, sustained when a patient falls from a height of eight feet or more and lands feet-first on a hard surface.

Treatment Treatment for anyone you suspect of having a bony injury of the neck or back depends on the position you find them in and if your physician is available. Treatment almost always includes calling EMS. If the patient is standing, they need to be fastened from head to toe to a special stretcher and then laid down flat. The last thing you would want to do for someone under that circumstance is to help them to squat and lie down, unless you have plenty of experienced help and the right equipment. If you find the patient already lying down, keep them right where they are until EMS arrives. Keep them as comfortable as you can without moving them.

Eventually, a patient with bony spinal injuries may need to see an orthopedist, and possibly a neurologist. Their jobs are easier and cheaper for the patient if a good history is available. Once you've made the patient comfortable and convinced them to lie still, determine their motor and sensory status. What happened, and how did they get to your office? Can they feel and move all of their fingers and toes? What are their vital signs? Do they hurt anywhere besides at the site of their injury? Record the times of your observations and the patient's body position throughout your assessment.

Fractured Jaw

The mandible and nose are probably the weakest structures in the face, and are commonly fractured in fist-fights as well as auto accidents in which the driver of a vehicle strikes his face on the steering wheel. They are painful, but only produce a real threat if the mandible is shattered. This is because it is the mandible and its muscular (hyoid) floor that keeps the tongue in place.

Findings A fractured mandible would not necessarily be unstable. If it were, the patient would consciously limit his speech and any movements of the mouth, and would not permit examination. Oral bleeding might be present, and if so it might be brisk. A caregiver should be concerned about the possibility of broken teeth, which could lead to airway obstruction and further lacerations of the oral mucosa. In addition, an impact great enough to shatter the mandible might also produce bony neck injury as well other facial injuries.

Treatment An unstable mandible will eventually require surgical repair. A painful mandible in a patient who is controlling his own secretions and in whom there is no bleeding may be left alone, or may be gently immobilized by the physician in the position of function (with the mouth closed) using a conforming bandage (preferably 5-1/2-inch Kerlix). The patient with this kind of injury will often complain about the teeth not fitting properly, because even the smallest dimensional change inside the mouth can seem very large.

Patients with more serious, less stable injuries should be warned not to swallow their secretions, should be offered a basin to drool or spit into, and should be allowed to choose whatever position permits their secretions to drain. Uncontrollable oral bleeding from such an injury should be left to a physician. If a physician is not available, contact EMS immediately and anticipate transport to a trauma center. As a last resort, it may be prudent to inform the patient that he is bleeding and instruct him as to where he should apply his own pressure dressing. (This may be the only way to secure the patient's cooperation.)

The paramedics may apply high-flow oxygenation by non-rebreather mask for any patient with severe bleeding, but the mask should be loosely applied. If the patient has trouble controlling bleeding and/or secretions, they will use suction as necessary, but do not discard the suction reservoir, in case it contains tooth fragments which may still be reused many hours later. Patients with severe facial injuries eventually require transport to trauma centers.

Heat and Cold Exposure (Hyperthermia and Hypothermia)

The human body normally controls its internal temperature very effectively, despite extreme variations in its surroundings (by as much as 100 degrees Fahrenheit). But when the body is exposed to a high or low temperature extreme for a long enough time, or when there is a breakdown in the body's internal heat-regulating ability, it can become hyperthermic (overheated) or hypothermic (its temperature can drop unacceptably). Either circumstance causes a systemic breakdown and can eventually result in death if not corrected.

Findings: Heat exhaustion The hyperthermic patient can suffer a wide assortment of disorders, ranging from a series of warning signs called simple heat exhaustion to a lethal condition called heat stroke. Heat exhaustion occurs when a patient is exposed to a hot environment and does not drink adequate amounts of fluids to maintain a healthy body temperature. Urine output falls, there is tachycardia, dizziness, nausea and vomiting, headache, muscle cramps and diarrhea, and the patient may faint when he tries to stand up.

Treatment This patient needs fluids and electrolytes, especially sodium. If he can drink and is not vomiting, any "sports drink" (like Gatorade) will resolve his discomfort within an hour. An ECG is important, even if there is a history of working in a hot environment, because these signs can mimic a heart attack. (Myocardial infarction can occur under the same circumstances as heat exhaustion.) If the patient does well, chances are he will not require transport to a hospital. If the patient cannot drink or is unresponsive, IV normal saline (0.9%) is the treatment of choice and the EMS should be called.

Findings: Heat stroke Heat stroke is caused by sufficient overheating (higher than 105° F centrally) for a long enough time to cause failure of the temperature control center in the medulla of the brain. The patient's skin may be red in color and will be very hot to the touch. The skin may be wet or dry, depending on what the patient was doing when he collapsed. He will be in shock, with a very low blood pressure and a rapid pulse which gradually becomes very slow. If he is still conscious, he may be very disoriented. If not, he may begin seizing and eventually become unresponsive to any stimuli.

Treatment Heat stroke is deadly if not corrected. This patient needs to be cooled as rapidly as possible using any means at your disposal, until his temperature reaches a level specified by your physician (probably around 102° F). If your physician is not available, contact EMS immediately while you continue cooling measures. Treat the patient for shock. Monitor the ECG, and if possible get the patient to accept fluids. Then reassess the vitals, and carefully record changes in the temperature. EMS will treat the patient with IV fluids en route to the ED.

Findings: Hypothermia Hypothermia is a state of body temperature lower than 95 degrees Fahrenheit. It is caused by decreased heat production, increased heat loss, or both. It can occur quickly in the case of cold water immersion, or slowly if a patient is exposed to cold outside temperatures over several hours.

The hypothermic patient may be found conscious and shivering (a sign of mild to moderate hypothermia), clumsy and slightly disoriented, or in severe hypothermia (86° F) he may be stiff and stuporous or even comatose. A slow, barely perceptible heart rate is a grave sign.

Note: Temperatures should be taken rectally or aurally. Standard thermometers normally do not register below 96° Fahrenheit. If you practice in an area where cold weather is commonplace, you will need special equipment in order to assess and treat hypothermia.

Treatment The patient in mild hypothermia (94°-97° F and shivering) can be treated in the office by removing cold or wet clothing and using warm liquids, heated oxygen (warmer than 99° F) and blankets. Do not administer nicotine, alcohol or caffeine. The patient should be kept horizontal and quiet. Avoid unnecessary or rough handling, as this can precipitate cardiac dysrhythmias. Monitor the ECG and the core temperature (as above). Be aware that rewarming can dilate the blood vessels in the extremities, which can lower the blood pressure. Although this patient can benefit from prompt treatment, he eventually needs to be hospitalized.

Treatment for the patient who is severely hypothermic needs to be done in the hospital, by a team of people who understand hypothermia and treat it routinely. Contact EMS. Begin gradual rewarming with blankets until EMS arrives.

Frostbite Frostbite is a cold injury of the distal extremities, usually beginning in the toes, fingers and nose, which is caused by such exposure to cold that ice crystals form in the cells. Exposure usually involves temperatures below zero.

Findings The patient who suffers from frostbite may or may not also be hypothermic. If he is, the hypothermia takes priority over the frostbite. Frostbite presents in many ways from patient to patient, but generally can be gauged on the basis of whether freezing has taken place. In severe frostbite, the affected parts will be white or gray and will be frozen solid.

Treatment The mechanism of injury in frostbite is the rupturing of cell membranes and other structures inside the cells when ice crystals form inside the cells. That is worsened by allowing the patient to use frozen extremities, or by rubbing the affected parts. Emergency treatment is limited to gentle rewarming, elevation of the affected parts, and treating for pain before thawing. This is all best done in a hospital setting.

Heart Attack Myocardial infarction, the death of heart muscle, can result either from an arrhythmia, from trauma, or from blockage of a coronary artery (initially with or without arrhythmias). It has been linked to a list of risk factors, such as smoking, high fat diet, and lack of exercise, none of which are important at the time of an emergency. Depending on the size of an infarction and the portion of the heart affected, a patient with a heart attack may present with a variety of signs and symptoms ranging from none at all to cardiac arrest.

Findings In the case of a silent MI, a patient may never notice any symptoms. Or, especially if the infarction is on the inferior side of the heart (prob-

ably because it is so close to the stomach), the patient may experience nausea with or without vomiting as the only clue that he or she has had a heart attack. The nausea may or may not be accompanied by diaphoresis, changes in the vital signs, and/or arrhythmias. The heart rate may be slower than normal, or bradycardic.

More commonly, an MI produces non-pleuritic (unaffected by breathing) dull, crushing substernal pain with or without shortness of breath. The pain may radiate into the left arm, the neck, the back, or the left side of the face, and be unrelieved by anything short of narcotics. Such a patient may appear to be in shock—anxious or frightened, pale, weak, sweaty, and cyanotic. The vital signs may vary. Caregivers should watch for signs of acute left ventricular failure (low blood pressure, shortness of breath, distended neck veins, and the sounds of crackling or wheezing as the patient breathes). Once you suspect that a patient may be infarcting, do not waste time with extensive assessment. Obtain a good set of vitals and a brief history and, if a physician is not available, contact EMS.

Any MI can produce any arrhythmia, anytime, including lethal ones such as asystole, V-fib or V-tach. If ventricular damage is sufficient, the patient may go into cardiogenic shock, which is a grave event. It is possible for a patient to be in cardiogenic shock following an MI with no symptoms other than weakness and no external signs of shock other than a low blood pressure.

Treatment An MI is a serious event, especially in the young; and it always requires aggressive treatment, supportive care and immediate hospitalization. Patients often know there is something very wrong, although many deny such a possibility and refuse to seek medical help.

Because of its potential consequences, any non-pleuritic chest pain in a patient of middle age or older should be suspected of cardiac origin; and any non-pleuritic chest pain that does not subside after nitroglycerin should be regarded as an MI until ruled out by a physician. A caregiver who suspects that a patient has had an MI should involve a physician immediately, and should activate EMS immediately if the physician is not available.

Do not leave this patient alone. Be prepared to provide CPR, if necessary. Always treat the patient with calm reassurance.

Hyperventilation

There are times when shortness of breath can be very frightening to a patient and still constitute only a minor problem, medically. Some patients are prone to a disorder called *hyperventilation syndrome*, in which strong emotional triggers can stimulate sudden changes in blood chemistry that produce extreme air hunger, diaphoresis, paresthesias, and emotional distress.

Findings Patients suffering from this condition are usually remarkable in their appearance, depending on how intense their symptoms. They commonly appear to be terrified. They may seem very tense, especially in their extremities and facial features, and are not usually found on the ground. Their respirations are typically rapid and deep, but not especially noisy. The heart rate may be elevated, the blood pressure may be either normal or slightly elevated, and there is no related fever.

Treatment Rebreathing from a paper bag sealed against the face around the nose and mouth seems to help some of these patients, but not without focused, sustained reassurance from supportive caregivers. Unfortunately, patients who hyperventilate sometimes do not receive this kind of support in a busy medical facility, where resources are often channeled instead to patients with more urgent physical needs.

It should be noted that hyperventilation syndrome is a physician's diagnosis. Patients can hyperventilate in response to causes that are much less benign, including diabetic coma, cerebral edema and poisoning—all of which warrant hyperoxygenation and hyperventilation instead of rebreathing treatment.

Open Wounds

Open wounds are seldom life-threatening, unless they penetrate the head, chest, throat or abdomen. Those cases are serious emergencies that warrant EMS transport to a trauma center. Most soft-tissue injuries are uncomplicated. They typically require irrigation, debridement (or surgical trimming), sutures and antibiotics. Wounds that involve important structures like nerve or muscle tissue, the genitalia, the eyes and possibly the hands require specialized care and will probably be referred. Figure 34-25 provides a classification of open wounds for injuries.

Findings Open soft tissue wounds can be superficial (penetrating only the skin) or deep (penetrating the fascia, or connective layer beneath the skin, and other structures that lie deeper still).

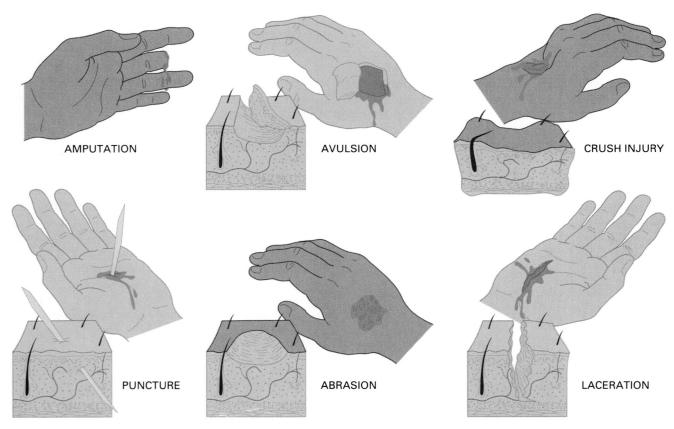

AMPUTATION   AVULSION   CRUSH INJURY

PUNCTURE   ABRASION   LACERATION

Figure 34-25   Classification of open injuries.

You may see some industrial soft tissue injuries that appear quite dramatic, but which will probably heal well after office treatment. The one thing that should matter to you most is something you can almost always control, and that is bleeding.

Wound Care Pointers You need a grasp of some basic concepts that relate to dressing wounds, and a functional list of them follows.

- A *dressing* is a piece of clean or sterile cloth, like cotton gauze, that you place over a wound. A *compress* is a thick dressing, like a stack of 25 or more 4×4-inch dressings, that you might use to absorb liquids or provide padding. Besides the common 2×2-inch and 4×4-inch sizes, an obstetrical pad is also a useful dressing. Larger sizes include 8×10 and 10×20 inches, used for large burns or abrasions.
- A *bandage* is a strip of binding material (like tape or Kling) that you would use to hold a dressing in place. A dressing or compress pre-fastened to a bandage is called a *bandage compress* (a Band-Aid is one example of a bandage compress). And a *pressure dressing* is a compress held in place by an *elastic bandage* (like an Ace bandage). All of these devices come in various widths. You would choose the sizes that fit the wound you need to care for. Figure 34-26 illustrates various types of elastic bandages and stockings.

What if you do not have a big enough sterile dressing for the injury you need to dress? Temporarily, use one or more clean towels. They're not sterile, but chances are they're cleaner than the wound. And as one of the ABCs, bleeding is a much higher priority than infection.

Treatment Simple direct pressure with a bulky dressing will usually stop bleeding from a soft tissue injury. Once you have determined that direct pressure is sufficient, keep the dressing in place with an elastic bandage. Use care, because an elastic bandage applied too tightly on an extremity can restrict venous blood flow out of the extremity. That can increase bleeding, not stop it.

Once bleeding is controlled, treat for shock—especially in the very young and the very old. Get the patient into a supine position. Raise the feet and legs slightly, along with the injured area if you

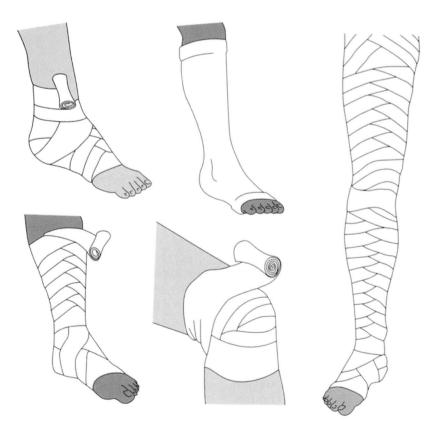

Figure 34-26 Elastic stockings and bandages.

can. Get a good set of vitals and check for other injuries. If there are signs of shock, do not underestimate them. Get your physician involved first and then contact EMS. Do not leave the patient alone.

If shock is not an issue, the priority will be to prevent infection by dressing the wound. That always begins with cleansing. Cleanse the wound from the center outward, beginning with vigorous irrigation using a disinfecting solution prescribed by your physician and followed by 0.9% normal saline solution. Wipe the edges of the wound in all directions away from the wound, then cover with a sterile dressing and fasten the dressing in place. The use or non-use of antibacterial ointments or creams should be specified by your employer.

It takes a fair amount of energy to inflict a laceration in the absence of a sharp instrument. When the history suggests that a laceration was caused by a blow or fall, especially if the laceration seems to be unusually painful for the patient, consider the possibility of a nearby fracture and report that to the physician.

The edges of jagged lacerations may require debridement by the physician prior to suturing. Deep wounds will eventually need to be irrigated by the physician and then sutured, possibly with removable drains in place. These will also need to be followed up by the physician, so anticipate making a future appointment for the patient.

Abrasions need to be examined closely and cleaned well. Look for embedded foreign materials. If not removed, they will eventually form permanent "tattoos", and they can produce nasty infections that leave scars. The physician will numb the area with topical lidocaine and abrade it as necessary with sterile gauze and your employer's preferred cleaning soap, to remove all traces of foreign matter.

Med Tip: Do not forget to inquire about the status of the patient's tetanus immunizations. That's important anytime someone suffers a break in the skin.

Poisoning

Poisonings account for 80% of all suicide attempts and 10% of all emergency responses every year. The vast majority of *accidental* poisonings involve children under the age of six. There are no figures to indicate how many poisonings are seen first in physicians' offices.

The world around us is full of poisons that we can absorb without knowing it. In addition, some people experiment or recreate by ingesting, injecting, and inhaling things that can kill them. Small children naturally and deliberately taste everything in their environment. Some individuals get deadly sick in response to things that do not bother other people at all. And even our most valuable medicines are poisons that can kill us in large enough doses. It seems impossible for a caregiver to mentally catalogue all of the substances and combinations of substances that are likely to hurt people.

Findings When the body absorbs a poison, it reacts in two ways. First, it responds to the chemistry of the poison itself—by slowing down, for instance, after absorbing sleeping pills. And second, it reacts by trying to get rid of the poison. Increased urine production, sweating, vomiting, diarrhea and respiratory and circulatory rates are all mechanisms the body can use to get rid of a toxin. Every caregiver still needs to know four things about what a patient has absorbed in order to choose the best treatment:

- What did the patient take?
- How much?
- When?
- How was it taken, and was it mixed with anything else?

The patient's age and weight are also important findings. All toxic substances act differently in the very old and the very young than they do in a healthy adult. And a 300-lb. male has a much larger liver and much bigger kidneys than a 90-lb. female. (Most toxins are broken down in the liver or the kidneys or in both.)

Pay special attention to the affect, or mood, of a person who has ingested a poison. Intentional poisoning always warrants psychiatric support. By the way, never completely trust anything you think you know about a patient. Addicts almost never tell the truth about their addictions, and that includes nicely dressed ones. Consider the possibility of an injection, ingestion or inhalation, anytime a patient's mental capacity seems impaired.

Finally, pay attention to what the patient's body is doing. Without knowing anything at all about what substances a patient has absorbed, you may notice breath odors that will later disappear. Likewise, there may be odors in the perspiration. If the patient voids urine or stool, collect specimens. All of these hints are important to the poison control center where this patient may eventually be seen.

Treatment Treating a poisoning patient begins before they ever come in your door—with the stickers on your office telephones, that tell you how to reach the poison control center. It continues with a good history. And finally, treatment for any kind of poison depends on the variables listed above. Although you may be able to administer the first few rounds of treatment to a toxic patient, chances are that even your physician will contact the poison center before doing anything else. The poison center has instant access to the best available information about poisons.

Shock

Circulation is the body's way of perfusing individual cells—supplying them with the nutrients they need and removing their wastes. Shock is the process of cell death that occurs anytime perfusion is not adequate. It can be caused by blood loss, nerve or brain damage, heart disease, a severe allergic reaction, diabetes, sepsis (infection), poisoning, and lung collapse or any major disruption of the pulmonary circulation.

Findings The outward appearance of a shock patient may not vary much by cause, but there are some general differences. Patients with most kinds of shock tend to be very cold to the touch and very pale, almost white. Those with disruption of their respiratory systems are almost always the color of blood that has not been oxygenated in a long time: blue. Almost all shock patients get dizzy (or they may just plain faint) when they stand up after sitting for a while. Almost all become diaphoretic (sweaty). An exception to the notion about pale, cold skin is the patient in anaphylactic (allergic) shock. These patients act just like other shock patients, only their skin color may be bright red.

Patients in cardiogenic (cardiac) shock just do not follow the rules. They vary a lot, both in appearance and in vital signs. They can remain awake and alert with no detectable pulse or blood pressure until they die. They often tell you they're going to die, and they tend to be very accurate about it. Their heart rates can be slow, normal, or fast. Their skin color may be pale, cyanotic, gray, or even normal to the very end.

Treatment Treatment *does* vary between shock patients, because the correct treatment is to support life while correcting the cause of shock. Always reassure the patient, helping him or her to lie down; always contact EMS and anticipate transport. Consult Table 34-8 for treatment specific to the probable cause of shock, and monitor the patient for changes.

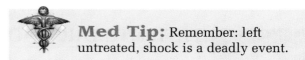

Med Tip: Remember: left untreated, shock is a deadly event.

Tourniquet What you need to know about tourniquets will be one of easiest of all the things you need to remember: *do not use one*. A tourniquet is a closed loop, with a stick shoved through it, that some people twist to stop bleeding in an extremity. When you use a tourniquet, everything underneath it and distal to it dies.

The body does a good job of controlling its own bleeding. When that fails, apply direct pressure to the site of bleeding. Direct pressure stops bleeding. In the rare event that direct pressure fails, try using one or more pressure points.

TABLE 34-8   **Treatment for Shock in the Physician's Office**

Cause	Treatment
Anaphylactic shock	Epinephrine.
Cardiogenic shock	IV dopamine, (pacemaker), stat transport to ED.
Hemorrhagic shock	Stop bleeding, replace volume, stat transport to ED.
Hypovolemic shock	Replace volume.
Insulin shock	Sugar, by any means tolerated (IV if patient unconscious).
Neurogenic shock	IV dopamine, stat transport, surgery (not likely to see in the office).
Poisoning	Consult poison center, treat specifically for poison.
Respiratory shock	ET intubation, stat transport, surgery.
Sepsis	Fluids, IV dopamine, transport to ED.

LEGAL AND ETHICAL ISSUES

As a medical assistant, you have three primary legal responsibilities in the face of an emergency. The first is obviously a duty to act within your scope of practice. Even though we all feel a little intimidated by the thought of an emergency, you are a medical professional. As such, in case of an emergency you are accountable to yourself, your employer and the public for actions that measure up to your degree of medical training.

Once you do receive medical training, your duty to act never really goes away. You will always be expected to act like someone who has had the same kind of training that you have. You will never be able to witness an accident in a public place without some responsibility to do the best you can to help.

Your second legal responsibility is to document the constant emergency readiness of the office you work in. You not only need to check your equipment when you come to work every day (an ethical responsibility), but you need to be able to prove that you did so (a legal responsibility). That means documentation, by means of timed, dated, and signed logs as required in your office. When a piece of equipment fails that you were supposed to check but did not, the failure is at least partially on your shoulders.

Your third legal responsibility, which you share with others in your workplace, is to do all you can to prevent emergencies, for example correcting things like loose carpet, spills and water leaks, electrical hazards. Educating patients and their families about their own safety is also part of emergency prevention.

Always stay within your scope of practice; know what is beyond your scope; and let your physician know.

PATIENT EDUCATION

One of the best things about being a good caregiver is that people trust you. They believe what you say, and that makes it possible for you to convince them to do or avoid things that will keep them healthy and safe.

There are a thousand little ways to make sure that people's lives are a little healthier without ever preaching to anyone or giving them unqualified medical advice. And you're just the one to do it. The best emergency medicine is preventive care. The medical assistant should be alert to the many opportunities to teach patients healthy habits in order to avoid burns, falls, fractures, and poisoning.

Summary

An understanding of what causes most medical emergencies, a knowledge of some basic first steps to take, and the will to help are essential elements of emergency first aid and of all emergency medicine.

Competency Review

1. Define and spell the glossary terms for this chapter.
2. Demonstrate what emergency care steps you would take if patients exhibiting the following symptoms came into your medical office and the physician was unavailable.
   (A) Respiratory distress (age 55).
   (B) Seizure
   (C) Allergic reactions
   (D) Spider bite
   (E) Hemorrhage
   (F) Chest pain
3. What do you say to a mother who tells you over the telephone that her child has just swallowed bleach?
4. Call a local emergency center or hospital emergency room and request to observe them as they respond to paramedics' communications from the ambulance.
5. Correctly perform both infant and adult CPR according to the protocol in your school or medical office (for example, American Heart Association).
6. Develop a protocol for handling emergencies in the medical office. Include how to do the primary assessment, determining the chief complaint, obtaining the medical history, gathering the medications, determining the allergies, and the components of the physical examination.
7. List on a chart the differences between diabetic coma and insulin shock.

PREPARING FOR THE CERTIFICATION EXAM

Test Taking Tip — Read all of the possible answers to the following review questions before choosing any answer. There are no trick questions and all of them are designed to help you.

Examination Review Questions

1. Heat stroke is usually defined by a number of signs, in addition to
   - (A) a temperature of 104° F
   - (B) a rectal temperature of 105° F
   - (C) any central temperature over 100° F
   - (D) high blood pressure
   - (E) none of the above

2. Your overall impression about the appearance of a patient in shock is
   - (A) not a very important consideration
   - (B) a very important finding
   - (C) not affected by your medical experience
   - (D) totally irrelevant
   - (E) none of the above

3. The best single question to ask any patient before you ask them anything else is
   - (A) what happened
   - (B) why they came in to the physician's office today
   - (C) their name
   - (D) which doctor they want to see
   - (E) none of the above

4. The first thing you need to do when you discover that a patient has arrested is:
   - (A) call for help
   - (B) check the airway
   - (C) contact EMS
   - (D) drag the patient somewhere where you have some room to work
   - (E) get the crash cart and charge the defibrillator paddles

5. Patients who have suffered a major amputation are very likely to
   - (A) be in a state of shock
   - (B) stop bleeding before a critical loss of blood occurs
   - (C) have other injuries which may be overshadowed at first glance
   - (D) be taken somewhere besides a physician's office
   - (E) all of the above

6. A patient in diabetic coma, if administered sugar
   - (A) will usually get worse because . . . .
   - (B) will have no response to the sugar
   - (C) will respond immediately
   - (D) should not be given insulin
   - (E) none of the above

7. The patient who has been bitten by a rattlesnake
   - (A) will have immediate pain and swelling
   - (B) does not need to go to the hospital if he receives antivenin
   - (C) can be treated with coral snake antivenin if rattlesnake antivenin is unavailable
   - (D) has a better chance for recovery if he is very young
   - (E) needs to have the venom sucked out of his wounds

8. The EMS includes
   - (A) you as first responder
   - (B) the hospital ED
   - (C) ambulance paramedics
   - (D) EMTs
   - (E) all of the above

9. The first thing you should do if a conscious patient appears to be choking is:
   - (A) stand behind them, encircle their abdomen with both arms and squeeze them
   - (B) help them to lie down so they do not fall
   - (C) ask them if they are choking
   - (D) look down their throat
   - (E) all of the above

10. Sunburn is
    - (A) not really a burn
    - (B) most often a first-degree burn
    - (C) most often a second-degree burn
    - (D) usually safe to treat with an ointment or cream and cool water.
    - (E) both B and D

ON THE JOB

Mary Ann, a medical assistant, works in a busy primary care office operated by two physicians, Dr. Johnson and Dr. Laskar. It is Saturday so the staff consists of just Mary Ann, Dr. Johnson, and another medical assistant named Valerie. On Saturdays, the office is only open until 1 PM.

When Mary Ann arrives to relieve one of the medical assistants who requested to leave at 11 AM, the office is extremely busy. Valerie has not had time to do her morning checks yet, and the reception room is full of crying children. As Mary Ann is looking over the schedule, she hears a commotion out front, followed by sudden quiet, and then Valerie's call for help.

When Mary Ann gets to the reception room, there is a worried-looking man bent over a 35-year-old woman who is supine on the floor. She is in her bathrobe and there is a blanket wrapped around her. She appears to be awake, but her eyes are closed in a grimace. She seems very short of breath. Her face is profusely diaphoretic and pale. Very pale.

"She had some indigestion last night when she went to bed," the man says, "and she did not sleep much last night. This morning when she got up to go to the bathroom, she just collapsed in a heap on the floor."

When asked, the lady responds with her name, and says she is having some really sharp pain in her right lower abdomen. She points to it with one finger. The office does not have a gurney, so the man picks her up and places her in a wheelchair. She immediately complains of dizziness and increased pain, and now her breathing becomes extremely labored. She cannot seem to talk at all in response to questions. Mary Ann and Valerie wheel her into an examining room.

What is your response?

1. What is your clinical impression of this lady?
2. Why do you think she got dizzy and short of breath when she was placed in the wheelchair?
3. What position should she be placed in?
4. What kind of history would you be especially curious about?
5. What would you expect this lady's vitals to be like?
6. What kind of initial treatment would you administer?
7. Considering the available resources and this patient's status, what would you like to see happen next?

References

Bledsoe, B., Cherry, R., and Porter, R. *Intermediate Emergency Care.* Upper Saddle River, NJ: Brady/Prentice Hall, 1995.

Bledsoe, B., Porter, R., and Shade, B. *Paramedic Emergency Care.* Upper Saddle River, NJ: Brady/Prentice Hall, 1997.

Campbell, J. *Basic Trauma Life Support.* Upper Saddle River, NJ: Brady/Prentice Hall, 1995.

Grant, H., Murray, R., Bergeron, J., O'Keefe, M., and Limmer, D. *Emergency Care.* Upper Saddle River, NJ: Brady/Prentice Hall, 1995.

Hafen, B., Karren, K., and Mistovich, J. *Prehospital Emergency Care.* Upper Saddle River, NJ: Brady/Prentice Hall, 1996.

Roberts, J. & Hedges, J. *Clinical Procedures in Emergency Medicine*, 2nd Ed. Philadelphia, PA: W. B. Saunders, 1991.

Stutz, D. & Janusz, S. *Hazardous Materials Injuries: A Handbook for Prehospital Care*, 2nd Ed. Beltsville, MD: Bradford Communications, 1988.

Taber's Cyclopedic Medical Dictionary, 18th Ed. Philadelphia, PA: F.A. Davis, 1997.

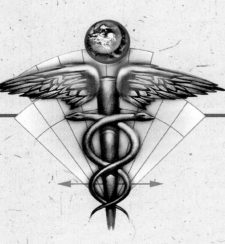

Unit Four

Career Assistance

MEDICAL ASSISTANT ROLE DELINEATION CHART

Highlight indicates material covered in this chapter

ADMINISTRATIVE

ADMINISTRATIVE PROCEDURES

- Perform basic clerical functions
- Schedule, coordinate, and monitor appointments
- Schedule inpatient/outpatient admissions and procedures
- Understand and apply third party guidelines
- Obtain reimbursement through accurate claims submission
- Monitor third-party reimbursement
- Perform medical transcription
- Understand and adhere to managed care policies and procedures
- *Negotiate managed care contracts (adv)*

PRACTICE FINANCES

- Perform procedural and diagnostic coding
- Apply bookkeeping principles
- Document and maintain accounting and banking records
- Manage accounts receivable
- Manage accounts payable
- Process payroll
- *Develop and maintain fee schedules (adv)*
- *Manage renewals of business and professional insurance policies (adv)*
- *Manage personal benefits and maintain records (adv)*

CLINICAL

FUNDAMENTAL PRINCIPLES

- Apply principles of aseptic technique and infection control
- Comply with quality assurance practices
- Screen and follow up patient test results

DIAGNOSTIC ORDERS

- Collect and process specimens
- Perform diagnostic tests

PATIENT CARE

- Adhere to established triage procedures
- Obtain patient history and vital signs
- Prepare and maintain examination and treatment areas

- Prepare patient for examinations, procedures, and treatments
- Assist with examinations, procedures, and treatments
- Prepare and administer medications and immunizations
- Maintain medication and immunization records
- Recognize and respond to emergencies
- Coordinate patient care information with other health care providers

GENERAL (TRANSDISCIPLINARY)

PROFESSIONALISM

- Project a professional manner and image
- Adhere to ethical principles
- Demonstrate initiative and responsibility
- Work as a team member
- Manage time efficiently
- Prioritize and perform multiple tasks
- Adapt to change
- Promote the CMA credential
- Enhance skills through continuing education

COMMUNICATION SKILLS

- Treat all patients with compassion and empathy
- Recognize and respect cultural diversity
- Adapt communications to individual's ability to understand
- Use professional telephone technique
- Use effective and correct verbal and written communications
- Recognize and respond to verbal and non-verbal communications
- Use medical terminology appropriately
- Receive, organize, prioritize, and transmit information
- Serve as liaison
- Promote the practice through positive public relations

LEGAL CONCEPTS

- Maintain confidentiality
- Practice within the scope of education, training, and personal capabilities
- Prepare and maintain medical records
- Document accurately
- Use appropriate guidelines when releasing information
- Follow employer's established policies dealing with the health care contract
- Follow federal, state, and local legal guidelines
- Maintain awareness of federal and state health care legislation and regulations
- Maintain and dispose of regulated substances in compliance with government guidelines
- Comply with established risk management and safety procedures
- Recognize professional credentialing criteria
- Participate in the development and maintenance of personnel, policy, and procedure manuals
- *Develop and maintain personnel, policy, and procedure manuals (adv)*

INSTRUCTION

- Instruct individuals according to their needs
- Explain office policies and procedures
- Teach methods of health promotion and disease prevention
- Locate community resources and disseminate information
- *Orient and train personnel (adv)*
- *Develop educational materials (adv)*
- *Conduct continuing education activities (adv)*

OPERATIONAL FUNCTIONS

- Maintain supply inventory
- Evaluate and recommend equipment and supplies
- Apply computer techniques to support office operations
- *Supervise personnel (adv)*
- *Interview and recommend job applicants (adv)*
- *Negotiate leases and prices for equipment and supply contracts (adv)*

SOURCE: Reprinted by permission of the American Association of Medical Assistants from the *AAMA Role Delineation Study: Occupational Analysis of the Medical Assisting Profession.*

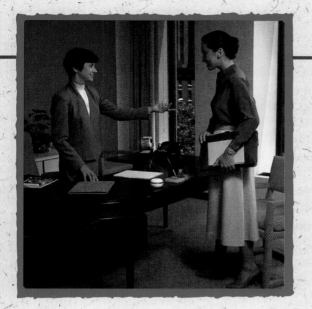

35

Externship and Career Opportunities

LEARNING OBJECTIVES

After completing this chapter, you should:
1. Define and spell the glossary terms for this chapter.
2. Discuss three advantages of an externship experience.
3. Describe what you would do if your program did not have an externship component.
4. Complete your own personal assessment.
5. State the purpose of a cover letter.)
6. Develop your own resumé.)
7. Write a letter in response to a classified advertisement from your local newspaper.
8. Discuss the steps used in preparing for an interview.
9. Develop a follow-up letter following an interview.

All indications are that job opportunities for medical assistants are expanding at a rapid rate. The United States Department of Labor estimates that the demand for medical assistants will grow by approximately 70% by the year 2010. This demand for health personnel means that a well-prepared medical assistant will have a secure future.

One of the best means to facilitate the transition between the classroom and the medical setting is through the externship experience. This experience can be a time of great challenge and learning since the student is able to gain experience while under supervision. In order to receive the most benefit from the experience, careful preparation needs to take place. The externship experience is also one of the most exciting components of a medical assisting program.

As the student's formal educational experience in school draws to a close, he or she will prepare for the certification examination offered by the American Association of Medical Assistants (AAMA). Most hiring physicians look for this certification. This credential, along with graduation from an accredited program, indicates that entry-level skills have been accomplished.

During this final stage of training the student will also begin the search for employment. This chapter discusses skills that are useful.

What Is An Externship?

An externship refers to a situation in which one leaves the confines of the classroom and works, without payment, in a health care setting using the newly acquired medical assisting skills under the supervision of someone at the site. This is also referred to as "on-the-job training." There is as wide a range of externships as there are medical facilities. An externship can be as short as four weeks or as long as one or two semesters of school. Schools that are accredited by the Council on Accreditation of Allied Health Education Programs (CAAHEP) in conjunction with the AAMA and AMA require an externship of a minimum of 160 hours. The externship experience should provide the medical assistant with ample experience in both administrative and clinical skills.

Your school and you will work together to select the right externship for you based on your skills, needs and residence location (Figure 35-1).

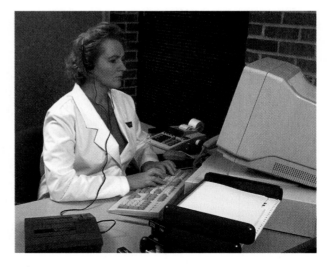

Figure 35-1   Medical assistant doing transcription work.

Ideally, the externship experience is carefully monitored by the clinical instructor/externship coordinator so that problems can be addressed when they arise.

The Externship Experience

Students generally find the externship experience to be the most rewarding part of their school experience. You will have the opportunity to see how a physician's office, ambulatory care setting, clinic, hospital or extended care facility operates on a day-to-day basis (Figure 35-2). In addition you will be exposed to a variety of different personalities in the work setting. Other advantages of the externship include gaining additional experience using your skills such as phlebotomy, taking EKG's and vital signs, conducting urinalysis and hematology testing, using the computer, interviewing patients, performing billing and insurance procedures, and scheduling patients. You will gain experience in budgeting your time and balancing your work day, school day and your home life.

Your performance and behavior will be carefully observed by your supervisor at the externship site. Some of the areas that will be evaluated are

- Administrative and clinical skills and technique
- Caring attitude
- Empathy for patients
- Enthusiasm
- Ethical standards

- Grooming/dress
- Initiative
- Integrity
- Interpersonal skills with patients and coworkers
- Language skills
- Poise under pressure
- Professionalism
- Punctuality/dependability

Student's Responsibilities

The student has an overall responsibility to prepare well in advance of the interview for the externship. This preparation includes a review of skills, updating the resumé, and planning on how to project a professional appearance.

Each externship site is somewhat unique and may have additional requirements. The externship requires the medical assistant to carry malpractice insurance. Documentation of a recent physical exam and immunizations including hepatitis and tetanus may also be required. A tuberculosis (TB) test is required if you are working near patients. Since some of the immunizations, particularly hepatitis, require several months to complete it is wise to begin this process 8-9 months before your expected externship. It is the student's responsibility to make sure that necessary physical examinations, paperwork and immunizations are completed on a timely basis.

You are being given a great responsibility and opportunity by being allowed to gain experience in the externship site. The physician or facility pro-

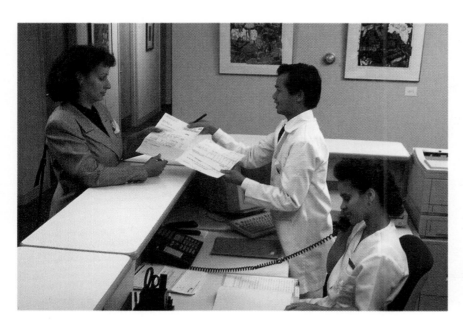

Figure 35-2 Medical assistant working in a front office area of a medical office.

viding an externship expects candidates will be extremely cautious regarding ethical and legal concerns. Errors can result in malpractice claims against the physician you are working with. If an error occurs, it should be reported immediately to the supervisor without alarming the patient. In many cases when errors are handled immediately, they can be corrected. If you cover up an error or mistake, it could result in immediate dismissal. Regular interviews with the office manager provide opportunities for the medical assistant to discuss issues that may need clarification (Figure 35-3).

Issues of confidentiality and patient privacy are of great concern to the physician and staff in all facilities. Discussion of information regarding any patient or the physician's practice with anyone outside of that facility is never allowed.

You will receive supervision from your on-the-job supervisor and your externship coordinator. Be sure to ask questions. The externship experience is meant to be a learning experience. If you find that you are not receiving the experience you require, bring this to the attention of your clinical supervisor.

Many students are able to take advantage of excellent externship opportunities simply because of a previous student's good performance in that externship. Remember: the behavior and work performance of the medical assistant during the externship is a direct reflection on the school that prepared him or her.

Finding the Right Site

Most schools have an externship coordinator who screens and selects health care sites that are appropriate for training. The screening process requires the coordinator to conduct an interview with the physician or office manager at the site to assure that the student will benefit from appropriate experiences and receive supervision on site. Often the school has an agreement with the externship site that is kept on file at the school. Ideally, the externship site will have a former graduate of your program in their employ who can identify what skills and situations are needed.

Generally, it is not a good idea for students to select externship sites without the assistance from the school or the externship coordinator in particular. The school has the responsibility to require that the students are well supervised (Figure 35-4).

The Preceptor Role

The medical assistant at an externship site always works under the supervision of the physician.

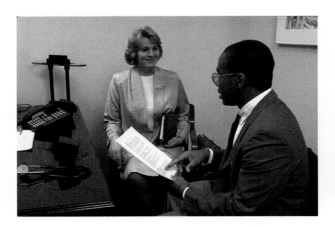

Figure 35-3 Medical Assistant during interview with the office manager.

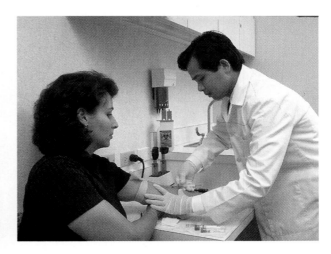

Figure 35-4 Drawing blood is one of the procedures the medical assistant performs in the medical office.

However, the physician may designate another member of the health care team as a supervisor for the student.

This person performs in the role of a preceptor. A preceptor provides additional instruction and guidance for a student by observing the performance of particular skills. The preceptor will also provide a formal written evaluation for the student, usually at the midpoint and final point. Table 35-1 lists several areas that are included on a typical evaluations form.

The preceptor is looking for continual improvement in skills as the student gains confidence. The student should make every attempt to establish a rapport, or comfortable work relationship, with the preceptor.

Externship Site Evaluation

At the end of the externship experience the student will be asked to provide an evaluation of the site. This evaluation may include the following types of questions:

- Was the overall externship experience positive or negative? Explain.
- Was the supervisor or preceptor approachable and available to answer questions?
- What, in your opinion, could be improved about this externship site/experience?
- Should this externship site be offered to other students?

Volunteer Services

If you are in a program without an externship component, then you may wish to gain experience through a volunteer program. In addition to gaining confidence in the work setting, an additional benefit of volunteer "work" is that you will be able to enter it on your resumé. It is wise for you to discuss malpractice insurance coverage with any facility in which you volunteer. They may advise you to carry some coverage of your own.

TABLE 35-1 Sample Student Externship Form

Areas Evaluated	Rating*				
Makes effective use of time	1	2	3	4	N/A
Ability to work well with others	1	2	3	4	N/A
Accepts suggestions/criticisms willingly	1	2	3	4	N/A
Expresses concern for patients	1	2	3	4	N/A
Protects confidentiality of physician and patients	1	2	3	4	N/A
Always on time for work	1	2	3	4	N/A
Willingly works until the job is completed	1	2	3	4	N/A
Able to work independently	1	2	3	4	N/A
Demonstrates skill as appropriate	1	2	3	4	N/A
Does not perform skills beyond scope of training, education, and personal capability	1	2	3	4	N/A
Practices principles of aseptic technique	1	2	3	4	N/A
Projects a positive attitude	1	2	3	4	N/A
Recognizes emergencies	1	2	3	4	N/A
Dresses appropriately	1	2	3	4	N/A
Practices good hygiene	1	2	3	4	N/A

*Rating: 1 = Excellent, 2 = Good, 3 = Average, 4 = Needs Improvement, N/A = Not Applicable

Preparing for the Certification Examination

The certification examination to become a certified medical assistant is offered by the American Association of Medical Assistants (AAMA) twice a year on the last Friday of January and June. The examination is given at numerous locations throughout the United States. It is a four hour examination which is scheduled from 9 AM until 1 PM. Beginning January 1998, the examination will only be available to medical assistants who have completed an accredited program in medical assisting. The certification examination is a comprehensive test which includes questions relating to general medical knowledge, administrative knowledge, and clinical knowledge. Table 35-2 describes the areas covered under each category.

The certification examination to become a Registered Medical Assistant (RMA) is given each March, June, and November. Eligibility to take this examination is either based on five years of work experience or a combined training and work program.

Preparation for this examination begins as soon as the student begins a training program. All the subject matter taught in a program is interrelated and forms the base of the student's knowledge. All class notes and information acquired during the training program should be maintained in an organized fashion so that preparation for the examination can be efficient. A variety of examination preparation courses are offered. In addition, several excellent review books provide the student with sample test questions. These review books should be purchased well before the actual date of the examination. The study questions are generally related to the three major categories covered on the examination: general, administrative, and clinical. Students should time themselves while answering these sample test questions since the actual examination is timed.

Med Tip: Examination review books are useful for study purposes during a medical assisting program since they help prepare students to take multiple choice type questions.

See Chapter 1 for a further discussion of the credentialing agencies.

The Job Search

Many offices that offer externship opportunities do not have a full-time position available. Do not think it is a reflection of your work if you are not

TABLE 35-2   Three Major Areas Tested on CMA Examination

Category	Topics Covered
General Medical	Medical terminology
	Anatomy and physiology
	Behavioral science; psychology
	Medical law and ethics
Administrative	Oral and written communication
	Records management
	Insurance and coding
	Computers and office machines
	Bookkeeping, collections, and credit
Clinical	Examination room techniques
	Laboratory procedures
	Pharmacology and medication administration
	Emergency procedures
	Specimen collection

offered a position at the end of your externship. If your externship experience did not lead to a permanent position, then you need to begin the job search in earnest. In some cases, a facility will not want to hire you as a medical assistant until you become credentialed after taking the required examination. However, some facilities will interview you for a permanent position with the understanding that you must pass the certification exam.

Any job search should begin with careful planning. You will need to prepare a list of information sources for identifying job opportunities, update your resumé, rehearse interviewing, and plan your professional attire for the interview process. Six reasons are cited as the most common job search mistakes. They are

1. Having no clear plan
2. Failing to inform others of your job search
3. Spending too much time answering classified ads
4. Looking for the perfect job
5. Limiting yourself to one field
6. Giving up the search too soon

There are several areas to pursue in your search for job opportunities. Some of these are listed in Table 35-3.

Personal Assessment

Before moving ahead with your job search, it is a good idea to perform a personal assessment or evaluation of your own strengths and weaknesses. While it is not a good idea to point out any weaknesses to potential employers, you must be cautious to avoid taking on tasks for which you are not qualified. Employers often ask about weaknesses. State one and indicate what you are doing about it. This shows you are not unaware of limitations but lets the employer know you are serious about improving yourself. By performing a personal assessment, you can determine in what fields you might enjoy working, which areas require more skill development, and for which positions you are qualified (Figure 35-5).

You can ask your instructors for guidance and observations on your appearance, attitude and skills. While it is never easy to accept criticism, a

TABLE 35-3 **Sources for Job Opportunities**

Source	Description/Explanation
Classified ads	Use local and out-of-town newspapers, professional journals and trade magazines. Use the local public library's access to national newspapers.
Employment agencies	Place your name with the agency and career consultants.
Health care facilities in your area	Contact hospitals, veteran's facilities, extended care facilities, ambulatory care sites.
Local medical society	Obtain a listing of physicians who are looking for help or a listing of all the medical practice offices in your area.
Parents, friends	Network within your own friends and relatives. Make sure they know you are looking for employment.
Personal physician	Your own physician may network for you and call his or her colleagues.
Publications	American Association of Medical Assistants (AAMA) and other local professional publications.
Professional	Use both state and local chapters of your own professional association and other allied health groups.
School placement service	One of the best sources since they know your training and skills well. In many cases the perspective employer will call the schools looking for new employees.
State employment office	After completing the required application forms your name will be on file for available positions.

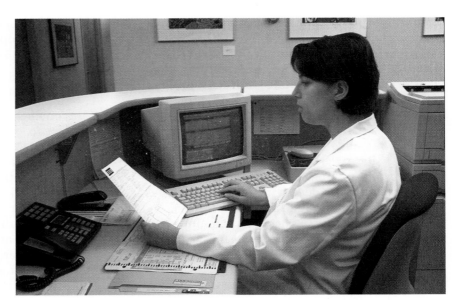

Figure 35-5 Medical assistants who do billing must know and use the proper codes to assure third party payments by insurance companies.

well-intentioned comment from someone you know about the need to bleach your uniforms, eliminate jewelry, change to a more professional hair style, or brush up on particular skills may help you obtain the job you are seeking.

You may wish to practice your interview skills with your instructors or in front of a mirror. Use every opportunity to speak up in class to further develop your communication skills. Work on smiling at every opportunity.

The Resumé

What is a resumé? The resumé is a summary of your credentials which include your employment history, experience, training, and education. For your first position the resumé is generally one page. Since you will create a first impression with your resumé it should be carefully written. You may wish to ask your career office for guidance when putting together a resumé for the first time.

Med Tip: Spend time working on your resumé. Remember that the purpose of a resumé is to obtain an interview. Keep a personal portfolio in which you gather the names, addresses, dates of schools and programs you attend. Record association membership and credentialing information, such as certification and/or registration numbers and expiration dates. This is particularly important if you have earned multiple credentials.

The most popular resumé format is chronological order. In other words, the events are placed in the order of their occurrence. Using this format education, work experience, and achievements are listed in reverse chronological order with the most recent events listed first. The chronological resumé format is illustrated in Figure 35-6.

Another resumé format is the skills resumé. This format is useful if you are just graduating from school and have not had extensive work experience. With this format you concentrate on administrative and clinical skills that have been learned while participating in a medical assisting program.

The resumé should be typed on 8 1/2″ × 11″ good quality white or off-white paper. Do not use bright colored paper. The resumé must be neatly typed and error free. If possible use a word processor for preparing your resumé so that you can easily go back and add updates. Print at least ten copies of your resumé so that you always have several copies available for distribution.

What Is Included in a Resumé?

Resumés vary somewhat based on the personal preferences of the writers but several items are standard. These include

- Heading
- Education
- Work experience
- Externship experience
- Licensing and credentials

Ralph Taylor
222 E. Main St.
Chicago, IL 60601
(312) 555-1212

EDUCATION

Associate Degree	Central State College, Hometown, Illinois. Expected date of graduation: June 19xx. Major in Health Science.
Medical Assistant	Central State College, Hometown, Illinois. February 19xx–June 19xx. Graduated with honors.

CERTIFICATES

Medical Assistant	Passed certification examination in January 19xx.
CPR	Certified by American Heart Association, December 19xx.

SPECIAL COMPETENCIES Fluent in Spanish.

EXPERIENCE

Medical Assistant	Dr. Earl Brown, Internal Medicine Externship, 2222 State St., Chicago, IL. Externship duties included: drawing blood, handling medical records, scheduling patients, and patient education. 19xx–19xx.
Nursing Assistant	Jane Young, M.D. Family Practice, 111 Hoyne Ave., Chicago, IL. Duties included taking vital signs, EKGs, assisting with well-baby visits and in treatment room. 19xx–19xx.

HONORS	National Honor Society.
INTERESTS	Tennis, Christian ministry to inner-city youth, Teach English As a Second Language to young adults.
REFERENCES	Furnished upon request.

Figure 35-6   An example of a resumé with a chronological format.

- Extracurricular activities and interests
- Statement regarding references

Your name all in capital letters, address, and telephone number are prepared as a heading at the top of the page. When this information is printed in slightly larger type than the rest of the text, it stands out and provides an easy reference for the reader.

If you are still a student or a recent graduate with limited work experience, then list your education first in reverse chronological order with the most recent school/program listed first. Add any educational experiences you have had, such as workshops or courses presented by the AAMA.

Your work experience is then listed in the same reverse chronological order. Include externship experience with a brief description of your duties. Many prospective employers also wish to see part-time employment listed. This is especially necessary and even beneficial if you have other experience in the health care field.

Include information about your professional credentials, such as CMA certification or RMA registration and professional memberships. Next list interests and only one or two extracurricular activities. Extracurricular refers to events or activities that are beyond the regular academic requirements. The presence of such activities is evidence of personal initiative and development. Be selective about your choices being sure to include volunteer work in this category. Indicate that references are available upon request.

Some Items Not Included on a Resumé
- Age
- General health
- Photograph
- Marital status
- Spouse and children's names
- Salary information
- Names and addresses of references
- Reasons for leaving previous positions.

You should continually update your resumé. For example, as you complete an externship, obtain certification, change positions, or perform volunteer work you will want to update your resumé so that it is always current.

Professional References

A professional reference is the statement of someone who has either worked with you or known you for a period of time. This person will be asked to attest to your skills and/or personal integrity or value system. For example, he or she may be asked if you are an honest and sincere person. A prospective employer will call your references before hiring you to ask questions about your work and attendance record.

State at the bottom of your resumé that references will be furnished upon request. You should type on a separate piece of paper a list of at least three references with their addresses and telephone numbers. Names of references are generally not included on the actual resumé.

You should obtain the permission to use a person's name as a reference. It is wise to include names of professional as well as personal references. Your instructors and dean might serve as professional references as well as your externship supervisor. A personal reference might include a friend or someone from your church. Parents and spouses do not generally serve as references. Of course, you would not include the name of anyone who may not provide you with an excellent reference.

The Cover Letter

What is the cover letter? A cover letter is intended to introduce you to the recipient—the person to whom you send your letter and, of course, your resumé. The cover letter should clearly state the purpose of your correspondence. Since health care institutions may have several positions they are advertising for at the same time, you will need to state clearly which position you are interested in.

The cover letter should be brief. It is not a restatement of everything that is in your resumé. Explain what you can do for the employer and why your qualifications are a good match for their requirements. Be sure to include an address and telephone number where you can be contacted. Do not add handwritten comments or additional information to your cover letter. Always update or revise information on your resumé and cover letter with a word processor.

Always check over the spelling of the employer's name and address carefully. Some of the most common typing errors are made with individual's names. A potential employer will judge you by your writing until they have had a chance to meet you in person. Your local library or college library will have references on sample resumé and cover letter writing. An example of a sample cover letter written in response to a classified ad is illustrated in Figure 35-7.

If you have word processing capability you may wish to draft several sample cover letters which you can then pull up from your computer and add the appropriate heading. For instance, different sample cover letters could be drafted to respond to "blind" ads, classified ads, and unsolicited interview requests at local medical facilities. A blind ad refers to an ad that does not identify the institution or facility that placed the ad. Unsolicited interview requests are requests for interviews initiated by the candidate or prospective employee not the institution or facility or individual representing the facility. Some of the most common mistakes to be avoided when writing a cover letter are:

Ralph Taylor
222 E. Main St.
Chicago, IL 60601
(312) 555-1212

May 20, 19xx

James Stark, M.D.
1450 N. Devonshire
Chicago, IL 60611

Dear Dr. Stark:

This letter is in response to your recent advertisement in the May 19, 19xx, Chicago Sun News for a certified medical assistant.

I believe that my qualifications are a good match for your position. During my medical assisting program at Central State College in Hometown, Illinois, I maintained a 3.6 GPA on a 4.0 scale.

My medical assisting program at Central State College was completed in December of 19xx. I passed the American Association of Medical Assistant's certification examination January 27, 19xx. Currently I am completing an associate degree program at CSC and plan to graduate in June, 19xx.

The enclosed resumé includes my experience as a part-time nursing assistant for Dr. Jane Young in her family practice office.

I look forward to meeting you to discuss your position needs and my qualifications.

Thank you for your consideration.

Sincerely,

Ralph Taylor, C.M.A.

Figure 35-7 An example of a cover letter sent in response to a classified ad.

- Not addressing the letter to a specific person in the organization. Be sure to check for name, title, and correct spelling.
- Failing to clearly state the position for which you are applying.
- Sending a cover letter that is too long. One page works best.
- Sending a letter that is poorly worded and/or has spelling or typing errors. Always send the original cover letter, never a copy.

See Figure 35-7 for an example of a cover letter in response to a classified ad.

The Interview

Your library will have reference material on what to expect during the interview process. All interviewers have standard questions which may include, "Tell me why you went into medical assisting?" or "Why do you want to work here?" You should practice responses to these questions before you go to the interview (Figure 35-8).

Preparing for Tough Interview Questions

In addition to the standard questions, there may be some difficult questions such as, "We all have our strengths and weaknesses. Tell me one of your weaknesses." It is always a good idea to highlight your strengths. Therefore, to answer a tough question select a strength. For instance, you might make the following response to the question about your weakness, "I am a perfectionist and may sometimes hold myself to a very high standard which is almost unobtainable" or "I care very deeply about people and must work to empathize with them rather than sympathize."

The interviewer may ask you questions regarding any "gaps" in the chronology. Answer all questions honestly using simple statements, such as "I did not work during that year because I was caring for an elderly relative" or "It has been six months since I finished school. I did not seek employment because I was studying for the CMA examination." It is not necessary to provide lengthy explanations for termination from a position. Be especially careful not to criticize the institution or individual who terminated you.

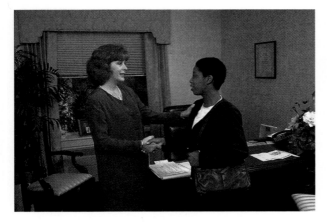

Figure 35-8 The job interview.

Be prepared to answer the difficult questions with great poise and professionalism. You will have only about 20 minutes to convince your potential employer that you should be the applicant hired. Be absolutely honest about your achievements. However, don't be afraid to talk positively

Guidelines: Successful Interviewing

1. Learn all you can about the organization. Interviewers are impressed by candidates who indicate knowledge of their facility or organization.
2. Have a specific job in mind when you interview so that you project the impression of self-assurance.
3. Know your qualifications for each specific job area/task requirement. Rehearse or review possible responses several times before going to the interview. You can role play with a friend or relative to build your confidence.
4. Prepare responses to possible "difficult questions" you might be asked or to respond to the request to tell the interviewer something about yourself.
5. Be prepared to discuss where you want to be in five years.
6. Carry extra copies of your resumé.
7. Arrive five to ten minutes before your scheduled appointment. You may wish to wait outside the facility if you arrive too early.
8. Dress conservatively to project a professional well-groomed appearance. Generally, a white uniform is not required for an interview.
9. Never ask for permission to smoke during an interview. Do not eat anything during an interview unless the interview takes place during a meal. Chewing gum is never acceptable during the interview.
10. Be alert and prompt in giving answers to the interviewer's questions. Do not offer information that isn't requested. Keep answers concise.
11. Ask questions about the position and the organization. It is generally not a good idea to inquire about benefits on the first interview.
12. Bring your social security number, a pen, driver's license number, extra resumés, and the names of three references with their telephone numbers.

about yourself. There is no one else present at the interview who knows you as well as you do. Refer to Guidelines: Successful Interviewing for additional interview tips.

Professionalism at the Interview

The day of the interview you will be judged immediately by your appearance. You should present a conservative, well groomed professional appearance. Wear little or no jewelry and avoid showy hair styles, heavy perfume, bright nail polish, and bright clothing. Of course, this is the same appearance that you will want to present on the job.

Women should wear a suit or dress. Slacks, pantsuits and open shoes are not appropriate at interviews. Men should wear a suit and tie. If you are still in a medical assisting program, you may wish to wear a clean pressed uniform with your school insignia.

No one should accompany you to an interview. Introduce yourself to the receptionist and wait quietly in the reception room until you are called for the interview. Be very courteous to all the office staff. Many physicians will have their entire office team assist in selecting new employees.

Med Tip: Remember that as a member of the health care team, you are always under observation. It is not a good idea to use the casual language that one might use at home. And always remember to smile!

Greet the person interviewing you with a firm handshake. Interviewers will generally take a few minutes to ask casual questions that will allow you to relax. Be prepared for such questions as, "Tell me about yourself." Have good eye contact with interviewer and answer all questions in a sincere and friendly manner.

Questions relating to age, ethnic origin, place of birth, marital status, and number of children are prohibited by law. Most interviewers are aware of this law and will not ask these questions. You do not have to answer them if they are asked. However, since you are interested in being employed it is not a good idea to create an issue over this.

Salary and benefits are not generally discussed in the first interview. If you are called back for a second interview or with a job offer then the topic of salary and benefits can be discussed. Remember to be pleasant when the interview is over. The interviewer will usually indicate the end of the interview by standing up and shaking your hand as you leave (Figure 35-9).

Every interview experience is an opportunity for personal growth. If you are not hired on the first or second interview do not become discouraged. Do a reassessment of your interviewing skills. Ask your instructor or friend to critique your skills to see how you might improve. Immediately send out more cover letters and resumés until you are hired. According to interviewers, the ten most common mistakes made in interviews are

1. Poor eye contact
2. Use of slang or improper grammar

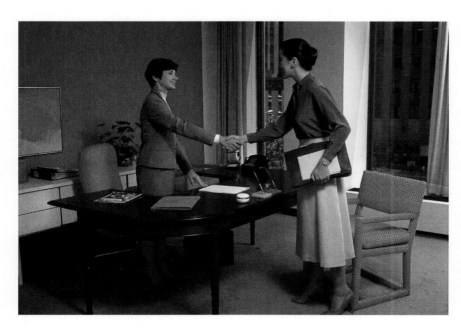

Figure 35-9 Medical Assistant shaking hands with the interviewer at the close of the interview.

3. Inappropriate dress or poor grooming
4. Lack of enthusiasm
5. Poor posture
6. Smoking or chewing gum
7. Talking too much or projecting an over-confident attitude
8. Arriving late
9. Speaking critically of previous employers
10. Inability to ask questions about the organization

The Application

If you have had work experience, there should be no "gaps" on your application or resumé from the time you began to work. You may have stopped working temporarily to complete your education. The employer will then expect the dates of employment and schooling to run consecutively. "Gaps" with no apparent work or schooling indicated should be clarified. If you were unemployed

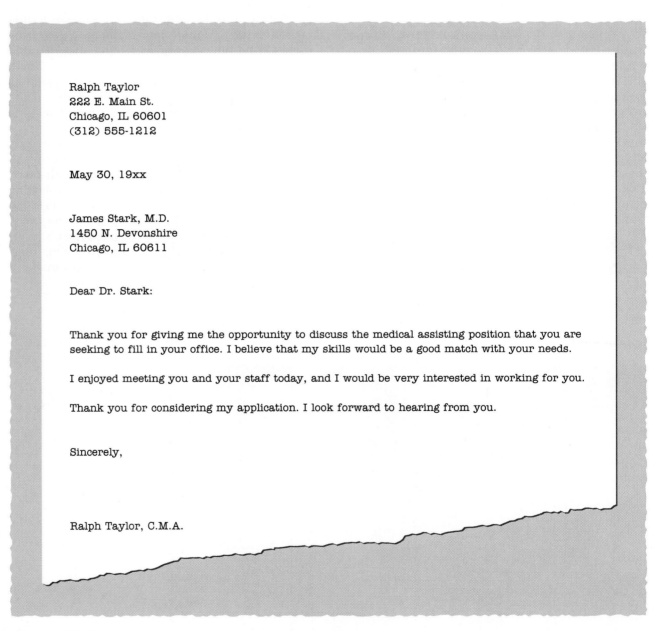

Ralph Taylor
222 E. Main St.
Chicago, IL 60601
(312) 555-1212

May 30, 19xx

James Stark, M.D.
1450 N. Devonshire
Chicago, IL 60611

Dear Dr. Stark:

Thank you for giving me the opportunity to discuss the medical assisting position that you are seeking to fill in your office. I believe that my skills would be a good match with your needs.

I enjoyed meeting you and your staff today, and I would be very interested in working for you.

Thank you for considering my application. I look forward to hearing from you.

Sincerely,

Ralph Taylor, C.M.A.

Figure 35-10   An example of a follow-up letter following an interview.

for a period of time, the potential employer will want to know why.

An application is usually completed at the time of the interview. Therefore bring along a folder containing all your documentation such as:

- Social security number
- Updated resumé and an extra copy for the interviewer
- List of three references with their addresses and telephone numbers
- A chronological list of all your work experience
- Driver's license number

The neatness of your handwriting and printing will be demonstrated on your application. Be careful to print if that is requested. Questions relating to age, ethnic origin, place of birth, and number of children are prohibited by law. However, some offices and institutions may still have these questions on their application forms. You do not have to answer these questions. Simply leave the questions blank.

Follow-up After the Interview

Immediately following the interview, the same day if possible, send a letter thanking the interviewer for his or her time. This is a good opportunity to again express your interest in the position. Be meticulous about proofreading your letter for mistakes. It is your final professional contact with the interviewer before the decision to hire is made.

You may wish to call the office a few days later to ask about the progress made on filling the position. If you are offered a position and decide not to accept it, you would use the same courtesy when turning down an offer as you use when accepting one. See Figure 35-10 for a sample of a follow-up letter.

If you are offered a position which you wish to accept then a letter of acceptance is sent within five days of the offer. Accept the offer and express your thanks. Clearly state the position you are accepting.

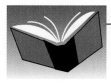

LEGAL AND ETHICAL ISSUES

You are responsible for providing complete and accurate information on application forms. Be sure all the facts surrounding your education and work experience are absolutely accurate. It is especially important to be honest about your skill level. Do not promise to perform procedures or tasks for which you are not trained. Lying on an application or a resumé is considered cause for termination. In some instances there may even be cause for prosecution.

PATIENT EDUCATION

Patients are not always clear regarding distinctions among the various health care workers credentials and responsibilities. During your externship, you may have to clarify that you are a student working under the direction of your supervisor. This is important in order to protect yourself from being expected to perform procedures of health care workers certified and/or licensed levels beyond your credentials. Always wear the insignia of your school and a name pin that designates your status.

Summary

One of the most valuable components of a medical assisting program is the externship since it provides an opportunity to practice skills that have been learned in school, under the direct supervision of the externship coordinator. This important stage of the training provides the student an opportunity to gain insight into strengths and weaknesses allowing students to work on or correct weaknesses before accepting employment.

The job interview process requires the medical assistant to be honest and sincere about capabilities and the desire to work diligently. A fulfilling career demands careful planning, the ability to arrive on time, and to work diligently for an employer while always keeping the patient's needs in mind.

Competency Review

1. Define and spell the glossary terms for this chapter.
2. Describe 5 areas of student responsibility concerning the externship.
3. List and discuss 3 externship opportunities in your area that you would like to pursue.
4. List and discuss 6 areas that your externship supervisor will be evaluating.
5. Write a resumé or update an existing resumé.
6. Select an advertisement for a medical assistant position from your local newspaper's classified section. Write a cover letter in response to that advertisement.
7. Write a follow-up letter after receiving an interview for the position mentioned in question 6.
8. What are three questions that you would ask a potential employer during an interview?
9. How would you respond to the questions, "What is your major strength?" and "What is your major weakness?"

PREPARING FOR THE CERTIFICATION EXAM

Test Taking Tip — Use the "plus-minus" strategy for taking a difficult examination. Answer easy questions immediately. Place a "+" next to any question/problem that seems solvable but time consuming. Make a guess and go on to the next question. Place a "−" next to any question that seems impossible. Act quickly to decide if a question is *plus* or *minus*. After completing all the questions you can do immediately, then go back and work on the "+" problems. If there is time left over when you finish, work on the "−" questions. Be sure to erase the *plus* and *minus* signs before handing in your exam/answer sheet since extraneous marks will count as wrong answers on machine graded exams.

Examination Review Questions

1. "On-the-job" training, as part of a medical assisting program is called a/an
   (A) clinical rotation
   (B) in-service
   (C) externship
   (D) internship
   (E) practicum

2. In accordance with the AAMA guidelines regarding "on-the-job" training, a minimum of how many hours must be successfully completed by a medical assistant?
   (A) 80
   (B) 100
   (C) 120
   (D) 140
   (E) 160

3. Some of the areas that are evaluated during this "on-the-job" training include
   (A) clinical skills
   (B) administrative skills
   (C) grooming

   (D) A and B
   (E) all of the above

4. In lieu of a more traditional "on-the-job" training arranged by a medical assisting program, how else could experience be gained and still fall within the AAMA guidelines?
   (A) volunteer work
   (B) a part-time job as a nursing assistant
   (C) a full-time job as a nursing assistant
   (D) a job as a medical receptionist
   (E) all of the above

5. Which of the following can be considered a job hunting mistake?
   (A) failing to network with others and tell them that you are looking
   (B) looking for the ideal job
   (C) defining a field and limiting yourself to that one
   (D) not having a clear plan
   (E) all of the above

(Continued)

6. The process by which a medical assistant self-evaluates one's strengths and weaknesses is referred to in the chapter as
   (A) ego identification
   (B) personal assessment
   (C) skill evaluation
   (D) self-reflection
   (E) self-assessment

7. What information is placed at the very top of a resumé?
   (A) name
   (B) name and address
   (C) name, address, and telephone number
   (D) name, address, telephone number, and social security number
   (E) all of the above

8. A statement from someone who has either worked with you or known you for a long time is called a
   (A) professional statement
   (B) professional reference

   (C) personal reference
   (D) A and B
   (E) A, B, and C

9. The name of the type of correspondence that is intended as a courtesy to introduce yourself is called a
   (A) cover letter
   (B) follow-up letter
   (C) resumé
   (D) interview letter
   (E) calling card

10. Which of the following is NOT considered one of the more common mistakes made in an interview?
   (A) shaking hands
   (B) being critical of a previous employer
   (C) not asking questions about the potential employer's organization
   (D) being extremely talkative
   (E) using very familiar language such as "yep" instead of "yes"

ON THE JOB

Stacy is the lead medical assistant in an ophthalmology practice of 10 physicians. The eye clinic sees patients, literally, from all over the world. Several of the physicians are premier in their specific area of ophthalmology like Dr. Keeler, who specializes in retinal diseases.

Today Stacy is going to interview a potential new employee, Sarah Banks. Sarah is currently finishing a CAAHEP-approved medical assisting program at a local college and is searching for full-time employment. She has some on-the-job experience dating back to when she was an after-school receptionist for a general practitioner, but that was more than 10 years ago.

The clinic tends to hire medical assistants who are certified, experienced, and very capable of dealing with patients from different age groups, races, and origins. However, Sarah is being considered for the position because, first of all, her father is a personal friend of Dr. Keeler's and, secondly, medical assistants, because of the high demand, are difficult to find. What should Stacy do to prepare for the interview with Sarah?

What is your response?

1. Consider that the practice is limited to ophthalmology, would any special requirements be warranted in a medical assistant that was going to work in this area?

2. Consider that the clinic patient population is very mixed by age and race. Would any special requirements in a medical assistant be warranted in this case?

3. Is it proper procedure for Sarah to be applying for this position given that she has not yet completed her medical assisting program?

4. Should Stacy, given the circumstances, invest a lot of time in interviewing Sarah? Why or why not?

5. Should the rather dated on-the-job experience be factored into Stacy's decision to hire Sarah or not?

6. If Stacy decides not to hire Sarah, does Stacy need to personally contact the reference and thank him anyway, given that he is a friend of Dr. Keeler's?

References

Badash, S. and Chesebro, D. *Introduction to Health Occupations.* Upper Saddle River, NJ: Brady/Prentice Hall, 1997.

Gieseking, H. and Plawin, P. *30 Days to a Good Job.* NY: Simon and Schuster, 1993.

Krannich, C. and Krannick, R. *Interview for Success.* Manassas Park, VA: Impact Publications, 1993.

"Results of the 1991 AAMA Employment Survey." *PMA.* November/December, 1991, pp. 23-26.

Slocum, J. and King, C. *How To Pack Your Career Parachute: A Guide to Successful Job Hunting.* Cincinnati: South-Western College Publishing, 1996.

Taber's Cyclopedic Medical Dictionary, 18th ed. Philadelphia, F.A. Davis Company, 1997.

US Department of Labor, Bureau of Labor Statistics, *Occupational Outlook Handbook.* Washington: US Government Printing Office, 1993.

Wirth, A. *Education and Work in the Year 2000.* San Francisco: Jossey-Bass Publishers, 1992.

Additional Sources

Office of Information and Consumer Affairs
US Department of Labor, Room C-4331
200 Constitution Ave. NW
Washington DC 20210

References

The Skeletal System

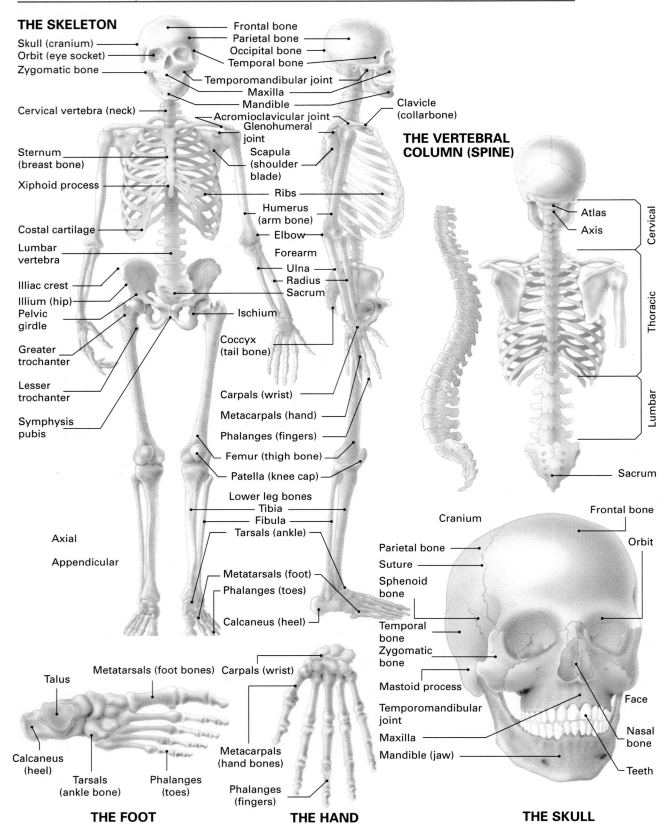

THE SKELETON

Skull (cranium)
Orbit (eye socket)
Zygomatic bone

Frontal bone
Parietal bone
Occipital bone
Temporal bone
Temporomandibular joint
Maxilla
Mandible

Cervical vertebra (neck)

Acromioclavicular joint
Glenohumeral joint
Scapula (shoulder blade)

Clavicle (collarbone)

Sternum (breast bone)

Xiphoid process

Ribs
Humerus (arm bone)
Elbow
Forearm
Ulna
Radius
Sacrum

Costal cartilage

Lumbar vertebra

Illiac crest
Illium (hip)
Pelvic girdle

Ischium

Coccyx (tail bone)

Greater trochanter

Lesser trochanter

Symphysis pubis

Carpals (wrist)
Metacarpals (hand)
Phalanges (fingers)
Femur (thigh bone)
Patella (knee cap)
Lower leg bones
Tibia
Fibula
Tarsals (ankle)
Metatarsals (foot)
Phalanges (toes)
Calcaneus (heel)

Axial

Appendicular

THE VERTEBRAL COLUMN (SPINE)

Atlas
Axis

Cervical

Thoracic

Lumbar

Sacrum

Cranium

Parietal bone
Suture
Sphenoid bone

Temporal bone
Zygomatic bone

Mastoid process

Temporomandibular joint

Maxilla

Mandible (jaw)

Frontal bone

Orbit

Face

Nasal bone

Teeth

Talus
Metatarsals (foot bones)

Calcaneus (heel)

Tarsals (ankle bone)

Phalanges (toes)

THE FOOT

Carpals (wrist)

Metacarpals (hand bones)

Phalanges (fingers)

THE HAND

THE SKULL

The Muscular System

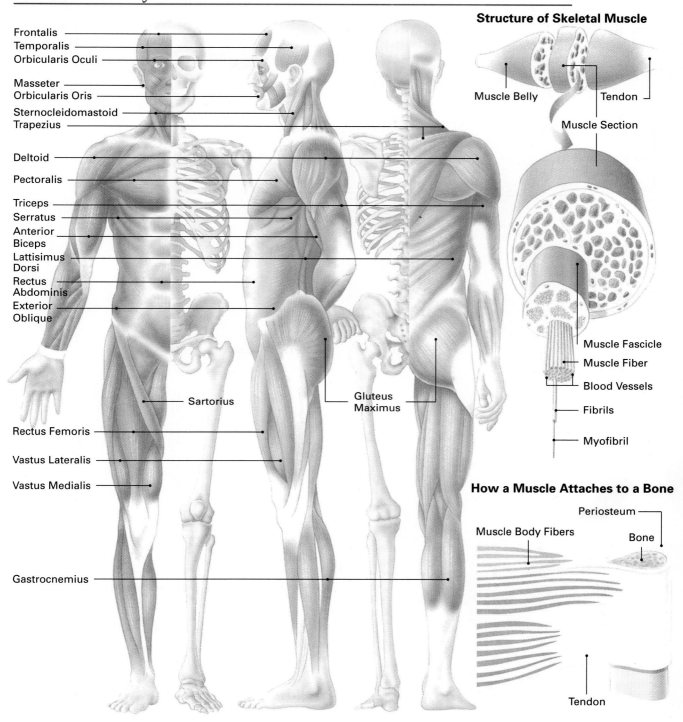

Frontalis
Temporalis
Orbicularis Oculi

Masseter
Orbicularis Oris
Sternocleidomastoid
Trapezius

Deltoid

Pectoralis

Triceps
Serratus
Anterior
Biceps
Lattisimus
Dorsi
Rectus
Abdominis
Exterior
Oblique

Sartorius

Rectus Femoris

Vastus Lateralis

Vastus Medialis

Gastrocnemius

Gluteus
Maximus

Structure of Skeletal Muscle

Muscle Belly
Tendon
Muscle Section

Muscle Fascicle
Muscle Fiber
Blood Vessels
Fibrils
Myofibril

How a Muscle Attaches to a Bone

Periosteum
Bone
Muscle Body Fibers

Tendon

THE BRAIN

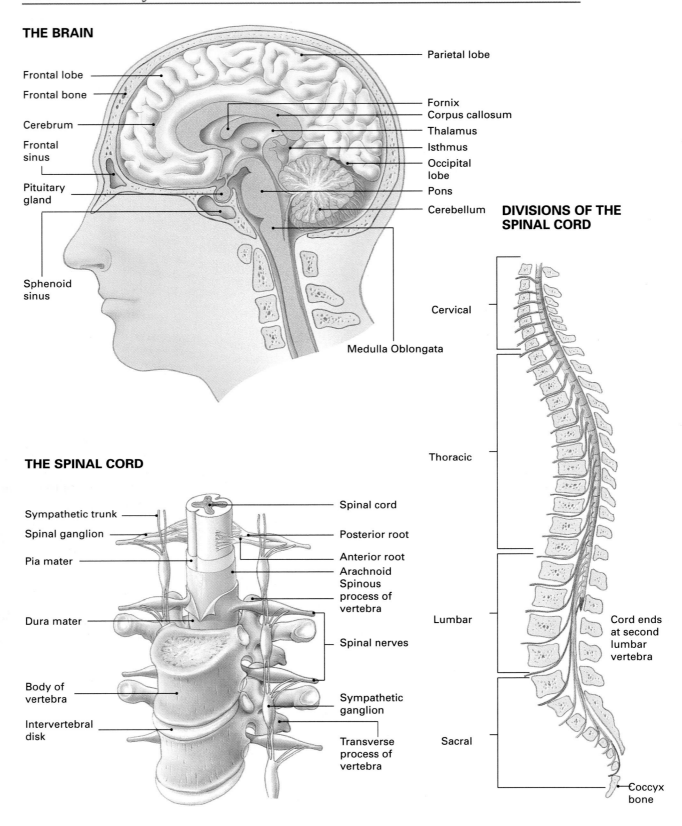

Frontal lobe

Frontal bone

Cerebrum

Frontal sinus

Pituitary gland

Sphenoid sinus

Parietal lobe

Fornix

Corpus callosum

Thalamus

Isthmus

Occipital lobe

Pons

Cerebellum

Medulla Oblongata

DIVISIONS OF THE SPINAL CORD

Cervical

Thoracic

Lumbar

Sacral

Cord ends at second lumbar vertebra

Coccyx bone

THE SPINAL CORD

Sympathetic trunk

Spinal ganglion

Pia mater

Dura mater

Body of vertebra

Intervertebral disk

Spinal cord

Posterior root

Anterior root

Arachnoid
Spinous process of vertebra

Spinal nerves

Sympathetic ganglion

Transverse process of vertebra

The Digestive System

ORGANS OF THE DIGESTIVE SYSTEM

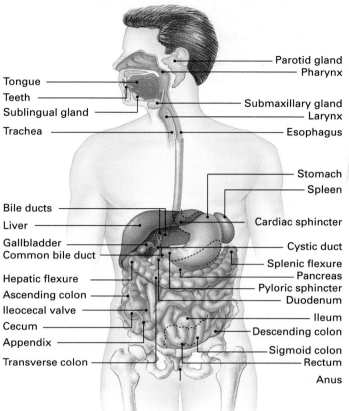

Parotid gland
Pharynx
Tongue
Teeth
Sublingual gland
Submaxillary gland
Larynx
Trachea
Esophagus
Stomach
Spleen
Bile ducts
Liver
Cardiac sphincter
Gallbladder
Common bile duct
Cystic duct
Splenic flexure
Hepatic flexure
Pancreas
Ascending colon
Pyloric sphincter
Ileocecal valve
Duodenum
Cecum
Ileum
Appendix
Descending colon
Transverse colon
Sigmoid colon
Rectum
Anus

LIVER, STOMACH, AND PANCREAS

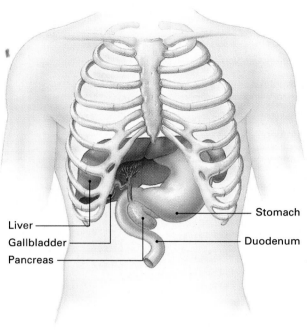

Liver
Gallbladder
Pancreas
Stomach
Duodenum

LARGE INTESTINE

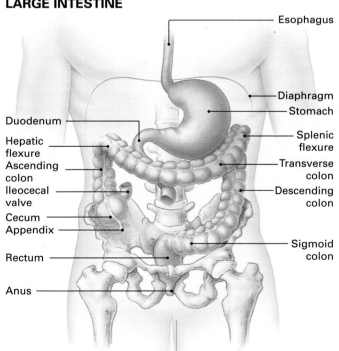

Esophagus
Duodenum
Diaphragm
Hepatic flexure
Stomach
Ascending colon
Splenic flexure
Ileocecal valve
Transverse colon
Cecum
Descending colon
Appendix
Rectum
Sigmoid colon
Anus

SMALL INTESTINE

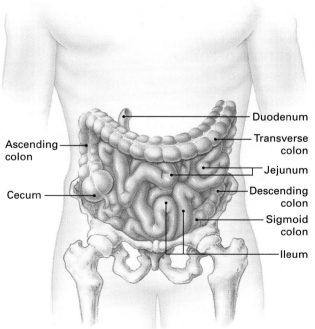

Duodenum
Transverse colon
Ascending colon
Jejunum
Cecum
Descending colon
Sigmoid colon
Ileum

The Urinary System

ORGANS OF THE URINARY SYSTEM

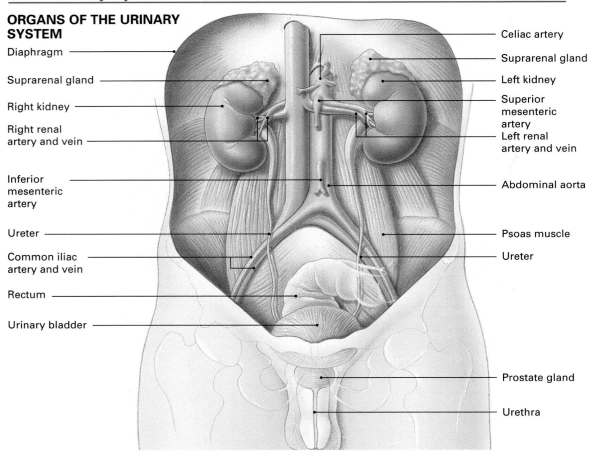

Diaphragm

Suprarenal gland

Right kidney

Right renal artery and vein

Inferior mesenteric artery

Ureter

Common iliac artery and vein

Rectum

Urinary bladder

Celiac artery

Suprarenal gland

Left kidney

Superior mesenteric artery

Left renal artery and vein

Abdominal aorta

Psoas muscle

Ureter

Prostate gland

Urethra

SECTIONED KIDNEY

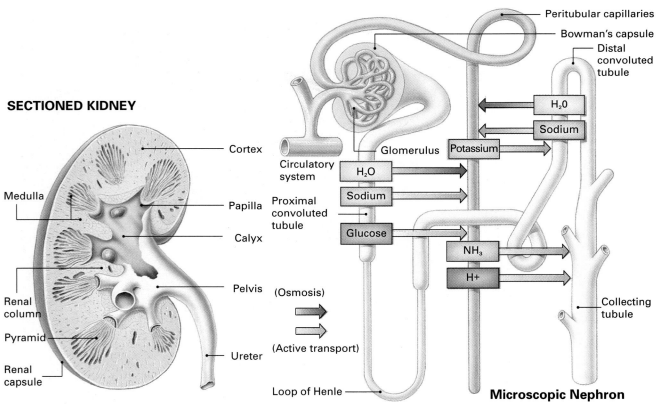

Cortex

Medulla

Papilla

Calyx

Pelvis

(Osmosis)

(Active transport)

Renal column

Pyramid

Renal capsule

Ureter

Loop of Henle

Peritubular capillaries

Bowman's capsule

Distal convoluted tubule

Glomerulus

Circulatory system

Proximal convoluted tubule

H_2O

Sodium

Potassium

H_2O

Sodium

Glucose

NH_3

$H+$

Collecting tubule

Microscopic Nephron

The Reproductive System

FEMALE

MALE

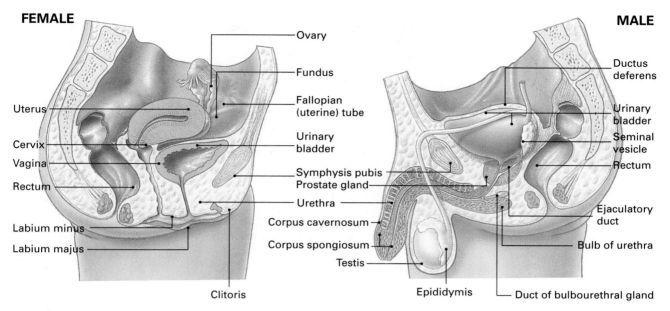

Ovary

Fundus

Fallopian (uterine) tube

Urinary bladder

Symphysis pubis

Prostate gland

Urethra

Corpus cavernosum

Corpus spongiosum

Testis

Uterus

Cervix

Vagina

Rectum

Labium minus

Labium majus

Clitoris

Ductus deferens

Urinary bladder

Seminal vesicle

Rectum

Ejaculatory duct

Bulb of urethra

Epididymis

Duct of bulbourethral gland

Labium minus (singular), Labia minora (plural)
Labium majus (singular), Labia majora (plural)

THE BREAST

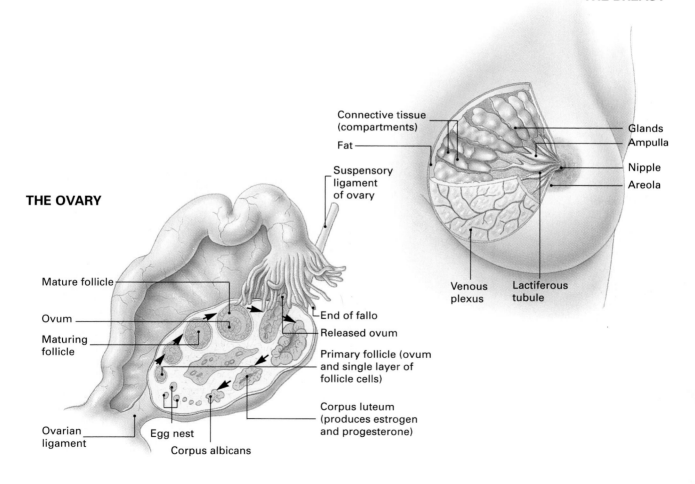

Connective tissue (compartments)

Fat

Suspensory ligament of ovary

Glands

Ampulla

Nipple

Areola

Venous plexus

Lactiferous tubule

THE OVARY

Mature follicle

Ovum

Maturing follicle

Ovarian ligament

Egg nest

Corpus albicans

End of fallo

Released ovum

Primary follicle (ovum and single layer of follicle cells)

Corpus luteum (produces estrogen and progesterone)

Membranes

THE SKIN

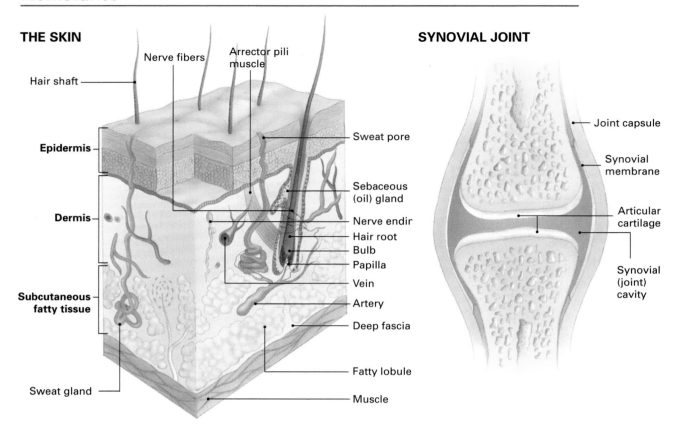

- Hair shaft
- Nerve fibers
- Arrector pili muscle
- Epidermis
- Dermis
- Subcutaneous fatty tissue
- Sweat gland
- Sweat pore
- Sebaceous (oil) gland
- Nerve endir
- Hair root
- Bulb
- Papilla
- Vein
- Artery
- Deep fascia
- Fatty lobule
- Muscle

SYNOVIAL JOINT

- Joint capsule
- Synovial membrane
- Articular cartilage
- Synovial (joint) cavity

THE PLEURA

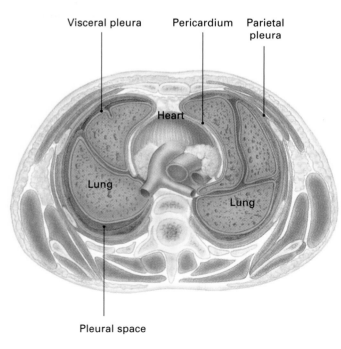

- Visceral pleura
- Pericardium
- Parietal pleura
- Heart
- Lung
- Lung
- Pleural space

THE PERITONEUM

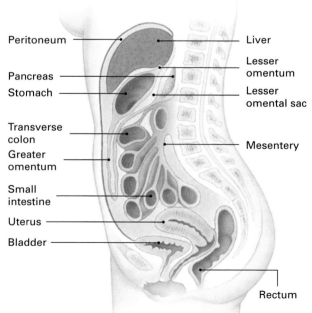

- Peritoneum
- Pancreas
- Stomach
- Transverse colon
- Greater omentum
- Small intestine
- Uterus
- Bladder
- Liver
- Lesser omentum
- Lesser omental sac
- Mesentery
- Rectum

THE EYE

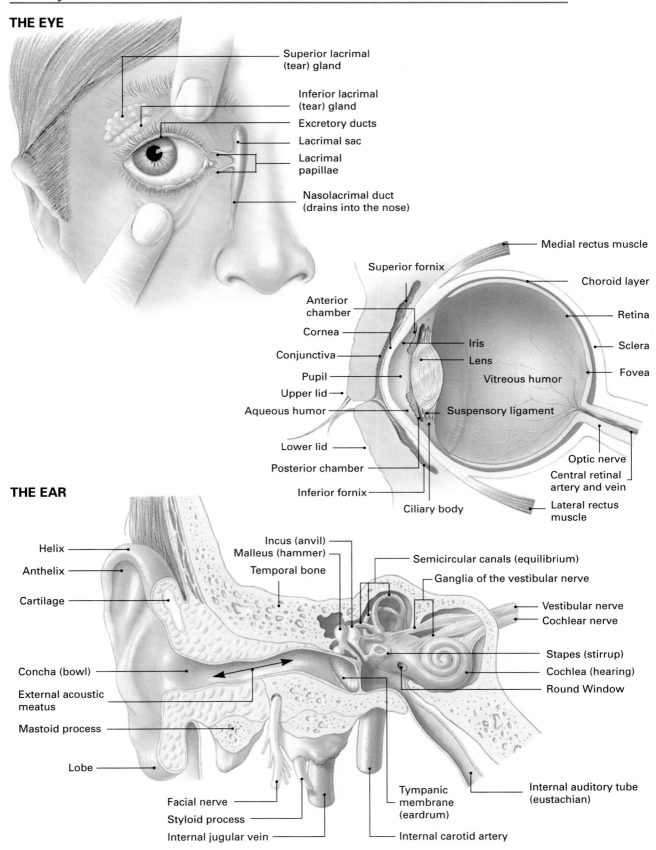

Superior lacrimal (tear) gland

Inferior lacrimal (tear) gland

Excretory ducts

Lacrimal sac

Lacrimal papillae

Nasolacrimal duct (drains into the nose)

Superior fornix

Medial rectus muscle

Choroid layer

Anterior chamber

Retina

Cornea

Sclera

Conjunctiva

Iris

Lens

Fovea

Pupil

Vitreous humor

Upper lid

Aqueous humor

Suspensory ligament

Lower lid

Posterior chamber

Optic nerve

Central retinal artery and vein

Inferior fornix

Ciliary body

Lateral rectus muscle

THE EAR

Helix

Anthelix

Cartilage

Incus (anvil)

Malleus (hammer)

Temporal bone

Semicircular canals (equilibrium)

Ganglia of the vestibular nerve

Vestibular nerve

Cochlear nerve

Concha (bowl)

External acoustic meatus

Mastoid process

Stapes (stirrup)

Cochlea (hearing)

Round Window

Lobe

Facial nerve

Styloid process

Internal jugular vein

Tympanic membrane (eardrum)

Internal carotid artery

Internal auditory tube (eustachian)

Assisting with Medical Specialties

TABLE 22-1   Common Types of Allergies

Allergy	Description
Allergic rhinitis	Inflammation of the nasal mucosa which results in nasal congestion, rhinorrhea (runny nose), sneezing and itching of the nose. Seasonal allergic rhinitis, such as seen in hay fever, occurs only during certain seasons of the year. Children suffering from this type of allergy may rub their nose in an upward movement, called the "allergic salute."
Asthma	A condition seen most frequently in early childhood in which wheezing, coughing, and dyspnea are the major symptoms. Asthmatic attacks may be caused by allergens inhaled from the air, food, and drugs. The patient's airway is affected by a constriction of the bronchial passages. Treatment is medication and control of the causative factors.
Contact dermatitis	Inflammation and irritation of the skin due to contact with an irritating substance, such as soap, perfume, cosmetics, plastic, dyes, and plants such as poison ivy. Symptoms include itching, redness, and skin lesions with blistering and oozing. Treatment consists of topical and systemic medications and removal of the causative item.
Eczema	A superficial dermatitis accompanied by papules, vesicles, and crusting. This condition can be acute or chronic.
Urticaria	A skin eruption of pale reddish wheals (circular elevations of the skin) with severe itching. It is usually associated with a food allergy, stress, or drug reactions. Also called hives.

TABLE 22-2   Common Skin Lesions

Type of Lesion	Description
Cyst	A fluid-filled sac or pouch under the skin.
Fissure	Crack-like lesion or groove in the skin.
Macule	Small, flat discolored area that is flush with the skin surface. An example would be a freckle and the flat rash of roseola.
Nodule	Solid, raised group of cells.
Papule	Small, solid, circular raised spot on the surface of the skin.
Polyp	Small tumor with a pedicle or stem attachment. They are commonly found in vascular organs such as the nose, uterus, and rectum.
Pustule	Raised spot on the skin containing pus.
Vesicle	Small, fluid-filled raised spot on the skin; blister.
Wheal	Small, round, raised area on the skin that may be accompanied by itching.

TABLE 22-3   Common Skin Infections

Infection	Description
Boil	Acute inflammation of the subcutaneous layer of skin, or hair follicle. Also called a furuncle. Treatment consists of the application of moist heat until the boil comes to a "head" or softens. An incision and drainage (I&D) may be performed to allow the purulent material to drain. Antibiotics may be prescribed.
Carbuncle	Inflammation and infection of the skin and hair follicle that may result from several untreated boils. They are most commonly found on the neck, upper back, or head. Treatment is similar to that for a single boil. Systemic antibiotics may be prescribed. A gauze bandage is applied when drainage is present.
Furuncle	Staphylococcal skin abscess with redness, pain and swelling. Also called a boil.
Herpes simplex	Infectious disease caused by the herpes simplex virus 1 and characterized by thin vesicles that tend to recur in the same area such as the lips or conjunctiva. Treatment consists of the drug acyclovir either locally or orally.
Herpes zoster	A painful, infectious viral disease which attacks the nerve endings. It is also called shingles and is caused by the same virus as chickenpox. Treatment consists of analgesics to relieve pain, and antiviral medications, such as acyclovir. In severe cases a nerve block may be necessary to relieve pain.
Impetigo	A highly contagious inflammatory skin disease with pustules that become crusted and rupture. Treatment consists of thorough cleansing using separate towels and wash cloths for the patient. These should be washed daily. Topical medications may be prescribed.
Scabies	Contagious skin disease caused by an egg-laying mite that causes intense itching. The lesions appear as small, red papules and vesicles between the fingers, toes, genitalia, and beneath the breasts. Treatment consists of a methrin cream from the neck down. All clothing and bedding need careful laundering.
Sebaceous cyst	Cyst filled with sebum (oil) from a sebaceous gland. This can grow to a large size and may need to be excised.

(continued)

TABLE 22-3   *(continued)*

Infection	Description
Tinea	A fungal skin disease resulting in itching, scaling lesions. Tinea pedis is also called athlete's foot. Diagnosis of tinea is made with the use of a Wood's light which are ultraviolet rays used to detect fluorescent materials in the skin and hair of patients with tinea. Topical treatment consists of fungicidal agents, such as griseofulvin.
Verruca	A benign neoplasm (tumor), which has a rough surface that is removed by chemicals and /or laser therapy, and is caused by a virus. Also called warts.

TABLE 22-4   Neoplasms

Benign (non-cancerous) Neoplasms	Description
Dermatofibroma	A fibrous tumor of the skin. It is painless, round, firm, red, and generally found on the extremities.
Hemangioma	Benign tumor of dilated vessels.
Keloid	The formation of a scar after an injury or surgery, which results in a raised, thickened, red area.
Keratosis	Overgrowth and thickening of cells in the epithelium located in the epidermis of the skin.
Leukoplakia	A change in the mucous membrane that results in thick, white patches on the mucous membrane of the tongue and cheek. It is considered precancerous and is associated with smoking.
Lipoma	Fatty tumor that generally does not metastasize (spread).
Nevus	A pigmented (colored) congenital skin blemish. It is usually benign but may become cancerous. Also called a birthmark or mole.

Malignant (cancerous) Neoplasms	Description
Basal cell carcinoma	An epithelial tumor of the basal cell layer of the epidermis. A frequent type of skin cancer that rarely metastasizes.
Kaposi's sarcoma	A form of skin cancer frequently seen in acquired immune deficiency syndrome (AIDS) patients. It consists of brownish-purple papules that spread from the skin and metastasize to internal organs.
Malignant melanoma	A dangerous form of skin cancer caused by an overgrowth of melanin in the skin. It may metastasize.
Squamous cell carcinoma	Epidermal cancer that may go into deeper tissue but does not generally metastasize.

TABLE 22-5   Diagnostic Procedures and Tests Relating to the Integumentary System

Procedure/Test	Description
Adipectomy	Surgical removal of fat.
Biopsy	Removal of a piece of tissue by syringe and needle, knife, punch, or brush to examine under a microscope as an aid in diagnosis.
Cauterization	The destruction of tissue with a caustic chemical, electric current, freezing, or hot iron.
Chemobrasion	Abrasion of the skin using chemicals. Also called a chemical peel.
Cryosurgery	The use of extreme cold to freeze and destroy tissue.
Curettage	The removal of superficial skin lesions with a curette or scraper.
Debridement	The removal of foreign material or dead tissue from a wound.
Dermabrasion	Abrasion or rubbing using wire brushes or sandpaper.
Dermatoplasty	The transplantation of skin. Also called skin grafting. May be used to treat large birthmarks (hemangiomas) and burns.
Electrocautery	To destroy tissue with an electric current.
Exfoliative cytology	Scraping cells from tissue and then examining them under a microscope.
Frozen section	Taking a thin piece of tissue from a frozen specimen for rapid examination under a microscope. This is often performed during a surgical procedure to detect the presence of cancer in a diseased organ.
Fungal scrapings (FS)	Scrapings taken with a curette or scraper of tissue from lesions are placed on a growth medium and examined under a microscope to identify fungal growth.
Incision and drainage (I & D)	Making an incision to create an opening for the drainage of material such as pus.
Laser therapy	Removal of skin lesions and birthmarks using a laser that emits intense heat and power at close range. The laser converts frequencies of light into one small beam.
Lipectomy	The surgical removal of fat.
Marsupialization	Creating a pouch to promote drainage by surgically opening a closed area, such as a cyst.
Needle biopsy	Using a sterile needle to remove tissue for examination under a microscope.
Plication	Taking tucks surgically in a structure to shorten it.
Rhytidectomy	Surgical removal of excess skin to eliminate wrinkles. Commonly referred to as a face lift.
Skin grafts	The transfer of skin from a normal area to cover another site. Used to treat burn victims and after some surgical procedures.
Sweat test	Test performed on sweat to see the level of chloride. There is an increase in skin chloride in some diseases, such as cystic fibrosis.

TABLE 22-6   Disorders of the Cardiovascular System

Disorder	Description
Anemia	A reduction in the number of circulating red blood cells per cubic millimeter of blood. It is not a disease but a symptom of disease.
Aneurysm	An abnormal dilation of a blood vessel, usually an artery, due to a congenital weakness or defect in the wall of the vessel.
Angina pectoris	Condition in which there is severe pain with a sensation of constriction around the heart. It is caused by a deficiency of oxygen to the heart muscle.
Angioma	Tumor, usually benign, consisting of blood vessels.
Angiospasm	Spasm or contraction of blood vessels.
Aortic aneurysm	Localized, abnormal dilation of the aorta, causing pressure on the trachea, esophagus, veins, or nerves. This is due to a weakness in the wall of the blood vessel.
Aortic insufficiency	A failure of the aortic valve to close completely which results in leaking and inefficient heart action.
Aortic stenosis	Condition caused by a narrowing of the aorta.
Arrhythmia	An irregularity in the heartbeat or action.
Arterial embolism	Blood clot moving within an artery. This can occur as a result of arteriosclerosis.
Arteriosclerosis	Thickening, hardening, and loss of elasticity of the walls of arteries.
Atherosclerosis	This is the most common form of arteriosclerosis. It is caused by the formation of yellowish plaques of cholesterol building up on the inner walls of the arteries.
Bradycardia	An abnormally slow heart rate (under 60 beats per minute).
Congenital heart disease	Heart defects that are present at birth, such as patent ductus arteriosus, in which the opening between the pulmonary artery and the aorta fails to close at birth. This condition requires surgery.
Congestive heart failure	Pathological condition of the heart in which there is a reduced outflow of blood from the left side of the heart. This results in weakness, breathlessness, and edema.
Coronary artery disease	A narrowing of the coronary arteries that is sufficient enough to prevent adequate blood supply to the myocardium.
Coronary thrombosis	Blood clot in a coronary vessel of the heart causing the vessel to close completely or partially.
Embolus	Obstruction of a blood vessel by a blood clot that moves from another area.
Endocarditis	Inflammation of the membrane lining the heart. May be due to microorganisms or to an abnormal immunological response.
Fibrillation	Abnormal quivering or contractions of heart fibers. When this occurs within the fibers of the ventricle of the heart, arrest and death can occur. Emergency equipment to defibrillate, or convert the heart to a normal beat, will be necessary.
Hypertensive heart disease	Heart disease as a result of persistently high blood pressure which damages the blood vessels and ultimately the heart.
Hypotension	A decrease in blood pressure. This can occur in shock, infection, anemia, cancer, or as death approaches.
Infarct	Area of tissue within an organ or part that undergoes necrosis (death) following the cessation of the blood supply.
Ischemia	A localized and temporary deficiency of blood supply due to an obstruction to the circulation.
Mitral stenosis	Narrowing of the opening (orifice) of the mitral valve which causes an obstruction in the flow of blood from the atrium to the ventricle on the left side of the heart.
Mitral valve prolapse (MVP)	Common and serious condition in which the cusp of the mitral valve drops back (prolapses) into the left atrium during systole.
Murmur	A soft blowing or rasping sound heard upon auscultation of the heart.
Myocardial infarction	Condition caused by the partial or complete occlusion or closing of one or more of the coronary arteries. Symptoms include a squeezing pain or heavy pressure in the middle of the chest. A delay in treatment could result in death. This is also referred to as MI or heart attack.
Myocarditis	An inflammation of the myocardial lining of the heart resulting in extremely weak and rapid beat, and irregular pulse.
Patent ductus arteriosus	Congenital presence of a connection between the pulmonary artery and the aorta that remains after birth. This condition is normal in the fetus.
Pericarditis	Inflammatory process or disease of the pericardium.
Phlebitis	Inflammation of a vein.
Reynaud's phenomenon	Intermittent attacks of pallor or cyanosis of the fingers and toes associated with the cold or emotional distress. There may also be numbness, pain, and burning during the attacks. It may be caused by decreased circulation due to smoking.
Rheumatic heart disease	Valvular heart disease as a result of having had rheumatic fever.
Tetralogy of Fallot	Combination of four symptoms (tetralogy), resulting in pulmonary stenosis, a septal defect, abnormal blood supply to the aorta, and the hypertrophy of the right ventricle. A congenital defect that is present at birth and needs immediate surgery to correct.
Thrombophlebitis	Inflammation and clotting of blood within a vein.
Thrombus	A blood clot.
Varicose veins	Swollen and distended veins, usually in the legs, resulting from pressure, such as occurs during a pregnancy.

TABLE 22-7 Diagnostic Procedures and Tests Relating to the Cardiovascular System

Procedure/Test	Description
Aneurysmectomy	The surgical removal of the sac of an aneurysm, which is an abnormal dilatation of a blood vessel.
Angiography	X-rays taken after the injection of an opaque material into a blood vessel. Can be performed on the aorta as an aortic angiogram, on the heart as an angiocardiogram, and on the brain as a cerebral angiogram.
Angioplasty	A surgical procedure of altering the structure of a vessel by dilating the vessel using a balloon inside the vessel.
Arterial blood gases	Measurement of the amount of oxygen (O_2), carbon dioxide (CO_2), and nitrogen in the blood. Also gives a pH reading of the blood. Blood gases are performed in emergency situations and provide valuable evaluation of cardiac failure, hemorrhage, and kidney failure.
Artery graft	A piece of blood vessel that is transplanted from a part of the body to the aorta to repair a defect.
Artificial pacemaker	Electrical device that substitutes for the natural pacemaker of the heart. It controls the beating of the heart by a series of rhythmic electrical impulses. An external pacemaker has the electrodes on the outside of the body. An internal pacemaker will have the electrodes surgically implanted within the chest wall.
Cardiac catheterization	Passage of a thin tube (catheter) through an arm vein and the blood vessels leading into the heart. It is done to detect abnormalities, to collect cardiac blood samples, and to determine the pressure within the cardiac area.
Cardiac enzymes	Complex proteins that are capable of inducing chemical changes within the body. Cardiac enzymes are taken by blood sample to determine the amount of heart disease or damage.
Cardiac magnetic resonance imaging (MRI)	A noninvasive procedure in which images of the heart and blood vessels are captured for examination to determine effects.
Cardiolysis	A surgical procedure to separate adhesions which involves a resection of the ribs and sternum over the pericardium.
Cardiorrhaphy	Surgical suturing of the heart.
Cardioversion	Converting a cardiac arrhythmia (irregular heart action) to a normal sinus rhythm using a cardioverter to give countershocks to the heart.
Commissurotomy	Surgical incision to change the size of an opening. For example in mitral commissurotomy, a stenosis or narrowing is corrected by cutting away at the adhesions around the mitral opening (orifice).
Coronary artery bypass surgery	Open-heart surgery in which a shunt is created to permit blood to travel around the constriction in coronary blood vessel(s).
Doppler ultrasonography	Measurement of sound-wave echoes as they bounce off tissues and organs to produce an image. Can assist in determining heart and blood vessel damage. Also called echocardiogram.
Electrocardiogram	Record of the electrical activity of the heart. Useful in the diagnosis of abnormal cardiac rhythm and heart muscle (myocardium) damage. This procedure is explained fully in Chapter 29.
Electrolytes	Measurement of blood sodium (Na), potassium (K), and chlorides (Cl).
Embolectomy	Surgical removal of an embolus or clot from a blood vessel.
Heart transplantation	Replacement of a diseased or malfunctioning heart with a donor's heart.
Holter monitor	Portable ECG monitor worn by the patient for a period of a few hours to a few days to assess the heart and pulse activity as the person goes through the activities of daily living. Used to assess a patient who experiences chest pain and unusual heart activity during exercise and normal activities when a cardiogram is inconclusive.
Lipoproteins	Measurement of blood to determine serum cholesterol and triglycerides.
Open-heart surgery	Surgery that involves the heart, coronary arteries, or the heart valves. The heart is actually entered by the surgeon.
Percutaneous balloon valvuloplasty	Insertion through the skin of a balloon catheter across a narrowed or stenotic heart valve. When the balloon is inflated, the narrowing or constriction is decreased.
Percutaneous transluminal coronary angioplasty (PTCA)	Method for treating localized coronary artery narrowing. A balloon catheter is inserted through the skin into the coronary artery and inflated to dilate the narrow blood vessel.
Phleborrhaphy	Suturing of a vein.
Prothrombin time	Measurement of the time it takes for a sample of blood to coagulate.
Stress testing	Method for evaluating cardiovascular fitness. The patient is placed on a treadmill or bicycle and then subjected to steadily increasing levels of work. An EKG and oxygen levels are taken while the patient exercises. The test is stopped if abnormalities occur on the EKG.
Treadmill test	Also called a stress test.
Valve replacement	Surgical procedure to excise a diseased heart valve and replace with an artificial valve.
Venography	X-ray of the veins by tracing the venous flow. Also called phlebography.

TABLE 22-8 Disorders of the Endocrine System

Disorder	Description
Acidosis	Excessive acidity of bodily fluids due to the accumulation of acids, as in diabetic acidosis.
Acromegaly	Chronic disease of middle-aged persons which results in an elongation and enlargement of the bones of the head and extremities. There can also be mood changes.
Addison's disease	A disease resulting from a deficiency in adrenocortical hormones. There may be an increased pigmentation of the skin, generalized weakness, and weight loss.
Adenoma	A neoplasm or tumor of a gland.
Cretinism	Congenital condition due to a lack of thyroid, which may result in arrested physical and mental development.
Cushing's syndrome	Set of symptoms which result from hypersecretion of the adrenal cortex. This may be the result of a tumor of the adrenal glands. The syndrome may present symptoms of weakness, edema, excess hair growth, skin discoloration, and osteoporosis.
Diabetes insipidus (DI)	Disorder caused by the inadequate secretion of the antidiuretic hormone ADH by the posterior lobe of the pituitary gland. There may be polyuria and polydipsia.
Diabetes mellitus (DM)	Chronic disorder of carbohydrate metabolism which results in hyperglycemia and glycosuria. Type I diabetes mellitus (IDDM) involves insulin dependency, which requires that the patient take daily injections of insulin. Type II (NIDDM) patients may not be insulin dependent.
Diabetic retinopathy	Secondary complication of diabetes mellitus (DM) which affects the blood vessels of the retina, resulting in visual changes and even blindness.
Dwarfism	Condition of being abnormally small. It may be the result of a hereditary condition or an endocrine dysfunction.
Gigantism	Excessive development of long bones of the body due to overproduction of the growth hormone by the pituitary gland.
Goiter	Enlargement of the thyroid gland.
Graves' disease	Disease that results from an over activity of the thyroid gland and can result in a crisis situation. Also called hyperthyroidism.
Hashimoto's disease	A chronic form of thyroiditis.
Hirsutism	Condition of having an excessive amount of hair on the body. This term is used to describe females who have the adult male pattern of hair growth. Can be the result of a hormonal imbalance.
Hypercalcemia	Condition of having an excessive amount of calcium in the blood.
Hyperglycemia	Having an excessive amount of glucose (sugar) in the blood.
Hyperkalemia	Condition of having an excessive amount of potassium in the blood.
Hyperthyroidism	Condition that results from over activity of the thyroid gland. Also called Graves' disease.
Hypothyroidism	Result of a deficiency in secretion by the thyroid gland. This results in a lowered basal metabolism rate with obesity, dry skin, slow pulse, low blood pressure, sluggishness, and goiter. Treatment is replacement with synthetic thyroid hormone.
Ketoacidosis	Acidosis due to an excess of ketone bodies (waste products) which can result in death for the diabetic patient if not reversed.
Myasthenia gravis	Condition in which there is great muscular weakness and progressive fatigue. There may be difficulty in chewing and swallowing and drooping eyelids. If a thymoma is causing the problem, it can be treated with removal of the thymus gland.
Myxedema	Condition resulting from a hypofunction of the thyroid gland. Symptoms can include anemia, slow speech, enlarged tongue and facial features, edematous skin, drowsiness, and mental apathy.
Thyrotoxicosis	Condition that results from overproduction of the thyroid gland. Symptoms include a rapid heart action, tremors, enlarged thyroid gland, exophthalmos, and weight loss.
von Rechlinghausen's disease	Excessive production of parathyroid hormone, which results in degeneration of the bones.

TABLE 22-9 Procedures and Tests Relating to the Endocrine System

Procedure/Test	Description
Basal metabolic rate (BMR)	Somewhat outdated test to measure the energy used when the body is in a state of rest.
Blood serum test	Blood test to measure the level of substances such as calcium, electrolytes, testosterone, insulin, and glucose. Used to assist in determining the function of various endocrine glands.
Fasting blood sugar	Blood test to measure the amount of sugar circulating throughout the body after a 12-hour fast.
Glucose tolerance test (GTT)	Test to determine the blood sugar level. A measured dose of glucose is given to a patient either orally or intravenously. Blood samples are then drawn at certain intervals to determine the ability of the patient to utilize glucose. Used for diabetic patients to determine their insulin response to glucose.
Parathyroidectomy	Excision of one or more of the parathyroid glands. This is performed to halt the progress of hyperparathyroidism.
Protein bound iodine (PBI) test	Blood test to measure the concentration of thyroxin (T4) circulating in the bloodstream. The iodine becomes bound to the protein in the blood and can be measured. This test is useful in establishing thyroid function.
Radioactive iodine uptake (RAIU) test	Test in which radioactive iodine is taken orally (PO) or intravenously (IV) and the amount that is eventually taken into the thyroid gland (the uptake) is measured to assist in determining thyroid function.

(continued)

TABLE 22-9 *(continued)*

Procedure/Test	Description
Radioimmunoassay (RIA) test	Test used to measure the levels of hormones in the plasma of the blood.
Serum glucose test	Blood test performed to assist in determining insulin levels and useful for adjusting medication dosage.
Thymectomy	Surgical removal of the thymus gland.
Thyroid echogram	Ultrasound examination of the thyroid which can assist in distinguishing a thyroid nodule from a cyst.
Thyroidectomy	Surgical removal of the thyroid gland. The patient is then placed on replacement hormone (thyroid) therapy.
Thyroid function tests	Blood tests used to measure the levels of T3, T4, and TSH in the bloodstream to assist in determining thyroid function.
Thyroparathyroidectomy	Surgical removal (excision) of the thyroid and parathyroid glands.
Thyroid scan	Test in which a radioactive element is administered which localizes in the thyroid gland. The gland can then be visualized with a scanning device to detect pathology such as tumors.
Total calcium	Blood test to measure the total amount of calcium to assist in detecting parathyroid and bone disorders.
Two-hour postprandial glucose tolerance test	Blood test to assist in evaluating glucose metabolism. The patient eats a high-carbohydrate diet and fasts overnight before the test. A blood sample is then taken two hours after a meal.

TABLE 22-10 **Disorders and Pathology of the Digestive System**

Disorder/Pathology	Description
Anorexia	Loss of appetite that can accompany other conditions such as a gastrointestinal (GI) upset.
Ascites	Collection or accumulation of fluid in the peritoneal cavity.
Bulimia	Eating disorder that is characterized by recurrent binge eating and then purging of the food with laxatives and vomiting.
Cholecystitis	Inflammation of the gallbladder.
Cholelithiasis	Formation or presence of stones or calculi in the gallbladder or common bile duct.
Cirrhosis	Chronic disease of the liver.
Cleft lip	Congenital condition in which the upper lip fails to come together. This is often seen along with cleft palate and is corrected with surgery.
Cleft palate	Congenital condition in which the roof of the mouth has a split or fissure. It is corrected with surgery.
Constipation	Experiencing difficulty in defecation or infrequent defecation.
Crohn's disease	Form of chronic inflammatory bowel disease affecting the ileum and/or colon. Also called regional ileitis.
Diverticulitis	Inflammation of a diverticulum or sac in the intestinal tract, especially in the colon.
Diarrhea	Passing of frequent, watery bowel movements. Usually accompanies gastrointestinal (GI) disorders.
Dyspepsia	Indigestion.
Emesis	Vomiting usually with some force.
Enteritis	Inflammation of only the small intestine.
Esophageal stricture	Narrowing of the esophagus which makes the flow of foods and fluids difficult.
Fissure	Cracklike split in the rectum or anal canal or roof of mouth.
Fistula	Abnormal tubelike passage from one body cavity to another.
Gastritis	Inflammation of the stomach which can result in pain, tenderness, nausea, and vomiting.
Gastroenteritis	Inflammation of the stomach and small intestine.
Halitosis	Bad or offensive breath, which is often a sign of disease.
Hepatitis	Inflammation of the liver.
Ileitis	Inflammation of the ileum of the small intestine.
Inflammatory bowel syndrome	Ulceration of the mucous membranes of the colon of unknown origin. Also known as ulcerative colitis.
Inguinal hernia	Hernia or outpouching of intestines into the inguinal region of the body. May require surgical correction.
Intussusception	Result of the intestine slipping or telescoping into another section of intestine just below it. More common in children.
Irritable bowel syndrome	Disturbance in the functions of the intestine from unknown causes. Symptoms generally include abdominal discomfort and an alteration in bowel activity.
Malabsorption syndrome	Inadequate absorption of nutrients from the intestinal tract. May be caused by a variety of diseases and disorders, such as infections and pancreatic deficiency.
Peptic ulcer	Ulcer occurring in the lower portion of the esophagus, stomach, and duodenum thought to be caused by the acid of gastric juices. Some peptic ulcers are now successfully treated with antibiotics.
Pilonidal cyst	Cyst in the sacrococcygeal region due to tissue being trapped below the skin.
Polyphagia	To eat excessively.
Polyps	Small tumors that contain a pedicle or footlike attachment in the mucous membranes of the large intestine (colon).
Reflux esophagitis	Acid from the stomach backs up into the esophagus causing inflammation and pain. Also called GERD (gastroesophageal reflux disease).

(continued)

TABLE 22-10 *(continued)*

Procedure/Test	Description
Regurgitation	Return of fluids and solids from the stomach into the mouth. Similar to emesis but without the force.
Ulcerative colitis	Ulceration of the mucous membranes of the colon of unknown source. Also known as inflammatory bowel disease.
Volvulus	Condition in which the bowel twists upon itself and causes an obstruction. Painful and requires immediate surgery.

TABLE 22-11   **Procedures and Tests Relating to the Digestive System**

Procedure/Test	Description
Abdominal ultrasonography	Using ultrasound equipment for producing sound waves to create an image of the abdominal organs.
Air contrast barium enema	Using both barium and air to visualize the colon on x-ray.
Anastomosis	Creating a passageway or opening between two organs or vessels.
Appendectomy	Surgical removal of the appendix.
Barium enema (Lower GI)	Radiographic examination of the small intestine, large intestine, or colon in which an enema containing barium is administered to the patient while the x-ray pictures are taken.
Barium swallow (Upper GI)	A barium mixture swallowed while x-ray pictures are taken of the esophagus, stomach, and duodenum used to visualize the upper gastrointestinal tract. Also called esophagram.
Colectomy	Surgical removal of the entire colon.
Cholecystectomy	Surgical excision of the gallbladder. Removal of the gallbladder through the laparoscope is a newer procedure with fewer complications than the more invasive abdominal surgery. The laparoscope requires a small incision into the abdominal cavity.
Cholecystogram	Dye given orally to the patient is absorbed and enters the gallbladder. An x-ray is then taken.
Choledocholithotomy	Removal of a gallstone through an incision into the bile duct.
Choledocholithotripsy	Crushing of a gallstone in the common bile duct. Commonly called lithotripsy.
Colonoscopy	A flexible fiberscope passed through the anus, rectum, and colon is used to examine the upper portion of the colon. Polyps and small growths can be removed during the procedure.
Colostomy	Surgical creation of an opening of some portion of the colon through the abdominal wall to the outside surface.
Diverticulectomy	Surgical removal of a diverticulum.
Endoscopic retrograde cholangiopancreatography (ERCP)	Using an endoscope to x-ray the bile and pancreatic ducts.
Esophagoscopy	The esophagus is visualized by passing an instrument down the esophagus. A tissue sample for biopsy may be taken.
Esophagram (barium swallow)	As barium is swallowed the solution is observed traveling from the mouth into the stomach over a television monitor.
Esophagogastrostomy	Surgical creation of an opening between the esophagus and the stomach. Also called Upper GI.
Esophagostomy	Surgical creation of an opening into the esophagus.
Exploratory laparotomy	Abdominal operation for the purpose of examining the abdominal organs and tissues for signs of disease or other abnormalities.
Fistulectomy	Excision of a fistula.
Gastrectomy	Surgical removal of a part of or whole stomach.
Gastrointestinal endoscopy	A flexible instrument or scope is passed either through the mouth or anus to facilitate visualization of the gastrointestinal (GI) tract.
Glossectomy	Complete or partial removal of the tongue.
Hemorrhoidectomy	Surgical excision of hemorrhoids from the anorectal area.
Hepatic lobectomy	Surgical removal of a lobe of the liver.
Ileostomy	Surgical creation of a passage through the abdominal wall into the ileum. The fecal material (stool) drains into a bag worn on the abdomen.
Intravenous cholangiogram	A dye is administered intravenously to the patient that allows for visualization of the bile vessels.
Intravenous cholecystography	A dye is administered intravenously to the patient that allows for visualization of the gallbladder.
Jejunostomy	Surgical creation of a permanent opening into the jejunum.
Lithotripsy	Crushing of a stone located within the gallbladder.
Liver biopsy	Excision of a small piece of liver tissue for microscopic examination. This is generally used to determine if cancer is present.
Liver scan	A radioactive substance is administered to the patient by an intravenous (IV) route. This substance enters the liver cells, and this organ can then be visualized. This is used to detect tumors, abscesses, and other hepatomegaly.
Supernumerary bone	An extra bone, generally a finger or toe, found in newborns.
Talipes	Congenital deformity of the foot. This is also referred to as a clubfoot.
Tumors: Benign	
• Epidermoid cyst	Cysts located in the skull and phalanges of the fingers.
• Ganglion cyst	Cyst found at the end of long bones.
• Giant cell tumor	Benign tumor that appears at the epiphysis but does not interfere with joint movement. It may become malignant or return after removal.

(continued)

TABLE 22-11 *(continued)*

Procedure/Test	Description
• Osteoblastoma	A benign lesion or tumor which is generally found on the spine, where it may result in paralysis.
• Osteochondroma	Tumor composed of both cartilage and bony substance.
• Osteoid osteoma	Painful tumor usually found in the lower extremities.
Malignant	
• Ewing's sarcoma	Malignant growth found in the shaft of the long bones that spreads through the periosteum. Removal is treatment of choice, as this tumor will metastasize or spread to other organs.
• Fibrosarcoma	Tumor that contains connective tissue that occurs in bone marrow. It is found most frequently in the femur, humerus, and jaw bone.
• Myeloma	Malignant neoplasm originating in plasma cells in the bone.
Whiplash	Injury to the bones in the cervical spine as a result of a sudden movement forward and backward of the head and neck. Can occur as a result of a rear-end auto collision.

TABLE 22-12   **Disorders and Pathology of the Lymphatic System**

Disorder/Pathology	Description
Acquired immune deficiency syndrome (AIDS)	A disease that involves a defect in the cell-mediated immunity system. A syndrome of opportunistic infections occur in the final stages of infection with the human immunodeficiency virus (HIV). This virus attacks T4 lymphocytes and destroys them, which reduces the person's ability to fight infection.
AIDS-related complex (ARC)	A complex of symptoms which appears in the early stages of AIDS. This is a positive test for the virus but only mild symptoms of weight loss, fatigue, skin rash, and anorexia.
Elephantiasis	Inflammation, obstruction, and destruction of the lymph vessels which results in enlarged tissues due to edema.
Epstein-Barr virus	Virus which is believed to be the cause of infectious mononucleosis.
Hodgkin's disease	Lymphatic system disease that can result in solid tumors in any lymphoid tissue.
Lymphadenitis	Inflammation of the lymph glands. Referred to as swollen glands.
Lymphangioma	A benign mass of lymphatic vessels.
Lyphoma	Malignant tumor of the lymph nodes and tissue.
Lymphosarcoma	Malignant disease of the lymphatic tissue.
Mononucleosis	Acute infectious disease with a large number of atypical lymphocytes. Caused by the Epstein-Barr virus. There may be abnormal liver function and spleen enlargement.
Multiple sclerosis	Autoimmune disorder of the central nervous system in which the myelin sheath of nerves is attacked.
Non-Hodgkin's lymphoma	Malignant, solid tumors of lymphoid tissue.
Peritonsillar abscess	Infection of the tissues between the tonsils and the pharynx. Also called quinsy sore throat.
Sarcoidoisis	Inflammatory disease of the lymph system in which lesions may appear in the liver, skin, lungs, lymph nodes, spleen, eyes, and small bones of the hands and feet.
Splenomegaly	Enlargement of the spleen.
Systemic lupus erythematosis (SLE)	A chronic autoimmune disorder of connective tissue that causes injury to the skin, joints, kidneys, mucous membranes, and nervous system.
Thymoma	Malignant tumor of the thymus gland.

TABLE 22-13   **Procedures and Tests Relating to the Lymphatic System**

Procedure/Test	Description
Bone marrow aspiration	Removing a sample of bone marrow by syringe for microscopic examination. Useful for diagnosing such diseases as leukemia. For example, a proliferation (massive increase) of white blood cells could confirm the diagnosis of leukemia.
ELISA	Enzyme immunoassay test used to test blood for an antibody to the AIDS virus. A positive test means that the person has been exposed to the virus. There may be a false-positive reading and then the Western blot test would be used to verify the results.
Lymphadenectomy	Excision of a lymph node. This is usually done to test for a malignancy.
Lymphangiogram	X-ray taken of the lymph vessels after the injection of dye into the foot. The lymph flow through the chest is traced.
Splenopexy	The artificial fixation of a movable spleen.
Tonsillectomy	The surgical removable of the tonsils. Usually the adenoids are removed at the same time. This procedure is known as a T & A.
Western Blot	The test that is used as backup to the ELISA blood test to detect the presence of the antibody to HIV (AIDS virus) in the blood.

TABLE 22-14 Disorders of the Musculoskeletal System

Disorder	Description
Arthritis	Inflammation of the bone joints.
Bunion	Enlargement of the joint at the base of the great toe caused by inflammation of the bursa of the great toe.
Bursitis	Inflammation of the bursa, the connective tissue surrounding a joint.
Carpal tunnel syndrome	Pain caused by compression of the nerve as it passes between the bones and tendons of the wrist.
Gout	Inflammation of the joints caused by excessive uric acid.
Kyphosis	Abnormal increase in the outward curvature of the thoracic spine. Also known as hunchback or humpback.
Lordosis	Abnormal increase in the forward curvature of the lumbar spine. Also known as swayback.
Muscular dystrophy	Inherited disease causing a progressive muscle weakness and atrophy.
Myasthenia gravis	An autoimmune disorder causing loss of muscle strength and paralysis.
Osteoarthritis	Noninflammatory type of arthritis resulting in degeneration of the bones and joints, especially those bearing weight.
Osteomalacia	Softening of the bones caused by a deficiency of phosphorus or calcium. It is thought that in children the cause is insufficient sunlight and vitamin D.
Osteomyelitis	Inflammation of the bone and bone marrow due to infection; can be difficult to treat.
Osteoporosis	Decrease in bone mass that results in a thinning and weakening of the bone with resulting fractures. The bones become more porous, especially in the spine and pelvis.
Paget's disease	A fairly common metabolic disease of the bone from unknown causes. It usually attacks middle-aged and elderly people and is characterized by bone destruction and deformity.
Polymyositis	A disease causing muscle inflammation and weakness from an unknown cause.
Rheumatoid arthritis	Chronic form of arthritis with inflammation of the joints, swelling, stiffness, pain, and changes in the cartilage that can result in crippling deformities.
Rickets	Deficiency in calcium and vitamin D in early childhood which results in bone deformities, especially bowed legs.
Ruptured intervertebral disk	Herniation or outpouching of a disk between two vertebrae—also called a slipped or herniated disk.
Scoliosis	Abnormal lateral curvature of the spine.
Spinal stenosis	Narrowing of the spinal canal causing pressure on the cord and nerves.

TABLE 22-15 Procedures and Diagnostic Tests Relating to the Musculoskeletal System

Procedure/Test	Description
Amputation	Partial or complete removal of a limb for a variety of reasons, including tumors, gangrene, intractable pain, crushing injury, or uncontrollable infection.
Anterior cruciate ligament (ACL) reconstruction	Replacing a torn ACL with a graft by means of arthroscopy.
Arthrocentesis	Removal of synovial fluid with a needle from a joint space, such as in the knee, for examination.
Arthrodesis	Surgical reconstruction of a joint.
Arthrography	Visualization of a joint by a radiographic study after injection of a contrast medium into a joint space.
Arthroplasty	Surgical reconstruction of a joint.
Arthroscopic surgery	Use of an arthroscope, a lighted instrument with camera/video capabilities, to facilitate performing surgery on a joint.
Arthrotomy	Surgically cutting into a joint.
Bone graft	Piece of bone taken from the patient that is used to take the place of a removed bone or a bony defect at another site, or to be wedged between bones for fusion of a joint.
Bone scan	Use of scanning equipment to visualize bones. It is especially useful in observing progress of treatment for osteomyelitis and cancer metastases to the bone.
Bunionectomy	Removal of the bursa at the joint of the great toe.
Carpal tunnel release	Surgical cutting of the ligament in the wrist to relieve nerve pressure caused by repetitive motion, for example typing (carpal tunnel disease).
Computerized axial tomography (CAT)	Computer-assisted x-ray used to detect tumors and fractures. Also referred to as CT-scan.
Electromyography	Study and record of the strength of muscle contractions as a result of electrical stimulation. Used in the diagnosis of muscle disorders and to distinguish nerve disorders from muscle disorders,.
Fasciectomy	Surgical removal of the fascia, which is the fibrous membrane covering and supporting muscles.
Laminectomy	Removal of the vertebral posterior arch to correct severe back problems caused by compression of the lamina.

(continued)

TABLE 22-15 *Continued*

Allergy	Description
Magnetic resonance imaging (MRI)	Medical imaging that uses radio-frequency radiation as its source of energy. It does not require the injection of contrast medium or exposure to ionizing radiation. The technique is useful for visualizing large blood vessels, the heart, brain, and soft tissues.
Menisectomy	Removal of the knee cartilage (meniscus).
Muscle biopsy	Removal of muscle tissue for pathological examination.
Myelography	Study of the spinal column after injecting opaque contrast material.
Photon absorptiometry	Measurement of bone density using an instrument for the purpose of detecting osteoporosis.
Reduction	Correcting a fracture by realigning the bone fragments. A closed reduction of the fracture is the manipulation of the bone into alignment and the application of a cast or splint to immobilize the part during the healing process. Open reduction is the surgical incision at the site of the fracture to perform the bone re-alignment. This is necessary when there are bone fragments to be removed.
Spinal fusion	Surgical immobilization of adjacent vertebrae. This may be done for several reasons, including correction of a herniated disk.
Total hip replacement	Surgical reconstruction of a hip by implanting a prosthetic or artificial joint.

TABLE 22-16 **Disorders and Diseases of the Nervous System**

Disorder/Disease	Description
Amnesia	Loss of memory in which people forget their identity as a result of head injury or a disorder, such as epilepsy, senility, and alcoholism. This can be either temporary or permanent.
Amyotrophic lateral sclerosis (ALS)	Disease with muscular weakness and atrophy due to degeneration of motor neurons of the spinal cord. Also called Lou Gehrig's disease, after the New York Yankees' baseball player who died from the disease.
Aneurysm	Localized abnormal dilatation of a blood vessel, usually an artery; the result of a congenital defect or weakness in the wall of the vessel.
Anorexia nervosa	Loss of appetite, which generally occurs in females between the ages of 12 and 21, due to a fear of obesity. The patient believes that she is fat even when thin. Psychiatric treatment may be necessary if the patient refuses to eat, since death can occur.
Aphasia	Loss of ability to speak.
Asthenia	Lack or loss of strength, causing extreme weakness.
Astrocytoma	Tumor of the brain or spinal cord that is composed of astrocytes.
Ataxia	Lack of muscle coordination as a result of a disorder or disease.
Autism	Form of mental introversion in which the patient, usually a child, shows no interest in anything or anyone except himself or herself.
Bell's palsy	One-sided facial paralysis caused by herpes simplex virus. The person cannot control salivation, tearing of the eyes, or expression but will usually recover.
Brain tumor	Intracranial mass, either benign or malignant. A benign tumor of the brain can be fatal since it will grow and cause pressure on normal brain tissue. The most malignant form of brain tumor in children is the glioma.
Cerebral palsy	Nonprogressive paralysis resulting from a defect or trauma at the time of birth.
Cerebrovascular accident (CVA)	Hemorrhagic lesion in the brain which can result in paralysis and the inability to speak.
Chorea	Involuntary nervous disorder that results in muscular twitching of the limbs or facial muscles.
Coma	Abnormal deep sleep or stupor resulting from an illness or injury.
Concussion	Injury to the brain that results from an illness or injury.
Convulsion (seizure)	Sudden severe involuntary muscle contractions and relaxations. These have a variety of causes, such as head injury, epilepsy, fever, and toxic conditions.
Encephalitis	Inflammation of the brain due to disease factors, such as rabies, influenza, measles, or smallpox.
Embolism	Obstruction of a blood vessel by a blood clot or foreign substance, such as air and/or fat.
Epidural hematoma	Mass of blood in the space outside the dura mater of the brain and spinal cord.
Epilepsy	A recurrent disorder of the brain in which convulsive seizures and loss of consciousness occurs.
• Grand mal	Severe seizures in which loss of consciousness and muscular contractions occur.
• Petit mal	Form of epilepsy in which there is an alteration in the level of consciousness but an absence of seizures or convulsions.
• Jacksonian	A localized form of epilepsy with spasms confined to one part or one group of muscles.
Glioma	Sarcoma of neurological origin.
Hematoma	Swelling or mass of blood confined to a specific area, such as in the brain.
Herniated nucleus pulposa	Protrusion of the nucleus pulposa of the intervertebral disk into the spinal canal. This is also called a herniated disk.
Huntington's chorea	Disease of the central nervous system that results in progressive dementia with bizarre involuntary movements of parts of the body.
Hydrocephalus	Accumulation of cerebrospinal fluid within the ventricles of the brain, causing pressure on the brain and for the head to be enlarged. It is treated by creating an artificial shunt for the fluid to leave the brain.
Meningioma	Slow-growing tumor in the meninges of the brain.
Meningitis	Inflammation of the membranes of the spinal cord and brain that is caused by a microorganism.

(continued)

TABLE 22-16 *(continued)*

Disorder/Disease	Description
Meningocele	Congenital hernia in which the meninges, or membranes, protrude through an opening in the spinal column or brain.
Multiple sclerosis	Degenerative, demyelination, inflammatory disease of the central nervous system in which there is extreme weakness and numbness.
Narcolepsy	Chronic disorder in which there is an extreme uncontrollable desire to sleep.
Neuritis	Inflammation of a nerve or nerves, causing pain.
Neuroblastoma	Malignant metastatic hemorrhagic tumor that originates in the sympathetic nervous system, especially in the adrenal medulla. Occurs mainly in infants and children.
Palsy	Temporary or permanent loss of the ability to control movement.
Paralysis	A temporary or permanent loss of the ability to control movement.
• Paraplegia	Paralysis of the lower portion of the body and both legs.
• Hemiplegia	Paralysis of only one side of the body. This is the same as hemiparesis.
• Quadriplegia	Paralysis of all four limbs. This is the same as tetraplegia.
Parkinson's disease	Chronic progressive disorder of the nervous system with fine tremors, muscular weakness, rigidity, and a shuffling gait.
Pica	An eating disorder in which there is a craving for material that is not food, such as clay, grass, wood, dirt, paper, soap, and plaster.
Reye's syndrome	A combination of symptoms that generally occurs in children under 15 years of age one week after they have had viral infection. It begins with a rash, vomiting, and confusion and may lead to coma, seizures, or respiratory arrest.
Shingles	Eruption of vesicles on the trunk of the body along a nerve path. Can be painful and generally occurs on only one side of the body. It is caused by the herpes zoster.
Spina bifida	Congenital defect in the walls of the spinal canal in which the laminae of the vertebra do not meet or close. May cause membranes and/or the spinal cord to herniate through the opening. This condition can also result in other defects such as hydrocephalus (fluid on the brain).
Subdural hematoma	Mass of blood forming beneath the dura mater of the brain.
Syncope	Fainting.
Tic douloureaux	Painful condition in which the trigeminal nerve is affected by pressure or degeneration. The pain is of a severe stabbing nature and radiates from the jaw and along the face.
Transient ischemic attack (TIA)	Temporary interference with blood supply to the brain, causing neurological symptoms, such as dizziness, numbness, and hemiparesis. May lead eventually to a full-blown stroke (CVA).

TABLE 22-17   Procedures and Tests Relating to the Nervous System

Procedure/Test	Description
Babinski's sign	Reflex test developed by John Babinski, a French neurologist, to determine lesions and abnormalities in the nervous system. The Babinski reflex is present, for a positive Babinski, if the great toe extends instead of flexes when the lateral sole of the foot is stroked. The normal response to this stimulation would be a flexion, or upward movement of the toe.
Brain scan	Injection of radioactive isotopes into the circulation to determine the function and abnormality of the brain.
Carotid endarterectomy	A surgical procedure for removing an obstruction within the carotid artery. It was developed to prevent strokes but is found to be useful only in severe stenosis with TIA.
Cerebral angiogram	X-ray of the blood vessels of the brain after the injection of radiopaque dye.
Cerebrospinal fluid shunts	Surgical creation of an artificial opening to allow for the passage of fluid. Used in the treatment of hydrocephalus.
Cordectomy	Removal of part of the spinal cord.
Craniotomy	Surgical incision into the brain through the cranium.
Cryosurgery	Use of extreme cold to produce areas of destruction in the brain. Used to control bleeding and treat brain tumors.
Echoencephalogram	Recording of the ultrasonic echoes of the brain. Useful in determining abnormal patterns of shifting in the brain.
Electromyogram	Written recording of the contraction of muscles as a result of receiving electrical stimulation.
Laminectomy	Removal of a vertebral posterior arch.
Lumbar puncture	Puncture with a needle into the lumbar area (usually the fourth intervertebral space) to withdraw fluid for examination and for the injection of anesthesia.
Nerve block	A method of regional anesthetic to stop the passage of sensory stimulation along a nerve path.
Pneumoencephalography	X-ray examination of the brain following withdrawal of cerebrospinal fluid and injection of air or gas via spinal puncture.
Positron emission tomography (PET)	Use of positive radionuclides to reconstruct brain sections. Measurement can be taken of oxygen and glucose uptake, cerebral blood flow, and blood volume.
Romberg's sign	Test developed to establish neurological function in which the person is asked to close their eyes and place their feet together. This test for body balance is positive if the patient sways when the eyes are closed.
Spinal puncture	Puncture with a needle into the spinal cavity to withdraw spinal fluid for microscopic analysis. Anesthetic is also administered by this route. This is also called a spinal tap.
Sympathectomy	Excision of a portion of the sympathetic nervous system. Could include a nerve or ganglion.
Transcutaneous electrical nerve stimulation (TENS)	Application of a mild electrical stimulation to skin electrodes placed over a painful area, causing interference with the transmission of the painful stimuli. Can be used in pain management to interfere with the normal pain mechanism.
Trephination	Process of cutting out a piece of bone in the skull to gain entry into the brain to relieve pressure.
Vagotomy	Surgical incision into the vagus nerve. Medication can be administered into the nerve to prevent its function.

TABLE 22-18   Common Disorders of the Eye

Disorder	Description
Achromatopsia	The condition of color blindness. This is more common in males.
Astigmatism	An eye disorder in which light rays are focused unevenly on the retina, resulting in a distorted image due to the abnormal curvature of the cornea.
Blepharitis	Inflammatory condition of the eyelash follicles and glands of the eyelids which results in swelling, redness, and crusts of dried mucus on the lids. This can be the result of allergy or infection.
Blepharochalasis	In this condition, the upper eyelid increases in size due to loss of elasticity, which is followed by swelling and recurrent edema of the lids. The skin may droop over the edges of the eyes when the eyes are open.
Cataract	Diminished vision resulting from the lens of the eye becoming opaque or cloudy. Treatment is usually surgical removal of the cataract.
Chalazion	A small, hard tumor or mass, similar to a sebaceous cyst, developing on the eyelid. This may require incision and drainage (I & D).
Conjunctivitis	An inflammation of the conjunctiva which is also called pinkeye.
Diabetic retinopathy	Small hemorrhages and edema that develop as a result of diabetes mellitus. Laser surgery and vitrectomy may be necessary for treatment.
Ectropion	Refers to an enversion (outward turning) of the eyelid, exposing the conjunctiva.
Entropion	Inversion (inward turning) of the eyelid.
Esotropia	Inward turning of the eye. An example of strabismus (muscle weakness of the eye).
Exophthalmus	Abnormal protrusion of the eyeball. Can be due to hyperthyroidism.
Esotropia	Outward turning of the eye. Also an example of strabismus (muscle weakness of the eye).
Glaucoma	Increase in intraocular pressure, which, if untreated, may result in atrophy (wasting away) of the optic nerve and blindness. Glaucoma is treated with medication and surgery. There is an increased risk of developing glaucoma in persons over 60 years of age, in people of African ancestry, after sustaining a serious eye injury, and in anyone with a family history of diabetes or glaucoma. Figure 22-8 [ID23-19] illustrates a glaucoma test.
Hemianopia	Loss of vision in half of the visual field. A stroke patient may suffer from this condition.
Hordeolum	Refers to a sty which is a small purulent inflammatory infection of a sebaceous gland of the eye. This is treated with hot compresses and, if necessary, surgical incision.
Hyperopia	With this condition a person can see things in the distance but has trouble reading material at close vision. It is also known as farsightedness.
Keratitis	Inflammation of the cornea.
Macular degeneration	Degeneration or deterioration of the macular area of the retina of the eye. It may be treated with laser surgery to destroy the blood vessels beneath the macula.
Myopia	With this condition a person can see things close up but distance vision is blurred. It is also known as nearsightedness.
Nystagmus	Jerky-appearing involuntary eye movement.
Presbyopia	Visual change due to aging, resulting in difficulty in focusing for near vision (such as reading).
Retinal detachment	A disorder that occurs when the two layers of the retina become separated or detached. The treatment is surgery.
Retinitis pigmentosa	Progressive disease of the eye which results in the retina becoming hard (sclerosed), pigmented, and atrophying (wasting away). There is no known cure for this condition.
Strabismus	An eye muscle weakness resulting in the eyes looking in different directions at the same time. (The eyes may be divergent or convergent). May be corrected with glasses, and/or surgery. Also called lazy eye, crossed eyes, or squint.
Trachoma	A chronic infectious disease of the conjunctiva and cornea caused by bacteria. This occurs more commonly in people living in hot, dry climates. Untreated, it may lead to blindness when the scarring invades the cornea. Trachoma can be treated with antibiotics.

TABLE 22-19   Procedures and Diagnostic Tests Relating to the Eye

Disorder	Description
Fluorescein angiography	The process of injecting a dye (fluorescein) to observe the movement of blood for detecting lesions in the macular area of the retina. This is used to determine if there is a detachment of the retina.
Gonioscopy	Use of an instrument called a gonioscope to examine the anterior chamber of the eye to determine ocular motility and rotation.
Keratometry	Measurement of the cornea using an instrument called a keratometer.
Laser Surgery	Surgical procedure performed with a laser handpiece that transfers light into intense, small beams capable of destroying or fixing tissue in place.
Slit lamp microscope	The instrument used in ophthalmology for examining the posterior surface of the cornea.
Tonometry	Measurement of the intraocular pressure of the eye using a tonometer to check for the condition of glaucoma. After a topical anesthetic is applied, the physician places the tonometer lightly upon the eyeball and a pressure measurement is taken. An air-puff tonometer similarly records the cornea's resistance to pressure, but uses more expensive equipment. This is generally part of a normal eye examination for adults.
Visual acuity	Measurements of the sharpness of a patient's vision. Usually a Snellen chart is used for this test and the patient identifies letters from a distance of 20 feet.
Vitrectomy	A surgical procedure for replacing the contents of the vitreous chamber of the eye.

TABLE 22-20 Common Disorders of the Ear

Disorder	Description
Acoustic neuroma	Benign tumor of the eighth cranial nerve sheath which can cause symptoms from pressure being exerted on tissues.
Anacusis	Total loss of hearing. Also called deafness.
Cerumen block	Ear wax causing a blockage in the external canal of the ear.
Conductive hearing loss	Loss of hearing as a result of the blocking of sound transmission in the middle ear or outer ear.
Meniere's disease	An abnormal condition within the labyrinth of the inner ear that can lead to a progressive hearing loss. The symptoms are dizziness or vertigo, hearing loss, and tinnitus (ringing in the ears).
Otitis media	Commonly referred to as a middle ear infection. This is seen frequently in children and is often preceded by an upper respiratory infection.
Otosclerosis	Progressive hearing loss caused by immobility of the stapes bone.
Presbycusis	Loss of hearing that can accompany the aging process.

TABLE 22-21 Procedures and Diagnostic Tests Relating to the Ear

Procedure/Test	Description
Audiogram	A chart that shows the faintest sounds a patient can hear during audiometry testing.
Audiometric test	A test of hearing ability by determining the lowest and highest intensity and frequencies that a person can distinguish. The patient may sit in a soundproof booth and receive sounds through earphones as the technician decreases and changes the volume or tones.
Falling test	A test used to observe balance and equilibrium. The patient is observed on one foot, then with one foot in front of the other, and then walking forward with eyes open. The same test is conducted with the patient's eyes closed. Swaying and falling with the eyes closed can indicate an ear and equilibrium malfunction.
Mastoid antrotomy	Surgical opening made in the cavity within the mastoid process to alleviate pressure from infection and allow for drainage.
Mastoid x-ray	X-ray taken of the mastoid bone to determine the presence of an infection, which can be an extension of a middle ear infection.
Myringoplasty	Surgical reconstruction of the eardrum.
Myringotomy	Surgical puncture of the eardrum with removal of fluid and pus from the middle ear, to eliminate a persistent ear infection and excessive pressure on the tympanic membrane. A tube is placed in the tympanic membrane to allow for drainage of the middle ear cavity.
Otoplasty	Corrective surgery to change the size of the external ear or pinna. The surgery can either enlarge or decrease the size of the pinna.
Otoscopy	The use of a lighted instrument (otoscope) to examine the external auditory canal and the middle ear.
Rinne and Weber tuning-fork tests	The physician holds a tuning fork, an instrument that produces a constant pitch when it is struck, against or near the bones on the side of the head. These tests assess both nerve and bone conduction of sound.
Sensorineural hearing loss	A type of hearing loss in which the sound is conducted normally through the external and middle ear but there is a defect in the inner ear or with the auditory nerve (eighth cranial nerve), resulting in the inability to hear.
Stapedectomy	Removal of the stapes bone to treat otosclerosis (hardening of the bone). A prosthesis or artificial stapes is implanted.
Tympanometry	Measurement of the movement of the tympanic membrane. Can indicate the presence of pressure in the middle ear.
Tympanoplasty	Another term for the surgical reconstruction of the eardrum. Also called myringoplasty.

TABLE 22-22 Common Disorders and Pathology of the Reproductive System

Disorder/Pathology	Description
Abruptio placenta	An emergency condition in which the placenta tears away from the uterine wall before the 20th week of pregnancy. This requires immediate delivery of the baby.
Amenorrhea	An absence of menstruation, which can be the result of many factors, including pregnancy, menopause, and dieting.
Breech presentation	Position of the fetus within the uterus in which the buttocks or feet are presented first for delivery rather than the head.
Carcinoma in situ	Malignant tumor that has not extended beyond the original site.
Cervical cancer	A malignant growth in the cervix of the uterus. This is an especially difficult type of cancer to treat, and causes 5 percent of the cancer deaths in women. PAP tests have helped to detect early cervical cancer.
Cervical polyps	Fibrous or mucous tumor or growth found in the cervix of the uterus. These are removed surgically if there is a danger that they will become malignant.
Cervicitis	Inflammation of the cervix of the uterus.

(continued)

TABLE 22-22 (continued)

Disorder/Pathology	Description
Choriocarcinoma	A rare type of cancer of the uterus which may occur following a normal pregnancy or abortion.
Condyloma	A wartlike growth on the external genitalia.
Cystocele	Hernia or outpouching of the bladder that protrudes into the vagina. This may cause urinary frequency and urgency.
Dysmenorrhea	Painful cramping that is associated with menstruation.
Eclampsia	Convulsive seizures and coma occurring between the 20th week of pregnancy and the first week of postpartum.
Ectopic	A fetus that becomes abnormally implanted outside the uterine cavity. This is a condition requiring immediate surgery.
Endometrial cancer	Cancer of the endometrial lining of the uterus.
Fibroid tumor	Benign tumor or growth that contains fiberlike tissue. Uterine fibroid tumors are the most common tumors in women.
Mastitis	Inflammation of the breast, which is common during lactation but can occur at any age.
Menorrhagia	Excessive bleeding during the menstrual period. Can be either in the total number of days or the amount of blood or both.
Ovarian carcinoma	Cancer of the ovary.
Ovarian cyst	Sac that develops within the ovary.
Pelvic inflammatory disease (PID)	Any inflammation of the female reproductive organs, generally bacterial in nature.
Placenta previa	When the placenta has become attached to the lower portion of the uterus and, in turn, blocks the birth canal.
Preeclampsia	Toxemia of pregnancy which if untreated can result in true eclampsia. Symptoms include hypertension, headaches, albumin in the urine, and edema.
Premature birth	Delivery in which the infant (neonate) is born before the thirty-seventh week of gestation (pregnancy).
Premenstrual syndrome (PMS)	Symptoms that develop just prior to the onset of a menstrual period, which can include irritability, headache, tender breasts, and anxiety.
Prolapsed uterus	A fallen uterus that can cause the cervix to protrude through the vaginal opening. It is generally caused by weakened muscles from vaginal delivery or as a result of pelvic tumors pressing down.
Rh factor	A condition developing in the baby when the mother's blood type is Rh-negative and the father's is Rh-positive. The baby's red blood cells can be destroyed as a result of this condition. Treatment is early diagnosis and blood transfusion.
Salpingitis	Inflammation of the fallopian tube or tubes.
Spontaneous abortion	Loss of a fetus without any artificial aid. Also called a miscarriage.
Stillbirth	Birth in which the fetus dies before or at the time of delivery.
Toxic shock syndrome	Rare and sometimes fatal staphylococcus infection that generally occurs in menstruating women.
Tubal pregnancy	Implantation of a fetus within the fallopian tube instead of the uterus. This requires immediate surgery.
Vaginitis	Inflammation of the vagina, generally caused by a microorganism.

TABLE 22-23 **Procedures and Diagnostic Tests Relating to the Female Reproductive System**

Procedure/Test	Description
Abortion	The termination of a pregnancy before the fetus reaches a viable point in development.
Amniocentesis	Puncturing of the amniotic sac using a needle and syringe for the purpose of withdrawing amniotic fluid for testing. Can assist in determining fetal maturity, development, and genetic disorders.
Cauterization	The destruction of tissue using an electric current, a caustic product, a hot iron, or freezing.
Cervical biopsy	Taking a sample of tissue from the cervix to test for the presence of cancer cells.
Cesarean section (C-section)	Surgical delivery of a baby through an incision into the abdominal and uterine walls.
Colposcopy	Visual examination of the cervix and vagina.
Conization	Surgical removal of a core of cervical tissue or a partial removal of the cervix.
Cryosurgery	Exposing tissues to extreme cold in order to destroy tissues. This procedure is used in treating malignant tumors, to control pain and bleeding.
Culdoscopy	Examination of the female pelvic cavity using an endoscope.
Dilation and curettage (D&C)	Surgical procedure in which the opening of the cervix is dilated and the uterus is scraped or suctioned of its lining or tissue. A D & C is performed after a spontaneous abortion and to stop excessive bleeding from other causes.
Doppler ultrasound	Using an instrument placed externally over the uterus to detect the presence of fibroid tumors to outline the shape of the fetus.
Endometrial biopsy	Taking a sample of tissue from the lining of the uterus to test for abnormalities.
Episiotomy	Surgical incision of the perineum to facilitate the delivery process. Can prevent an irregular tearing of tissue during birth.
Fetal monitoring	Using electronic equipment placed on the mother's abdomen to monitor the baby's heart rate and strength of uterine contractions during labor.
Hymenectomy	Surgical removal of the hymen.

(continued)

TABLE 22-23   *(continued)*

Procedure/Test	Description
Hysterectomy	Surgical removal of the uterus.
Hysterosalpingography	Taking an x-ray after injecting radiopaque material into the uterus and oviducts.
Hysteroscopy	Inspection of the uterus using a special endoscope instrument.
Intrauterine device (IUD)	A device inserted into the uterus by a physician for the purpose of contraception.
Kegel exercises	Exercises named after A.H. Kegel, an American gynecologist, who developed them to strengthen female pelvic muscles. The exercises are useful in treating incontinence and as an aid in childbirth.
Laparoscopy	Examination of the peritoneal cavity using an instrument called a laparoscope. The instrument is passed through a small incision made by the surgeon into the peritoneal cavity.
Laparotomy	Making a surgical opening into the abdomen.
Oophorectomy	Surgical removal of an ovary.
Panhysterectomy	Excision of the entire uterus, including the cervix.
Panhysterosalpingo-oophorectomy	Surgical removal of the entire uterus, cervix, ovaries, and fallopian tubes. Also called a total hysterectomy.
PAP (Papanicolaou) smear	Test for the early detection of cancer of the cervix named after the developer of the test, George Papanicolaou, a Greek physician. A scraping of cells is removed from the cervix for examination under a microscope.
Pelvic examination	The physical examination of the vagina and adjacent organs performed by a physician by placing the fingers of one hand into the vagina. A visual examination is performed using a speculum.
Pelvimetry	Measurement of the pelvis to assist in determining if the birth canal will allow the passage of the fetus for a vaginal delivery.
Pelvic ultrasonography	The use of ultrasound waves to produce an image or photograph of organ or fetus.
Pregnancy test	A chemical test on urine that can determine pregnancy during the first few weeks. This can be performed in the physician's office or with an at-home test.
Salpingo-oophorectomy	Surgical removal of the fallopian tube and ovary.
Tubal ligation	Surgical tying off of the fallopian tube to prevent conception from taking place. This results in the sterilization of the female.

TABLE 22-24   Disorders of the Male Reproductive System

Disorder	Description
Anorchism	A congenital absence of one or both testes.
Aspermia	The lack of, or failure to, eject sperm.
Azoospermia	Absence of sperm in the semen.
Balanitis	Inflammation of the skin covering the glans penis.
Benign prostatic hypertrophy	Enlargement of the prostate gland commonly seen in males over 50.
Carcinoma of the testes	Cancer of one or both testes.
Cryptorchidism	Failure of the testes to descend into the scrotal sac before birth. Generally, the testes will descend permanently before the boy is one year old. A surgical procedure called an orchidopexy may be required to bring the testes down into the scrotum permanently and secure them permanently. Failure of the testes to descend could result in sterility in the male.
Epididymitis	Inflammation of the epididymis which causes pain and swelling in the inguinal area.
Epispadias	Congenital opening of the male urethra on the dorsal surface of the penis.
Hydrocele	Accumulation of fluid within the testes.
Hypospadias	Congenital opening of the male urethra on the underside of the penis.
Impotent	Inability to copulate due to inability to maintain an erection or to achieve orgasm.
Perineum	In the male, the external region between the scrotum and the anus.
Phimosis	Narrowing of the foreskin over the glans penis which results in difficulty with hygiene. The condition can lead to infection or difficulty with urination. The condition is treated with circumcision, the surgical removal of the foreskin.
Prostate cancer	A slow-growing cancer that affects a large number of males after 50. The PSA (prostate-specific antigen) test is used to assist in early detection of this disease.
Prostatic hyperplasia	Abnormal cell growth within the prostate.
Prostatitis	An inflamed condition of the prostate gland which may be the result of infection.
Varicocele	Enlargement of the veins of the spermatic cord which commonly occurs on the left side of adolescent males. This seldom needs treatment.

TABLE 22-25 Procedures and Diagnostic Tests Relating to the Male Reproductive System

Procedure/Test	Description
Castration	Excision of the testicles in the male or the ovaries in the female.
Cauterization	Destruction of tissue with an electric current, a caustic agent, hot iron, or by freezing.
Circumcision	Surgical removal of the end of the prepuce or foreskin of the penis. Generally performed on the newborn male at the request of the parents. The primary reason is for ease of hygiene. Circumcision is also a ritual practiced in some religions.
Orchidopexy	Surgical fixation to move undescended testes into the scrotum, and attaching them to prevent retraction.
Prostatectomy	Surgical removal of the prostate gland.
Sterilization	Process of rendering a male or female sterile or unable to conceive children.
Transurethral resection of the prostate (TUR)	Surgical removal of the prostate gland by inserting a device through the urethra and removing prostate tissue.
Vasectomy	Removal of a segment or all of the vas deferens to prevent sperm from leaving the male body. Used for contraception purposes. A bilateral vasectomy would render the male sterile.
Semen analysis	This procedure is used when performing a fertility workup to determine if the male is able to produce sperm. Sperm is collected by the patient after abstaining from sexual intercourse for a period of three to five days. Also used to determine if a vasectomy has been successful. After a period of six weeks, no further sperm should be present in a sample from the patient.

TABLE 22-26 Sexually Transmitted Diseases

Disease	Description
Acquired immune deficiency syndrome (AIDS)	The final stage of infection from the human immunodeficiency virus (HIV). At present there is no cure.
Candidiasis	A yeastlike infection of the skin and mucous membranes which can result in white plaques on the tongue and vagina.
Chancroid	Highly infectious nonsyphilitic ulcer.
Chlamydial infection	Parasitic microorganism causing genital infections in males and females. Can lead to pelvic inflammatory disease (PID) in females and eventual infertility.
Genital herpes	Growths and elevations of warts on the genitalia of both males and females which can lead to cancer of the cervix in females. These painful vesicles on the skin and mucosa erupt periodically and can be transmitted through the placenta or at birth.
Genital warts	Growths and elevations of warts on the genitalia of both males and females which can lead to cancer of the cervix in females. There is currently no cure.
Gonorrhea	Sexually transmitted inflammation of the mucous membranes of either sex. Can be passed on to an infant during the birth process.
Hepatitis	Infectious, inflammatory disease of the liver. Hepatitis B and C types are spread by contact with blood and bodily fluids of an infected person.
Syphilis	Infectious, chronic, venereal disease that can involve any organ. May exist for years without symptoms.
Trichomoniasis	Genitourinary infection that is usually without symptoms (asymptomatic) in both males and females. In women the disease can produce itching and/or burning, a foul-smelling discharge, and results in vaginitis.

TABLE 22-27 Genetic Disorders

Procedure/Test	Description
Alopecia	Baldness in particular patterns, especially on the head.
Cooley's anemia	A rare form of anemia or a reduction of red blood cells which is found in some people of Mediterranean origin.
Cystic fibrosis	A disorder of the exocrine glands which causes these glands to produce abnormally thick secretions of mucus. The disease affects many organs, including the pancreas and the respiratory system. One reliable diagnostic test in children is the sweat test, which will show elevated sodium and potassium levels. There is presently no known cure for the disease, which can shorten the life span.
Down syndrome	A disorder which produces moderate-to-severe mental retardation and multiple defects. The physical characteristics of a child with this disorder are a sloping forehead, flat nose or absent bridge to the nose, low-set eyes, and a general dwarfed physical growth. The disorder occurs more commonly when the mother is over 40. Also called Trisomy 21.
Duchene muscular dystrophy	A muscular disorder in which there is progressive wasting away of various muscles, including leg, pelvic, and shoulder muscles. Children with this disorder have difficulty climbing stairs and running. They may eventually be confined to a wheelchair. Other complications relating to the heart and respiratory system can be present. It is caused by a recessive gene and is more common in males. This disorder often results in a shortened life-span.

(continued)

TABLE 22-27 *(continued)*

Procedure/Test	Description
Hemophilia	A bleeding disorder in which there is a deficiency in one of the factors necessary for blood to clot. There is an abnormal tendency to bleed, and victims of this disorder may require frequent blood transfusions. The female (mother) carries this recessive gene and it is passed on to males. Therefore, it is found almost exclusively in boys.
Huntington's chorea	A rare condition characterized by bizarre involuntary movements called chorea. The patient may have progressive mental and physical disturbances, which generally begin around 40.
Retinitis pigmentosa	Chronic progressive disease that begins in early childhood and is characterized by degeneration of the retina. This can lead to blindness by middle age.
Sickle cell anemia	Severe, chronic, incurable disorder that results in anemia and causes joint pain, chronic weakness, and infections. Occurs more commonly in people of Mediterranean and African heritage. The blood cell in this disease is sickle shaped.
Spina bifida	A congenital disorder that results in a defect in the walls of the spinal column, causing the membranes of the spinal cord to push through to the outside. It may be associated with other defects, such as hydrocephalus, which is an enlarged head as a result of the accumulation of fluid on the brain.
Tay-Sachs disease	A disorder caused by a deficiency of an enzyme, which can result in mental and physical retardation and blindness. It is transferred by a recessive trait and is most commonly found in families of Eastern European Jewish decent. Death generally occurs before the age of 4.

TABLE 22-28   Respiratory Disorders and Pathology

Procedure/Test	Description
Asthma	Disease caused by various conditions, such as allergens, and resulting in constriction of the bronchial airways and labored respirations. It can cause violent spasms of the bronchi (bronchospasms) but is not generally life-threatening. Medication can be very effective.
Atelectasis	A condition in which the lung tissue collapses, which prevents the respiratory exchange of oxygen and carbon dioxide. It can be caused by a variety of conditions, including pressure upon the lung from a tumor or other object.
Bronchiectasis	An abnormal stretching of the bronchi which results from a dilation of a bronchus or the bronchi that can be the result of an infection. The major symptom is a large amount of purulent (pus-filled) sputum. Rales (bubbling chest sounds) and hemoptysis (spitting up blood) may be present. This can be irreversible and may result in destruction of the bronchial walls.
Bronchitis	Inflammation of the mucous membranes of the bronchial tubes which results in a typical barking cough, fever, and **malaise** or discomfort.
Bronchogenic carcinoma	Malignant lung tumor that originates in the bronchi. It is usually associated with a history of cigarette smoking.
Chronic obstructive pulmonary disease (COPD)	Progressive, chronic, and usually irreversible condition in which the lungs have a diminished capacity for inspiration (inhalation) and expiration (exhalation). The patient may have difficulty breathing upon exertion (dyspnea) and a cough. Also called chronic obstructive lung disease.
Croup	An acute respiratory condition found in infants and children which is characterized by a barking type of cough or stridor.
Emphysema	Pulmonary condition that can occur as a result of long-term heavy smoking. Air pollution also worsens this disease. The patient may not be able to breath except in a sitting or standing position.
Empyema	Pus within the plural space, usually the result of infection.
Epistaxis	Nosebleed.
Histoplasmosis	A pulmonary disease from dust in the droppings of pigeons and chickens.
Hyaline membrane disease	Condition seen in premature infants whose lungs have not had time to develop properly. The lungs are not able to expand fully and a membrane (hyaline membrane) actually forms which causes extreme difficulty in breathing and may result in death. It is also known as infant respiratory distress syndrome (IRDS).
Laryngitis	Inflammation of the larynx (voicebox) causing difficulty in speaking.
Legionnaires' disease	Severe, often fatal disease characterized by pneumonia and gastrointestinal symptoms. It is caused by a gram-negative bacillus and named after people who came down with it at an American Legion Convention in 1976.
Paroxysmal nocturnal dyspnea	Attacks of shortness of breath (SOB) which occur only at night and awaken the patient.
Pertussis	Commonly called whooping cough, due to the "whoop" sound made when coughing. It is an infectious disease which children receive immunization against as part of their DPT shots.
Pleural effusion	The abnormal presence of fluid or gas in the pleural cavity. Physicians can detect the presence of fluid by tapping the chest (percussion) or listening with a stethoscope (auscultation).
Pleurisy	Inflammation of the pleura surrounding the lungs. The patient will experience pain upon inspiration due to friction caused by a rubbing of the pleural lining.
Pneumonia	Inflammatory condition of the lung which can be caused by bacterial and viral infections, diseases, and chemicals.
Pneumoconiosis	A condition that occurs as a result of inhaling environmental particles that become toxic. Can be the result of inhaling coal dust (anthracosis), or asbestos (asbestosis).

(continued)

TABLE 22-28 *(continued)*

Procedure/Test	Description
Pneumonomycosis	A disease of the lungs caused by a fungus.
Pneumothorax	Collection of air or gas in the pleural cavity which may result in collapse of the lung.
Pulmonary edema	Condition in which lung tissue retains an excessive amount of fluid. This results in labored breathing.
Pulmonary embolism	Blood clot or air bubble that moves to the pulmonary artery or one of its branches.
Respiratory distress syndrome (RDS)	Impairment of the respiratory function in premature infants due to immaturity.
Silicosis	A form of respiratory disease resulting from the inhalation of silica (quartz) dust. It is considered an occupational disease.
Sudden infant death syndrome (SIDS)	Unexpected and unexplained death of an apparently well infant.
Tracheostenosis	A narrowing and stenosis of the lumen or opening into the trachea.
Tuberculosis	An infectious disease caused by the tubercle bacillus, Mycobacterium tuberculosis. It most commonly affects the respiratory system and causes inflammation and calcification of the system. Tuberculosis is again on the uprise and is seen in many patients who have an impaired immune system, such as in AIDS.

TABLE 22-29 Procedures and Tests Relating to the Respiratory System

Procedure/Test	Description
Arterial blood gases	Testing for the gases present in the blood. This test is generally used to assist in determining the levels of oxygen (O_2) and carbon dioxide (CO_2) in the blood.
Bronchography	X-ray of the lung after a radiopaque substance has been inserted into the trachea or bronchial tube.
Bronchoplasty	The surgical repair of a bronchial defect.
Bronchoscopy	Using an instrument, the bronchoscope, to visualize the bronchi. During this procedure, tissue can be obtained for biopsy and foreign bodies can be removed.
Bronchotomy	A surgical incision of a bronchus, larynx, or trachea.
Cardiopulmonary resuscitation (CPR)	Emergency treatment provided by persons trained in CPR given to patients when their respirations and heart stop. CPR provides oxygen to the brain, heart, and other vital organs until medical treatment can restore a normal heart and pulmonary function. See an illustration of adult and infant CPR in Chapter 35.
Chest x-ray	Taking a radiographic picture of the lungs and heart from the back and front of the patient.
Endotracheal intubation	Placing a tube through the mouth to create an airway.
Heimlich maneuver	A technique for removing a foreign body from the trachea or pharynx by exerting diaphragmatic pressure.
Hyperbaric oxygen therapy	The use of oxygen under greater than normal pressure to treat cases of smoke inhalation, carbon monoxide poisoning, and other conditions. In some cases, the patient is placed in a hyperbaric oxygen chamber for this treatment.
Intermittent positive pressure breathing (IPPB)	A method for assisting the breathing of patients with a mask that is connected to a machine that produces an increased pressure.
Laryngectomy	The surgical removal of the larynx. This procedure is most frequently performed for excision of cancer.
Laryngoplasty	Surgical repair of the larynx.
Laryngoscopy	Examination of the interior of the larynx with a lighted instrument.
Lobectomy	Surgical removal of a lobe of the lung. Often the treatment of choice for lung cancer.
Pneumonectomy	The surgical removal of lung tissue.
Postural drainage	Drainage of secretions from the bronchi by placing the patient in a position that uses gravity to promote drainage. It is used for the treatment of cystic fibrosis, bronchiectasis, and before lobectomy surgery. May be combined with clapping and vibrating maneuvers to dislodge secretions.
Pulmonary angiography	Injecting dye into a blood vessel for the purpose of taking an x-ray of the arteries and veins of the lungs.
Pulmonary function test (PFT)	Breathing equipment used to determine respiratory function and measure lung volumes and gas exchange. Also called spirometry.
Rhinoplasty	Plastic surgery of the nose performed for cosmetic reasons and to facilitate breathing.
Sinus x-ray	An x-ray view of the sinus cavities from the front of the head.
Spirometry	Using a device to measure the breathing capacity of the lungs.
Sputum culture and sensitivity (CS)	Testing sputum by placing it on a culture medium and observing any bacterial growth. The specimen is then tested to determine antibiotic effectiveness.
Sputum cytology	Testing for malignant cells in sputum.
Throat culture	Removing a small sample of tissue or material from the pharynx and placing it upon a culture medium to determine bacterial growth.
Thoracentesis	The surgical puncture of the chest wall for the removal of fluids.
Thoracostomy	An insertion of a tube into the chest for the purpose of draining off fluid or air.
Tracheotomy	Surgical incision into the trachea to provide an airway. This is generally performed as an emergency procedure to provide oxygen.
Tuberculin skin tests (TB test)	Applying a chemical agent (Tine or Mantoux tests) under the surface of the skin to determine if the patient has been exposed to tuberculosis.

TABLE 22-30   Disorders and Diseases of the Urinary System

Disorder/Disease	Description
Anuria	No urine formed by the kidneys and a complete lack of urine excretion.
Bladder neck obstruction	Blockage of the bladder outlet.
Dysuria	Abnormal secretion of large amounts of urine.
Enuresis	Involuntary discharge of urine after the age by which bladder control should have been established. This usually occurs by the age of 5. Also called bed-wetting at night.
Glomerulonephritis	Inflammation of the kidney (primarily of the glomerulus). Since the glomerular membrane is inflamed, it becomes more permeable and this results in protein (proteinuria) and blood (hematuria) in the urine.
Hematuria	A condition of blood in the urine. This is a symptom of disease process.
Hypospadius	A congenital opening of the male urethra on the underside of the penis.
Interstitial cystitis	Disease of an unknown cause in which there is inflammation and irritation of the bladder. It is most commonly seen in middle-aged women.
Lithotomy	Surgical incision to remove kidney stones.
Meatotomy	A surgical enlargement of the urinary opening (meatus).
Nocturia	Excessive urination during the night. This may or may not be abnormal.
Pyelitis	Inflammation of the renal pelvis.
Pyelonephritis	Inflammation of the renal pelvis and the kidney. This is one of the most common types of kidney disease. It may be the result of a lower urinary tract infection that moved up to the kidney via the ureters. There may be large quantities of white blood cells and bacteria in the urine. Hematuria may also be present. This condition can occur whenever there is an untreated or persistent case of cystitis.
Pyuria	Presence of pus in the urine.
Renal colic	Pain caused by a kidney stone. This type of pain can be excruciating and generally requires medical treatment.

TABLE 22-31   Procedures and Tests Relating to the Urinary System

Procedure/Test	Description
Catheterization	The insertion of a sterile tube through the urethra and into the urinary bladder for the purpose of withdrawing urine. This procedure is used to obtain a sterile urine specimen and also to relieve distension when the patient is unable to void on their own. See Chapter 26 for procedure.
Cystography	The process of instilling a contrast material or dye into the bladder by catheter to visualize the urinary bladder.
Cystoscopy	Visual examination of the urinary bladder using an instrument called a cystoscope. The patient may receive a general anesthetic for this procedure.
Dialysis	The artificial filtration of waste material from the blood. It is used when the kidneys fail to function.
Excretory urography	Injection of dye into the bloodstream followed by taking an x-ray to trace the action of the kidney as it excretes the dye.
Hemodialysis	Use of an artificial kidney that filters the blood of a person to remove waste products. Use of this technique in patients who have defective kidneys is lifesaving.
Intravenous pyelogram (IVP)	An x-ray examination of the kidneys, ureters, and bladder by injecting a radiopaque dye into the circulatory system and tracing its route as it is excreted.
Lithotripsy	Destroying or crushing kidney stones in the bladder or urethra with a device called a lithotriptor.
Peritoneal dialysis	The removal of toxic waste substances from the body by placing warm chemically balanced solutions into the peritoneal cavity. This is used in treating renal failure and in certain types of poisonings.
Renal transplant	Surgical placement of a donor kidney.
Urinalysis	A laboratory test that consists of the physical, chemical, and microscopic examination of urine.
Urography	The use of a contrast medium to provide an x-ray of the urinary tract.

Abbreviations

AB,Ab	abortion	baso	basophil	CPD	cephalopelvic disproportion
ABG	arterial blood gases	BBB	bundle branch block (L for left; R for right)	CPR	cardiopulmonary resuscitation
AC	air conduction	BC	bone conduction	CRF	chronic renal failure
a.c.	before meals	BE	barium enema	CS	cesarean section
ACAT	automated computerized axial tomography	b.i.d.	twice a day	C&S	culture and sensitivity
Acc.	accommodation	BM	bowel movement	C-section	cesarean section (surgical delivery)
ACL	anterior cruciate ligament	BMR	basal metabolic rate	CSF	cerebrospinal fluid
ACLS	advanced cardiac life support	BP	blood pressure	C-spine	cervical spine film
ACTH	adrenocorticotropic hormone	BPH	benign prostatic hypertrophy	CTA	clear to auscultation
AD	right ear (O)	Broncho	bronchoscopy	CTS	carpal tunnel syndrome
ADH	antidiuretic hormone	BS	breath sounds; bowel sounds; blood sugar	CUC	chronic ulcerative colitis
ADL	activities of daily living	BUN	blood urea nitrogen	CV	cardiovascular
AF	atrial fibrillation	BX, bx	biopsy	CVA	cerebrovascular accident
AH	abdominal hysterectomy			CVP	central venous pressure
AI	aortic insufficiency	C1, C2, etc.	first cervical vertebra, second cervical vertebra, etc.	CWP	childbirth without pain
AIDS	acquired immune deficiency syndrome			Cx	cervix
AIH	artificial insemination homologous	Ca	calcium; cancer	CXR	chest x-ray
ALL	acute lymphocytic leukemia	CABG	coronary artery bypass graft	cyl.	cylindrical lens
ALS	amyotropic lateral sclerosis	CAD	coronary artery disease	cysto	cystoscopic exam
AMI	acute myocardial infarction	CAPD	continuous ambulatory peritoneal dialysis	D	diopter (lens strength)
AML	acute myelogenous leukemia	CAT, CT	computerized axial tomography	dB	decibel
Angio	angiogram	cath	catheterization	D/C	discontinue
ANS	autonomic nervous system	CBC	complete blood count	D&C	dilatation and curettage
A&P	auscultation and percussion	CBD	common bile duct	Derm	dermatology
AP, AP view	anterior-posterior; anteroposterior view	CC	clean-catch urine specimen	DI	diabetes insipidus
APB	atrial premature beat	CCU	coronary care unit; cardiac care unit	diff	differential
ARC	AIDS-related complex	CD4	protein on T-cell helper lymphocyte	DM	diabetes mellitus
ARD	acute respiratory disease			DOA	dead on arrival
ARDS	acute respiratory distress syndrome	CDH	congenital dislocation of the hip	DOB	date of birth
ARF	acute respiratory failure; acute renal failure	CGL	chronic granulocytic leukemia	DOE	dyspnea upon exertion
ARMD	age-related macular degeneration	c.gl.	correction with glasses	DPT	diphtheria, pertussis, tetanus injection
AROM	active range of motion	CHD	congestive heart disease	DSA	digital subtraction angiography
AS	aortic stenosis; arteriosclerosis; left ear (X)	chemo	chemotherapy	DTR	deep tendon reflex
		CHF	congestive heart failure	DT's	delerium tremens
ASCVD	arteriosclerotic cardiovascular disease	CHO	carbohydrate	DUB	dysfunctional uterine bleeding
ASD	atrial septal defect	chol	cholesterol	DVA	distance visual acuity
ASHD	arteriosclerotic heart disease	CIC	coronary intensive care	DVT	deep vein thrombosis
ASL	American Sign Language	CIS	carcinoma in situ	EBV	Epstein-Barr virus
Astigm.	astigmatism	CL	chloride	ECC	endocervical curettage
AU	both ears	CLL	chronic lymphocytic leukemia	ECCE	extracapsular cataract extraction
AV, A-V	atrioventricular	CNS	central nervous system	ECG; EKG	electrocardiogram
		c/o	complains of	E. coli	Escherichia coli
Ba	barium	CO2	carbon dioxide	EDC	estimated date of confinement
BaE	barium enema	COLD	chronic obstructive lung disease	EEG	electroencephalogram
				EENT	eyes, ears, nose, throat
		COPD	chronic obstructive pulmonary disease	EGD	esophagogastroduoden- oscopy
		CP	cerebral palsy; chest pain	ELISA	enzyme-linked immunosorbent assay
				EM	emmetropia (normal vision)

EMG	electromyography	h.s.	at bedtime	LP	lumbar puncture
ENT	ear, nose, and throat	HSG	hysterosalpingography	LUE	left upper extremity
EOM	extraocular movement	HSO	hysterosalpingoophrectomy	LUL	left upper lobe
eosin	eosinophil	HSV	herpes simplex virus	LUQ	left upper quadrant
ERCP	endoscopic retrograde cholangiopancreatography	HTN	hypertension	LVAD	left ventricular assist device
ERT	estrogen replacement therapy; external radiation therapy	Hz	Hertz	lymph	lymphocyte
		IBD	inflammatory bowel syndrome	mA	milliampere
ESR, SR	erythrocyte sedimentation rate	IC	intracardiac	MBC	minimal breathing capacity
EST	electric shock therapy	ICCE	intracapsular cataract cryoextraction	mCi	millicurie
ESWL	extracorporeal shock-wave lithotripsy	ICU	intensive care unit	mets	metastases
		I&D	incision and drainage	MH	marital history
ET	endotracheal	IDDM	insulin-dependent diabetes mellitus	MI	myocardial infarction; mitral insufficiency
FBS	fasting blood sugar	Ig	immunoglobins (IgA, IgD, IgE, IgG, IgM)	MICU	mobile intensive care unit
FEF	forced expiratory flow			mL	milliliter
FEKG	fetal electrocardiogram	IM	intramuscular	mmHg	millimeters of mercury
FEV	forced expiratory volume	I&O	intake and output	mono	mononucleosis; monocyte
FHR	fetal heart rate	IOL	intraocular pressure	MR	mitral regurgitation
FHT	fetal heart tone	IPD	intermittent peritoneal dialysis	MRI	magnetic resonance imaging
FS	frozen section				
FSH	follicle-stimulating hormone	IPPB	intermittent positive pressure breathing	MS	musculoskeletal; mitral stenosis; multiple sclerosis
FTND	full-term normal delivery	IRDS	infant respiratory distress syndrome	MSH	melanocyte-stimulating hormone
5-FU	5-fluorouracil	IRT	internal radiation therapy	MTX	methotrexate
FVC	forced vital capacity	IRV	inspiratory reserve volume	MV	minute volume
FX, fx	fracture	IUD	intrauterine device	MVA	motor vehicle accident
		IV	intravenous	MVP	mitral valve prolapse
Ga	gallium	IVC	intravenous cholangiogram	MVV	maximal voluntary ventilation
GB	gallbladder	IVCD	intraventricular conduction delay		
GH	growth hormone			MY	myopia
GI	gastrointestinal	IVP	intravenous pyelogram		
grav I	first pregnancy	IVU	intravenous urogram	Na	sodium
GSW	gunshot wound			NAD	no apparent distress
GTT	glucose tolerance test	JVP	jugular venous pulse	NB	newborn
GU	genitourinary			NCU	nongonococcal urethritis
gyn, gyne	gynecology	K	potassium	NED	no evidence of disease
		KB	knee bearing	NG	nasogastric (tube)
HAA	hepatitis-associated antigen	KS	Kaposi's sarcoma	NGU	nongonococcal urethritis
		KUB	kidneys, ureters, bladder	NHL	non-Hodgkin's lymphoma
HAV	hepatitis A virus	kV	kilovolt	NICU	neonatal intensive care unit
HBIG	hepatitis B immune globulin	kW	kilowatt	NIDDM	non-insulin-dependent diabetes mellitus
HBOT	hyperbaric oxygen therapy	L1, L2, etc.	first lumbar vertebra, second lumbar vertebra, etc.	NMR	nuclear resonance imaging
HBV	hepatitis B virus			NPDL	nodular, poorly differentiated lymphocytes
HCG	human chorionic gonadotropin	L&A	light and accommodation		
		LAC	laceration	NPH	neutral protamine Hegedorn (insulin)
HCI	hydrochloric acid	LAT, lat	lateral		
HCT, Hct, crit	hematocrit	LB	large bowel	NPO	nothing by mouth (nil per os)
		LBW	low birth weight		
HCV	hepatitis C virus	LDL	low-density lipoproteins	NSR	normal sinus rhythm
HD	hemodialysis; Hodgkin's disease	LE	left eye; lupus erythematosus; lower extremity	n&v	nausea and vomiting
				NVA	near visual acuity
HDL	high-density lipoproteins				
HgB, Hb, Hgh	hemoglobin	LGI	lower gastrointestinal series	O₂	oxygen
HGH	human growth hormone			OB	obstetrics
HIV	human immunodeficiency virus (causes AIDS)	LIF	left iliac fossa	OCG	oral cholecystography
		L K & S	liver, kidney, and spleen	OD	right eye (oculus dexter)
		ll	left lateral	OM	otitis media
HMD	hyaline membrane disease	LLE	left lower extremity	O&P	ova and parasites
HNP	herniated nucleus pulposa (herniated disk)	LLL	left lower lobe	ophth.	ophthalmology
		LLQ	left lower quadrant	ortho	orthopedics
H₂O	water	LMP	last menstrual period	OS	left eye (oculus sinister)
HRT	hormone replacement therapy	LOM	limitation of motion	Oto	otology

OU	each eye	RAI	radioactive iodine	T4	thyroxine; fourth thoracic vertebra; T-cell lymphocyte
		RAIU	radioactive active uptake		
P	pulse	RBC	red blood cell	T7	free thyroxine index; seventh thoracic vertebra
PA	posteroanterior view (radiology)	RD	respiratory disease		
		RDA	recommended daily allowance (dietary allowance)	T8	T-cell lymphocyte (cytotoxic or killer cell)
PAP	pulmonary arterial pressure; Papanicolaou test			T&A	tonsillectomy and adenoidectomy
para I	first delivery	RDS	respiratory distress syndrome	TAH	total abdominal hysterectomy
PAT	paroxysmal atrial tachycardia	RE	right eye	TB	tuberculosis
PBI	protein bound iodine	REM	rapid eye movement	TENS	transcutaneous electrical nerve stimulation
p.c.	after meals	RIA	radioimmunoassay		
PCP	*Pneumocystis carinii* pneumonia	RIF	right iliac fossa	TFS	thyroid function test
		RL	right lateral	THR	total hip replacement
PCV	packed cell volume (hematocrit)	RLL	right lower lobe	TIA	transient ischemic attack
		RLQ	right lower quadrant	t.i.d.	three times a day
PEG	percutaneous endoscopic gastrostomy; pneumoencephalogram	RML	right middle lobe; right mediolateral (episiotomy)	TKA	total knee arthroscopy
				TKR	total knee replacement
		ROM	range of motion	TLC	total lung capacity
PERLA	pupils equal, react to light and accommodation	RP	retrograde pyelogram	TNM	tumor, nodes, metastases
		RUL	right upper lobe	TPN	total parenteral nutrition
PET	positron emission tomography	RUQ	right upper quadrant	TSH	thyroid-stimulating hormone
Pe tube	polyethylene tube placed in the eardrum	S1	first heart sound		
		S2	second heart sound	TSS	toxic shock syndrome
PFT	pulmonary function test	SA, S-A	sinoatrial	TUR	transurethral resection
PGH	pituitary growth hormone	SBE	subacute bacterial endocarditis	TX	traction; treatment
pH	acidity or alkalinity of urine				
PID	pelvic inflammatory disease	SCLE	subacute cutaneous lupus erythematosus	U/A	urinalysis
PKU	phenylketonuria			UC	urine culture; uterine contractions
PMN, seg, poly	polymorphonuclear neutrophil	SEE-2	Signing Exact English		
		SG	skin graft; specific gravity	UCHD	usual childhood diseases
PMP	previous menstrual period	s. gl.	without correction or glasses	UE	upper extremity
PMS	premenstrual syndrome			UGI	upper gastrointestinal (x-ray) series
PND	paroxysmal nocturnal dyspnea; postnasal drip	SGOT	serum glutamic oxaloacetic transaminase		
				ung	ointment
PNS	peripheral nervous system	SIDS	sudden infant death syndrome	URI	upper respiratory infection
P.O.	per os (by mouth)			u/s	ultrasound
PP	postprandial (after meals)	SK	streptokinase	UTI	urinary tract infection
PPD	purified protein derivative (tuberculin test)	SLE	systemic lupus erythematosus	UV	ultraviolet
				UVR	ultraviolet radiation
prn	as required; as needed	SMD	senile macular degeneration		
PROM	passive range of motion			VA	visual acuity
prot.	protocol	SOB	shortness of breath	VC	vital capacity
PSA	prostate specific antigen	SOM	serous otitis media	VF	visual field
PT	prothrombin time	SPP	suprapublic prostatectomy	VLDL	very low-density lipoproteins
PTC	percutaneous transhepatic cholangiography	st	stage		
		stat	immediately	VPB	ventricular premature beat
PTCA	percutaneous transluminal coronary angioplasty	STD	skin test done; sexually transmitted diseases	VS	vital signs
				VSD	ventricular septal defect
PTH	parathyroid hormone	STSG	split-thickness skin graft		
PVC	premature ventricular contraction	Subcu	subcutaneous	WBC	while blood cell
		Subq	subcutaneous	WPW	Wolff-Parkinson-White syndrome
		SVT	supraventricular tachycardia		
q.d.	daily				
q.i.d.	four times a day			XRT	radiation therapy
		T1, T2, etc.	first thoracic vertebra, second thoracic vertebra, etc.	XX	female sex chromosomes
R	roentgen; also respiration			XY	male sex chromosomes
RA	rheumatoid arthritis; radium; right arm	T3	triiodothyronine; third thoracic vertebra	+	plus/convex
rad	radiation absorbed dose			−	minus/concave

Glossary

ABA number Code number on right upper corner of printed check to identify bank. (16)

abandonment To desert or leave a person, for example, when a physician discontinues treatment of a patient without providing coverage or sufficient notice of withdrawal. (5)

accession Record of numbers assigned to each new patient name. (13)

accounting The art or science of reporting the financial results of a business. (15)

accounts receivable Money owed to the physician/medical practice. (15, 16)

accreditation Process in which an institution (school) voluntarily completes an extensive self-study after which an accrediting association visits the school to verify the self-study statements. (1)

acquired immune deficiency syndrome (AIDS) Series of infections that occur as a result of infection by the human immunodeficiency virus (HIV) which causes the immune system to break down. (3)

active Medical files of patients who are currently being seen by the physician. These may cover from 1 to 5 years, depending on the office policy. (13)

active voice The subject of the sentence performs the action. (11)

acuity Clearness, sharpness (as of vision). (21)

acute condition Illnesses or injuries that come upon the patient suddenly and require treatment. (9)

addiction An acquired physical and psychological dependence on a drug. (31)

administrative Relating to the business functions of the physician's office. (1)

aerobes Microorganisms that are able to live only in the presence of oxygen. (25)

aerobic Microorganism which is able to live only in the presence of oxygen. (19)

affect A patient's mood or emotional state. (34)

age analysis A procedure for evaluating accounts receivable by age. (14)

agent Person who represents or acts on behalf of another person. (4)

agglutination Clumping. (25)

aggressive The practice of using a bold or pushy style when trying to convince the other person to agree with you. (7)

agranulocyte Type of white blood cell with a clear cytoplasm. (27)

alleged Asserted or declared without proof. (4)

allergen Any substance that triggers an allergic reaction. (34)

alphabetic Filing system based on the letters of the alphabet. (13)

alveoli Minute air sacs in lungs through which gas exchange takes place between alveolar air and pulmonary capillary blood. (20)

ambulatory care Refers to health service/facility which provides health care to individuals who are not hospitalized. (3)

ambulatory surgery A method for performing surgical procedures which allows the patient to walk into and out of the surgical facility on the same day. (23)

American Association of Medical Assistants (AAMA) Professional association for medical assistants that oversees program accreditation, graduate certification, and provides a forum for issues of concern to the physician. (1)

American Medical Association (AMA) Professional association for physicians which maintains directories of all qualified physicians, evaluates prescription and nonprescription drugs, advises congressional and state legislatures regarding proposed health care laws, and publishes a variety of scientific journals. (1)

American Medical Technologists (AMT) Professional association that oversees the registration of medical technologists. (1)

amplify To make more powerful, increase sound. (21)

amplitude Degree of variation from zero or the baseline, up or down, in recording electrical output of the heart. Also called voltage. (29)

anaerobes Microorganisms able to survive without oxygen. (25)

anaerobic Microorganism which thrives best or lives without oxygen. (19)

anaphylactic shock A life-threatening reaction to certain foods, drugs, and insect bites in some people. This can cause respiratory distress, edema, rash, convulsions, and eventually unconsciousness and death if emergency treatment is not given. (22, 31)

anemia Decrease in the number of circulating red blood cells. (27)

anesthesia Partial or complete loss of sensation. (2, 23)

aneurysm A weakening or out-pouching in the wall of an artery. (34)

angiography X-ray visualization of the heart and blood vessels after the injection of a radiopaque material into the blood vessels. (28)

anorexia Loss of appetite. (21)

antecubital fossa/space Area formed at the inside bend of the elbow. (20)

anthrax A deadly infectious disease caused by *Bacillus anthracis*. Humans contract the disease from infected animal hair, hides, or waste. (2)

anthropometric Refers to measurements of the human body such as height and weight. (21)

anthropometry Science of measuring the human body as to size of component parts, height, and weight. (20)

antibodies Proteins that defend the body against infection. (27)

anticoagulant Substance which prevents blood from clotting (EDTA and heparin). (27)

antigen Foreign substance which stimulates the production of antibodies. (27)

antipyretic Substance that reduces fever. (20)

apothecary system A system of weights and measures, used by physicians and pharmacists, that is based on these basic units of measurements: grain (gr.), gram (g), and dram (℥), for example. This system has been replaced by the metric system whenever possible. (32)

appellant A person who appeals a court decision by going to a higher court. (5)

archived File or information that has been placed in storage. (9)

archives Records that are no longer needed, such as when a patient dies, but must be kept for legal purposes. (13)

aromatic Pleasant, natural odor. (26)

arraignment Calling someone before a court of law to answer a charge. (5)

arrhythmia Irregular pulse or heart rate. (20, 29)

artifact(s) In reference to EKGs, these are deflections caused by electrical activity other than from the heart; irregular and erratic markings. (29)

artificial insemination Placement of semen into the vagina by means other than through sexual intercourse. (4)

artificial insemination donor (AID) An insemination procedure that uses the semen of a man other than the husband or partner. (4)

artificial insemination husband (AIH) An insemination procedure that uses the husband's semen. (4)

aseptic Germ free. (19)

asphyxia Suffocation, inability to breathe. (34)

aspirated Drawn in or out, by means of a vacuum. For example, a substance or an object being aspirated, or sucked, into the lungs. (34)

assertive The practice of declaring a point in a positive manner. (7)

assessment Evaluation. (7)

assignment of benefits Patient's written authorization giving the insurance company the right to pay the physician directly for billed charges. (14, 17)

asymptomatic Without having any symptoms; symptom free. (20)

attitude Refers to behavior indicating a specific mental attitude, either positive or negative, for example caring and supportive or overbearing and critical. (36)

atypical Unusual; out of the ordinary. (20)

audit An examination, usually by an accountant, of financial records of a medical practice for the purpose of determining the accuracy of the records. (15)

aural Pertaining to the ear or hearing. (20)

auscultatory gap Total loss of sound during phase II of the Korotkoff sounds while taking blood pressure. The sound later reoccurs. This is considered abnormal. (20)

autopsy An examination of organs and tissues in a deceased body to determine the cause of death. (2)

axilla The armpit. (21)

axillary Pertaining to the armpit or area under the arm. (20)

bacteria Microorganism capable of causing disease. (2)

bactericidal Ability to destroy disease-causing bacteria. (19)

baseline No electrical charge or activity; return to zero; flat on electrocardiogram recording. Also known as isoelectric line. (29)

benefit period Period of time for which payments for Medicare inpatient hospital benefits are available. (17)

benign Non-threatening, non-cancerous. (22, 34)

biopsy The removal of tissue for purposes of determining the presence of cancerous (malignant) cells. (23)

bipolar disorder Manic-depressive mental disorder. (24)

blind ad Classified advertisement for a position in which only a post office box number is listed. (36)

block Style of letter writing in which all lines are flush with the left margin. (11)

blood culture Culture used in the diagnosis of specific diseases, which consists of withdrawing blood from a vein, placing it in or upon suitable culture media to promote growth, and determining if there is actual growth. (25)

blood relative Related to another person by direct birth lineage. (21)

blood stasis Lack of circulation due to a stoppage of blood flow. (20)

bloodborne pathogens Disease producing microorganisms transmitted by means of blood and body fluids containing blood. (10, 19)

body mechanics Methods of standing and lifting objects in order to avoid injury and fatigue. (10)

bookkeeping Process of maintaining the accounts for the medical office. (15)

borderline hypertension Blood pressure which becomes gradually elevated over a period of time until it borders the edge of high blood pressure. A blood pressure of approximately 140/88 is considered borderline hypertension. (21)

bradycardic Pertaining to an abnormally slow heart rate (< 60 beats/minute). (34)

breach of contract Failure to comply with all the terms in a valid contract. (5)

breach (neglect) of duty Neglect or failure to perform an obligation. (5)

broad-spectrum The ability of a drug to be effective against a wide range of microorganisms. (31)

buffy coat The white colored layer which forms between the packed red blood cells and the plasma after centrifuging a whole blood sample; composed of white blood cells and platelets. (37)

bulimia Eating disorder characterized by recurrent binge eating and then purging the food with laxatives and vomiting. (21)

Bureau of Narcotics and Dangerous Drugs (BNDD) An agency of the federal government, used to enforce drug control. (31)

cadaver A dead body; a corpse. (2)

caduceus Symbol for healing made up of a staff with two snakes coiled around it which has become the recognized symbol for medicine. (2)

canceled checks Deposited checks that have been processed by the bank. (16)

capillaries Tiny blood vessels which connect arterioles and venules. (27)

cardiac cycle Time from the beginning of one beat of the heart to the beginning of the next beat, including the systole (contraction) and diastole (relaxation). (20); One heartbeat, designated arbitrarily as P, Q, R, S, and T, consisting of contraction and relaxation of both atria and ventricles; one pulse. (29)

cardiac rate Pulse rate, number of beats or contractions per minute. (29)

cardiogenic Pertaining to the heart. For example, shock related to heart failure. (34)

carrier(s) Individual who is unaware he or she has a disease but is capable of transmitting it to someone else. (For example "Typhoid Mary," who legend has it, spread the disease typhoid.) (19)

case law Law that is based on precedent—principles established in prior cases. (5)

catheterization Inserting a sterile tube into the bladder to withdraw urine or into a vein for a procedure. (26)

caustic Capable of burning or eating away tissue. (10)

censure To find fault with, criticize, or condemn. (4)

centigrade or Celsius Scale for measurement of temperature in which 0° C is the freezing point of water and 100° C is the boiling point of water at sea level. (20)

centrifuge An instrument used to separate blood into its liquid and solid components. (27)

cerebrovascular accident (CVA) Hemorrhage within the brain which may result in paralysis and loss of speech. (24)

certification The issuance by an official body of a certificate to a person indicating that he or she has been evaluated and has met certain standards. (1)

certified Guaranteed. (16)

certified medical assistant (CMA) A multiskilled health care professional who assists providers in an allied health care setting and who has successfully completed the CMA certification examination validating his or her credentials. (1)

channel(s) On a machine capable of receiving more than one signal at once, a channel is the pathway for one signal. (29)

chemotherapy Use of chemicals, including drugs, to treat or control infections and diseases; commonly used to treat cancer by killing the cells. (2, 31)

cholera Acute infection involving the small bowel which causes severe diarrhea. (2)

chronological Arrangement of events in the order of their occurrence. (36)

circumcised Foreskin surrounding the glans penis has been removed surgically. (26)

citation To quote an authority. (18)

civil case Court action between private parties, corporations, or government bodies not involving a crime. (5)

claim Written and documented request for reimbursement of an eligible expense under an insurance plan. (17)

claustrophobia Fear of closed-in or narrow spaces. (28)

clinical Relating to the medical treatment and care of patients. (1)

closed Medical files of patients who have indicated that they are no longer patients or who have died. These files are kept in storage for legal reasons. (13)

code of ethics Statement of principles or guidelines for moral behavior. (4)

coding Transferring narrative description of diseases and procedures into number coinsurance insurance plan pays a percentage of eligible benefits after a deductible has been paid. (17)

coinsurance A cost-sharing provision requires the insured to assume a portion of the cost of covered services.

collating Collect in one file all materials pertaining to a patient, and group this information by category, for example, progress notes and laboratory reports. (8)

colleague(s) A fellow member of a profession. (18)

colostomy An artificial opening created surgically into the large bowel for the removal of waste (feces). (24)

competent Qualified to make decisions about one's affairs. (5)

complex Multiple waves or deflections occurring in a group. (29)

condescending To assume an air of superiority. (7)

confidentiality Keeping private information about a person (patient) and not disclosing it to a third party without the patient's written consent. (1)

consent To give permission, approve, or allow as when a person gives permission to be examined and/or treated by authorized medical personnel. Consent may be written, verbal, informed, or implied (for example, rolling up one's sleeve to have blood drawn). (5)

consent, implied Inference by signs, inaction, or silence that consent has been granted. (5)

consent, informed Patient's consent to undergo surgery or treatment based on knowledge and understanding of the potential risks and benefits provided by the physician before the procedure is performed. (5)

consideration Inducement or benefit that compels a person to enter into a contract. (5)

contagious Diseases which can be transmitted from one person to another. (22)

continuing education units (CEUs) Credit awarded for additional course work beyond certification in order to remain current in one's field or for recertification. (1)

contract Agreement between two or more persons which creates an obligation to perform or not perform some action or service. (5)

contraindicated A condition in which the use of a drug should not be used. (31)

convulsions Involuntary muscle contractions that may alternate between contraction and relaxation of muscles. May be generalized or localized (focal) and may be followed by a period of unresponsiveness. (34)

copay A medical insurance plan which requires the patient pay a designated amount or percentage (for example $10 or 20%) of a bill for medical services or medication. This amount is usually collected at time of service. The rest of the bill (in this example 80%) is paid by the insurance company. (8)

copayment (copay) Amount specified by an insurance plan that the patient must pay before the plan pays (commonly used in managed care plans). (17)

CPU Central processing unit. (12)

credit(s) Funds added to an account. (16)

criminal case Court action brought by the state against persons or groups of people accused of committing a crime, resulting in a fine or imprisonment if found guilty. (5)

criteria Standards against which something is compared to make a decision or judgment. (6)

crossover claim Patient is eligible for both Medicare and Medicaid (also called Medi/Medi.). (17)

croup An acute viral infection of the upper and lower respiratory tract in children which may result in difficult, noisy breathing. (20)

cryosurgery Use of freezing temperatures from a probe to destroy abnormal cells. (23)

culture(s) The propagation of microorganisms or of living tissue cells in special media that are conducive to their growth, and/or the process by which organisms are grown on media and identified. (25)

Culturette Self-contained culturing packet system that readily adapts to most office specimen collections from the throat, nose, eye, ear, rectum, wound, and urogenital sites; it has a sterile, disposable plastic tube containing a cotton-tipped applicator swab and a sealed ampule of

Stuart's holding medium. (25)

cumulative Each exposure to a substance is added to the effect of all previous exposures. (28)

cumulative action The action that occurs in the body when a drug is allowed to accumulate or stay in the body. (31)

currency Paper money. (16)

cyanosis Bluish discoloration of the skin and mucous membranes due to oxygen deprivation; Bluish coloration to the skin or mucous membranes due to insufficient oxygen getting to the lungs. This may be caused by heart or respiratory disease. (20, 21)

cytology The science that deals with the formation, structure, and function of cells. (25)

damages Compensation for a loss or injury. (5)

data Statistics, figures, or information. (6)

debit(s) Charges against an account. (16)

deductible Amount of eligible charges each patient must pay each calendar year before the plan begins to pay benefits. (17)

defendant Person or group of persons who are accused in a court of law. (5)

defensive behavior Conscious or unconscious reaction to a perceived threat. (7)

deflection Deviation, up or down, from zero or the isoelectric line.

dehydration Loss of body water which can become life-threatening if not corrected. (27)

demographic Data relating to descriptive information such as age, gender, ethnic background, and education. (8)

depolarization, atrial Discharge of electrical activity in the upper heart chambers. (29)

depolarization, ventricular Discharge of electrical activity in the lower chambers. (29)

depolarized (depolarization) Discharge of electrical activity that precedes contraction. (29)

deposit To place money (cash and/or checks) into a bank account. (16)

deposition Written statement of oral testimony that is made before a public officer of the court to be used in a lawsuit. (5)

diagnose To determine the cause and nature of a pathological condition. (21)

diagnostic A type of test, series of tests, or an evaluation to determine the extent of an illness or disease. (30)

Diagnostic Related Groups (DRGs) Designations used to identify reimbursement per condition in a hospital. Used for Medicare patients. (3)

diaphragm Musculofibrous partition

that separates the thoracic and abdominal cavities. (20)

diastole   Period in the cardiac cycle during which the heart is relaxed and the heart cavities are being refilled with blood. (20)

diathermy   Use of heat-inducing wavelengths to provide muscle relaxation and therapy. (30)

differential diagnosis   A distinction between two or more alternative diagnoses. (21)

digestion   The process by which food is broken down mechanically and chemically in the alimentary canal. (33)

dilute   To weaken the strength of a substance by the addition of something else. (31)

disbursement   Payment of funds (money). (16)

discriminatory   To set someone apart or act with prejudice against a group. (18)

disk   Storage medium for data and software. (12)

dot matrix printers   Impact printers that produce characters by impacting small dots onto the paper's surface; capable of producing graphic images as well as text material. (12)

draft   A preliminary version of a writing. (18)

drug tolerance   A decrease in susceptibility to a drug after the continued use of the drug. (31)

duty   Obligation or responsibility. (5)

dyspnea   Difficult or labored breathing. (21)

dysuria   Painful urination. (21)

editing   Rearranging or restatement of a word or group of words in a document. (13)

electrocardiogram   Record of electrical activity of the heart; voltage with respect to time. (29)

electrocardiograph   Machine used to record electrical activity of the heart. (29)

electrode   Device that detects electrical charges. Also know as sensor. (29)

electrolyte(s)   Ionized salts in the blood, such as Na, K, and Cl. (27); Material applied to the skin to enhance contact between skin and the sensor. (29)

emancipated minor   Person under the age of 18 who is free of parental care and financially responsible for herself or himself. (5)

embezzlement   To take money by breach of trust. (16)

empathy   The ability to imagine how another person is feeling. (7)

emphysema   Abnormal pulmonary condition with loss of lung elasticity resulting in overinflation of the lungs and difficulty exhaling—"barrel chest." (20)

endocardium   Lining of the heart. (29)

erythemia   Redness of the skin. (30)

erythrocyte   A red blood cell (RBC). (27)

Escherichia coli (E. coli)   A bacillus present in the colon or intestinal tract. Can cause infections when it is present in the urinary tract. (26)

ethics   Principles and guides for moral behavior. (4)

evaluation   Assessment or judgment. (6)

expert witness   A medical practitioner who through education, training, or experience has special knowledge about a subject and gives testimony about that subject in court, usually for a fee. (5)

expulsion   The act of forcing out. (4)

externship   On-the-job training without payment generally performed while still attending school. (36)

extracurricular   Activities performed in addition to the usual academic requirements. (36)

exudate   Accumulation of fluid, pus, or serum in a cavity or tissue which may become hard and crusty. (30)

facsimile (fax)   An electronically transmitted document containing print and/or graphic information. (8)

Fahrenheit   Scale for measurement of temperature in which the boiling point of water is 212° F and the freezing point of water is 32° F at sea level. (20)

feces   Evacuation of the bowels. Also referred to as stool. (25)

fee schedule   Schedule of the amount paid by a specific insurance company for each procedure or service. Amounts are determined by a claims administrator and applied to claims subject to the fee schedule of a provider's managed care contract. (17)

fee splitting   Unethical sharing of a fee with another physician based on services other than medical services performed, for example, patient referral. (4)

feedback   Any response to a communication. (7)

felony   A crime more serious than a misdemeanor carrying a penalty of death or imprisonment. (5)

ferrous   Containing iron. (34)

fetid   Foul odor. (26)

fire extinguisher   Canister containing material capable of putting out many types of fires including paper, electrical, wood, and cloth. (10)

first morning specimen   The first voided urine of the day upon arising. (26)

fiscal   Relating to financial matters. (16)

fixative   Substance that serves to make firm, fixed, or preserved. Used for lab specimens to maintain stability during transport. (21)

floppy disk   Magnetic disks with a magnetic oxide coating over a thin slice of plastic used as a storage medium. (12)

fluoroscope   Device used to project an x-ray image on a special screen to allow for visual examination. (28)

fluoroscopy   Visual examination of internal body structures using a fluoroscope. Many fluoroscopy procedures require the use of a contrast medium. (28)

Food and Drug Administration (FDA)   The official federal agency with responsibility for the regulation of food, drugs, cosmetics, and medical devices. It is a part of the US Department of Health and Human Services. (31)

frenulum linguae   Longitudinal fold of mucous membrane connecting the floor of the mouth to the underside of the tongue. (20)

gag reflex   Closure of the glottis and constriction of its associated musculature in response to stimulation of the posterior pharynx by an object or substance in that area. (34)

gelatin culture   The culture of bacteria on a gelatin medium, such as agar. (25)

gender bias   Indicating either male or female by the type of language used. (11)

gender neutral   Unable to determine which gender is referred to based on the language used. (11)

gene therapy   Replacement of a defective or malfunctioning gene with one that functions properly. Gene therapy is being researched as a means of correcting medical conditions caused by defective genes. (4)

generalized   Involving the entire body or system; widespread. (34)

generic name   Common name by which a drug or product is known (for example, aspirin). (31)

gerontology   Scientific study of the effects of aging and age-related diseases. (24)

glomerulonephritis   Kidney disease which involves inflammation and lesions of the glomeruli. (26)

glucosuria/ glycosuria   The presence of sugar (glucose) in the urine. (26)

granulocyte   Type of white blood cell in which the cytoplasm contains granules. (27)

grievance   Real or imaginary wrong regarded as cause for complaint or resentment. (18)

gross annual wage   Salary calculated before taxes and withholdings are taken out. (15)

grounded   Connected to an electrical current or circuit with the ground through a conductor or other solid connection. (10)

group practice   A practice in which at least three physicians are joined in order to share the workload and expenses. (1)

guardian ad litem   Court-appointed guardian to represent a minor or unborn child in litigation. (5)

gynecology   The branch of medicine that deals with diseases and disorders of the female reproductive system. (22)

habituation   The development of an emotional dependence on a drug due to repeated use. (31)

halo effect   A white halo appearing around lights which may be an indication of an eye disorder such as glaucoma. (21)

handbreadth   Use of the size and surface of one's hand to measure distance on a patient for injection purposes. (32)

health care consumer   Individual who engages the services of a physician or other health care practitioner. (6)

health maintenance organization (HMO)   An organization established to provide comprehensive health care to an enrolled group of people at a fixed price. (1)

heart sounds   Normal noise produced within the heart during the cardiac cycle. (20)

hemacytometer   Instrument used to count red and white blood cells. (27)

hematology   Study of blood and blood-forming tissues. (27)

hematoma   Collection of blood underneath the skin, for example, a bruise. (27)

hematopoiesis   Formation of blood cells. (27)

hematuria   The presence of blood in the urine. (21, 26)

hemiplegia   Paralysis on one side of the body. (24)

hemoglobin   Carries oxygen and an iron containing pigment which gives an RBC its color. (27)

hemolyzed   Refers to the destruction (hemolysis) of blood cells. (27)

hemoptysis   Coughing up blood. (21)

hemostatic   Any drug, medicine, or blood component that stops bleeding, such as vasopressin, vitamin K, or whole blood. (31)

hernia   The protrusion of an organ through the wall of a cavity in which it is usually located. (21)

high-power field (hpf)   High power magnification of the microscope. (26)

histology   The study of the microscopic structure of tissue. (25)

hives   Peculiar raised patches of skin surrounded by reddened areas, triggered by the release of histamine. Also called urticaria. (34)

holistic   Viewing the human body as a whole organism. (24)

homeopathy   Treatment and prevention of disease based on the premise that large doses of drugs which cause symptoms in healthy people will cure the same symptoms when given in small doses. (2)

homeostasis   The human body in balance. (20)

homophones   Words which sound alike but have different meanings and spellings. (11)

honorarium   Small payment for a service (for example, a speaking engagement). (18)

hospice   Patient-centered interdisciplinary program of care and supportive services for terminally ill patients and their families. (3)

hydrogenation   A process of changing an unsaturated fat to a solid saturated fat by the addition of hydrogen. (33)

hyfrecators   Small electrocautery units used to perform minor cautery procedures in the medical office. (23)

hypertension   Elevated blood pressure. (20)

hypotension   Blood pressure which is below normal. (20)

hypothalamus   Portion of brain in the lateral wall of the third ventricle which controls autonomic nervous system functions, such as body temperature, sleep, and appetite. (20)

idiosyncrasy   An unusual or abnormal response to a drug or food by an individual. (31)

ileostomy   An artificial opening created surgically into the small intestine for the removal of waste. (24)

immunity   Resistance to disease. (19)

immunology   Study of immunity—resistance to or protection from disease. (2)

inactive   Medical files for patients who have not been seen, according to the time period set up by the office policy (generally 1 to 5 years). (13)

incident report   Formal written description of an incident, such as a patient falling, occurring in a medical setting. (6, 10)

incision(s)   Surgical cut into tissue. (23)

incontinent   Unable to control the passing of urine or feces. (26)

incubation   Period of time during which a disease develops after the person is exposed. (19); In bacteriology, this is the period of culture development or the time it takes from placing an inoculated agar plate in an incubator or "oven" to when the microorganisms start to grow. (25)

indemnity schedule   List of determined amounts to be paid for specific services by the insurance carrier on behalf of the insured. (17)

infarction   Death of tissue, as in myocardial infarction or heart attack. (34)

ingested   Food or drink taken orally. (33)

inguinal   The area of flexion in the groin area between the hips and legs. (21)

inoculate   To inject or transfer a microorganism, serum, or toxic material into the body, culture, medium, or slide. (25)

inpatient   Patient who remains within the medical facility at least overnight for care and/or treatment. (3)

inspiration   Inhalation. (34)

insured   Individual(s) who is covered under an insurance plan. (17)

integrity   Adherence to a code of moral values; usually found along with honesty. (36)

intermittent pulse   Skipping an occasional heart beat. (20)

interrogation   Questioning by authorities of a person, often a witness, to obtain information. (5)

interval   Time between beginning of one phase and beginning of the next phase. (29)

intravenous   Inserting a medication or fluid into the vein via a needle or tube. (24)

invasive   Enters the skin. (23)

inventory   A list of articles with a description and quantity of each. (10)

isoelectric line   *See baseline.*

jaundice   Yellowish cast to the skin and eye sclera. Usually caused by liver disease or damage, dehydration of the newborn, and bile duct obstruction. (21)

K   *See kilobyte.* (12)

kilobyte(s) (K)   A measure of storage capacity or memory. (12)

kilograms   Metric weight.

labia   Two folds of tissue on either side of the female vaginal opening. (26)

laryngitis   Inflammation of the larynx (voice box) causing temporary loss of voice. (21)

lead(s)   An electrical connection to the body to receive data from a specific combination of sensors. (29)

ledger card   A record for each patient of charges, payments, and current balance. (14)

legally binding   Form of contract that must be honored by law. (4)

Legionnaires' disease   Severe, sometimes fatal disease, caused by a bacillus that is inhaled. First occurrence was at the Legionnaires' convention in 1976. (3)

leukemia   Cancerous condition with elevated numbers of white blood cells. (27)

leukocyte   A white blood cell (WBC). (27)

leukoplakia   White patches on mucous membranes which may become cancerous. (21)

leukorrhea   White discharge. (21)

liable   Compelled or responsible under the law to make satisfaction, restitution, or compensation because a wrong has occurred. (5)

libel   False statements placed in writing about another person. (5)

licensure   An authorization to practice one's profession usually issued after successful completion of an examination. (4)

litigation   Lawsuit tried in court. (5)

localized   Limited to a definable area of the body; focal. (34)

low-power field (lpf)   Low power magnification of the microscope. (26)

lumen   Space/cavity within an object or organ. (20)

Magnetic Ink Character Recognition (MICR)   Characters and letters printed on the bottom of the check used as routing information to identify the bank and number of the individual account. (16)

main memory   That part of the central processing unit which stores data and program instructions; it does not perform any of the logical operations, for example, computations, sorting. (12)

maker (of check)   Person who signs the check (or corporation who pays it). This is the same as the payer. (16)

malaise   Discomfort, uneasiness which is often indicative of an infection. (22)

malignant   Cancerous. (22)

malpractice   Professional negligence. (5)

mammogram   X-ray of breasts in women to detect early cancer. (21)

managed care organization (MCO)   An organization that acts as a "gatekkeeper" such as the insurance company to approve all non-emergency services, hospitalization, or tests before they can be provided. (1)

mandate(s)   Require. (10, 15)

manometer   Device for taking a measurement (for example, pressure). (20)

massage   To apply pressure with hands. (30)

matrix   Base upon which to build, for example, to develop a shape or format for the daily schedule. (9)

mature minor   Person, usually under 18 years of age, who possesses an understanding of the nature and consequences of proposed treatment. (5)

Mayo stand   Small portable tray/table used to hold surgical instruments during a procedure. (23)

media   A substance on which microor-

ganisms may grow; those most commonly used are broth, gelatin, and agar. (25)

medical asepsis   Killing organisms after they leave the body. (19)

medical emergency   A patient condition which may be life-threatening if not treated. (8)

medical ethics   Moral conduct based on principles regulating the behavior of health care professionals. (4)

medical etiquette   Courtesy physicians extend to one another. (4)

medical privileges   Ability of a physician to admit patients and practice medicine at a particular hospital. (3)

medically indigent   Person without insurance coverage and with no funds. (17)

Medicare   Federal health care insurance program for adults over 65 and disabled persons who qualify. (6)

medicinal   Plants and other substances that have a therapeutic value for the body. (2)

medulla oblongata   Most vital part of the brain which contains the respiratory, cardiac, and vasomotor centers of the brain. (20)

menstrual   Relating to menstruation or monthly uterine blood flow in women. (21)

mensuration   Measurement. (21)

metastasize   Cancerous cells or tumors that spread to another location or organ. (22)

metric system   A system of weights and measures based upon the meter as the unit of measurement. This system uses the decimal system. (32)

microbes   One-celled form of life such as bacteria. (2); Small organisms including bacteria, protozoa, algae, fungus, and defined viruses. (25)

microbiology   The scientific study of microorganisms. (25)

microcomputer   Small computer systems designed to be portable, including desktop, laptop notebook, and handheld computers. (12)

microfiche   Sheets of microfilm. (13)

microfilm   Miniaturized photographs of records. (13)

microorganisms   Minute living organisms such as bacteria, virus, protozoa, and fungus that are not visible to the human eye without a microscope. (2, 25)

microprocessor   A small chip that does the work of processing data in a microcomputer. (12)

microscopic   Visible only by using a microscope. (25)

minor   Person under the age of 18. (5)

misdemeanor   Crime that is less serious

than a felony carrying a penalty of up to one year imprisonment and/or a fine. (5)

modified block   Style of letter writing in which the date, complimentary close, and signature line begin in the center with all other lines at the left margin. (11)

modified wave   Flexible scheduling in which each hour is divided into segments of time with each patient arriving within 10 to 15 minutes of each other. Time is allowed at the end of the hour for "catch up." (9)

monitor   Screen which allows the user to see input and output. (12)

monosaccharides   A simple sugar that cannot be decomposed further, such as fructose or glucose. (33)

morale   Positive or negative state of mind of employees (as regards a feeling of well being) with relationship to their work or work environment. (10)

morbidity rate   Number of sick persons or cases of a disease within a certain population. (2)

mortality rate   Death rate; the ratio of the number of deaths in a given population. (2, 6)

mouse   Pointing and selection device to input data. (12)

myocardial   Heart muscle, especially referring to the ventricles. (29)

myocardium   Heart wall composed of muscle and fibrous tissue. (29)

necrotic   Refers to death of tissue, such as occurs with venoms of pit vipers and the brown recluse spider. (34)

negative   Culture that fails to reveal the suspected organism. (25)

neglect   Failure to perform some action. (5)

negligence   Injury or harm to a patient caused by the performance of an act that a responsible and prudent physician would not have done or the failure to do some act that a responsible and prudent physician would have done. (5)

negotiable   To transfer money to another person (for example, through an endorsement on a check). (16)

network   A circle of friends and relations or professionals who communicate to provide support and information for varying purposes, frequently as a source of job opportunities. (36)

neuroses   Mild emotional disturbances that impair judgment. (24)

no-show   Patient's failure to keep an appointment without notifying the physician's office personnel. (8)

non-invasive procedure   Procedure or treatment in which the skin and body is not entered or invaded. (6)

non-pleuritic   Not related to the pleura,

or membranes that lubricate the outer surfaces of the lungs. A pleuritic chest pain worsens when the patient takes a deep breath, and is not characteristic of a cardiac disorder. (34)

nonparticipating provider Provider who decides not to accept an allowable charge as the full fee for care. (17)

nonverbal communication The information conveyed by the way a person acts over and above (or in place of) the message conveyed by his words. (7)

norm Standard, criterion, or the ideal measure for a specific group. (6)

normal value(s) The amount of a substance that is normally present. There can also be a range for normal value. (26)

nosocomial infection Infection that is acquired after a person has entered the hospital. It is caused by the spread of an infection from one patient or person to another. (19); Infection acquired in a hospital. (26)

nuclear medicine Medical discipline that uses radioactive isotopes in the diagnosis and treatment of disease. (28)

numeric Filing system which assigns an identification number to each person's name. (13)

nutrient(s) Food or any substance that supplies the body with elements necessary for metabolism. (33)

obesity An abnormal amount of fat on the body of an individual who is 20% over the average weight for his or her age, sex, or height. (33)

obstructive lung disease Those diseases that obstruct the flow of air out of the lungs characterized by generally slow expiratory rate and increased residual volume. (29)

occult Hidden, as in hidden bleeding. (34)

occult blood Blood in such small quantity that it can only be seen under a microscope or detected by a specific test (for example, Multistix test). (26)

occurrence Any event or incident out of the norm. (6)

oliguria Reduced production of urine; Reduction of urine, scant amount. (21)

open-ended questions Questions which require an explanatory answer rather than a *yes* or *no* response. (7)

opportunistic infections Infections, such as pneumonia, that occur in a body with a reduced immune system (for example, as seen in AIDS). (19)

optional May or may not be used. (15)

orifice Opening of a part of the body, such as the mouth. (21)

orifices Openings, especially naturally occurring body surface openings. (34)

orthopnea Difficulty breathing when lying down. Breathing is easier in a straight sitting position. (21)

outpatient Patient undergoing medical treatment which does not necessitate staying overnight in the facility. Also referred to as ambulatory or a "23 hour hold." (3)

outpatient surgery Surgical procedures, which usually requires less than 60 minutes, performed in a setting in which the patient is ambulatory and does not stay in the facility overnight. (23)

outstanding deposits Checks that have been deposited to one's account but not yet processed by the bank. (16)

overbooking The practice of scheduling more than one patient in the same time slot. This practice is not recommended. This is also referred to as double or triple booking. (8)

oxyhemoglobin Combination of oxygen and hemoglobin; carries oxygen to the tissues. (27)

pacemaker The portion of cardiac electrical tissue that establishes the beat; the sinoatrial node; also the artificial equipment used when the natural pacemaker fails. (29)

palpatory method To determine by using the sense of touch. (20)

PAP smear Also called Papanicolaou test. Used for cytology testing including early detection of cervical and vaginal cancer cells. (21)

parasites An organism that lives within another organism. (26)

parenteral Medication route other than the alimentary canal (oral and rectal). Parenteral routes include subcutaneous, intravenous, and intramuscular. (10, 31)

participating provider One who accepts assignment and is paid directly by the plan. (17)

passive voice The subject of the sentence receives the action. (11)

password A word or phrase that identifies a person and that allows access or entry to a program or records. (12)

pasteurization Process of heating substances, such as milk or cheese, to a certain temperature in order to destroy bacteria. (2)

pathogens Disease producing microorganisms. (10, 19, 25)

pathologic Pertaining to a condition of disease or injury. (34)

pathology Study of the nature and cause of disease; Disease process. (2, 26)

payee Person or company named as the receiving party to whom the amount on the check is payable. (16)

payer Person signing a check to release money. (16)

pediatrics The branch of medicine which involves the development, diagnosis, and treatment of diseases and disorders in children. (22)

Peer Review Organization (PRO) A professional organization that reviews a physician's conduct. (6)

perfusion The process of bathing cells in healthy blood which is rich in nutrients, especially oxygen and glucose. (34)

pericardium A double-walled sac that encloses the heart. (29)

perineal care Cleansing the area between the vulva and the anus and within the vulva in a female and between the scrotum and the anus in a male. (26)

periosteum A membrane that covers the shaft of a long bone; promotes growth and healing. (34)

peripheral edema Swelling of the extremities (especially the legs) due to fluid retention. (21)

permeable Material that allows something to penetrate or pass through. (19)

personal assessment Examination of one's own strengths and weaknesses. (36)

phagocytosis Process of engulfing, digesting, and destroying pathogens (19); Process in which white blood cells (WBCs) ingest and digest foreign material. (27)

pharmacist A druggist or one who is licensed to prepare and dispense drugs. (31)

pharmacology The study of drugs, their origins, nature, properties, and effects on the living organism. (31)

phenylketonuria (PKU) A recessive hereditary disease caused by the lack of an enzyme, phenylalanine hydroxylase, which results in severe mental retardation in children if not detected and treated soon after birth. (22)

phlebotomy Blood collection using the venipuncture method. (27)

photophobia Sensitivity to light. (21)

physiatrist A physician specializing in physical medicine and rehabilitation. (30)

physiatry Medical specialty of physical medicine and rehabilitation. (30)

***Physician's Desk Reference* (PDR)** A book used as a quick reference on drugs. (31)

placebo An inactive, harmless substance used to satisfy a patient's desire for medication. This is also used in research when given to a control group of patients in a study in which another group receives the actual drug. The effect of the placebo versus the drug is then observed. (31)

plaintiff Person or group of persons who bring an action into litigation. (5)

plasma The liquid portion of blood, contains fibrinogen. (27)

platelet   A cell which aids in the blood clotting process, for example thrombocyte. (27)

polarized   State of electrical charge in living cells. (29)

polycythemia   A condition where there are too many red blood cells (RBCs) in blood. (27)

positive   Culture that reveals the suspected organism. (25)

post(ed)   Enter amounts into a record. (15)

postdate   To write a future date on a check and then sign it. (16)

pre-register   Refers to the process by which patient information such as name, address, age, social security number, and health insurance information, is given to a medical assistant or secretary over the telephone prior to admission to a health care facility or insurer for prior approval. It may also be done just prior to the patient's visit. (9)

preauthorization   A requirement of Medicare and insurance companies to obtain prior approval for surgery and other procedures performed in order to receive reimbursement. (17)

precedent   Law that is established in a prior case. (5)

predisposes   The tendency or susceptibility to develop a certain disease or condition. (33)

premium   Amount paid for insurance coverage. (17)

prepaid plan   A group of physicians or other health care providers who have a contractual agreement to provide services to subscribers on a negotiated fee-for-service or capitated basis (also called managed care plan). (17)

primary care   Basic or general health care a person receives for common illnesses. A primary care physician is the one to whom the patient and/or family will go to seek most medical care. (3)

printer(s)   An output device for hard copy; classified as impact and nonimpact. (12)

probationary period   A trial period during the early months of employment to see if there is a fit between the employee and the position. It is usually 3 months in length. During this period the employee can be dismissed without cause. (18)

procedure manual   A collection of policies and procedures for carrying out day-to-day operations in an office or facility. (6)

prognosis   Prediction of the course and outcome of a disease. (22)

program   A set or sets of programmed instructions that tell the computer hardware what to do in order to complete the required data processing (also called software). (12)

prompt   A reminder or hint to the user that some action must be taken by the user before processing of data can continue. (12)

proofreading   Reviewing or reading printed, typed, or written material for correct content (grammar, spelling, style) and mechanical (typing, printing) errors. (11)

prophylaxis   The prevention of disease. A medication, such as an antibiotic, can be used to prevent the occurrence of an infection prior to surgery (as opposed to antibiotics given to *treat* an infection). (31)

proprietary hospital   A hospital that operates on a for-profit basis. (3)

prosthesis   An artificial body part. (30)

protocol   The standard (for example, a protocol for behavior). (18)

proximate cause   Natural continuous sequence of events, without any intervening cause, which produces an injury. Also referred to as the direct cause. (5)

psychoses   Severe mental disorders that interfere with a perception of reality. (24)

public duty   Physician's responsibility to provide birth and death certificates and report cases of communicable diseases and abuses. (5)

puerperal sepsis   Severe infection of the genital tract during the postpartum period or as a complication of an abortion. Also called childbed fever. (2)

pulmonary volume tests   Under constant conditions, the patient breathes with extreme inhalations and exhalations, and the amount of gas inhaled or exhaled is recorded. (29)

pulse deficit   Difference between the rate of the apical pulse and the radial pulse. Normally there is no difference. (20)

pulse pressure   Difference between systolic and diastolic readings of blood pressure. (20)

pure culture   Culture of a single form of microorganism uncontaminated by other organisms. (25)

pyrexia   Abnormally elevated body temperature; fever. (20)

quality assurance program (QAP)   A program in which hospitals and medical practices evaluate the services they provide by comparing their services with accepted standards. (6)

radiation   Use of radioactive substances for the diagnosis and treatment of disease. (28)

radioactive   Ability to give off radiation as the result of the disintegration of the nucleus of an atom. (28)

radiologist   Physician who specializes in the practice of radiology. (28)

radiology   Branch of medicine which uses radioactive substances and visual-ization techniques for the diagnosis and treatment of disease. (28)

radiopaque   Substance which does not allow the passage of x-rays or other radiant materials. Bones are considered radiopaque and show up as white on exposed x-ray film. (28)

RAM   Random-access memory. (12)

random sample   The selection of one sample from a large group. In urinalysis it means any sample taken throughout the day. (26)

reading   Interpretation of data. (20)

receptionist   A physician's staff employee, often a medical assistant, who greets and assists patients as they come into the office. The receptionist usually sits in an area where the waiting patients can be observed. (8)

reconciliation (of bank statement)   To adjust one's banking records against a bank statement so that both are in agreement. (16)

redundant   Repetitive. (11)

reflecting   Directing the conversation back to the patient by repeating the words. Also called mirroring. (7)

refractometer   Used to measure the specific gravity of urine. (26)

regimen   A systematic plan of activities. (33)

Registered Medical Assistant (RMA)   A multiskilled health care professional who assists providers in an allied health setting, has taken and successfully completed the RMA examination, and is registered with a national association. (1)

rehabilitation   Process of assisting patient to regain a state of health and the highest level of function position. (30)

reimplantation   Reattachment of a severed limb or portion of a severed limb. (34)

renal colic   Pain in kidney area usually due to kidney stones. (21)

repolarization   Return to polarization from the depolarized state; return to rest. (29)

repolarization, atrial   Return to polarization of the upper heart chambers. (29)

repolarization, ventricular   Return to polarization of the lower chambers. (29)

res ipsa loquitur   Latin phrase which means "The thing speaks for itself." This is a doctrine of negligence law. (5)

reservoir   Source of the infectious pathogen. (19)

respondeat superior   Latin phrase which means "Let the master answer." This means the physician/employer is responsible for acts of the employee. (5)

restating   Directing the conversation back to the patient by stating what the patient has said in different terms. (7)

restrictive lung disease Those diseases that prevent the expansion of the lungs, diminish the total lung capacity, vital capacity, and inspiratory capacity. (29)

resumé Document that sums up one's work and educational experiences. (36)

reticulocyte An immature red blood cell containing a nucleus. Red blood cells containing granules or filaments in an immature stage of development. (27)

revocation The act of taking away or recalling, for example, taking away a license to practice medicine. (4)

rheumatoid arthritis Form of arthritis with inflammation of the joints, stiffness, swelling, and pain. Called crippling, deforming arthritis. (21)

rider A written exception to an insurance contract, expanding, decreasing, or modifying coverage of an insurance policy. (17)

ROM Read-only memory. (12)

rosacea Chronic disease of the skin of the face in middle aged and older patients. Resembles butterfly rash of lupus erythematosis. (21)

rule of discovery The statute of limitations begins to run at the time the injury is discovered or when the patient should have known of the injury. (5)

salivation Production of fluid (saliva) in the mouth. (21)

scheduling system A method that is used in a particular physician's practice to provide efficient services. (8)

scrub assistant A sterile assistant who passes instruments, swabs (sponges) bodily fluids from the operative site, retracts incisions, and cuts sutures. (23)

sediment The substance settling to the bottom of a fluid. (26)

segment Time from the end of one phase to the beginning of another phase. (29)

seizures Same as convulsions. (34)

seniority Refers to the person who has been with the organization longest. (18)

sensitivity Ability of the equipment to detect a change in amplitude; normally a state of one. (29)

sensor *See electrode.* (29)

serologic Pertaining to the study of the serum component of the blood. (25)

serum The liquid portion of blood which contains no fibrinogen. (27)

settle Act of determining the outcome of a case outside a courtroom. Settling a case is not an indication of guilt or innocence. (5)

side effect(s) A response to a drug other than the effect desired. (31)

signee Person who signs a check or document. (16)

slander False, malicious spoken words

about another person. (5)

smears Bacteria spread on a surface, such as a microscopic slide or a culture medium. (25)

smear fixation Holding or fastening a bacterial specimen to a slide; adhering a smear to a glass slide by a fixative or heat. (25)

software A set or sets of programmed instructions that tell the computer hardware what to do in order to complete the required data processing (also called a program). (12)

solo practice A physician practicing alone. (1)

solvent Having sufficient assets (money) to pay debts. (18)

specific gravity (S.G.) Weight of a substance compared with an equal volume of water. (26)

specific time Refers to a type of scheduling in which a particular time slot is assigned to one person. (9)

specimen(s) A part of something intended to show the kind and quality of the whole, as a specimen of urine. (25)

speculum Instrument used to examine canals and body orifices. (21)

sputum The substance expelled by coughing or clearing the bronchi. Can be used as a specimen for culturing to discover possible causative agents of respiratory disease. (25)

squamous epithelial cells Flattened scale like cells attached at the edges which line the bladder. Commonly seen in microscopic examinations. (26)

standard of care The ordinary skill and care that medical practitioners such as physicians, nurses, and medical assistants must use which is commonly used by other medical practitioners when caring for patients. (5)

standardization Test performed to document a machine's compliance with the international agreement. (29)

statute of limitations Maximum time period set by federal and state governments during which certain legal actions can be brought forward. (5, 14)

statutes Laws and regulations. (4); Acts of a federal, state, or county legislature. (5)

sterile All microorganisms and spores are killed. (19)

sterile field Work area in surgery in which the area is prepared using sterile drapes (cloths) to cover nonsterile areas. (23)

stool Evacuation of the bowels; waste matter used as a specimen for culturing to discover possible diseases. Also referred to as feces. (25)

stop payment Procedure in which the

maker of a check instructs the bank (in writing) not to honor the payment of a check. There is a charge for this service. (16)

streak culture Spreading of the bacteria by drawing a wire containing the inoculum across the surface of the medium. (25)

sublingual Beneath the tongue. (34)

sublingual(ly) Under the tongue. (20)

subnormal Abnormally lowered body temperature. (20)

subpoena Court order for a person to appear in court. Documents as well as persons may be subpoenaed. (4, 5)

subpoena duces tecum Court order requiring a witness to appear in court and to bring certain records or other material to a trial or deposition. (5)

subscriber Person who holds a health benefit plan/contract. This plan, contract, or policy may include other family members. (14, 17)

superbill Record of services for billing and for insurance processing. Also called a charge slip or encounter form. (14)

suppuration Process of pus formation due to infection. (30)

surgical asepsis A technique practiced to maintain a sterile environment. (19, 23)

surgical schedule A list of surgery appointments maintained by a secretary (surgical scheduler) in the surgery department. (9)

swab Cotton or gauze on the end of a slender stick used for cleansing, applying remedies, or obtaining tissue or secretions for bacteriologic examination. (25)

sympathy Feeling sorry for a patient. (7)

symptom(s) An objective (observable) or subjective (perceived or felt by the patient) change in the body, for example vomiting or muscle soreness, that indicates disease or a phase of a disease. (21)

syncope Sudden loss of consciousness, which may be transient. Also called fainting. (34)

syndrome A set of symptoms or disorders which occur together and indicate the presence of a disease. (19)

syphilis An infectious, chronic, venereal disease with lesions that can affect many organs. It is treated with antibiotics. (2)

systemic Pertaining to the body as a whole; affects the entire body. (34)

systemic lupus erythematosis (SLE) Chronic, progressive inflammatory disease of the connective tissue and skin which resembles rheumatoid arthritis. The characteristic butterfly rash resembles rosacea. (21)

systole Period during the cardiac cycle when the atria and ventricles contract and eject the blood out of the heart. (20)

tax withholding   Amounts of salary withheld from payroll check for the purpose of paying government taxes. (15)

terminal   Also called a monitor or dumb terminal; allows the computer operator to see input and output. (12)

terminal digit filing   Medical record filing system based on the last digits of the ID number. (13)

terminal disease   A disease which is expected to end with death. (10)

terminal illness   Illness that is expected to end in death. (19, 24)

termination   End as in the end of a contract. (5)

thesaurus   Reference book that lists words alphabetically and gives synonyms for each entry word. (11)

third party payer(s)   A party other than the patient who assumes responsibility for paying the patient's bills (for example, insurance company). (14)

third-party check   Check written to the payment of another payee but presented to you as payment (the third payee). (16)

thready pulse   Pulse rate that is barely perceptible. (20)

thrombocyte   *See platelet.* (27)

tidal volume   The volume of air inspired and expired during one normal respiratory cycle. (34)

tinnitus   Ringing in the ears. (21)

tort   Wrongful act (other than a breach of contract) committed against another person or property that results in harm. (5)

toxicity   The extent or degree to which a

substance is poisonous. (31)

tracing   Recording. (29)

transcription   Listening to dictation of a medical record while typing it into a written record. (11)

triage   To determine the priority for handling patients with severe conditions or injuries. For example, the most severely injured patient with a chance for survival will be treated first. (9, 34)

turbidity   Having a cloudy appearance. (26)

two hour postprandial   Two hours after eating a meal. (26)

tympanic membrane   Thin semitransparent membrane separates the outer ear and the middle ear. Also called eardrum. (20, 21)

***United States Pharmacopeia-National Formulary* (USP-NF)**   A drug book listing all the official drugs that are authorized for use in the United States. This is used in medical facilities and physicians' offices as a reference. (31)

unsolicited   Something that is not sought out or invited. (36)

untoward effect   An undesirable side effect; an unexpected or adverse reaction of a patient to a medication. (31, 32)

urinalysis (U/A)   Refers to the testing of urine for the presence of infection or disease. The testing may be physical, chemical, or microscopic. (26)

urinary meatus   Opening from the urethra to the outside of the body. (26)

urinary retention   Inability to urinate. (26)

urinometer   Used to measure specific

gravity of urine. (26)

urticaria   Itchy skin rash, commonly called "hives." (21)

usual, customary and reasonable (UCR)   Refers to the usual fee a physician would charge for the services, the customary fee a majority of physicians would charge for the same service, and a reasonable fee that the patient might expect to pay. Used to determine medical benefits. (14)

vendor   One who supplies goods and services. (10, 15)

venipuncture   The process of withdrawing blood from a vein. (27)

viable   Capable of living. (25)

virulent   Relating to transmission of disease. Exceedingly harmful. (10)

visual acuity   Sharpness of vision. (22)

void   To pass urine. (26)

voltage   *See amplitude.* (29)

warrant   Written non-negotiable evidence that a debt (money) is due to a person. The warrant can then be used to collect the money. (16)

wave   Flexible scheduling in which each hour is divided into segments of time. All patients who will be seen during that hour arrive at the beginning of the hour. (9); *See deflection.* (29)

x-rays   Electromagnetic radiation of shorter wavelength than visible light rays; able to pass through opaque bodies. (28)

xiphoid process   The piece of cartilage that forms the lowermost tip of the sternum, and which functions as a major point of attachment for the abdominal muscles. (34)

Index

A

Abandonment, 74, 78–79
ABA number, checks, 294
Abbreviations, 204–5, 883–85
    pharmacological, 697–99
Abdominal pain, 793–94
Abdominal sutures, 504
Abnormal cell growth, 508
Abnormalities, in electrocardiogram, 634
Abnormal psychology, 525
Abrasions, 501, 826
Absorbable sutures, 485
Acceptance stage, grief, 525
Accepting cash, 301
Accepting checks, 296–97
Accessibility parameter, health care, 98
Accession, 234
Accountant, hiring, 299
Accounting, 268
Accounting systems, 268–70
Accounts payable, 270
Accounts receivable, 268, 269–70
Accounts receivable control, 280
Accounts receivable insurance, 262
Accounts receivable ratio, 280
Accreditation, 4
Accrediting Bureau of Health Education
    Schools (ABHES), 11
Accrediting Commission of Career Schools
    and Colleges of Technology (ACCSCT), 11
Acne vulgaris, 445
Acquired immune deficiency syndrome
    (AIDS), 42, 48, 173, 368–71, 449, 526, 714
    AIDS antibody test, 370
    AIDS-related complex (ARC), 369
    human immunodeficiency virus (HIV), 48,
        173, 353, 368–71
    and opportunistic infections, 369
    transmission of, 369
    See also Human immunodeficiency
        virus (HIV)
Acquired immunity, 350
Active assist range of motion (AAROM), 653
Active immunity, 350
Active listening, 119
Active range of motion (AROM), 653, 658
Active records, 234, 235
Active resistance, 658
Active voice, 190, 192
Activities of daily living (ADL), 51
Acuity, 418
Acute conditions, 152, 161–62
Adaptive equipment, 670–72
    canes, 670
    special furniture, 672
    walkers, 670
    wheelchairs, 670–71, 673
Addiction, 680, 682
Adjustments, and pegboard system, 277
Administering medications:
    equipment for, 718–21
    intradermal injection, 729
    intramuscular injections, 721–26
    oral, 714–15
    OSHA standards, 713–15
    parenteral, 715–29
    parenteral injections, 729, 732–33

rectal/vaginal suppository, 717–18
subcutaneous injections, 726–28
sublingual/buccal, 716
weights/measures, 706
Administrative, use of term, 4
Administrative equipment, 181
Administrative responsibilities, 5, 7
Adolescent medicine, 31
Adult learning, 748
Advance booking, 158–59
Aerobes, 536
Aerobic, use of term, 344
Aerobic exercise, 653
Affect, 782
Age analysis, 254, 259
Agent, 60, 69
Agglutination, 536, 549–50
Agglutination inhibition test, 550–51
Agranulocytes, 580, 598
Agranulocytic white cells, 598
Aided exercise, 658
AIDS antibody test, 370
AIDS-related complex (ARC), 369
Airborne precautions, 351
Airway obstruction, 790–93
    Heimlich maneuver, 791–92
    infant, 792
    small child, 792
    variations, 792
Albee, George, 527
Alcohol, 433, 776
Alcohol method of disinfection, 362
Alcohol wipes, 433
Alleged, use of term, 60, 62
Allergy/allergic reactions, 442–43, 794
    allergy testing, 443
    anaphylactic shock, 442–43
    determining in medical emergency, 789
    and immunology, 31
    sensitization, 443
    treatment, 794
Allied-health careers, 49–50
Alphabetic filing system, 234, 238–40
Alpha-Z system (Smead Manufacturing
    Company), 241
Alveoli, 376
Alzheimer's disease, 522, 523, 609
Ambulatory care, 42, 47–48, 51
    clinics, 47
    laboratories, 47–48
Ambulatory surgery, 474–75
American Academy of Pediatrics, 457
American Association of Blood Services, 53
American Association of Medical Assistants
    (AAMA), 4, 5, 10–11, 69, 834
    Code of Ethics, 63, 65
    Creed of, 66
    DACUM curriculum, 8–9
American Association for Medical
    Transcription (AAMT), *AAMT Book of
    Style for Medical Transcription,* 244
American Board of Medical Specialties, 30–31
American Cancer Society:
    breast self-examination
        recommendations, 461–62
    endometrial cancer guidelines, 509
    mammography recommendations, 607
American College of Physicians, 31

American College of Surgeons, 31
American Medical Association (AMA), 4,
    5, 313
    coding system, 313
    Council on Ethical and Judicial Affairs, 62
    essentials of quality care, 98–99
    principles of medical ethics, 62–63
American Medical Technologists (AMT), 4, 11
American Occupational Therapy Association
    (AOTA), 51
American Sign Language (ASL), 674
American Society of Clinical Pathologists
    (ASCP), 52
Amino acids, 761
Amplification, 418
Amplitude, 622, 625
Ampule, 721
Amputation, 651, 794–95
AMT Institute for Education (AMTIE), 11
Anaerobic, use of term, 344
Anaphylactic shock, 442–43, 680, 692, 827
Anatomic position, 427
Ancient civilizations, contributions to
    medical history, 19
Andwin Safetex One PAP Smear Kit, 465
Anemia, 580
Aneroid sphygmomanometer, 403–4
Anesthesia, 18, 23, 474, 499–501
Anesthesiology, 31–32
Aneurysm, 782
Angiography, 604, 610–11, 614
Angry patients, handling, 121–22
Annual tax returns, 286
Anorexia, 418
Answering service, using, 127–28
Antecubital fossa/space, 376
Anthrax, 18
Anthropometry, 376, 408
Antibodies, 549, 580–81
Anticoagulant, 580, 582
Antidepressants, 529
Antigen, 580
Antigen-antibody reaction, 350
Antipsychotics, 529 ,
Antipyretic, use of term, 376
Antisocial reactions, 528
Anxiety, 426, 527
Apical heart rate, 392
Apical-radial pulse, 392, 394–95
Apothecary system, 706
Appellant, 74
Application, 846–47
    legal/ethical issues, 847
Appointment book, 157–58
Appointment cards, 158–59
Appointment list, 136
Appointment scheduling, 151–65
    for admission to hospital, 159–60
    advance booking, 158–59
    appointment book, 157–58
    appointment cards, 158–59
    cancellations, 155–57
    computer-assisted scheduling, 158
    double booking patients, 154
    exceptions to appointment system, 161
    follow-up calls, 159
    free time, scheduling for physician, 155
    grouping procedures, scheduling by, 154

Bulimia, 418
Bureau of Narcotics and Dangerous Drugs (BNDD), 680–81
Burns, 651, 804–6
    classification of, 805
    Rule of Nines, 804–5
    treatment of, 806
Business letters, 197–201
    body, 200
    closing, 200
    copy notation, 200
    courtesy titles, 199
    date, 198
    enclosure notation, 200
    heading, 197–98
    inside address, 198–99
    reference initials, 200
    salutation, 199–200
    two-page letters, 200–201
Business responsibilities, 5, 7

C

Cadaver, 18
Caduceus, 18, 19
Calculator, 181
Calorie content diet, 773
Calories, 770–71
    in food, calculating, 771
    supplied by fat, calculating, 771
Cancellations, 155–57
Cancer, 32, 445, 517
Canes, 670
Capillaries, 580
Capillary puncture (manual), 588, 590
Capital equipment, 181
Capitalization, 193, 197
Carbohydrates, 759, 760–61
Cardiac arrest, 806–7
Cardiac cycle, 376, 622
Cardiac rate, 622
Cardiogenic, use of term, 782, 827
Cardiology, 32, 445
Cardiology abnormalities, caused by cardiac pathology, 635
Cardiology specials, 634–36
    exercise tolerance testing, 636
Cardiopulmonary resuscitation (CPR), 47, 807–10
Cardiovascular disease, 651
Cardiovascular surgery, 35
Cardiovascular system, 856
Career opportunities, for medical assistant, 12
Carriers, 344, 347
Case law, 74
Cash, accepting, 301
Cash control proof, 273, 275
Cash disbursement, 301
Cashier's checks, 294
Cash payment journal, 270–71
Casts:
    care of, 519–22
    in urine, 570
Cathartic, 606
Catheterization, 556, 558–59
Cautery (electrosurgery), 507–8
CBC, See Complete blood count (CBC)
CDC, See Centers for Disease Control (CDC)
CD-ROM, 221–22
Cellulitis, 444
Celsius, 376, 379
Celsius/Fahrenheit conversions, 379
Censure, use of term, 60
Centers for Disease Control (CDC), 48, 350–52, 368, 457, 538
Centigrade, 376, 379
Centrifuge, 580, 592, 594
Cerebral embolism, 516
Cerebral palsy, 651
Cerebrospinal fluid (CSF), 449

Cerebrovascular accident (CVA), 516, 611, 810–13
Certificate of mailing, 209–10
Certification, 4
    medical assistant, 91
Certification examination, 838
Certified checks, 294
Certified mail, 208–9
Certified Medical Assistant (CMA), 4, 10, 842
Certified nursing assistant (CNA), 50
Certified registered nurse anesthesiologists (CRNA), 31
Certified respiratory therapy technician (CRTT), 51
Cervical collars, 821
CHAMPUS (Civilian Health and Medical Program of the Uniformed Services), 312
CHAMPVA (Civilian Health and Medical Program of the Veterans Administration, 312
Channels, 622, 627
Charge slips, 140
    and pegboard system, 275–76
Chart, 135, 141
    color vision, 452
    medication, 736
    Snellen, 451–52, 454
    SOAP charting, 424–25
    visual acuity testing chart, 451
Checks, 293–99
    ABA number, 294
    accepting, 296–97
    advantages of, 293
    check writing, 295
        errors in, 295–96
    endorsement of, 297–98
    Magnetic Ink Character Recognition (MICR), 294–95
    mailing, 298
    returned, 298–99
    stub, 297
    types of, 293–94
    warrants, 294
    write-it-once system, 295
Checkwriter, 181
Chemcard Cholesterol Test, 551
Chemical burns, 805
Chemical cold packs, 663–64
Chemical disinfectants, 358, 360
Chemical hazards, 172
Chemical wastes, 172
Chemotherapy, 18, 23, 445, 680
Chest pain, 813–15
Chief complaint (CC), 419–21
    determining, 787
Childbirth, emergency, 795–96
Children:
    airway obstruction in, 792
    breathing rate in, 396
    CPR for, 810
    giving injections to, 730–36
    leaving unattended, 426
    in waiting room, 142
    See also Pediatrics
Chiropractor, 29
Chlorine, 362
Chlorophenyl, 358
Chloroprocaine, 500
Cholecystogram (GB series), 607, 614
Cholera, 18
Cholesterol, 764
Christian Scientists, 84
Chronic obstructive pulmonary disease (COPD), 397
Chronological, use of term, 834
Circulatory system, 857
Circumcised, use of term, 556, 559
Citation, 336
Civil case, 74, 76
Civil law, 76–80
    contract law, 78–80

tort law, 76–78
Claim, 308
Claims processing, 315–21
    accuracy, review for, 320
    birthday rule, 320
    claim form, example of, 317, 319
    and continuing education, 320–21
Clamping instruments, 482
Clark's rule, for pediatric doses, 712
Claustrophobia, 604, 610
Clean-catch midstream specimen, 558–59
Clear liquid diet, 772
Clear writing, tips for, 753
Clinical, defined, 4, 13
Clinical Laboratory Improvement Act (CLIA), 104, 538
Clinical Laboratory Technician (CLT), 52
Clinical responsibilities, 5, 8
Clinics, 47
Clinitest, 564
Closed records, 234, 235–36
Closing, business letters, 200
Closing the office, 143
Clozaril, 529
Cocci, 544
Code of ethics, 60
Code of Hammurabi, 60, 69
Coding, 308, 313–15
Coding books, 205
Coinsurance, 308, 310
Collating records, 134, 135–36
Collect calls, 126
Collection letters, 261
Collections, 259–62
    accounts receivable insurance, 262
    aging accounts receivable, 259
    bankruptcy, 262
    collection agency, using, 262
    collection letters, 261
    delinquent accounts, 259
    legal/ethical issues, 263
    patient education, 263
    process, 259
    regulations, 260
    special problems, 261–62
    statute of limitations, 262
    techniques, 259–60
    telephone, 260
Color-coded filing systems, 240–42
Colorectal surgery, 35
Color vision chart, 452
Colostomy, 516, 517–18
    patient education for, 521
Colposcope, 465–66
Colposcopy, 508
Commercial carriers (insurers), 310–11
Commission on Accreditation of Allied Health Education Programs (CAAHEP), 10, 11
Communication, 111–31, 328
    answering service, using, 127–28
    assertive vs. aggressive behavior, 117–19
    in breathing emergencies, 800
    channels of, 113–14
    directive communication techniques, 116
    emergency telephone call, handling, 128–29
    feedback, 117
    legal/ethical issues, 129
    listening, 119
    local calls, 125
    long distance calls, 125–27
    loyalty to employer, 118
    patient education, 129
    patients:
        discussing sensitive issues with, 118
        greeting, 118
    positive attitude, conveying, 115
    prescription refill requests, 125
    process of, 112–15
    S-M-C-R acronym, 112
    telephone techniques, 122–25
    verbal/nonverbal information, 114–15

Doctor's bag *(con't.)*
    legal/ethical issues, 185
    patient education, 185
Doctors of osteopathy (DOs), 28–29
Documentation, 86–89, 303
    court testimony, 87–89
    and medical assistant, 91
    medical records:
        notice of use of, 87
        use in litigation, 87
Domagk, Gerhard, 23
Do not resuscitate (DNR) order, 47
Dorsogluteal (gluteus medius) muscle,
    725–26
Dosages, calculating, 710–11
Dosimeter, 615
Dot matrix printers, 218, 221
Double booking patients, 154
Double-entry bookkeeping, 270–72
Draping, 426, 433, 499
Dressings, 433, 502–3, 825
Droplet precautions, 351–52
Drug classifications, 682–90
    controlled substances, 682–83
    general classes of drugs, 683–86
    nonprescription drugs, 682
    prescription drugs, 682
Drug Enforcement Agency (DEA), 682
Drug regulations, 89
    and medical assistant, 91
Drug samples, 183
Drug tolerance, 680, 692–94
Dry heat, 662
Durable power of attorney, 86
Duty, 74
    and negligence, 77
Dyspnea, 418
Dysuria, 418

E

Early medicine, 19–20
Ears, 453–57, 863
    audiometry, 457
    components of, 454
    foreign bodies in, 818–19
    hearing impairments, 522
    irrigation, 455, 456
    removal of foreign body from, 455
E codes, 315
Editing, 234
    and medical transcription, 244
Effeurage, 652
Ehrlich, Paul, 22
Eighteenth-century medicine, 20–21
Einthoven's triangle, 628, 631
Elastic bandages, 825
Elderly patients, 426, 522–23
    decreased dexterity, 754
    decreased short-term memory, 754
    increased anxiety, 754–55
    slowed processing time, 753
    teaching, 753–55
Elective surgery, 474
    scheduling, 160
Electrical burns, 805
Electrical safety, 171
Electrocardiogram, 433, 622, 625–34
    abnormalities, 634
    adjustments, making, 632
    artifacts, 632–33
    ECG machines, 626–27, 813
    mounting, 634
    normal rhythm, defined, 634
    paper, 627
    patient preparation, 628–30
    procedure, 630–32
    recording, 633
    sensor placement, 628
    time and cardiac cycle, 626
Electrocardiograph, 622, 625

Electrocardiograph technologist, 50
Electrocoagulation, 507
Electroconvulsive therapy (ECT), 529
Electrodes, 622, 625
Electrodessication, 507
Electroencephalograph technologist, 50
Electrofulguration, 508
Electrolytes, 580, 581, 622, 759
Electromyography (EMG), 669
Electronic claims submission, 224–27
Electronic mail (e-mail), 210–11
Electronic Tabulator, 595
Electronic thermometers, 386–88
Electrosection, 508
Electrosurgery, 507–8
Electrosurgical unit (ESU), 508
ELISA (Enzyme-Linked ImmunoSorbent
    Assay), 370
Emancipated minors, 74, 79, 85
Emergencies:
    abdominal pain, 793–94
    airway obstruction, 790–93
    allergic reactions, 794
    amputation, 794–95
    asphyxia, 795
    birth, 795–96
    bites/stings, 796–99
    breathing emergencies, 800–803
    burns, 804–6
    cardiac arrest, 806–7
    cerebrovascular accident (stroke), 810–13
    chest pain, 813–15
    convulsions (seizures), 815–16
    CPR (cardiopulmonary resuscitation),
        807–10
    diabetic crisis, 816–19
    epistaxis (nosebleed), 817
    fainting, 817–18
    foreign bodies in nose/ear/eye, 818–19
    fractures, 819–21
        jaw, 821–22
        neck/back, 821
    heart attack, 823
    heat and cold exposure, 822–23
    hyperventilation, 823–24
    open wounds, 824–26
    poisoning, 826–27
    severe bleeding, 799
    shock, 827
    tourniquet, 827
    See also Emergencies, assisting in
Emergencies, assisting in, 128, 134, 162,
    784–90
    first aid kit, 790
    office emergency crash cart, 790
    primary assessment, 785–90
    in waiting room, 142
    See also Emergencies; Emergency first aid
Emergency crash cart, 790
Emergency first aid, 781–830
    emergency medical services (EMS) system,
        783–84
    first aid kit, 790
    guidelines for providing, 784
    legal/ethical issues, 828
    medical emergencies, 784–90
    patient education, 828
    See also Medical emergencies
Emergency medical services (EMS) system,
    783–84
Emergency medical technicians
    (EMTs)/paramedics, 47, 50, 783–84
Emergency medicine, 32, 47
Emergency surgery, 475
Emergency telephone call, handling, 128–29
Emesis basin, 433
Empathy, of medical assistant, 9
Emphysema, 376
Employee handbook, 332
Employee records, 327–28
Employee safety, 172

Enclosure notation, business letters, 200
Encounter form, *See* Superbill
Endocardium, 622, 624
Endocervical curettage (ECC), 508
Endocrinology, 23, 445
Endometrial biopsy (EMB), 508–9
Endorsement, checks, 297–98
Envelopes:
    formats, 207
    inserting letters into, 206–7
    Number 6 3/4 envelope, 207
    Number 10 envelope, 206–7
Environment, office, 143–45
Eosinophil, 598
Epinephrine, 500
Epistaxis (nosebleed), 817
Equal Credit Opportunity Act (1975), 80
Equipment, laboratory, 538–40
Equipment inventory record, example of, 184
Error correction, in office correspondence,
    194–97
Erythema, 650, 658
Erythrocytes, 580
Erythrocyte sedimentation rate (ESR), 598–99
Escherichia coli (E. coli), 346, 556, 569
Escorting patient into examination room, 141
Ethics, definition of, 60
Evaluations, 98, 99
Evaluative listening, 119
Evoked potential studies, 669
Examination room, 180–81
    escorting patient into, 141
    preparing, 431–36
    supplies, 431, 433
Exclusive Provider Organizations (EPOs), 49
Exercise tolerance testing, 636
Expendable office supplies, 183
Expert witness, 74, 88
Expulsion, 60, 62
    See also Medical ethics
Extended-care facilities (ECF), 45–46
External billing, 255–56
Externship, 834–38
    finding site for, 836
    patient education, 847
    preceptor role, 836–37
    site evaluation, 837
    student responsibilities, 835–36
Extracurricular, use of term, 834, 842
Exudate, 650
Eye protective equipment, 174
Eyes, 47, 451–53, 863
    foreign bodies in, 818–19
    irrigation of, 453
    See also Ophthalmology

F

Facial sutures, 504
Facility and equipment management, 328
Facsimile (fax) machine, 134, 136, 181
    transmission of medical records, 87
Fahrenheit/Celsius conversions, 379
Fahrenheit (F), 376, 377
Fainting, 817–18
Fair Credit Reporting Act (1971), 80
Fair Debt Collection Practices Act (1978),
    80, 260
Fallopius, Gabrielle, 20
False imprisonment, as intentional tort, 77
Family medical history, 421
Family practice, 32
Family therapy, 529
Fats, 759, 761
FDA, *See* Food and Drug Administration
    (FDA)
Feces, 536, 540
Federal Communications Commission,
    notice on "Use of Telephone for Debt
    Collection," 80
Federal Unemployment Tax Act (FUTA), 285

Medical office, *See* Office
Medical Patients Rights Act, 67
Medical practice, 25–31
  acts, 25–27
  endorsement, 27
  examination, 7
  licensure, 27
  medical education, 25
  medical license, suspending/revoking, 28
  reciprocity, 28
  registration, 28
  residency, 28
  title of doctor, 28–29
  types of, 29–30
    associate practice, 29
    group practice, 29
    partnership, 29
    professional corporation, 30
    solo practice, 29
Medical privileges, 42, 45
Medical records, 233–43, 435
  contents of, 234
  FAX transmission of, 87
  file system, selection of, 235
  as legal document, 234–35
  legal/ethical issues, 249
  notice of use of, 87
  patient education, 249
  releasing, 242–43
  statute of limitations, 243
  supplies/equipment, 235–38
  use in litigation, 87
  See also File system
Medical records technician, 53
Medical science, 17–39
  history of medicine, 18–25
Medical social workers, 53–54
Medical specialties, 31–34, 441–71
  allergy, 442–45
  cardiovascular system, 445
  dermatology, 442–45
  endocrinology, 445
  gastrointestinal system, 445
  gynecology, 460–67
  legal/ethical issues, 469
  lumbar puncture, assisting with, 449–51
  lymphatic (immune) system, 449
  male reproductive system, 467–68
  musculoskeletal system, 449
  nervous system, 449
  ophthalmology, 451–53
  patient education, 469
  pediatrics, 457–60
  respiratory system, 468
  sigmoidoscopy, 446–47
  urinary system, 468
Medical terminology:
  use of, 121
    as communication barrier, 121
Medical transcription, 53, 190, 243–48
  and computers, 247
  editing, 244
  equipment, 245–47
    for the physically challenged, 247
  reference materials for, 248
  reminders, 244–45
  reports, types of, 247–48
  sound-alike words, 244
  transcribers, 245–46
  transcriptionists, 243–45
  voice recognition technology (VRT), 247
  word processing, 246
Medicare, 42–43, 45, 98, 138, 159, 282, 310,
  311–12, 321
  and hospice facilities, 46
Medications:
  administering, 705–45
  charting, 736
  drug calculation, 706–7
  injectable drugs in medical office,
    730–36, 741

  legal/ethical issues, 742
  math principles review, 707–11
    conversion rules, 711
  patient education, 743
  pediatric doses, calculating, 712–13
  See also Administering medications
Medication side effects, 691–95
Medicinal, defined, 18
Medicine and the law, 73–95
Medi-jector insulin delivery system, 721–22
Medulla oblongata, 376, 394
Membranes, 862
Memory, computers, 200
Menstrual, use of term, 418
Mensuration, 418, 429
Mentally incompetent, 79
Mepivacaine, 500
Mercury sphygmomanometer, 402–4
Mercury thermometers, 381–82
  cleaning/storing, 387
  oral temperature using, 384
Message taking, 124
Metabolism, 759
Metastasize, use of term, 442
Metric system, 706–7
Microbes, 18, 22, 536–37
Microbiology, 535–53
  culture growth, 544–49
  culture preparation, 544
  legal/ethical issues, 551
  patient education, 551
  serological testing, 549–51
Microcomputer, 218
Microfiche, 234
Microhematocrit procedure, 589–92, 593
Microorganisms, 18, 345–47, 501, 536,
  537, 541
  disease-producing, 348
Microprocessor, 218
Microscopes, 538–40, 571–72
  care/maintenance of, 540
  using, 541
Military medical benefits, 312
Mind-body connection, 525–26
Minerals, 759, 764, 765–67
Minicomputers, 219
Minors, 74, 79
  billing, 258
  legal implications to consider when
    treating, 85
  rights of, 84–85
Minor surgery, 473–513
  ambulatory surgery, 474–75
  anesthesia, 499–501
  colposcopy, 508
  cryosurgery, 508
  draping, 426, 499
  electrosurgery, 507–8
  endometrial biopsy (EMB), 508–9
  foreign bodies/growths, removal of, 509
  incision and drainage (I & D), 509
  informed consent, 499
  legal/ethical issues, 510
  patient education, 511
  patient's skin, preparation of, 501, 503–4
  positioning, 499
  postoperative patient care, 501–7
  preoperative/postoperative
    instructions, 497
  preparing patient for, 495–501
  surgical asepsis, 475–78
  surgical assisting, 493–97
  surgical instruments, handling, 478–93
  surgical setup, 495
  suture materials/needles, 484–93
  suturing, assisting with, 498–99
  vasectomy, 509–10
  See also Surgical asepsis; Surgical
    instruments
Misdemeanor, 74
Missed appointments, *See* No-shows

Missing files, locating, 242
Modesty of patient, protecting, 141
Modified block style, 190, 201–2
Modified wave scheduling, 152, 154
Money order, 294
Monitors, 218, 221
Monocytes, 598
Monosaccharides, 748
Monounsaturated fat, 761
Monthly planning, 329
Morbidity rate, 18, 23
Morning specimens, 556, 558
Mortality rate, 18, 23, 98
Morton, William, 23
Mouse, 218
Movement produced by muscles,
  terminology for, 659
Mueller-Hinton agar, 547
Multi-dose vials, 721
Multiple sclerosis, 651
Muscular dystrophy, 651
Musculoskeletal injuries, 819–21
Musculoskeletal system, 449, 852–53
Mycardium, 622
Myleogram, 614
Myocardial, use of term, 782
Myocardial infarction, 611, 823
Myocardium, 624

N

Name pins/tag, receptionist, 135
Narcissistic behavior, 528
Narcotics log, 682
Nasopharyngeal culture, collecting using
  Culturette system, 543
National Board Medical Examination
  (NBME), 27
National Certification Agency for Medical
  Laboratory Personnel, 52
Neck, fraction of, 821
Neck trauma, 651
Necrotic, use of term, 782
Needle holder forceps, 482
Needles, 490–93
  gauge, 718
  length, 718–19
Negative, use of term, 536, 550
Neglect, 74
Neglect of duty, 74
Negligence, 74, 76
  contributory, 78
  and duty, 77
  four D's of, 77
Neoplasms, 445
Nerve blocks, 500
Nervous system, 449, 854–55
Network, 834
Neurology, 47, 449
Neuroses, 52, 516
Neurosurgery, 35
New patients, registering, 138–40
Niacin, 763
Nightingale, Florence, 24
Nineteenth-century medicine, 21–23
Nitrites, 569
No charge (N/C) notation, 140
Nonabsorbable sutures, 485
Noncompliance, handling, 755
Non-invasive procedure, 98
Nonparticipating provider, 308, 319–20
Non-patient visitors, scheduling
  appointments with, 161–62
Non-pleuritic, use of term, 782
Nonprescription drugs, 682
Nonsterile gown technique, 357
Non-venomous bites/stings, 798–99
Norm, 98
Normal values, 556, 562–63
Nose, foreign bodies in, 818–19
Nosebleed, 817

No-shows, 134, 142–43, 153, 157–58
Nosocomial infection, 344, 347, 556, 559
Nova 16 Analyzer, 594
Novocain, 500
Nuclear medicine, 32, 604, 612
Number 6 3/4 envelopes, 207
Number 10 envelopes, 206–7
Numbers, in letter writing, 194, 198
Numeric filing system, 234, 238–40
   middle digit filing, 238
   serial numbering, 240
   straight numeric filing, 238
   terminal digit filing, 238
   unit numbering, 238–40
Nurse practitioner (NP), 51
Nurses, 50–51
   certified nursing assistant (CNA), 50
   licensed practical nurse (LPN), 50
   nurse practitioner (NP), 51
   registered nurse (RN), 50–51
Nursing homes, 45–46
Nutrients, 748
Nutrition, 755–76
   alcohol, 776
   balanced diet, 764–69
   calories, 770–71
   carbohydrates, 760–61
   cholesterol, 764
   dietary guidelines, 772
   dietary modifications, 772–76
   digestion, 758–59
   fats, 761
   food pyramid, 764–68, 771
   food supplements, 776
   legal/ethical issues, 777
   metabolism, 759
   minerals, 764, 765–67
   nutrient classification, 759–64
   patient education, 777
   proteins, 761
   Recommended Dietary Allowances
     (RDAs), 769–70
   vitamins, 763–67
   water, 763
   See also Diets
Nylon suture, 487

O

Oath of Hippocrates, 60, 69
Obesity, 748
Obsession, 527
Obstetrics, 32
Obstructive lung disease, 622, 639
Occult, use of term, 782
Occult blood, 541, 556, 567
Occult fracture, 821
Occupational Safety and Health
   Administration (OSHA), 104, 145, 537
   administration standards, 713–15
   Occupational Exposure to Bloodborne
     Pathogens Standards, 173–74, 352–53
Occupational therapist (OT), 51, 672–74
Office:
   bathrooms, 181
   closing, 143
   doctor's bag, 184–85
   drug samples, 183
   environment, 143–45
   equipment, 181–82
   examination room, 180–81
   facilities planning, 180
   housekeeping, 145
   injectable drugs in, 730–36
   opening, 135–36
   supplies, 182–83
   temperature, 180
Office emergency crash cart, 790
Office equipment, 181–82
   administrative equipment, 181
   warranties, 182

Office management, 325–40
   definition of, 53
   legal/ethical issues, 337
   and medical assistant, 91
   medical meetings/speaking
     engagements, 336
   office procedures manual, 332
   patient education, 337
   patient information booklet, development
     of, 336–37
   personnel management responsibilities,
     326–28
   personnel policy manual, 332
   systems approach to, 326–28
   time management, 330–31
   See also Office manager; Personnel
     management
Office manager, 328–30
   monthly planning, 329
   staff meetings, 329–30
Office procedures, time estimates for, 156
Office procedures manual, 332
Office safety, 168–72
Office security, 176–79
   incident report, 176–79
Oliguria, 418, 556, 562
Once-a-month billing, 258
Oncology, 32, 445
ONE TOUCH Profile Diabetes Tracking
   System, 592
Open-ended questions, 116
Opening the office, 135–36
Open office hours system, 154
Open wounds, 824–26
Operating scissors, 481
Operative note, 248
Operator-assisted calls, 126
Ophthalmology, 47, 451–53
   Ishihara test, 451, 453
   Snellen chart, 451–52, 454
   visual acuity testing charts, 451
   See also Eyes
Ophthalmoscope, 430
Opportunistic infections, 344, 369
Opthalmologist, 32–33
Optional, use of term, 268
Optional surgery, 475
Oral administration, 686
Oral medications, administering, 714–15
Oral method of temperature
   measurement, 379
Oral surgery, 35
Orientation/training, 327
Orifice, 418, 782
Orthopedic instruments, 492
Orthopedics, 33, 47, 449
Orthopnea, 418
Osteopaths, 28–29
Osteoporosis, 651
Ostomy patients, 517–18
Otolaryngology, 453
Otology, 453–57
Otorhinolaryngologist (ENT), 33
Otorhinolaryngology, 453
Otoscope, 430
Outgoing mail, preparing, 206–8
Outpatient, 42, 43
Outpatient surgery, 474–75
Outpatient surgical/procedure forms, 84
Overbooking, 154
Over-the-counter (OTC) drugs, 682
Oximeter, 644
Oxygen delivery system, preparing, 803–4
Oxyhemoglobin, 344, 580, 581

P

Pacemaker, 622, 625
Palpation, 429
Palpatory method, 376
   of measuring radial pulse, 408

PAP smear, 418, 431, 465
PAP test, assisting with, 467
Paragraph length, 191
Paramedics, 47, 50, 783–84
Paranoia, 528
Paraplegia, 651
Parasites, 556, 571
Parenteral, use of term, 680
Parenteral administration, 686, 691, 715–29
Parenteral injections, 729, 732–34
Parkinson's disease, 651
Part A, Medicare, 43
Part B, Medicare, 43, 46
Participating provider, 308, 319
Partnership, 29
Parts of speech, 194, 198
Passive immunity, 350
Passive listening, 119
Passive range of motion (PROM), 653, 658
Passive voice, 190, 192
Password, 218
Pasteurization, 18
Pasteur, Louis, 21, 344, 537
Past medical history, 421, 788
Pathogenic bacteria, 548
Pathogens, 344, 536, 537, 544
Pathologic, 782
Pathology, 18, 33, 556, 561
Pathology report, 248
Patient:
   angry, handling, 121–22
   credit information, confidentiality of, 263
Patient accounts, 269–70
Patient assessment, 116
Patient care careers, 50–52
Patient education, 13, 36, 747–55
   adult learning, 748
   banking, 304
   billing, 263
   collections, 263
   colostomy, 521
   communication, 129
   computers, 228
   doctor's bag, 185
   emergency first aid, 828
   financial management, 287
   hematology, 599
   infection control, 371
   insurance, 321
   medical assisting, 13
   medical records, 249
   medical specialties, 469
   medications, 743
   microbiology, 551
   minor surgery, 511
   noncompliance, handling, 755
   nutrition, 777
   office management, 337
   patient reception, 146
   pharmacology, 700
   physical therapy, 674
   pulmonary function, 645
   radiology, 616
   special patient needs, 530
   teaching methods/strategies, 548–53
   teaching older adults, 753–55
   teaching plan, developing, 755, 756–58
   vital signs, 413
   written communication, 212
Patient history, 419–22
Patient information booklet, development of,
   336–37
Patient/physician relationship, 83–86
   informed consent, 74, 83–84
   patient rights, 83
   physician rights, 83
Patient preparation, for physical
   examinations, 425–26
Patient reception, 133–49
   charge slips, 140
   closing the office, 143

Respiration, 394–98
  breath sounds, 397
  characteristics of, 396–97
  depth, 397
  measuring, 398
  physiology of, 394
  rate, 396
  rhythm, 396
  See also Breathing; Breathing emergencies
Respiratory Care Specialist, 639
Respiratory system, 468, 858
Respiratory therapist (RT), 51
Respiratory tract specimens, 542–43
Respondeat superior, 75, 80–81
Restrictive lung disease, 622, 639
Resume, 834, 840–42
  components of, 840–41
  cover letter, 842–43
  legal/ethical issues, 847
  professional reference, 842
  See also Career opportunities; Interview
Reticulocyte, 580, 595
Retinoblastoma, 612
Retrograde pyelogram, 614
Returned checks, 298–99
Returned mail, 210
Review of systems (ROS), 421, 423
Revocation, 60, 62
Rheumatoid arthritis, 418, 652
Rheumatology, 34
Rhonchi, 397
Rickettsia, 346
Rider, 308
Right lateral recumbent position, 427–28
Rights of minors, 84–85
Ritter M11 Ultra Clave Automatic
  Sterilizer, 364
Roget's International Thesaurus, 205–6
Role delineation, 8–9
ROM (read-only memory), 218, 220
Rosacea, 418
Rule of discovery, 75
Rule of Nines, 804–5

S
Sabin, Albert, 23
Safety:
  biological hazards, 172–73
  body mechanics, 175–76
  chemical hazards, 172
  disaster plan, 168
  electrical, 171
  employee, 172
  fire, 170–71
  general safety measures, 168–72
  housekeeping, 174–75
  laboratory, 537
  mechanical, 172
  and medical assistant, 92
  office, 168–72
  OSHA Occupational Exposure to
    Bloodborne Pathogens Standards,
    173–74
  patient, 145
  personal protective equipment, 174
  physical hazards, 168–70
  physicians' office laboratories (POLs),
    537–38
  quality assurance, 538
  quality control, 538
  radiation, 171–72
  universal precautions, 174
  See also Asepsis; Handwashing; Standard
    Precautions; Surgical asepsis
Safety needs, 526
Salary review, 327
Salespersons, scheduling appointments with,
  161–62
Salivation, 418
Salk, Jonas, 23

Salt, 776
  low-sodium/low-salt diet, 774
Salutation, business letters, 199–200
Sanitization, 358
Saturated fat, 761
Savings accounts, deposits to, 300–301
Scales, 408–10
  calibration of, 409
Scalpels, 479, 485
Scanners, 181
Schedule book, *See* Appointment book
Scheduling process, 328
Scheduling system, 134
Schizophrenia, 527
Scientific discovery, and medical ethics, 68
Scissors, 481, 486
Scleroderma, 445
Scope, 482
Screening telephone calls, 123–25
Scrotum, 467
Scrub assistants, 474
  sterile technique for, 494
Seating, waiting room, 144
Second-degree burns, 805
Security, computers, 224
Sediment, 556, 569–70
Sedimentation rate, 433
Segment, 622
Seizures, 782, 815–16
Self-actualization, 526
Semi-Fowler's position, 427
Semmelweiss, Ignaz, 22, 344
Sensitivity, 622
Sensitivity testing, 547–49
Sensitization, 443
Sensor placement, electrocardiogram, 628
Sensors, 622, 625, 628–30
Sentence length, 191
Serial numbering filing system, 240
Serologic, use of term, 536, 549
Serological testing, 549–51
  pregnancy tests, 550–51
  strep tests, 549–50
Serum, 580, 581
Settle, use of term, 75, 81
Severe bleeding, 799–80
Sexually transmitted diseases (STDs), 468
Shelf-life, 367
Shock, 799, 825–26, 827
  and irritability, 801
Side effects, 680, 691–95
Sigmoidoscopy, 446–47
Signature on File notation, 316, 319
Signing Exact English (SEE-2), 674
Signing-in, 137–38
Silk suture, 487
Simplified letter style, 201–2
Sims' position, 427–28
Single-dose vials, 721
Single-entry bookkeeping, 270
Site evaluation, externship, 837
Sitting position, 427, 432
Skilled nursing facilities (SNF), 45–46
Skin cancer, 445
Skin disorders and treatments, 444–45
Slander, 75
Slide preparation, 596
S-M-C-R acronym, 112
Smear fixation, 536
Smears, 536, 538, 597
  preparing, 546
Snakebites, 798
Snellen chart, 451–52, 454
SOAP charting, 424–25
Soap dispenser, 433
Social needs, 526
Social Security taxes, 282
Social work, 53–54
Software, 218, 221–23
Solid wastes, 172
Solo practice, 4, 7

Somatosensory evoked peripheral nerves
  (SEP), 669
Sound-alike words, 244
Speaking engagements, *See* Medical
  meetings/speaking engagements
Special delivery, 210
Special furniture, 672
Special handling, 210
Special patient needs, 515–33
  Alzheimer's disease, 523
  blind patients, 522
  casts, care of, 519–22
  CVA patients, 516
  elderly patients, 522–23
  health habits, 526
  hearing impairments, 522
  intravenous therapy (IV), 499, 518–19
  legal/ethical issues, 530
  mind-body connection, 525–26
  ostomy patients, 517–18
  patient education, 530
  psychological disorders, 526–29
    treatments, 529
  psychology, 525
  terminally ill patients, 523–25
  tube feeding, 519
Special postal services, 208–10
Species immunity, 350
Specific gravity (S.G.), 556, 562–63, 565
Specified time scheduling, 152–53
Specimen collection, 540–44
  respiratory tract, 542–43
  stool, 540–42
  in urinalysis, 557–60
Specimens, 536
Speculum, 418, 430, 433, 482, 488–89
Speech, parts of, 194, 198
Speech therapy, 674
Spelling, 192–93, 196
Spermatozoa, 571
Sphygmomanometers, 401–4, 433
Spider bites, 798
Spirillum, 544
Spirometry procedure, 642–44
Splinter forceps, 482
Splints, 820
Sponge forceps, 482
Spores, 544
Sprain, 652
Sputum, 536, 543
  specimen, obtaining, 545
Squamous epithelial cells, 556
Staff communications, communication
  barriers in, 121–22
Staff meetings, 329–30
Standard of care, 75, 81
Standardization, 622, 626
Standard Precautions, 350–52, 379
  and HIV, 370
  summary of, 353
  Universal Precautions compared
    to, 352
"Standards for Blood Banks and Transfusion
  Services," 53
Standing position, 432
Staphlococcus bacterium, 48, 345
Staples, 493
  steel, 487–88
State disability insurance, 286
State unemployment tax, 285
Statute of limitations, 75, 82
  and collections, 262
  for keeping medical records, 243
Statutes, 60, 75
Steam sterilization, 173
Steel, in staples, 487–88
Sterile, 344, 354
Sterile dressing, changing, 505
Sterile field, 474, 478
  transferring sterile solutions onto, 484
Sterile gloving technique, 363